W9-AUY-048

# CANCER
## Principles & Practice of Oncology

# ANNUAL ADVANCES IN ONCOLOGY

## VOLUME 1

*Editors:*

### Vincent T. DeVita, Jr., MD

Amy and Joseph Perella Professor of Medicine
Yale Comprehensive Cancer Center and Smilow Cancer
  Hospital at Yale New Haven
Yale University School of Medicine
Professor of Epidemiology and Public Health
Yale School of Public Health
New Haven, Connecticut

### Theodore S. Lawrence, MD, PhD

Isadore Lampe Professor and Chair
Department of Radiation Oncology
University of Michigan
Ann Arbor, Michigan

### Steven A. Rosenberg, MD, PhD

Chief of Surgery, National Cancer Institute
National Institutes of Health
Professor of Surgery
Uniformed Services of the Health Sciences School
  of Medicine
Bethesda, Maryland
Professor of Surgery
George Washington University School of Medicine
Washington, DC

 Wolters Kluwer | Lippincott Williams & Wilkins
Health
Philadelphia · Baltimore · New York · London
Buenos Aires · Hong Kong · Sydney · Tokyo

*Senior Executive Editor:* Jonathan W. Pine, Jr.
*Senior Product Manager:* Emilie Moyer
*Vendor Manager:* Alicia Jackson
*Senior Manufacturing Manager:* Benjamin Rivera
*Senior Marketing Manager:* Angela Panetta
*Senior Designer:* Stephen Druding
*Production Service:* Aptara, Inc.

**Library of Congress Cataloging-in-Publication Data**

Cancer : principles & practice of oncology : annual advances in oncology / editors,
Vincent T. DeVita Jr., Theodore S. Lawrence, Steven A. Rosenberg.
     p. ; cm. – (Advances in oncology ; v. 1)
  Includes bibliographical references and index.
  ISBN 978-1-4511-0314-4 (alk. paper)
  1. Cancer.   I. DeVita, Vincent T.  II. Lawrence, Theodore S.  III. Rosenberg, Steven A.
IV. Series: Advances in oncology ; v. 1.
  [DNLM: 1. Neoplasms.  QZ 200 C21537 2010]
  RC261.C27395 2010
  616.99′4–dc22                          2010017159

# Section Editors

**Kenneth C. Anderson, MD**
Division of Hematologic Neoplasia
Dana Farber Cancer Institue
Harvard Medical School
Boston, Massachusetts
*New Therapies for Myeloma: Impact on Survival*

**Sharon L. Bober, PhD**
Sexual Health Program
Lance Armstrong Adult Survivorship Clinic
Dana Farber Cancer Institute
Boston, Massachusetts
*Sexuality After Cancer*

**Tito Fojo, MD, PhD**
Center for Cancer Research
National Cancer Institute
Bethesda, Maryland
*Monitoring of Therapeutic Response to Cancer Treatment*

**Olivier Glehen, MD, Phd**
Surgical Oncology Department
Centre Hospitalo-Universitaire Lyon Sud
Hospices Civils de Lyon
Pierre Bénite, France
Peritoneal Carcinomatosis Laboratory
Université Lyon-1
Ouillins, France
*Management of Peritoneal Carcinomatosis From Colorectal and Appendiceal Malignancy*

**Theodore S. Lawrence, MD, PhD**
Isadore Lampe Professor and Chair
Department of Radiation Oncology
University of Michigan
Ann Arbor, Michigan
*Charged Particle Therapy*

**Dan L. Longo, MD**
Clinical Research Branch
National Institute on Aging
National Institutes of Health
Baltimore, Maryland
*Hodgkin's Lymphoma*

**Benjamin Movsas, MD**
Department of Radiation Oncology
Henry Ford Health System
Detroit, Michigan
*Charged Particle Therapy*

**Paul H. Sugarbaker, MD, FACS, FRCS**
Program in Peritoneal Surface Malignancy
Washington Cancer Institute
Washington Hospital Center
Washington, D.C.
*Management of Peritoneal Carcinomatosis From Colorectal and Appendiceal Malignancy*

# Contributors

**Susan Allen, PhD**
Department of Community Health
Brown University
Providence, Rhode Island

**Barbara L. Andersen, PhD**
The Department of Psychology and the Comprehensive Cancer
    Center and Solove Research Institute
The Ohio State University
Columbus, Ohio

**William F. Anderson, MD, MPH**
The Division of Cancer Epidemiology and Genetics
National Cancer Institute
National Institutes of Health
Bethesda, Maryland

**Kenneth C. Anderson, MD**
The Division of Hematologic Neoplasia
Dana Farber Cancer Institute
Harvard Medical School
Boston, Massachusetts

**James O. Armitage, MD**
Section of Hematology and Oncology
University of Nebraska Medical Center
Omaha, Nebraska

**Jean Francois Baladi**
Novartis Pharmaceuticals Corporation
Florham Park, New Jersey

**Udai Banerji, MD, MRCP, PhD**
Cancer Research UK Centre for Cancer Therapeutics
The Institute of Cancer Research
Haddow Laboratories
Drug Development Unit
Section of Medicine
The Institute of Cancer Research and The Royal Marsden Hospital
    NHS Trust
Sutton, United Kingdom

**Philip Bao, MD**
Division of Surgical Oncology
University of Pittsburgh Medical Center
Pittsburgh, Pennsylvania

**Rachel E. Barnett, MS**
Cancer Genetic Counseling
Yale Cancer Center
New Haven, Connecticut

**David Bartlett, MD**
The Division of Surgical Oncology
University of Pittsburgh Medical Center
Pittsburgh, Pennsylvania

**Susan E. Bates, MD**
Medical Oncology Branch
National Cancer Institute
National Institutes of Health
Bethesda, Maryland

**Fernando Bazan, MD**
Department of Oncology, University Hospital J. Minjoz, and
    Institut National de la Santé et de la Recherche Médicale
Besançon, France

**William Berg, MD**
Novartis Pharmaceuticals Corporation
Florham Park, New Jersey

**Eleanor A. Blakely, PhD**
Life Sciences Division
Lawrence Berkeley National Laboratory
Berkeley, California

**Sharon L. Bober, PhD**
Sexual Health Program
The Lance Armstrong Foundation Adult
    Survivorship Clinic
Perini Family Survivors' Center
Dana-Farber Cancer Institute/Harvard Medical School
Boston, Massachusetts

**Ulrike Boehmer, PhD**
Department of Social and Behavioral Sciences
Boston University
Boston, Massachusetts

**Deborah J. Bowen, PhD**
Department of Social and Behavioral Sciences
Boston University
Boston, Massachusetts

**Michael Brada, BSc, FRCP, FRCR**
The Institute of Cancer Research and The Royal Marsden NHS
    Foundation Trust Sutton
Surrey, United Kingdom

**Penelope Bradbury, MB BCh, FRACP, MD**

NCIC Clinical Trials Group
Queen's University
Kingston, Ontario, Canada

**Marc Buyse, ScD**

International Drug Development Institute
Louvain-la-Neuve, Belgium
Center for Statistics, I-BioStat
Hasselt University
Diepenbeek, Belgium

**Neil E. Caporaso, MD**

The Division of Cancer Epidemiology and Genetics
National Cancer Institute
National Institutes of Health
Bethesda, Maryland

**Polly Y. Chang, PhD**

BioSciences Division, Molecular and Genetic Toxicology
    Department
SRI International
Menlo Park, California

**Diana Cirstea, MD**

Leebow Institute of Myeloma Therapeutics and Jerome Lipper
    Multiple Myeloma Disease Center
Dana-Farber Cancer Institute
Harvard Medical School
Boston, Massachusetts

**Joseph M. Connors, MD**

The Department of Medicine
Division of Medical Oncology
University of British Columbia and the British Columbia
    Cancer Agency
Vancouver, British Columbia, Canada

**David W. Coon, PhD**

College of Nursing and Healthcare Innovation
Arizona State University
Phoenix, Arizona

**Eddy Cotte, MD**

Surgical Oncology Department
Centre Hospitalo-Universitaire Lyon Sud, Hospices Civils de Lyon,
    Pierre Bénite, France
Peritoneal Carcinomatosis Laboratory, Université Lyon-1,
    Oullins, France

**Marc Dahlke, MD, PhD**

University Medical Center
Department of Surgery
Regensburg, Germany

**Johann S. de Bono, MD, FRCP, MSc, PhD**

Cancer Research UK Centre for Cancer Therapeutics
The Institute of Cancer Research
Haddow Laboratories
Drug Development Unit
Section of Medicine
The Institute of Cancer Research and The Royal Marsden Hospital
    NHS Trust
Sutton, United Kingdom

**Dirk De Ruysscher, MD, PhD**

The Institute of Cancer Research and The Royal Marsden NHS
    Foundation Trust Sutton
Surrey, United Kingdom

**Vincent T. DeVita, Jr., MD**

Amy and Joseph Perella Professor of Medicine
Yale Comprehensive Cancer Center and Smilow Cancer
    Hospital at Yale New Haven
Yale University School of Medicine
Professor of Epidemiology and Public Health
Yale School of Public Health
New Haven, Connecticut

**James J. Driscoll, MD, PhD**

Medical Oncology Branch
National Cancer Institute
National Institutes of Health
Bethesda, Maryland

**Christine Duffy, MD, MPH**

Division of General Internal Medicine
Rhode Island Hospital
Warren Alpert Medical School of Brown University
Providence, Rhode Island

**Andrew Dwyer, MD**

Department of Imaging Sciences
National Institutes of Health
Bethesda, Maryland

**Franziska C. Eberle, MD**

The Hematopathology Section
Laboratory of Pathology
Center for Cancer Research
National Cancer Institute
National Institutes of Health
Bethesda, Maryland

**Maureen Edgerly, RN**

Medical Oncology Branch
National Cancer Institute
National Institutes of Health
Bethesda, Maryland

**Jason A. Efstathiou, MD, DPhil**
Department of Radiation Oncology
Massachusetts General Hospital
Harvard Medical School
Boston, Massachusetts

**Dominique M. Elias, MD, PhD**
Department of Oncologic Surgery
Institut Gustave Roussy
Villejuif, France

**Yusri A. Elsayed, MD, PhD**
Clinical Oncology Research
Ortho Biotech Oncology Research and Development
Unit of Johnson & Johnson Pharmaceutical
    Research & Development
Raritan, New Jersey

**Andreas Engert, MD, PhD**
Department I of Internal Medicine and the German
    Hodgkin's Study Group (GHSG) University Hospital
Cologne, Germany

**Jesus Esquivel, MD, FACS**
Surgical Oncology
Peritoneal Surface Malignancy Program
St. Agnes Hospital
Baltimore, Maryland

**Jacob Flanz, PhD**
Department of Radiation Oncology
Massachusetts General Hospital
Francis F. Burr Proton Therapy Center
Boston, Massachusetts

**Patricia Fobair, LCSW, MPH**
Supportive Care Program
Stanford Hospital Cancer Center
Stanford, California

**Tito Fojo, MD, PhD**
Medical Oncology Branch
Center for Cancer Research
National Cancer Institute
National Institutes of Health
Bethesda, Maryland

**Alfredo Garofalo, MD**
Department of Surgical Oncology
Digestive Branch
National Cancer Center "Regina Elena"
Rome, Italy

**Michelle D. Garrett, BSc (Hons), PhD**
Cancer Research UK Centre for Cancer Therapeutics
The Institute of Cancer Research
Haddow Laboratories
Sutton, United Kingdom

**François Noël Gilly, MD, PhD**
Surgical Oncology Department
Centre Hospitalo-Universitaire Lyon Sud
Hospices Civils de Lyon
Pierre Bénite, France
Peritoneal Carcinomatosis Laboratory
Université Lyon-1, Oullins, France

**Olivier Glehen, MD, PhD**
Surgical Oncology Department
Centre Hospitalo-Universitaire Lyon Sud
Hospices Civils de Lyon
Pierre Bénite, France
Peritoneal Carcinomatosis Laboratory
Université Lyon-1
Oullins, France

**Gabriel Glockzin, MD**
University Medical Center
Department of Surgery
Regensburg, Germany

**Lynn R. Goldin, PhD**
The Division of Cancer Epidemiology and
    Genetics
National Cancer Institute
National Institutes of Health
Bethesda, Maryland

**Luis González-Bayón, MD, PhD**
Peritoneal Surface Oncology Program
Departments of Surgical Oncology
M.D. Anderson International España
Madrid, Spain

**Concepción González-Hernando, MD**
Department of Diagnostic Imaging
M.D. Anderson International España
Madrid, Spain

**Santiago González-Moreno, MD, PhD**
Peritoneal Surface Oncology Program
Departments of Surgical Oncology and Diagnostic
    Imaging
M.D. Anderson International España
Madrid, Spain

**Mary K. Gospodarowicz, MD, FRCPC, FRCR (Hon)**
Department of Radiation Oncology
University of Toronto
Princess Margaret Hospital
Toronto, Ontario, Canada

**Norma C. Gutierrez, MD, PhD**
Servicio de Hematología
Hospital Universitario de Salamanca, Spain
CIC IBMCC (USAL-CSIC)
Salamanca, Spain

**Jean-Luc Harousseau, MD**
Cancer Center René Gauducheau
Saint Herblain, France

**Stacey L. Hart, PhD**
Department of Psychology
Ryerson University
Toronto, Ontario, Canada

**Ming-Ann Hsu, MPH**
Global Outcomes Research
Oncology, Pfizer Inc
New London, Connecticut

**Hui Huang, MD**
Medical Oncology Branch
National Cancer Institute
National Institutes of Health
Bethesda, Maryland

**Elaine S. Jaffe, MD**
The Hematopathology Section
Laboratory of Pathology
Center for Cancer Research
National Cancer Institute
National Institutes of Health
Bethesda, Maryland

**John E. Janik, MD**
Clinical Trials Team
Metabolism Branch
Center for Cancer Research
National Cancer Institute
National Institutes of Health
Bethesda, Maryland

**Anne Katz, RN, PhD**
Cancer Care Manitoba
Winnipeg, Manitoba, Canada

**Jonathan Kaufman, MD**
Winship Cancer Institute
Emory University
Atlanta, Georgia

**Andrea Kay, MD**
Novartis Pharmaceuticals Corporation
Florham Park, New Jersey

**Stan B. Kaye, BSc, MD, FRCP, FRCR, FRSE, FMedSci**
Cancer Research UK Centre for Cancer Therapeutics
The Institute of Cancer Research, Haddow
    Laboratories
Drug Development Unit
Section of Medicine
The Institute of Cancer Research and The Royal Marsden Hospital
    NHS Trust
Sutton, United Kingdom

**Karen Kayser, MSW, PhD**
Graduate School of Social Work
Boston College
Chestnut Hill, Massachusetts

**Beate Klimm, MD**
Department I of Internal Medicine and the German
    Hodgkin's Study Group (GHSG) University Hospital
Cologne, Germany

**Sara J. Knight, PhD**
University of California
San Francisco Comprehensive Cancer Center
Departments of Psychiatry and Urology
Genitourinary Cancer Epidemiology and Populations Sciences
    Program
San Francisco VA Medical Center
San Francisco, California

**Andre Konski, MD, MBA**
Department of Radiation Oncology
Wayne State University School of Medicine
Detroit, Michigan

**Herb Kotz, MD**
Medical Oncology Branch
National Cancer Institute
National Institutes of Health
Bethesda, Maryland

**Gerhard Kraft, PhD**
GSI Biophysik
Darmstadt, Germany

**Sigurdur Yngvi Kristinsson, MD, PhD**

Division of Hematology
Department of Medicine
Karolinska University Hospital Solna and Karolinska
    Institutet
Stockholm, Sweden

**Ola Landgren, MD, PhD**

Division of Cancer Epidemiology and Genetics
Division of Medical Oncology
Medical Oncology Branch
Center for Cancer Research
National Cancer Institute
National Institutes of Health
Bethesda, Maryland

**David M. Latini, PhD**

Scott Department of Urology and Dan L. Duncan Cancer Center
Baylor College of Medicine, and Health Services
    Research and Development Center of Excellence
Michael E. DeBakey VA Medical Center
Houston, Texas

**Theodore S. Lawrence, MD, PhD**

Isadore Lampe Professor and Chair
Department of Radiation Oncology
University of Michigan
Ann Arbor, Michigan

**David Lebwohl, MD**

Novartis Pharmaceuticals Corporation
Florham Park, New Jersey

**Jeremie H. Lefevre, MD**

Department of Oncologic Surgery
Institut Gustave Roussy
Villejuif, France

**Antony J. Lomax, PhD**

Centre for Proton Radiotherapy
Paul Scherrer Institute
Villingen, Switzerland

**Dan L. Longo, MD**

Clinical Research Branch
National Institute on Aging
National Institutes of Health
Baltimore, Maryland

**Sagar Lonial, MD**

Winship Cancer Institute
Emory University
Atlanta, Georgia

**Valeria Magarotto, MD**

Divisione de Ematologia dell'Università di Torino
A.O.U. S. Giovannia Battista
Torino, Italy

**Michael L. Maitland, MD, PhD**

Section of Hematology/Oncology
University of Chicago Medical Center
Chicago, Illinois

**Haresh Mani, MD**

The Hematopathology Section
Laboratory of Pathology
Center for Cancer Research
National Cancer Institute
National Institutes of Health
Bethesda, Maryland

**M. Victoria Mateos, MD, PhD**

Servicio de Hematología
Hospital Universitario de Salamanca
Salamanca, Spain

**Ellen T. Matloff, MS**

Cancer Genetic Counseling
Yale Cancer Center
Department of Genetics
Yale School of Medicine
New Haven, Connecticut

**Peter M. Mauch, MD**

Department of Radiation Oncology
Brigham and Women's Hospital and Dana-Farber Cancer
    Institute
Harvard Medical School
Boston, Massachusetts

**Richard McQuellon, PhD**

Department of Internal Medicine
Section of Hematology and Oncology
Wake Forest University School of Medicine
Winston-Salem, North Carolina

**Michael Menefee, MD**

Division of Hematology and Oncology
Mayo Clinic
Jacksonville, Florida

**Thomas E. Merchant, DO, PhD**

Department of Radiation Oncology
St. Jude Children's Research Hospital
Memphis, Tennessee

**Faheez Mohamed, MD, FRCSEd (Gen Surg)**
The Pseudomyxoma Peritonei Centre
Colorectal Research Unit
Basingstoke and North Hampshire Hospital
    Foundation Trust
Hampshire, United Kingdom

**Brendan J. Moran, MCh, FRCS**
The Pseudomyxoma Peritonei Centre
Basingstoke and North Hampshire Hospital
    Foundation Trust
Hampshire, United Kingdom

**Benjamin Movsas, MD**
Department of Radiations Oncology
Henry Ford Health System
Detroit, Michigan

**Andrea K. Ng, MD, MPH**
Department of Radiation Oncology
Brigham and Women's Hospital and Dana-Farber
    Cancer Institute
Harvard Medical School
Boston, Massachusetts

**Ajay Nooka, MD, MPH**
Winship Cancer Institute
Emory University
Atlanta, Georgia

**Rebecca L. Norris, BA**
Department of Psychiatry
University of Massachusetts
Boston, Massachusetts

**Gloria Ortega-Pérez, MD**
Peritoneal Surface Oncology Program
Departments of Surgical Oncology
M.D. Anderson International España
Madrid, Spain

**Antonio Palumbo, MD**
Divisione de Ematologia dell'Università di Torino
A.O.U. S. Giovannia Battista
Torino, Italy

**Elyse R. Park, PhD, MPH**
Department of Psychiatry and the Institute for
    Health Policy
Massachusetts General Hospital
Harvard Medical School
Boston, Massachusetts

**Guillaume Passot, MD**
Surgical Oncology Department
Centre Hospitalo-Universitaire Lyon Sud
Hospices Civils de Lyon
Pierre Bénite, France
Peritoneal Carcinomatosis Laboratory
Université Lyon-1
Oullins, France

**Madelon Pijls-Johannesma, MSc, PhD**
Department of Radiation Oncology (MAASTRO)
GROW, University Hospital Maastricht
Maastricht, The Netherlands

**Pompiliu Piso, MD, PhD**
University Medical Center
Department of Surgery
Regensburg, Germany

**Xavier Pivot, MD, PhD**
Department of Oncology
University Hospital J. Minjoz, and Institut National de la Santé
    et de la Recherche Médicale
Besançon, France

**Felix Popp, MD**
University Medical Center
Department of Surgery
Regensburg, Germany

**Jennifer Potter, MD**
Harvard Medical School
Boston, Massachusetts

**Fahd Quddus, MD**
Section of Hematology and Oncology
University of Nebraska Medical Center
Omaha, Nebraska

**Noopur Raje, MD**
Leebow Institute of Myeloma Therapeutics and Jerome Lipper
    Multiple Myeloma Disease Center
Dana-Farber Cancer Institute
MGH-Cancer Center
Massachusetts General Hospital
Harvard Medical School
Boston, Massachusetts

**Vincent S. Rajkumar, MD**
Division of Hematology
Mayo Clinic
Rochester, Minnesota

**Mark J. Ratain, MD**
Section of Hematology/Oncology
University of Chicago Medical Center
Chicago, Illinois

**Tiffany A. Richards**
Division of Cancer Medicine
Department of Lymphoma/Myeloma
University of Texas
M.D. Anderson Cancer Center
Houston, Texas

**Oliver Rixe, MD, PhD**
Division of Hematology and Oncology
University of Cincinnati College of Medicine
Cincinnati, Ohio

**Jesus San-Miguel, MD, PhD**
Servicio de Hematología
Hospital Universitario de Salamanca, Spain
CIC, IBMCC (USAL-CSIC)
Salamanca, Spain

**Hans Juergen Schlitt, MD, PhD**
University Medical Center
Department of Surgery
Regensburg, Germany

**Daniela Schulz-Ertner, MD**
Radiological Institute
MVZ (Medical Care Center)
Markus Hospital
Frankfurt/Main, Germany

**Jennifer L. Scott, MCP, PhD**
School of Psychology
University of Tasmania
Hobart, Tasmania, Australia

**Pamela Seam, MD**
Clinical Trials Team
Metabolism Branch
Center for Cancer Research
National Cancer Institute
National Institutes of Health
Bethesda, Maryland

**Lesley Seymour, MD, PhD**
NCIC Clinical Trials Group
Queen's University
Kingston, Ontario, Canada

**Manish R. Sharma, MD**
Section of Hematology/Oncology
University of Chicago Medical Center
Chicago, Illinois

**Richard Simon, PhD**
Biometrics Research Branch
National Cancer Institute
National Institutes of Health
Bethesda, Maryland

**Alfred Smith, PhD**
Department of Radiation Oncology
University of Texas MD Anderson Cancer Center
Center for Global Oncology
Houston, Texas

**David Spiegel, MD**
Department of Psychiatry and Behavioral Sciences
Stanford University School of Medicine
Stanford, California

**Walter Stadler, MD, FACP**
Departments of Medicine and Surgery
Sections of Hematology/Oncology and Urology
University of Chicago
Chicago, Illinois

**Wilfred D. Stein, PhD**
Medical Oncology Branch
National Cancer Institute
National Institutes of Health
Bethesda, Maryland
Department of Biological Chemistry
Silberman Institute of Life Sciences
Hebrew University
Jerusalem, Israel

**Michael L. Steinberg, MD**
Department of Radiation Oncology
David Geffen School of Medicine
University of California–Los Angeles
Los Angeles, California

**Oswald A. Stuart, BS**
Washington Cancer Institute
Washington Hospital Center
Washington, D.C.

**Paul H. Sugarbaker, MD, FACS, FRCS**
Program in Peritoneal Surface Malignancy
Washington Cancer Institute
Washington Hospital Center
Washington, D.C.

**Talal Sulaiman**
University Medical Center
Department of Surgery
Regensburg, Germany

**Liang-Liang Sun, MD**
Department of Endocrinology and Metabolism
Changzheng Hospital
Second Military Medical University
Shanghai, People's Republic of China

**Karen L. Syrjala, PhD**
Clinical Research Division
Biobehavioral Sciences
Survivorship Program
Fred Hutchinson Cancer Research Center
Department of Psychiatry and Behavioral Sciences
University of Washington
Seattle, Washington

**Daniel S. W. Tan, BSc (Hons), MRCP**
Drug Development Unit
Section of Medicine
The Institute of Cancer Research and The Royal Marsden Hospital
    NHS Trust
Sutton, United Kingdom

**Antoine Thierry-Vuillemin, MD**
Department of Oncology
University Hospital J. Minjoz, and Institut National
    de la Santé et de la Recherche Médicale
Besançon, France

**George V. Thomas, MRCPI, MD**
Translational Molecular Oncology Team
Section of Cell and Molecular Biology
Chester Beatty Laboratories
London, United Kingdom
Translational Molecular Oncology Team
Section of Medicine
The Institute of Cancer Research
Haddow Laboratories
Sutton, United Kingdom

**Sheeba K. Thomas**
The Division of Cancer Medicine
Department of Lymphoma/Myeloma
University of Texas MD Anderson Cancer Center
Houston, Texas

**Anthony W. Tolcher, MD, FACP**
START-South Texas Accelerated Research Therapeutics
San Antonio, Texas

**Peter C. Trask, PhD, MPH**
Global Outcomes Research
Oncology, Pfizer Inc.
New London, Connecticut

**Alexei V. Trofimov, PhD**
Department of Radiation Oncology
Massachusetts General Hospital
Harvard Medical School
Boston, Massachusetts

**Mario Valle, MD**
The National Cancer Center "Regina Elena"
Rome, Italy

**Sonia Vallet, MD**
MGH Cancer Center
Massachusetts General Hospital
Harvard Medical School
Boston, Massachusetts

**Kurt Van der Speeten, MD**
Department of Surgical Oncology
Ziekenhuis Oost-Limburg
Genk, Belgium

**Delphine Vaudoyer, MD**
Surgical Oncology Department
Centre Hospitalo-Universitaire Lyon Sud
Hospices Civils de Lyon
Pierre Bénite, France

**Vic J. Verwaal, MD, PhD**
The Netherlands Cancer Institute-Antoni van Leeuwenhoek Hospital
Amsterdam, The Netherlands

**Tatiana Vidaurre, MD**
Medical Oncology Branch
National Cancer Institute
National Institutes of Health
Bethesda, Maryland

**Cristian Villanueva, MD**
Department of Oncology
University Hospital J. Minjoz, and Institut National
    de la Santé et de la Recherche Médicale
Besançon, France

**Phillip von Breitenbuch, MD**
University Medical Center
Department of Surgery
Regensburg, Germany

**Uli Weber, PhD**
Rhön-Klinikum AG
Universitäts-Kliniken Giessen
Marburg, Germany

**Donna M. Weber**
Division of Cancer Medicine
Department of Lymphoma/Myeloma
University of Texas
M.D. Anderson Cancer Center
Houston, Texas

**Julia Wilkerson**
Medical Oncology Branch
National Cancer Institute
National Institutes of Health
Bethesda, Maryland

**Julia Wilkerson**
The Medical Oncology Branch
Center for Cancer Research
National Cancer Institute
National Institutes of Health
Bethesda, Maryland

**Paul Workman, BSc (Hons), PhD, DSc (Hon) FMedSci, FIBiol**
Cancer Research UK Centre for Cancer Therapeutics
The Institute of Cancer Research
Haddow Laboratories
Sutton, United Kingdom

**Liang Xiu, PhD**
Clinical Oncology Research
Ortho Biotech Oncology Research and Development
Unit of Johnson & Johnson Pharmaceutical
    Research & Development
Raritan, New Jersey

**Joachim Yahalom, MD**
The Memorial Sloan-Kettering Cancer Center
Weill Medical College of Cornell University
New York, New York

**James Yang, MD**
Surgical Oncology Branch
National Institutes of Health
Bethesda, Maryland

**Jean C. Yi, PhD**
Clinical Research Division
Biobehavioral Sciences
Fred Hutchinson Cancer Research Center
Seattle, Washington

**Qing Yi, MD, PhD**
Division of Cancer Medicine
Department of Lymphoma and Myeloma
Center for Cancer Immunology Research
The University of Texas
M.D. Anderson Cancer Center
Houston, Texas

**Ji Zheng**
Novartis Pharmaceuticals Corporation
Florham Park, New Jersey

**Sen H. Zhuang, MD, PhD**
Clinical Oncology Research
Ortho Biotech Oncology Research and
    Development
Unit of Johnson & Johnson Pharmaceutical
    Research & Development
Raritan, New Jersey

**Anthony L. Zietman, MD**
The Department of Radiation Oncology
Massachusetts General Hospital
Harvard Medical School
Boston, Massachusetts

# Preface

We live in challenging times for publishing textbooks. We are in an age when information is everywhere. You can search any subject on the Internet in minutes from your computer or handheld device and be deluged with a long list of replies. The real issues, though, are the quality of the information, not the quantity—the interpretation of the data, not the listing of information or newly published papers on a subject. This is where the opinion of experts excels.

Coincident with the publication of the eighth edition of *Cancer: Principles & Practice of Oncology*, the editors decided to use the vehicle of our companion journal, *The Cancer Journal: Principles & Practice of Oncology* to freshen the text on a continuous basis.

We asked experts to focus on areas of special importance to oncologists of all persuasions and distill the literature on important advances in oncology into manageable pieces of information.

We have been pleased with the results. And readers of the *Journal* have suggested we package these publications into a convenient monograph for easy access.

Lippincott Williams & Wilkins, we are pleased to announce, has enthusiastically agreed to do this on a regular basis.

The result lies before you: a wealth of medical literature, properly vetted for quality and leavened by the wisdom and judgment of experts in each of the special areas of special focus. We hope you find it as useful and informative as we have.

*Vincent T. DeVita, Jr., MD*
*Theodore S. Lawrence, MD, PhD*
*Steven A. Rosenberg, MD, PhD*

# Contents

## PART 6: New Therapies For Myeloma: Impact On Survival

CHAPTER

# 1

# Out in the Open

## Addressing Sexual Health After Cancer

Sharon L. Bober

Sexuality is an organic, life-affirming component of human experience. It is also one of the first elements of daily living disrupted by a cancer diagnosis; a disruption the majority of cancer patients feel unprepared for.[1] Recent advances in cancer care now mean that the majority of newly diagnosed cancer survivors will "live beyond cancer." Survival rates have been steadily increasing since 1990, and the number of cancer survivors is expected to double in the coming decade. However, it is imperative to acknowledge that the range of life-saving cancer treatments at our disposal (eg, surgery, chemotherapy, radiation, and hormonal therapies) often result in severe and devastating effects on patients' experiences of sexuality and intimacy. Although there has been increasing attention on quality of life both during and after cancer, there is, for many patients, a deafening silence when it comes to the topic of sexuality.

This reality is particularly unfortunate because the effects of cancer treatment on sexuality are not only short-term, but also potentially enduring and distressing long after treatment ends. Patients' sexual functioning is often initially disrupted by a wide range of treatments from the impact of invasive or disfiguring surgery to the acute and often devastating effects of chemotherapy, radiation, and hormonal therapies. Beyond the short-term, many long-term effects of treatment are permanent. For example, young women who undergo sudden and marked treatment-induced menopause are at high risk for menopause-related sexual dysfunction as well as fertility-related distress, problems that are still salient on long-term follow-up. Despite efforts to reduce the debilitating side effects of radical prostatectomy and radiation therapy, the overwhelming majority of men treated for prostate cancer are left with erectile dysfunction long after treatment ends. Prostate cancer patient treated with antiandrogen therapy have described themselves as feeling "neutered" and struggling not only with issues around masculinity but also with feelings of guilt and shame. Sometimes, the devastating changes in sexuality are not always obvious. There are also a variety of more subtle ways in which cancer treatment affects sexuality over time. For example, the rhythm of normal sexuality may be severely disrupted when a patient is told not to have sex when they are on certain chemotherapy regimen or when they are immunosuppressed. As one stem-cell transplant survivor explained over a year-off therapy, "How am I supposed to feel comfortable having sex again when I was told that I could not even ride a city bus without potentially catching a germ that might kill me."

And sex is not easy to talk about. Despite living in a culture that is saturated with overtly sexual images, graphic lyrics, and explicit advertising, most of us do not have experience talking about sex and intimacy in a frank, direct, and authentic manner, whether it is in our role as a physician, family-member, patient, or spouse. As it has been recently pointed out, there are greatly mismatched expectations when it comes to doctor-patient communication about patient sexuality. Patients often have significant needs for education, support, and practical help with managing sexual changes after treatment yet this topic is routinely unaddressed or only barely touched on.[2] Starting with standard medical school curricula, there is a significant lack of formal sexual health curricula[3] and clinicians only rarely receive any kind of formal training in how to communicate about sexuality with patients.

With great appreciation to our contributors, this issue of *The Cancer Journal* features 11 articles that discuss various aspects on the topic of sexuality after cancer. Many of our papers will focus on topics that have, to date, received very little, yet much needed, attention such as sexual functioning in sexual minority women, sexuality in the context of cancer recurrence, and sexuality with BRCA1/2 mutation carriers. We have also attempted to present articles with an emphasis on intervention such as the articles that overview sexual rehabilitation with prostate cancer survivors, intervention with gynecologic cancer survivors, and novel approaches to working with couples after cancer.

In the words of another long-term cancer survivor, "Sure it is important to still be alive, but it is also important to reclaim my sexuality. The changes in my sex life continue to represent an immense and often ignored loss." Although there are a myriad of reasons why we do not talk about sex, the proverbial elephant in the consulting room, it is imperative to start. As the numbers of cancer survivors continue to grow, it is critical to learn how to best help patients and families to manage the potentially devastating effects that cancer treatment can have on their sexual and intimate experience. This issue will hopefully provide the reader with a broad overview of the topic of sexuality after cancer that understandably may raise as many questions as there are answers. But in a sense, that is part of the purpose, as this issue is meant to start the conversation, not finish it.

## REFERENCES

1. Schover L. *Sexuality and Fertility after Cancer.* New York: Wiley; 1997.
2. Hordern A, Street A. Communicating about patient sexuality and intimacy after cancer: mismatched expectations and unmet needs. *Med J Aust.* 2007;186:224–227.
3. Mahotra S, Khurshid A, Hendricks KA, et al. *J Natl Med Assoc.* 2008;100:1097–1106.

# Unraveling the Next Chapter

## Sexual Development, Body Image, and Sexual Functioning in Female BRCA Carriers

Ellen T. Matloff • Rachel E. Barnett • Sharon L. Bober

The hereditary breast and ovarian cancer genes, *BRCA1* and *BRCA2*, were cloned in the early 90s and clinical testing became available in 1996.[1,2] Mutations in these 2 genes are found in the majority of autosomal dominant hereditary breast and ovarian cancer families.[3]

Female mutation carriers have a high lifetime risk of both breast (55%–85%) and ovarian cancer (15%–40%).[4-7] Research in the last decade has centered on the psychologic impact of genetic testing on patients and the medical efficacy of surveillance, chemoprevention, and prophylactic surgery on cancer risk reduction for female carriers. The focus of this research has been, appropriately, on ascertaining the most effective ways for female BRCA carriers to reduce their risks of developing breast and ovarian cancers. Prophylactic bilateral mastectomy (BM) has been shown to reduce the risk of breast cancer in BRCA carriers by greater than 90%.[8] Prophylactic bilateral salpingo-oophorectomy (BSO) significantly reduces the risk of ovarian cancer (~80%–85%) and also the risk of breast cancer (~50%–72%) in BRCA carriers, particularly in premenopausal women.[9-11] *BRCA1* carriers seem to benefit most from the reduction in ovarian cancer risk after BSO, whereas *BRCA2* carriers benefit most from the reduction in breast cancer risk because the majority of breast cancers in these women are estrogen receptor positive.[11,12] It is recommended that female *BRCA1* carriers have their ovaries and fallopian tubes removed prophylactically by age 35 to 40 years. The majority of *BRCA2* carriers may be able to defer this surgery until their early to mid-40s because the average age of ovarian cancer development is later, although they will lose some of the risk reduction benefit of this surgery on the risk to develop breast cancer.[11,12] However, with a decade of clinical experience under our belts, it is becoming clear that predisposition genetic testing, and the decision-making that follows, brings with it a plethora of complex emotional, physical, and body image and sexuality issues for BRCA carriers and their children.[13-17] The sequelae of this process for the individual and her family continue to be unearthed as we move forward in this new age of predictive testing and risk reduction. This article will focus on some of the complicated issues around sexuality and intimacy faced by healthy women who are known to carry a BRCA mutation.

## Sexual Development and Self-Image

The roots of sexual self-image and sexuality begin in early childhood and include a young girl's observations of her mother's body in comparison to her own. In families with BRCA mutations, the course of this developmental stage is often altered. Breasts may represent not just breast-feeding, lingerie, and sexual maturity, but too often cancer, illness, anxiety, scars, reconstruction, and fear of death. Puberty in an average girl is marked by the development of breast buds, shopping for a first bra, excitement and anxiety about the beginning of menstruation, and the changing self-image from prepubescence

to womanhood. In a cancer-prone family, such physical development may spark anxiety in family members and the girl herself, who fear that sexual maturity may be the gateway to the "the family curse." The development of breast buds is often misconstrued as a "breast lump" by young pubescents, and some young girls (and boys) may hide this finding from their parents, not wishing to alarm them. One 15-year-old boy at 50% risk to carry his mother's *BRCA2* mutation confided to his mother's genetic counselor that he felt lumps on his chest, but did not tell his mother because he knew she would worry. The development of breasts may also mark the beginning of heightened breast cancer surveillance. Young girls who have watched their own relatives undergo prophylactic or treatment-based breast surgery may view breast development as the first step in a campaign of aggressive and worrisome monitoring before moving toward having their "cancer targets" removed at some point in the future.

For these reasons, BRCA carriers may well be vulnerable to an array of anxiety, fear, anger, depression, and ambivalence in the context of breast development and sexual maturation.[18] Young girls from families in which other women no longer have their breasts may experience guilt about their breast development and their young, healthy bodies. They often struggle with balancing excitement about pubertal development with fear and anxiety about their risk for cancer. Indeed, and perhaps even more pronounced is the tenable, yet often unspoken fear that parents develop as their daughters mature into young women, now at risk for breast and ovarian cancer. Some young women pronounce that they plan to have their breasts removed if they test positive for the BRCA mutation in their family. This decision can be empowering and may parallel decisions made by their mothers or female relatives. For others it is fear-based or imposed by well-meaning relatives or healthcare providers, who insist that this is the only way to stave off the imposing threat of breast cancer that has ravaged generations of the family. Whatever the underlying rationale, these young women at-risk certainly have a different experience of their breasts and their bodies than the majority of their peers.

## Genetic Testing

The decision of when to pursue genetic testing is a controversial one, although all professional recommendations state that testing for adult onset genetic diseases should be deferred until after the age of 18, when the child is an adult and can provide informed consent.[18-20] Genetic testing by the age of 25, or 10 years before the first cancer diagnosis in the family, is often recommended because that is when surveillance would begin; therefore, these young BRCA carriers enter into the cancer world, whereas their peers are seeking medical attention only for pap smears and birth control.[21] Some young women want to be tested before the age of 25 years, often because they hope for the 50% chance that they do not carry the mutation in their family.

For women who instead learn that they do carry the mutation in their family, this can be disappointing and frightening.

## Dating, Relationships, and Marriage

Testing positive for a BRCA mutation can affect a young woman's outlook on dating, relationships, and marriage. Some young women have, remarkably, been advised by healthcare providers to get married and have children as soon as possible so they can have their breasts and ovaries removed. Patients note that they have received this type of "life counseling" as though it is a treatment plan comparable with the more straightforward recommendation of beginning yearly breast magnetic resonance imaging (MRIs) at 25 years of age.[22] These weighty pieces of advice are of questionable benefit, and may actually do more harm than good.

Deana, a 23-year-old woman who recently tested positive, explains, "It (testing positive) suddenly put a time limit on things for me. I think its good, like, I don't want to waste my time on someone who isn't worth it. I'm looking for someone fun, but also compassionate. Someone who *wants* to understand this and support me." Deana admits that she has recently felt "bitter" toward people her own age who are in love, because she wants that too. "I don't want to be one of those women whose clock is ticking, but kind of, mine is."

Carrie, a 37-year-old woman who is now married with children, recalls that when she tested positive in her 20s, she felt the need to "expose my flaw" early in relationships with men. "Looking back, I probably told people too early, because I had this need to get it out there." She also discusses thinking about when and how to tell new boyfriends her "secret," and wondering whether they will still be interested in her after this disclosure.

Sandra, a 53-year-old woman who tested positive 7 years ago and has since divorced, recalls knowing that she was at risk to develop cancer based on her family history since age 3 or 4—decades before *BRCA1* and *BRCA2* were cloned. "I've been worrying about this since childhood. I was in such a *rush* to get married. I wanted to have children and have them grow up before I died. It made me marry someone who wasn't right for me, because I had a limited time on earth."

## Prophylactic Surgery

### Decision Making

The options of prophylactic BM or BSO also raise unique issues and choices for female BRCA carriers. When a woman is suspected to have cancer, she is immediately given an action plan: mammogram, MRI, biopsy, surgery, chemotherapy, radiation, and/or hormonal therapy. The situation is imminent, and the focus is survival; no one questions whether or not immediate action is necessary or prudent. The situation is quite different for an unaffected BRCA carrier. An unaffected carrier, of any age, is given a host of options for managing her risk. These most often include breast surveillance (mammogram, MRI), chemoprevention (tamoxifen, evista), and bilateral prophylactic mastectomy.[8,11,12,23–26] For ovarian cancer risk, she may also be offered surveillance (transvaginal ultrasound, CA-125), chemoprevention (oral contraceptives), and bilateral salpino-oophorectomy or total hysterectomy.[11,27–31]

Many of these options are not appropriate or practical for young, unaffected women who are premenopausal and have not started or completed childbearing. Other options are not appropriate for older, unaffected women who are poor surgical candidates or have comorbidities. Some options, like BSO are recommended almost uniformly for all healthy female BRCA carriers who are 40 years of age or older.[32] However, these choices are generally presented as options to female carriers, and the ultimate decisions and the timing of those de-cisions falls into their laps. Different professionals provide differing information about the actual risks associated with BRCA mutations, as well as the efficacy of each surveillance and risk reduction option. The ambiguity of this information has become greater in an age when the genetic testing company that owns the patent on BRCA testing is pushing healthcare providers not well-versed in genetic counseling to order testing themselves.[33] Many patients, therefore, do not receive adequate counseling and receive little, if any, accurate assistance with decision-making.

## Sexual Self-Image and Sexual Functioning

The sole focus of discussion on prophylactic surgery is often cancer risk reduction, whereas other issues are pushed to the back burner or are ignored. Prophylactic BSO is highly effective in reducing the risk of both ovarian and breast cancer; however, the risks of these cancers for BRCA carriers are not 100%.[4–7] The risk of early, immediate, surgical menopause after the procedure, however, is 100%. And although the risk:benefit ratio still favors this surgery for most carriers, the decision-making discussion with healthcare providers often lacks a balanced discussion of the menopausal symptoms that may follow, the pros and cons of hormone replacement therapy, and the impact on bone and heart health. Many women report having received little or no discussion about the impact of this surgery on vaginal dryness and their libido, body image, and achievement of orgasm during preoperative visits. In the anonymity of BRCA discussion groups and listservs, carriers frequently describe their fears that this surgery will make them "asexual," "castrated," "shriveled," or will cause them to develop male secondary sexual characteristics, like a deep voice and facial hair. Many BRCA carriers report that they do not raise these fears with their physicians, because they sound trivial and ridiculous in contrast to the benefits of this cancer risk-reducing measure. Guilt is often described in being concerned about surgical side effects because these women believe they should feel only "lucky" and "fortunate" for having the opportunity to "dodge cancer," particularly because many of their relatives were not so fortunate (Yale Cancer Genetic Counseling, unpublished data, 2008). And, while they often do feel fortunate, it is just one of the emotions they experience.

Sheryl, a 42-year-old woman who had a prophylactic BSO last year, describes, "The procedure is life-saving, and that trumps everything else; but it also represents an enormous amount of loss—not just future childbearing, but femininity, sexuality. It's like you've got a gun to your head and there is no other option. In preop I was crying—not scared, but angry that there is no better option. Let's face it, this is pretty primitive. I was panicked that it would end my sex life and experienced a lot of anticipatory grief leading up to the procedure." Sheryl describes that she felt "surprisingly well" after the surgery, since she had done much of her grieving preop, but that her husband had a very difficult time after the procedure. "It became very real to him and he had his own grief, loss. We definitely wouldn't be having more kids and maybe our sex life wouldn't ever be the same." She points out that there is no counseling for the partner going through this process, as there now is for many spouses of cancer survivors.

Amber, who had a prophylactic BSO at 40 years, also describes that her husband had a harder time with the surgery than she did, which was, in turn, hard for her. "He would say to me, 'Why would you cut open your perfect body?' The negative pressure was hard on me, but now he is relieved that I did it. I was afraid I'd fall apart and go to wrinkles. I do think my libido is lower, although I didn't have a change in vaginal dryness or orgasm. But it has boosted my confidence and sexuality, and my body image has increased. Worrying is more paralyzing than anything."

Sandra, who had a prophylactic BSO in her mid-40s was concerned about aging and her sex drive after surgery. The surgery was not as bad as she feared, although it was harder to achieve orgasm and she lost the "sex fog" she would enjoy right before her period each month. But, she can still get in the mood and enjoy sex. Sandra is now contemplating prophylactic BM. She is nervous about the surgery and is "scared of waking up in a body I don't know and I don't like" although she admits that she has a hard time enjoying intimacy and sex when it comes to her breasts. "I don't like it when people touch my breasts. It reminds me that I have breasts, and breasts get cancer."

Gretchen, a 34-year-old newly divorced single mother, chose to have a prophylactic BM this year. She felt that she could not afford to develop breast cancer or to die because she needs to raise her young daughter. She was very worried about losing her breasts because they were central to her self-image, but calls the decision to have a BM "the best decision I ever made." "This is a constant reminder of how strong I am," and she feels proud to have shown her young daughter, and even her friends, that you can survive adversity. She now has peace of mind and feels good about the way she looks in tiny, sexy shirts. "Sexuality is more about how you feel about yourself than how people feel about you." She has had to balance dating this year with issues like how many bandages she would have at the time of a date, but says its been manageable. Gretchen describes that she has also learned that "Everyone has something. This is my thing. And if this is the worst problem I have, I'm doing pretty well."

In contrast, Carrie chose a prophylactic BM at 30 years of age and does not feel good about her reconstruction. "I'm not happy with the way I look, I feel grotesque. I don't change in public anymore, like at the pool, and I don't take baths anymore because I don't like to look at my body." She describes still having an active sex life with her husband, even after a recent prophylactic BSO, but things have changed. "I find myself fantasizing more during sex than I ever did before. I've developed techniques to remove myself from my body during sex so that I'm not hung up on how my body looks." She describes that her husband has been very supportive and loving through the entire process.

Rosie, a 61-year-old breast cancer survivor, chose to have a contralateral mastectomy 15 years after her breast cancer diagnosis and original unilateral mastectomy and reconstruction. She never felt good about the original reconstruction and felt that this surgery would both reduce her cancer risks and help her to feel better about her body. The surgery and recovery were much more difficult than she anticipated, but she reports, "I look better and feel better about myself."

## External Reactions

Women who have tried to discuss prophylactic decision making with family, friends, and even healthcare providers are often met with resistance, shock, misinformation, and negative responses. One woman described that her in-laws referred to her upcoming prophylactic BM as her "boob job" and chided her for what they considered a narcissistic and paranoid decision. Another woman who requested a BSO described that her physician decisively, and incorrectly, told her that *BRCA2* mutations increased risk for breast and colon cancer, and that ovarian cancer was not associated with this mutation. A 43-year-old patient who elected to have both prophylactic BSO and BM described that her decision was met with opposition, instead of support, by her younger sister. Her sister had already been diagnosed with breast cancer and felt that prophylactic surgery was drastic and ridiculous; sadly, that sister has since died of her disease. Other patients describe increasing familial pressure to have prophylactic surgery as they reach the age at which their family members were diagnosed with cancers (Yale Cancer Genetic Counseling, unpublished data, 2008). The plethora of inaccurate and negative opinions that these women face can be overwhelming and is in direct contrast to the warm, widespread support that many women now receive when diagnosed with cancer, both individually and globally (eg, cancer walks, support groups, ribbons).

## Fertility and Childbearing

Women who learn they carry a BRCA mutation before having children, or before completing their family, face many issues and dilemmas. A common thread is that women and couples who are still toying with the idea of having more children realize that having a prophylactic BSO will prematurely and permanently close that door. Although many carriers in their late 30s and 40s report that they probably would not have had more children, there is a profound sense of loss when that option is taken away. This loss does not necessarily end after menopause. Felicia, a vibrant 69-year-old woman who tested positive last year and reluctantly agreed to a BSO, said that the surgery has had no impact on her sex life or body image. She was, however, "reluctant to have surgical intervention on a healthy body." Although she was clearly postmenopausal, losing her ovaries represented a loss of parts of her body that had served her well. Felicia recalls that her surgeon told her that her ovaries were "old and shriveled" and that she would not notice they were gone. Although this may have been true biologically, it was not true emotionally or psychologically and was hurtful. She eventually came to peace with BSO by imagining that she was "releasing the energy from these ovaries back into the universe, to a woman who needs them now to have a baby."

A less common, but still prevalent, topic of discussion is the 50% risk of passing a mutation, and the legacy of cancer, on to their children. One 39-year-old lesbian patient just out of a serious partnership was contemplating having a child on her own and chose not to after testing positive for the *BRCA2* mutation in her family. She described that she did not want to risk passing the mutation on to her children, did not want to be exposed to the hormones used in fertility treatments or associated with pregnancy, and was afraid to bring a child into the world by herself if her cancer risks were high. She instead chose to have a prophylactic BSO to reduce her risks of both ovarian and breast cancers and may adopt a child in the future. Another married 30-year-old woman chose to have a prophylactic BM before starting a family because she was so worried about developing breast cancer during pregnancy and possibly being faced with either postponing treatment or having a therapeutic abortion to start treatment. Sandra recalls when her first baby was born by Cesearean section and the doctor told her it was a girl. "My husband said, 'You must be so happy, you wanted a girl!' and I thought to myself, 'Why would I want a girl?' They develop breasts."

Some patients have preimplantation genetic diagnosis to reduce the risk of passing on a BRCA mutation to offspring. Others may elect for sperm separation to increase the likelihood of having a male fetus, which would be less affected by carrying a mutation.[34] However, the minority of BRCA carriers elect to have these procedures or prenatal testing for these mutations.[35]

## CONCLUSIONS

Genetic counseling and testing for *BRCA1* and *BRCA2* allows women and their healthcare providers to effectively tailor their surveillance and medical management plans. However, as we move forward with a new generation of women who know their high-risk status from childhood, it is imperative to explore the impact of the information on sexual development and self-imagery by developing future research protocols in this area. Information regarding how to manage menopausal side-effects, as well as pre- and postsurgical sexual rehabilitation counseling, should be available to patients and partners. Although prophylactic BSO and BM are highly-effective tools in reducing cancer risk in female BRCA carriers, the effects of these choices on sexual self-image and sexual functioning should not be underestimated.

## REFERENCES

1. Miki Y, Swenson J, Shattuck-Eidens D, et al. A strong candidate for the breast and ovarian cancer susceptibility gene BRCA1. *Science.* 1994;266:66–71.
2. Wooster R, Bignell G, Lancaster J, et al. Identification of the breast cancer susceptibility gene BRCA2. *Nature.* 1995;378:789–792.
3. Claus E, Risch N, Thompson W, et al. Autosomal dominant inheritance of early-onset breast cancer. *Cancer.* 1994;73:643–651.
4. Struewing J, Hartge P, Wacholder S, et al. The risk of cancer associated with specific mutations of BRCA1 and BRCA2 among Ashkenazi Jews. *N Engl J Med.* 1997;336:1401–1408.
5. Ford D, Easton D, Stratton, M, et al. Genetic heterogeneity and penetrance analysis of the BRCA1 and BRCA2 genes in breast cancer families: the Breast Cancer Linkage Consortium. *Am J Hum Genet.* 1998;62:676–689.
6. Antoniou A, Pharoah P, Narod S, et al. Average risks of breast and ovarian cancer associated with BRCA1 or BRCA2 mutations detected in case series unselected for family history: A combined analyses of 22 studies. *Am J Hum Genet.* 2003;72:1117–1130.
7. King M, Marks J, Mandell J. Breast and ovarian cancer risks due to inherited mutations in BRCA1 and BRCA2. *Science.* 2003;302:643–646.
8. Rebbeck T, Friebel T, Lynch H, et al. Bilateral prophylactic mastectomy reduces breast cancer risk in BRCA1 and BRCA2 mutation carriers: the PROSE Study Group. *J Clin Oncol.* 2004;15:1055–1062.
9. Finch A, Beiner M, Lubinski J, et al. Salpingo-oophorectomy and the risk of ovarian, fallopian tube, and peritoneal cancers in women with a BRCA1 or BRCA2 mutation. *JAMA.* 2006;296:185–192.
10. Eisen A, Lubinski J, Klijn J. Breast cancer risk following bilateral oophorectomy in BRCA1 and BRCA2 mutation carriers: an international case-control study. *J Clin Oncol.* 2005;23:7491–7496.
11. Kauff N, Domchek S, Friebel T, et al. Risk-reducing salpingo-oophorectomy for the prevention of BRCA1 and BRCA2 associated breast and gynecologic cancer: a multicenter, prospective study. *J Clin Oncol.* 2008;26:1331–1337.
12. Domchek S, Friebel T, Neuhausen S, et al. Mortality reduction after risk-reducing bilateral salpingo-oophorectomy in a prospective cohort of BRCA1 and BRCA2 mutation carriers. *Lancet Oncol.* 2006;7:223–229.
13. Brandberg Y, Sandelin K, Erikson S, et al. Psychological reactions, quality of life, and body image after bilateral prophylactic mastectomy in women at high risk for breast cancer: a prospective 1-year follow-up study. *J Clin Oncol.* 2008;26:3943–3949.
14. Besser P, Synaeve C, Van Gool A, et al. Satisfaction with prophylactic mastectomy and breast reconstruction in genetically predisposed women. *Plast Reconstr Surg.* 2006;117:1675–1682.
15. Van Oostrom I, Meijers-Heijboer H, Lodder L, et al. Long-term psychological impact of carrying a BRCA1/2 mutation and prophylactic surgery: a 5-year follow-up study. *J Clin Oncol.* 2003;21:3867–3874.
16. Robson M, Hensley M, Barakat R, et al. Quality of life in women at risk for ovarian cancer who have undergone risk-reducing oophorectomy. *Gynecol Oncol.* 2003;89:281–287.
17. Tercyak K, Peshkin B, Streisand R, et al. Psychosocial issues among children of hereditary breast cancer gene (BRCA1/2) testing participants. *Psychooncology.* 2001;10:336–346.
18. Biesecker B, Boehnke M, Calzone K, et al. Genetic counseling for families with inherited susceptibility to breast and ovarian cancer. *JAMA.* 1993;269:1970–1974.
19. American Society of Clinical Oncology: ASCO policy statement update: genetic testing for cancer susceptibility. *J Clin Oncol.* 2003;21:2397–2406.
20. American Society of Human Genetics Board of Directors & American College of Medical Genetics Board of Directors: Points to consider: ethical, legal, and psychosocial implications of genetic testing in children and adolescents. *Am J Hum Genet.* 1995;57:1233–1241.
21. National Comprehensive Cancer Network Clinical Practice Guidelines in Oncology: Genetic/Familial High-Risk Assessment: Breast and Ovarian V.1.2008. Available at: http://www.nccn.org/professionals/physician_gls/PDF/genetics_screening.pdf. Accessed September 12, 2008.
22. Matloff E, Moyer A, Shannon K, et al. Healthy women with a family history of breast cancer: impact of a tailored genetic counseling intervention on risk perception, knowledge, and menopausal therapy decision-making. *J Women's Health.* 2006;15:843–856.
23. Warner E, Plewes D, Hill K, et al. Surveillance of BRCA1 and BRCA2 mutation carriers with magnetic resonance imaging, ultrasound, mammography, and clinical breast examination. *JAMA.* 2004;202:1317–1325.
24. Metcalfe K, Lynch H, Ghadirian P, et al. Contralateral breast cancer in BRCA1 and BRCA2 mutation carriers. *J Clin Oncol.* 2004;22:2328–2335.
25. Gronwald J, Tung N, Foulkes W, et al. Tamoxifen and contralateral breast cancer in BRCA1 and BRCA2 carriers: an update. *Int J Cancer.* 2006;118:2281–2284.
26. Narod S, Brunet J, Ghadirian P, et al. Tamoxifen and risk of contralateral breast cancer in BRCA1 and BRCA2 mutation carriers: a case-control study. *Lancet.* 2000;356:1876–1881.
27. Stirling D, Evans D, Pichert G, et al. Screening for familial ovarian cancer: failure of current protocols to detect ovarian cancer at an early stage according to the International Federation of Gynecology and Obstetrics System. *J Clin Oncol.* 2005;23:5588–5596.
28. McLaughlin J, Risch H, Lubinski J, et al. Reproductive risk factors for ovarian cancer in carriers of BRCA1 or BRCA2 mutations: a case-control study. *Lancet Oncol.* 2007;8:26–34.
29. McGuire V, Felberg A, Mills M, et al. Relation of contraceptive and reproductive history to ovarian cancer risk in carriers and noncarriers of BRCA1 gene mutations. *Am J Epidemiol.* 2004;160:613–618.
30. Whittemore A, Balise R, Pharoah P, et al. Oral contraceptive use and ovarian cancer risk among carriers of BRCA1 and BRCA2 mutations. *Br J Cancer.* 2004;91:1911–1915.
31. Rebbeck T, Lynch H, Neuhausen S, et al. Prophylactic oophorectomy in carriers of BRCA1 or BRCA2 mutations. *N Engl J Med.* 2002;346:1616–1622.
32. Kauff N, Barakat R. Risk-reducing salpingo-oophorectomy in patients with germline mutations in BRCA1 or BRCA2. *J Clin Oncol.* 2007;25:2921–2927.
33. Matloff E, Caplan A. Direct to confusion: lessons learned from marketing BRCA testing. *Am J Bioeth.* 2008;8:5–8.
34. Microsort. Available at: www.microsort.net. Vol 2008, 2008.
35. Menon U, Harper J, Sharma A. Views of BRCA gene mutation carriers on preimplantation genetic diagnosis as a reproductive option for hereditary breast and ovarian cancer. *Hum Reprod.* 2007;22:1573–1577.

# Concerns About Sexuality After Breast Cancer

Patricia Fobair  •  David Spiegel

"Sexuality is an integral part of human life with the potential to create new life, foster intimacy and shared pleasure in a relationship. It is an important part of health and general well-being that cancer and cancer treatment can alter significantly."[1]

"A key feature of sexual desire is the positive anticipation and belief that sex is a satisfying part of life and the relationship."[2]

Cancer treatment, especially chemotherapy, creates changes in the female body that abruptly affects sexual desire, sexual problems, and emotional relationships.[3,4] Although healthy women also experience physiological changes due to low estrogen leading to menopause, these changes happen to them gradually leaving women sexually active, 5 to 10 years longer and with fewer problems in sexual functioning[3,5-8] (Table 1).

Breast cancer accounts for 33% of new cancers diagnosed among women in North America[9] and 22% of all cancer survivors.[10] Survival rates of breast cancer have improved from 60% in 1954 to 95% or better for localized disease in 2004.[11] Although patients are grateful for improved survival, they often face unpleasant changes in sexual functioning as a result of treatment.[9] Sexual problems have been reported since 1983, after treatment.[12] Definitive studies have associated chemotherapy with sexual problems, since 1994.[13,14] Survivors of breast cancer discuss sexual problems with each other and would like to talk about them with their physicians. Some have complained that they were inadequately prepared for chemotherapy-induced menopause and were surprised by the abruptness of onset.[15] They would like to find solutions for hot flashes, vaginal dryness, dyspareunia, including painful vaginal entry and pain with intercourse, as well as loss of sexual desire, but not at the expense of promoting further disease.[16,17] This article summarizes what is known about sexual problems after treatment for breast cancer, and enumerate solutions that lie within the control of the patient and her physician.

Ovarian toxicity is a predictable side effect of alkylating agent-based chemotherapy and is influenced by the cumulative dose and duration of therapy.[8,18]

A recent review on the impact of premature ovarian failure in young women with breast cancer concluded that menopause symptoms have a negative effect on quality of life.[19] There is a good deal of evidence that breast cancer patients treated with chemotherapy experience vaginal dryness and early menopause resulting in less sexual activity with their partners than patients treated by other means.[9,19-22] Loss of desire for sexual activity has consequences for relationships, and increases chances for "partner misunderstanding."[23] Vaginal dryness, a physiological disappointment for women over 50 years, is even more difficult for younger breast cancer patients, diagnosed during the most sexually active years of their lives.

"Silence about sexual problems can hurt relationships."[24] There are benefits when physicians talk with their patients about the challenges facing them after treatment. The benefit of knowing in advance that sexual changes frequently follow treatment provides the patient with an opportunity to regain control by anticipating problems ahead of time, and planning ways to cope. Patients can choose to talk with their partners before problems begin, locate group or individual support, and improve communication with her partner. She can also purchase supplements and lotions that could accord her greater physical comfort in love making.

## SEXUAL PROBLEMS AMONG BREAST CANCER PATIENTS

Problems with body image and sexuality occur during or after treatment.[3,20,25,26] While problems with body image, like "feeling less feminine," tend to improve, sexual problems, like "lack of sexual interest," persist over time among women with breast cancer.[4,9,21,25,27-29] The percentage of patients concerned with their body image varies from 31% to 67%.[3,30-34] The percentage of survivors reporting sexual problems varied from 50% to 56%[3,4,31,32] in 4 studies, leaving 44% to 50% of the breast cancer survivors less affected. Although problems with body image improved with time, (Table 1) sexual problems continued 5 years after treatment.[3,4] This article concerns the 50% or more patients struggling with sexual problems that did not improve with time.[9]

The extent of the patient's treatment affects the percent reporting sexual problems after treatment. Ganz et al[9,20] looked at the impact of breast cancer on the patients' sex life, and found that those who had a lumpectomy or mastectomy followed by chemotherapy were more likely to report a negative impact on their sex life (48% lumpectomy, 51% mastectomy) than patients with surgery only (18% lumpectomy, 25% mastectomy). In addition to "lack of interest," sexual problems included "difficulty in becoming sexually aroused," "unable to relax and enjoy sex," and "difficulty in reaching a climax."

Extent of treatment also made a difference on the impact in patients' sexual lives. Exploring sexual dysfunction among breast cancer survivors, Bukovic et al[32] found that 70% or more patients rated their sex lives as satisfying before cancer, with satisfaction dropping to 56% among patients with breast conserving surgery, and to 50% among patients with adjuvant treatment.[31,32] As Ganz and Greendale[35] noted premature menopause secondary to chemotherapy, radiation, or oophorectomy can complicate sexual functioning through vaginal atrophy and dyspareunia or painful intercourse. Other potential disruptions from treatment to the sexual response cycle in women may include fatigue, depression, pain, and changes in body image.[23,35-37]

Although surgery and radiation are also responsible for problems that breast cancer patients experience after treatment, studies

**TABLE 1.** Comparison of Breast Cancer Survivors With Women Without Cancer on Sexual Issues and Body Image

| Sexual Issues | Cancer Free[7] | 0–7 mo, After Diagnosis[3] | 5 yr Later[4] | Results |
|---|---|---|---|---|
| Age span | 35–49 | 22–50 | 27–55 | |
| Number | n = 6318 | n = 360 | n = 185 | |
| Sexual activity | 80% | 67% | 69% | Sexual activity improved slightly (2%) during 5 yr |
| Problems with sexual interest, desire | 35% | 56% | 56% | Problems with sexual interest, desire persisted over time |
| Difficulty in becoming sexually aroused | 30% | 47% | 46% | Problems with sexual arousal improved slightly (1%) w/time |
| Unable to relax and enjoy sex | 27% | 40% | 35% | Difficulties to relax and enjoy sex improved slightly (5%) w/time |
| Problems w/orgasm | 29% | 35% | 38% | Problems w/orgasm became slightly worse (3%) w/time |
| Hot flashes | 26% | 41% | 63% | Hot flashes got worse (22%) w/time |
| Vaginal dryness | — | 34% | 49% | Vaginal dryness got worse (15%) w/time |
| Postmenopausal | — | 40% | 75% | 35% increase in women postmenopausal 5 yr later |
| Unhappy w/body image | 60% | 67% | 46% | Body image improved with time for survivors |

Data from healthy women who were free of cancer. Ganz et al.[7], Breast Cancer Prevention Trial, Base-line quality of life assessment, from sexually active women 35–49 yr of age. Data on Breast Cancer Patients, 0–7 mo after diagnosis (n = 549) includes only partnered women (n = 360),[3] and at 5 yr (n = 185) includes both partnered and single women,[4] from the San Francisco Greater Bay Area Cancer Registry; Breast Cancer in Young Women: A Population Based Approach.
In both the Fobair et al. (2006) and Bloom (2004) articles, the proportion of sexually active women applies to the partnered women, and the proportion with various types of sexual problems applies to sexually active women.

have shown that sexual problems were worse for women who received chemotherapy.[3,4,9,14,20,22,23,25,27,28,36,38]

Two studies looked at the sexual experience of breast cancer patients in the greater San Francisco Bay Area (Table 1). Fobair et al[3] found that 67% of the 360 sexually active younger women, ages 22 to 50, reported sexual problems; 52% reported having one or more problems in sexual functioning. Variables associated with sexual problems were "vaginal dryness," "poor mental health," "body image," "being married," and having a "partner who has difficulty understanding my feelings." Five years later, 185 women in the same study group were reinterviewed, and 69% were sexually active, with 56% reporting problems with sexual desire or interest. In the time between interviews, hot flashes increased from 41% to 63%, and patients in menopause increased from 40% to 73%.[4] (Table 1) Other studies have also found that sexual problems continue to be severe at follow-up in women treated with chemotherapy for premenopausal breast cancer.[19,21,23,39]

The frequency of sexual activity declined after treatment, whereas sexual problems increased with time, in studies by Ganz et al [40,41] Among the 763 disease-free survivors interviewed an average of 6.3 years earlier, hot flashes were less frequent, but vaginal dryness increased with time, while sexual activity declined with partners between the 2 assessments (from 65% to 55%, $P = 0.001$.)[40] In a previous study, Ganz et al [41] found that sexual functioning showed deterioration between the 1st and 2nd year evaluation, whereas marital and sexual functioning showed a significant decline between the 1st and 3rd evaluations in a study of 139 breast cancer survivors interviewed over 3 points of time.[41]

Sexual problems have had an impact on marriages that were associated with partner misunderstanding in several studies. Marital status and partner's difficulty understanding were associated with sexual problems in studies by Lasry et al[42]; Ganz et al[36,41,43]; Lindley et al[44]; Meyerowitz et al[45]; Speer et al[46]; and Fobair et al.[3] In the work of Speer et al[46], it was the level of "relationship distress" that was the most significant variable affecting arousal, orgasm, lubrication, satisfaction, and sexual pain. Mental health and the quality of the partnership relationship, ie, "partner has difficulty in understanding," were independently associated with body image and sexual

problems.[3] There is a close relationship between variables like body image, mental health, depression, having had a mastectomy without reconstruction, and younger age that predict sexual problems in several studies.[3,23] For example, research on depression among breast cancer patients found that decreased libido, poor self-image, and relationship problems were common among those who are found to be depressed. Depression is a treatable problem with medication and psychotherapy.[47]

## EFFECTS OF BREAST CANCER TREATMENT VERSUS NORMAL AGING ON SEXUAL FUNCTION

How do breast cancer survivors differ from comparison groups and healthy women without cancer? In a study from Brazil,[48] 97 women with breast cancer were compared with 85 without breast cancer. The women with breast cancer reported less sexual activity (51.5%) compared with healthy women (62.4%, $P < 0.01$) without cancer.[48] Comparing symptoms and sexual activity between young (22–50 years) breast cancer patients, 0 to 7 months postdiagnosis[3] with healthy women in a similar age group, (35 to 49 years),[7] the breast cancer survivors reported more problems with hot flashes (41% vs. 26%), body image (67% vs. 60%), and lack of sexual interest (56% vs. 35%). Cancer patients had more sexual problems like difficulty in becoming sexually aroused (47% vs. 30%) compared with healthy women, had more trouble "relaxing and enjoying sex" (40% vs. 27%), and greater "difficulty in having orgasm" (35% vs. 29%) compared with healthy women. More (80%) of the healthy women (35–49 years) were sexually active, compared with the sexually active (22–50 years) breast cancer patients (67%), 0–7 months from treatment[7] (Table 1).

Healthy older women, 40 to 69 years of age[49] were more sexually active and had fewer sexual problems compared with the women in breast cancer studies mentioned above.[3,4] Data from healthy middle-aged and older women (40–69 years) reported by Addis et al[49] at Kaiser Permanente, indicated that 75% of the 2109 women were sexually active, 60% at least monthly, and 33% reported a sexual problem in 1 or more areas. These results are similar to those obtained by Sadovsky et al[50] who found that 34% of healthy minority women reported sexual problems in a primary care practice.[50] In the multiethnic

Study of Women's Health Across the Nation study of 3262 healthy women, 42 to 52 years of age, 79% had engaged in sex with a partner during the last 6 months.[51]

Comparing the 75% sexually active Kaiser patients, or the 79% of multiethnic women in the Study of Women's Health Across the Nation study who reported being sexually active, with the 67% of the recently diagnosed breast cancer patients age 50 year or less,[3] or the 69% of women interviewed at 5 years later,[4] and one can see that treatment played an important role in the patients' outcome. A chemotherapy-induced menopause is more abrupt than natural menopause and can have a more profound physiologic and psychologic effect.[8,35]

Sexual activity for most women declines gradually during the later decades of life. As age increases, the percent of sexually active women in each group declines. This was demonstrated in a study of healthy older women by Lindau et al,[6] 62% of women, 57 to 64 years of age, reported sexual activity with their partners during the last year, compared with 40% of women 65 to 74 years and 17% of women 75 to 85 years. Healthy women also report problems with sexual functioning, but less often, (35% to 43%)[7,52,53] than among women recently treated for breast cancer (67%).[3] While 35% to 43% of healthy women complain of 1 or more sexual problems in studies,[7,52,53] sexual problems persist at follow-up among women treated with chemotherapy for premenopausal breast cancer."[4,19]

A key feature of sexual desire is the positive anticipation and belief that sex is a satisfying part of life and the relationship. When either party loses the cycle of positive anticipation for pleasure-oriented intercourse, a regular rhythm of sexual contact may be replaced by a cycle of anticipatory anxiety, and tense unsuccessful intercourse, hitting a snag in the sexual connection. When sex becomes an awkward experience, it may be easier to avoid it.[2,54] Menopausal symptoms were believed by 56% of 200 patients in a study by Gupta et al[55] to affect their spouse's quality of life. The strongest correlations concerned severity of sexual symptoms and vaginal dryness.

## EFFECTS OF SEXUAL PROBLEMS ON INTIMATE RELATIONSHIPS

Interpersonal relationships can be vulnerable after a cancer diagnosis. The patient needs to talk about her feelings over changes in life, changes that present new challenges for everyone, patients, family and friends. Mages et al,[56,57] write about the patient's need to maintain continuity in life. In their study of cancer patients over time, patients reported that they had been changed by the experience of cancer and had developed new attitudes towards time, mortality, work, personal relationships, and their priorities in life. "The adaptive task is to understand and communicate one's changed attitudes, needs, and limitations in a way that permits formation of a new balance with the environment," wrote Mages and Mendelsohn.[56] Many scenarios threaten to change communication patterns among family and friends. The patient may feel isolated by the news of the diagnosis. Although the spouse or family member remains helpful and attentive, the patient may feel that "they just don't get it!" When patients feel "wounded" after hearing they have a malignant disease, they often feel separate from others. They feel that their life will never be the same again. Some partners pull away or distance themselves from the patient leading to new problems in the relationship. Younger women who received chemotherapy reported concerns about menopause, fertility, body image, sexuality, and partner relationship.[39] Couples facing breast cancer reported greater decreases in their marital and family functioning, more uncertain appraisals, and more adjustment problems associated with the illness when compared with couples adjusting to benign breast disease.[58]

The patient's ability to be open in her communication with her partner predicted outcome, in 2 studies.[59,60] In a study of 58 couples coping with the wives' breast cancer, Walker[59] concluded "Overall, the amount of communication about the illness explained the most variance in adjustment for both spouses." Wimberly et al[60] found that, "partner initiation of sex predicted greater marital satisfaction." among breast cancer survivors. In a second part of this study, they found that the partner's reactions to his wife or partner were important in conveying subtle messages as well. For example, an adverse reaction to the patient's surgical scar by the partner predicted less marital satisfaction.[60]

Spouses also experience mood changes and depression after their partner's diagnosis. Northouse et al[50,58,61,62] found in several studies that "Couples facing breast cancer reported greater decreases in their marital and family functioning, more uncertain appraisals, and more adjustment problems associated with the illness when compared with couples adjusting to benign breast disease."[58] In a small study of 50 Israeli men whose wives had been diagnosed with breast cancer, 75% of the men noted changes in their relationship, and more than a third experienced a reduction in communication within their families.[63]

Some couples become closer after breast cancer. Dorval et al[64] found that 42% of 282 couples said breast cancer brought them closer. What helped that happen? When the spouse found the patient confident, and (accepted) received advice from her in the first 2 weeks about how he should cope with breast cancer, when he accompanied her to surgery, and provided more affection, then at 3 months after her diagnosis, both partners agreed that the disease brought them closer.[64] Spouses affect each others' adjustment over time, Northouse et al[65] found husbands' and wives' levels of adjustment at 1 year had a significant direct effect on each other's adjustment.

## WHAT KINDS OF INTERVENTIONS ARE HELPFUL?

Multiple approaches to supporting breast cancer survivors can be effective, educational tools,[66] group[47,67] and individual interventions, using sex education,[68] supportive-expressive techniques,[69,70] cognitive behavioral and coping skills,[71] and relaxation and meditation techniques.[72] Offering interventions following treatment can be helpful for patients seeking their, "new normal self." More distressed patients do well in group interventions, particularly when they are led by experienced therapists.[73]

Both patients and their physicians have difficulty in being open about sexual issues. A recent international study found that initiating a conversation about sexual issues during a medical visit was not a high priority for either patient or physician.[74] The Global Study of Sexual Attitudes and Behaviors interviewed 27,500 men and women, 40 to 80 years of age, and found that although 50% experienced at least 1 sexual problem, less than 19% had attempted to ask for medical help. Only 9% of physicians asked the men and women in their practice about their sexual health during a routine visit during the past 3 years.[74] In the United Kingdom, a small study of 27 doctors and 16 nurses found that most healthcare professionals thought that the majority of women with ovarian cancer would experience a sexual problem, but only a 25% of the doctors and 20% of the nurses actually discussed sexual issues with the women.[75] A feeling that, "It's not my responsibility," or personal "embarrassment," "lack of knowledge and experience," or "lack of resources to provide support if needed" were cited as reasons.[75] Mismatched expectations between patients and health professionals were cited as the problem in a study in Melbourne, Australia.[76] Patients sought information, support, and practical strategies about how to live with intimate and sexual changes after treatment for cancer, while physicians assumed that patients shared their professional focus on combating the disease, irrespective of the emotional and physical costs to the patient.[76]

In Japan, physicians did a little better. Among the 318 breast cancer surgeons interviewed, 32% had been consulted about sexual issues by patients or families.[77] When the surgeon believed that it was his/her responsibility to raise the topic, they were significantly more likely to be consulted. When they felt it was up to the patient to initiate discussion, they were less likely to be consulted.[77]

## STARTING THE CONVERSATION WITH YOUR PATIENT

Before the end of treatment, physicians can give the patient permission to talk about sexual issues with questions like: "Women undergoing this procedure often have questions or concerns about sexuality. Is there anything you would like to talk about?"[78] or "What changes have you noticed sexually?" "Tell me about any sexual changes." "Sexually, how are things going?" "How has this affected you, sexually?" Questions can open the topic,[1] and give the patient permission to talk and think about sexuality and cancer at the same time.

It is helpful when physicians tell patients that there are sexual side effects to chemotherapy for many women, problems like low libido, vaginal dryness, and menopausal symptoms. This, "difficult to hear" information can be usefully followed with specific suggestions, such as the importance of "looking after yourself," "staying physically fit," "staying emotionally connected with your spouse," and "obtaining vaginal lubricants and moisturizers." It is important to counsel patients, when appropriate, that sexual activity is not harmful. Staying sexually active is an appropriate part of recovery from cancer and its treatment. And that, there are other support programs available like group therapy, individual counseling, or marital therapists, and sexual therapists or psychotherapists.[1] Patients will appreciate your openness, honestly disclosing anticipated changes from treatment along with possible solutions. Here are a few recommendations.

## DIALOGUE BETWEEN PHYSICIANS AND SURVIVORS

1. Consider telling the patient and her partner there are possibly going to be changes in the way her body responds to sexual encounters during and after chemotherapy, and these changes could affect her intimate relationship.[3]
2. Advise your patient to create and maintain open communication with her partner; look after her health, pay attention to her diet, and general well-being including her emotional health, use vaginal creams to cope with vaginal dryness; and remain sexually active as much as possible, as engaging in sexual activity actually helps maintain sexual desire.[79] Ganz has suggested that health care providers who wish to assist their breast cancer survivors with diminished sexual desire should take notice of the partner relationship and its quality, the woman's body image and mental health, as well as vaginal dryness and dyspareunia, as these problems can provide aversive conditioning for engaging in sexual activity and may decrease desire.[79]
3. Be ready to refer your patient for brief counseling or group support, as major changes like she is going through often need to be discussed with others who understand from a personal point of view.[3,80] Schover has suggested that many patients and their partners can benefit from brief counseling, with elements including education on how cancer treatment impacts sexual functioning; suggestions on how to resume sex without anxiety; skills to improve sexual communication; and suggestions on

overcoming specific sexual problems, for example, pain with intercourse or loss of desire for sex[80]

Physicians are encouraged to learn about counseling and the pharmaceutical and over the counter solutions. Many styles of education, individual and group counseling for patients and/or partners have been found to be effective.[46,50,69,81-86]

## TYPES OF COUNSELING

An educational booklet, "Sexuality and Cancer: For the Woman Who Has Cancer and Her Partner (2007)" by The American Cancer Society can be helpful. It is distributed (free) to patients and family members in the offices of the American Cancer Society throughout the country. It discusses sensitive topics, including how orgasm is achieved; the importance of touching; effects of cancer treatment on sexual desire and response; pain; how chemotherapy drugs irritate mucous membranes in the body; learning how to relax vaginal muscles, kegel exercises; using a vaginal dilator, lubricants; and the importance of talking with one's partner to keep one's sexual life going.[66]

Several brief sexual counseling interventions have been found helpful. Schover et al offered individual sexual counseling to 76 women cancer patients referred at the Cleveland Clinic. Most counseling consisted of one or two-session evaluation. Where it was longer, the median time between first and last session was 5 months. After treatment, problems, like "loss of desire" and "difficulty with orgasm" improved.[81] In their book, "Sexuality and Chronic Illness: A Comprehensive Approach," Schover and Jensen[82] discuss sex therapy and behavioral techniques.

Ganz et al[87] at University of California in Los Angeles demonstrated a brief intervention that was successful in helping women with menopausal symptoms, and problems with sexual functioning. Using a self-report screening instrument distressed women were referred for counseling. The intervention took place over a 4-month period. Patients receiving the intervention demonstrated statistically significant improvement ($P = 0.0004$) in both menopausal symptoms and sexual functioning ($P = 0.04$) in the treatment group compared with the usual-care group.

Partners of breast cancer patients also benefited from support at critical moments, as their coping abilities are also be taxed by their wife's cancer. Baider and Bengal[88] found that "Being a passive bystander is as stressful as being a cancer patient." In a study by Bultz et al, 36 patients and their partners participated in a randomized controlled trial of a brief psycho-educational group program. Three months after the intervention, the partners had less mood disturbance, ie, less anxiety or depression, than did controls. Patients whose partners received the intervention also reported less anxiety or depression, greater confidant support and greater marital satisfaction.[83]

When there is a sense of isolation and distancing from a partner, emotionally focused marital therapy like that offered by Johnson and Talitman[84] offer support to couples dealing with post-traumatic stress or recurrent anxiety from the diagnosis and treatment for breast cancer. Their approach may offer something fresh and positive to couples with cancer in the family. Emotionally focused marital therapy focuses on the creation of secure attachment.[85] An attachment injury occurs when one partner violates the expectation that the other will offer comfort and caring in times of danger or distress. There is particular disappointment when spouses fail to communicate their concern or withdraw from the patient after diagnosis or treatment. The injurious incident defines the relationship as insecure and maintains relationship distress because it is continually used as a standard for the dependability of the offending partner.[86] Johnson and Talitman[84] found that among the couples dealing with trauma, the female partners' trust, her faith in her husband predicted the couples' satisfaction at follow-up. The female partners' faith in her husband also significantly predicted males' level of intimacy at follow-up. When wives showed trust and faith in their husband, husbands were more comfortable with physical intimacy in the relationship. Interventions that encourage emotional self-disclosure and interpersonal trust may be specifically helpful for cancer patients after treatment.

Support groups are probably the most available source of assistance to breast cancer survivors throughout the country. Usually available in hospitals and cancer centers, 1 to 2 hour groups with an experienced professional leader offer breast cancer patients a chance to learn, through supportive-expressive group therapy, or cognitive behavior stress management from leaders and others in the group.[89–91]

Weekly physical activity is very important. Encouraging patients to be physically active has benefits for their longevity, and quality of life, plus exercise improves a woman's body image and sexuality. Women who engaged in greater levels of physical activity (3 to 5 miles per week) had a significantly lower risk of dying from breast cancer,[92,93] and had better cardiopulmonary function,[94] and improved quality of life when compared with control groups.[95] Regular exercisers also reported higher body self-esteem and more positive attitudes towards their sexual attractiveness than sedentary breast cancer survivors.[96]

## WHAT KIND OF HELP IS AVAILABLE FOR HOT FLASHES AND SEXUAL COMFORT IN LOVEMAKING?

Menopausal symptoms, such as hot flashes, are reported to take place more often, and are considered to be more distressing, severe and longer in duration in women with breast cancer than in controls.[97,98] Therapeutic options include centrally acting agents such as, venlafaxine, paroxetine, gabapentin, and clonidine.

1. Venlafaxine (Effexor), used mainly for depression, has been found to be helpful with hot flashes in menopausal women. It's contraindicated for women already taking an monomine oxidase inhibitor oral route, those with heart, liver, thyroid or kidney problems. It may increase high blood pressure. Effexor may reduce sexual desire.[99]
2. Paroxetine (Paxil) primarily used to treat major depression, obsessive compulsive disorder and post-traumatic stress disorder, has also been found to be helpful with hot flashes. Side effects, such as headache, nausea, dry mouth or sweating, usually develop during the first 1 to 4 weeks as the body adapts to the drug. It is safe and easy to discontinue the drug. Paxil may also reduce libido and create an inability to achieve orgasms.[100]
3. Gabapentin (Neurontin) has been recommended when venlafaxine is contraindicated or is not effective. It is an anticonvulsant drug, which also may prevent migraine headaches and neuropathic pain following shingles, and hot flashes. It's adverse effects include dizziness, drowsiness, an peripheral edema in extremeties.[101,102]
4. Clonidine Catapres-TTS (transdermal patch) is used as an antihypertensive agent, for migraine headaches and hot flashes associated with menopause. It may cause drowsiness, lightheadedness, dry mouth or constipation. It may cause hypotension and inhibit orgasm in women.[102,103]

Each remedy for hot flashes has been found useful in some studies for women with breast cancer, although venlaxafine is far more effective than the other, and has fewer side effects. However, with the exception of gabapentin, each interferes with some aspect of sexual functioning, desire, reduced libido, or orgasm. The patient may choose "hot flashes" as the problem to cope with first.

For some women, a well-known antidepressant, bupropion (Wellbutrin) may be worth considering as an aid to increasing sexual arousal and satisfaction. Sustained-release bupropion (Wellbutrin SR) 300 mg daily used for 4 weeks has been shown to increase sexual arousal, orgasm completion and sexual satisfaction in nondepressed, premenopausal women. For women already using an antidepressant that has increased their sexual dysfunction, sustained release bupropion 300 mg daily used for 4 weeks has been shown to increase sexual desire and frequency of sexual activity in patients.[98]

Sildenafil (50 mg, adjustable from 25 mg to 100 mg) (Viagra) has been shown to increase vaginal lubrication, genital sensation, ability to achieve orgasm, and overall satisfaction in a 12-week double-blind placebo-controlled study of 202 postmenopausal women, by Berman et al[104] An industry study with 614 patients found a dose-dependent effect favoring 100 mg of sildenafil citrate. In this study, Claret et al[105] found that the treatment effect in postmenopausal women was larger than in premenopausal women. An earlier study by Basson et al took place in multiple centers. It was a placebo-controlled trial examining the efficacy and safety of sildenafil 10 to 100 mg taken 1 hour before sexual activity in 2 groups of women (estrogen-replete, n = 577 and estrogen-deficient, n = 207). Basson et al found no increase in sexual arousal at any dose. Side effects included headache, flushing, rhinitis, visual disturbance, and dyspepsia.[106] Very recently, sildenafil was found to improve the sexual dysfunction women experience while on antidepressant medications, although the effect was modest.[107] Sildenafil may be helpful for some women.

Emerging therapies for female sexual dysfunction include a topical vasodilatory agent called, alprostadil. In-clinic application of alprostadil increased genital vasocongestion, vaginal erythema, and some patient-assessed indices of sexual arousal; however, these effects have not been consistently superior to placebo. Two formulations of topical alprostadil are in phase II clinical trials. Kielbasa and Daniel[108] conclude that the results of ongoing clinical studies are needed to further define the role of topical alprostadil.

Alternative therapies worth some consideration include 400 mg of vitamin E. Vitamin E is an antioxidant, which can reduce free radicals. There is some evidence that vitamin E can help to moderate hot flash symptoms, if taken in 400 international units daily. Doses over 1000 mg units are not recommended as they may cause bleeding.[109]

ArginMax[110] is a supplement containing L-arginine, ginseng, ginkgo, damiana, multivitamins, and minerals. It has been found effective in increasing sexual desire and satisfaction with overall sex life with among women, ages 22 to 73 years of age, who were pre-, peri- or postmenopausal in life stage, compared with controls. Dr. Ito and his group at the School of Medicine in Hawaii, observes that, "since ArginMax for women has been shown to exhibit no estrogen activity, it may be a desirable alternative to hormone therapy for sexual concerns."[110]

Younger women will be especially concerned about the possibility of vaginal atrophy. Derzko et al[85] discusses how treatment options range from lifestyle modifications to nonhormonal and hormonal interventions. A lifestyle recommendation, regular vaginal coital activity, has the benefit of increasing blood circulation to the pelvic organs. It is good to avoid contact dermatitis of the vulva from irritants like dyed toilet tissue, or tight-fitting garments. Pure cranberry juice concentrates help to avoid urinary tract infections.[85]

Vaginal moisturizers like Replens, a nonhormonal moisturizing gel, used 3 times weekly has proven effective in increasing vaginal moisture and in decreasing vaginal itching and irritation. Schover et al[82] recommends liquid lubricants that are water or silicone based rather than gel lubricants, and suggests that vaginal dilators used several times a week have reduced pain during intercourse in some women. Locally applied vitamin E in daily doses of 100 to 600 international units has been found to increase vaginal lubrication and relieve the dryness and irritation that accompany atrophic and other forms of vaginitis. Placing a vitamin E capsule in the vagina will help as the vitamin membrane melts with the body's pH balance. KY Jelly with vitamin E is another possibility.[111] The Canadian Consensus Conference on Menopause and 2006 guidelines indicate that local treatment with intravaginal estrogen offers relief for urogenital and vulvovaginal atrophy. Because the minimal systemic absorption occurs with use of the recommended doses, it is their opinion that women who with a history of breast cancer, who are not taking adjuvant aromatase inhibitor therapy, may use low-dose forms of intravaginal estrogen, like the Estring, or Vagi-fem suppositories.[85,112]

As Ganz and Greendale[35,87] note, "Management of vaginal dryness with nonestrogen or low-dose vaginal estrogen preparations may be an important first step that all clinicians can institute in their symptomatic patients."

Each of the pharmaceuticals and over the counter supplements have advantages and disadvantages, requiring that the individual medical picture in each case be evaluated, with suggestions about choice of solutions discussed with information and agreement on the risks.

## CONCLUSIONS

The success in cancer treatment for breast cancer is offset by the problems women face after treatment, especially chemotherapy. The rate of sexual dysfunction is higher among breast cancer patients than healthy women, and it happens at a younger age, complicating the patient's self-image, and personal relationships. Physicians can help their patient by choosing to discuss these problems along with possible solutions. A straightforward discussion of the predictable sexual problems, can lead to patients to be more frank with their spouses, choose to participate in brief psycho-educational support, group therapy, sexual counseling, marital counseling or intensive psychotherapy, all known to be helpful. In addition, there are pharmacologic and over the counter supplements for problems like depression, hot flashes, vaginal dryness, and pain with lovemaking that can prevent or ameliorate problems with sexual function.

## ACKNOWLEDGMENTS

*The authors thank, Drs. Patricia Ganz, Joan Bloom, and Susan Stewart, for their help in confirming data for Table 1, Leslie Schover for her thoughtful comments, Susan Brain for her critique from the patient's point of view.*

## REFERENCES

1. Hughes MK. Quick reference for oncology clinicians: the psychiatric and psychological dimensions of cancer symptom management. In: Holland JC, Greenberg DB, Hughes MK, ed. *Sexual Dysfunction.* Charlottesville: IPOS Press; 2006.
2. McCarthy B, Ginsberg RL, Fucito LM. Resilient sexual desire in heterosexual couples. *Fam J.* 2006;14:59–64.
3. Fobair P, Stewart SL, Chang S, et al. Body image and sexual problems in young women with breast cancer. *Psychooncology.* 2006;15:579–594.
4. Bloom JR. Then and now: quality of life of young breast cancer survivors. *Psychooncology.* 2004;13:147–160.
5. Conde DM, Pinto-Neto AM, Cabello C, et al. Menopause symptoms and quality of life in women aged 45–65 years with and without breast cancer. *Menopause.* 2005;12:436–443.
6. Lindau ST, Schumm LP, Laumann EO, et al. A study of sexuality and health among older adults in the United States. *N Engl J Med.* 2007;357:762–774.
7. Ganz PA, Day R, Ware JE Jr, et al. Base-line quality-of-life assessment in the National Surgical Adjuvant Breast and Bowel Project Breast Cancer Prevention Trial. *J Natl Cancer Inst.* 1995;87:1372–1382.
8. Knobf MT. The influence of endocrine effects of adjuvant therapy on quality of life outcomes in younger breast cancer survivors. *Oncologist.* 2006;11:96–110.
9. Ganz PA. Breast cancer, menopause, and long-term survivorship, critical issues for the 21st century. *Am J Med.* 2005;118:136–141.
10. Cancer Survivorship, United States, National Cancer Institute Cancer Survivorship Research. In: Office of Cancer Survivorship CCPS. Vol 53. Available at http://survivorship.cancer.gov, *MMWR* 2004:526–529.
11. Surveillance E, and End Results (SEER) Program, SEER17 Registries, 1973–2004. Female Breast Cancer-US, 1996–2003. In: 2007–2008 BCFF, ed. *American Cancer Society, Surveillance Research,* 2007. Atlanta: American Cancer Society; 2007.
12. Beckmann J, Johansen L, Richardt C, et al. Psychological reactions in younger women operated on for breast cancer. Amputation versus resection of the breast with special reference to body-image, sexual identity and sexual function. *Dan Med Bull.* 1983;30 (Suppl 2):10–13.
13. Shapiro CL, Recht A. Late effects of adjuvant therapy for breast cancer. *J Natl Cancer Inst Monogr.* 1994;16:101–112.
14. Schover LR, Yetman RJ, Tuason LJ, et al. Partial mastectomy and breast reconstruction. A comparison of their effects on psychosocial adjustment, body image, and sexuality. *Cancer.* 1995;75:54–64.
15. Wilmoth MC. The aftermath of breast cancer: an altered sexual self. *Cancer Nurs.* 2001;24:278–286.
16. Breastcancer.org. "You and your partner". Available at http://breastcancer.org/tips/intimacy/partner.jsp.
17. OncoLink. Meeting sexuality needs of women with breast cancer. Web Page. Available at http://www.oncolink.upenn.edu/coping/article.cfm. Accessed on July 2, 2008.
18. Averette HE, Boike GM, Jarrell MA. Effects of cancer chemotherapy on gonadal function and reproductive capacity. *CA Cancer J Clin.* 1990;40:199–209.
19. Schover LR. Premature ovarian failure and its consequences: vasomotor symptoms, sexuality, and fertility. *J Clin Oncol.* 2008;26:753–758.
20. Ganz PA, Kwan L, Stanton AL, et al. Quality of life at the end of primary treatment of breast cancer: first results from the moving beyond cancer randomized trial. *J Natl Cancer Inst.* 2004;96:376–387.
21. Ganz PA, Greendale GA, Petersen L, et al. Breast cancer in younger women: reproductive and late health effects of treatment. *J Clin Oncol.* 2003;21:4184–4193.
22. Schover LR. The impact of breast cancer on sexuality, body image, and intimate relationships. *CA Cancer J Clin.* 1991;41:112–120.
23. Ganz PA, Desmond KA, Belin TR, et al. Predictors of sexual health in women after a breast cancer diagnosis. *J Clin Oncol.* 1999;17:2371–2380.
24. Hwang MY. Silence about sexual problems can hurt relationships. *JAMA.* 1999;281:584.
25. Arora NK. Impact of surgery and chemotherapy on the quality of life of younger women with breast carcinoma: a prospective study. *Cancer.* 2001;92:1288–1298.
26. Yurek D, Farrar W, Andersen BL. Breast cancer surgery: comparing surgical groups and determining individual differences in postoperative sexuality and body change stress. *J Consult Clin Psychol.* 2000;68:697–709.
27. Ganz PA. Quality of life in long-term, disease-free survivors of breast cancer: a follow-up study. *J Natl Cancer Inst.* 2002;94:34–49.
28. Avis NE. Psychosocial problems among younger women with breast cancer. *Psychooncology.* 2004;13:295–308.
29. Gupta P SD, Palin SL. Menopausal symptoms in women treated for breast cancer: the prevalence and severity of symptoms and their perceived effects on quality of life. *Climacteric.* 2006;9:49–58.
30. Figueiredo MI, Cullen J, Hwang YT, et al. Breast cancer treatment in older women: does getting what you want improve your long-term body image and mental health? *J Clin Oncol.* 2004;22:4002–4009.
31. Bukovic D, Fajdic J, Strinic T, et al. Differences in sexual functioning between patients with benign and malignant breast tumors. *Coll Antropol.* 2004;28 (Suppl 2):191–201.
32. Bukovic D, Fajdic J, Hrgovic Z, et al. Sexual dysfunction in breast cancer survivors. *Onkologie.* 2005;28:29–34.
33. Avis NE, Crawford S, Manuel J. Psychosocial problems among younger women with breast cancer. *Psychooncology.* 2004;13:295–308.
34. Avis NE, Crawford S, Manuel J. Quality of life among younger women with breast cancer. *J Clin Oncol.* 2005;23:3322–3330.
35. Ganz PA, Greendale GA. Female sexual desire—beyond testosterone. *J Natl Cancer Inst.* 2007;99:659–661.

36. Ganz PA, Rowland JH, Desmond K, et al. Life after breast cancer: understanding women's health-related quality of life and sexual functioning. *J Clin Oncol.* 1998;16:501–514.

37. Bower JE, Ganz PA, Desmond KA, et al. Fatigue in breast cancer survivors: occurrence, correlates, and impact on quality of life. *J Cllin Oncol.* 2000;18:743–753.

38. Schover LR. Premature ovarian failure and its consequences: vasomotor symptoms, sexuality, and fertility. *J Clin Oncol.* 2008;26:753–758.

39. Spencer SM, Lehman JM, Wynings C, et al. Concerns about breast cancer and relations to psychosocial well-being in a multiethnic sample of early-stage patients. *Health Psychol.* 1999;18:159–168.

40. Ganz PA, Desmond KA, Leedham B, et al. Quality of life in long-term, disease-free survivors of breast cancer: a follow-up study. *J Natl Cancer Inst.* 2002;94:39–49.

41. Ganz PA, Coscarelli A, Fred C, et al. Breast cancer survivors: psychosocial concerns and quality of life. *Breast Cancer Res Treat.* 1996;38:183–199.

42. Lasry JC, Margolese RG, Poisson R, et al. Depression and body image following mastectomy and lumpectomy. *J Chronic Dis.* 1987;40:529–534.

43. Ganz PA. Impact of quality of life outcomes on clinical practice. *Oncology (Huntingt).* 1995;9 (11 Suppl):61–65.

44. Lindley C, Vasa S, Sawyer WT, et al. Quality of life and preferences for treatment following systemic adjuvant therapy for early-stage breast cancer. *J Clin Oncol.* 1998;16:1380–1387.

45. Meyerowitz BE, Desmond KA, Rowland JH, et al. Sexuality following breast cancer. *J Sex Marital Ther.* 1999;25:237–250.

46. Speer JJ, Hillenberg B, Sugrue DP, et al. Study of sexual functioning determinants in breast cancer survivors. *Breast J.* 2005;11:440–447.

47. Spiegel D, Bloom JR. Group therapy and hypnosis reduce metastatic breast carcinoma pain. *Psychosom Med.* 1983;45:333–339.

48. Conde DM, Pinto-Neto AM, cabello c, et al. Menopause symptoms and quality of life in women aged 45 to 65 years with and without breast cancer. *Menopause.* 2005;12:436–443.

49. Addis IB, Van Den Eeden SK, Wassel-Fyr MS, et al. Sexual activity and function in middle-aged and older women. *Obstet Gynaecol.* 2006;107:755–764.

50. Sadovsky R, Enecilla M, Cosiquien R, et al. Sexual problems among a specific population of minority women, aged 40–69 attending a primary care practice. *J Sex Med.* 2006;3:795–803.

51. Cain V, Johannes CB, Avis NE, et al. Sexual functioning and practices in a multi-ethnic study of midlife women: baseline results from SWAN. *J Sex Res.* 2003;40:266–276.

52. Rosen RC, Taylor JF, Leiblum SR, et al. Prevalence of sexual dysfunction in women: results of a survey study of 329 women in an outpatient gynecological clinic. *J Sex Marital Ther.* 1993;19:171–188.

53. Laumann EO, Paik A, Rosen RC. Sexual dysfunction in the United States: prevalence and predictors. *JAMA.* 1999;281:537–544.

54. Basson R. Sexual desire and arousal disorders in women. *N Engl J Med.* 2006;354:1497–1506.

55. Gupta P, Sturdee DW, Palin SL, et al. Menopausal symptoms in women treated for breast cancer: the prevalence and severity of symptoms and their perceived effects on quality of life. *Climacteric.* 2006;9:49–58.

56. Mages NL, Mendelsohn GA. *Effects of Cancer on Patients' Lives: A Personological Approach.* San Francisco: Jossey-Bass, Inc.; 1979.

57. Mages NL, Castro JR, Fobair P, et al. Patterns of psychosocial response to cancer: can effective adaptation be predicted? *Int J Radiat Oncol Biol Phys.* 1981;7:385–392.

58. Northouse LL, Templin T, Mood D, et al. Couples' adjustment to breast cancer and benign breast disease: a longitudinal analysis. *Psychooncology.* 1998;7:37–48.

59. Walker BL. Adjustment of husbands and wives to breast cancer. *Cancer Pract.* 1997;5:92–98.

60. Wimberly SR, Carver CS, Laurenceau JP, et al. Perceived partner reactions to diagnosis and treatment of breast cancer: impact on psychosocial and psychosexual adjustment. *J Consult Clin Psychol.* 2005;73:300–311.

61. Northouse LL, Swain MA. Adjustment of patients and husbands to the initial impact of breast cancer. *Nurs Res.* 1987;36:221–225.

62. Northouse LL, Schafer JA, Tipton J, et al. The concerns of patients and spouses after the diagnosis of colon cancer: a qualitative analysis. *J Wound Ostomy Continence Nurs.* 1999;26:8–17.

63. Kadmon I, Ganz FD, Woloski-Wruble AC. Social, marital, and sexual adjustment of Israeli men whose wives were diagnosed with breast cancer. *Oncol Nurs Forum.* 2008;35:131–135.

64. Dorval M, Guay S, Mondor M, et al. Couples who get closer after breast cancer: frequency and predictors in a prospective investigation. *J Clin Oncol.* 2005;23:3588–3596.

65. Northouse L, Templin T, Mood D. Couples' adjustment to breast disease during the first year following diagnosis. *J Behav Med.* 2001;24:115–136.

66. ACS. *Sexuality and Cancer: For the Woman Who Has Cancer and Her Partner.* Atlanta: American Cancer Society; 2007.

67. Spiegel D. Mind matters—group therapy and survival in breast cancer. *N Engl J Med.* 2001;345:1767–1768.

68. Helgeson V, Cohen S, Schulz R, et al. Long term effects of educational and peer discussion group interventions on adjustment to breast cancer. *Health Psychol.* 2001;20:387–392.

69. Spiegel D, Bloom JR, Yalom I. Group support for patients with metastatic cancer. A randomized outcome study. *Arch Gen Psychiatry.* 1981;38:527–533.

70. Spiegel D, Bloom JR, Kraemer HC, et al. Effect of psychosocial treatment on survival of patients with metastatic breast cancer. *Lancet.* 1989;2:888–891.

71. Cruess D, Antoni MH, McGregor BA, et al. Cognitive-behavioral stress management reduces serum cortisol by enhancing benefit finding among women being treated for early stage breast cancer. *Psychosom Med.* 2000;62:304–308.

72. Carlson LE, Speca M, Patel K, et al. Mindfulness-based stress reduction in relation to quality of life, mood, symptoms of stress, and immune parameters in breast and prostate cancer outpatients. *Psychosom Med.* 2003;65:571–581.

73. Stanton AL. Psychosocial concerns and interventions for cancer survivors. *J Clin Oncol.* 2006;24:5132–5137.

74. Moreira EJ, Brock G, Glasser DB, et al. Help-seeking behaviour for sexual problems: the global study of attitudes and behaviors. *Int J Clin Pract.* 2005;59:6–16.

75. Stead M, Brown JM, Fallowfield L, et al. Lack of communication between healthcare professionals and women with ovarian cancer about sexual issues. *Br J Cancer.* 2003;88:666–671.

76. Hordern A, Street AF. Communicating about patient sexuality and intimacy after cancer: mismatched expectations and unmet needs. *Med J Aust.* 2007;186:224–227.

77. Takahashi M, Kai I, Hisata M, et al. Attitudes and practices of breast cancer consultations regarding sexual issues: a nationwide survey of Japanese surgeons. *J Clin Oncol.* 2006;24:5763–5768.

78. Katz A. The sounds of silence: sexuality information for cancer patients. *J Clin Oncol.* 2005;23:238–241.

79. Ganz PA, Greendale GA. Female sexual desire—beyond testosterone. *J Natl Cancer Inst.* 2007;99:659–661.

80. Schover L. Counseling cancer patients about changes in sexual function. *Oncology (Williston Park).* 1999;13:1585–1591.

81. Schover LR, Evans DA, von Eschenbach AC. Sexual rehabilitation in a cancer center: diagnosis and outcome in 384 consultations. *Arch Sex Behav.* 1987;16:445–461.

82. Schover LR, Jensen SB. *Sexuality and Chronic Illness: A Comprehensive Approach.* New York: The Guilford Press; 1988.

83. Bultz BD, Speca M, Brasher PM, et al. A randomized controlled trial of a brief psychoeducational support group for partners of early stage breast cancer patients. *Psychooncology.* 2000;9:303–313.

84. Johnson SM, Talitman E. Predictors of success in emotionally focused marital therapy. *J Marital Fam Ther.* 1997;23:135–152.

85. Johnson SM, Williams-Keeler L. Creating healing relationships for couples dealing with trauma: the use of emotionally focused marital therapy. *J Marital Fam Ther.* 1998;24:25–40.

86. Johnson SM, Makinen JA, Millikin JW. Attachment injuries in couple relationships: a new perspective on impasses in couples therapy. *J Marital Fam Ther.* 2001;27:145–155.

87. Ganz PA, Greendale GA, Petersen L, et al. Managing menopausal symptoms in breast cancer survivors: results of a randomized controlled trial. *J Natl Cancer Inst.* 2000;92:1054–1064.

88. Baider L, Bengel J. Cancer and the spouse: gender-related differences in dealing with health care and illness. *Crit Rev Oncol Hematol.* 2001;40:115–123.

89. Fobair P. Cancer support groups and group therapies: Part I, Historical and theoretical background and research on effectiveness. *J Psychosoc Oncol.* 1997;15:63–81.

90. Fobair P. Cancer support groups and group therapies:, Part II: Process, organizational, leadership, and patient issues. *J Psychosoc Oncol.* 1997;15:123–147.

91. Antoni MH, Wimberly SR, Lechner SC. Reduction of cancer-specific thought intrusions and anxiety symptoms with a stress management intervention among women undergoing treatment for breast cancer. *Am J Psychiatry.* 2006;163:1791–1797.

92. Holick CN, Newcomb PA, Trenthan-Dietz A, et al. Physical activity and survival after diagnosis of invasive breast cancer. *Cancer Epidemiol Biomarkers Prev.* 2008;17:379–386.

93. Irwin ML, Smith AW, McTiernan A, et al. Influence of pre-and postdiagnosis physical activity on mortality in breast cancer survivors: the health, eating, activity, and lifestyle study. *J Clin Oncol.* 2008;26:3958–3964.
94. Courneya LS, Mackey JR, Bell GJ, et al. Randomized controlled trial of exercise training in postmenopausal breast cancer survivors: cardiopulmonary and quality of life outcomes. *J Clin Oncol.* 2003;21:1651–1652.
95. Aiello EJ, Yasui Y, Tworoger SS. Effect of a yearlong, moderate-intensity exercise intervention on the occurrence and severity of menopause symptoms in postmenopausal women. *Menopause.* 2004;11:382–388.
96. Pinto BM, Trunzo JJ. Body esteem and mood among sedentary and active breast cancer survivors. *Mayo Clin Proc.* 2004;79:181–186.
97. Bordeleau L, Pritchard K, Goodwin P, et al. Therapeutic options for the management of hot flashes in breast cancer survivors: an evidence-based review. *Clin Ther.* 2007;29:230–241.
98. Derzko C, Eliott S, Lam W. Management of sexual dysfunction in postmenopausal breast cancer patients taking adjuvant aromatase inhibitor therapy. *Current Oncology.* 2007;14(Suppl 1):S20–S40.
99. Wikipedia. Venlafaxine. Available at http://en.wikipedia.org/wiki/Effexor_xr; 2007.
100. Wikipedia tfe. Paroxetine. Available at http://en.wikipedia.org/wiki/Paroxetine; 2007.
101. Wikipedia TFE. Gabapentin, from the wikipedia, the free encyclopedia. Available at http://en.wikipedia.org/wiki/Gabapentin; 2008.
102. Hot flashes: minimize discomfort during menopause. Available at *MayoClinic.com*; 2007.
103. Wikipedia. Clonidine. Available at http://en.wikipedia.org/wiki/Clonidine; 2008.
104. Berman JR, Berman LA, Toler SM, et al. Safety and efficacy of sildenafil citrate for the treatment of female sexual arousal disorder: a double-blind, placebo controlled study. *J Urol.* 2003;170:2333–2338.
105. Claret L, Cox EH, McFadyen L, et al. Modeling and simulation of sexual activity daily diary data of patients with female sexual arousal disorder treated with sildenafil citrate (Viagra). *Pharm Res.* 2006;23:1756–1764.
106. Basson R, McInnes R, Smith MD, et al. Efficacy and safety of sildenafil citrate in women with sexual dysfunction associated with female sexual arousal disorder. *J Womens Health Gend Based Med.* 2002;11:367–377.
107. Nurnberg GH, Hensley PL, Heiman JR, et al. Sildenafil treatment of women with antidepressant-associated sexual dysfunction: a randomized controlled trial. *JAMA.* 2008;300:395–399.
108. Kielbasa LA, Daniel KL. Topical alprostadil treatment of female sexual arousal disorder. *Ann Pharmacother.* 2006;40:1369–1376.
109. Stephan KD. Vitamin E lowers breast cancer risk and moderates hot flashes. Available at http://breastcancer.about.com/od/lifeduringtreatment/p/vitamin_E.htm;.
110. Ito TY, Polan ML, Whipple B, et al. The enhancement of female sexual function with ArginMax, a nutritional supplement, among women differing in menopausal status. *J Sex Marital Ther.* 2006;32:369–378.
111. Fugh-Berman A. Use vitamin E for vaginal dryness-Ask the experts: answers to your questions from the Leaders in Natural Medicine-Brief Article. *Natural Health.* 2003. Available at http://findarticles.com/p/articles/mi_m0NAH/is_7_33/ai_107637374.
112. Belisle S, Blake J, Basson R. Canadian consensus conference on menopause, 2006 update. *J Obstet Gynaecol Can.* 2006;28 (Suppl 1):S7–S94.

# Medical and Psychosocial Aspects of Fertility After Cancer

Christine Duffy • Susan Allen

Nearly 100,000 women between the age of 20 and 49 are diagnosed with cancer every year. Fortunately, survival for cancer has improved significantly in the last 25 years with excellent overall 5-year and 10-year survival rates (79% and 74%, respectively) for all cancers in women in this age range.[1] Hence, the majority of young women diagnosed with cancer can expect to live for decades, making quality of life issues such as fertility increasingly important.

Many premenopausal women diagnosed with breast cancer today are still contemplating conception of their first child, or have not completed their child-bearing. Recent estimates from the Office for National Statistics have shown that the average age of women for all births in the United States has gradually increased from 24.6 years in 1972 to 27.2 years in 2000.[2] In addition, the first birth rate for women between the age of 40 and 44 years has more than doubled since 1981.[3] A diagnosis of cancer at a young age threatens the developmental tasks that characterize a woman's reproductive years such as building intimate relationships and having children.[4,5] Young women diagnosed with cancer before the age of 50 experience greater psychologic morbidity than their older counterparts,[4,6–9] with fertility issues among the most troubling of the issues they face.[10–13]

## RISKS OF INFERTILITY WITH CANCER TREATMENT

The risk of infertility with cancer treatments varies widely, and is dependent on the age of the patient as well as the types and combinations of treatment received.[14] Difficulties with fertility increase with age and are much more common for women >40 years versus women ≤40.[15–18] Unfortunately, there is no clinically useful predictive test to reliably assess ovarian reserve,[19] making it difficult to predict risk of amenorrhea for an individual woman. Table 1 reviews some common treatments for various cancers and the associated risks of amenorrhea on a population level.

Certain classes of chemotherapy agents are quite toxic to the ovaries, such as alkylating agents, which include cyclophosphamide and procarbazine,[20,21] and are frequently used cancer-treatment regimens. High-dose chemotherapy administered in preparation for stem-cell transplant is also associated with high rates of ovarian failure.[21,22] There are a number of new chemotherapy agents for which data is lacking or not conclusive such as the monoclonal antibodies, the taxanes, and tyrosine kinase inhibitors.[20] It should be noted that even women who do not experience ovarian failure immediately but continue menstruating after chemotherapy will have reduced ovarian reserve, and high rates of premature ovarian failure.[16,23]

Damage to the ovaries from radiotherapy is dependent on the dose, irradiation field, and the age of the woman.[24] The ovaries are exposed to significant doses of irradiation when radiotherapy is used to treat pelvic or abdominal disease, such as cervical and rectal cancer. Women aged <40 years usually require 20 Gy for permanent ovarian failure, whereas the dose is only 6 Gy in older women.[23] In addition, whole body radiation, spinal radiation, whole brain radiation, and pelvic radiation combined with chemotherapy are associated with high rates of amenorrhea. Radiation to the pelvis also affects the uterus. Uterine radiation is associated with increased risk of spontaneous abortion, preterm labor, and low birth rate, likely due to changes in the musculature and blood flow from radiation.[25] Very young women are more susceptible to the damage from radiation to their uterus.[24]

Surgical treatments that remove the reproductive organs, as in treatment of ovarian cancer, advanced cervical or uterine cancer, typically leave a woman infertile because standard treatment generally involves total abdominal hysterectomy with oophorectomy. However, depending on the stage and type of gynecologic cancer, conservative treatment, which preserves the reproductive organs, can sometimes be attempted. Observational studies following women receiving conservative surgical treatment for cervical cancer suggest radical trachelectomy (which spares the uterus and ovaries), does not appear to increase the risk of recurrence or mortality when patients are early stage, properly screened for the procedure, and undergo surgery at a center experienced with performing the procedure.[26–29] Women with early stage (stage I) and low-grade (I-II) ovarian cancer also appear to have no increased risk of recurrence when treated with conservative unilateral oophorectomy,[30–32] although the potential for a second primary malignancy in the other ovary must be considered.[33] Women with early-stage (stage I) endometrial cancer can often be treated successfully with a progestational agent, rather than abdominal hysterectomy. In fact, younger women with endometrial cancer tend to have better differentiated lesions and higher survival rates.[34] About three-fourths of women will respond to hormonal therapy, and those who do not can then proceed to more aggressive treatment if needed.[35–37]

## FERTILITY PRESERVATION OPTIONS

Several options for patients with cancer entering chemotherapy treatment who wish to preserve fertility are available. These options range from clinically well-established techniques such as embryo cryopreservation to more experimental techniques such as egg freezing and ovarian tissue cryopreservation.[17,38] Descriptions of these options are listed in Table 2.

Embryo cryopreservation is a widely established procedure that is commonly used in many infertility clinics around the world.[17] It involves stimulation of the ovaries to produce eggs that can be fertilized by sperm and stored as embryos for future implantation and pregnancy. Cumulative pregnancy rates can be >50%.[39,40] The procedure can take from 2 to 6 weeks, however, so it can delay the start of treatment. Women who have estrogen-sensitive tumors are generally not considered as candidates for traditional in vitro fertilization (IVF) before cancer treatment because stimulation of the ovaries to produce

**TABLE 1.** Risk of Amenorrhea With Treatments in Common Cancers Among Premenopausal Women

| | Therapy | Age | Risk |
|---|---|---|---|
| Breast cancer | AC | <40 | Low |
| | | 40+ | Intermediate |
| | CMF | <30 | Low |
| | | 30–39 | Intermediate |
| | | 40+ | High |
| | CEF | <30 | Low |
| | | 30–39 | Intermediate |
| | | 40+ | High |
| | CAF | <30 | Low |
| | | 30–39 | Intermediate |
| | | 40+ | High |
| | Trastuzumab | All ages | Unknown |
| | Taxanes | All ages | Unknown |
| Hematologic malignancies | | | |
| General therapies | BMT | All ages | High |
| | Whole body irradiation, spinal radiation, pelvic radiation | All ages | High |
| Lymphomas | | | |
| Hodgkin's | ABVD | All ages | Low |
| | Protocols with procarbazine (MOPP, BEACOPP) | All ages | High |
| Non-Hodgkin's lymphoma | ABVD, CHOP | All ages | Low |
| | Cyclophosphamide (7.5 g/m$^2$) | All ages | High |
| Leukemias | | | |
| Acute myeloid leukemia | Anthracycline, cytarabine | All ages | Low |
| Acute lymphoblastic leukemia | Cyclophosphamide (7.5 g/m$^2$) | All ages | High |
| Colorectal | Irotecan, cetuximab, bevacizumab | All ages | Unknown |
| | Alkylating agents | All ages | High |
| | Pelvic radiation (rectal cancer) | All ages | High |
| Ovarian | Alkylating agents plus radiation | All ages | High risk |

Data primarily from *J Clin Oncol.* 2006;24:2917–2931 and *Gynecol Oncol.* 2006;103:1109–1121.
High risk >80%, intermediate 20%–80%, low <20%.
BMT, bone marrow transplant; AC, adriamycin, cyclophosphamide; CMF, cyclophosphamide, methotrexate, fluorouracil; CEF, cyclophosphamide, epirubicin, fluorouracil; CAF, cyclophosphamide, adriamycin, fluorouracil; ABVD, adriamycin, bleomycin, vinblastine, dacarbazine; CHOP, cyclophosphamide, adriamycin, vincristine, prednisone; MOPP, mechlorethamine, vincristine, prednisone, procarbazine; BEACOPP, cyclophosphamide, adriamycin, etoposide, vincristine, bleomycin, procarbazine, prednisone.

embryos results in high levels of circulating estrogen. Alternative cycles using aromatase inhibitors, which result in lower circulating estrogen, are increasingly being used in women who have hormone-sensitive tumors.[41,42] Women must have a male partner or be willing to use donor sperm for IVF, an important limitation. In addition, creation of embryos may conflict with moral or religious beliefs.

Women who can delay chemotherapy treatment for fertility preservation but do not have partners and do not wish to use sperm donation may opt for freezing mature oocytes. At a later date, these oocytes can then be thawed and fertilization with sperm attempted. Success rates for fertilization of cryopreserved oocytes are much lower than for cryopreserved embryos and only several hundred offspring have been produced world-wide.[38,43] The mean pregnancy rate per thawed oocyte is low (1.5%–4%), and the safety record for oocyte cryopreservation is not as extensive as it is for embryos.[17] A recent meta-analysis suggests that pregnancy rates from oocytes are about one quarter the pregnancy rates achieved from embryos.[42] However, technical advances in freezing and thawing oocytes are evolving.[20]

Cryopreservation of ovarian tissue does not involve stimulation of the ovaries (and hence high levels of circulating estrogen), but is still experimental and should be done only at reproductive research centers under monitoring by the Institutional Review Boards of participating institutions.[44] Ovarian tissue is harvested, usually laparoscopically, and cryopreserved (frozen) for later use. Tissue can be transplanted with the hope of regaining ovarian function. Successful reimplantation and harvesting of mature oocytes have been achieved,[17] and a total of 12 live births from cryopreserved ovarian tissue have been reported it the literature.[45] In the future, as advances occur in the field, mature eggs ready for transplantation or implantation may be coaxed from the immature eggs in a woman's frozen ovarian tissue. These approaches are highly experimental and women should understand this when considering cryopreservation. However, this procedure does not require weeks of hormonal stimulation and can be done immediately, both aspects that may be attractive to women who wish to prevent substantial delay in cancer treatment.

Some small studies have suggested that women whose ovarian function was suppressed during chemotherapy were less likely to experience ovarian failure,[46–48] but others have not.[49] Gonadotropin-releasing hormone agonists and antagonists are used to achieve ovarian suppression, but this also puts a woman in chemical menopause. Prospective randomized trials of sufficient power have not been

**TABLE 2.** Fertility Preservation Options

| | In-Vitro Fertilization Options[*][†] | | | Ovarian Cryopreservation | Ovarian Suppression | Radical Trachelectomy | Oophoropexy |
| --- | --- | --- | --- | --- | --- | --- | --- |
| | Embryo Freezing | Egg Freezing | Donor Embryos/Eggs | | | | |
| What is it? | IVF cycle—creating embryo from egg and sperm and freezing them for later implantation into patient or into a gestational carrier[†] | Harvesting eggs, which are later used to create embryos for implantation into patient or a gestational carrier | Embryos or egg donated, patient could then carry the pregnancy. Other option would be to obtain a surrogate, whereby another woman would both provide egg and carry the pregnancy | Freezing ovarian tissue and reimplantation after treatment | Shutting down of ovaries using GnRH analogues or antagonists | Modified cervical cancer surgery to preserve the uterus | Moving ovaries out of field of pelvic radiation |
| When? | Best results before treatment | Best results before treatment | After treatment | Best results before treatment | During treatment | Must be performed as part of cancer treatment | Before radiation |
| Time and effort required | 3–6 wk for IVF, which includes daily hormonal injections, frequent blood draws, multiple vaginal ultrasounds, and outpatient surgical procedure | ~One quarter that of traditional IVF | None before cancer treatment, but requires finding a suitable donor, and then undergoing IVF | Outpatient surgical procedure to obtain ovarian tissue; possible second procedure to reimplant tissue | Appointment for monthly injections | Surgery recovery similar to traditional radical hysterectomy with Lymph node dissection | Laparoscopic surgery |
| Risks | Potential delay of cancer treatment Hyperstimulation syndrome[§] Risks of anesthesia and infection Unclear risks of IVF on cancer recurrence Pregnancy could theoretically increase risk of recurrence for hormone-sensitive cancers, although observational data suggest safe | | Risks of anesthesia and infection Unclear risks of IVF on cancer recurrence Pregnancy could theoretically increase risk of recurrence for hormone-sensitive cancers, although observational data suggest safe | Risks of anesthesia and infection | Symptoms of menopause such as night sweats, sleep and mood disturbances | Surgical risks similar to traditional cervical cancer surgery Limited data suggest risk of recurrence similar as well | Risks of anesthesia and infection May require IVF to become pregnant Surgery can cause disruptions in ovarian blood supply which can damage ovaries, cyst formation |
| Success rates | ~40% per transfer; varies by age and center | ~One quarter that of traditional IVF | Slightly higher than embryo freezing | 12 live births reported world-wide Experimental | Unknown: conflicting results reported- Experimental | ~70% who try to conceive are successful, but only small percentage of women attempt | ~60%–90% will resume menses (range 16%–90%) |
| Misc | Need partner or donor sperm: may be religious objections | Do not need sperm at time of harvesting | Can use partner sperm: may be religious objections; if choose surrogacy (other woman carries child), laws in each state differ | Advanced breast cancer, some lymphomas not suitable due to concern for ovarian mets | Puts you into chemical menopause (reversible) | Increased risk of premature labor and 2nd trimester loss: requires surgeon is trained in technique, may require travel | Does nothing to protect from chemotherapy, which is often part of cancer treatment regimen |

[*]IVF, process of stimulating ovaries to produce many eggs, then extracting them surgically and creating embryos.
[†]Woman can choose to carry pregnancy herself, or use a surrogate (a woman who carries a baby for another couple or individual) for any of the IVF options.
[†]Gestational carrier, a woman carries a child that is genetically not related to her (implanted embryo) for another person/couple.
[§]Hyperstimulation syndrome occurs when the ovaries produce excessive mature egg follicles and results in abdominal pain, bloating, aborted IVF cycle and extremely rarely surgical intervention to relieve the condition. IVF, in-vitro fertilization.

performed to determine whether ovarian suppression is protective, and this cannot be solely relied upon to preserve ovarian function.[17,50] A large randomized controlled trial is on-going to address the role of ovarian suppression in protecting fertility.

Finally, women may choose their chemotherapy regimen based on its impact on ovarian function. For instance, in breast cancer treatment, 4 cycles of adriamycin and cytoxan therapy () result in very low rates of amenorrhea (10%–15%) when compared with 6 cycles of cyclophosphamide, methotrexate, and fluorouracil therapy (20%–60%),[51–53] with no difference in survival. Choice of treatment for ovarian[54] and hematologic cancers[33] can also be tailored to reduce the risk of infertility, with equivalent clinical responses. Women may decide to forgo chemotherapy entirely, if the absolute gains in survival are small. Although the number of young women who alter their treatment based on fertility concerns is not known, Partridge et al[13] found that fertility concerns affected treatment choices in 28% of their web-based sample of young breast cancer survivors.

Protecting the ovaries from pelvic radiation can be attempted by oophoropexy. Oophoropexy is a surgical procedure that moves the ovaries out of the field of pelvic radiation. It can be done laparoscopically just before radiation is initiated, or by laparotomy at the time of primary treatment for cancer. The effectiveness of the procedure varies greatly, and estimates of efficacy range from 16% to 90%.[23,55] Even when ovarian function is preserved, IVF may be required to restore fertility because of the position of the ovaries. In addition, oophoropexy does not protect the ovaries from whole body or spine radiation, chemotherapy, or injury to the vasculature during the surgery itself.

## PREGNACY OUTCOMES IN CANCER SURVIVORS

Rates of pregnancy among cancer survivors are generally lower than age-matched peers.[56] This may reflect both higher rates of infertility, as well as reduced attempts at conception. Pregnancy does not appear to increase the risk of cancer recurrence.[57] However, there has been considerable concern and debate regarding the safety of pregnancy in women with hormone-sensitive tumors. The high levels of circulating sex hormones could theoretically increase the chances of recurrence. Studies among breast cancer survivors do not suggest an increased risk of recurrence with pregnancy.[58–60] In fact, several studies suggest a decreased risk of recurrence,[58,59] but there are methodological problems with these studies including selection bias (only healthy women with the best prognosis pursue pregnancy) and publication bias (studies are unpublished because they are small studies or case series).

Patients with cancer also report concerns regarding the risks of chemotherapy to their offspring and the safety of pregnancy itself.[61,62] Chemotherapy does not appear to increase the risk of abnormalities in offspring, as long as pregnancy is delayed at least 6 months after treatment.[60,63] However, Tamoxifen, used as adjuvant chemotherapy in premenopausal women with estrogen receptor-positive breast cancer tumors to prevent recurrence, does increase the risk of fetal abnormalities and pregnancy is contraindicated while on therapy.[60,64] There is no evidence that a history of cancer increases cancer risk in offspring, a concern many cancer survivors have regarding pregnancy.[65] An exception is individuals who harbor autosomal dominant genetic mutations such as BRCA-1 or BRCA-2, whose offspring have a 50% chance of inheriting the gene. Radiation to the pelvis does increases the risk of premature delivery, and birth weight is lower in women who have received pelvic radiation.[65] A pregnancy in a woman who has received pelvic radiation should be considered a high-risk pregnancy.

For women who cannot become pregnant naturally, IVF can be attempted. IVF after cancer treatment is an unusual occurrence and experience is extremely limited. However, one case series by Ginsburg et al[66] suggested women with early breast cancer can be stimulated successfully, though the number of oocytes and embryos retrieved is lower. Several researchers[59,60,63] have called for national registries to help quantify and study these issues in female cancer survivors.

## THE PSYCHOSOCIAL IMPACT OF FERTILITY IN CANCER SURVIVORS

Infertility alone is associated with significant psychologic distress with levels of depression twice that of the normal population, and quality of life is reduced in areas of emotional well-being, relationships, and sexuality.[67,68] When infertility is superimposed on cancer, there can be great stress on the patient, partner, and family.[69] Even for persons who may have not planned to have children, the threat of infertility can result in a deep sense of loss and anger.

Women diagnosed with cancer must process complex information regarding cancer treatment options. The process of diagnosis and treatment decision-making has long been recognized as a particularly difficult and challenging time for women. Fertility preservation options are also very complex, requiring women to weigh their desire for preserving childbearing potential against the possible treatment delays and uncertain risks of fertility preservation options. Given that physicians often do not discuss these issues with their cancer patients, women may perceive physician failure to raise the issue as an implicit dismissal of its importance or feasibility. Some women may feel that they should be grateful just to survive their cancer.

However, we know that issues related to fertility remain very important to women in the short[13,62] and long term.[70] The loss of fertility is sometimes felt as painfully as the cancer diagnosis itself.[63,71] In qualitative studies that have inquired as to the motivations for having children after cancer among breast cancer survivors, women cite a sense of reclaiming their lives, a wish to feel normal again, and a desire to achieve the goals they set before their cancer diagnosis.[71,72] Surveys of breast cancer survivors have found that infertility is an important long-term survivorship issue, which has a negative impact on women's quality of life.[7,73]

Schover et al[61] surveyed a sample of 100 young female cancer survivors age 14 and older who were free of disease, specifically addressing issues of fertility. The average age of young women in the sample was 26 and the mean time since diagnosis was 5 years. They found that the experience of cancer did not decrease the desire to have children, and in fact it actually increased the value placed on parenthood and family ties. Of those childless at the time of the questionnaire, 76% wanted children in the future, and over 30% of those who already had children at diagnosis wanted additional children.

Zanagnolo et al[74] examined attitudes of 75 women who underwent conservative treatment for ovarian cancer and found that cancer did not diminish their desire to have children in 78% of women, and over half of women were concerned about the effects of removing one ovary on infertility risk. The authors also found that infertility concerns were associated with increased distress in these women, regardless of whether they already had children. A review of the psychosocial outcomes in women with gestational trophoblastic disease found that women had persistent fears regarding their ability to carry a normal pregnancy to term and also worried about pregnancy increasing the risk of disease recurrence.[75] Women who had children before their diagnosis, and women who bore children after their diagnosis had the highest quality of life scores.

In a cross-sectional study of 231 women diagnosed between ages 17 to 45 with cervical cancer, gestational trophoblastic tumors, or lymphoma, Wenzel et al[76] found that greater reproductive concerns were associated with significantly lower quality of life and increased cancer-specific distress. Women unable to conceive after cancer treatment reported significantly more reproductive concerns, poorer mental health, and lower psychologic well-being than women who were able to have children. Cervical cancer survivors reported the most reproductive concerns. Carter et al[67] examined quality of life measures in 20 women aged 29 to 49 with known infertility due to gynecologic cancer treatment, and found 40% met the clinical criteria for depression on the CES-D. Approximately, half of the women experienced trouble accepting infertility, yearning to give birth, or anger over their infertility.

Regardless of the type of cancer women face, the limited research conducted to date indicates that fertility concerns are prevalent, and negatively impact on a woman's quality of life. The consistency of these findings points to the importance of discussing fertility issues with premenopausal women in the clinical setting before the initiation of cancer treatment. Fertility changes and options to preserve fertility must be discussed before treatment is begun, when options to prevent fertility loss are still feasible. However, there are a number of potential barriers to discussing fertility issues.

## BARRIERS TO DISCUSSING FERTILITY OUTCOMES

Research regarding oncologists' discussions with premenopausal women regarding fertility changes associated with breast cancer treatment suggests that between one third to two thirds of women are not counseled regarding the impact of cancer treatment on their fertility.[13,77] Rates for other cancers are even lower.[78] Qualitative studies have indicated that women want information both about the risks of becoming infertile, as well as options for protecting or preserving their fertility.[10] Yet even when counseled, the information received is often not adequate from the patient's perspective.[13,62,79]

Limited research has examined the barriers and facilitators of fertility discussions from a medical provider's perspective.[80–82] These studies suggest that awareness and comfort in discussing fertility issues, as well as knowledge of available resources, play a role in either facilitating discussions or hindering the discussion of fertility. In addition, providers rated the importance of fertility to their patients as low, in contrast to patients, who rate fertility issues as quite important.[81] Often, providers do not raise fertility issues unless the patient herself raises them.[82]

Time constraints are also an often-cited barrier to fertility discussions. In the United States, there is an increasing pressure to see more and more patients within defined periods of time to offset decreasing reimbursement and increasing administrative costs. In the context of visits before cancer treatment, providers are challenged to discuss the many cancer treatment options available to women, with their associated risks and benefits. To many providers, adding a discussion of potential threats to fertility associated with treatment, as well as fertility preservation options, may seem overwhelming. The use of oncology nurses and social workers to provide much of the counseling regarding fertility and cancer has been proposed as a solution to this issue.[83] Resources such as Fertile Hope, Susan G. Komen Foundation, and Lance Armstrong Foundation all provide information in web and print form, which can assist women with cancer and their providers in discussing fertility issues.

Characteristics of the cancer, such as advanced stage, may also impact whether fertility issues are discussed. Providers may neglect to discuss fertility issues in women with a poor prognosis. However, it is impossible to know which women will survive and which women will not—even among women diagnosed with advanced stage cancer, some women will live. In addition, personal characteristics, such as financial status, marital status, or age, may also present barriers to oncologists' raising fertility issues with premenopausal women. However, findings from a study of young breast cancer survivors indicated that these characteristics were not associated with interest in fertility information.[13] Only the desire for children at time of diagnosis, number of previous pregnancies, and previous infertility were associated with concern regarding infertility. The safest and most equitable approach is to raise fertility issues with every patient.

Fertility issues in premenopausal women diagnosed with cancer present important challenges to the provider and to the patient. However, failure to discuss these options adequately can have lasting negative consequences on a woman's quality of life. Physician education interventions should seek to improve the knowledge of fertility preservations options, and of locally and nationally available resources. In addition, incorporating fertility issues into oncology training programs would both improve comfort and knowledge, and would be an important signal of the importance of the topic.

## REFERENCES

1. SEER. Surveillance Research Program, 2008. National Cancer Institute. Available at http://seer.cancer.gov/faststats/selections.php#Output.
2. Mathews TJ, Hamilton BE. Mean age of mother, 1970–2000. *Natl Vital Stat Rep.* 2002;51:1–13.
3. Hamilton BE, Martin JA, Sutton PD. Births: preliminary data for 2003. *Natl Vital Stat Rep.* 2004;53:1–17.
4. Mor V, Malin M, Allen S. Age differences in the psychosocial problems encountered by breast cancer patients. *J Natl Cancer Inst Monogr.* 1994:191–197.
5. Braun M, Hasson-Ohayon I, Perry S, et al. Motivation for giving birth after breast cancer. *Psychooncology.* 2005;14:282–296.
6. Vinokur AD, Threatt BA, Caplan RD, et al. Physical and psychosocial functioning and adjustment to breast cancer. Long-term follow-up of a screening population. *Cancer.* 1989;63:394–405.
7. Ganz PA, Greendale GA, Petersen L, et al. Breast cancer in younger women: reproductive and late health effects of treatment. *J Clin Oncol.* 2003;21:4184–4193.
8. Bloom JR, Stewart SL, Johnston M, et al. Intrusiveness of illness and quality of life in young women with breast cancer. *Psychooncology.* 1998;7:89–100.
9. Bloom JR, Kessler L. Risk and timing of counseling and support interventions for younger women with breast cancer. *J Natl Cancer Inst Monogr.* 1994:199–206.
10. Thewes B, Meiser B, Rickard J, et al. The fertility- and menopause-related information needs of younger women with a diagnosis of breast cancer: a qualitative study. *Psychooncology.* 2003;12:500–511.
11. Schover LR. Psychosocial aspects of infertility and decisions about reproduction in young cancer survivors: a review. *Med Pediatr Oncol.* 1999;33:53–59.
12. Schover LR. *Sexuality and Fertility After Cancer.* New York: Wiley; 1997.
13. Partridge AH, Gelber S, Peppercorn J, et al. Web-based survey of fertility issues in young women with breast cancer. *J Clin Oncol.* 2004;22:4174–4183.
14. Shapiro CL, Recht A. Side effects of adjuvant treatment of breast cancer. *N Engl J Med.* 2001;344:1997–2008.
15. Simon B, Lee SJ, Partridge AH, et al. Preserving fertility after cancer. *CA Cancer J Clin.* 2005;55:211–228; quiz 63–64.
16. Partridge AH, Burstein HJ, Winer EP. Side effects of chemotherapy and combined chemohormonal therapy in women with early-stage breast cancer. *J Natl Cancer Inst Monogr.* 2001:135–142.
17. Oktay K, Sonmezer M. Ovarian tissue banking for cancer patients: fertility preservation, not just ovarian cryopreservation. *Hum Reprod.* 2004;19:477–480.
18. Dow KH, Kuhn D. Fertility options in young breast cancer survivors: a review of the literature. *Oncol Nurs Forum.* 2004;31:E46–E53.
19. Lutchman Singh K, Davies M, Chatterjee R. Fertility in female cancer survivors: pathophysiology, preservation and the role of ovarian reserve testing. *Hum Reprod Update.* 2005;11:69–89.

20. Lee SJ, Schover LR, Partridge AH, et al. American Society of Clinical Oncology recommendations on fertility preservation in cancer patients. *J Clin Oncol.* 2006;24:2917–2931.

21. Meirow D. Ovarian injury and modern options to preserve fertility in female cancer patients treated with high dose radio-chemotherapy for hematooncological neoplasias and other cancers. *Leuk Lymphoma.* 1999;33:65–76.

22. Apperley JF, Reddy N. Mechanism and management of treatment-related gonadal failure in recipients of high dose chemoradiotherapy. *Blood Rev.* 1995;9:93–116.

23. Meirow D, Nugent D. The effects of radiotherapy and chemotherapy on female reproduction. *Hum Reprod Update.* 2001;7:535–543.

24. Mitwally MF. Effect of cancer and cancer treatment on human reproduction. *Expert Rev Anticancer Ther.* 2007;7:811–822.

25. Critchley HO, Wallace WH. Impact of cancer treatment on uterine function. *J Natl Cancer Inst Monogr.* 2005:64–68.

26. Dursun P, LeBlanc E, Nogueira MC. Radical vaginal trachelectomy (Dargent's operation): a critical review of the literature. *Eur J Surg Oncol.* 2007;33:933–941.

27. Plante M, Renaud MC, Hoskins IA, et al. Vaginal radical trachelectomy: a valuable fertility-preserving option in the management of early-stage cervical cancer. A series of 50 pregnancies and review of the literature. *Gynecol Oncol.* 2005;98:3–10.

28. Plante M, Renaud MC, Roy M. Radical vaginal trachelectomy: a fertility-preserving option for young women with early stage cervical cancer. *Gynecol Oncol.* 2005;99 (3 Suppl 1):S143–S146.

29. Ramirez PT, Schmeler KM, Soliman PT, et al. Fertility preservation in patients with early cervical cancer: radical trachelectomy. *Gynecol Oncol.* 2008;110 (3 Suppl 2):S25–S28.

30. Colombo N, Parma G, Lapresa MT, et al. Role of conservative surgery in ovarian cancer: the European experience. *Int J Gynecol Cancer.* 2005;15 (Suppl 3):206–211.

31. Schilder JM, Thompson AM, DePriest PD, et al. Outcome of reproductive age women with stage IA or IC invasive epithelial ovarian cancer treated with fertility-sparing therapy. *Gynecol Oncol.* 2002;87:1–7.

32. Park JY, Kim DY, Suh DS, et al. Outcomes of fertility-sparing surgery for invasive epithelial ovarian cancer: oncologic safety and reproductive outcomes. *Gynecol Oncol.* 2008;110:345–353.

33. Maltaris T, Boehm D, Dittrich R, et al. Reproduction beyond cancer: a message of hope for young women. *Gynecol Oncol.* 2006;103:1109–1121.

34. Wang CB, Wang CJ, Huang HJ, et al. Fertility-preserving treatment in young patients with endometrial adenocarcinoma. *Cancer.* 2002;94:2192–2198.

35. Chiva de Agustin L, Lapuente Sastre F, Corraliza Galan V, et al. Conservative management of patients with early endometrial carcinoma: a systematic review. *Clin Transl Oncol.* 2008;10:155–162.

36. Ramirez PT, Frumovitz M, Bodurka DC, et al. Hormonal therapy for the management of grade 1 endometrial adenocarcinoma: a literature review. *Gynecol Oncol.* 2004;95:133–138.

37. Gotlieb WH, Beiner ME, Shalmon B, et al. Outcome of fertility-sparing treatment with progestins in young patients with endometrial cancer. *Obstet Gynecol.* 2003;102:718–725.

38. Falcone T, Attaran M, Bedaiwy MA, et al. Ovarian function preservation in the cancer patient. *Fertil Steril.* 2004;81:243–257.

39. Wang JX, Yap YY, Matthews CD. Frozen-thawed embryo transfer: influence of clinical factors on implantation rate and risk of multiple conception. *Hum Reprod.* 2001;16:2316–2319.

40. Son WY, Yoon SH, Yoon HJ, et al. Pregnancy outcome following transfer of human blastocysts vitrified on electron microscopy grids after induced collapse of the blastocoele. *Hum Reprod.* 2003;18:137–139.

41. Azim A, Oktay K. Letrozole for ovulation induction and fertility preservation by embryo cryopreservation in young women with endometrial carcinoma. *Fertil Steril.* 2007;88:657–664.

42. Oktay K, Hourvitz A, Sahin G, et al. Letrozole reduces estrogen and gonadotropin exposure in women with breast cancer undergoing ovarian stimulation before chemotherapy. *J Clin Endocrinol Metab.* 2006;91:3885–3890.

43. Tucker M, Morton P, Liebermann J. Human oocyte cryopreservation: a valid alternative to embryo cryopreservation? *Eur J Obstet Gynecol Reprod Biol.* 2004;113 (Suppl 1):S24–S27.

44. Ethics Committee of the American Society for Reproductive Medicine. Fertility preservation and reproduction in cancer patients. *Fertil Steril.* 2005;83:1622–1628.

45. Meirow D. Fertility preservation in cancer patients using stored ovarian tissue: clinical aspects. *Curr Opin Endocrinol Diabetes Obes.* 2008;15:536–547.

46. Recchia F, Sica G, De Filippis S, et al. Goserelin as ovarian protection in the adjuvant treatment of premenopausal breast cancer: a phase II pilot study. *Anticancer Drugs.* 2002;13:417–424.

47. Blumenfeld Z, Haim N. Prevention of gonadal damage during cytotoxic therapy. *Ann Med.* 1997;29:199–206.

48. Blumenfeld Z. Ovarian rescue/protection from chemotherapeutic agents. *J Soc Gynecol Investig.* 2001;8 (1 Suppl Proceedings):S60–S64.

49. Waxman JH, Ahmed R, Smith D, et al. Failure to preserve fertility in patients with Hodgkin's disease. *Cancer Chemother Pharmacol.* 1987;19:159–162.

50. Blumenfeld Z, Eckman A. Preservation of fertility and ovarian function and minimization of chemotherapy-induced gonadotoxicity in young women by GnRH-a. *J Natl Cancer Inst Monogr.* 2005:40–43.

51. Goodwin PJ, Ennis M, Pritchard KI, et al. Risk of menopause during the first year after breast cancer diagnosis. *J Clin Oncol.* 1999;17:2365–2370.

52. Burstein HJ, Winer EP. Primary care for survivors of breast cancer. *N Engl J Med.* 2000;343:1086–1094.

53. Bryce C, Shenkier T, Gekman K, et al. Menstrual disruption in premenopausal breast cancer patients receiving CMF (IV) versus AC adjuvent chemotherapy [abstract]. *Breast Cancer Res Treat.* 1998;50:284.

54. Kang H, Kim TJ, Kim WY, et al. Outcome and reproductive function after cumulative high-dose combination chemotherapy with bleomycin, etoposide and cisplatin (BEP) for patients with ovarian endodermal sinus tumor. *Gynecol Oncol.* 2008;111:106–110.

55. Sonmezer M, Oktay K. Fertility preservation in female patients. *Hum Reprod Update.* 2004;10:251–266.

56. Magelssen H, Melve KK, Skjaerven R, et al. Parenthood probability and pregnancy outcome in patients with a cancer diagnosis during adolescence and young adulthood. *Hum Reprod.* 2008;23:178–186.

57. Fossa SD, Dahl AA. Fertility and sexuality in young cancer survivors who have adult-onset malignancies. *Hematol Oncol Clin North Am.* 2008;22:291–303, vii.

58. Kroman N, Jensen MB, Wohlfahrt J, et al. Pregnancy after treatment of breast cancer—a population-based study on behalf of Danish Breast Cancer Cooperative Group. *Acta Oncol.* 2008;47:545–549.

59. Partridge A, Schapira L. Pregnancy and breast cancer: epidemiology, treatment, and safety issues. *Oncology (Williston Park).* 2005;19:693–697; discussion 697–700.

60. Upponi SS, Ahmad F, Whitaker IS, et al. Pregnancy after breast cancer. *Eur J Cancer.* 2003;39:736–741.

61. Schover LR, Rybicki LA, Martin BA, et al. Having children after cancer. A pilot survey of survivors' attitudes and experiences. *Cancer.* 1999;86:697–709.

62. Thewes B, Meiser B, Taylor A, et al. Fertility- and menopause-related information needs of younger women with a diagnosis of early breast cancer. *J Clin Oncol.* 2005;23:5155–5165.

63. Surbone A, Petrek JA. Childbearing issues in breast carcinoma survivors. *Cancer.* 1997;79:1271–1278.

64. Barthelmes L, Gateley CA. Tamoxifen and pregnancy. *Breast.* 2004;13:446–451.

65. Sankila R, Olsen JH, Anderson H, et al. Risk of cancer among offspring of childhood-cancer survivors. Association of the Nordic Cancer Registries and the Nordic Society of Paediatric Haematology and Oncology. *N Engl J Med.* 1998;338:1339–1344.

66. Ginsburg ES, Yanushpolsky EH, Jackson KV. In vitro fertilization for cancer patients and survivors. *Fertil Steril.* 2001;75:705–710.

67. Carter J, Rowland K, Chi D, et al. Gynecologic cancer treatment and the impact of cancer-related infertility. *Gynecol Oncol.* 2005;97:90–95.

68. Lukse MP, Vacc NA. Grief, depression, and coping in women undergoing infertility treatment. *Obstet Gynecol.* 1999;93:245–251.

69. Loscalzo MJ, Clark KL. The psychosocial context of cancer-related infertility. *Cancer Treat Res.* 2007;138:180–190.

70. Zebrack BJ, Mills J, Weitzman TS. Health and supportive care needs of young adult cancer patients and survivors. *J Cancer Surviv.* 2007;1:137–145.

71. Dow KH. Having children after breast cancer. *Cancer Pract.* 1994;2:407–413.

72. Dunn J, Steginga SK. Young women's experience of breast cancer: defining young and identifying concerns. *Psychooncology.* 2000;9:137–146.

73. Avis NE, Crawford S, Manuel J. Psychosocial problems among younger women with breast cancer. *Psychooncology.* 2004;13:295–308.

74. Zanagnolo V, Sartori E, Trussardi E, et al. Preservation of ovarian function, reproductive ability and emotional attitudes in patients with malignant ovarian tumors. *Eur J Obstet Gynecol Reprod Biol.* 2005;123:235–243.

75. Garner E, Goldstein DP, Berkowitz RS, et al. Psychosocial and reproductive outcomes of gestational trophoblastic diseases. *Best Pract Res Clin Obstet Gynaecol.* 2003;17:959–968.

76. Wenzel L, Dogan-Ates A, Habbal R, et al. Defining and measuring reproductive concerns of female cancer survivors. *J Natl Cancer Inst Monogr.* 2005: 94–98.
77. Duffy CM, Allen SM, Clark MA. Discussions regarding reproductive health for young women with breast cancer undergoing chemotherapy. *J Clin Oncol.* 2005;23:766–773.
78. Strong M, Peche W, Scaife C. Incidence of fertility counseling of women of child-bearing age before treatment for colorectal cancer. *Am J Surg.* 2007;194:765–767; discussion 767–768.
79. Zebrack B. Information and service needs for young adult cancer patients. *Support Care Cancer.* 2008;16:1353–1360.
80. Quinn GP, Vadaparampil ST, Gwede CK, et al. Discussion of fertility preservation with newly diagnosed patients: oncologists' views. *J Cancer Surviv.* 2007; 1:146–155.
81. Vadaparampil S, Quinn G, King L, et al. Barriers to fertility preservation among pediatric oncologists. *Patient Educ Couns.* 2008;72:402–410.
82. King L, Quinn GP, Vadaparampil ST, et al. Oncology nurses' perceptions of barriers to discussion of fertility preservation with patients with cancer. *Clin J Oncol Nurs.* 2008;12:467–476.
83. Canada AL, Schover LR. Research promoting better patient education on reproductive health after cancer. *J Natl Cancer Inst Monogr.* 2005:98–100.

# Sexual Rehabilitation After Localized Prostate Cancer

## Current Interventions and Future Directions

David M. Latini • Stacey L. Hart • David W. Coon • Sara J. Knight

Prostate cancer is the most common cancer among American men, with an estimated 186,320 new cases expected in 2008. It represents 25% of all new cancer diagnoses in men, has an incidence comparable with that of breast cancer in women, and continues to disproportionately affect minority men.[1] Patients with early localized prostate cancer have a number of treatment options, including surgical removal of the prostate, radiation therapy (external beam or implantation of radioactive "seeds"), hormonal therapy, cryoablation, or expectant monitoring ("active surveillance").[2,3] However, most of these currently available treatments carry the risk of a number of treatment-related side-effects, including urinary incontinence, erectile dysfunction (ED), and others that vary, depending on the treatment received.[4] The issue of treatment-related side-effects is particularly important because the prognosis of men with prostate cancer, relative to other cancers, is good; and potential treatment-related symptoms can have important implications for health-related quality of life (HRQOL). Because early prostate cancer has a long natural history, men who develop treatment-related side-effects experience them for years.[5]

Beginning in 1995 with the publication of the University of California Los Angeles CLA Prostate Cancer Index by Litwin et al,[4] much has been learned about HRQOL in men treated for localized prostate cancer. Many articles have been published from large disease registries, such as the Cancer of the Prostate Strategic Urologic Research Endeavor study, a 13,000-man national study primarily drawn from community urology practices[6] and the Prostate Cancer Outcomes Study, a study that obtained follow-up HRQOL data from men who were part of the National Cancer Institute's Surveillance, Epidemiology, and End Results Program.[6,7] A large number of publications from smaller studies also have documented the changes in HRQOL experienced by men treated for localized prostate cancer.[8-10] Recent reviews have summarized the patterns in HRQOL over time.[11,12]

The recent Institute of Medicine (IOM) report, *From Cancer Patient to Survivor: Lost in Transition,*[13] highlights the growing number of persons now living far beyond treatment for their cancer, and the particular needs of cancer survivors for research and interventions that can improve symptom management and other aspects of quality of life. In particular, the IOM report recommends "intervention for consequences of cancer and its treatment, for example: medical problems such as lymphedema and sexual dysfunction; symptoms, including pain and fatigue; psychologic distress experienced by cancer survivors, and their caregivers."[13] Among men with localized prostate cancer, the number of descriptive studies carried out has grown quite large and documents the ongoing burden of treatment-related symptoms; however, the literature contains relatively few intervention studies.[14]

Early general interventions for men with prostate cancer have included support-group programs,[15] diet and lifestyle interventions,[16-18] cognitive-behavioral stress-management programs,[19]

psychoeducational groups,[9] nurse case management,[20] and uncertainty management.[21] In a study of the unmet information needs for men with prostate cancer, Boberg et al[22] found the greatest need for improvement in prostate-cancer education programs related to treatment-related symptoms and cancer recurrence. Among the published intervention studies, most have not provided specific information about managing treatment-related symptoms that are an important concern of men treated for localized disease and that address the IOM recommendations. The purpose of this article was to identify and briefly review published reports of sexual-rehabilitation and symptom-management interventions for men with localized prostate cancer, using PubMed and the recently published Cochrane reports on interventions for ED and sexual dysfunction after cancer treatment,[23,24] that sought to manage treatment-related side-effects or reduce the level of sexual-symptom distress or bother.

## GENERAL INTERVENTIONS THAT REPORTED SEXUAL REHABILITATION OUTCOMES

### Uncertainty Management

One of the earliest interventions that included sexual rehabilitation after prostate cancer was conducted by Mishel et al[21] (Table 1) at the University of North Carolina School of Nursing. The program was delivered by trained nurse educators over the phone and focused on psychologic outcomes, such as problem-solving, cognitive reframing, cancer knowledge, and patient-provider communications, and disease-specific outcomes that included symptom distress, number of symptoms, urinary and sexual functioning, and satisfaction with sexual functioning. Participants were assigned to 1 of 3 groups: intervention for prostate-cancer survivor alone, intervention for prostate-cancer survivor alone plus modified intervention for a family member, or a usual-care control condition. The intervention included both techniques to assess and reduce uncertainty about prostate cancer, and didactic information about various concerns, including symptom management. The intervention was offered in weekly telephone calls over 8 consecutive weeks. Most intervention effects were from baseline to 4 months. Men in the 2 uncertainty-management arms reported significantly better scores on the cognitive reframing and problem-solving scales at 4 months than men in the control arm, but this effect did not hold up at the 7-month assessment. As would be expected, given what is known in the prostate-cancer-symptom literature, men in all 3 groups reported fewer symptoms over time. A significant difference in urinary incontinence and satisfaction with sexual functioning was seen at 4 months between men in the 2 intervention groups combined versus control-group men. However, no significant differences between groups were found in cancer knowledge, patient-provider communication, or erectile functioning.[21]

**TABLE 1.** Psychosocial Interventions for Sexual Rehabilitation After Treatment for Localized Prostate Cancer

| Author | Publication Year | Number of Participants | Randomized | Intervention Type | Partner Included | Outcomes | Results |
|---|---|---|---|---|---|---|---|
| Mishel et al[21] | 2002 | 239 | Yes | Psychoeducational telephone sessions with patient and designated person | Patient could designate person to be included in intervention (ie, partner, family member, etc) | SDS, SWOG QOL, nonstandard urinary function, and sexual function and satisfaction questions | Significant improvement in sexual satisfaction, trend toward interaction between sexual functioning and ethnicity |
| Lepore et al[9] | 2003 | 250 | Yes | 6 educational sessions vs. 6 educational sessions plus discussion group | No | PCI, SF-36 | Sexual bother reduced for men in the education-plus-discussion arm |
| Maliski et al[26] | 2004 | 7 nurse case managers' notes on 30 patients | No | Case management | No | Not specified | Not specified |
| Weber et al[27] | 2004 | 30 | Yes | In-person peer support | No | PCI, GDS | Significantly less sexual bother in treatment group participants at follow-up |
| Canada et al[30] | 2005 | 51 couples | Yes | 4 sessions of psychoeducation for patient and partner | Some | IIEF, DAS, FSFI, PCI, SF-36, BSI | Significant improvements for treatment men in all IIEF domains and for treatment women in all FSFI domains |
| Giesler et al[31] | 2005 | 99 | Yes | Monthly sessions (2 in person, 4 by telephone) with patient and partner | Some | PC-QoL, DAS, CES-D, SF-36 | Significant gains in sexual functioning and significant reductions in how much sexual dysfunction limited role activities at 7 and 12 mo post-treatment |
| Titta et al[32] | 2006 | 57 | Yes | Short-term psychodynamic therapy in person and on the phone | Yes | IIEF | Significant improvements in erectile functioning over time for both groups but men in the sexual counseling plus injection group reported significantly better erectile functioning at 18-mo follow-up |
| Molton et al[33] | 2008 | 101 | Yes | 10-wk cognitive behavioral stress-management intervention | No | PCI | Men with greater interpersonal sensitivity reported greater increases in sexual functioning than men lower on this personality characteristic |

BSI indicates Brief Symptom Index; CES-D, Center for Epidemiologic Studies—Depression; DAS, Dyadic Adjustment Scale; EDITS, Erectile Dysfunction Inventory of Treatment Satisfaction; FSFI, Female Sexual Function Inventory; GDS, Geriatric Depression Scale; IIEF, International Index of Erectile Function; PCI, University of California Los Angeles Prostate Cancer Index; PC-QoL, Prostate Cancer Quality of Life; SDS, Symptom Distress Scale; SF-36, MOS Short Form-36; SWOG QOL, Southwest Oncology Group Quality of Life Measure.

This study included information about managing symptoms, such as sexual functioning. However, data were collected before the introduction of sildenafil and similar oral medications and focused on facilitating insertive sexual practices, mainly through the use of mechanical devices that helped participants develop erections. One reason participants who received the intervention did not show significant improvements in sexual functioning is that they also reported being troubled by the intrusiveness of the erectile aids. Another important lesson from the Mishel et al study is that symptom-management education may be more effective if it is available over an extended period (Mishel et al offered participants telephone sessions over 8 consecutive weeks). This is an important distinction as symptoms vary over time, based on the type of treatment selected.[25]

## Psychoeducational Groups

Another intervention that focused on disease-specific outcomes, and general HRQOL, randomized men to 1 of 3 groups: education, education plus discussion, or usual care.[9] Education sessions were offered over 6 weeks and consisted of 1-hour lectures on prostate-cancer biology, epidemiology, follow-up treatment, symptom management, and partner issues. Men also received printed materials summarizing the lectures. Men in the education plus discussion group received an additional 45-minute discussion group after each lecture, facilitated by a male clinical psychologist. The study focused on general and disease-specific HRQOL, prostate-cancer knowledge, an index of positive health behaviors mentioned in the lectures, and a standard measure of depression. The education plus discussion intervention was generally more effective than the control condition. Men in the education conditions reported significantly better outcomes for prostate-cancer knowledge, physical functioning, positive health behaviors, and sexual bother. No significant differences were found in sexual or urinary functioning. There was a differential effect by educational level, with less educated men benefiting more from the intervention.[9]

## Nurse Case-Manager Intervention

Maliski et al[26] provided an intervention for low-income men with prostate cancer, using a nurse case-manager format. They based their intervention on Self-Efficacy Theory, with the primary goal of empowering patients by increasing self-efficacy. Unlike other studies reviewed in this article, the 7 nurse case managers were not providing patients with a standard intervention. As a first step toward developing a standardized intervention, Maliski et al used retrospective record review to examine characteristics of intervention strategies used by nurse case managers. The interventions employed by the nurse case managers included assessment of patient needs and the best strategy to meet those needs, facilitation of successful self-action by patients, advocacy for patients' needs and concerns, coordination between care providers, teaching new knowledge and skills (including sexual rehabilitation), emotional support, collaborative problem-solving, and tracking patients. Although this is an important and promising approach to describe intervention strategies currently in use, it would be difficult to replicate the intervention with other patients until it has been better specified.

## Dyadic Support

Another nurse-led intervention study focused on the impact of dyadic support for men who had not attended a prostate-cancer support group.[27] This study is particularly important because many men are unwilling or unable to seek support for psychosocial or physical concerns from a support group.[28,29] Men who provided support to study participants were prostate-cancer survivors who had attended prostate-cancer support groups and were experienced in giving and receiving support about prostate-cancer concerns. The primary purpose of the intervention was to provide social support and lessen depression related to prostate-cancer treatment and side-effects. Results showed improvements in depression at 4 weeks for treatment-group subjects and significantly better self-efficacy at 8 weeks for treatment-group men, who also reported significantly less sexual bother and a trend toward better sexual functioning at 8 weeks than men in the control group.

## INTERVENTIONS THAT SPECIFICALLY TARGET SEXUAL REHABILITATION

### Psychoeducational Intervention for Men and Their Partners

Canada et al[30] developed a 4-session psychoeducational intervention for men treated for localized prostate cancer with surgery or radiation and their partners. Each session included both didactic information about sexual side-effects, and behavioral homework and skill-building exercises to improve couple communication and increase sexual stimulation. Men were randomized to attend either with their partner or alone. Partners in the patient-only condition still completed homework. Results were not affected by the partner's attendance. Men completing the intervention experienced significant reductions in male overall distress and male global sexual function, and their female partners increased global sexual function at 3 months. Over time, these improvements lessened. Men who completed the intervention reported increasing use of ED treatments over time.

### Nurse-Led Computerized/Telephone Intervention

Another patient-education program led by nurses used a computerized questionnaire to determine which symptoms required intervention.[31] Men and their partners were randomized to receive the intervention or standard care. Intervention sessions were scheduled monthly. The first 2 sessions were completed in person, and the 4 remaining sessions were completed by telephone. Sessions included both the patient and his partner. Sexual symptoms and side-effects were the most commonly reported concern among men in the study. Men in the treatment group were offered a videotape that offered models of how to discuss sexual problems with a partner. The nurse interventionist offered further information about communication skills and ED treatments. Treatment-group participants reported significant improvements in sexual functioning and bother at 4, 7, and 12 months postbaseline compared with control-group men.

### Sexual Counseling for Erectile Rehabilitation

A unique study by Titta et al[32] focused specifically on facilitating intracavernous injection therapy for ED in men treated for localized prostate cancer or muscle-invasive bladder cancer. Participants in this intervention were offered didactic information about how to use injections and randomized to receive either didactic information alone or didactic information plus telephone-based, short-term psychodynamic sexual counseling. Over time, men in the sexual-counseling group were significantly less likely to stop using injection therapy, even though rates of side-effects (eg, pain or bruising) were similar in the 2 groups. Both groups had good response to injections and significantly improved erectile functioning scores over the 18-month follow-up period.

### Group-Based Stress Management

On the basis of their work with patients living with other chronic illnesses, Molton et al[33] adapted their cognitive behavioral stress-management program to assist men treated for localized prostate cancer to improve their sexual functioning, whereas also improving psychosocial outcomes. The intervention included 10 group sessions encompassing both information about the restoration of sexual functioning, and relaxation exercises, and cognitive, behavioral, and interpersonal skills necessary to cope with life stressors. Sexual functioning was measured at baseline and postintervention. Men receiving the intervention reported significantly better sexual functioning than men in the control condition, who completed a 4-hour workshop that taught the same stress-management skills as the longer intervention. Interpersonal sensitivity, described by Molton et al as "a problematic interpersonal style characterized by being "too sensitive" to others, a tendency to perceive and elicit criticism, and a chronic perception of rejection and abandonment," moderated the intervention effects. Post hoc analysis showed that men with greater interpersonal sensitivity showed greater pre-postimprovement in sexual functioning after completing the 10-week intervention, compared with men in the intervention group with lower interpersonal sensitivity.

## COMMON THEMES

### Global Versus Specific Goals

A number of common themes emerged from the studies reviewed here. First, most interventions have focused primarily on psychosocial outcomes. For example, Mishel et al based their intervention on Uncertainty in Illness Theory and emphasized the reduction of uncertainty in patients and their partner or other designated person. Such programs have had mixed effects on sexual outcomes. Mishel et al[21] reported that their intervention reduced sexual bother and improved urinary functioning, but they did not find significant differences in sexual functioning. Lepore et al[9] also reported significant decreases in sexual bother but no effect of their intervention on urinary or sexual functioning.

Interventions involving sexual rehabilitation as the primary goal have had better results than interventions focusing on more general goals. Short-term changes in sexual functioning were reported by Canada et al[30] and Molton et al.[33] In the intervention by Canada et al, improvements in sexual functioning faded over time. Molton et al did not report long-term results. Both Titta et al[32] and Giesler et al[31] reported continued improvements in sexual functioning at 12 months or longer after baseline. Giesler et al offered their intervention over a 6-month period. It may be that offering patient education over an extended period increases the efficacy of the intervention.

### Treatment Implementation Characteristics (Intensity, Frequency, and Duration)

Adherence to ED treatment recommendations can be problematic. Many studies have reported the necessity of trying successive treatments to achieve better sexual functioning and rates of ED treatment use as time since prostate-cancer treatment increases.[34,35] Thus, it was particularly gratifying that Canada et al reported higher rates of ED treatment use 6 months after enrollment in men who completed their intervention.[30] In the case of the study by Titta et al,[32] the investigators focused on intracavernous injection. Most studies and general practice in ED clinics start with less invasive treatments (ie, oral medications) and progress to more invasive treatments when patients fail oral medications. However, such an approach offers men the negative experiences of either obtaining no response to ED treatment or having a positive response that then diminishes over time. Such experiences could be problematic from the perspective of Self-Efficacy Theory because they may reduce a man's confidence that ED treatment can be successful, Bandura's concept of outcome efficacy.[36] The intervention reported by Titta et al bypassed treatment approaches that may

or may not be effective for men treated for localized prostate cancer, bypassing the possible negative consequences of ED-treatment failure.

Interventions varied in length, from 4 to 10 sessions spread over a month to 6 months. Although the length of the intervention was the same for all participants, Giesler et al described a program that was adaptive in that it focused on the symptoms most problematic for each participant. The particulars are unclear; however, the intervention described by Maliski et al was also tailored to each participant's concerns. Other studies offered the same interventions to each participant. In times when resources are hard to find, longer interventions that address multiple symptoms (eg, Molton et al) might be difficult to sustain. In other conditions, a stepped-care approach, motivated in part by cost considerations, has been shown to work.[37–39] The approach by Giesler et al could be further adapted to adapt not just intervention content but also amount of intervention received to a patient's needs for sexual rehabilitation.

### Moderators of Treatment

A participant's response to an intervention is based not only on clinical characteristics such as whether he had a nerve-sparing prostatectomy or not, but also on sociodemographic and psychologic characteristics. Lepore et al found men with little education benefited more from the psychosocial intervention than men with more education. In particular, less-educated men showed significantly greater improvements in physical functioning, positive health behaviors, and sexual bother. Similarly, a study using Cancer of the Prostate Strategic Urologic Research Endeavor data from 3 Veterans Affairs medical centers showed that men with limited formal education had poorer HRQOL over a 2-year period after prostate-cancer treatment, after controlling for other sociodemographic and clinical variables, than men with a high level of education.[40] Thus, men with limited education may be in greater need of sexual-rehabilitation interventions than men with a high level of education, but it is important to ensure that patient-education materials are targeted to the appropriate reading level. Readability of materials and health literacy of the target audience are particularly a concern with men treated for prostate cancer. African American men, a group with a significantly high prevalence of prostate cancer, are over-represented among lower-health-literacy men with prostate cancer.[41,42]

Low sexual desire may result from some prostate cancer treatments. The level of desire in men treated with surgery generally remains unchanged but is typically lower for men on androgen deprivation therapy.[10,43] Some studies also have reported reductions in level of desire for men treated with radiation.[44] Low desire is difficult to treat, particularly for prostate cancer survivors because pharmacologic treatment usually involves testosterone, which is controversial because of the possibility of cancer recurrence, and because low desire is sometimes mistaken for ED.[45–47]

Other personal characteristics also may be important predictors of response to sexual-rehabilitation programs or predictive of the need for intervention. Molton et al showed that men with high levels of interpersonal sensitivity reported greater gains in sexual functioning than men with low levels. Dahn et al reported significantly poorer HRQOL among men treated for prostate cancer who had high sexual desire and low erectile functioning than among men with low desire and low erectile functioning.[8] Thus, another feasibility consideration may be targeting sexual-rehabilitation efforts to men who are the most likely to benefit from such interventions (men with high interpersonal sensitivity) or men who may be most likely to report poor general HRQOL—those who have a substantial mismatch between level of desire and erectile ability. Though other areas of disease management have benefited from research trying to understand how to match patients to the optimal treatment, little has been done in cancer survivorship. The work by Molton et al and Dahn et al provides an excellent start in understanding who might benefit most from sexual-rehabilitation efforts.

## Missing Voices

Another area of sexual rehabilitation in need of further research and clinical efforts is in helping gay men reestablish their sexual lives after cancer.[48] No published data suggest that gay men are diagnosed with prostate cancer at any different rate than their heterosexual counterparts. Estimates suggest that approximately 5000 gay men may be diagnosed with prostate cancer in a year and that 50,000 or more gay men are living with prostate cancer and its treatment-related side-effects.[48] Prostate cancer affects gay men in many of the same ways as heterosexual men, but some of their concerns may differ. For example, the average age of men diagnosed with prostate cancer is 70 years old.[49] Thus, gay men with prostate cancer are typically older and may have more concerns about disclosing their sexuality to healthcare providers than younger gay men who may feel more comfortable being open about their sexuality.[50] Such reluctance may also preclude gay men diagnosed with prostate cancer from involving their partners in healthcare decisions and treatment planning, in contrast with their heterosexual counterparts. Many gay men report that healthcare providers fail to ask about sexual orientation during initial consultations and assume they are heterosexual.[50] Older gay men might be less likely than younger gay men to insist on including partners in the face of opposition or even lack of support for inclusion by healthcare providers.[51] Gay men who are not partnered may lack not only a supportive partner but also other family-support systems enjoyed by heterosexual men. Such men also have the same challenges that single heterosexual men face when seeking sexual rehabilitation of not having a primary partner with whom they have long-established trust and affection.[52] Support from peers also may be difficult to obtain. The number of support groups specifically for gay men with prostate cancer is limited to half a dozen in large cities. Gay men in other areas are forced to find a support group open to having gay men participate, remain closeted, rely on internet-based support groups, or be socially isolated.[51] After treatment, some sexual functioning and dysfunction may be similar for gay and straight men; but gay men have some particular concerns. For example, sexual rehabilitation may be focused on creating erections rigid enough for vaginal penetration. However, anal penetration requires a greater degree of rigidity than vaginal intercourse.[51,53] Moreover, research on communication between gay men with prostate cancer and their partners is lacking to inform whether or not, and if so how, sexual risk taking for HIV infection changes with cancer treatment-related sexual dysfunction.

## A BIOPSYCHOSOCIAL MODEL OF CANCER-SYMPTOM MANAGEMENT

Keeping in mind the reports of sexual-rehabilitation interventions already in the literature, we now shift our focus to proposing a biopsychosocial model of prostate-cancer symptom management. It is based on 2 theoretical and conceptual frameworks, the University of California San Francisco Symptom Management Model (SMM) and Self-Efficacy Theory and informed by results from the studies reviewed above.[36,54] The original SMM was published in 1994 and revised in 2001.[55,56] The symptom experience includes an individual's perception of a symptom, evaluation of the meaning of the symptom, and response to a symptom. The symptom-management-strategies dimension includes the specifics of the intervention (ie, what, when, why, where, how much, and to whom). The outcomes dimension specifies that outcomes emerge from the symptom-management strategies, and from the symptom experience. The outcome dimension focuses on 8 factors (ie, functional status, emotional status, self-care, costs, HRQOL, morbidity and comorbidity, and mortality).

Self-Efficacy Theory has been used in numerous psychosocial interventions for patients with chronic diseases[57-59] and is highly compatible with the SMM. It holds that 2 important determinants of behavior are outcome efficacy (confidence that an outcome can be affected) and self-efficacy (confidence that one can personally accomplish an outcome).[36] In the SMM, self-efficacy would be considered part of the symptom experience; for example, men who repeatedly fail to have an erection sufficient for intercourse are likely to have low confidence in their ability to have an erection the next time they want to have sex. This experience of ED erodes their confidence and makes it less likely that they will attempt sex in the future. For some men, their ED limits showing affection to their partner for fear their partner will want intercourse, which the man cannot provide.[34]

Figure 1 shows our adaptation of the SMM and Self-Efficacy Theory to the specific case of prostate-cancer symptom management,

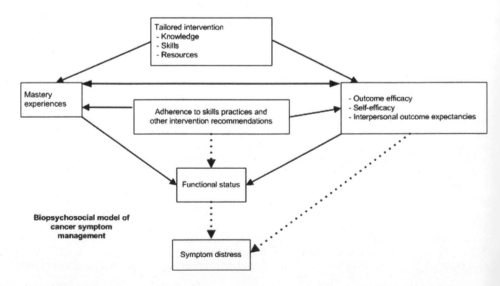

**FIGURE 1.** A biopsychosocial model of prostate cancer symptom management.

including sexual rehabilitation. Interventions derived from this model should provide participants with the knowledge, skills, and resources that will lead to a set of mastery experiences as participants begin to manage their symptoms effectively, leading to stronger beliefs that prostate-cancer symptoms can be managed (Bandura's concept of outcome efficacy) and that they are capable of managing their symptoms (self-efficacy). Staff providing rehabilitation interventions can help patients increase their sense of a supportive environment by assisting them with their symptom management work (interpersonal outcome expectancies). Like the interventions published by Maliski et al,[26] Weber et al,[27] and Lepore et al,[9] our model views increasing self efficacy as an integral part of symptom management.

As participants master symptom-management tasks, they improve their functional status. We hypothesize that men who improve their functional status will have reduced symptom distress and that men who are adherent with interventions are more likely to reduce their symptom distress than men who are not adherent with the intervention. Adherence also is likely to increase the number of mastery experiences that a participant has and his sense of outcome and personal efficacy. Previous work in men with advanced cancer suggests that men with a large number of symptoms report more distress than men with fewer symptoms.[60] Our model is based on the premise that this relationship between functional status and symptom distress exists and that providing rehabilitation for treatment-related side-effects and other symptoms will reduce both symptom distress and general levels of distress. Similar to the approaches by Mishel et al and Giesler et al, our model is focused on reducing symptom distress.

## CONCLUSIONS

Many studies have described the substantial impact of prostate-cancer treatment on sexual functioning. In this article, we have summarized the limited number of intervention studies developed for sexual rehabilitation of prostate-cancer survivors. A number of common themes emerged. Several interventions have focused primarily on psychosocial symptoms, with sexual rehabilitation as a secondary goal. Interventions that focused on sexual rehabilitation as a primary goal had better results. One intervention was tailored to address the symptoms of greatest concern to the participants. Developing such tailored interventions may be a way to increase "face validity" of the intervention with participants by closely linking the intervention to what they report as their primary concerns and could be linked with a stepped-care approach to increase the likelihood of developing cost-effective interventions that can be sustained past the end of a funded study.

Although clinical characteristics are important, others such as personality traits, literacy level, or the lack of congruence between sexual desire and functioning, may be important determinants of who needs rehabilitation efforts the most and who is most likely to benefit from them. Research is needed to understand how gay men are affected by prostate cancer and its treatment, and how sexual-rehabilitation efforts could be tailored to their particular needs. Finally, we have proposed a conceptual model for prostate-cancer–symptom research informed by psychologic and nursing theories and the published research on sexual rehabilitation in prostate-cancer survivors.

Further work is needed to build on the published work reviewed here to encourage sexual-rehabilitation efforts to focus on populations with greatest need because of psychologic makeup, low health literacy, or other characteristics that may put a prostate-cancer survivor at risk for low HRQOL. Physicians should recognize the importance of sexual rehabilitation programs and actively refer their patients to such programs. Mental health providers and nurses should provide sexual rehabilitation interventions to patients and work with their physician

colleagues to provide effective medical interventions supported by patient education materials at the appropriate reading level. Such efforts will address concerns raised in the IOM report by helping men move smoothly from being a patient to a survivor, armed with the necessary tools and support needed to live well after cancer.

## REFERENCES

1. American Cancer Society. *Cancer Facts and Figures 2008.* Atlanta, GA: American Cancer Society; 2008.
2. Lynch JH, Batuello JT, Crawford ED, et al. Therapeutic strategies for localized prostate cancer. *Rev Urol.* 2001;3(suppl 2):S39–S48.
3. Speight JL, Roach M. New techniques and management options for localized prostate cancer. *Rev Urol.* 2006;8(suppl 2):S22–S29.
4. Litwin MS, Hays RD, Fink A, et al. Quality-of-life outcomes in men treated for localized prostate cancer. *JAMA.* 1995;273:129–135.
5. Talcott JA. Quality of life in early prostate cancer: do we know enough to treat? *Hematol Oncol Clin North Am.* 1996;10:691–701.
6. Lubeck DP, Litwin MS, Henning JM, et al. The CaPSURE database: a methodology for clinical practice and research in prostate cancer. CaPSURE Research Panel. Cancer of the prostate strategic urologic research endeavor. *Urology.* 1996;48:773–777.
7. Potosky AL, Harlan LC, Stanford JL, et al. Prostate cancer practice patterns and quality of life: the Prostate Cancer Outcomes Study. *J Natl Cancer Inst.* 1999;91:1719–1724.
8. Dahn JR, Penedo FJ, Gonzalez JS, et al. Sexual functioning and quality of life after prostate cancer treatment: considering sexual desire. *Urology.* 2004;63:273–277.
9. Lepore SJ, Helgeson VS, Eton DT, et al. Improving quality of life in men with prostate cancer: a randomized controlled trial of group education interventions. *Health Psychol.* 2003;22:443–452.
10. Schover LR. Sexual rehabilitation after treatment for prostate cancer. *Cancer.* 1993;71:1024–1030.
11. Eton DT, Lepore SJ. Prostate cancer and health-related quality of life: a review of the literature. *Psychooncology.* 2002;11:307–326.
12. Penson DF. Quality of life after therapy for localized prostate cancer. *Cancer J.* 2007;13:318–326.
13. Institute of Medicine. *From Cancer Patient to Cancer Survivor: Lost in Transition.* Washington, DC: National Academies Press; 2005.
14. Visser A, van Andel G. Psychosocial and educational aspects in prostate cancer patients. *Patient Educ Couns.* 2003;49:203–206.
15. American Cancer Society. *Man to Man.* Vol. 2001. Atlanta, GA: American Cancer Society; 1999. Available at http://www3.cancer.org/cancerinfo/Documents/cancer_36/m2m_background.asp.
16. Demark-Wahnefried W, Morey MC, Clipp EC, et al. Leading the way in exercise and diet (Project LEAD): intervening to improve function among older breast and prostate cancer survivors. *Control Clin Trials.* 2003;24:206–223.
17. Carmack Taylor CL, Smith MA, De Moor C, et al. Quality of life intervention for prostate cancer patients: design and baseline characteristics of the active for life after cancer trial. *Control Clin Trials.* 2004;25:265–285.
18. Berglund G, Petersson LM, Eriksson KR, et al. "Between men": patient perceptions and priorities in a rehabilitation program for men with prostate cancer. *Patient Educ Couns.* 2003;49:285–292.
19. Penedo FJ, Dahn JR, Molton I, et al. Cognitive-behavioral stress management improves stress-management skills and quality of life in men recovering from treatment of prostate carcinoma. *Cancer.* 2004;100:192–200.
20. Maliski SL, Kwan L, Krupski T, et al. Confidence in the ability to communicate with physicians among low-income patients with prostate cancer. *Urology.* 2004;64:329–334.
21. Mishel MH, Belyea M, Germino BB, et al. Helping patients with localized prostate carcinoma manage uncertainty and treatment side effects: nurse-delivered psychoeducational intervention over the telephone. *Cancer.* 2002;94:1854–1866.
22. Boberg EW, Gustafson DH, Hawkins RP, et al. Assessing the unmet information, support and care delivery needs of men with prostate cancer. *Patient Educ Couns.* 2003;49:233–242.
23. Miles CL, Candy B, Jones L, et al. Interventions for sexual dysfunction following treatments for cancer. *Cochrane Database Syst Rev.* 2007;4:CD005540.
24. Melnik T, Soares BG, Nasselo AG. Psychosocial interventions for erectile dysfunction. *Cochrane Database Syst Rev.* 2007;3:CD004825.
25. Lubeck DP, Litwin MS, Henning JM, et al. Changes in health-related quality of life in the first year after treatment for prostate cancer: results from CaPSURE. *Urology.* 1999;53:180–186.
26. Maliski SL, Clerkin B, Letwin MS. Describing a nurse case manager intervention to empower low-income men with prostate cancer. *Oncol Nurs Forum.* 2004;31:57–64.

27. Weber BA, Roberts BL, Resnick M, et al. The effect of dyadic intervention on self-efficacy, social support, and depression for men with prostate cancer. *Psychooncology.* 2004;13:47–60.

28. Deans G, Bennett-Emslie GB, Weir J, et al. Cancer support groups—who joins and why? *Br J Cancer.* 1988;58:670–674.

29. Katz D, Koppie TM, Wu D, et al. Sociodemographic characteristics and health related quality of life in men attending prostate cancer support groups. *J Urol.* 2002;168:2092–2096.

30. Canada AL, Neese LE, Sui D, et al. Pilot intervention to enhance sexual rehabilitation for couples after treatment for localized prostate carcinoma. *Cancer.* 2005;104:2689–2700.

31. Giesler RB, Given B, Given CW, et al. Improving the quality of life of patients with prostate carcinoma: a randomized trial testing the efficacy of a nurse-driven intervention. *Cancer.* 2005;104:752–762.

32. Titta M, Tavolini IM, Moro FD, et al. Sexual counseling improved erectile rehabilitation after non-nerve-sparing radical retropubic prostatectomy or cystectomy—results of a randomized prospective study. *J Sex Med.* 2006;3:267–273.

33. Molton IR, Siegel SD, Penedo FJ, et al. Promoting recovery of sexual functioning after radical prostatectomy with group-based stress management: the role of interpersonal sensitivity. *J Psychosom Res.* 2008;64:527–536.

34. Latini DM, Penson DF, Colwell HH, et al. Psychological impact of erectile dysfunction: validation of a new health related quality of life measure for patients with erectile dysfunction. *J Urol.* 2002;168:2086–2091.

35. Schover LR, Fouladi RT, Warneke CL, et al. The use of treatments for erectile dysfunction among survivors of prostate carcinoma. *Cancer.* 2002;95:2397–2407.

36. Bandura A. *Social Foundations of Thought and Action: A Social Cognitive Theory.* Englewood Cliffs, NJ: Prentice-Hall, 1986.

37. Newman MG. Recommendations for a cost-offset model of psychotherapy allocation using generalized anxiety disorder as an example. *J Consult Clin Psychol.* 2000;68:549–555.

38. Otto MW, Pollack MH, Maki KM. Empirically supported treatments for panic disorder: costs, benefits, and stepped care. *J Consult Clin Psychol.* 2000;68:556–563.

39. Wilson GT, Vitousek KM, Loeb KL. Stepped care treatment for eating disorders. *J Consul Clin Psychol.* 2000;68:564–572.

40. Knight SJ, Latini DM, Hart SL, et al. Education predicts quality of life among men with prostate cancer cared for in the Department of Veterans Affairs: a longitudinal quality of life analysis from CaPSURE. *Cancer.* 2007;109:1769–1776.

41. Bennett CL, Ferreira MR, Davis TC, et al. Relation between literacy, race, and stage of presentation among low-income patients with prostate cancer. *J Clin Oncol.* 1998;16:3101–3104.

42. Wolf MS, Knight SJ, Lyons EA, et al. Literacy, race, and PSA level among low-income men newly diagnosed with prostate cancer. *Urology.* 2006;68:89–93.

43. Schover LR. Sexuality and fertility in urologic cancer patients. *Cancer.* 1987;60:553–558.

44. Helgason AR, Fredrikson M, Adolfsson J, et al. Decreased sexual capacity after external radiation therapy for prostate cancer impairs quality of life. *Int J Radiat Oncol Biol Phys.* 1995;32:33–39.

45. Meuleman EJ, van Lankveld JJ. Hypoactive sexual desire disorder: an underestimated condition in men. *BJU Int.* 2005;95:291–296.

46. Khera M, Lipshultz LI. The role of testosterone replacement therapy following radical prostatectomy. *Urol Clin North Am.* 2007;34:549–553.

47. Brand TC, Canby-Hagino E, Thompson IM. Testosterone replacement therapy and prostate cancer: a word of caution. *Curr Urol Rep.* 2007;8:185–189.

48. Blank TO. Gay men and prostate cancer: invisible diversity. *J Clin Oncol.* 2005;23:2593–2596.

49. Hankey BF, Feuer EJ, Clegg LX, et al. Cancer surveillance series: interpreting trends in prostate cancer. I. Evidence of the effects of screening in recent prostate cancer incidence, mortality, and survival rates. *J Natl Cancer Inst.* 1999;91:1017–1024.

50. Mitteldorf D. Psychotherapy with gay prostate cancer patients. In: Perlman G, Drescher J, eds. *A Gay Man's Guide to Prostate Cancer.* Binghamton, NY: The Haworth Medical Press; 2005:57–67.

51. Cornell D. A gay urologist's changing views of prostate cancer. In: Perlman G, Drescher J, eds. *A Gay Man's Guide to Prostate Cancer.* Binghamton, NY: The Haworth Medical Press; 2005:29–41.

52. McCarthy BW. Treatment of erectile dysfunction with single men. In: Rosen RC, Leiblum SC, eds. *Erectile Disorders: Assessment and Treatment.* New York: Guilford Press; 1992:313–340.

53. Goldstone SE. The ups and downs of gay sex after prostate cancer treatment. In: Perlman G, Drescher J, eds. *A Gay Man's Guide to Prostate Cancer.* Binghamton, NY: The Haworth Medical Press; 2005:43–55.

54. Bandura A. Self-efficacy: the exercise of control. New York: W.H. Freeman; 1997.

55. UCSF Faculty Group in Symptom Management. A model for symptom management. *Image J Nurs Sch.* 1994;26:272–276.

56. Dodd M, Janson S, Facione N, et al. Advancing the science of symptom management. *J Adv Nurs.* 2001;33:668–676.

57. Lorig KR, Ritter P, Stewart AL, et al. Chronic disease self-management program: 2-year health status and health care utilization outcomes. *Med Care.* 2001;39:1217–1223.

58. Lorig KR, Sobel DS, Stewart AL, et al. Evidence suggesting that a chronic disease self-management program can improve health status while reducing hospitalization: a randomized trial. *Med Care.* 1999;37:5–14.

59. Wilson SR, Latini D, Starr NJ, et al. Education of parents of infants and very young children with asthma: a developmental evaluation of the Wee Wheezers program. *J Asthma.* 1996;33:239–254.

60. Ullrich PM, Carson MR, Lutgendorf SK, et al. Cancer fear and mood disturbance after radical prostatectomy: consequences of biochemical evidence of recurrence. *J Urol.* 2003;169:1449–1452.

# Sexual Side Effects and Prostate Cancer Treatment Decisions

## Patient Information Needs and Preferences

Sara J. Knight • David M. Latini

Each year in the United States, several hundred thousand men are diagnosed with prostate cancer and asked what they would prefer: To possibly give up some degree of sexual function? To probably experience some level of urinary incontinence? To live with cancer without treatment? Treatment options differ in side effects, but for most men no alternative is clearly advantageous in prolonging survival. The choice of management strategy involves complex trade-offs that represent difficult decisions for men, their significant others, and their clinicians.[1,2] The common primary treatments (ie, radical prostatectomy, external beam radiation therapy, brachytherapy) have associated side effects including sexual dysfunction, urinary incontinence, and bowel problems.[3,4] Anxiety about cancer progression and recurrence is frequently a concern in the trade-off along with side effects.[5-7] Among all the considerations that patients weigh in making prostate cancer treatment decisions, concern about sexual function is central in the choice of treatment for localized prostate cancer.[8,9]

It is clear that patients would like to have their goals and values related to their sexuality considered in prostate cancer treatment decision making.[10,11] Typically, models of prostate cancer decision making include sexual function, urinary function, bowel function, and anxiety about survival as the important preferences for prostate cancer treatment decision making.[12,13] Most conceptual models of prostate cancer treatment decisions place sexual function centrally as a concern of most patients. As shown in Figure 1, these models assume that the choice of treatment for prostate cancer can only be judged in reference to the patient's goals and values for treatment. The patient's goals and values for treatment are defined as the patient's treatment-related preferences that are associated with attributes of treatment outcomes (eg, disease-free time, survival), treatment-related side effects (eg, urinary incontinence, sexual dysfunction), and other qualities of the treatment itself (eg, invasiveness of the procedure, recovery time). The figure shows the influence of these domains of concerns or preferences (ie, sexual function, urinary function, bowel function, anxiety) on the choice of treatment in Section A. In addition to these domains of patient preferences, the physician recommendation, based on the physician's understanding of patient preferences and clinical factors, such as the patient's age and comorbid conditions, has a reciprocal relationship with patient preferences (Section B). We assume that ultimately both the patient's preferences and the physician's recommendation influence treatment choice. The treatment choice, in turn, contributes to both treatment choice outcomes such as satisfaction or regret with the decision and treatment outcomes such as quality of life (Section C).

Although sexual function is widely thought to be important in prostate cancer treatment decisions, the physician alone is not the best judge of how a man may value sexuality in making this choice. Studies of patients and urologists have found that treatment priorities differ across these groups. For example, both patients and urologists identified treatment effectiveness as the most important treatment goal, but patients noted quality of life issues such as sexual function (45%) as the top concern in selecting treatment in contrast to urologists who noted treatment efficacy.[14] Physician characteristics, such as specialty, have also been shown to influence their perspectives on prostate cancer treatment recommendations.[15] Physician judgments of their own patients' preferences do not correspond to patient judgments of their own preferences when assessed either by utilities or rank order elicitation methods.[16-19] There is little correlation between patient-rated utilities and physician ratings when utilities are elicited by a time trade-off (TTO) method and the physicians were asked to complete the TTO as they thought their patients would. When patients and physicians were asked to rank order attributes associated with prostate cancer treatment (ie, sexual function, bowel and bladder problems) in terms of their importance to the patient there was little relationship between patient and physician ratings. This relationship did not increase even when patients perceived that their physicians had actively solicited their preferences.[16-19] Therefore, to understand how a patient's concern about sexuality is weighed with other potential treatment outcomes, such as survival and urinary function, it is necessary to ask the patient directly.

Thus, to know how to support men in making prostate cancer treatment decisions, it is critical to understand men's need for information about sexuality and prostate cancer and men's preferences for maintaining sexual function as compared with other aspects of well-being, such as urinary function and anxiety. In this article, we discuss the research findings on the need for information about sexuality among men making prostate cancer treatment decisions and the value that men place on sexual function in their choices of treatment for prostate cancer. We examine the potential for current decision aids to inform patients and clarify values, and we point to directions for future research.

## INFORMATION NEEDS AND SEXUALITY

Although a man's goals and values are critical considerations in prostate cancer treatment, men need information about the treatments and their expected outcomes to fully understand or predict their own preferences. For example, information about how several treatments influence erectile dysfunction or sexual desire would be expected to influence a man's preferences with respect to those treatments. A number of studies have identified information needs among men diagnosed with prostate cancer and suggest that information on sexual function is important in prostate cancer treatment decisions. However, the relative importance of information on sexuality varies considerably, compared with information on urinary function and survival.[20]

Feldman-Stewart et al[21] identified a wide range of information needs among men recently diagnosed with prostate cancer

**FIGURE 1.** Conceptual framework for understanding patient preferences and outcomes. Section A depicts the contribution of attribute domains to patient preferences. Sexual function is included in most models of prostate cancer treatment decisions. Section B shows the relationship between patient preferences and treatment choice, and the effect of physician recommendation on preferences and choice. Section C illustrates several potential outcomes associated with treatment choice.

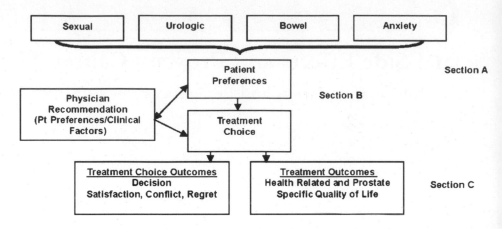

(6–12 months). Among the many questions that men raised, those concerning sexuality that were evaluated as essential to address in making prostate cancer treatment decisions were options to manage impotence (61%) and the impact of treatment on sexual function (55%). In contrast, questions about survival, cure, recurrence, and spread of prostate cancer were rated as essential to address before making a treatment decision by 80% or more of the sample. Questions about loss of bladder control were rated as essential to address by 74% of the sample.

Other studies suggest that information on sexuality is an unmet need among men diagnosed with prostate cancer. For example, in a study of 500 men diagnosed with localized prostate cancer in the United States, the 3 most frequently endorsed support needs were related to the impact of prostate cancer and its treatment on sexual activity or sexuality (ie, support/counseling on when/how to return to sexual activity, support in dealing with your loss of interest in sex, support in dealing with the cancer's impact on your sex life, support in dealing with feelings of "loss of manhood").[22] In a qualitative study of informational needs among men treated for prostate cancer, Maliski et al[23] similarly found that men were not prepared for sexual side effects such as penile numbness, perineal soreness, and dry ejaculation.

## THE VALUE OF SEXUALITY IN PROSTATE CANCER TREATMENT DECISIONS

Compared with the literature on information needs, a more extensive body of empirical work exists that has examined the relative value of sexual function compared with other preferences that influence the choice of prostate cancer treatment. Conventional measures of preferences yield utilities, numbers that range from 0.0 to 1.0 where a health state of 1 is equivalent to perfect health and those near 0.0 represent states near death. Utilities provide a means to compare preferences across health states (eg, sexual function, urinary function) and people. Most studies that have measured utilities using methods such as the standard gamble (SG), time trade off (TTO), and visual analog scale have found that both sexual functioning and urinary functioning are valued highly. Albertsen et al[24] studied 50 men diagnosed with prostate cancer and, using TTO, found utilities of 0.91 for current health, 0.898 for sexual function, 0.892 for urinary function, and 0.978 for bowel function. Another study of men diagnosed with prostate cancer obtained utilities of 0.91 for current health, 0.95 for sexual function, 0.98 for urinary function, and 0.99 for bowel function.[25] Other findings are similar for men diagnosed with prostate cancer.

In contrast to studies of men diagnosed with prostate cancer, both men who have not been diagnosed with prostate cancer and men diagnosed with prostate cancer and asked to predict utilities for future health states provide markedly lower utilities.[25,26] Utilities of 0.71 for sexual function and 0.62 for urinary function have been found for men seen in primary care clinics with no history of prostate cancer.[26] In a study using SG to elicit utilities in a sample of older men 52% of whom had been previously diagnosed with prostate cancer, impotence (0.89) was evaluated as better than urinary difficulty (0.88), urinary incontinence (0.83), and bowel problems (0.71).[27] Despite the relative important of sexual function in prostate cancer treatment decision, concern about survival and removal of the prostate cancer is an important driving factor in decisions to seek active treatment and this seems to outweigh concerns about sexual function.[28]

Thus, whether or not men are diagnosed with prostate cancer influences how they value sexual functioning compared with other side effects associated with prostate cancer treatment. Studies of which men value what prostate cancer outcomes more highly than others suggest that some predictors influence utilities across all domains, including the domain of sexual function. For example, men diagnosed with prostate cancer who are generally healthy have higher utility for quantity of life as compared with men who are less healthy who value quality of life concerns such as sexual function.[25] In another study, older men, compared with younger, showed a greater concern about maintaining quality of life domains relative to living longer.[15] However, Smith et al[29] have reported that age, race, and comorbid conditions did not predict utilities in their study of 209 men who had surgical treatment for prostate cancer.

While general health seems to be related to utilities for sexual function and other potential side effects associated with prostate cancer treatment, a related question is whether current sexual function influences how sexual function is valued. In a study of predictors of prostate cancer utilities, Saigal et al[25] found little relationship between sexual functioning and the utility of maintaining sexual function. In contrast, other studies have showed a relationship between sexual behavior and utilities for sexual function. Men who reported more frequent sexual activity had lower utilities for living with erectile dysfunction than did those reporting less activity.[15] Similarly, Smith et al found a relationship between sexual function and how men value sexuality. In this study, those with increased urinary and sexual bother and those with only sexual bother were willing to give up more life years to obtain perfect sexual function than those reporting less current burden due to sexual side effects.[29]

Qualitative research, as compared with utilities, provides a more nuanced view of the importance of sexuality in prostate cancer treatment choices. A study of prostate cancer narratives in men who had undergone definitive treatment for prostate cancer identified 4 domains of sexuality—sexual intimacy, interactions with women, sexual fantasy, and perceptions of masculinity—that are profoundly impacted by prostate cancer treatment.[8] These impacts on sexuality are broad and it is not clear that they are well articulated to men during the treatment decision-making process. Rather than guided by careful assessment of the risks of side effects such as sexual dysfunction, another study found that men's preferences relevant to prostate cancer treatment options were based on initial uninformed assumptions and fear about prostate cancer.[6] These fears motivated rapid treatment with post-treatment sexual side effects justified by earlier misunderstandings about treatment benefits and harms. Diefenbach et al reported similar findings in a quantitative study of beliefs and perceptions in 654 men diagnosed with localized prostate cancer. Those seeking surgical treatment were more likely than men selecting radiation therapy to see prostate cancer as serious and as likely to spread.[30]

It should be noted that the studies reviewed for the most part have investigated localized disease. Adjuvant treatment for localized prostate cancer and treatments for locally advanced and advanced disease often involve the addition of hormone therapies. These involve sexual side effects such as reduced sexual interest and desire that have not been evaluated extensively in studies of patient preferences for prostate cancer treatment outcomes. Similarly, little is known about how other hormone therapy side effects such as gynecomastia and hot flashes influence sexual function and how these outcomes are valued in the treatment decision-making trade-offs.

## DECISION AIDS AND SEXUALITY IN PROSTATE CANCER TREATMENT CHOICES

Based on the evidence of unmet educational needs among men making prostate cancer treatment decisions, a variety of decision aids have been developed and disseminated to provide information on prostate cancer, its treatments, treatment outcomes, and the risks and benefits of the options available to manage prostate cancer.[31-34] The standards for the development of decision aids advocate that an assessment of patient values related to treatment outcomes be included in the decision aid, either through a formal preferences assessment or a task used to clarify patient values.[35,36] Several decision aids have been developed for prostate cancer treatment decisions and include information on the impact of prostate cancer treatment on sexuality.[2,18,32,34,37-39]

In a 2004 review of materials used for decision making in early-stage prostate cancer, Fagerlin et al[40] identified 44 sets of patient education materials publicly available in print, video, electronic media, and Web-based formats. These materials include descriptions of the sexual side effects expected to occur with common treatments for prostate cancer. Information on sexual side effects were included in 84% of the materials for radical prostatectomy, 81% for radiation therapy, and 72% for hormone therapy. These rates are similar to that for the inclusion of information on urinary function. Few of the materials distinguished the temporary and permanent sexual side effects (34% for radical prostatectomy, 30% for radiation therapy, and 7% for hormone therapy). None of the materials included ways to help patients understand their preferences or values related to sexual function and other outcomes. Because of the absence of preference assessment and values clarification methods, these investigators concluded that these materials could not be considered as decision aids.

## CONCLUSIONS

The results of studies of the relative value of maintaining sexual function compared with prolonging life and avoiding other side effects are mixed, but several limited conclusions may be drawn from this work. First, sexual function seems to be an important consideration for men making prostate cancer treatment decisions. It is clear that men value maintaining sexual function at levels similar to how they value maintaining urinary function. For many men, survival seems to

be the most highly valued factor influencing prostate cancer treatment decisions. Thus, although sexual problems are important to men in prostate cancer treatment decisions, and sexual difficulties impact the lives of men deeply when they occur, fears about cancer survival, recurrence, and progression can overshadow considerations related to sexuality out of proportion of the actual risk.[41] Inadequate understanding of the risk of sexual problems or a man's lack of insight into the importance of sexual functioning in his life can contribute to poorly informed decisions about prostate cancer treatment.[42] Unfortunately, regret about prostate cancer treatment is not rare and has been related to post-treatment concern about sexual function.[4,43] Second, despite inconsistencies in findings on the predictors of utilities for sexual function, several findings stand out including the influence of general health and current sexual function on how important men feel it is to maintain sexual function after prostate cancer treatment. Men in good general health and those experiencing increased sexual bother due to prostate cancer treatment place a higher value on maintaining sexual function.

It is important to note that a limitation of studies of patient preferences is the incomplete conceptualization of sexuality as a value. For many persons, sexuality is a highly personal and nuanced experience. As a biopsychosocial construct, sexuality is complex and multifaceted. It encompasses a variety of constructs including, but not limited to, self-concepts, attitudes, preferences, desires, behaviors, activities, relationships, and functions. In contrast to the construct of sexuality, most measures of patient preferences for sexual function are one-dimensional and therefore limited in their ability to assess preferences. A related measurement issue is that most utilities elicitation approaches ask about impotence, erectile function, or sexual function. Treatments can be disruptive to a variety of sexual functions (eg, erectile, ejaculatory), to sexual desire and interest, and to sexual relationships. It is difficult to know what research participants are thinking about when they answer questions about trade-offs concerning sexual function. Like measures of preferences for sexual function, existing decision aids are limited in terms of the presentation of sexual side effects. Some content is covered by most educational programs, but this does not distinguish among the variations of sexual experience that are impacted by prostate cancer treatment. Qualitative studies suggest that consideration of sexuality as a complex construct may provide important insights about how men's concerns about sexuality influence the choices that are made in prostate cancer treatment. Decision aids have yet to incorporate the more nuanced information on sexuality suggested by studies of men's narratives.

In conclusion, for many men, next to survival, sexuality is one of the most important considerations in prostate cancer treatment decision making. It is clear that men value sexuality as highly as urinary control, and these concerns are more important than many other side effects and treatment characteristics that influence the final choice of management strategy. However, there are unmet needs for information about sexuality among men diagnosed with prostate cancer, and this is particularly concerning because of the potential for regret about the decision. Additional research is needed to better understand how to educate men about prostate cancer and its treatments, so that men are able to make informed decisions that fully incorporate their values about sexuality as a multidimensional experience.

## ACKNOWLEDGMENTS

*S.J.K. is supported by a Veterans Administration (VA) Health Services Research and Development award (IIR02-142-1) and her work on this article was supported by the resources and facilities of the interdisciplinary Program to Improve Care for Veterans with Complex Comorbid Conditions at the San Francisco VA Medical Center.*

*This material is partly the result of work supported with re-sources and the use of facilities at the Health Services Research & Development Center of Excellence (HFP90-020), Michael E. De-Bakey Veterans Affairs Medical Center. D.M.L. is supported by Mentored Research Scholar Grant 06-083-01-CPPB from the American Cancer Society.*

*The contents of this work are solely the responsibility of the author and do not necessarily represent the official views of the Department of Veterans Affairs.*

## REFERENCES

1. Cox J, Amling CL. Current decision-making in prostate cancer therapy. *Curr Opin Urol.* 2008;18:275–278.
2. Wei JT, Uzzo RG. Shared decision-making strategies for early prostate cancer. *Semin Urol Oncol.* 2002;20:74–78.
3. Chen RC, Clark JA, Manola J, et al. Treatment 'mismatch' in early prostate cancer: do treatment choices take patient quality of life into account? *Cancer.* 2008;112:61–68.
4. Clark JA, Inui TS, Silliman RA, et al. Patients' perceptions of quality of life after treatment for early prostate cancer. *J Clin Oncol.* 2003;21:3777–3784.
5. Dale W, Bilir P, Han M, et al. The role of anxiety in prostate carcinoma: a structured review of the literature. *Cancer.* 2005;104:467–478.
6. Denberg TD, Melhado TV, Steiner JF. Patient treatment preferences in localized prostate carcinoma: the influence of emotion, misconception, and anecdote. *Cancer.* 2006;107:620–630.
7. Latini DM, Hart SL, Knight SJ, et al. The relationship between anxiety and time to treatment for patients with prostate cancer on surveillance. *J Urol.* 2007;178(3 Pt 1):826–831; discussion 831–822.
8. Bokhour BG, Clark JA, Inui TS, et al. Sexuality after treatment for early prostate cancer: exploring the meanings of "erectile dysfunction." *J Gen Intern Med.* 2001;16:649–655.
9. Penson RT, Gallagher J, Gioiella ME, et al. Sexuality and cancer: conversation comfort zone. *Oncologist.* 2000;5:336–344.
10. Davison BJ, Goldenberg SL. Decisional regret and quality of life after participating in medical decision-making for early-stage prostate cancer. *BJU Int.* 2003;91:14–17.
11. Davison BJ, Parker PA, Goldenberg SL. Patients' preferences for communicating a prostate cancer diagnosis and participating in medical decision-making. *BJU Int.* 2004;93:47–51.
12. Kattan MW, Cowen ME, Miles BJ. A decision analysis for treatment of clinically localized prostate cancer. *J Gen Intern Med.* 1997;12:299–305.
13. Lubeck DP, Grossfeld GD, Carroll PR. A review of measurement of patient preferences for treatment outcomes after prostate cancer. *Urology.* 2002;60(3 Suppl 1):72–77; discussion 77–78.
14. Crawford ED, Bennett CL, Stone NN, et al. Comparison of perspectives on prostate cancer: analyses of survey data. *Urology.* 1997;50:366–372.
15. Sommers BD, Beard CJ, D'Amico AV, et al. Predictors of patient preferences and treatment choices for localized prostate cancer. *Cancer.* 2008;113:2058–2067.
16. Elstein AS, Chapman GB, Chmiel JS, et al. Agreement between prostate cancer patients and their clinicians about utilities and attribute importance. *Health Expect.* 2004;7:115–125.
17. Elstein AS, Chapman GB, Knight SJ. Patients' values and clinical substituted judgments: the case of localized prostate cancer. *Health Psychol.* 2005;24(4 Suppl):S85–S92.
18. Knight SJ, Nathan DP, Siston AK, et al. Pilot study of a utilities-based treatment decision intervention for prostate cancer patients. *Clin Prostate Cancer.* 2002;1:105–114.
19. Knight SJ, Siston AK, Chmiel JS, et al. Ethnic variation in localized prostate cancer: a pilot study of preferences, optimism, and quality of life among black and white veterans. *Clin Prostate Cancer.* 2004;3:31–37.
20. Carvalhal GF, Smith DS, Ramos C, et al. Correlates of dissatisfaction with treatment in patients with prostate cancer diagnosed through screening. *J Urol.* 1999;162:113–118.
21. Feldman-Stewart D, Brundage MD, Hayter C, et al. What questions do patients with curable prostate cancer want answered? *Med Decis Making.* 2000;20:7–19.
22. Boberg EW, Gustafson DH, Hawkins RP, et al. Assessing the unmet information, support and care delivery needs of men with prostate cancer. *Patient Educ Couns.* 2003;49:233–242.
23. Maliski SL, Connor S, Fink A, et al. Information desired and acquired by men with prostate cancer: data from ethnic focus groups. *Health Educ Behav.* 2006;33:393–409.
24. Albertsen PC, Nease RF Jr, Potosky AL. Assessment of patient preferences among men with prostate cancer. *J Urol.* 1998;159:158–163.
25. Saigal CS, Gornbein J, Nease R, et al. Predictors of utilities for health states in early stage prostate cancer. *J Urol.* 2001;166:942–946.
26. Cowen ME, Miles BJ, Cahill DF, et al. The danger of applying group-level utilities in decision analyses of the treatment of localized prostate cancer in individual patients. *Med Decis Making.* 1998;18:376–380.
27. Stewart ST, Lenert L, Bhatnagar V, et al. Utilities for prostate cancer health states in men aged 60 and older. *Med Care.* 2005;43:347–355.
28. Mazur DJ, Hickam DH. Patient preferences for management of localized prostate cancer. *West J Med.* 1996;165:26–30.
29. Smith DS, Krygiel J, Nease RF Jr, et al. Patient preferences for outcomes associated with surgical management of prostate cancer. *J Urol.* 2002;167:2117–2122.
30. Diefenbach MA, Dorsey J, Uzzo RG, et al. Decision-making strategies for patients with localized prostate cancer. *Semin Urol Oncol.* 2002;20:55–62.
31. Barry MJ. Health decision aids to facilitate shared decision making in office practice. *Ann Intern Med.* 2002;136:127–135.
32. Feldman-Stewart D, Brundage MD, Van Manen L. A decision aid for men with early stage prostate cancer: theoretical basis and a test by surrogate patients. *Health Expect.* 2001;4:221–234.
33. Myers RE, Kunkel EJ. Preparatory education for informed decision-making in prostate cancer early detection and treatment. *Semin Urol Oncol.* 2000;18:172–177.
34. Gomella LG, Albertsen PC, Benson MC, et al. The use of video-based patient education for shared decision-making in the treatment of prostate cancer. *Semin Urol Oncol.* 2000;18:182–187.
35. Holmes-Rovner M, Nelson WL, Pignone M, et al. Are patient decision aids the best way to improve clinical decision making? Report of the IPDAS Symposium. *Med Decis Making.* 2007;27:599–608.
36. O'Connor AM, Bennett C, Stacey D, et al. Do patient decision aids meet effectiveness criteria of the international patient decision aid standards collaboration? A systematic review and meta-analysis. *Med Decis Making.* 2007;27:554–574.
37. Diefenbach MA, Butz BP. A multimedia interactive education system for prostate cancer patients: development and preliminary evaluation. *J Med Internet Res.* 2004;6:e3.
38. Kim SP, Knight SJ, Tomori C, et al. Health literacy and shared decision making for prostate cancer patients with low socioeconomic status. *Cancer Invest.* 2001;19:684–691.
39. McGregor S. Information on video format can help patients with localised prostate cancer to be partners in decision making. *Patient Educ Couns.* 2003;49:279–283.
40. Fagerlin A, Rovner D, Stableford S, et al. Patient education materials about the treatment of early-stage prostate cancer: a critical review. *Ann Intern Med.* 2004;140:721–728.
41. Fagerlin A, Zikmund-Fisher BJ, Ubel PA. Cure me even if it kills me: preferences for invasive cancer treatment. *Med Decis Making.* 2005;25:614–619.
42. Fagerlin A, Ubel PA, Smith DM, et al. Making numbers matter: present and future research in risk communication. *Am J Health Behav.* 2007;31(Suppl 1):S47–S56.
43. Diefenbach MA, Mohamed NE. Regret of treatment decision and its association with disease-specific quality of life following prostate cancer treatment. *Cancer Invest.* 2007;25:449–457.

# Interventions for Sexuality After Pelvic Radiation Therapy and Gynecological Cancer

Anne Katz

## INTERVENTIONS FOR SEXUALITY AFTER PELVIC RADIATION THERAPY AND GYNECOLOGICAL CANCER

Gynecologic cancer affects almost 78,000 women each year in the United States. Because this cancer affects the organs intimately involved in sexual functioning, treatments for this cancer almost always affect one or more stages of the female sexual response cycle.[1]

## EFFECT OF GYNECOLOGIC CANCER ON SEXUALITY

The diagnosis of any kind of cancer can have a deleterious effect on sexual functioning. After a cancer diagnosis, women may experience alterations in how they see themselves as sexual beings, their body image, and their role in their intimate relationship.[1] Changes in body image are a central aspect of the cancer experience for women and may have long lasting effects. The loss of reproductive potential resulting from treatment of these cancers can also impact on how women view themselves.[2]

Gynecologic cancer may be treated with surgery, radiation, chemotherapy, or some combination of the three. Any and all of these treatments may result in genital and pelvic pain, loss of sensation and sensitivity of sexual tissue, decrease in sexual desire, shortening and stenosis of the vagina and atrophic vaginitis.[3] These may be due to anatomic changes and/or loss of ovarian hormones. Overlying all of this is the experience of fatigue, a common side effect of radiation therapy.[4]

## CERVICAL CANCER

Radiation therapy may be used to treat cervical cancer and has far reaching effects on sexual functioning. Radiation causes changes in the blood vessels in the walls of the vagina leading to fibrosis.[5] In fact, the vaginal epithelium may be completely destroyed during the active phase of treatment.[6] Changes to the walls of the vagina may reduce the length of the vagina, resulting in pain with penetration. Loss of epithelial tissues results in lack of lubrication, which compounds this. Collateral radiation damage to the ovaries leads to estrogen deficiency, which in turn leads to further thinning of the vaginal walls.[7] Women have reported extreme sensitivity to touch at the vaginal introitus, friable tissues, and a burning sensation when the vagina was exposed to semen during intercourse.[8]

The bladder and bowel may be exposed to some radiation scatter and this can also affect sexual functioning.[9] Cystitis and rectal pain or diarrhea interferes with sexual desire and pain with penetration may be felt in both the rectum and urethra. Women with cervical cancer state that their sexual functioning is altered and while some improvement may be seen over time, they never go back to pretreatment levels of sexual activity or satisfaction.[10] These women also report feeling sexually unattractive, experience pain with intercourse,

and are fearful that sexual activity may cause a recurrence of their disease[11] or local spread.[12]

Many women report a general dissatisfaction with their sex lives after this treatment and distress about the changes that they have to deal with. Radiation causes vaginal atrophy and a resultant loss of lubrication, which in turn leads to dyspareunia. Women report that the vagina feels smaller and less elastic and does not react normally to sexual stimulation.[13] These problems may persist for 5 to 10 years after treatment[14] and ultimately affect the way the woman views herself as a sexual being.[15] Some women may choose not to resume sexual activity after treatment or may avoid it because of pain or lack of interest; this has the potential to cause problems in their intimate relationship.[16]

Women describe the numerous diagnostic and treatment-related examinations as invasive. For women with a history of sexual abuse, this may reactivate latent psychologic trauma.[13]

## OVARIAN CANCER

Ovarian cancer is often diagnosed when the disease has progressed and usually requires aggressive multimodal treatment with poor outcomes. Most of the research on gynecologic cancer and sexuality has not separated participants with ovarian cancer from the sample and so little is known about the effects of this cancer and its treatments on sexuality. The seriousness of the disease and the late diagnosis may lead to the assumption that sexuality is not an issue for women with ovarian cancer.

But treatment for this cancer usually involves removal of the ovaries, which immediately causes menopausal symptoms that can be very severe. This is of particular significance for the younger pre-menopausal woman. Typical symptoms include hot flashes, vagina atrophy, fatigue, irritability, and increased incidence of urinary tract infections.[17] Debulking of any visible tumor during surgery, sampling of lymph nodes and omentum[18] contributes to internal scar tissue development, which may interfere with the anatomy of the pelvis and cause pain. For those women who are diagnosed early, an unaffected ovary may be spared, which will alleviate or reduce some of the symptoms.[19]

Most women will require chemotherapy after surgery and the side effects of this further impacts on well being and energy levels.[18] Fatigue may persist well after completion of treatment and is associated with anxiety, depression, and overall lower quality of life; the impact on sexuality is obvious.[20] The loss of body hair, which often accompanies chemotherapy has a profound effect on body image.[21] Women may not expect to lose their pubic hair too, and this can have a significant effect on sexual self-image. Women with ovarian cancer report that they are distressed by feelings of inadequacy in their roles as wife, mother, and sexual partner.[22] Others are afraid that lack of sexual activity after treatment may cause problems in their relationship.[23]

The life-threatening aspects of this cancer impact on psychologic and emotional well being. But this does not mean that women are concerned about quality of life, including sexuality. Younger women are reported to be concerned about sexual issues and are afraid that they will be sexually unattractive after treatment.[24] The woman who has been treated for this cancer will have scars from surgery, may have lost weight during chemotherapy; all these impact on body image. It is not uncommon for women to avoid appearing naked in front of a partner; this can lead to distancing between them.

## Cancer of the Vulva or Vagina

Although primary cancer of the vagina is rare and cancer of the vagina is usually metastatic from the cervix or endometrium, these cancers have profound effects on sexuality. Even though cancer of the vulva is also rare and mostly effects women older than 60 years of age, the sexual effects of this cancer also impacts sexuality.[25] In the past, radical surgery was performed that profoundly affects sexual functioning and sexual and body image.[26] Surgery usually causes lack of interest in sex resulting in less frequent sexual activity, pain in the genital area, and changes to body image.[27] More recently, tissue sparing surgery is performed, especially for early-stage cancers of the vagina and vulva.[28]

## INTERVENTIONS IN THE CARE OF WOMEN WITH GYNECOLOGIC CANCER

There are a limited number of interventions for the woman who has been treated for gynecologic cancer with radiation. These focus on the provision of information and some specific suggestions related to treating vaginal dryness, the need for vaginal dilatation after radiation therapy, and management of fatigue.

As with any cancer, an important intervention should always be the provision of information about the treatments and any and all side effects that may occur. Informing the woman about sexual side effects is something that traditionally has not been done well. It is important to assess what the woman needs and wants to know as well as her knowledge and attitudes about sexuality and sexual functioning. Healthcare providers often assume that women have a clear understanding of how the body works and what the different parts do; this in not always the case.[29]

## Information Sharing

In the crisis of diagnosis, many women are not able to fully understand the vast amounts of information that they are given. This should be an ongoing process with numerous opportunities for the healthcare provider to give information and for the patients to ask questions. Many women say that sexuality is not important in the early days after the diagnosis and treatment. The partner may have an entirely different opinion about this, and the woman may change her mind as time goes by. Offering opportunities to talk about this important quality of life issue, even if refused, shows the patient and partner that this is regarded as important by the healthcare provider and that he/she is willing to talk about it. Many people subscribe to myths about cancer itself and especially sexuality; 2 common myths are that sexual activity caused the cancer or that sexual activity can spread the cancer to the partner. The healthcare provider is an important source of accurate information that can reduce anxiety for both the patient and her partner.

## Interventions for Treatment-Related Side Effects

Women are often bothered by vaginal atrophy after radiation therapy. This will cause pain on any kind of sexual touching, even without penetration. A reflex cycle of muscle tension in anticipation of the pain results and is called vaginismus. The woman contracts the pubococcygeal muscle in anticipation of the pain and this narrows the opening to the vagina. It is notoriously difficult to treat and often precludes pelvic examinations so prevention of this is of utmost importance. Treatment of vaginismus usually requires a multimodal approach with pharmacotherapy and sex therapy and may take years to treat but some women do return to satisfying sexual activity.[30]

The most effective treatment for vaginal atrophy is local estrogen in the form of a cream (Premarin), pessary (vagifem), or ring (Estring). There is little systemic absorption with this form of estrogen, but some oncologists or women themselves may want to avoid any exposure to estrogen.

If the woman is experiencing itching and burning of vulval and vaginal tissue outside of sexual activity, a vaginal moisturizer such as Replens may help. This is a polycarbophil that carries up to 60 times its weight in water and restores moisture levels in the vaginal walls.

If the women is desirous of sexual activity and complains of lack of lubrication, a lubricant should be suggested. There are a number of these on the market and are essentially of 2 kinds: water-based or silicone based. Oil-based lubricants are not recommended. Water-based lubricants (KY jelly) are the easiest to find as they are usually available in drug stores and supermarkets. They tend to dry out quite quickly and need to be reapplied or reactivated with the addition of some water. One water-based lubricant is called Astroglide and it has the ability to remain slick for an extended period of time. Many of these water-based lubricants contain glycerine and may predispcose some women to vaginal yeast infections. Silicone-based lubricants are available on line or in sex stores. These lubricants are not absorbed into the tissues and sit on top of the skin or mucus membranes, remaining slick for a long time. Any excess needs to be removed with soap and water. Women should avoid anything that has perfume or dyes and should never use anything that has a caution about avoiding the eyes; if a substance cannot go into the eyes it should not go near the vagina!

## Vaginal Dilatation

To maintain the patency of the vagina, women are recommended to perform regular vaginal dilatation. There is little consensus on when to begin dilatation, how often it should be performed, and for how long.[31] But the general recommendation is to start as soon as it is comfortable but within 4 weeks of completion of radiation therapy. There are a number of dilators available from medical supply stores and many institutions provide their patients with dilators that have been manufactured in-house by the engineering department. These tend to be made of stainless steel or a hard plastic and may not be all that comfortable to use. An alternative is silicone dilators that are available in a variety of sizes (and colors) from Soul Source Enterprises (http://soulsourceenterprises.com). The woman should start with a small dilator (0.5–1 in) and progress to a dilator with a maximum diameter of 1.5 in. Women should use the dilators at least 3 times a week. The dilator should be inserted into the vagina and moved side ways and in and out for about 10 to 15 minutes per session. This should continue for at least 3 years and possibly for ever.[31] Using a lubricant will ease insertion and many women use an estrogen cream for this purpose; it acts as a lubricant for insertion and has the added benefit of treating vaginal atrophy. Penetrative intercourse at least 3 times a week may be substituted for this. It is doubtful that women would be interested in intercourse during or shortly after treatment but this may be preferable in the long term.

It is important for the value of this intervention to be repeated with each interaction with the patients. Research has shown that an intervention that includes education, motivation, and behavioral skills was more effective in promoting and sustaining the use of dilators than written material.[32]

## Management of Fatigue

Fatigue is an extremely common experience for patients undergoing radiation therapy for any kind. This affects general quality of life and sexuality. The fatigue experienced as a result of radiation therapy affects libido. Fatigue as a result of radiation therapy is often cumulative and usually appears a few weeks into treatment; it may persist for weeks or months after completion of treatment.[33]

## CONCLUSION

Gynecologic cancer and its treatments can have a profound effect on sexual functioning in all phases of the sexual response cycle as well as on body image and sexual self-concept. A diagnosis of cancer and the associated distress may have a profound effect on the emotional status of both the woman and her partner. This psychologic impact combined with the physical sensations of the disease itself and treatment side effects may lower both interest in sex and frequency of sexual activity.

## REFERENCES

1. Lagana L, McGarvey E, Classen C, et al. Psychosexual dysfunction among gynecological cancer survivors. *J Clin Psychol Med.* 2001;8:73–84.
2. Wilmoth MC, Spinelli A. Sexual implications of gynecologic cancer treatments. *J Obstet Gynecol Neonatal Nurs.* 2000;29:413–421.
3. Weijmar Schultz W, van de Wiel H. Sexuality, intimacy, and gynecological cancer. *J Sex Marital Ther.* 2003;29:121–128.
4. de Groot JM, Mah K, Fyles A, et al. The psychosocial impact of cervical cancer among affected women and their partners. *Int J Gynecol Cancer.* 2005;15:918–925.
5. Katz A, Njuguna E, Rakowsky E, et al. Early development of vaginal shortening during radiation therapy for endometrial or cervical cancer. *Int J Gynaecol Cancer.* 2001;11:234–235.
6. Pras E, Wouda J, Willemse P, et al. Pilot study of vaginal plethysmography in women treated with radiotherapy for gynecological cancer. *Gynecol Oncol.* 2003;91:540–546.
7. Lamb M. Questions women ask about gynecologic cancer and sexual functioning. *Develop Support Cancer Care.* 1998;1:11–13.
8. Jenkins B. Sexual healing after pelvic irradiation. *Am J Nurs.* 1986;86:920–922.
9. Burke L. Sexual dysfunction following radiotherapy for cervical cancer. *Br J Nurs.* 1996;5:239–244.
10. Andersen B, Anderson B, deProsse C. Controlled prospective longitudinal study of women with cancer. I. Sexual functioning outcomes. *J Consult Clin Psychol.* 1989;6:683–691.
11. Cull A, Cowie V, Farquharson D, et al. Early stage cervical cancer: psychosocial and sexual outcomes of treatment. *Br J Cancer.* 1996;68:1216–1220.
12. Kritcharoen S, Suwan K, Jirojwong S. Perceptins of gender roles, gender power relationships, and sexuality in Thai women following diagnosis and treatment for cervical cancer. *Oncol Nurs Forum.* 2005;32:682–688.
13. Bergmark K, vall-Lundqvist E, Dickman PW, et al. Synergy between sexual abuse and cervical cancer in causing sexual dysfunction. *J Sex Marital Ther.* 2005;31:361–383.
14. Wenzel L, DeAlba I, Habbal R, et al. Quality of life in long-term cervical cancer survivors. *Gynecol Oncol.* 2005;97:310–317.
15. Bukovic D, Strinic T, Habek M, et al. Sexual life after cervical carcinoma. *Coll Antropol.* 2003;27:173–180.
16. Corney R, Crowther M, Everett H, et al. Psychosexual dysfunction in women with gynaecological cancer following radical pelvic surgery. *Br J Obstet Gynaecol.* 1993;100:73–78.
17. Carmack Taylor CL, Basen-Engquist K, Shinn EH, et al. Predictors of sexual functioning in ovarian cancer patients. *J Clin Oncol.* 2004;22:881–889.
18. Mannix J, Jackson D, Raftos M. Ovarian cancer: an update for nursing practice. *Int J Nurs Pract.* 1999;5:47–50.
19. Fitch MI, Turner F. Ovarian cancer. *Can Nurse.* 2006;102:17–20.
20. Holzner B, Kemmler G, Meraner V, et al. Fatigue in ovarian carcinoma patients: a neglected issue? *Cancer.* 2003;97:1564–1572.
21. Fitch MI. Psychosocial management of patients with recurrent ovarian cancer: treating the whole patient to improve quality of life. *Semin Oncol Nurs.* 2003;19:40–53.
22. Lammers SE, Schaefer KM, Ladd EC, et al. Caring for women living with ovarian cancer: recommendations for advanced practice nurses. *J Obstet Gynecol Neonatal Nurs.* 2000;29:567–573.
23. Sun CC, Bodurka DC, Weaver CB, et al. Rankings and symptom assessments of side effects from chemotherapy: insights from experienced patients with ovarian cancer. *Support Care Cancer.* 2005;13:219–227.
24. Stewart D, Wong FW, Duff S, et al. "What doesn't kill you makes you stronger": an ovarian cancer survivor survey. *Gynecol Oncol.* 2001;83:537–542.
25. Goodman A. Primary vaginal cancer. *Surg Oncol Clin N Am.* 1998;7:347–361.
26. Carter J, Auchincloss S, Sonoda Y, et al. Cervical cancer: issues of sexuality and fertility. *Oncology (Williston Park).* 2003;17:1229–1234.
27. Green M, Naumann W, Elliot M, et al. Sexual dysfunction following vulvectomy. *Gynecol Oncol.* 2000;77:73–77.
28. Gotlieb W. The assessment and surgical management of early-stage vulvar cancer. *Best Pract Res Clin Obstet Gynecol.* 2003;17:557–569.
29. Juraskova I, Butow P, Robertson R, et al. Post-treatment sexual adjustment following cervical and endometrial cancer: a qualitative insight. *Psychooncology.* 2003;12:267–279.
30. Amsterdam A, Krychman M. Sexual dysfunction in patients with gynecologic neoplasms: a retrospective pilot study. *J Sex Med.* 2006;3:646–649.
31. Lancaster L. Preventing vaginal stenosis after brachytherapy for gynaecological cancer: an overview of Australian practices. *Eur J Oncol Nurs.* 2004;8:30–39.
32. Robinson JW, Faris PD, Scott CB. Psychoeducational group increases vaginal dilation for younger women and reduces sexual fears for women of all ages with gynecological carcinoma treated with radiotherapy. *Int J Radiat Oncol Biol Phys.* 1999;44:497–506.
33. Maher KE. Radiation therapy: toxicities and management. In: Yarbo C, Frogge C, Goodman M, et al., eds. *Cancer Nursing: Principles and Practice.* 5th ed. Boston, MA: Jones and Bartlett Publishers; 2000:323–351.

# A Review of Couple-Based Interventions for Enhancing Women's Sexual Adjustment and Body Image After Cancer

Jennifer L. Scott • Karen Kayser

"Being deeply loved by someone gives you strength while loving someone deeply gives you courage." Lao Tzu

In response to reminders of our mortality, a very strong human instinct is to seek affiliation with loved ones, to combat feelings of anxiety by seeking solace and courage in our intimate attachments.[1] People often express their needs for attachment through a heightened desire for physical and/or sexual intimacy with their romantic partner and in emotional commitment to this relationship.[2] Physical comfort, even barely discernable acts of support from someone close to us might also have biologic relevance for our adaptation to stressful situations.[3] Functional magnetic resonance imaging research with women has shown that even the simple act of holding hands with their partner when they face a threatening situation reduces the neural activity that underpins emotional and behavioral responses characteristic of the stress response.[3]

Conditions involving corporeal danger also heighten people's body awareness, leading to greater scrutiny of their body and appearance. Their physical body takes on greater significance, with their bodies serving as markers of vitality, and of their existence in the world; the body symbolically representing the self.[3,4] Increases in the desire for closeness with loved ones, and body consciousness occur even in situations when the danger is only an imagined life-threatening scenario.[5] Fundamentally, our close relationships and our sense of self, serve as psychologic protections against anxiety about death,[1,2] they are important potential sources of coping.

It is understandable then, that in the face of the very real threat that cancers pose to women's lives, many women report a heightened need for emotional and physical closeness with their spouse.[6,7] For some couples, sexual intimacy is also an important way of coping. It can reaffirm life and vitality and bring a reassuring sense of normalcy in their lives at a time when many other things may seem "unreal."[8] However, physical intimacy and women's body image are highly vulnerable to disruption after cancer diagnosis and treatments.[9] High rates of sexual dysfunction are common[10] and treatments can impair women's sense of femininity and body image, particularly with breast and gynecologic cancers. Difficulties often arise in the first year after treatment, and women's sexual well-being can remain impaired even if disturbance to mood and disruption to routines and roles have resolved.[9,11]

## INTERVENTIONS TO ENHANCE WOMEN'S BODY IMAGE AND SEXUAL FUNCTIONING

Consequently, psycho-oncology interventions that hope to help women adjust fully to their cancer experiences should aim to improve their recovery of sexual functioning and body image because these aspects of their life are most at risk for impairment after cancer.

Furthermore, if problems in these areas of functioning are left untreated, they may undermine women's psychosocial recovery more broadly, via their impact on women's coping.[12] Disruptions to women's sense of self or wholeness, and feelings of closeness and connectedness with partners and loved ones, can impede their coping self-regulation and ability to derive benefit from social support.[13]

We conducted a literature review to ascertain the extent and effectiveness of interventions that have attempted to address women's recovery of their sexual well being and body image after cancer. Multiple search strategies were used to maximize the probability of locating as many relevant articles as possible. First, the computerized databases, Medline, Psyclit, Science Direct, Proquest, Ovid, Scopus, Healthplan, and PubMed, were searched, using the search terms cancer, neoplasm, oncology and psychologic therapy, psychotherapy, counseling, sexual counseling/therapy, group support, peer groups, relaxation, imagery, coping skills training, cognitive therapy or psychosocial support, body-image concerns, sexual adjustment/difficulties/functioning problems, and intimacy problems. Second, the references from relevant articles located through database searchers were examined for additional potential articles. Third, references were identified through citations from meta-analytic and review articles and relevant book chapters.[14-28]

The review excluded studies that primarily aimed to increase women's knowledge of disease or treatments, improve compliance or adjustment to medical treatments, manage physical symptoms such as pain, or enhance immune function and prolong survival. Interventions that exclusively focused on improving general cancer coping and/or mood were also excluded. Although such interventions may indirectly improve aspects of women's sexual functioning and/or body image, this review focuses instead on studies that have purposively investigated the impact of intervention on women's sexual adjustment and/or body image.

The review includes trials that randomly assign participants to conditions, and compare one or more psychologic intervention conditions with a control condition. Quasi-experimental nonequivalent control group studies that assign participants to only one condition at a time are also included, provided the studies involved at least preintervention and postintervention assessments, and that all participants were drawn from the same recruitment setting. Such quasi-experimental studies have higher interpretability than posttest-only designs because comparability between conditions before intervention can be examined. On the basis of these criteria, 2 often-cited studies,[29,30] both concerning female patients with cancer, are also excluded from the review. These studies, involving 97 women diagnosed with gynecologic cancers[30] and 200 women diagnosed with breast cancer,[29] did assess the effect of intervention on sexual or body image adjustment. However, in both studies preintervention data were not collected from control group participants.[23,31]

Furthermore, 7 couple-focused studies (all involving women with breast cancer)[32-37] and one study[38] that included women with mixed cancer diagnoses and their nominated significant-other were also excluded. Although these studies used either randomized or wait-list control condition designs, the studies either did not include intervention components that aimed to enhance women's sexual or body image adjustment,[32,33,34-39] or did not measure the impact of intervention on body image and/or sexual functioning as discrete indices, separate from other quality of life domains.[34,40]

The interventions included in this review are reported in Table 1. There have been 12 studies that evaluated the efficacy of psychologic interventions for enhancing psychosexual adjustment in female patients with cancer. Eight studies are randomized control trials.[41-48] Two studies report findings from pilot randomized control trials,[49,50] and another 2 studies involve quasi-experimental designs.[51,52]

## Patient Sample

Women with breast cancers have been the exclusive focus of 7 studies,[41,43,45,47,49-51] and have been included in 2 other studies[44,52] that involved samples with heterogeneous cancer diagnoses. One intervention was developed specifically for women with either breast or gynecologic cancers.[48] Despite the high prevalence of sexual functioning difficulties in women with gynecologic cancers,[53] only one study has focused exclusively on this diagnostic group.[42]

Beyond breast and gynecologic cancers, women with other types of cancers have not been the focus of interventions to promote psychosexual recovery. One trial[46] did include a small number of patients diagnosed with other cancers,[35] though their sex was not reported. There are commonalities across cancer diagnoses in some aspects of women's reactions to their cancer experience, particularly their levels of reported body image concerns.[8,54] Thus, some of the results reported in this review may generalize somewhat to women with cancers other than breast and gynecologic cancers.

Almost half the studies included in Table 1 do not specify patients' staging classifications, particularly the pioneering studies conducted during the 1980s.[42,44,50-52] These studies tended to report broad descriptions of disease status, such as "nonmetastatic," "local," or "curative," or patients' estimated survivorship duration, such as "survival expectancy greater than one year." Most of the other studies involved women with stage I or II disease, although women with advanced stage disease comprised a small proportion (<10%) of participants in one study,[44] and approximately half of the sample in another study.[46]

One trial[46] involved selected or targeted intervention meaning therapy was provided only to patients identified as experiencing elevated levels of distress or psychologic morbidity. The authors[46] operationalized psychologic morbidity as elevated levels of depression, anxiety, or avoidant coping, or any combination of these difficulties.

In terms of when in the trajectory of women's disease experience interventions are delivered, most studies describe recruiting "newly diagnosed patients." However, with several studies it is difficult to ascertain precisely when interventions were delivered. Some researchers do not report time since diagnosis[45,49,51,52] and others report only duration since completion of cancer treatments such as mastectomy[43,50] or unspecified treatment(s).[44] It seems that most interventions are delivered to women when they are some months into their cancer journey, with the exception of 2 studies[47,48] that provided therapy very close to the time of diagnosis (<2 weeks postdiagnosis) and before women commencing any cancer treatment(s).

## Types of Interventions Investigated

Interventions have usually been delivered to women individually[42,51,52] or in peer-group formats.[41-44] In this type of interventions, the aim is to enhance women's adjustment, and support is derived either from peers and/or from health professionals who deliver the therapy.

Two studies delivered the intervention to women individually, but also offered them the option that their partners could participate if they so desired.[45,46] The partners' role was to serve as a "coach," helping women with their acquisition of therapy skills. These partner-assistant type studies[55] do not involve a focus on enhancing partners' mood, coping, or support skills. These studies did not specify the number of sessions male partners attended, and did not collect outcome data related to males' adjustment.

In contrast to therapies where partners' presence is optional, there have been 4 couple-based studies.[47-50] These interventions take a couple-level approach,[55,56] which involves conjoint therapy session with the woman and her partner, and actively includes both partners in sessions. The focus of therapy is to enhance both partners' adjustment, and their relationship, in the context of their cancer experience. The 4 couple-based trials all delivered therapy to individual couples, not in group formats.

There have been 3 studies that have involved treatment comparison designs. Two studies compared the efficacy of different types of interventions, or modes for therapy delivery, for enhancing women's psychosexual functioning. Cain et al[42] compared peer-group to patient-only formats for delivery of an educational and emotional support intervention. Helgeson et al[43] compared the efficacy of educational with emotion-support interventions. Finally Scott et al compared couple-based therapy to patient-only therapy for the delivery of coping training intervention.

Most interventions have involved therapy sessions ranging from 1 to 2 hours in length, though 3 studies did not specify session length.[47,50,51] Intervention programs have usually been brief in duration with over half of the interventions in Table 1 described as 8 weeks or less in duration. Two studies did not specify therapy duration.[41,51] Two interventions were markedly longer in therapy length (6 months),[48,52] although in the Scott et al[48] intervention (CanCOPE) most therapy components were delivered in 5 sessions over an 8-week period. A brief (30 minutes) telephone call was made at 3-month follow-up, and one face-to-face booster session was held 6 months postintervention, to review progress and problem solving difficulties.

The majority of interventions have been multifaceted. Common across all studies was some form of components, which taught women about their disease and treatments. This was often combined with some form of emotional support enhancement whereby therapists encouraged women to express their feelings, with discussion and normalization of their reactions.

In contrast to these approaches, the focus of emotional support components in the 4 couple-based interventions,[47-50] was to enhance the quality of mutual support partners provided each other. As such, these interventions all included communication skills training, to varying degrees, as the conduit or foundation for promoting effective partner support.

Several studies in Table 1 also included a coping skills training component, which ranged in complexity from merely providing training in a relaxation exercise[44,52] to teaching them skills in cognitive[41] and/or behavioral coping (CBT),[46] or problem solving.[45] Only 2 of couple-based interventions included coping training components. Although both studies aimed to promote coping at the couple-level, to

**TABLE 1.** Summary of Control-Trial Evaluations of Interventions to Improve Body Image and/or Sexual Adjustment in Women's Cancers

| Study | N, Diag, stage | N, Cond. | INT Timing (F/up End Point) | Sessions Frequency, No., Length (Duration) | Treatment Format Components | Coping (ES) | Mood (ES) | Body Image (ES) | Partner Related Body Image (ES) | Sexual Adjust (ES) | Relationships (ES) |
|---|---|---|---|---|---|---|---|---|---|---|---|
| **Randomized - patient only interventions** | | | | | | | | | | | |
| Berglund et al[44] | 199, 80 Br, mixed | 1 SC, 1 INT | 2-mo PT, (3 mo) | 11 × 2 h (7 wk) | Peer Group ED + RT + ES | 0 | 0 | 0 | | 0 | 0 |
| Cain et al[42] | 59 Gyn, ? | 1 UC, 2 INT | 1-mo PD (6 mo) | 8 × 2 h (8 wk) | Patient-only ED + ES / Peer Group ED + ES | | + (ID) / + (ID) | | | + (ID) / + (ID) | 0 / 0 |
| Helgeson et al[43] | 312, Br, early | 1 C, 3 INT | 4-mo PS (3 yr) | 8 × 45–105 min (8 wk) | Peer Group / ED / ES / ED + ES | x | x / 0 / 0 | x | | | + (0.11) / 0 / 0 |
| **Quasi-experimental - patient only interventions** | | | | | | | | | | | |
| Narvaez, A et al[51] | 38 Br | 1 C, 1 INT | <3-yr PD (Post) | 9 × 1.5 h (?) | Peer Group CogR + CS | 0 | + (ID) | + (ID) | | 0 | 0 |
| Gordon et al[52] | 308 mixed, 71 Br, mixed | 1 C, 1 INT | ? PD (6 mo) | 13 × 20 min (6 mo) | Patient-only ED + ES + RT | 0 | x | 0 | | 0 | + (ID) |
| Maguire et al[51] | 152, Br | 1 UC, 1 INT | ? PD (18 mo) | ? | Patient-only ED + ES | | + (ID) | | | + (ID) | |
| **Randomized - partners included in intervention to some degree** | | | | | | | | | | | |
| Allen et al[45] | 164, Br, early | 1 C, 1 INT | ? mo PD (8 mo) | 2 × 2 h + 4 × ? min ph calls (12 wk) | Patient + support person ED + PS | x | x | 0 | | 0 | 0 |
| Greer and Moorey et al (1992; '94)[75] | 137 (82 Br; mixed 19 gyn) mixed | 1 SC, 1 INT | 4–12 wk PD (12 mo) | 6 × 1 h (8 wk) | Patient + Spouse ED + CogR + CS + RT | X | + (0.35) | | | 0 | 0 |
| **Randomized—specifically couple-focused** | | | | | | | | | | | |
| Kalaitzi et al[47] | 40 Br, ? | 1 C, 1 INT | 2 d PreS (Post) | 6 × ? (3 wk) | Patient + Spouse ED + CT + SexC + SexT | + | + (ID) | + (ID) | + (ID) | + (ID) | + (ID) |
| Scott et al[54] | 94 women (57 br 37 gyn) early | 1 MI, 2 INT | <1 wk PD (12 mo) | 5 × 2 h + 2 × 30 min calls (6mths) | Patient + Spouse ED + CT + MS + SBF + SCogR + SexT + CCS / Patient only ED + CogR + SexC + CS | + / 0 | + / 0 | + / 0 | + / 0 | + / 0 | |
| **Pilot Randomized trial - specifically couple-focused, 10 or fewer couples per condition** | | | | | | | | | | | |
| *Baucom et al[55] | 14 Br, early | 1 UC, 1 INT | ? (1 yr) | 6 (bi-weekly) × 1.2 h | Patient + Spouse CT + ProbS + MS + SBF + SexC | + (3 wk) | + (3 wk) | + | + | + | + |
| Christensen[50] | 20 Br, early | 1 C, 1 INT | 2–3 mo PS (1 wk) | 4 × ? (4 wk) | Patient + Spouse ED + CT + ES + SexC | 0 | + | 0 | + | + | 0 |

*Reported between group effect sizes, not statistical significance.

Br indicates breast cancer; C, no-treatment control; CC, couple cancer communication; CCS, couple coping skills; CogR, cognitive coping skills; CS, coping skills training; CT, communication training; Diag, diagnosis; ED, disease/treatment education, with or without coping information; ES, emotional support such as psychotherapy and or ventilation; Gyn, gynecological cancers; ID, insufficient data (means and/or standard deviations not reported); PreS, pre-surgery; INT, intervention; MI, minimal intervention control; MS, mutual support skills; NS, not specified; PD, post-diagnosis; ph, phone calls; ProbS, problem solving skills; PS, post-surgery; PT, post-radiotherapy and/or chemotherapy treatment(s); RT, relaxation training in range of exercises; SC, standard-care control; SCogR, shared cognitive coping skills; SBF, shared benefit finding; SexC, sex counseling; SexT, sex therapy techniques (eg sensate focus); +, significant differences between intervention and control; x, statistically significant difference (at $P < 0.05$ or lower) between conditions at follow-up, but not maintained to final assessment; 0, no significant difference between intervention and control conditions; blank spaces, outcomes not measured; ?, not specified.

strengthen partners' skills in mutually supporting the 2 studies differed considerably in the methods used for promoting couple coping. The CanCOPE intervention of Scott et al[48] first targeted enhancing the cognitive and behavioral coping skills of each partner. Next, at the couple level, components focused on training in shared cognitive coping and mutual support, to help partner's understand and support each other's ways of coping. The ultimate aim of the coping training components was to help couples develop a unified approach to coping with their cancer experience to cope as a team.

In contrast, the relationship enhancement (RE) intervention of Baucom et al,[49] where it shares similarities with CanCOPE, does not aim to expand or strengthen each partner's repertoire of cancer-specific coping skills. Rather, RE aims to foster couple coping by intervening at the level of the relationship. For example, partners are taught problem-solving skills and ways to share their thoughts and feeling about their cancer experience. The aim of these approaches is to reduce the impact that their cancer journey may have on their relationship functioning and satisfaction.

Finally, only the couple-based interventions implemented evidence-based techniques that were found in the broader clinical psychology literature to be effective in treating sexual and body image disorders.[57-59] The sexual therapy techniques included sensate focus,[47,48] guided exposure to mastectomy scar,[50] and specific psycho-education counseling and discussion around sexuality and body image.[48,49] The techniques are designed to provide couples with cognitive and behavioral skills to help them; reduce anxiety about the resumption of sexual activity, manage sexual difficulties (eg, lowered sexual desire or coital pain), and improve women's sense of attractiveness and femininity. The techniques delivered early in the disease experience and were preventative in focus, aiming to reduce the occurrence and impact of psychosexual problems on the quality of couple's relationship intimacy.

## The Processes for Therapy Delivery

The delivery of intervention content varied markedly across studies. Processes included unstructured or structured, insight-orientated discussions,[42,43,51,52,] and didactic seminars,[43] to varying degrees. One study predominately involved telephone call sessions.[45] The majority of interventions used CBT training techniques to promote skills acquisition, such as modeling, in-session rehearsal and role-play of skills, homework practice, and monitoring and shaping of skills acquisition.[41,44-50]

Most studies do not provide details about the control or comparison conditions. Five studies compared the efficacy of interventions with "standard" or "usual" care conditions. Ostensibly, women in these conditions received information and support routinely offered by nursing, medical, or allied health staff working in participating oncology recruitment sites. Unfortunately, the nature and extent of patients' contact with oncology clinic staff is rarely reported. Furthermore, only one study[46] reported on patients' receipt of counseling or professional support external to the trial.

## Outcome Measures Related to Sexual Adjustment

### Sexual Well-Being

Five studies assessed global sexual difficulties[42,44-46,52] and one measured overall sexual satisfaction.[50] These studies used generic measures of sexual adjustment that summed difficulties occurring across a range of diverse problems, such as arguments with partners about sexual issues, reduction in frequency of sexual activities, general relationship difficulties, and body image dissatisfaction or concerns. Only 2 studies, both couple-based, assessed the effect of intervention

on sexual dysfunctions that can occur across the phases of the male and female sexual response cycles.[48,49]

### Body Image

Five studies assessed body image outcomes separately from indices of sexual functioning.[41,43,48,49,51] Of these one study[51] reported nurses' ratings of women's adjustment to changes their appearance, whereas the remaining studies assessed women's body-image satisfaction.[41,43,48,49]

Women's formulation of their body image does not occur in isolation. It is shaped within the context of their relationship, and their interactions with their partners.[60] Women's perceptions about their partners' reactions to their appearance after cancer consistently predict their own acceptance of their appearance and sense of femininity.[54,61] Ultimately, how a partner seems to respond to them can influence a woman's broader adjustment to cancer[61,62] via its impact on her self-esteem[63] and coping.[12,13] In this regard, 2 couple-based studies also assessed the impact of intervention on women's partner-related body image, that is, women's perceptions of their partners' reactions to their body and appearance.[48,49]

Women's views about sexual aspects of themselves also predict a range of sexual attitudes, behaviors, and cognition, including the development of sexual difficulties and concerns in women with breast[64] and gynecologic cancers.[65] Thus, Scott et al[48] also assessed the impact of CanCOPE on women's sexual self-concept.[66]

## EFFICACY OF INTERVENTIONS

The findings from 4 studies need to be interpreted with caution when making conclusions about the efficacy of interventions for reducing women's sexual and body image problems after cancer.[23] These studies showed serious methodological limitations such as, significant baseline differences between conditions on dependent measures that were not controlled statistically in analyses,[51] or marked differences between conditions in the timing of follow-up assessment data collection[45] (ie, greater than 1 month duration). In 2 studies the results could be explained by differential attrition between conditions.[46,52]

It is also difficult to draw conclusions about the magnitude of beneficial effects for the dependent measures because effect sizes cannot be calculated for almost half the studies.[41,42,47,51,52] A related issue is that it is difficult to determine the clinical significance of statistically significant findings for sexual and body image outcomes. Two thirds of the studies used experimenter-derived instruments with unknown reliability and validity, and body image was usually not assessed separately from sexual functioning. This was the case even in more recent trials that ordinarily would be expected to demonstrate greater experimental rigor than trails conducted in the 1980s.[41,43-45,47]

Finally, the findings from Baucom et al[49] should be treated with caution. The authors acknowledge that because of the small sample size, between-group effect sizes are not statistically significant. Hence the results might be due to chance, though the consistent pattern of results favoring their RE intervention over the control condition lends some support for the conclusions that are drawn from this pilot.

## Effects on Sexual Functioning

Interventions that do not systematically involve women's partners have mostly produced weak effects on women's sexual adjustment. The majority of studies report no effects, or short-term effects that were not maintained to follow-up.[41,44-46,52] In 2 studies, educational support interventions improved global sexual satisfaction for women with gynecologic[42] and breast cancers.[51] However, the magnitude of these effects is not known.

These weak results are likely due to a combination of methodological limitations. First, 2 studies reporting no effects involved a mixed cancer diagnoses sample.[46,52] Their severity of sexual difficulties and rates of recovery in sexual functioning varies markedly across cancer sites.[8] Heterogeneity in these variables in these samples may have reduced sensitivity for detecting intervention effects, and researchers did not investigate possible differential intervention effects on sexual outcomes across diagnostic subgroups. Second, most studies reporting no effects use experimenter-derived instruments that may not have been sensitive to intervention effects. Third, these studies did not report the proportions of premorbidly sexually active women and may have had reduced power to detect effects of intervention on sexual outcomes. Fourth, interventions producing null effects on sexual outcomes may not have adequately addressed women's sexual difficulties. None of these interventions involved sexual therapy components that counseled couples about sexual techniques. Furthermore, some delivery formats (eg, group settings or telephone counseling) may not have been conducive to women discussing intimate sexual matters.

Alternatively, it may be that interventions need to actively include women's partners to produce a benefit on sexual functioning. In support of this premise it is noticeable that all of couple-based interventions reported significant effects of intervention on indices of sexual adjustment, albeit that for 2 studies these were only short term effects.[47,50] Positive moderate size effects of couple-based intervention have been found for women's sexual drive and satisfaction in the first few months after diagnosis and surgery.[47,49,50] The RE intervention was also beneficial for women's sexual drive and satisfaction in the longer term, though effects had decreased at 12 month follow up ($d = 0.34$). Noticeably, the RE program produced stronger effects for male partners' sexual drive and satisfaction than for women's, especially 12 months postintervention ($d = 1.04$). Across all studies reviewed in Table 1, this intervention is the only one to report benefits for male partner's sexual adjustment.

The CanCOPE intervention[48] produced strong effects ($d = 0.91$) on women's sense that sexual intimacy was preserved in their relationship in the 12 months after their cancer diagnosis. The intervention also produced large ($d = 0.80$) long-term benefits for women's cognitive appraisals of their sexual selves. CanCOPE women reported significantly more positive sexual self-schemas than women in either patient-only therapy or the control. However, CanCOPE had no effect on sexual functioning in either women, or their partners. This may have been due to a floor effect with low rates of sexual dysfunction in the women in this trial. Across all assessments their sexual functioning was comparable with healthy women.[48]

## Effects on Body Image

Interventions that have focused primarily on only women-only produced either no effects[44,45,52] or small short-term effects that were not maintained to follow-up (eg, $d = 0.21$:42, 57). Though Maguire et al[51] report a significant long-term benefit of intervention on women's body image, the size of this effect is unknown. Furthermore, the clinical significance of improvement is also unclear, and the results should be interpreted with caution. Body-image satisfaction was based upon nurses' judgment about women's reactions to breast loss and postoperative scars, not women's self-reports, and nurse assessors may not have been blind to participants' condition assignment.

In contrast, the couple-based interventions show promise for enhancing body image as all 4 studies report short-term treatment benefits. However, the clinical significance of findings must be considered in the context of the various measurement problems inherent with 2 of the studies that have been described.[47,50] For example, the results from these studies are difficult to interpret as they are based

upon measures that pool women's responses across sexual and body image items.[47,50] Furthermore, both studies did not assess women beyond immediate postintervention. Hence, the sustainability of effects is unknown.

In spite of this, there is some evidence from 2 studies for long-term benefits of couple-based interventions on women's body image. The RE intervention produced long-term improvement (12 months) in women's satisfaction with their body image ($d = 1.02$), and their perceptions of their attractiveness to their partners ($d = 0.80$). The Can-COPE intervention[48] also produced improvement in partner-related body image across the 12 month after diagnosis. CanCOPE women reported their partners as more positive and accepting of their body ($d = 0.44$) than did women in either patient-only therapy or control conditions. Patient-only therapy and control conditions were equivalent in their effects on partner-related body image.

However, unlike the RE intervention, CanCOPE did not produce significant effects on women's self-acceptance of their body image. The reasons why these similar interventions produced disparate effects for females' body image satisfaction are not immediately apparent as the studies report comparable levels of women's preintervention body-image satisfaction. One possible explanation might be due to differences between the studies in the intensity of treatments women underwent. In the CanCOPE trial twice as many women (57%) received adjunctive medical treatments (ie, radiation therapy, chemotherapy, or a combination of these treatments) than women in the RE trial (28%). CanCOPE treatment components focused on developing couples' mutuality in coping and support, and less on women's personal journeys. There may need to be more time dedicated to self- and body-acceptance strategies[67] to help women come to terms with bodily changes after invasive or intense medical treatments.

A plausible alternative explanation is that women's self-acceptance might be better nurtured by fostering their feelings of connectedness and closeness with partners. RE focused directly on enriching couples' relationships in this way where as CanCOPE did not. This premise is consistent with findings from clinical and psychooncology research showing that body image satisfaction in healthy women,[68] and women with cancer,[69] is predicted by their satisfaction with the quality of their relationships with their partners. Furthermore, in couples coping with lung cancer, conversations about their relationship in the context of their cancer experiences predicted less psychologic distress and higher relationship satisfaction in both partners over time.[70]

## Effects on Secondary Outcomes

### Mood

Two thirds of the psychologic interventions to promote sexual and/or body adjustment in women with cancers also produced small benefits for their psychologic adjustment or mood. Relative to control conditions, both emotional support and coping skill-based interventions significantly reduce women's levels of global distress, anxiety, and/or depression. However, effect sizes in many studies are generally small ranging from $d = 0.22$[48] to $d = 0.45$.[49]

Findings for the effect of intervention on reducing trauma symptoms are limited and contradictory. An educational and problem-solving training intervention[45] found no significant effect of intervention. In contrast women in CanCOPE[48] reported significantly fewer trauma symptoms than women in either the patient-only coping skills or control conditions. This pattern of findings suggests training couples in shared cognitive coping is modestly ($d = 0.34$) more effective for assisting women to challenge unhelpful intrusive thoughts about stressful cancer experiences than training women individually in either cognitive coping or problem-solving skills. Unfortunately the small sample size in the CanCOPE trial precluded exploration of the mechanisms of intervention effects. There are other CanCOPE components, such as enhanced partner emotional support, that might also account for the findings.

More broadly, the pattern of results of weak effects for psychologic adjustment is consistent with meta-analyses indicate interventions for women and men cancer, across a range of diagnoses and stages of disease generally produce statistically small effects on mood.[22] Stronger effects for mood are found for interventions that are "selected" or "targeted," meaning therapy is only provided to patients identified as experiencing elevated levels of distress.[23] In the current review, the only targeted intervention[46] did not produce stronger effects on mood. Possibly, heterogeneity in cancer type and gender in the study sample reduced power to detect effects for women.

The large effect (d = 0.74) for depression reported in the Christensen et al study[50] is likely the result of women's high initial distress. Compared with women with breast cancer in other psycho-oncology trials, women in this study showed elevated levels of depression on the Beck Depression Inventory.[71] Perhaps the method of recruitment was biased towards women with elevated stress. Women were referred to the intervention by doctors or nurses involved in their care, rather than participation being offered to all consecutive women who met study criteria. It is possibly that women who displayed overt signs of upset were more likely to be referred to the study by oncology staff.

There is limited evidence from 2 studies[49,43] for long-term benefits of intervention on enhancing positive psychologic adjustment, as opposed to preventing disorder. In one trial[43] an educational intervention demonstrated small but significant benefits over support interventions for increasing women's positive affect, and these benefits were maintained to 6-month follow-up (d = 0.20). Moderately large short-term benefits in posttrauma growth are reported for both women (d = 0.63) and their partners (d = 0.66) after the RE couple-based intervention.[49] These benefits remained at 12-month follow-up, although the effects had reduced markedly for the women (d = 0.22) and to a lesser extent for partners (d = 0.41).

### Social Support

As seen in Table 1, focusing therapy primarily on the women with cancer does not seem effective for improving their relationships with their or other people in their social networks. One study[52] found a benefit of intervention on women's reported martial satisfaction. However, the clinical significance of this finding is questionable as it is based on an experimenter-derived measure that combined sexual, body image, and relationship difficulties.

There was evidence from one trial that peer-group interventions can increase women's use of support from people in their social network. Helgeson et al's[43] educational intervention increased the amount of cancer-related discussions that the women engaged in with people close to them. However, these effects had faded by 6-month follow-up, and there was no effect of intervention on women's perceptions of people's responsiveness during these conversations. Further the sources of support that women assessed are not known.

The couple-based interventions seem to hold greater potential for enhancing the quality of women relationships with their partners. Two of three trials assessing this outcome found moderate (d = 0.48) to large size (d = 0.77) benefits of couple-focused therapy on women's relationship satisfaction in the short[47,49] and longer term.[49] One of these studies[49] also found that couple-level therapy promoted relationship satisfaction in women's partners. Moderately large effects

(d = 0.64) were produced in the short term, although by 12-month follow-up the magnitude of the effect was small (d = 0.34).

Unfortunately no studies assessed the impact of intervention on women's satisfaction with support for their cancer experience from others generally, or partners' support. The results from one study[48] suggest that the quality of emotional support women give to, and receive from their partners, might be enhanced by couple-based intervention. CanCOPE produced significant improvements in couples' supportive communication about their cancer experience that was maintained over the 6-month follow-up period. Specifically, there were large increases in partners' observed couple-coping statements (d = 1.23) and a trend (P = 0.05) to reduce partners' withdrawal during cancer-related discussion.

### Coping

Generally, women only studies show no benefits for coping. One study increased women's coping through support seeking[46] but found no effect for intervention on other coping skills. Similarly, 3 studies found no sustained effects of intervention on women's sense of control.[43,50,52] The strongest effects for coping were seen in the Scott et al.[48] CanCOPE couples, compared with couples in the other 2 conditions, showed a greater reduction in their coping-effort in the year after diagnosis and intervention, and significantly lower coping effort at 12-month follow-up (d = 0.64). However, coping-effort is a marker of coping burden or strain, and the impact of the intervention on specific individual, or couple-level, cognitive behavioral coping skills is not know.

### Effects on Physical Recovery

The most consistent and sustained effects of intervention are seen for women's physical recovery, though again, the magnitude of effects is mostly small or unknown. The common treatment component across studies with significant effects was provision of information about diagnosis and treatments. Educational interventions increased women's knowledge about medical aspects of their cancer,[43,44] return of stamina, physical functioning, and vitality[42,49] with effects on vitality maintained between 6[42,43] and 12 months (d = 1.1450). One trial[43] reported intervention effects on vitality maintained to 3-year follow-up, though by this stage the magnitude of effect was very small (d = 0.16).

Interventions are generally effective in improving women's physical recovery. The significant benefits on role functioning seem to be associated with interventions delivered whereas the women were still receiving cancer treatments,[51] usually in the immediate postoperative period[42,43,52] and positive effects of intervention were maintained to 6-month follow-up. The 2 studies finding no effects of intervention were delivered months after women's diagnoses and surgical treatments were complete.[44,46] At this point in their recovery many women may have resumed usual activities and there may have been a ceiling effect that made it difficult to detect any added effect of intervention.

## METHODOLOGICAL ISSUES

Clearly there is a paucity of trials from which to draw firm conclusions about the efficacy of interventions for enhancing women' body image and sexual adjustment after cancer. Serious methodological problems in many of the existing trials also render interpretations difficult. To advance knowledge in the field it is imperative that future trials are conceived and conducted in accordance with the revised CONSORT (Consolidated Standards of Reporting Trials) statement.[72,73] Studies that omit CONSORT elements risk bias in estimates of intervention effects, and the reliability and relevance of findings is questionable.

Research in the future should particularly aim to use strategies to improve the statistical rigor and clinical integrity inherent in trial design.

## Strategies to Improve Future Research

Studies need to attend to measurement selection, statistical analysis, and reporting of results, in a manner that enables findings to be understood from a broader public health perspective.[74] Some significant effects reported in Table 1 may be attributable to inflation of type I error rates, as half the studies involved a large number of analyses conducted on correlated variables.[42,46,47,50,52] In addition, 2 studies found significant differences between conditions at baseline on dependent measures[44,50] that the researchers attempted to control statistically using covariance analyses. However, the results may be explained by regression to the mean.[25] Measures need to be selected in consideration of their psychometric properties and sensitivity to clinical change. There should be separate measures for body image, sexual satisfaction, and sexual dysfunction. Future studies should report effect sizes and clinical significance to enable comparisons across psycho-oncology, clinical, and chronic illness intervention research.[74]

## Treatment Integrity and Fidelity

The potential for replication and dissemination of trials found to efficacious could be enhanced by attention to treatment integrity and fidelity strategies. For example, most studies do not report whether they monitor or control for the important potential confound of women/and or their partners receiving counseling from sources external to the study.[23] A further problem is that, although there seem to be commonalities across interventions in treatment components, information about the precise content and processes involved in therapy delivery was often limited and vague, especially with early studies.[42,50–52] Most studies do not report therapists' levels of training and experience. Only 3 research teams have published treatment manuals[8] or detailed descriptions of therapy used in their trials.[75,76] Thus, the extent of replicated results for similar intervention types cannot be ascertained.

## Improving the Clinical Utility of Interventions

A key criteria for interventions to be considered "empirically supported"[17] is that they are generalizable and acceptable more broadly beyond the trial setting. In many of the studies the generalizability of results is constrained by the high rates of refusal. Some studies fail to report refusal rates and seem purposive in approach[47,50] rather than offering intervention to all consecutive women who meet study criteria. Typically the rates of reported refusal for women-only interventions are 30%.[43,44] In studies that invite women's partners to participate to some extent, refusal rates are even higher ranging from 40%[46] to 87%.[49] This high level of refusal is consistent with refusal rates (around 70%) found in psychooncology intervention and descriptive studies generally that have attempted to recruit males, either as partners of women with cancer or as patients.[34]

Greater male participation is found in psycho-oncology studies that deliver intervention in patients' homes. For example, a family-based intervention for women with recurrent breast cancer and their family caregivers reported an 80% recruitment rate. This figure is similar to the recruitment rates for the CanCOPE trial, which also involved in home therapy delivery. However, therapies delivered face-to-face in women's home are very expensive to provide and most health care systems could not financially sustain such services.

An alternative approach to enhance engagement with interventions might be delivering self-help programs via flexible delivery formats (eg, internet, DVD, or telephone-therapy). These types of programs show promise across a range of other chronic and mental illnesses.[77–79] There is also tentative evidence from pilot randomized control trials that couple-coping programs can be delivered effectively via the telephone to couples coping with prostate[80] breast, or gynecologic cancers.[81]

## CLINICAL IMPLICATIONS AND FUTURE DIRECTIONS

There is much to be done in the field. Interventions almost exclusively involved women diagnosed with breast cancer who were 50 years and older, well educated, and Caucasian. Little is known about the best way to enhance sexual health and well being after cancer for couples who are younger or from minority or less-educated groups. It is also not clear whether findings would generalize to women confronting other types of cancer diagnoses, such as colon[82,83] or head and neck cancers.[84] Some surgical procedures associated with these cancers, such as stomas or changes to facial appearance, may present unique challenges to self or partner acceptance of body image, compared with conservative surgeries for breast cancer, that largely preserves breast appearance. Furthermore, the needs of women with advanced or progressive disease have not been explored. Although they may not be physically well and have reduced desire for sexual activity, their need for emotional and physical intimacy may actual heighten as their disease progresses. Changes in their physical appearance and sense of self or body integrity may also be distressing for them and their partner.[85] No studies have assessed women with advanced disease and how to assist them with these challenges.

We currently know little about the best ways to treat sexual dysfunction, but more about how to improve global sexual functioning and body image in women after cancer. Interventions that produce stronger effects tend to be couple focused and include treatment components that (1) educate both partners about the woman's diagnosis and treatments, (2) promote couples' mutual coping and support processes, and (3) include specific sexual therapy techniques to address sexual and body-image difficulties.

There were little differences among couple, individual, or peer-group interventions for effects on most secondary outcomes, especially mood. This might be due to the low rate of psychologic morbidity or traumatic stress in most samples. Furthermore, couple's psychologic distress levels are generally moderate, comparable with community and primary care populations. Thus, their distress may not be due to the challenges posed by their cancer experience per se, but rather due to precancer relationship issues, or other chronic stressors, that interventions to cope specifically with cancer may not adequately address.[28]

Across all domains of recovery, interventions were more effective if they were delivered nearer to the time of diagnosis and commencement of treatments, when emotional distress and coping support needs in women and their partners are highest.

The effectiveness of interventions for enhancing recovery of sexual and body image in women in maritally distressed relationships is unknown. There is a high level of marital satisfaction in couples involved in psych-oncology studies more broadly[86] and the couple-based interventions reviewed here. In the CanCOPE trial women with low marital satisfaction relationships were more likely to drop out. The techniques for improving sex and body image adjustment may not generalize to martially distressed couples. Interventions may need to intervene first to improve relationship functioning and satisfaction before cancer-specific coping can be addressed. In reality, recruiting martially distressed couples into face-to-face interventions, especially early on in the disease experience when couples might be in crisis, is highly unlikely to be successful.

In summary, individual and peer-group studies have often produced no or few significant benefits for enhancing women's body image and sexual functioning after cancer. There is tentative evidence that couple-based interventions may lead to stronger sustained effects in these domains of recovery than offering therapy to women on their own. This question warrants further investigation in treatment comparison trials with larger sample sizes. However, researchers should be aware of potential obstacles to feasibility that they might encounter when attempting intervention research with couples at times of stress, and of the importance of finding ways to increase the clinical utility of interventions, especially for actively involving the partners of women with cancer.

## REFERENCES

1. Hart J, Shaver PR, Goldenberg LJ. Attachment, self-esteem, worldviews, and terror management: evidence for a tripartite security system. *J Pers Soc Psychol.* 2005;88:999–1031.
2. Victor F, Mikulincer M, Gilad H. The anxiety-buffering function of close relaitonships: evidence that relationship commitment acts as a terror management mechanism. *J Pers Soc Psychol.* 2002;82:527–542.
3. Coan JA, Schaefer HS, Davidson RJ. Lending a hand: social regulation of the neural response to threat. *Psychol Sci.* 2006;17:1032–1039.
4. Goldenberg JL, McCoy SK, Pyszczynski T, et al. The body as a source of self-esteem: the effect of mortality salience on identification with one's body, interest in sex, and appearance monitoring. *J Pers Soc Psychol.* 2000;79:118–130.
5. Mikulincer M, Florian V. Exploring individual differences in reactions to mortality salience: does attachment style regulate terror management mechanisms. *J Pers Soc Psychol.* 2000;79:260–273.
6. Schover LR. *Sexuality and Fertility After Cancer.* New York: Wiley; 1997.
7. Makar K, Cumming CE, Lees AW, et al. Sexuality, body image and quality of life after high dose or conventional chemotherapy for metastatic breast cancer. *Can J Hum Sex.* 1997;6:1–8.
8. Kayser K, Scott JL. *Helping Couples Cope with Women's Cancers.* New York: Springer; 2008:229.
9. Andersen BL, Anderson B, DeProsse C. Controlled prospective longitudinal study of women with cancer. I. Sexual functioning outcomes. *J Consult Clin Psychol.* 1989;57:683–691.
10. Andersen BL, van der Does E. Surviving gynecological cancer and coping with sexual morbidity: an international problem. *Int J Gynecol Cancer.* 1994;4: 225–240.
11. Fobair P, Stewart SL, Chang S, et al. Body image and sexual problems in young women with breast cancer. *Psychooncology.* 2006;15:579–594.
12. Sedikidies C, Skowronski JJ. The symbolic self in evolutionary context. *Pers Soc Psychol Rev.* 1997;1:80–102.
13. Norton TR, Manne SL, Rubin S, et al. Ovarian cancer patient's psychological distress: the role of physical impairment, perceived unsupportive family and friend behaviors, perceived control, and self-esteem. *Health Psychol.* 2005;24:143–152.
14. Andersen BL. Psychological interventions for cancer patients to enhance the quality of life. *J Consult Clin Psychol.* 1992;60:552–568.
15. Andersen BL. Biobehavioral outcomes following psychological interventions for cancer patients. *J Consult Clin Psychol.* 2002;70:590–610.
16. Baum A, Andersen BL, eds. *Psychosocial Interventions for Cancer.* Washington, DC: American Psychological Association; 2001:446.
17. Chambless DL, Ollendick TH. Empirically supported psychological interventions: controversies and evidence. *Annu Rev Psychol.* 2001;52:685–716.
18. Compas BE, Haaga DA, Keefe FJ, et al. Sampling of empirically supported psychological treatments from health psychology: smoking, chronic pain, cancer, and bulimia nervosa. *J Consult Clin Psychol.* 1998;1:89–112.
19. Devine EC, Westlake SK. The effects of psychoeducational care provided to adults with cancer: meta-analysis of 116 studies. *Oncol Nurs Forum.* 1995;22:1369–1381.
20. Edelman S, Craig A, Kidman DA. Group interventions with cancer patients: efficacy of psychoeducational versus supportive groups. *J Psychosoc Oncol.* 2000;18:67–85.
21. Fawzy FI, Fawzy NW. Psychoeducational interventions. In: Holland J, ed. *Textbook of Psycho-Oncology.* New York: Oxford University Press; 1998:676–693.
22. Meyer TJ, Mark MM, Effects of psychosocial interventions with adult cancer patients: a meta-analysis of randomized experiments. *Health Psychol.* 1995;14:101–108.
23. Newell SA, Sanson-Fisher RW, Savolainen JN. Systematic review of psychological therapies for cancer patients: overview and recommendations for future research. *J Natl Cancer Inst.* 2002;94:558–584.
24. Tapper VJ. Psychotherapeutic trials specific to women with breast cancer: the state of the science. *J Psychosoc Oncol.* 1999;17:85–99.
25. Trijsburg RW, van Knippenberg FCE, Rijpma SE Effects of psychological treatment on cancer patients: a critical review. *Psychosom Med.* 1992;54:489–517.
26. Berg CA, Upchurch R. A developmental-contexuall model of couples coping with chronic illness across the adult life span. *Psychol Bull.* 2007;133:920–954.
27. Cochrane BB, Lewis FM. Partner's adjustment to breast cancer: a critical analysis of intervention studies. *Health Psychol.* 2005;24:327–332.
28. Hagedoorn M, Sanderman R, Bolks HN, et al. Distress in couples coping with cancer: a Meta analysis and critical review of role and gender effects. *Psychol Bull.* 2008;134:1–30.
29. Burton MV, Parker RW, Farrell A, et al. A randomized controlled trial of preoperative psychological preparation for mastectomy. *Psychooncology.* 1995;4: 1–19.
30. Capone MA, Good RS, Westie KS, et al. Psychosocial rehabilitation of gynecologic oncology patients. *Arch Phys Med Rehabil.* 1980;61:128–132.
31. Fawzy FI, Fawzy NW, Arndt L, et al. Critical review of psychosocial interventions in cancer patients. *Arch Gen Psychiatry.* 1995;52:100–113.
32. Badger T, Segrin C, Dorros SM, et al. Depression and anxiety in women with breast cancer and their partners. *Nurs Res.* 2007;56:44–53.
33. Budin WC, Hoskins CN, Haber J, et al. Breast cancer: education, counseling, and adjustment among patients and partners: a randomised clinical trial. *Nurs Res.* 2008;57:199–213.
34. Manne SL, Ostroff JS, Winkel G, et al. Couple-focused group intervention for women with early stage breast cancer. *J Consult Clin Psychol.* 2005;73:634–646.
35. Hoskins C, Budin W, Haber J, et al. Breast Cancer: education, couseling and adjustment among patients and their partners—a randomised controlled trial. *Psychooncology.* 2008;17:S13.
36. Kuijer RG, Buunk BP, De Jong GM, et al. Effects of a brief intervention program for patients with cancer and their partners on feelings of inequity, relationship quality and psychological distress. *Psychooncology.* 2004;13:321–334.
37. Northouse L, Kershaw T, Mood D, et al. Effects of a family intervention on the quality of life of women with recurrent breast cancer and their family caregivers. *Psychooncology.* 2005;14:478–491.
38. Nezu A, Nezu CM, Felgoise SH, et al. Project Genesis: assessing the efficacy of problem-solving therapy for distressed adult cancer patients. *J Consult Clin Psychol.* 2003;71:1036–1048.
39. Kayser K. Enhancing dyadic coping during a time of crisis: a theory-based intervention with breast cancer patients and their partners. In: *Couples Coping with Stress: Emerging Perspectives on Dyadic Coping.* Revenson TA, Kayser K, Bodenmann G, eds. Washington, DC: American Psychological Association; 2005:175–194.
40. Kayser K. An evaluation of a couples-based intervention on the psychosocial adjustment to breast cancer. *Psychooncology.* 2005;S1–S104:v2.
41. Narvaez A, et al. Evaluation of effectiveness of a group cognitive-behavioral therapy on body image, self-esteem, sexuality and distress in breast cancer patients. *Psicooncologia.* 2008;5:93–102.
42. Cain EN, Kohorn EI, Quinlan DM, et al. Psychosocial benefits of a cancer support group. *Cancer.* 1986;57:183–189.
43. Helgeson V, Cohen S, Schulz R, et al. Education and peer discussion group interventions and adjustment to breast cancer. *Arch Gen Psychiatr.* 1999;56:340–347.
44. Berglund G, Bolund C, Gustafsson UL, et al. A randomized study of a rehabilitation program for cancer patients: the 'starting again' group. *Psychooncology.* 1994;3:109–120.
45. Allen SM, Shah AC, Nezu AM, et al. A problem-solving approach to stress reduction among young women with breast carcinoma: a randomized controlled trial. *Cancer.* 2002;94:3089–3100.
46. Greer S, Moorey S, Baruch JD, et al. Adjuvant psychological therapy for patients with cancer: a prospective randomised trial. *Br Med J.* 1992;304:675–680.
47. Kalaitzi C, Papadopoulos VP, Michas K, et al. Combined brief psychosexual interventions after mastectomy: effects of sexuality, body image, and psychological well-being. *J Surg Oncol.* 2007;96:235–240.
48. Scott JL, Halford WK, Ward BG. United we stand? The effects of a couple-coping intervention on adjustment to breast or gynaecological cancer. *J Consult Clin Psychol.* 2004;72:1122–1135.
49. Baucom D, Porter LS, Kirby JS, et al. A couple-based intervention for female breast cancer. *Psychooncology.* 2008 [Epub ahead of print].
50. Christensen DN. Postmastectomy couple counselling: an outcome study of a structured treatment protocol. *J Sex Marital Ther.* 1983;9:266–275.
51. Maguire GP, Tait A, Brooke M, et al. Effect of counselling on the psychiatric morbidity associated with mastectomy. *Br Med J.* 1980;281:1454–1456.
52. Gordon WA, Freidenbergs I, Diller L, et al. Efficacy of psychosocial intervention with cancer patients. *J Consult Clin Psychol.* 1980;48:743–759.

53. Nelson EL, Wenzel LB, Osann K, et al. Stress, immunity, and cervical cancer: biobehavioral outcomes of a randomized clinical trial [corrected]. *Clin Cancer Res* 2008;14:2111–2118.

54. Scott JL, Brough P. Does sharing the burden help? An examination of couples' observed communication about cancer diagnosis. Presented in Combined Abstracts of the Australian and New Zealand Psychological Society Joint Conference. Auckland, NZ: 2006.

55. Baucom DH, Shoham V, Mueser KT, et al. Empirically supported couple and family interventions for marital distress and adult mental health problems. *J Consult Clin Psychol.* 1998;66:53–88.

56. Snyder DK, Castellani AM. Current status and future directions in couple therapy. *Annu Rev Psychol.* 2006;57:317–344.

57. Heiman JR, Meston CM. *Emperically Validated Treatments for Sexual Dysfunction, in Emperically Supported Therapies: Best Practice in Professional Psychology.* Dobson SK, Craig KD, eds. New York: Sage; 1998:259–303.

58. McCarthy BW. *Sexuality, Sexual Dysfunction, and Couple Therapy, in Clinical Handbook of Couple Therapy.* Gurman SA, Jacobson NS, eds. New York: Guilford Press; 2002:629–652.

59. Spence SH. *Sex and Relationships, in Clinical Handbook of Marriage and Couples Interventions.* Halford KW, Markman HJ, eds. Chichester: Wiley; 1997:73–105.

60. Drigotas SM, Rusbult CE, Wieselquist J, et al. Close partner as sculptor of the ideal self-behavioral affirmation and the michelangelo phenomenon. *J Pers Soc Psychol.* 1999;77:293–323.

61. Stanton AL, Estes MA, Estes NC, et al. Treatment decision making and adjustment to breast cancer: a longitudinal study. *J Consult Clin Psychol.* 1998;66:313–322.

62. Manne SL. Intrusive thoughts and psychological distress among cancer patients: the role of spouse avoidance and criticism. *J Consult Clin Psychol.* 1999;67:539–546.

63. Baumeister RF, DeWall CN, Ciarocco NJ, et al. Social Exclusion impairs self-regulation. *J Pers Soc Psychol.* 2005;88:589–604.

64. Yurek DL, Farrar WB, Andersen LB. Breast cancer surgery: comparing surgical groups and determining individual differences in postoperative sexuality and body change stress. *J Consul Clin Psychol.* 2000;38:697–709.

65. Andersen BL, Woods XA, Copeland JL. Sexual self-schema and sexual morbidity among gynecologic cancer survivors. *J Consult Clin Psychol.* 1997;65:221–229.

66. Andersen BL, Cyranowski JM. Women's sexual self-schema. *J Pers Soc Psychol.* 1994;67:1079–1100.

67. Cash TF. *The Body Image Workbook: An 8-Step Program for Learning to Like you Looks.* Oakland, CA: New Harbinger Publications; 1997:221.

68. Weller JE, Dziegielewski SF. The relationship between romantic partner support styles and body image disturbance. *J Hum Behav Soc Environ.* 2004;10:71–92.

69. Abend TA, Williamson GM. Feeling attractive in the wake of breast cancer: optimism matter, and so do interpersonal relationships. *Pers Soc Psychol Bull.* 2002;28:427–436.

70. Badr H, Acitelli LK, Taylor C. Does talking about their relationship effect couples' marital and psychological adjustment to lung cancer? *J Cancer Surviv.* 2008;2:53–64.

71. Beck AT, Ward CH, Mendelson M, et al. An inventory for measuring depression. *Arch Gen Psychiatr.* 1961;4:561–571.

72. Moher D, Schulz KF, Altman GD. The CONSORT statement: revised recommendations for improving the quality of reports of parallelgroup randomized trials. *Ann Intern Med.* 2001;134:657–662.

73. Coyne JC. Improving the reporting of couples interventions in health psychology: some data and a plea. *Psychol Health.* 2005;20(suppl 1)54.

74. Fidler F, Cumming G, Thomason N, et al. Toward improved statistical reporting in the journal of consulting and clinical psychology. *J Consult Clin Psychology.* 2005;73:136–143.

75. Greer S, Moorey S. Adjuvant psychological therapy for cancer patients. *Palliat Med.* 1997;11:240–244.

76. Nezu AM. *Helping Cancer Patients Cope: A Problem-solving Approach.* Washington, DC: American Psycholoogical Association; 1998.

77. Tate DF, Zabinski MF. Computer and internet applications for psychological treatment: update for clinicians. *J Clin Psychol.* 2004;60:209–220.

78. Lehrer PM, Sargunaraj D, Hochron MS. Psychological approaches to the treatment of asthma. *J Consult Clin Psychol.* 1992;60:639–643.

79. Fekete EM, Antoni MH, Schneiderman N. Psychosocial and behavioural interventions for chronic medical conditions. *Curr Opin Psychiatr.* 2007;20:152–157.

80. Campbell LC, Keefe FJ, Scipio C, et al. Facilitating research participation and improving quality of life for african american prostate cancer survivors and their intimate partners a pilot study of telephone-based coping skills training. *Cancer.* 2007;109:414–424.

81. Scott JL, et al. How can we disseminate psycho-oncology interventions to oncology and community settings? Results from a trial of a self-directed coping training program for women with cancer and a closer support persons. *Aust J Psychol.* 2003;55:211.

82. Northouse LL, Mood D, Templin T, et al. Couples' patterns of adjustment to colon cancer. *Soc Sci Med.* 2000;50:271–284.

83. Wasteson E, Nordin K, Hoffman K, et al. Daily assessment of coping in patients with gastrointestinal cancer. *Psychooncology.* 2002;11:1–11.

84. De Leeuw JRJ, de Graeff A, Ros W, et al. Negative and positive influences of social support on depression in patients with head and neck cancer: a prospective study. *Psychooncology.* 2000;9:20–28.

85. LeMay K, Wilson KG. Treatment of existential distress in life threatening illness: a review of manualized interventions. *Clin Psychol Rev.* 2008;28:472–493.

86. Manne SL, Ostroff JS, Winkel G. Social-cognitive processes as moderators of a couple-focused group intervention for women with early stage breast cancer. *Health Psychol.* 2007;26:735–744.

# Sexuality After Hematopoietic Stem Cell Transplantation

Jean C. Yi • Karen L. Syrjala

As survival rates for hematopoietic stem cell transplantation (HSCT) have grown in the past 2 decades with improved management of acute toxicities,[1,2] attention to long-term complications has become more salient to clinicians, researchers, and survivors themselves. Sexual dysfunction has been defined as one of the most common long-term issues after HSCT.[3,4] Prospective studies have described the extent and nature of sexual difficulties in this population,[4-6] and have also documented elevated problem rates relative to healthy controls.[3,4,7,8] The aims of this article are to review the state of knowledge about sexual dysfunction following HSCT, to examine issues related to sexual dysfunction, and to address strategies to treat these long-term problems.

HSCT is a procedure designed primarily for hematologic malignancies, such as leukemia and lymphoma, although some solid tumors and nonmalignant diseases, such as aplastic anemia, are also treated with this aggressive treatment method. Before the transplant, to prepare the body to receive stem cells, the conditioning regimens always include chemotherapy, usually supralethal doses of an alkylating agent such as cyclophosphamide or busulfan, and often including total body irradiation (TBI) at a dose of 1200 cGy or higher. This process lowers immune defenses so that stem cells from either marrow or peripheral blood, donated from oneself (autologous) or from another person (allogeneic) can be infused. If the transplant is allogeneic, survivors are at risk for chronic graft-versus-host disease (GVHD), where the donor immune cells identify the body as foreign and attack it. Chronic GVHD can manifest anywhere in the body and often involves the skin, liver, eyes, mouth, sinuses, and gut.[2] For women, vaginal mucosal tissues are particularly susceptible. Chronic GVHD is managed with the use of immunosuppressants that often include high-dose corticosteroids along with a calcineurin inhibitor, such as cyclosporine or other newer agents, that suppress immune recovery and bring a host of potential additional complications.

Recent efforts to reduce the toxicities of HSCT have used very low-dose chemotherapies and TBI in attempts to optimize a "graft versus leukemia" effect. This increasingly widely used methodology for treating hematologic malignancies seems to spare gonadal function along with other organ systems, but risks for chronic GVHD remain.

The population of HSCT survivors who receive high-dose treatment is usually well under the age of 50, and most often relatively healthy until their diagnosis. Because treatment is so arduous and potentially toxic, major comorbidities are exclusions for eligibility for transplant. Thus women are frequently premenopausal and many men and women report active sex lives until the start of cancer treatment. Although some transplant recipients have had several cycles of treatment before HSCT, others may have had little exposure to previous chemotherapy effects. The dramatic changes brought by treatment can make sexual adjustments more challenging than those of older adults already experiencing adaptations to aging-related physiological changes. This context begins to explain some of the deficits seen even many years after treatment in these HSCT survivors.

## MEDICAL FACTORS CONTRIBUTING TO SEXUAL DYSFUNCTION

Numerous components of medical treatment impact sexual function, including chemotherapy, TBI, medications for chronic GVHD, and the other treatments for symptoms or side effects that are commonly used in patients with cancer such as antidepressants. Alkylating agents are particularly toxic to gonadal function and consequently nearly all HSCT recipients are infertile after treatment (although infertility is not guaranteed, leaving a level of uncertainty unless confirmed with fertility testing). TBI is also toxic to gonadal function and can contribute to genital tissue sensitivity, atrophy or scarring. These treatments impair the production of testosterone at least for the first year for males, and induce ovarian failure for most women.[9-13]

Effects are not solely gonadal. Treatments are known to permanently damage function of the hypothalamic-pituitary-gonadal axis.[14,15] Luteinizing hormone is elevated in most female survivors and normal in most males. Follicle stimulating hormone is elevated in over 90% of females and most males. Most females have primary ovarian failure with consequent low endogenous estrogen levels, and vaginal tissue atrophy is a risk. Chronic GVHD may also contribute to vaginal introital stenosis and mucosal changes that contribute to dyspareunia, vaginal irritation, and increased sensitivity of genital tissues.[16] Male sexual problems have been attributed to gonadal and cavernosal arterial insufficiency with resulting libido and erectile dysfunction.[17,18] TBI or chronic GHVD may contribute to scarring or adhesions in the blood vessels of the penis. Chronic GVHD can also cause inflammation, rash, and sensitivity in the skin of the penis. Most males recover Leydig cell function by 1 year, returning testosterone levels to within normal range.[14,15] However, males with sexual problems have been noted to have testicular insufficiency and diminished libido or erectile dysfunction even when serum testosterone levels are within normal range.[17-20] Thus, they may require dynamic testing of pituitary-gonadal function or empirical testing of testosterone supplementation if levels are low-normal. Ideally male testosterone levels would be tested before beginning treatment as a baseline indicator of an individual's "norm."

The type and dose of chemotherapy are factors to consider when identifying potential effects of treatment.[13,21] In some studies comparing chemotherapy alone with HSCT, those patients who have received only chemotherapy report less sexual dysfunction in all phases of the sexual response cycle.[22] However, this differential effect has not been confirmed in other research.[23]

High-dose corticosteroids are a common component of chronic GVHD treatment and can continue for years. This treatment not only suppresses endogenous hypothalamic and adrenal hormones, but also has major impacts on physical features and body image, along with potential for emotional lability and depression. Over time it creates cushingoid features with weight and fat gain along with loss of muscle. Major joint problems are not uncommon and include avascular necrosis that can require joint replacement. With all of these changes, it is not surprising that feelings of attractiveness and sexual responsiveness suffer. For many survivors who experience this treatment and its effects, sexual activity is put on hold for years and can consequently be difficult to reinitiate without intervention. In this circumstance, a combination of medical and behavioral treatments may be needed.[24]

Chronic GVHD can impact sexual functioning for women through a number of symptoms and physiological changes.[5,22,25,26] Vaginal dryness, irritation, pain, and bleeding can be because of chronic GVHD as well as to ovarian failure.[27,28] At times, as GVHD diminishes in other parts of the body, medication doses may be lowered but then GVHD in the vaginal area develops after resolving in other organs.[29] In a medical chart review of 11 patients with vaginal chronic GVHD, women had been on a regimen of systemic cyclosporine and hormone therapy, yet developed chronic GVHD in the vulva and vagina.[28] Onset occurred on average 10 months posttransplant but some women developed GVHD of the vulva/vagina as much as 2 years after HSCT. The pattern of GVHD of the vulva/vagina was most similar to GVHD found in the skin. Although, the severity of GVHD of the vagina did not correlate with the severity of GVHD

found elsewhere. The work to date in this area has focused on women and evidence of chronic GVHD effects specific to male genital tissue or sexual functioning has been very limited.

When addressing sexual dysfunction in research or clinical care, it is important to consider contributions from biologic effects on psychosocial factors. For example, low levels of testosterone (in both males and females) and years of high-dose corticosteroid treatments for chronic GVHD are associated with decreased sexual desire and depressed mood.[5,30] Calcineurin inhibitors or interferon treatments can affect cognitive function and mood.[31] Fatigue related to cancer and its treatment is likely to impact sex drive if it has other functional impacts.[22,32] Hypothyroidism, diabetes, cardiovascular health problems, and significant loss of muscle mass are all frequent after HSCT and can contribute to sexual performance problems and loss of libido. Depression and antidepressant use along with insomnia are known risk factors for sexual dysfunction in the general population and occur widely in transplant recipients. Thus a full medical examination is needed for HSCT survivors who report sexual dysfunction.

## PSYCHOLOGIC FACTORS CONTRIBUTING TO SEXUAL DYSFUNCTION

As noted above, common symptoms after HSCT have both physiological and psychologic components. Consequently, separation of these factors is somewhat artificial. Figure 1 contains a conceptual model

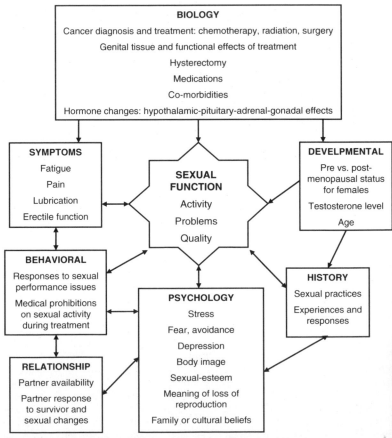

**FIGURE 1.** Conceptual model of sexual dysfunction causes and effects in cancer survivors.

of sexual dysfunction that includes physiological and psychologic aspects. Fatigue, depression, insomnia, body changes, even pain or other physical discomforts may have biologic roots, but they also have cognitive and emotional consequences that can actively contribute to inhibiting sexual activity or responsiveness. If one barely has the energy to maintain mandatory daily activities to promote health, it can be hard to imagine saving time and energy for sex. For survivors of HSCT, this is a common experience in the months after treatment. In addition, appearance changes in hair loss, muscle loss, skin rashes, skin sensitivity or dryness, scars, and weight changes influence body image, which in turn contributes to sexual self-consciousness.[30,32,33] Fear of pain or discomfort, and even fear of failing to become aroused can become barriers to trying again for both survivors and their partners. Another barrier to return to sexual activity is the expectation that responsiveness should return to as it was before diagnosis. Lack of communication about what has changed, what feels good or not, and insecurities about appearance can inhibit couple's attempts at intercourse. These worries and lack of communicating concerns are often also reflected in reduced intimacy, because emotional intimacy and physical expressions of closeness for many couples are seen as precursors to intercourse. Patterns set in the months after returning home can turn into habits that continue for many years.

## ASSESSMENT OF SEXUAL FUNCTIONING

To be able to confidently measure a construct, it is important to have measures that are well validated within the population being tested. The timing of assessments also becomes important as assessing sexual functioning before treatment[32] allows evaluation of changes from an individual or couple's norms. Since sexual function varies so greatly across the population even within the United States,[34] individuals' norms constitute a better reference than population averages. In a study with gynecologic cancers, prior sexual functioning predicts 24% of the variance in sexual outcomes.[35] After HSCT, our data indicate that pretransplant sexual function predicts 19% of the variance in sexual function after 5 years, whereas 1 year sexual function predicts 36% of the variance after 5 years.[4] Thus baseline and 1 year function are strong indicators of how a survivor's function will be long term for both males and females. These results also provide evidence that intervention needs to be timed to intercede, if possible before 1 year after transplant. In a 1-year longitudinal study of sexual functioning of HSCT patients who had received high dose chemotherapy as part of their conditioning regimen, just under half of the patients reported sexual dysfunction before treatment.[36] This finding has been supported in another study of male HSCT survivors.[21] To decrease potential hesitation to raise questions or discuss sexual problems, routine assessment of sexual function by designated health care providers needs to be provided to all patients.[9,22] Reluctance to engage in these discussions is often as great on the part of health care professionals as for patients, in part because providers do not see themselves as knowledgeable and able to treat the problems that patients raise.[37–39] Having a standard assessment tool can decrease these barriers and give survivors and their health care providers a way to start a conversation about sexuality. This standardized measurement then becomes a reference tool for explaining both problems and progress. Thus assessment not only provides a reference marker for change but also the terminology that facilitates clinical communications.[40]

Recent reviews of sexuality after cancer[40,41] indicate a need for further research into assessing sexual function. A limited number of tools have been developed for or tested with cancer patients and survivors. Those that do exist have focused on gynecologic cancer[42,43] and erectile dysfunction after prostate cancer.[44,45] Several broad qual-

ity of life measures contain sexual functioning subscales but may be limited to one-to-three questions and not have been tested with long-term cancer survivors in mind. Thus, there has been a need to devise a measure targeted to HSCT survivors for their specific needs and to do rigorous psychometric testing of sexual function measures in this population.

To meet this need, we tested the Sexual Functioning Questionnaire (SFQ) in a sample of 400 cancer survivors and their matched noncancer controls who were of the same gender, ethnicity, and within 5 years of age of the cancer survivors.[7] The questions were based on the Brief Index of Sexual Functioning for Women.[46] The initial form of the SFQ was tested with 200 HSCT recipients before and after their treatment. The instrument was revised to delete items that did not load on any factor and to add items that participants had written in the open-ended questions. In its final form, the SFQ is a gender-specific measure with 30 items. It has 9 subscales and 2 overall scores (overall SFQ score and SFQ treatment impact). The 9 subscales correspond to the sexual response cycle plus specific sexual behaviors or difficulties are as follows: interest, desire, arousal, orgasm, satisfaction, masturbation, relationship, activity, and problems.

The SFQ asks about sexual practices in the past month. The measure does not depend on the participant having a partner, the sexual orientation of the participant, or the medical condition of the respondent. However, there is a treatment-impact scale that can be scored separately so that the impact of specific treatments on sexuality can be assessed. Principal components analyses were conducted separately for men and women. No item factor loading differences were found by gender; therefore for the final factor analysis both males and females were combined. Factor loadings for each item were above 0.5. Reliabilities were above 0.8 for each of the subscales and for the total score. There was also high test-retest reliability when comparing pre and posttransplant. The SFQ had very good psychometric properties as evidenced by the reliabilities and validation confirmed with content, construct, and criterion validity. Discriminant validity was also established with the ability of the measure to distinguish between survivors and controls.

With the National Institutes of Health and the Patient-Reported Outcomes Measurement System Network,[47] there is a unique opportunity to have an item bank specifically for sexual functioning. Measures for fatigue, distress, pain, social function, and physical function have already been developed through the Patient-Reported Outcomes Measurement System initiative. A sexual function item bank will be available in the near future for use. An additional need in this area is to validate a measure for same sex couples as the work to date has been primarily with heterosexual couples.[41]

## EVIDENCE ON SEXUALITY AFTER HSCT

Lower sexual activity and satisfaction after HSCT in comparison with the time before transplantation or relative to the general population is a consistent finding across time points after HSCT, and across ages at time of transplantation, in both prospective longitudinal and cohort comparison studies.[5,8,22,33,48–53] Numerous cross-sectional studies have documented declines in sexual satisfaction and functioning of HSCT survivors.[3,5,33] Survivors of both genders report a loss of sexual desire.[54] Nonetheless, reported rates of sexual satisfaction vary quite widely perhaps because of different measures used or adequacy of sampling. As few as 22% of participants have reported sexual dissatisfaction,[33] whereas in most studies half or more of the participants report dissatisfaction.[53,55] Few studies have continued to followed HCST survivors long term to assess their sexual functioning after full recovery. However, decrements in sexual

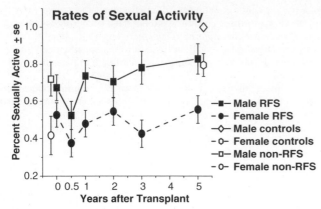

**FIGURE 2.**    Percent of males and females who were sexually active, among responding relapse-free-survivors (RFS) from before transplant (N = 109) to 5 years after transplant (N = 80). Rates are also graphed for non-RFS patients before transplant (N = 49) and controls at 5 years (N = 77). Both males and females declined in rates of being sexually active from pretransplant to 6 months ($P = 0.05$). On average, males improved compared with 6 month levels by 1 year ($P = 0.02$); females improved by 2 years ($P = 0.03$), but both remained below their respective controls at 5 years.

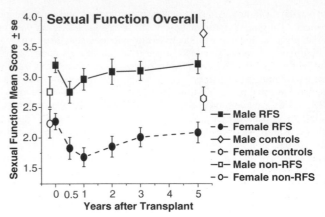

**FIGURE 3.**    Sexual function means for responding male and female relapse-free-survivors (RFS) from before transplant (N = 109) to 5 years after transplant (N = 80), measured on the same scale, though with different problem items content. Means are also graphed for non-RFS patients before transplant (N = 49) and controls at 5 years (N = 77). Both males and females declined in average sexual function from pretransplant to 6 months ($P < 0.01$). Females did not improve from 6-month posttransplant levels by 5 years ($P = 0.17$) and remained below matched controls ($P = 0.03$). Males improved by 2 years ($P = 0.02$), but remained below their respective controls at 5 years ($P = 0.01$).

functioning have been found in long-term survivors past 5 years after treatment.[4]

Since differences, both in problem rates and satisfaction, are marked between males and females it is necessary to consider effects on these survivors separately. Before HSCT, 42% of females and 14% of males report 1 or more sexual problems compared with 17% to 35% of the general population of females and up to 19% of males.[5] By 3 years after HSCT, the prevalence of problems increases to 80% of females and 29% of males. Also by 3 years posttransplant, a majority of women report difficulties with lubrication and desire, whereas the most prevalent problems for men include obtaining and maintaining erections and desire.[5,25,55–57]

In a 5 year prospective, longitudinal examination of sexual functioning, almost 20% of women between 6 months and 5 years reported a lack of interest, whereas lack of interest for men decreased from 14% at 6 months after treatment to 6% after 5 years.[4] As indicated by our research (Fig. 2), men and women who had relapse-free survival were able to recover their sexual activity to their pretreatment levels but remained lower than controls at 5 years.[4] Women continued to have lower rates of sexual activity than men across time, and at all times over 40% of female HSCT survivors were sexually inactive. A similar picture emerges for the quality of overall sexual functioning, as can be seen in Figure 3. In general, women report more problems than men do,[22,30] and men report higher levels of sexual satisfaction than women.[26] However, both males and females generally note that their difficulties are not in their sexual relationships but rather with desire and specific sexual problems.

Because of the high levels of ovarian failure in women who had HSCT, it is common for women to experience menopausal symptoms. For example, vaginal dryness is highly prevalent and this can make intercourse uncomfortable.[5,10,28,55] Women also report pain[58] during intercourse and, less often, bleeding after intercourse.[28] An-

other problem for women that seems to increase with time is the ability to achieve an orgasm.[5]

These findings to date with HSCT survivors highlight that, while physical and emotional functioning may return to normal with the passage of time for most survivors,[3,59] sexual functioning does not follow a similar trajectory.[4,57] A finding that highlights the importance of assessing sexual functioning early after treatment is that, for women in particular, if sexual activity has not returned by 1 year, these problems can persist for 5 years and possibly indefinitely.[5] Our research also highlights that if women are not taking HRT by 1 year, their sexual problems are more likely to continue.

## RISK FACTORS FOR SEXUAL DYSFUNCTION AFTER HSCT

Other than gender, few clear risk factors for poorer sexual function have been identified. In part, this is because these difficulties are so prevalent and most treatments have some impact on sexual problems. Men and women are at risk for enduring sexual problems, regardless of the type of transplant received.[6] Age is also a variable to consider, as younger women and those who are premenopausal before transplant report more problems with lubrication and other menopausal symptoms.[5] Other risk factors for women include initiation of hormone therapy after 1 year posttransplantation, being premenopausal before transplant and chronic GVHD. For men risk factors include older age, chronic GVHD, and psychologic function before HSCT.[5,7,22] Prospective cohort studies indicate that hormone therapy with oral estrogen improves or prevents more serious decline in sexual function in women after HSCT, but does not eliminate problems.[5,19,26]

## RELATED ISSUES: SEXUAL RELATIONSHIPS AND OTHER UNDERLYING ISSUES

Clearly, most sex does not happen in a relationship vacuum and most people prefer to have sex with another person. A partner's needs and responses are relevant in determining both participants' sexual satisfaction. Numerous relationship issues after HSCT can disrupt the psychologic responsiveness of 1 or both partners.

Preoccupation with health-focused tasks or worry by a partner, or a change in relationship balance, will potentially influence the couple's intimacy and, in turn, their sexual interest and responsiveness to sexual signals or approaches. Two aspects of this balance that are predictable after HSCT include the issue of infertility and the changes in roles. Any couple or individual who does not yet have children at the time of transplantation can be expected to have concerns about how they will manage infertility.[60] Our research has documented that these concerns do not resolve with time and take active discussion and problem solving by couples. Role changes caused by a patient's focus on survival and the need for a spouse to move into a caregiving position in the relationship can inhibit return to sexual activity. In addition, survivors and spouses may engage in protective buffering[61] and not express sexual interests or concerns about infertility issues for fear of upsetting or burdening their partner.

For single individuals, the issues can be somewhat different than for those who are in a stable couple relationship. It can be difficult to explain to a new partner, or partners, the effects of chemotherapy and/or chronic GVHD on genital tissues and sexual responsiveness. This is especially true for young women who may be prematurely postmenopausal or young men whose erections are not as firm as expected. Guidance in raising these issues with new dating situations can be helpful for young adults especially, who may avoid relationships out of fear of not meeting their partner's expectations for sexual behavior.

## MEDICAL TREATMENT OPTIONS

Medical treatments exist for the treatment of sexual dysfunction. However, health care professionals are usually untrained to have the relevant discussions needed to appropriately prescribe care.[38] Training of these health care providers is needed to improve outcomes in sexual function for HSCT and other cancer survivors. Patients need careful assessment and discussion of their sexual functioning before the initiation of chemotherapy, not only when problems are entrenched.[23] This can prepare patients and partners for the sexual changes that are common and can initiate a discussion of potential treatment options. Further, it alerts patients and partners of the need to plan for and act on their return to sexual activity before years pass. For both men and women, randomized controlled trials need to be conducted to determine which biologic treatments are efficacious and safe.

If a woman is premenopausal, discussion of hormone therapy options is needed so that these can begin as soon after transplant as medically safe. The risks and benefits of hormone therapy need to be discussed, along with a plan for when hormone therapy would be discontinued and under what conditions. In a nonrandomized study of younger women who did versus did not take hormone therapy, taking hormones did not effect chronic GVHD in allogeneic survivors.[19] Nonetheless, hormone therapy would not be an option for women with elevated risks for hormone-sensitive tumors or those who have chronic GVHD of the liver.[5,12] Hormone therapy will sometimes restore ovarian function[62] and not just alleviate symptoms. A study that assessed the relationship between hormones and sexual functioning found that women still experienced sexual dissatisfaction while taking estrogen therapy.[26] This could be because of the reduced effectiveness of the hormones because of decreased absorption in the intestinal tract.[12] Testosterone therapy has been thought to increase sexual libido, but was not found to do so in a group of female cancer survivors who were not also on estrogen therapy.[63] Randomized controlled trials have yet to be conducted on the efficacy of hormones for sexual dysfunction in women after HSCT, and more research is needed on the risk-benefit ratio of hormone therapy to be able to recommend this option with appropriate safety and efficacy qualifications. Still the abnormal and premature cessation of endogenous hormones for a young adult female is equally untested for consequences, safety and efficacy. In short, a balance of empirical testing of hormones and thoughtful weighting of risks and benefits for the individual is the best recommendation possible at this point.

Women may find topical estrogen to be helpful in the treatment of vaginal dryness or constriction, and for women who have vaginal or vulva chronic GVHD, topical cyclosporine may be another treatment to consider.[28] Some women use vaginal dilators to reduce constriction and sensitivity to penile penetration. In more extreme cases, women with vaginal stenosis may need surgery.[28,29] However, the use of estrogen creams or dilators may obviate the need for surgery to correct stenosis. The research in this area has small sample sizes and, possibly for that reason, data are conflicting. One study has described the use of topical estrogen as helpful in relieving chronic GVHD symptoms,[28] and another found it ineffective.[29]

Male sexual problems center on libido and erectile dysfunction.[56] Results from a small case series of 8 patients, 6 months after HSCT, suggested that testosterone injections and sildenafil 1 to 2 times per week improved sexual performance for men with erectile dysfunction, low libido, and ejaculatory disorders.[56] However, other data indicate that most males recover testosterone levels and sexual function between 6 months and 1 year after transplantation.[64] Thus without controlled clinical trials, it is unclear whether sexual function in the treated men would have recovered without treatment so caution is needed when interpreting the results and in applying them in practice. If medications do not work, men can consider external vacuum devices or penile implants, but very few elect mechanical solutions to erectile problems.[65,66]

A drug that has shown promise in treating ED in men and lack of arousal in women is a class of drugs called melanocortins.[67] Bremelanotide, a type of drug in this class, has been used in healthy men and was found to be effective in treating ED. This drug may have a safer profile than that of sildenafil because melanocortins can be used in conjunction with nitrates, which is not the case for sildenafil and other drugs like it. In women, bremelanotide has been associated with increases in self-reported arousal. More research needs to be done with melanocortins and to also test the drug in a group of cancer survivors as the samples to date have used healthy people.

As noted earlier, sexuality involves both biologic and psychologic responses. Although medical factors and medications may inhibit sexual response, the cognitive and psychologic responses to these biologic factors will have a major impact on sexual satisfaction. As a major component of this psychologic response, relationship quality and the response of a partner to the physiologic changes after transplant will positively or negatively affect sexual functioning.[22,54]

## BEHAVIORAL TREATMENT OPTIONS

A majority of sexual changes after HSCT are managed with behavioral strategies and, for women, topical agents or devices rather than medical treatment. A combination of approaches is likely to be most effective, utilizing education, hormone evaluation, hormone therapy where indicated, topical or behavioral strategies, and couples intervention. No study has tested this combination of therapies to address sexual dysfunction after HSCT.

A few interventions that are likely applicable to HSCT survivors have been tested with other cancer populations. Robinson et al[68] used a group intervention for women who were diagnosed with gynecologic cancer and were treated with radiation therapy. Women were randomized to 1 of 2 groups as follows: an intervention that included education about how to use lubricants and vaginal dilators or a control group. The intervention group consisted of two 1.5-hour group sessions. Women were informed about sexuality and cancer, encouraged to talk about their fears, and educated about the use of dilators and lubricants. Women in the control condition met with a counselor and were given a book on sexuality. Women of all ages reported a decrease in the fear of sexual activity, and women under the age of 50 in the experimental group were more adherent to the recommendations regarding the use of lubricants and dilators than were older women. This trial is a promising start in testing strategies to teach women how return to sexuality after treatment but also demonstrates that compliance is an issue with behavioral treatment recommendations. Behavioral treatments after breast cancer have also demonstrated improvements in sexual functioning. Scott et al[69] tested a couple-based intervention for patients who were diagnosed with either early stage breast or gynecologic cancers. The couple-based intervention was more effective at improving sexual adjustment than an individually-based intervention. A major strength of this study was the use of pre- and post-test measurements, along with a 1 year follow-up. Although the findings are promising, these interventions need to be tested with HSCT survivors.

Although traditional sex therapy such as sensate focus treatment[70] and medications are available to treat sexual dysfunction, there are other important issues to consider. After cancer and HSCT, in our clinical practice we find that a communication and intimacy-based approach is remarkably effective for many couples in facilitating return to satisfying sexual activity. In addition to addressing fears and overcoming avoidance, we encourage gradual reintroduction of sexual activity beginning with scheduling of time for "dating" and intimacy without intercourse. Even 1 or 2 couples counseling sessions focused on communication around appearance, fears or barriers, and changes in sensation can facilitate readiness to engage in intimacy and return to sexual practice. Because vaginal dryness is so common, we recommend lubricants for all women after HSCT until experience informs them whether continued use of lubricants is needed. When avoidance, fear or negative experiences have added to sexual problems, we urge women alone or couples to try vibrators and dilators until they are comfortable with their physical responses. Helping couples to decide on hand signals or other brief communication cues can facilitate their feeling safe to try sexual activity after a long period of abstinence and numerous psychologic and physical adjustments.

Depression or fear, fatigue, loss of muscle mass, antidepressant use or other medications that impact libido and arousal, as well as relationship conflict are just a few factors that need to be assessed when considering behavioral approaches to sexual dysfunction.[54] When deciding on treatment strategies, it is important to consider the multiple pathways to sexual dysfunction along with the many ways that people can increase their sexual satisfaction beyond traditional intercourse. For most people this involves a gradual return to intercourse with a partner, but not infrequently, full erections, orgasm or sexual responsiveness are not achieved at the same level as before diagnosis.

Nonetheless many survivors find satisfaction from renewed intimacy and sexual function that is rewarding if not fully at the level they would wish for.

## DEFICITS IN RESEARCH ON UNDERSTANDING AND TREATING SEXUAL DYSFUNCTION AFTER HSCT

Although we know from survey and longitudinal research that sexuality is a major concern for many HSCT survivors, there are gaps in the research that need to be filled. Much of the research has been conducted with white, heterosexual, middle or upper economic class couples. Little is known about the sexual functioning, needs or concerns of people who are not in committed relationships, have cultural or other differences from the usual research samples, or are in same sex relationships. In addition, little is known about HSCT survivors who are sexually inactive for many years after treatment. We do not yet know much about the sexual outcomes of survivors who received reduced intensity chemotherapies followed by HSCT. Although descriptive studies have been recently published, mechanism and treatment studies are severely lacking. The need for studies of treatment in this area cannot be overstated given the prevalence of problems, the conflicting or uncertain data from those outcomes that are published, and the questions of safety for some of the hormonal treatments frequently described.

## CONCLUSIONS

As more people survive cancer and its associated treatments, it becomes imperative to monitor survivors for long-term and late effects. This is especially the case for sexual function after HSCT. These generally young adult survivors have typically undergone high-dose treatments to cure their malignancies, and sexual dysfunction is one of the most prevalent long-term complications of treatment. Survivors and their partners should be assessed for their sexual functioning before treatment, so that any changes may be tracked over time and the appropriate treatment recommendations can be made. Although medical and behavioral treatments similar to those used in other populations who experience dramatic changes in sexual response can be used, the safety and efficacy of these treatments in the long-term HSCT survivor population remains to be tested and documented.

## ACKNOWLEDGMENTS

*The authors thank Allison Stover for her assistance with manuscript preparation.*

### REFERENCES

1. Socie G, Stone JV, Wingard JR, et al. Long-term survival and late deaths after allogeneic bone marrow transplantation: late effects working committee of the international bone marrow transplant registry. *NEJM.* 1999;341:14–21.
2. Syrjala KL, Martin P, Deeg J, et al. Medical and psychosocial issues in transplant survivors. In: Chang AE, Ganz PA, Hayes DF, et al, eds. *Oncology: An Evidence-Based Approach.* New York, NY: Springer Science + Business Media, Inc., 2006:1902–1928.
3. Syrjala KL, Langer SL, Abrams JR, et al. Late effects of hematopoietic cell transplantation among 10-year adult survivors compared with case-matched controls. *J Clin Oncol.* 2005;23:6596–6606.
4. Syrjala KL, Kurland BF, Abrams JR, et al. Sexual function changes during the 5 years after high-dose treatment and hematopoietic cell transplantation for malignancy, with case-matched controls at 5 years. *Blood.* 2008;111:989–996.
5. Syrjala KL, Roth-Roemer SL, Abrams JR, et al. Prevalence and predictors of sexual dysfunction in long-term survivors of marrow transplantation. *J Clin Oncol.* 1998;16:3148–3157.
6. Lee SJ, Fairclough D, Parsons SK, et al. Recovery after stem-cell transplantation for hematologic diseases. *J Clin Oncol.* 2001;19:242–252.

7. Syrjala KL, Schroeder TC, Abrams JR, et al. Sexual function measurement and outcomes in cancer survivors and matched controls. *J Sex Res.* 2000;37:213–225.

8. Andrykowski MA, Bishop MM, Hahn EA, et al. Long-term health-related quality of life, growth, and spiritual well-being after hematopoietic stem-cell transplantation. *J Clin Oncol.* 2005;23:599–608.

9. Schover LR, Schain WS, Montague DK. Sexual problems of patients with cancer. In: DeVita V, Hellman S, Rosenberg SA, eds. *Principles and Practice of Oncology.* 3rd ed. Philadelphia, Pennsylvania: J.B. Lippincott; 1989:2206–2225.

10. Cust MP, Whitehead MI, Powles R, et al. Consequences and treatment of ovarian failure after total body irradiation for leukemia. *Br Med J.* 1989;299:1494–1497.

11. Lee SJ, Schover LR, Partridge AH, et al. American Society of Clinical Oncology recommendations on fertility preservation in cancer patients. *J Clin Oncol.* 2006;24:2917–2931.

12. Tauchmanova L, Selleri C, Rosa GD, et al. High prevalence of endocrine dysfunction in long-term survivors after allogeneic bone marrow transplantation for hematologic diseases. *Cancer.* 2002;95:1076–1084.

13. Apperley JF, Reddy N. Mechanism and management of treatment-related gonadal failure in recipients of high dose chemoradiotherapy [review]. *Blood Rev.* 1995;9:93–116.

14. Sanders JE, Buckner CD, Leonard JM, et al. Late effects on gonadal function of cyclophosphamide, total-body irradiation, and marrow transplantation. *Transplantation.* 1983;36:252–255.

15. Kauppila M, Koskinen P, Irjala K, et al. Long-term effects of allogeneic bone marrow transplantation [BMT] on pituitary, gonad, thyroid and adrenal function in adults. *Bone Marrow Transplant.* 1998;22:331–337.

16. Schubert MA, Sullivan KM, Schubert MM, et al. Gynecological abnormalities following allogeneic bone marrow transplantation. *Bone Marrow Transplant.* 1990;5:425–430.

17. Chatterjee R, Kottaridis PD, McGarrigle HH, et al. Management of erectile dysfunction by combination therapy with testosterone and sildenafil in recipients of high-dose therapy for haematological malignancies. *Bone Marrow Transplant.* 2002;29:607–610.

18. Heaton RK, Grant I, Matthews CG. *Comprehensive Norms For an Expanded Halstead-Reitan Battery.* Odessa, FL: Psychological Assessment Resources, Inc.; 1992.

19. Balleari E, Garre S, van Lint MT, et al. Hormone replacement therapy and chronic graft-versus-host disease activity in women treated with bone marrow transplantation for hematologic malignancies. *Ann N Y Acad Sci.* 2002;966:187–192.

20. Chatterjee R, Kottaridis PD. Treatment of gonadal damage in recipients of allogeneic or autologous transplantation for haematological malignancies. *Bone Marrow Transplant.* 2002;30:629–635.

21. Monti M, Rosti G, De Giorgi U, et al. Sexual functions after high-dose chemotherapy in survivors of germ cell tumors. *Bone Marrow Transplant.* 2003;32:933–939.

22. Watson M, Wheatley K, Harrison GA, et al. Severe adverse impact on sexual functioning and fertility of bone marrow transplantation, either allogeneic or autologous, compared with consolidation chemotherapy alone: analysis of the MRC AML 10 trial. *Cancer.* 1999;86:1231–1239.

23. Socie G, Salooja N, Cohen A, et al. Nonmalignant late effects after allogeneic stem cell transplantation. *Blood.* 2003;101:3373–3385.

24. Shadiack AM, Sharma SD, Earle DC, et al. Melanocortins in the treatment of male and female sexual dysfunction [review]. *Curr Top Med Chem.* 2007;7:1137–1144.

25. Baruch J, Benjamin S, Treleaven J, et al. Male sexual function following bone marrow transplantation. *Bone Marrow Transplant.* 1991;7(suppl 2):52.

26. Heinonen H, Volin L, Uutela A, et al. Gender-associated differences in the quality of life after allogeneic BMT. *Bone Marrow Transplant.* 2001;28:503–509.

27. Hayes EC, Rock JA. Treatment of vaginal agglutination associated with chronic graft-versus-host disease. *Fertil Steril.* 2002;78:1125–1126.

28. Spiryda LB, Laufer MR, Soiffer RJ, et al. Graft-versus-host disease of the vulva and/or vagina: diagnosis and treatment. *Biol Blood Marrow Transplant.* 2003;9:760–765.

29. Spinelli S, Chiodi S, Costantini S, et al. Female genital tract graft-versus-host disease following allogeneic bone marrow transplantation. *Haematologica.* 2003;88:1163–1168.

30. Humphreys CT, Tallman B, Altmaier EM, et al. Sexual functioning in patients undergoing bone marrow transplantation: a longitudinal study. *Bone Marrow Transplant.* 2007;39:491–496.

31. Couriel D, Carpenter PA, Cutler C, et al. Ancillary therapy and supportive care of chronic graft-versus-host disease: national institutes of health consensus development project on criteria for clinical trials in chronic graft-versus-host

32. Mumma GH, Mashberg D, Lesko LM. Long-term psychosexual adjustment of acute leukemia survivors: impact of marrow transplantation versus conventional chemotherapy. *Gen Hosp Psychiatry.* 1992;14:43–55.

33. Wingard JR, Curbow B, Baker F, et al. Sexual satisfaction in survivors of bone marrow transplantation. *Bone Marrow Transplant.* 1992;9:185–190.

34. Laumann EO, Paik A, Rosen RC. Sexual dysfunction in the United States: prevalence and predictors. *JAMA.* 1999;281:537–544.

35. Andersen BL. Surviving cancer: the importance of sexual self-concept. *Med Pediatr Oncol.* 1999;33:15–23.

36. Marks DI, Friedman SH, Carpini LD, et al. A prospective study of the effects of high-dose chemotherapy and bone marrow transplantation on sexual function in the first year after transplant. *Bone Marrow Transplant.* 1997;19:819–822.

37. Stead ML, Brown JM, Fallowfield L, et al. Lack of communication between healthcare professionals and women with ovarian cancer about sexual issues. *Br J Cancer.* 2003;88:666–671.

38. Vadaparampil S, Quinn G, King L, et al. Barriers to fertility preservation among pediatric oncologists. *Patient Educ Couns.* 2008;72:402–410.

39. Hordern AJ, Street AF. Communicating about patient sexuality and intimacy after cancer: mismatched expectations and unmet needs. *Med J Aust.* 2007;186:224–227.

40. Corona G, Jannini EA, Maggi M. Inventories for male and female sexual dysfunctions [review]. *Int J Impot Res.* 2006;18:236–250.

41. Arrington R, Cofrancesco J, Wu AW. Questionnaires to measure sexual quality of life [review]. *Qual Life Res.* 2004;13:1643–1658.

42. Jensen PT, Klee MC, Thranov I, et al. Validation of a questionnaire for self-assessment of sexual function and vaginal changes after gynaecological cancer. *Psychooncology.* 2004;13:577–592.

43. Bransfield D, Horiot JC, Nabid A. Development of a scale for assessing sexual function after treatment for gynecologic cancer. *J Psychosoc Oncol.* 1984;2:3–19.

44. Wei JT, Dunn RL, Litwin MS, et al. Development and validation of the expanded prostate cancer index composite (EPIC) for comprehensive assessment of health-related quality of life in men with prostate cancer. *Urology.* 2000;56:899–905.

45. Litwin MS, Hays RD, Fink A, et al. The UCLA Prostate Cancer Index: development, reliability, and validity of a health-related quality of life measure. *Med Care.* 1998;36:1002–1012.

46. Taylor JF, Rosen RC, Leiblum SR. Self-report assessment of female sexual function: psychometric evaluation of the brief index of sexual functioning for women. *Arch Sex Behav.* 1994;23:627–643.

47. Garcia SF, Cella D, Clauser SB, et al. Standardizing patient-reported outcomes assessment in cancer clinical trials: a patient-reported outcomes measurement information system initiative [review]. *J Clin Oncol.* 2007;25:5106–5112.

48. Bush NE, Donaldson GW, Haberman MH, et al. Conditional and unconditional estimation of multidimensional quality of life after hematopoietic stem cell transplantation: a longitudinal follow-up of 415 patients. *Biol Blood Marrow Transplant.* 2000;6:576–591.

49. Zittoun R, Suciu S, Watson M, et al. Quality of life in patients with acute myelogenous leukemia in prolonged first complete remission after bone marrow transplantation [allogeneic or autologous] or chemotherapy: a cross—sectional study of the EORTC—GIMEMA AML 8 A trial. *Bone Marrow Transplant.* 1997;20:307–315.

50. Chiodi S, Spinelli S, Ravera G, et al. Quality of life in 244 recipients of allogeneic bone marrow transplantation. *Br J Haematol.* 2000;110:614–619.

51. Howell SJ, Radford JA, Smets EM, et al. Fatigue, sexual function and mood following treatment for haematological malignancy: the impact of mild Leydig cell dysfunction. *Br J Cancer.* 2000;82:789–793.

52. Schimmer AD, Ali V, Stewart AK, et al. Male sexual function after autologous blood or marrow transplantation. *Biol Blood Marrow Transplant.* 2001;7:279–283.

53. Molassiotis A, van den Akker OB, Milligan DW, et al. Gonadal function and psychosexual adjustment in male long-term survivors of bone marrow transplantation. *Bone Marrow Transplant.* 1995;16:253–259.

54. Schover L. Reproductive complications and sexual dysfunction in cancer survivors. In: Ganz P, ed. *Cancer Survivorship: Today and Tomorrow.* New York: Springer; 2007:251–271.

55. Claessens JJ, Beerendonk CC, Schattenberg AV. Quality of life, reproduction and sexuality after stem cell transplantation with partially T-cell-depleted grafts and after conditioning with a regimen including total body irradiation. *Bone Marrow Transplant.* 2006;37:831–836.

56. Chatterjee R, Kottaridis PD, McGarrigle HH, et al. Patterns of Leydig cell insufficiency in adult males following bone marrow transplantation for haematological malignancies. *Bone Marrow Transplant.* 2001;28:497–502.

57. Schover LR. Sexuality and fertility after cancer. *Hematology*. 2005;523–527.

58. Winer EP, Lindley C, Hardee M, et al. Quality of life in patients surviving at least 12 months following high dose chemotherapy with autologous bone marrow support. *Psychooncology*. 1999;8:167–176.

59. Syrjala KL, Langer SL, Abrams JR, et al. Recovery and long-term function after hematopoietic cell transplantation for leukemia or lymphoma. *JAMA*. 2004;291:2335–2343.

60. Hammond C, Abrams JR, Syrjala KL. Fertility and risk factors for elevated infertility concern in 10-year hematopoietic cell transplant survivors and case-matched controls. *J Clin Oncol*. 2007;25:3511–3517.

61. Langer SL, Rudd ME, Syrjala KL. Protective buffering and emotional desynchrony among spousal caregivers of cancer patients. *Health Psychol*. 2007;26:635–643.

62. Liu J, Malhotra R, Voltarelli J, et al. Ovarian recovery after stem cell transplantation. *Bone Marrow Transplant*. 2008;41:275–278.

63. Barton DL, Wender DB, Sloan JA, et al. Randomized controlled trial to evaluate transdermal testosterone in female cancer survivors with decreased libido. *J Natl Cancer Inst*. 2007;99:672–679.

64. Kauppila M, Viikari J, Irjala K, et al. The hypothalamus-pituitary-gonad axis and testicular function in male patients after treatment for haematological malignancies. *J Intern Med*. 1998;244:411–416.

65. Glasgow M, Halfin V, Althausen AF. Sexual response and cancer. *CA Cancer J Clin*. 1987;37:322–333.

66. Miller DC, Wei JT, Dunn RL, et al. Use of medications or devices for erectile dysfunction among long-term prostate cancer treatment survivors: potential influence of sexual motivation and/or indifference. *Urology*. 2006;68:166–171.

67. Schover LR. Premature ovarian failure and its consequences: vasomotor symptoms, sexuality, and fertility [review]. *J Clin Oncol*. 2008;26:753–758.

68. Robinson JW, Faris PD, Scott CB. Psychoeducational group increases vaginal dilation for younger women and reduces sexual fears for women of all ages with gynecological carcinoma treated with radiotherapy. *Int J Radiat Oncol Biol Phys*. 1999;44:497–506.

69. Scott JL, Halford WK, Ward BG. United we stand? The effects of a couple-coping intervention on adjustment to early stage breast or gynecological cancer. *J Consult Clin Psychol*. 2004;72:1122–1135.

70. Masters WH, Johnson VE. Human sexual response. Boston, MA: Little, Brown, 1966.

# Sexual Functioning After Cancer in Sexual Minority Women

Ulrike Boehmer • Jennifer Potter • Deborah J. Bowen

Global and persistent sexual problems or sexual dysfunction have been documented in at least 50% of women treated for breast, colorectal, or gynecologic cancer.[1] Common presentations of sexual dysfunction include loss of sexual desire, difficulty feeling arousal and pleasure, decreased ability to achieve orgasm, pain, sexual inactivity, and sexual dissatisfaction.[2] These various dimensions of sexual dysfunction have been reviewed for different cancer sites, with breast cancer predominating[3-8] and have been studied in survivors who are diverse with respect to cancer stage or time since diagnosis and demographic factors, such as age.[9,10] Unlike other side effects of cancer and its treatment, sexual problems do not tend to resolve after several years of disease-free survival. Rather sexual problems persist and have been recognized as a long-term outcome that impacts the lives of survivors.[3,11-13]

The recent increase in research and information about the impact of cancer and its treatments on women's sexuality has been limited to heterosexual women or women who were assumed to be heterosexual as sexual orientation is generally not assessed in these studies. One author of a review article on sexuality and body image of breast cancer survivors noted, "the voices of homosexual women with cancer are missing from the literature."[4] Sexual minority women, defined here as women who identify as lesbian or bisexual women, or women who report a preference for a female partner, who receive a cancer diagnosis, are also at risk for suffering from sexual problems after cancer and its treatment. For this reason, we aim to review what is known about sexual minority women's sexual functioning after cancer, explore reasons why the sexual functioning of these women may differ from heterosexual women's, and point to critical areas that need further research attention.

## What Is Currently Known About the Sexual Functioning of Sexual Minority Women After Cancer?

A search of Medline and Psychinfo for articles on the postcancer sexual functioning of sexual minority women using the search terms, sexual orientation, lesbian, homosexuality, female, cancer, neoplasm, and sexual dysfunction yielded zero publications, pointing to a gap in knowledge. In the absence of published studies that focus explicitly on the sexual sequelae of cancer in sexual minority women, we report on unpublished data[14] and 2 published studies on sexual minority women with cancer that include measures of sexual functioning among their main outcome of psychological adaptation.[15,16] Each of these studies focused on breast cancer and compared SMW with heterosexual women. Fobair et al[16] compared 29 lesbians and 246 heterosexual women: participants had completed surgical treatment, but could still be in the process of undergoing adjuvant therapy. The authors' hypothesis that lesbians have fewer sexual problems was not confirmed, because their comparative analysis indicated no sig-

nificant differences in the frequency of sexual activity and sexual satisfaction between lesbian and heterosexual women. Among a subgroup of women who were not currently sexually active, lesbians were more likely than heterosexual women to indicate that they were not interested in sex.[16] The finding that lesbians do not differ from heterosexual women with respect to the frequency of sexual activity and sexual satisfaction was confirmed in a sample of lesbian and heterosexual women with DCIS or stage I or II breast cancer who were matched by age and time since diagnosis.[15] This study also found that lesbians reported less disruption in their sexual relationships after diagnosis and treatment compared with heterosexual women.[15] Our own analyses also revealed significant differences, with heterosexual women reporting more sexual problems than lesbians.[14] Specifically, heterosexual women reported greater difficulty with vaginal dryness and achieving orgasm than lesbians, whereas there were no significant differences between the groups on sexual interest or arousal.[14]

## What About Sexual Minority Women Without Cancer?

These limited findings on the sexual functioning of lesbians compared with heterosexual women raise larger questions about which aspects of sexual functioning are likely to differ between SMW and heterosexual women. Research on SMW who do not have cancer is helpful in addressing these questions. Studies of the general population corroborate the findings regarding frequency of sexual activity found in the aforementioned studies of women who have had cancer. In particular, the national probability sample of Laumann et al[17] concluded that there are no differences between women with same-sex and those with opposite-sex partners; 2 subsequent studies that compared community samples of lesbian and heterosexual women confirmed this finding.[18,19]

Few studies have assessed the qualitative dimensions of sexual functioning among sexual minority women. In 2 community samples comparing lesbians and heterosexual women, no differences were found with respect to the perceived importance of sex, frequency of achieving orgasm, or overall sexual satisfaction.[18,19] However, another study found that lesbian/bisexual women reported less problems with desire, arousal, and pleasure/orgasm compared with heterosexual women.[20] Given these contradictory results, it is clear that more research is needed to determine whether there are important differences between sexual minority and heterosexual women in qualitative aspects of sexual functioning.

## Why Do We Expect Differences in Sexual Functioning by Sexual Orientation?

The degree to which a woman experiences sexual difficulties after cancer depends on the cancer site and the extent to which she develops physical side effects related to the surgical and medical modalities used to treat the cancer. Not surprisingly, treatment for breast and gynecologic cancers impacts sexual functioning differently than cancers at anatomic sites unrelated to the genitalia and other erogenous zones. Chemotherapy and hormonal therapies used to treat cancer can also impact sexual functioning profoundly via endocrine, vascular, and neurologic systems involved in women's sexual response. At the purely biologic-physiological level, there is no reason to expect the bodies of SMW and heterosexual women to react any differently to insults caused by cancer therapies. Yet sexual problems likely result from an interaction between physiological, psychologic, and interpersonal factors.[3,14,20,21] That is, sexuality is about much more than the functional and genital ability to engage in sexual acts; rather, in addition to physical functionality, sexual satisfaction encompasses eroticism, pleasure, and intimacy.[22] It is within these psychologic and social explanatory factors that impact sexual functioning, including intimacy and pleasure on which sexual minority women are expected to differ from heterosexual women. In particular, evidence suggests differences in body image, psychologic well-being, and relationship-related issues between sexual minority and heterosexual women, which are psychosocial processes that have been consistently linked to sexual functioning.

## Body Image Might Be a Source of Disparities

A more positive body image is linked to better sexual functioning after breast cancer.[21] Cancer treatments, in particular surgical treatments such as gynecologic and breast surgery, cause changes in body image. Sexual orientation has an important impact on the body image of women with breast cancer. For example, lesbians reported fewer problems with their body image and were significantly more comfortable showing their body to others both before and after breast cancer and its treatments.[16] Similarly, Arena et al[15] found that lesbians had less concerns about their physical appearance compared with heterosexual women with breast cancer, yet they found no differences between these 2 groups in body integrity, which was measured using questions such as "When something goes wrong inside your body, you're never really the same person again." Another difference is the perceived importance ascribed to having breasts before a cancer diagnosis, in that heterosexual women endorse a greater value than lesbians.[14] Similarly, a qualitative study that focused on decision making about breast reconstruction after mastectomy in a group of SMW found that, regardless of whether they decided for or against reconstruction, participants prioritized a sense of wellbeing, defined by body strength, survival, and physical functioning, over normative beauty standards.[23] Another closely related factor that may further compound women's perceptions of their body image and appearance is weight gain, which is caused by receiving chemotherapy treatment for cancer.[24] Thus far, no studies have yet compared pre- and post-weight changes in SMW and heterosexual women. However, there is ample evidence of differences in weight by sexual orientation, indicating a higher prevalence of overweight and obesity among lesbians than all other female sexual orientation groups, that is, bisexual and heterosexual women.[25,26] Given this strong evidence, differences in weight after cancer, is likely another distinction between lesbian and heterosexual women.

## Mental Health Differences as a Possible Source of Disparities

A sizable group of cancer survivors suffer from depression, anxiety, and post-traumatic stress, despite being disease free,[27–29] These mental health problems have adverse effects on quality of life, including sexual functioning. Considerable research has established the existence of differences in mental health of lesbians compared with heterosexual women.[30,31] Lesbians experience, more acute mental health symptoms, a higher prevalence of generalized anxiety disorder, and a higher utilization of mental health services compared with their heterosexual counterparts.[32,33] One might therefore assume that cancer diagnosis and treatments would tend to exacerbate psychologic problems among SMW. Lesbian and heterosexual women do seem to differ significantly in their use of various coping styles. For example, lesbians have less fighting spirit[16] and lower perception of benefit finding from having cancer.[15] Despite these differences, studies to date have found that, overall, lesbian survivors do not differ from heterosexual women with respect to depression or level of emotional distress,[14–16] thereby refuting the hypothesis that lesbians with cancer have worse mental health outcomes than heterosexual women.

Subgroups of SMW who have had cancer may be more vulnerable to the effects of psychosocial stress. Two studies that examined sexual minority women with breast cancer without a heterosexual reference group[34,35] identified risk factors for poor psychologic outcomes. Both found no significant association between disclosure of sexual identity and distress. However, Mc Gregor et al[34] found that internalized homophobia was associated with a higher level of distress in lesbians with breast cancer. Boehmer et al[35] studied a sample of SMW with breast cancer that included self-identified lesbians, self-identified bisexual women, and women who reported their sexual minority status as having a relationship with another woman, rather than embracing a sexual identity as lesbian or bisexual. In this study, women who reported partnering with women reported more cognitive avoidance coping compared with both lesbian and bisexual women. Furthermore, women who partnered with women experienced significantly greater distress compared with women who embraced a lesbian sexual identity.[35] Future studies are needed that link these explanatory factors of distress to sexual functioning after cancer. To date, internalized homophobia has been linked to sexual satisfaction among lesbian and bisexual women, yet only in a sample without cancer.[20]

## Relationship Structure and Function Might Explain Disparities in Sexual Functioning

Having a partner and relationship dynamics are inextricably linked to women's sexual functioning.[3,11,21] Studies point to differences between lesbian and heterosexual women with respect to partners. Fobair et al[16] found that lesbians were significantly more likely than heterosexual women to report that their partner made them feel loved and cared for, were willing to listen, and could be counted on to help with daily tasks. In contradistinction, Arena et al[15] found no differences between lesbians and heterosexual women with respect to overall relationship satisfaction or in reports of how much affection their partners demonstrated toward them, how bothered their partners were by their surgical scar, the extent to which their partners reacted to breast cancer as a threat to their life, or whether there was increased fighting or friction between the couple. Given these inconsistent findings, relationship dynamics will be an important issue for further studies.

In our earlier study of SMW with breast cancer, participants were asked to identify the most significant support person with respect to their breast cancer experience.[36] The majority (79%) named their partner; others identified friends or female relatives. In this sample, 77% of the women had a support person on whom to rely, and those who did were more likely to be partnered and to have a higher level of perceived social support compared with women who did not identify a support person.[36] Although subsequent analyses did not distinguish between support providers who were partners versus those who were friends or family members, survivors were more distressed if there was discordance between themselves and their support person in the level of disclosure of sexual orientation, in that the support provider was more open than the woman with breast cancer.[36] These results provide important insights into potentially problematic relationship issues that may occur among SMW with cancer. A qualitative study that focused on decision making about breast reconstruction among SMW concluded that partners played an important role in reaching and then supporting the decision made about breast reconstruction and suggested that the SMW with breast cancer had great confidence that their partner would love them regardless of their physical appearance after mastectomy.[23] Future studies are needed to more fully explore the roles and responses of partners, and how having a partner and the quality of the relationship affect sexual well-being of SMW.

## Medical Care Systems Might Be a Source of Disparities for Survivors

Another critical area of potential difference between sexual minority and heterosexual women is the role of medical professionals in providing information and support about sexual functioning. A review of studies that dealt with presumed heterosexual women's sexuality after cancer concluded that women lament that medical professionals are lacking in willingness to engage in frank and honest discussions about sexuality with their patients, which results in women's unresolved need for information about these issues and a perception of lacking support from medical professionals.[22] For example, in one study of 126 women with breast cancer,[7] the majority (87%) received no counseling regarding the potential impact of treatment on sexual function. All of the participants had sexuality issues they wanted to discuss with their provider; however, only one-third felt comfortable raising the issue themselves, and those who did do so felt that the response was inadequate. There is considerable evidence to support the notion that the problem of obtaining support and information about sexuality from medical providers is compounded for sexual minority women.

The relationship of sexual minority women with breast cancer is marked by apprehension: it has been suggested that providers do not inquire about the sexual orientation of their breast cancer patients but that patients chose between actively disclosing their sexual orientation or passively refusing disclosure.[37] From studies on women without cancer, we know that SMW are less likely than heterosexual women to raise sexual concerns spontaneously due to fear of negative consequences after they disclose their sexual orientation.[38] Compounding the problem, few providers (11%–37%) obtain comprehensive sexual histories routinely,[39] due to fear of being intrusive; ignorance regarding clinical relevance; lack of knowledge about what and how to ask; concern about how to respond to the information that is divulged; and time constraints. Consequently, many are unaware that they have SMW patients in their practice: some report reluctance to discuss sexual issues with this population due to lack of knowledge about specific sexual practices and embarrassment.[40]

SMW are extremely sensitive to nonverbal cues that signal acceptance.[41] Although clinicians may initially be reticent, skills can easily be developed to enhance the sensitivity with which physicians relate to SMW: research demonstrates that doing so enhances patient satisfaction among SMW with breast cancer.[42] Several simple measures can be used to create a welcoming environment, including a prominent display of a statement that the office does not discriminate on the basis of sexual orientation, use of an intake form that acknowledges the full range of sexual expression, and availability of pamphlets that address sex after cancer in a manner that does not assume the reader is heterosexual.[43] During the interview, it is best to use gender-neutral language, such as "Do you have a partner?" or "Are you in a relationship?" rather than "Do you have a boyfriend/husband?" As with heterosexual cancer survivors, the sexual history should begin by asking whether an SMW is sexually active, and, if so, with whom she is having sex, and whether and how cancer has affected the way she feels about herself as a woman, her relationship, and her sexual function. When sexual problems are reported, it is important to obtain specific information about the patient's satisfaction with her level of sexual interest, responsiveness (arousal), orgasmic capacity, and comfort during sexual activity. Questions posed should be free of heterosexual assumptions: for example, "Do you experience any discomfort during sexual activity?" is better than "Do you experience pain during intercourse?" For a complete discussion of the evaluation and management of sexual problems in female cancer survivors, the reader is referred to an excellent review article.[44]

## Where Do We Need to Go From Here? Recommendations for Clinicians and Researchers

Based on this review of the limited relevant literature on sexual functioning in sexual minority women with cancer a still rather incomplete picture emerges. This review points to the need for additional research to unanswered questions regarding to what extent, how, and why sexual functioning of sexual minority survivors differs from that of heterosexual women who have had cancer. Studies done to date indicate that there are some similarities and differences between these populations, and suggests tentatively that SMW may enjoy several advantages compared with heterosexual women. Areas of potential strengths of sexual minority women are less disruption in their sexual relationship, fewer sexual problems such as lubrication, achieving orgasm, better body image, and more understanding and supportive partners compared with heterosexual women.

However, there might be areas of disparity for sexual minority women as well. Areas of greater vulnerability and risk for sexual minority women survivors compared with heterosexual survivors consist of some maladaptive coping and problems obtaining information and support from medical professionals with respect to sexual functioning. In addition there are indications of unique factors for sexual minority women, such as internalized homophobia and discordance in disclosure about sexual orientation between women with breast cancer and their partners who may put SMW at risk for worse outcomes. However, these findings are preliminary and mostly derived from small convenience samples, indicating that central aspects of this topic remain unexplored.

## Methodological Issues for Future Research

Currently, there is little research that assesses the prevalence of sexual dysfunction in sexual minority women with cancer. Because of this, it is unknown whether the level of sexual dysfunction is higher or lower compared with heterosexual women. It may be that the true picture of disparity (or not) is mixed, but the current literature does not allow for such conclusions. In addition, among heterosexual women, we have an emerging body of literature that compares the sexual functioning of women with cancer to their peers, which are defined as the women in the general population. This raises the question about the appropriate reference group for sexual minority women. Most studies on this topic to date approached the sexual functioning of SMW by comparing these women with heterosexual women with the same type of cancer and who possibly share further similarities with respect to the time since diagnosis, stage of the disease, and age.[14–16] Another much needed approach for understanding these women's sexual functioning is to compare SMW with cancer and SMW without cancer. The argument for conducting case and control studies of SMW with and without cancer is the existence of greater similarity between these 2 groups, while considerable differences exist between heterosexual and SMW with respect to the gender of their sexual partner, the number of sex partners, their sexual practices, and their perception of happiness.[17] Therefore, comparing SMW and heterosexual female survivors may result in findings that are more influenced by the differences in sexual expression rather than explaining the impact of cancer on sexual minority women's sexual functioning. This is not to suggest that one approach replaces the other, rather both approaches are needed to more comprehensively assess sexual functioning in SMW survivors.

Another methodological issue for this field are the current measures that assess sexual functioning, all of which have been developed using a heterosexual or presumed heterosexual sample. A comprehensive review of the available measures of sexual functioning identified 57 instruments suitable to measure patients' perceptions.[45] The authors concluded that only 28% of these instruments could be used in homosexual patients. They noted a general lack of adequate testing for reliability and validity and more specifically a lack of testing among sexual minorities.[45] Many instruments of sexual functioning include questions about pain during intercourse. This question may be understood differently by sexual minority than heterosexual women. Furthermore, the frequency with SMW engage in penetrative vaginal sexual activities is not known. SMW who enjoy insertive vaginal and/or anal stimulation may use sex toys to achieve that stimulation. Research shows that lesbians are more likely to engage in autosexual activities,[46] suggesting the possibility of a different relevance of various dimensions of sexual functioning between sexual minority and heterosexual women. Greater comfort with self-stimulation may facilitate adjustment to a body that has been changed by cancer treatment, in that directed masturbation helps women become aware of the location and intensity of stimulation they need to increase sexual arousal and pleasure.[47] This calls for formative work about the meaning and importance of sexuality among sexual minorities to ensure that the assessment of sexual functioning in this population reflects the most crucial dimensions of sexual minorities' sexual expression.

## CONCLUSIONS

Areas for future research on this topic are not unlike the work that remains to be done to more fully understand sexual functioning among women with cancer in general. So far, studies have focused on the sexual functioning after breast cancer. Currently, no information is available on sexual minority women with other types of cancer. Schover's[3] review of sexual dysfunction after cancer laments the need for interventions that would prevent sexual dysfunction in cancer survivors and psychotherapeutic approaches to increase rehabilitation of sexual functioning after cancer and its treatment. Only one intervention study of lesbians with cancer has been conducted. The intervention consisted of a supportive–expressive group therapy, which showed no significant impact on sexuality.[48] As with so many areas of research, it is most desirable for future studies, including interventions, to consider sexual orientation as one factor to be specified, so study results on sexual functioning specify from which sexual orientation group they are derived and the development of interventions shall accommodate the perspectives of various sexual orientations, whenever possible or appropriate.

## REFERENCES

1. Schover LR. Sexuality and fertility after cancer. *Hematology.* 2005;2005:523–527.
2. Frank JE, Mistretta P, Will J. Diagnosis and treatment of female sexual dysfunction. *Am Fam Physician.* 2008;77:635–642.
3. Schover LR. Reduction of psychosexual dysfunction in cancer patients. In: Miller S, Bowen D, Croyle R, et al., eds. *Handbook of Behavior and Cancer.* Washington, DC: APA; 2008:379–389.
4. Pelusi J. Sexuality and body image. Research on breast cancer survivors documents altered body image and sexuality. *Am J Nurs.* 2006;106:32–38.
5. Krychman ML, Pereira L, Carter J, et al. Sexual oncology: sexual health issues in women with cancer. *Oncology.* 2006;71:18–25.
6. Bodurka DC, Sun CC. Sexual function after gynecologic cancer. *Obstet Gynecol Clin North Am.* 2006;33:621–630, ix.
7. Huber C, Ramnarace T, McCaffrey R. Sexuality and intimacy issues facing women with breast cancer. *Oncol Nurs Forum.* 2006;33:1163–1167.
8. Stead ML. Sexual dysfunction after treatment for gynaecologic and breast malignancies. *Curr Opin Obstet Gynecol.* 2003;15:57–61.
9. Andersen BL, Carpenter KM, Yang HC, et al. Sexual well-being among partnered women with breast cancer recurrence. *J Clin Oncol.* 2007;25:3151–3157.
10. Kornblith AB, Powell M, Regan MM, et al. Long-term psychosocial adjustment of older vs younger survivors of breast and endometrial cancer. *Psychooncology.* 2007;16:895–903.
11. Ganz PA, Rowland JH, Desmond K, et al. Life after breast cancer: understanding women's health-related quality of life and sexual functioning. *J Clin Oncol.* 1998;16:501–514.
12. Thors CL, Broeckel JA, Jacobsen PB. Sexual functioning in breast cancer survivors. *Cancer Control.* 2001;8:442–448.
13. Ganz PA. Psychological and social aspects of breast cancer. *Oncology (Williston Park).* 2008;22:642–646, 50; discussion 50, 53.
14. Matthews AK, Boehmer U. Biopsychosocial predictors of sexual dysfunction in a community sample of lesbian and heterosexual breast cancer survivors. In press.
15. Arena PL, Carver CS, Antoni MH, et al. Psychosocial responses to treatment for breast cancer among lesbian and heterosexual women. *Women Health.* 2006;44:81–102.
16. Fobair P, O'Hanlan K, Koopman C, et al. Comparison of lesbian and heterosexual women's response to newly diagnosed breast cancer. *Psychooncology.* 2001;10:40–51.
17. Laumann EO, Gagnon JH, Michael RT, et al. *The Social Organization of Sexuality. Sexual Practices in the United States.* Chicago: University of Chicago Press; 1994.
18. Matthews AK, Hughes T, Tartarto J. Sexual behavior and sexual dysfunction in a community sample of lesbian and heterosexual women. In: Omoto AM, Kurtzman HS, eds. *Sexual Orientation and Mental Health: Examining Identity and Development in Lesbian, Gay, and Bisexual People.* Washington, DC: American Psychological Association Books; 2005:185–206.
19. Matthews AK, Tartaro J, Hughes TL. A comparative study of lesbian and heterosexual women in committed relationships. *J Lesbian Stud.* 2003;7:101–114.
20. Henderson A, Lehavot K, Simoni J. Ecological models of sexual satisfaction among lesbian/bisexual and heterosexual women. *Arch Sex Behav.* In press.
21. Ganz PA, Desmond KA, Belin TR, et al. Predictors of sexual health in women after a breast cancer diagnosis. *J Clin Oncol.* 1999;17:2371–2380.
22. Hordern A. Intimacy and sexuality after cancer: a critical review of the literature. *Cancer Nurs.* 2008;31:E9–E17.
23. Boehmer U, Linde R, Freund KM. Breast reconstruction following mastectomy for breast cancer: the decisions of sexual minority women. *Plast Reconstr Surg.* 2007;119:464–472.
24. Wilmoth MC, Coleman EA, Smith SC, et al. Fatigue, weight gain, and altered sexuality in patients with breast cancer: exploration of a symptom cluster. *Oncol Nurs Forum.* 2004;31:1069–1075.
25. Boehmer U, Bowen DJ, Bauer GR. Overweight and obesity in sexual minority women: evidence from population-based data. *Am J Public Health.* 2007;97:1134–1140.
26. Bowen DJ, Balsam KF, Ender SR. A review of obesity issues in sexual minority women. *Obesity (Silver Spring).* 2008;16:221–228.
27. Institute of Medicine, ed. *From Cancer Patient to Cancer Survivor: Lost in Transition.* Washington, DC: Committee on Cancer Survivorship: Improving Care and Quality of Life, Institute of Medicine and National Research Council; 2006.
28. National Institute of Mental Health (NIMH). *Depression and cancer.* National Institutes of Health, U.S. Department of Health and Human Services; 2002.
29. Simon A, Palmer S, Coyne J. Cancer and depression. In: Steptoe A, ed. *Depression and Physical Illness.* Cambridge: Cambridge University Press; 2006.
30. Kerr SK, Emerson AM. A review of lesbian depression and anxiety. *J Psychol Human Sex.* 2004;15:143–162.
31. Oetjen H, Rothblum ED. When lesbians aren't gay: factors affecting depression among lesbians. *J Homosex.* 2000;39:49–73.
32. Cochran SD, Mays VM, Sullivan JG. Prevalence of mental disorders, psychological distress, and mental health services use among lesbian, gay, and bisexual adults in the United States. *J Consult Clin Psychol.* 2003;71:53–61.

33. Sandfort TG, Bakker F, Schellevis FG, et al. Sexual orientation and mental and physical health status: findings from a Dutch population survey. *Am J Public Health.* 2006;96:1119–1125.

34. McGregor BA, Carver CS, Antoni MH, et al. Distress and internalized homophobia among lesbian women treated for early stage breast cancer. *Psychol Women Quart.* 2001;25:1–9.

35. Boehmer U, Linde R, Freund KM. Sexual minority women's coping and psychological adjustment after a diagnosis of breast cancer. *J Women's Health.* 2005;14:214–224.

36. Boehmer U, Freund KM, Linde R. Support providers of sexual minority women with breast cancer: who they are and how they impact the breast cancer experience. *J Psychosom Res.* 2005;59:307–314.

37. Boehmer U, Case P. Physicians don't ask, some patients tell: disclosure of sexual orientation among women with breast cancer. *Cancer.* 2004;101:1882–1889.

38. Eliason MJ, Schope R. "Don't ask don't tell" Apply to health care? Lesbian, gay, and bisexual people's disclosure to health care providers. *J Gay Lesbian Med Assoc.* 2001;5:125–134.

39. Diamant AL, Wold C, Spritzer K, et al. Health behaviors, health status, and access to and use of health care: a population-based study of lesbian, bisexual, and heterosexual women. *Arch Fam Med.* 2000;9:1043–1051.

40. Hinchliff S, Gott M, Galena E. 'I daresay I might find it embarrassing': general practitioners' perspectives on discussing sexual health issues with lesbian and gay patients. *Health Soc Care Commun.* 2005;13:345–353.

41. Potter J, Goldhammer H, Makadon H. Clinicians and the care of sexual minorities. In: Makadon H, Mayer K, Potter J, et al., eds. *The Fenway Guide to Lesbian, Gay, Bisexual, and Transgender Health.* Philadelphia: American College of Physicians; 2007:3–24.

42. Boehmer U, Case P. Sexual minority women's interactions with breast cancer providers. *Women Health.* 2006;44:41–58.

43. McGarry K, Hebert M, Kelleher J, et al. Taking a comprehensive history and providing relevant risk reduction counseling. In: Makadon H, Mayer K, Potter J, et al., eds. *The Fenway Guide to Lesbian, Gay, Bisexual, and Transgender Health.* Philadelphia: American College of Physicians; 2007:419–439.

44. Derzko C, Elliott S, Lam W. Management of sexual dysfunction in postmenopausal breast cancer patients taking adjuvant aromatase inhibitor therapy. *Curr Oncol.* 2007;14(Suppl 1):S20–S40.

45. Arrington R, Cofrancesco J, Wu AW. Questionnaires to measure sexual quality of life. *Qual Life Res.* 2004;13:1643–1658.

46. Burleson MH, Trevathan WR, Gregory WL. Sexual behavior in lesbian and heterosexual women: relations with menstrual cycle phase and partner availability. *Psychoneuroendocrinology.* 2002;27:489–503.

47. Heiman JR, Meston CM. Empirically validated treatment for sexual dysfunction. *Annu Rev Sex Res.* 1997;8:148–94.

48. Fobair P, Koopman C, Dimiceli S, et al. Psychosocial intervention for lesbians with primary breast cancer. *Psychooncology.* 2002;11:427–438.

# In Sickness and in Health

## Maintaining Intimacy After Breast Cancer Recurrence

Barbara L. Andersen

Longitudinal study of patients with recurrence suggests that multiple aspects of life are initially disrupted[1] and may remain impaired for months.[2] Decades ago Silberfarb et al[3] noted the sexual difficulties of those with recurrence. They interviewed 52 women with recurrent but stable disease, 59 with recurrent, end-stage disease, and 50 with initial diagnoses. Patients with recurrent disease were 50% more likely to experience significant disruptions in sexual desire and frequency of coitus than were their newly diagnosed counterparts. In the ensuing 30+ years, few studies of patients coping with recurrence have been conducted in comparison with many studies with the initially diagnosed, with no further examination of sexuality, except one report.[4] The dearth of data may be due to the assumption that, in the context of recurrence, sexuality might be the least of a patient's concerns. However, heightened symptomatology, treatment side effects, and impaired functional status adversely affect sexual activity, desire, and responding for women with cancer.[5] More recently, we have contributed empirical studies from patients coping with breast cancer recurrence. We will quickly summarize these findings. However, new data will show the sexual responses of patients before their recurrence diagnosis and their responses thereafter. In combination, these data detail the struggles of breast cancer patients coping with the sexual changes that inevitably occur with cancer diagnosis.

Before discussing recurrence, we note that the initial breast cancer diagnosis and the ensuing treatments introduce significant sexual changes. There is an extensive literature on the sexual morbidities after breast cancer, most of which focuses on the newly diagnosed coping with mastectomy and adjuvant treatments. For them, there is an immediate reduction in sexual activity and responsiveness that we[6] and others[7–9] have noted. Unfortunately, this disruption does not, for the majority, resolve. In Figures 1 and 2 we provide data for 163 patients followed longitudinally [see Stress and Immunity Breast Cancer Project (SIBCP) description below]. Those with partners provided estimates of the frequency of sexual intercourse (Fig. 1) and their global evaluation of their sexual life (Fig. 2) for the 2 months before diagnosis. Assessments were then repeated every 6 months for the next 5 years. Before diagnosis, patients reported the frequency of intercourse being approximately once per week, as shown in Figure 1. The frequency dropped by one half (1–2 times per month) when chemotherapy was initiated, and during the 5 years that followed there was no return to pre-cancer levels and little improvement overall. The same trajectory is found with data on sexual satisfaction provided in Figure 2. The level falls from a rating that is above average (4) before diagnosis and below average, thereafter. Thus, sexuality has already significantly changed when recurrence occurs.

## PSYCHOLOGIC RESPONSES TO RECURRENCE DIAGNOSIS

Our descriptive studies of patients with breast cancer recurrence come from 2 sources. The first (sample I) are patients (N = 227) followed from a prior randomized clinical trial (SIBCP) testing the effectiveness of a psychologic intervention to reduce the risk for breast cancer recurrence and death. Patients were randomized to either intervention and assessment or assessment only study arms. Previously reported, the intervention produced significant gains across secondary outcomes [distress, social adjustment, health behaviors (diet and smoking cessation), treatment adherence, and health] and enhanced T-cell immunity.[10,11] After a mean of 11 years of follow-up, intervention patients had a reduced risk of disease progression, ie, breast cancer recurrence (hazard ratio, 0.55, $P = 0.034$) and death from breast cancer (hazard ratio, 0.44, $P = 0.016$).[12]

All patients were followed for upward of 13 years, including those who were subsequently diagnosed with recurrence. These data provided for the following recurrence studies: (a) prospective (ie, before recurrence) longitudinal analyses; (b) repeated measures studies comparing the responses of individuals to their initial and recurrence diagnoses; and (c) comparison of those with recurrence with matched trial participants who did not recur. Our discussion is also informed by accrual of a second sample (II), who did not participate in the trial but who were recently diagnosed with breast cancer recurrence (N = 80) and also followed longitudinally.

We have previously reported that at recurrence cancer-related traumatic stress symptoms are significant, much like they are at the initial diagnosis.[13] We compared patients' biobehavioral data (stress, distress, quality of life, physical functioning, and physical symptoms) at recurrence to their own data from the initial diagnosis.[14] We studied the first 30 patients in the trial who recurred and analyses showed that cancer-specific stress for the 2 diagnoses was equivalent.

These findings were extended.[15] Patients with newly diagnosed recurrent (n = 69) or initial (n = 113) breast cancer were compared. All patients were assessed shortly after diagnosis (baseline) and 4, 8, and 12 months later. Mixed-effects models with appropriate sociodemographic, disease, and cancer treatment controls were conducted. Replicating the previous study, all patients—initial or recurrence diagnosis—had comparable, high levels of cancer-specific stress and stress levels equivalent to those of patients seeking psychiatric treatment for anxiety disorders. Although cancer-related stress declined, it remained at or above the clinical cutoff for patients as long as 8 months after diagnosis. In contrast, general stress showed a trend to decline more quickly for recurrence patients. These data suggest a shift in the experience of the stress after cancer diagnosis. That is, patients' learn to cope and general feelings of stress decline

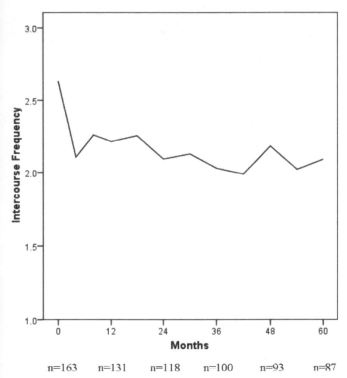

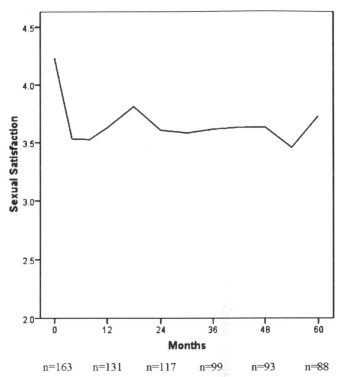

**FIGURE 1.** Reports of intercourse frequency by partnered women with breast cancer (N = 163) at diagnosis and across 5 years of follow-up. The initial data point indicates patients' retrospective estimate of intercourse frequency for the 2 months before diagnosis.

**FIGURE 2.** Global evaluations of sexual life from partnered women with breast cancer (N = 163) at diagnosis and across 5 years of follow-up. The initial data point indicates patients' retrospective evaluation for the 2 months before diagnosis.

but patients do not acclimate to the trauma of the diagnosis itself. Another important difference between the samples was the treatment and symptom context. After an initial breast cancer diagnosis, adjuvant treatment is completed within the next 6 to 8 months, but recurrence patients often receive medical treatments through the next 12 months. We found that patients with recurrence experienced greater fatigue and slower recovery over the year of follow-up.

Recurrence may also be remarkable by patients' heightened risk for depressive symptoms. In surveys, both dated and recent, it is estimated that 30% to 50% of cancer patients meet criteria for mood or anxiety disorders,[16] with depression being the most common.[17] Estimates for major depressive disorder are 22% to 29% for patients with early stage (stage I) disease,[18] upwards of 40% for patients with advanced disease (stage II/III or IV),[16] and the rates increase further with recurrence.[19] We examined predictors of depressive symptoms in women diagnosed with a recurrence.[20] Patients (N = 67) were assessed at diagnosis and 4 months later. Controlling for physical symptoms and baseline depression, hopelessness at diagnosis was a significant predictor of the maintenance of depressive symptoms. Also, structural social support (ie, presence/absence of a romantic partner) was also important and interacted with hopelessness. That is, women feeling hopelessness and who were alone (ie, without a partner) were especially vulnerable to depressive symptoms. In summary, the diagnosis and treatment for an initial diagnosis of cancer can be seen as a series of time-limited stressors, whereas stress with

recurrence is chronic. The experience of recurrence is qualitatively different from that of the initial diagnosis.

## FROM HEALTH TO SICKNESS: SEXUAL CHANGES WITH RECURRENCE

We have previously reported data comparing breast cancer patients with recurrence (R; n = 60) assessed at diagnosis (baseline) and 4-, 8-, and 12-months later compared with patients who remained disease-free (DF; n = 120) and matched to R sample on age, stage of disease at initial diagnosis, and duration of follow-up.[21] Using linear mixed modeling, group comparison revealed differences in their trajectories of change on measures of sexuality, relationship satisfaction, cancer-specific stress, and physical functioning. Data showed that the R group at baseline had significantly lower intercourse frequency and physical functioning compared with the DF group and these differences were maintained though the period of follow up. There were no significant differences in the frequencies of kissing or sexual and relationship satisfaction. Sexual changes were notable for younger patients. These data provided the first longitudinal and the first controlled study of sexuality for women coping with recurrence.

We provide here a more detailed look at the sexuality trajectory of recurrence. SIBCP patients (N = 123) who recurred (R; n = 41) were matched to patients remaining DF (n = 82) on demographic and prognostic characteristics, duration of DF follow-up, and study arm. A unique perspective is offered. Namely, we display the sexual

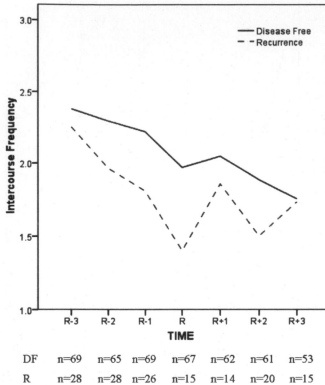

DF     n=69    n=65    n=69    n=67    n=62    n=61    n=53

R      n=28    n=28    n=26    n=15    n=14    n=20    n=15

**FIGURE 3.** Frequency of sexual intercourse reported by partnered women diagnosed with recurrence (R; n = 28) at time R. A matched sample of partnered women previously diagnosed with breast cancer who remained DF (n = 69) is provided. A timeline relevant for the R group is used. R − 3, R − 2, and R − 1 correspond to 18, 12, and 6 months before the recurrence diagnosis, with R, R + 1, R + 2, and R + 3 corresponding to the time of recurrence diagnosis and 4, 8, and 12 months after diagnosis. Equivalent disease-free follow-up time points for the DF are used.

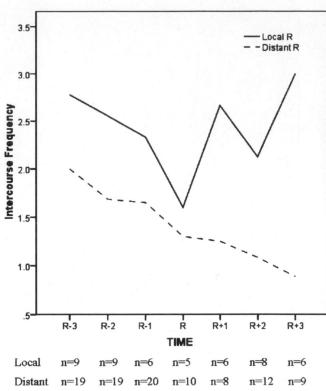

Local    n=9     n=9     n=6     n=5     n=6     n=8     n=6

Distant  n=19    n=19    n=20    n=10    n=8     n=12    n=9

**FIGURE 4.** Frequency of sexual intercourse reported by partnered women with recurrent breast cancer (N = 28), contrasting patients with localized (n = 9) and distant (n = 19) metastases. R − 3, R − 2, and R − 1 indicate 18, 12, and 6 months before recurrence diagnosis and R, R + 1, R + 2, and R + 3 indicate recurrence diagnosis and 4, 8 and 12 months after diagnosis, respectively.

trajectory of patients 18, 12, and 6 months before recurrence diagnosis and the trajectory, 4, 8, and 12 months after the recurrence diagnosis. Equivalent time points for the DF group are provided for reference.

Of the 123, data from the patients who had partners and completed sexuality measures were analyzed and sample sizes at each time point are reported in the figures. Figure 3 displays data for the frequency of intercourse. Both groups reported a frequency equivalent to twice per month at 18 months (R − 3). However, at recurrence diagnosis (R), intercourse frequency for the R group declined to less than once per month whereas the DF group maintained their level of intercourse frequency. During the subsequent months, intercourse frequency for the R group increased and eventually reached to that of the DF group by 12 months (R + 3). Similar trajectories were observed for sexual satisfaction (data not shown).

However, the view of DF and R group equivalence at 12 months (R + 3) is moderated by the extent of disease for the recurrence patients. Figure 4 shows data for the R group only and reveals that the trajectory of improvement in intercourse frequency (and sexual

satisfaction) at 12 months (R + 3) in Figure 3 occurred primarily among patients with localized disease (32%), as there was a steady decline in intercourse frequency for patients with distant metastases (68%). At 12 months after recurrence (R + 3), both intercourse frequency and sexual satisfaction were significantly higher for the patients with a local recurrence than the patients with distant metastases ($Ps < 021$).

The data also revealed an important perspective on intimacy among couples. When intercourse (or an equivalent activity) becomes difficult or impossible, the need for affection and intimacy remains. The stress of recurrence is great, both for the patient and partner. The prospect of losing one's spouse is one of the most stressful events that can be experienced.[22,23] Given and Given[24] found that caregivers, primarily partners of women with recurrent breast cancer, had more depressive symptoms than caregivers of patients with newly diagnosed cancer; depressive symptoms also increased across time. Thus, as both individuals are struggling with recurrence, our data on the frequency of kissing conveys an important message (Fig. 5). With illness, intercourse becomes more difficult for many, but the need for affection remains, and couples respond with an immediate and steady increase in the frequency of kissing after recurrence diagnosis (ie, R to R + 3).

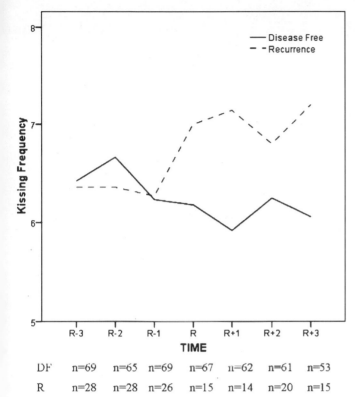

DF    n=69    n=65    n=69    n=67    n=62    n=61    n=53

R     n=28    n=28    n=26    n=15    n=14    n=20    n=15

**FIGURE 5.**   Frequency of kissing reported by partnered women diagnosed with breast cancer recurrence (R; n = 28). A matched sample of partnered women previously diagnosed with breast cancer who remained DF (n = 69) is provided. A timeline relevant for the R group is used. R − 3, R − 2, and R − 1 correspond to 18, 12, and 6 months before the recurrence diagnosis, with R, R + 1, R + 2, and R + 3 corresponding to the time of recurrence diagnosis and 4, 8, and 12 months after diagnosis. Equivalent disease-free follow-up time points for the DF are used.

## SUMMARY

In conclusion, we provide empirical detail on the trajectory of sexuality in the months leading to and after diagnosis of breast cancer recurrence. General health plays a major role in the extent to which women can maintain a sexual life. We previously reported that younger patients might be most vulnerable to sexual disruption as are patients with disseminated disease. Women coping with recurrence are attempting to maintain their quality of life and physical and emotional intimacy with their partner. The evidence suggests that they are able to do so despite the chronic stress and ongoing health challenges of recurrence.

## ACKNOWLEDGMENTS

*The author thanks the patients for their continuing support, Dr. Hae-Chung Yang, and the research staff of the Stress and Immunity Cancer Projects.*

## REFERENCES

1. Oh S, Heflin L, Meyerowitz BE. Quality of life of breast cancer survivors after a recurrence: a follow-up study. *Breast Cancer Res Treat.* 2004;87:45–57.
2. Thornton AA, Madlensky L, Flatt SW, et al. The impact of a second breast cancer diagnosis on health related quality of life. *Breast Cancer Res Treat.* 2005;92:25–33.
3. Silberfarb PM, Maurer LH, Crouthamel CS. Psychosocial aspects of neoplastic disease. I. Functional status of breast cancer patients during different treatment regimens. *Am J Psychiatry.* 1980;137:450–455.
4. Hanson Frost M, Suman VJ, Rummans TA, et al. Physical, psychological and social well-being of women with breast cancer: the influence of disease phase. *Psychooncology.* 2000;9:221–231.
5. Wolberg WH, Romsaas EP, Tanner MA, et al. Psychosexual adaptation to breast cancer surgery. *Cancer.* 1989;63:1645–1655.
6. Yurek D, Farrar W, Andersen BL. Breast cancer surgery: comparing surgical groups and determining individual differences in postoperative sexuality and body change stress. *J Consult Clin Psychol.* 2000;68:697–709.
7. Ganz P, Rowland JH, Desmond KA, et al. Life after breast cancer: understanding women's health-related quality of life and sexual functioning. *J Clin Oncol.* 1998;16:501–514.
8. Ganz PA, Desmond KA, Belin TR, et al. Predictors of sexual health in women after a breast cancer diagnosis. *J Clin Oncol.* 1999;17:2371–2380.
9. Henson H. Breast cancer and sexuality. *Sexuality Disability.* 2002;20:261–275.
10. Andersen BL, Farrar WB, Golden-Kreutz DM, et al. Psychological, behavioral, and immune changes after a psychological intervention: a clinical trial. *J Clin Oncol.* 2004;22:3570–3580.
11. Andersen BL, Farrar WB, Golden-Kreutz DM, et al. Distress reduction from a psychological intervention contributes to improved health for cancer patients. *Brain Behav Immun.* 2007;21:953–961.
12. Andersen BL, Yang H-C, Farrar WB, et al. Psychological intervention improves survival for breast cancer patients: a randomized clinical trial. *Cancer.* 2008;113:3450–3458.
13. Andersen BL, Farrar WB, Golden-Kreutz D, et al. Stress and immune responses after surgical treatment for regional breast cancer. *J Natl Cancer Inst.* 1998;90:30–36.
14. Andersen BL, Shapiro CL, Farrar WB, et al. Psychological responses to cancer recurrence: a controlled prospective study. *Cancer.* 2005;104:1540–1547.
15. Yang H-C, Thornton LM, Shapiro CL, et al. Surviving recurrence: psychological and quality of life recovery. *Cancer.* 2008;112:1178–1187.
16. Zabora JR, Brintzenhofeszoc K, Curbow B, et al. The prevalence of psychological distress by cancer site. *Psychooncology.* 2001;10:19–28.
17. Raison CL, Miller AH. Depression in cancer: new developments regarding diagnosis and treatment. *Biol Psychiatry.* 2003;54:283–294.
18. Burgess C, Cornelius V, Love S, et al. Depression and anxiety in women with early breast cancer: five year observational cohort study. *Br Med J.* 2005;330:1–4.
19. Hotopf M, Chidgey J, Addington-Hall J, et al. Depression in advanced disease: a systematic review, Part 1: Prevalence and case finding. *Palliat Med.* 2002;16:81–97.
20. Brothers BM, Andersen BL. Hopelessness as a predictor of depressive symptoms for cancer patients coping with recurrence. *Psychooncology.* 2008 [Epub ahead of print].
21. Andersen BL, Carpenter KM, Yang H-C, et al. Sexual well-being among partnered women with breast cancer recurrence. *J Clin Oncol.* 2007;25:3151–3157.
22. Chekryn J. Cancer recurrence: personal meaning, communication, and marital adjustment. *Cancer Nurs.* 1984;7:491–498.
23. Lewis FM, Deal LW. Balancing our lives: a study of the married couple's experience with breast cancer recurrence. *Oncol Nurs Forum.* 1995;22:943–953.
24. Given B, Given CW. Patient and family caregiver reaction to new and recurrent breast cancer. *JAMA.* 1992;47:201–206.

# Sexual Health Communication During Cancer Care

## Barriers and Recommendations

Elyse R. Park • Rebecca L. Norris • Sharon L. Bober

The Institute of Medicine report, "Cancer Care for the Whole Patient: Meeting Psychosocial Health Needs," calls for a new standard of cancer care that tackles often unaddressed psychosocial issues; sexual functioning was not among the identified issues. This omission is surprising, given that many cancer patients have significant issues related to sexual functioning, body image, and intimacy. Sexual problems often result from the physical and psychologic side effects associated with cancer and cancer treatment regimens.[1] Surgery may cause temporary or permanent physical disfigurement and hormonal changes to the body. Effects of chemotherapy can be both short and long term. Nausea, fatigue, weight changes, and hair loss may contribute to sexual problems that resolve over time, whereas side effects such as premature menopause may result in ongoing sexual dysfunction long after chemotherapy treatment ends. Radiation may cause fatigue, damage to organs, and loss of potency for men. Hormone manipulation therapy can exacerbate women's menopause symptoms and deplete men's testosterone levels. Overall, cancer treatment may cause individuals to feel less sexually attractive and more self-conscious about their physical appearance. Many cancer patients and survivors experience psychologic responses such as grief, loss, fear, depression, and anxiety about cancer,[2,3] all of which can affect their capacity for intimacy and sexuality.

Considering the wide range of side effects that cancer treatment can have on sexual functioning, it is surprising that conversations about sexual health are frequently missing during cancer care. This article will explain why discussions about sexual health are important during cancer care. It will cover the frequency of patient and clinician communication about sexual health. Patients' and physicians' perspectives of the importance of and barriers to sexual health communication will be discussed. Finally, recommendations on how medical professionals can help cancer patients will be presented.

## WHY ARE THESE CONVERSATIONS IMPORTANT?

With improved medical treatments, cancer survivors are living longer. It is becoming increasingly important to focus on quality of life issues, such as sexuality, throughout all stages of cancer treatment. Sexuality and intimacy can help to lessen emotional distress and improve psychosocial adjustment in the face of cancer.[4,5] Physical pleasure in the face of life-threatening illness can relieve stress and provide an experience that is life affirming during a tenuous time. For patients who endure the challenges of managing cancer treatment, the additional loss of sexuality and intimacy can add a profound burden that is often magnified by the lack of discussion about this problem.

There are now many treatments for sexual dysfunction, ranging from psychologic and behavioral to pharmacological, which can be effective at tackling sexual dysfunction or cancer-related symptoms (eg, fatigue), that negatively impact sexual functioning. But for patients to be identified to receive these treatments, conversations about sexual dysfunctions must be initiated in the medical setting. These conversations can help normalize concerns for patients, debunk myths, provide a basis for brief counseling or serve as an entree for a referral. Whether it is a matter of simply reassuring a patient that sexual difficulties are common or identifying a patient who really needs a referral for sexual rehabilitation counseling, it is imperative that these conversations become an integral part of cancer care.

## FREQUENCY OF SEXUAL HEALTH COMMUNICATION BETWEEN CANCER PATIENTS AND MEDICAL PROFESSIONALS

To date, a pervasive theme in research is that the communication between cancer patients and their medical team concerning sexual functioning is less than adequate.

### Patients' Reports

Cancer patients report that they seldom remember discussing sexual risks before treatment or treatment options for sexual dysfunction after treatment.[3,6–9] In a small focus group study in the United States of women's experiences after cancer therapy for breast and gynecologic malignancies, all participants expressed that their sexual concerns were not addressed.[3] Barni and Mondin[7] conducted a study with 50 breast cancer survivors in Italy; 10% of these women had talked to a doctor about sexual disorders that may arise as a result of their treatment. A recent multicenter study in the United Kingdom of the informational needs of 394 cancer patients revealed that only 37% of respondents recalled having discussions about sexual well-being with any member of their multidisciplinary care team.[10]

### Medical Professionals' Reports

Similar to patients' reports, oncology physicians and nurses acknowledge that conversations about sexual health usually do not occur during the course of cancer treatment. A survey of members of the New England Association of Gynecologic Oncologists found that although nearly all surveyed reported that they were comfortable taking a sexual history, only 49% reported that they take a sexual history greater than or equal to 50% of the time.[11] Stead et al[12] conducted a study involving 27 doctors and 16 nurses treating women with ovarian cancer and found that although most acknowledged that ovarian cancer patients would experience a sexual problem, only 1 of 4 doctors and 1 of 5 nurses actually discussed sexual issues with these women. Park et al[13] found that, among 216 primary care physicians surveyed, 62% reported that they "never" or "rarely" address sexual dysfunction with their patients, and 54% reported that they are "not at all likely" or "a little likely" to initiate conversations about sexual dysfunction with their patients.

When queried as to the relative importance of these issues, medical professionals' beliefs about what should be done often contrast with what they are doing. For example, 91% of oncologists reported that sperm banking should be offered to all men at risk for infertility as a result of cancer treatment, but 48% either never bring it up or mention it to less than a quarter of eligible men.[14] In-depth interviews with doctors and nurses treating women with ovarian cancer demonstrated that almost all felt that sexual issues should be discussed, but many did not know which member of the team should take responsibility for this discussion.[12]

Furthermore, when these conversations do occur, they are limited in scope. In an Australian study of healthcare professionals who work with cancer and palliative care patients, medical professionals acknowledged that they typically limit their understanding of patient sexuality to medical information (eg, fertility or menopausal status for women or erectile status for men).[15,16] In interviews with 15 women treated for ovarian cancer, no women received written information, and only 2 women reported having brief conversations.[12]

## WHAT DO PATIENTS WANT?

Patients in general do not anticipate that physicians would react well if asked about sexual issues. In the general population, a poll of 500 adults in the United States showed that 85% would be willing to talk to their physician if they had a sexual problem, but 71% did not think that their doctor would be responsive or helpful.[17] Seventy-one percent were concerned that their physician would dismiss their concerns, and 68% were concerned that their physician would be uncomfortable discussing a problem that was sexual in nature. This is disappointing, since patients seem to hope for much more from medical professionals.

A repeated theme in the cancer patient literature is the desire of patients to have open communication and frank discussions about sexual issues with medical professionals.[3,18] Cancer patients want permission to discuss their sexual concerns with members of their medical team[9,12] and are interested in being asked about their sexuality (eg, the impact of therapy on their sexual relationship) and not just their sexual functioning.[3] In a recent qualitative work, conducted by Hordern and Street in Australia,[15] semistructured interviews with 50 cancer patients revealed that most of these patients, across many different cancer types, desired practical information about how to live with intimacy and sexual changes after treatment for cancer.

Cancer patients want basic information about their sexual functioning and reassurance that their sexual health issues are not unique.[9,12] In qualitative interviews among women who had been treated for cervical and endometrial cancer,[18] participants said that at treatment initiation they wanted more information about female anatomy and physiology as well as information about the long-term physical and emotional effects of treatment that affected their sexual functioning. Patients also want reassurance about safety of sexual activity.[12]

## BARRIERS TO SEXUAL HEALTH COMMUNICATION

Many survivors do not feel that they were prepared to cope with sexual changes after cancer treatment. Currently, assessment and counseling around sexual issues are not integrated into routine care, despite patients' desires and needs. Candid conversations about sex are not easy, and this is not a problem endemic only in the United States—studies have shown a dearth of these conversations in patient care in many countries.[19] Physicians and patients do not know who should be initiating these conversations, and each fear embarrassing the other. Physicians are often unsure about what to say and do not know if patients want to discuss this quality of life issue during their treatment for a life threatening illness; patients do not know if it is appropriate to bring up sexual concerns and are unsure if their physicians will be able to help them.

## Patients' Perspectives

Patients' relationships with their oncology providers, knowledge about their cancer treatment, and beliefs about sexuality can be barriers to sexual health communication. Positive relationships with physicians are necessary for women with cancer to be able to voice their sexual concerns, and patients who do not feel respected by their physicians are particularly vulnerable to missed opportunities to address their sexual health.[20] Ironically, another barrier to these discussions is having implicit trust in one's physician; many patients hold the belief that if a physician does not bring an issue up, then it is not a valid concern.[15,16,20] Thus, if sexual health conversations are not physician-initiated then they are unlikely to happen.

The second factor is patients' knowledge; at diagnosis, many patients may not fully understand their normal body anatomy and sexual function.[20] During high-stress periods such as diagnosis and treatment phases, patients may not be able to fully comprehend all of the medical information imparted.[21] Patients may be overwhelmed with basic information about their treatment regimen and unable to ask about or process additional information about treatment side effects such as sexual dysfunction.

Finally, patients may hold beliefs about cancer and sexuality that deter them from broaching this topic with anyone in their treatment team. They may fear that cancer is contagious through sexual activity, sex may promote a recurrence or exacerbate cancer, side effects from cancer treatments may also affect the partner during sex, or that giving up sex will help cure cancer.[1,22] Unfortunately, these erroneous beliefs may deter patients from discussing their sexual health.

## Medical Professionals' Perspectives

Studies examining medical professionals' barriers to sexual health communication revealed 3 types of barriers: patient characteristics, provider characteristics, and systems issues. Certain patient characteristics may deter medical professionals from asking about sexual health. Medical professionals may make assumptions about the patients' desires for sexual health information based on patients' age, gender, prognosis, race/ethnicity, sexual orientation, and partner status.[12,15,16] If patients are perceived as anxious, physicians are less likely to initiate conversations about sexual dysfunction.[13] Physicians may also assume that patients with a poor prognosis are more concerned about survival than sexual functioning. Hordern and Street[15,16] found that medical professionals in palliative care settings assumed that patients would have a "uni-dimensional" focus on their prognosis and not be concerned with the physical and emotional treatment effects.

Providers' training, knowledge, and attitudes may serve as barriers. Lack of experience and knowledge are repeated explanations for these conversations not happening;[12,13,15,23] professionals often lack the confidence to discuss these issues with their patients. Medical professionals may be uncertain whether it is their responsibility to inform their patients about sexual side effects before, during, and after treatment. It is often not clear whose responsibility it is to initiate discussions about sexuality, and providers may feel that "somebody else" in the team will address this issue.[12,15,16] Medical professionals also admit to being uncomfortable or embarrassed when discussing sexual issues,[12,15,22] and acknowledge that they therefore avoid intimate discussions.[15,16]

Finally, systems issues are often reported as barriers. Oncology professionals report that they do not have adequate time to discuss sexual functioning with their patients.[9,11,22] Furthermore, there are concerns about the lack of resources available if patients acknowledge experiencing sexual dysfunctions,[9,11] particularly for patients whose insurance would not provide coverage for mental health or sexual dysfunction issues.[22]

## RECOMMENDATIONS FOR COMMUNICATION ABOUT SEXUAL HEALTH

It is important to let patients know that sexual dysfunction is an issue that they might encounter and that discussions on the topic are welcomed. These conversations should ideally begin as early into treatment as possible, so that patients could be prepared for potential changes in sexual functioning. Prior knowledge of treatment-related sexual side effects could help patients to make better informed decisions about treatment options. Practical information could be provided to patients to set expectations in the future, and then this information should be repeated at multiple time points if necessary. Finally, it is important to revisit these issues when patients are transitioning to being off treatment and during the survivorship phase of cancer care.

Building on the 5 A's model[24] used for the behavioral health counseling, we propose a framework for sexual health communication with cancer patients. This model extends the PLISSIT MODEL[25,26] for sexual communication to medical settings. The PLISSIT model involves asking permission (P) is to raise the topic of sexuality, providing limited information (LI) to address patient concerns, giving individually tailored specific suggestions (SS) about resuming sexual activity, and referring for intensive therapy (IT) if needed. We present a 5 A's comprehensive model, targeted to an oncology team setting. We recommend that sexual health conversations are worked out among the care team, to designate roles and responsibilities within the oncology team, the institution/hospital setting, and the community. This model thus relies on a multidisciplinary approach; different clinicians may take on different components of the 5 A's.

### Ask

The first step is Ask—to simply bring the topic up. To begin, it is important for oncologists to note that they may need to further explain patients' sexual, anatomic, and physiologic functioning to help them understand how sexual side effects are connected to their treatment. This will give the patient an opening to discuss any concerns and relieves confusion about who is supposed to lead this conversation. A clinician-initiated discussion would allay any patient concerns about embarrassing his/her care team.

All patients should be asked about this issue, repeatedly, throughout treatment. It is important to designate who within the care team (eg, physician, nurse, social worker) is doing the asking. Whoever is asking about sexuality needs to be aware of the common assumptions that may or may not be true (eg, patients who are older, single, or receiving palliative care are not sexually active). Hordern and Street[4] provided practical strategies to assist healthcare professionals to communicate effectively about sex and intimacy, including creating a conducive atmosphere, initiating the topic, using open-ended questions and a nonjudgmental approach, and avoiding medical jargon.

This kind of inquiry is open ended and there are different strategies that clinicians can use to frame these questions. For example, a clinician may ask directly, "How has your treatment affected your sex life?" Or a clinician may ask about treatment-related symptoms that may affect sexual functioning (eg, fatigue, depression, pain). For some clinicians and patients, it may be more comfortable to initially focus on these symptoms as an indirect way to lead into a more direct conversation about sexuality.

### Advise

This step provides an opportunity to convey a strong, brief message about the importance of the problem. It is the time to normalize symptoms for patients—to acknowledge that many cancer patients struggle with sexual dysfunctions. This is the time to reinforce that sexual functioning is an important quality of life issue and to reassure patients that they can get help.

### Assess

Although asking about sexuality requires an investment of time, a brief assessment can determine who needs more services and therefore save time in the long run. Professionals may find it easier to begin by conducting standardized sexual assessments with their patients to ask about symptoms to initiate discussions about sexual problems and treatment recommendations.[19] In 1981, Derogatis and Kourlesis[27] wrote a landmark article in which they proposed the following approach to evaluating sexual problems: take a history of sexual functioning, assess current problems, and formulate the treatment plan. Currently, many resources exist on how oncology professionals can conduct sexual health assessments.[1,26,28,29]

### Assist

Patients should be informed about available electronic resources. The American Cancer Society website includes information on "Sexuality for Men/Women and Their Partners" (http://www.cancer.org). The Lance Armstrong Foundation provides electronic resources on "Male/Female Sexual Dysfunction" (http://www.livestrong.org). The National Cancer Institute website has information on "Sexuality and Reproductive Issues" (http://www.cancer.gov).

On the basis of the assessment, a determination is made as to what is most helpful for the patient and a treatment plan can be carried out. Does the patient just need reassurance about the safety of sexual activity? Does the patient need a referral to counseling, physical therapy, or further medical evaluation?

Many patients primarily need education and information (eg, lubricants, vaginal moisturizers). Others may benefit from brief counseling that can be offered by a clinician in the unit, perhaps a nurse or social worker. Schover[22] provided an overview of content areas in brief sexual counseling, which included educating patients about treatment-related sexual problems, encouraging patients to resume sex during and after treatment, encouraging open sexual communication between partners, helping patients cope with physical handicaps, and advising patients on overcoming specific sexual dysfunctions.

Some patients will benefit from a referral. One determination to be made is if the patient will benefit from a psychologic or medical referral (peer counselors, social workers, psychologists, psychiatrists, physical therapist, nurse, endocrinologist, gynecologist, or urologist). Collaborative relationships should be developed within the unit, hospital, and community so that once a patient acknowledges having a problem there are established resources available.

### Arrange Follow-up

It is imperative for patients to receive follow-up at subsequent visits. Check to see if patients read informational pamphlets given to them or if they followed up with a referral. Check in to see how a patient is doing with his/her sexual health. This will reinforce the importance of it for the patient and reassure the patient that it is an issue that he/she can discuss.

## ADDITIONAL TRAINING

Regardless of who is doing the 5 A's, medical professionals need to know how to open conversations about sex in a frank and skilled manner so that it can be treated like any other quality of life issue of cancer treatment. Currently, sexuality issues are not emphasized in medical training curricula.[26] Medical professionals could receive additional training to help prepare them to approach discussions about sexual health with their patients. Unfortunately, one of the ongoing challenges is the limited access for continuing medical education in this area. However, as the focus on cancer survivorship continues to grow, presumably sexual functioning after cancer will also continue to garner more attention. As Schover noted,[22] if oncology healthcare professionals invest the time, they can become more comfortable and knowledgeable about sexual counseling. However, perhaps the most important way to become comfortable is to practice asking patients about their sexuality and learning where to refer patients if there are problems.

## REFERENCES

1. Schover LR, Jensen SB. *Sexuality and Chronic Illness: A Comprehensive Approach.* New York, NY: Guilford Press; 1988.
2. Andersen BL, Woods XA, Copeland LJ. Sexual self-schema and sexual morbidity among gynecologic cancer survivors. *J Consult Clin Psychol.* 1997;65:221–229.
3. Bruner DW, Boyd CP. Assessing women's sexuality after cancer therapy: checking assumptions with the focus group technique. *Cancer Nurs.* 1999;22:438–447.
4. Hordern AJ, Currow DC. A patient-centred approach to sexuality in the face of life-limiting illness. *Med J Aust.* 2003;179(6 Suppl):S8–S11.
5. Wimberly SR, Carver CS, Laurenceau JP, et al. Perceived partner reactions to diagnosis and treatment of breast cancer: Impact on psychosocial and psychosexual adjustment. *J Consult Clin Psychol.* 2005;73:300–311.
6. Hendren SK, O'Connor BI, Liu M, et al. Prevalence of male and female sexual dysfunction is high following surgery for rectal cancer. *Ann Surg.* 2005;242:212–223.
7. Barni S, Mondin R. Sexual dysfunction in treated breast cancer patients. *Ann Oncol.* 1997;8:149–153.
8. Cox A, Jenkins V, Catt S, et al. Information needs and experiences: an audit of UK cancer patients. *Eur J Oncol Nurs.* 2006;10:263–272.
9. Stead ML, Fallowfield L, Brown JM, et al. Communication about sexual problems and sexual concerns in ovarian cancer: qualitative study. *BMJ.* 2001;323:836–837.
10. Catt S, Fallowfield L, Jenkins V, et al. The informational roles and psychological health of members of 10 oncology multidisciplinary teams in the UK. *Br J Cancer.* 2005;93:1092–1097.
11. Wiggins DL, Wood R, Granai CO, et al. Sex, intimacy, and the gynecologic oncologists: survey results of the new England association of gynecologic oncologists (NEAGO). *J Psychosoc Oncol.* 2007;25:61–70.
12. Stead ML, Brown JM, Fallowfield L, et al. Lack of communication between healthcare professionals and women with ovarian cancer about sexual issues. *Br J Cancer.* 2003;88:666.
13. Park ER, Bober S, Campbell EG, et al. Primary care physician assessment of sexual function after cancer. Presentation at the 4th biennial survivorship research conference. June 2008; Atlanta, GA.
14. Schover LR, Brey K, Lichtin A, et al. Oncologists' attitudes and practices regarding banking sperm before cancer treatment. *J Clin Oncol.* 2002;20:1890–1897.
15. Hordern AJ, Street AF. Communicating about patient sexuality and intimacy after cancer: mismatched expectations and unmet needs. *Med J Aust.* 2007;186:224–227.
16. Hordern AJ, Street AF. Constructions of sexuality and intimacy after cancer: patient and health professional perspectives. *Soc Sci Med.* 2007;64:1704–1718.
17. Marwick C. Survey says patients expect little physician help on sex. *JAMA.* 1999;281:2173–2174.
18. Juraskova I, Butow P, Robertson R, et al. Post-treatment sexual adjustment following cervical and endometrial cancer: a qualitative insight. *Psychooncology.* 2003;12:267–279.
19. Hartmann U, Burkart M. Erectile dysfunctions in patient-physician communication: optimized strategies for addressing sexual issues and the benefit of using a patient questionnaire. *J Sex Med.* 2007;4:38–46.
20. Butler L, Banfield V, Sveinson T, et al. Conceptualizing sexual health in cancer care. *West J Nurs Res.* 1998;20:683, 99; discussion 700–705.
21. Mallinger JB, Griggs JJ, Shields CG. Patient-centered care and breast cancer survivors' satisfaction with information. *Patient Educ Couns.* 2005;57:342–349.
22. Schover LR. *Sexuality and Fertility After Cancer.* New York, NY: Wiley; 1997.
23. Tsimtsiou Z, Hatzimouratidis K, Nakopoulou E, et al. Predictors of physicians' involvement in addressing sexual health issues. *J Sex Med.* 2006;3:583–588.
24. Fiore MC, Bailey WC, Cohen SJ, et al. Treating tobacco use and dependence. In: *Clinical Practice Guideline.* Rockville, MD: U.S. Department of Health and Human Services, Public Health Service; 2000.
25. von Eschenbach AC, Schover LR. The role of sexual rehabilitation in the treatment of patients with cancer. *Cancer.* 1984;54(11 Suppl):2662–2667.
26. Penson RT, Gallagher J, Gioiella ME, et al. Sexuality and cancer: conversation comfort zone. *Oncologist.* 2000;5:336–344.
27. Derogatis LR, Kourlesis SM. An approach to evaluation of sexual problems in the cancer patient. *CA Cancer J Clin.* 1981;31:46–50.
28. McKee AL Jr, Schover LR. Sexuality rehabilitation. *Cancer.* 2001;92(4 Suppl):1008–1012.
29. Burbie G, Polinsky M. Intimacy and sexuality after cancer treatment: restoring a sense of wholeness. *J Psychosoc Oncol.* 1992;10:19–33.

# Hodgkin's Lymphoma

## An Overview

Dan L. Longo

Hodgkin's lymphoma was once a uniformly fatal disease. However, today at least 80% to 85% of all patients are cured. No stage of disease is beyond cure. Patients may even be cured after they have relapsed. Indeed, anecdotal data make it difficult to ever throw in the towel in managing patients with Hodgkin's lymphoma. When one sees a patient who has been in her fifth complete remission for 26 years, it makes one reluctant to ever say "never." Even when the physician has exhausted the conventional curative approaches, palliative therapy may also produce long periods of symptom-free survival. The paradoxical outcome from this success is that it makes the death of a patient with Hodgkin's lymphoma much more difficult to bear. For many advanced cancers, death is the expected outcome and when it comes, it is painful to be sure, but the physician has been preparing himself or herself, the patient, and the patient's family for the event. When a patient with Hodgkin's lymphoma dies, it is often an even more devastating blow because the course of treatment was embarked upon with such high hopes.

Despite the enormous progress that has been made in successfully treating patients with Hodgkin's lymphoma, our knowledge about the disease is far from comprehensive. Furthermore, even the information we know about Hodgkin's lymphoma and its treatment is not agreed upon. Controversy surrounds the decision on the best treatment approach. In this issue of *The Cancer Journal*, I have been fortunate to collect the thoughts of many of the leading figures in Hodgkin's lymphoma in the world. Their contributions here will bring the reader up to date on the facts and opinions of many experienced thought leaders.

What causes Hodgkin's lymphoma? We don't know. However, in these pages, Neil Caporaso and his colleagues from the National Cancer Institute (NCI) discuss what has been revealed from studies of the epidemiology of the disease. Genetic factors contribute to the disease, but we do not know precisely what genes are involved or how they lead to the tumor. A higher incidence occurs in westernized populations including those who emigrate from low-incidence sites to the United States. Efforts to find an infectious etiologic agent have been largely unsuccessful, though a role for Epstein-Barr virus has been implicated in some cases.

How does Hodgkin's lymphoma present and progress? Fortunately, we have Joseph Connors, a master clinician and clinical researcher at the British Columbia Cancer Agency, to draw on his own vast experience and the world literature on the clinical manifestations and natural history of Hodgkin's lymphoma. The disease has a predilection for lymph nodes. If only a single site is involved, it is usually the left supraclavicular node region. The disease marches progressively from one lymph node-bearing group to the next. When it spreads to the abdomen, usually the spleen is the first site involved. Because the spleen lacks afferent lymphatics, this may argue for hematogenous spread with selective growth in the fertile soil of the spleen. Fever, weight loss, and night sweats reflect systemic effects from tumor-induced cytokines. The disease may also be associated with important alterations in other organs including nephrotic syndrome and neurologic symptoms.

What is Hodgkin's lymphoma? As discussed in detail by the NCI's Franziska Eberle, Haresh Mani, and Elaine Jaffe, Hodgkin's lymphoma currently seems to be at least 2 diseases, as reflected in the World Health Organisation classification of lymphoid malignancies: the more common classic Hodgkin's lymphoma and the much less common nodular lymphocyte predominant Hodgkin's lymphoma. However, more recent evidence suggests that classic Hodgkin's lymphoma may be a heterogeneous category with at least 2 diseases, nodular sclerosis representing 1 subset and mixed cellularity and lymphocyte depleted types forming a continuum on the other. Reliably distinguishing these entities is the first step toward sorting out their pathogenesis and perhaps defining new therapeutic targets for the subset of patients not cured by existing approaches.

The staging of the extent of disease has undergone changes through the years as therapy has produced better results and nearly all patients receive some systemic therapy. Thus, removed from the evaluation is the exploratory laparotomy that was formerly an essential component of treatment decision making. However, novel evaluation methods, particularly positron emission tomography scanning, have taken on new significance in patient management. We are fortunate to have Mary Gospodarowicz from Princess Margaret Hospital in Toronto to summarize the current state of the art of patient evaluation. As she explains, the notion of adapting therapeutic strategy to risk factors is complicated by the fact that the factors were defined as affecting outcome at an earlier time when treatment was not so successful. As treatment improves, fewer factors influence outcome. We must modify old habits in light of new information to assure that our patients have the best chance of achieving cure with a minimized risk of late complications.

The next 4 articles in this volume deal with treatment. Beate Klimm and Andreas Egert of the German Hodgkin Study Group based at the University of Koln summarize data from studies of combined modality therapy. Pamela Seam, John Janik, Vincent DeVita, and I (all current or former NCI researchers) discussed combination chemotherapy as a sole modality of therapy. Joachim Yahalom from Memorial Sloan-Kettering Cancer Center makes a case for radiation therapy. Fahd Quddus and James Armitage from the University of Nebraska discuss treatment options for patients whose initial treatment has failed to cure the disease.

Finally, Andrea Ng and Peter Mauch from Harvard review what is known about the late complications of Hodgkin's lymphoma treatment. It was these careful investigators who first noted that more people died of treatment complications (especially second cancers and fatal cardiovascular disease) than from Hodgkin's lymphoma. The documentation of late effects in people cured of Hodgkin's lymphoma has received too little attention. The late effects of mechlorethamine, vincristine, prednisone, procarbazine chemotherapy and radiation therapy have been well defined, but little has been published on late effects of doxorubicin, bleomycin, vinblastine, dacarbazine (ABVD) chemotherapy. This could be because ABVD is not associated with serious late complications or that ABVD-treated patients have not yet been followed sufficiently to have the effects documented.

Now embracing my role as editor, it is difficult for me to understand the current widespread use of combined modality therapy to treat nearly every patient with Hodgkin's lymphoma. It has been amply demonstrated that subtotal nodal radiation therapy produces an unacceptable rate of late toxicity and fatality. Similar data do not exist for ABVD chemotherapy. Perhaps there are late effects from ABVD, but those effects could not possibly be of the magnitude seen with radiation therapy and have gone unnoticed. Therefore, the approach has been the creation of treatment programs that administer less than curative chemotherapy (either lower doses or fewer cycles or both) plus lower doses and smaller fields of radiation therapy. The reasoning seems to be that radiation therapy will have fewer late effects if it is delivered to smaller fields at lower doses. However, long-term follow-up data documenting that hope are not widely available. It remains unclear why it is thought that the late effects of ABVD require amelioration. The chemotherapy is being reduced because of a phantom; fear of not-yet-documented late effects. Does it make sense to use less than curative doses of 2 modalities rather than curative doses of 1 modality?

To their credit, these combined modality approaches achieve excellent short-term results, but no data have been published with follow-up into the second decade, when the effects of radiation begin to emerge with a vengeance. Will second malignancies be reduced? Will the combination of radiation and an anthracycline have less serious effects on the heart and vasculature? No one knows. Regardless of one's feelings (because there are no data), the safest dose of radiation therapy is zero. Thus, the onus should be on those who want to use radiation therapy to justify its use at all. Does it produce better long-term survival when added to chemotherapy than does chemotherapy alone? The available data suggest not. I wish there were more data. More studies should directly assess long-term survival of patients treated with chemotherapy alone versus combined modality therapy. But several studies that have addressed the question have found no value in adding radiation therapy to curative combination chemotherapy.

It would be my preference that we acknowledge that not all the bad effects of radiation therapy can be eliminated by reducing the field and giving 2400 rather than 4400 cGy. I would prefer that we acknowledge that chemotherapy alone is highly effective treatment in all stages of Hodgkin's lymphoma. And finally, I would prefer that we acknowledge that the best approach would be to cure as many people as possible with chemotherapy alone and reserve radiation therapy (and its late effects) for the subset that actually need it to be cured. This would include those, whose best chemotherapy response is a partial response and possibly those with slow clearance of positron emission tomography-positive disease. We do not need to expose every single patient to radiation therapy to cure him/her.

Although a substantial amount of territory is covered here, we have not been comprehensive. Important work has been omitted. A substantial amount of information is now available on the malignant cell of Hodgkin's lymphoma, the Reed-Sternberg cell. For example, it is known that the cell is of B-cell origin based on the rearrangement of its immunoglobulin genes. However, unlike any other malignancy of B cells, the rearranged genes are not transcribed into mRNA and immunoglobulin proteins are not synthesized. The essential transcription factors for immunoglobulin transcription are not expressed. This is similar to a phenomenon observed in the laboratory many years ago by investigators working with somatic cell fusion. A phenomenon called extinction made any cell fusion between a B cell and another type of somatic cell unable to transcribe the immunoglobulin genes. Although we know the missing transcription factor in Reed-Sternberg cells, we do not know why it is not expressed or whether its downregulation is an integral part of the neoplastic process. Much remains to be learned about the molecular pathogenesis of the disease.

Similarly, we devote little to no attention here to important aspects of the host-tumor relationship in Hodgkin's lymphoma. It has long been noted that patients with Hodgkin's lymphoma have defects in cellular immunity that are not fully characterized. Indeed, some evidence suggests that the immune defect may precede the development of overt Hodgkin's lymphoma. We do not understand the basis for this immune dysfunction and have not defined the degree to which it contributes to later problems in patients cured of the disease. These and other fascinating aspects of Hodgkin's lymphoma will likely be further elucidated over the coming years.

I would like to make one final comment about fads. Two fads have made an impact on Hodgkin's lymphoma in the past decade. It has been 177 years since the original report of the disease by Thomas Hodgkin. It has been 144 years since Samuel Wilks proposed naming the disorder Hodgkin's disease in the year before Hodgkin's death. Throughout that time, the condition has been known to affect lymph nodes primarily, even though the fundamental nature of the malignant cells was not defined with precision until more recently. The disease has always been taught along with the other lymphomas. I am unhappy with the fad of changing Hodgkin's disease to Hodgkin's lymphoma. I would argue that Hodgkin's lymphoma is not better than Hodgkin's disease as a descriptor. Everyone recognizes that at least 3 distinct entities currently comprise Hodgkin's lymphoma and it is expected that further research will better define the discrete illnesses currently lumped together as well as their relationship to one another and to other lymphomas. In other areas of medicine, it has not been the standard practice to rename the disease as one gets closer to its pathogenesis. Pernicious anemia is still pernicious anemia, not intrinsic factor deficiency anemia. Peptic ulcer disease is still peptic ulcer disease, not *Helicobacter pylori*-induced duodenal erosion. Alzheimer's disease is still Alzheimer's disease, not $\beta$-amyloid deposition neurodegenerative disease. In the grand scheme of things, knowing that Hodgkin's disease is a malignancy of lymphoid cells is not particularly insightful and certainly does not represent a grand leap forward in our understanding that would justify changing

144 years of tradition. Furthermore, it is confusing. I have had trainees who asked me how Hodgkin's lymphoma is different from Hodgkin's disease. When I explain that they are the same, I can't answer the next question: why the change? It isn't to distinguish this from some other disease that Hodgkin described. It isn't because some revolutionary new insight taught us that the disease is not a sarcoma or a carcinoma. The change is just because. To follow suit, we should expect Cushing's syndrome to become Cushing's endocrinopathy and Alzheimer's disease to become Alzheimer's neurodegenerative cognitive decline. I suppose that is one way to stamp out "disease."

Although I resent this particular fad, I have acquiesced to it in this volume. The second fad I shall not follow; the omission of apostrophe "s" as an indicator of the possessive form of a proper noun. It has become all the rage to list eponym-associated tests, signs, and diseases in medicine without the apostrophe s. Thus, it has become Alzheimer disease, Cushing disease (not to be confused with Cushing syndrome), and, alas, Hodgkin lymphoma. I won't do it. I won't go along with this fad. It seems to me to be a form of intellectual laziness to try to eliminate apostrophe s. Is there some sort of war on apostrophes? Will we soon omit them from contractions? That would be confusing. Some words have different meaning without an apostrophe (won't versus wont; can't versus cant). It is my understanding from my former colleague, Jean Wilson, a paragon of scholarship, that the practice of omitting possessive apostrophes originated innocently with Victor McKusick when he began using a computer to revise his great work, *Mendelian Inheritance in Man*. Apparently, his first computer was primitive and the keyboard did not have an apostrophe key. Therefore, he left apostrophe s off when he designated eponym-associated disease. From there, medical journal editors got a hold of the idea (it saves space) and apostrophe s became history; but their use was eliminated selectively. Some medical journals retain them even in their name (eg, Bailliere's family of publications). Classic medical texts continue to use them (eg, *Braunwald's Heart Disease*, *Harrison's Principles of Internal Medicine*). People continue to use possessive eponyms when they speak to each other and in talks at scientific and medical meetings. It is my hope that the effort to eliminate apostrophe s goes the way of certain other suggestions through the years such as adopting the metric system and SI units.

# Current Insight on Trends, Causes, and Mechanisms of Hodgkin's Lymphoma

Neil E. Caporaso • Lynn R. Goldin • William F. Anderson • Ola Landgren

In 1832 Thomas Hodgkin (1798–1866) published his article entitled "On some morbid appearances of the adsorbent glands and spleen," describing the postmortem appearance of 7 patients with lymph node and spleen enlargements.[1] More than 30 years later, based on some 15 additional cases, Wilks published his article entitled "Cases of enlargement of the lymphatic glands and spleen, (or Hodgkin's disease) with remarks" which ultimately named the disease after Thomas Hodgkin.[2] In 2001, the World Health Organization lymphoma classification system designated Hodgkin (sic) disease to Hodgkin (sic) lymphoma.[3]

Hodgkin's lymphoma (HL)[4,5] has drawn attention from clinicians, pathologists, and researchers in part due to its generally unusual biology and epidemiology, but also because it is one of the first malignancies to exhibit curative response to chemotherapy. Its symptomatic features (such as recurrent cycles of fever, night sweats, and lymphadenopathy) which at times emerge clinically like an infectious disease and preferential targeting of young adults have influenced many clinicians and researchers to suspect an infectious cause of the malignancy.

Etiologic clues about HL have been suggested by the bimodal age distribution with one peak occurring in the third decade of life and a second peak after age 50 years; by elevated risks in men, in individuals with higher socioeconomic status and in smaller families; and by the occurrence of Epstein-Barr virus (EBV) in HL tumor cells.[6,7] Interestingly, after the introduction of highly active antiretroviral therapy in 1996 for HIV-infected persons, AIDS non-HL (NHL) has declined substantially; however, the incidence of HL has been observed to increase simultaneously.[8] In the past decade, increased risk of HL among individuals who have undergone organ transplant or bone marrow transplant[9,10] has been reported. More recently, autoimmune and related conditions have drawn attention to a potential role for immune-related and inflammatory conditions in the etiology and pathogenesis of the malignancy.[11] A role for genetic factors is unequivocal based on evidence from multiply-affected families from case series, a twin study, a case-control study, and population-based registry studies.[12–17] Emerging data from Eastern Asia and among Chinese immigrants in North America indicate increasing incidence trends for HL associated with westernization, which emphasizes the importance of lifestyle and environmental risk factors even in a short-term perspective.[18,19]

## CLASSIFICATIONS OF HODGKIN'S LYMPHOMA

### Classification Systems

Jackson and Parker[20] and Harris[21] were the first to propose a comprehensive classification of HL. However, this classification was subsequently found to be clinically irrelevant because most of the patients belonged to the granuloma subtype with a huge variation in response

to therapy and outcome. In 1956, Smetana and Cohen[22] identified a variant of granuloma characterized by sclerotic changes and a better prognosis. Lukes and Butler suggested a histologic classification distinguishing 6 types of HL based on the varying degree of lymphocytic infiltration.[23–25] At the Rye symposium in 1965 the number of separate histologic groups was reduced from 6 to 4 and thereafter applied routinely for several decades because of the high reproducibility and good clinicopathological correlations. In 1994, in the light of morphologic, phenotypic, genotypic, and clinical findings, HL was listed in the Revised European-American Lymphoma classification and subdivided into 2 main types: nodular lymphocyte predominant and classic HL.[3,26] Classic HL was further divided into 4 histologically and clinically defined subtypes: nodular sclerosis, mixed cellularity, lymphocyte rich, and lymphocyte depleted. This approach has been adopted by the most recent World Health Organization classification of lymphomas,[3] which promoted classic HL from a provisional to an accepted entity.

### Origin of Neoplastic Cells

Nodular lymphocyte predominant and classic HL[3,26] share certain pathognomonic characteristics. For example, affected tissues contain only small number of neoplastic Hodgkin's and Reed-Sternberg cells (typically less than 1%) in a background of non-neoplastic inflammatory and accessory cells,[3] suggestive of a chronic inflammatory process. Several lines of evidence indicate that the neoplastic cells of HL originate from a germinal center or immediate postgerminal B-cell which has been selected and stimulated by antigen.[27–32] Furthermore, immunohistochemical studies have found neoplastic cells of nodular lymphocyte predominant HL (popcorn cells) to be of BCL6+/CD138– phenotype which is typical for germinal center cells. For the classic HL subtype; however, the neoplastic cells (Reed-Sternberg cells) have been observed to be typically BCL6+/CD138–, but sometimes they can be BCL6–/CD138+, which suggests that classic HL is a heterogeneous entity including both tumors of germinal center and postgerminal center B-cell origin.[33–35] In rare cases of classic HL, tumor cells have been observed to be derived from peripheral (post-thymic) T-cells.[36,37]

## DESCRIPTIVE EPIDEMIOLOGY

### Incidence and Mortality in Western Countries

HL comprises about 30% of all lymphomas in western countries and has a unique bimodal (sometimes trimodal) age-incidence shape (Fig. 1). It is currently estimated by the American Cancer Society that there will be about 8220 new cases (55% men) and 1350 (72% men) deaths of HL in the United States in 2008.[38] Also, the United States National Cancer Institute's Surveillance, Epidemiology, and End Results (SEER) and European-based International Agency for Research

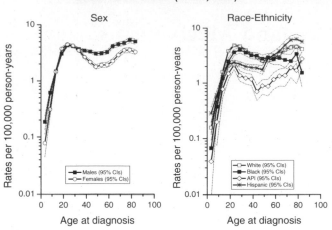

### SEER 1992-2005 (*n=20,309*)

**FIGURE 1.**    Age-specific incidence rates with 95% confidence intervals in the National Cancer Institute's SEER Database for Hodgkin's lymphoma by sex and Race-Ethnicity. API, Asian or Pacific Islander; Hispanic races are not mutually exclusive from white, black, API. Statistics for Hispanics are based on the NHIA (NAACCR Hispanic Identification Algorithm) and exclude cases from the Alaska Native Registry and Kentucky.[115,116]

on Cancer population-based cancer registries have estimated the incidence of HL in the United States and in Europe to be around 2.3 to 3.1 per 100,000 men and 1.6 to 2.3 per 100,000 women, which underscores the fact that HL is a rare malignancy in the general population.[4,5] Although the risk of developing HL is small (a life time risk of 0.24% for men and 0.20% for women),[5] it accounts for approximately 15% of all cancers in young adult ages (15–24 years). In terms of racial variation within the United States, a previous study on cancer incidence in California found the highest HL rates among whites, followed by African Americans and Hispanics, and the lowest incidence was observed among persons of Asian descent.[39] This pattern is consistent with currently available data from the SEER database (Fig. 1).[5]

The introduction of modern staging procedures and advances in both radiotherapy and chemotherapy have significantly contributed to improved survival of patients with HL over the past decades.[40] Clinical trials have observed long-term failure-free survival of 60% to 70% among patients treated with doxorubicin-, bleomycin-, vinblastine-, and dacarbazine-based therapies.[41,42] The German Hodgkin's Study Group has reported further improved outcomes using their dose-escalated BEACOPP regimen (including cyclophosphamide, doxorubicin, etoposide, procarbazine, prednisone, vincristine, and bleomycin) developed for patients with advanced stage HL.[43] Consistent with results from clinical trials, data from 2000 to 2003 in the population-based SEER database reveal mortality rates for HL patients of 0.4 per 100,000 and 0.3 per 100,000 for men and women, respectively.[5] However, if one restricts the estimates to patients that are 65 years or older, the mortality rates are 2.1 per 100,000 (men) and 1.4 per 100,000 (women). By using 5-year relative survival rates as the measure of outcome the same pattern can be seen: the 5-year relative survival rates for all HL is about 85% while the corresponding relative survival rate for older patients (65 years or older) is only 53%.[5] Thus, the outcomes of elderly (>50–60 years)

patients still remain unsatisfactory, with inferior complete remission rates and overall survival.[44–46] Because older patients generally are not included in clinical trials the information on this topic is sparse. However, population-based data from Scandinavia show that the 5-year overall survival for younger patients (diagnosed below the age of 50) increased from about 55% to 90% between the 2 calendar periods 1926–1955 and 1972–1994; while the corresponding improvement for patients diagnosed at 50 years or older improved from 20% to 50% during the same calendar periods.[47,48] Currently, the underlying mechanisms for the clinically well-known poor prognosis of older HL patients treated with chemotherapy[49–53] remain unclear. HL in older patients is clinically more aggressive in that anemia, increased erythrocyte sedimentation rate, advanced stage, and B-symptoms are significantly more frequent at diagnosis among the elderly,[50,54] which supports the hypothesis of age-related disease differences in HL. Alternatively, aging itself and associated factors (such as increased comorbidity,[55] reduced tolerability of conventional therapy,[49,56] more severe toxicity and treatment-related deaths,[57,58] and poorer outcome after relapse[59]) may contribute to the worse prognosis of elderly patients. Future research is needed to explore disease mechanisms for HL patients by age.[60] Clinically, more accurate markers of outcome in combination with less toxic novel therapies are needed.[44–46]

## International Variation and Westernization

The incidence of HL varies between westernized countries versus economically disadvantaged countries (Fig. 2). In the early 1970s, 3 epidemiological patterns were described by Correa and O'Conor: Type I in developing countries (a first incidence peak in male children and a second peak in older age around 50 years, with a predominance of histopathologic subtypes mixed cellularity and lymphocyte-depleted); Type II in rural areas of developed countries (an intermediate pattern with high male childhood incidence and a second decade peak among women); Type III in developed urbanized countries (a bimodal age distribution with a pronounced peak in young adults experiencing nodular sclerosis as the most frequent histopathologic subtype, and a continuously rising incidence above 40 years).[61] Correa and O'Conor[61] suggested that the observed variation in international patterns of disease reflected differences in economic development (ie, correlated for example with the level of public hygiene). More recent data from the mid-1990s have shown that the incidence rates for young adults have increased in less developed countries while remaining static in western countries.[62] A recent study from Japan, where historically HL has been rare before the age of 50 years, reported increasing incidence of HL in recent decades.[63] For HL, the number of cases between 1998 and 2002 is small (n = 122), making interpretation of the time trend difficult. However, there is evidence of an upward trend of the malignancy over the past decade.[19]

In a recent study on incidence trends for HL among immigrant of Chinese descent in British Columbia in Canada, Au et al found the incidence of HL among Chinese immigrants to be significantly lower than expected from the British Columbia background population (standardized incidence ratio = 0.34; P < 0.0001).[18] However, at the same time the incidence was significantly higher than that expected by extrapolating from the Hong Kong Chinese population (standardized incidence ratio = 2.81; P < 0.0001).[18] Interestingly, the difference was mainly accounted for by young immigrants diagnosed with nodular sclerosis HL subtype. Although that study was restricted in terms of size, it supports the hypothesis of a combined contribution of genetic, lifestyle, and environmental factors in the pathogenesis of HL. Importantly, the results indicate that extrinsic factors can exert their influence over a relatively short period of time. Taken together, there is need for studies designed to quantify incidence trends for

## GLOBOCAN 2002

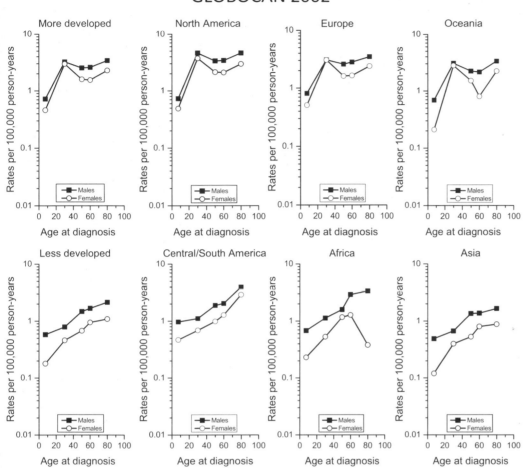

**FIGURE 2.** Age-specific incidence rates in GLOBOCAN 2002 for Hodgkin's lymphoma by sex and geographic regions. More developed regions have been calculated as the population-weighted average of Northern America, Japan, Eastern Europe, Northern Europe, Southern Europe, Western Europe, and Ocean (Australia/New Zealand). Less developed regions have been calculated as the population-weighted average of Eastern Africa, Middle Africa, Northern Africa, Southern Africa, Western Africa, Caribbean, Central America, South America, Eastern Asia (less Japan), South Eastern Asia, South Central Asia, Western Asia, Melanesia, Micronesia, and Polynesia.[117]

lymphomas in countries under the influence of westernization. Such results might provide opportunities to generate hypotheses regarding risk factors for the development of lymphomas and also are useful measures for healthcare planners who are responsible for future allocation of health care resources in these regions.

## Late Effects

As discussed earlier, developments in modern therapy have dramatically improved survival significantly for HL patients the past decades. The improved outcomes have been accompanied by long-term toxicity, such as elevated risks of second primary malignancies,[64,65] cardiovascular disease,[66] and infections.[66,67] Second malignant neoplasms now comprise the leading cause of death among long-term survivors of HL,[68] with breast cancer being the most common solid tumor among women.[69] Risk of breast cancer is greatest among women diagnosed with HL at age 30 years or younger[69–71] and is strongly associated with chest radiotherapy for HL. Risk increases up to 8-fold with increasing given radiation dose.[69,71,72] Other reported second cancers include acute nonlymphocytic leukemia, non-HL, lung cancer, stomach cancer, and melanoma.[73] Very similar to the pattern of elevated risk for breast cancer, risks for other second cancer sites are highest among patients treated for HL at younger ages. Also, most solid tumors have been found to start within or at the edge of the

irradiated field. Importantly, elevated radiation-related risks for second tumors have been found to increase even 20 to 30 years after therapy.[73] Finally, several studies have reported increased mortality of cardiac disease after mediastinal radiotherapy for HL.[66,67] Anthracycline chemotherapy significantly adds to the elevated risks of congestive heart failure (HR = 2.8) and valvular disorders (HR = 2.1) from mediastinal radiotherapy.[74]

## ETIOLOGICAL FACTORS

### EBV and Other Candidate Viruses

The EBV has been the major candidate for an infectious etiologic agent causing HL. There is evidence that individuals with a personal history of infectious mononucleosis are at elevated risk of developing HL; that risk is greater among persons infected at older ages and weaker with time since infection.[75] Hypothetically, the observed association with infectious mononucleosis could be due to as yet unidentified factors associated with higher socio-economic status resulting in relatively late infections with EBV. However, based on Scandinavian data, there is no elevated risk of HL among first-degree relatives of cases with infectious mononucleosis, strengthening the case for increased risk with infectious mononucleosis itself.[75]

Previous studies investigating serum have reported altered EBV antibody patterns in HL patients[76,77] including higher mean antibody titers to EBV viral capsid antigen than control subjects, consistent with prior infection. Also, there is serological evidence of elevated antibodies to early antigen and Epstein-Barr nuclear antigen among individuals subsequently diagnosed with HL.[78]

Evidence of EBV genome has been reported in malignant cells of about one third to half of the HL cases.[78] Almost all studies have demonstrated that EBV is more likely to be associated with the mixed cellularity subtype than with the nodular sclerosis subtype.[79] The association of EBV with HL is strongest in children, the elderly, men, and those living in disadvantaged social conditions. The frequency of an EBV association is higher in Asian and Central/Middle American countries than in the United States and Europe.[80,81] In situ hybridization and immunohistochemistry studies of affected tissues have demonstrated that EBV is localized to neoplastic Reed-Sternberg cells, which express EBV latent genes. Southern blot analysis of the fusion pattern of the EBV terminal repeat have shown that EBV in Reed-Sternberg cells is clonal. All this evidence plausibly argues for the role of EBV in the pathogenesis of HL. However, the EBV genome has only been found within the tumor in about 20% to 40% of HL cases with a prior diagnosis of infectious mononucleosis[82,83] and in around 30% to 40% of young adult cases.[79] The association between infectious mononucleosis and HL has been found to be strongest for EBV-positive (vs. EBV-negative) tumors.[79,82] It has also been hypothesized that EBV is etiologic in cases without viral genomic material within the tumor via a hit-and-run mechanism. However, recent studies have not found evidence to support that hypothesis.[84]

A number of other viruses (such as cytomegalovirus, human herpesviruses 6, 7, and 8, polyoma viruses JC and BK, SV40, lymphotropic papovavirus, adenoviruses, human T-lymphotropic virus 1, and measles virus) have been examined as potential candidates or cofactors for involvement in HL. However, there is no consistent evidence indicating that these viruses are important in the etiology of HL.[85] The risk of HL has been found to be elevated among persons infected with human immunodeficiency virus (HIV).[86] Furthermore, it has been observed that HIV-associated HL cases are more likely to be of mixed cellularity or lymphocyte-depletion subtype and 80% to 100% of the cases have been reported to be EBV positive.[87] In a recent study investigating lymphoma trends in relation to highly active antiretroviral therapy, it was found that the dramatic decrease of non-HL has been paralleled by an increase of HL.[8] Currently, the underlying mechanisms for that observation remain unknown.

## Autoimmunity and HL

Autoimmune diseases are characterized by dysregulated lymphocyte reactivity against self-antigens and the production of autoantibodies, leading to damage of the targeted tissues, such as joints or skin.[88] Previous studies have shown that there is an increased risk of mainly non-HL subsequent to autoimmune conditions including rheumatoid arthritis, Sjögren syndrome, and systemic lupus erythematosus.[89–100] Recent studies focusing on underlying pathophysiologic mechanisms related to lymphomagenesis have provided new evidence establishing differences in the risk of NHL development associated with various autoimmune disorders.[101] Recently, a wide range of autoimmune conditions was evaluated for subsequent risk of HL.[11] Elevated risk of HL was found for personal histories of several autoimmune conditions, including rheumatoid arthritis, systemic lupus erythematosus, sarcoidosis, and immune thrombocytopenic purpura. Also, a significant increased risk of HL was associated with family histories of sarcoidosis and ulcerative colitis. The association between both personal and family history of sarcoidosis and a statistically significant

increased risk of HL suggests a degree of shared susceptibility for these conditions.

## Transplant and HL

Allogeneic bone marrow transplantation is associated with an elevated risk of developing posttransplant lymphoproliferative disorders (PTLD). Although HL after transplantation is rare, an elevated risk has been reported.[10] Five of 6 assessable cases contained EBV genome. Differences from posttransplant lymphoproliferative disease after bone marrow transplantation were later onset ($>2.5$ years) and lack of association with established risk factors (such as T-cell depletion and human leukocyte antigen disparity). Rowlings et al[10] pointed out that the long latency of HL after transplant and lack of association with risk factors for posttransplant lymphoproliferative disorders are remarkable and should be explored further for possible insights into pathogenesis.

Previous studies of solid organ transplant patients have not generally found a raised risk of HL. The Israel Penn Transplant Tumor Registry lists HL as the lymphoid malignancy in 2.5% (31 cases) among 1252 diseases after solid organ transplant.[102] EBV nuclear material has been demonstrated in some of the cases of HL after transplantation.[103,104]

## Genetic Factors

The importance of genetic factors in HL is indicated by reports of multiply-affected families from case series, a twin study, a case-control study, and population-based registry studies carried out in Utah, Denmark, Israel, and Sweden.[12–17] Our group recently analyzed data from registries in Scandinavia and found significant familial aggregation of HL (RR = 3.1) and other lymphoproliferative tumors.[13] Relative risks were higher in men compared with women, and in siblings of cases compared with parents and offspring. Relatives of earlier onset cases were at higher risk for HL and for all lymphoproliferative tumors and were also at higher risk for developing early onset tumors themselves.

Currently, it is not known whether (or how) extrinsic risk factors interact with genetic susceptibility. Identifying inherited susceptibility genes is an important step towards defining the pathways leading to development of HL and understanding its complex etiology. Until recently, there have been no comprehensive searches of the genome for HL genes, largely due to the difficulty in assembling informative samples. In 2005, we conducted a genome-wide linkage study in 44 informative high risk HL families. No significant linkages were identified but several regions of the genome including on chromosomes 4, 2, and 11 were strongly suggestive.[105] The findings from this investigation are consistent with recessive inheritance. We recently conducted a candidate gene association study including unrelated familial HL patients and found associations with the genes IL6, IL4R, IL1R, and $LMO_2$ (unpublished data). Other studies have also implicated polymorphisms in IL6 as being important in HL etiology.[106–108] Importantly, these results are early steps in the discovery of germ line susceptibility genes and delineation of the pathways involved in development of HL. Future work is needed to better define pathways and to determine their interactions with environmental factors.

## Other Factors

On the basis of the shape of the incidence curve for HL by age and gender, Glaser[109] proposed in the mid-1990s that that childbearing potentially could be protective against HL in adult women. Results from Norwegian studies have supported this hypothesis[110,111] but the difference in the shape of the incidence curves between the sexes was not seen in England and Wales.[112]

Prior studies examining occupational exposures and subsequent cancer risk have reported on HL risk. The results on HL risk in relation to exposure to wood, wood dust and chemicals are generally inconsistent and based on small numbers. Phenoxy herbicides and chlorophenols have also been investigated but, again, consistent evidence of a causal association is lacking.[113] There is no evidence of an association of ionizing radiation with risk of HL. Some studies have found elevated risk of HLs after tonsillectomy, however, the results are inconsistent. Many studies of clustering have been reported, however, a review by Mueller and Grufferman concludes "there is no persuasive evidence of meaningful time-space clustering of HL." In general, studies of environmental, chemical, and occupational risk factors in HL generally reveal only weak and inconsistent evidence.[114]

## REFERENCES

1. Hodgkin T. On some morbid experiences of the absorbent glands and spleen. *Med Chir Trans.* 1832;17:69–97.
2. Wilks S. Cases of enlargement of the lymphatic glands and spleen (or Hodgkin's disease), with remarks. *Guy's Hosp Rep.* 1865;11:56–67.
3. Jaffe ES, Harris NL, Stein H, et al, eds. World Health Organization Classification of Tumours. Pathology and Genetics of Tumours of Haematopoietic and Lymphoid tissues. Lyon: IARC Press; 2001.
4. Parkin DM, Whelan SL, Ferlay J, et al. *Cancer Incidence in Five Continents.* Vol. I–VIII. IARC CancerBase No. 7. Lyon: International Agency for Research on Cancer (IARC); 2005.
5. Ries LAG, Harkins D, Krapcho M, et al. *SEER Cancer Statistics Review, 1975–2003.* Bethesda, MD: National Cancer Institute; 2006.
6. O'Grady J, Stewart S, Elton RA, et al. Epstein-Barr virus in Hodgkin's disease and site of origin of tumour. *Lancet.* 1994;343:265–266.
7. Diepstra A, Niens M, Vellenga E, et al. Association with HLA class I in Epstein-Barr-virus-positive and with HLA class III in Epstein-Barr-virus-negative Hodgkin's lymphoma. *Lancet.* 2005;365:2216–2224.
8. Biggar RJ, Jaffe ES, Goedert JJ, et al. Hodgkin lymphoma and immunodeficiency in persons with HIV/AIDS. *Blood.* 2006;108:3786–3791.
9. Bierman PJ, Vose JM, Langnas AN, et al. Hodgkin's disease following solid organ transplantation. *Ann Oncol.* 1996;7:265–270.
10. Rowlings PA, Curtis RE, Passweg JR, et al. Increased incidence of Hodgkin's disease after allogeneic bone marrow transplantation. *J Clin Oncol.* 1999;17:3122–3127.
11. Landgren O, Engels EA, Pfeiffer RM, et al. Autoimmunity and susceptibility to Hodgkin lymphoma: a population-based case-control study in Scandinavia. *J Natl Cancer Inst.* 2006;98:1321–1330.
12. Goldgar DE, Easton DF, Cannon-Albright LA, et al. Systematic population-based assessment of cancer risk in first-degree relatives of cancer probands. *J Natl Cancer Inst.* 1994;86:1600–1608.
13. Goldin LR, Pfeiffer RM, Gridley G, et al. Familial aggregation of Hodgkin lymphoma and related tumors. *Cancer.* 2004;100:1902–1908.
14. Lindelof B, Eklund G. Analysis of hereditary component of cancer by use of a familial index by site. *Lancet.* 2001;358:1696–1698.
15. Paltiel O, Schmit T, Adler B, et al. The incidence of lymphoma in first-degree relatives of patients with Hodgkin's disease and non-Hodgkin lymphoma: results and limitations of a registry-linked study. *Cancer.* 2000;88:2357–2366.
16. Shugart YY, Hemminki K, Vaittinen P, et al. A genetic study of Hodgkin's lymphoma: an estimate of heritability and anticipation based on the familial cancer database in Sweden. *Hum Genet.* 2000;106:553–556.
17. Westergaard T, Melbye M, Pedersen JB, et al. Birth order, sibship size and risk of Hodgkin's disease in children and young adults: a population-based study of 31 million person-years. *Int J Cancer.* 1997;72:977–981.
18. Au WY, Gascoyne RD, Gallagher RE, et al. Hodgkin's lymphoma in Chinese migrants to British Columbia: a 25-year survey. *Ann Oncol.* 2004;15:626–630.
19. Seow A, Koh WP, Chia KS, et al. *Trends In Cancer Incidence in Singapore 1968–2002, 6.* Singapore: Singapore Cancer Registry; 2004.
20. Jackson J, Parker J. *Hodgkin's Disease and Allied Disorders.* New York: Oxford University Press; 1947.
21. Harris NL. Hodgkin's lymphomas: classification, diagnosis, and grading. *Semin Hematol.* 1999;36:220–232.
22. Smetana HF, Cohen BM. Mortality in relation to histologic type in Hodgkin's disease. *Blood.* 1956;11:211–224.
23. Rosenthal S. Significance of tissue lymphocytes in the prognosis of lymphogranulomatosis. *Arch Path.* 1936;21:628–646.
24. Lukes RJ. Relationship of histologic features to clinical stages in Hodgkin's disease. *Am J Roentgenol Radium Ther Nucl Med.* 1963;90:944–955.

25. Lukes RJ, Butler JJ. The pathology and nomenclature of Hodgkin's disease. *Cancer Res.* 1966;26:1063–1083.
26. Harris NL, Jaffe ES, Diebold J, et al. Lymphoma classification—from controversy to consensus: the R.E.A.L. and WHO classification of lymphoid neoplasms. *Ann Oncol,* 2000;11 (Suppl 1):3–10.
27. Cossman J, Annunziata CM, Barash S, et al. Reed-Sternberg cell genome expression supports a B-cell lineage. *Blood.* 1999;94:411–416.
28. Brauninger A, Hansmann ML, Strickler JG, et al. Identification of common germinal-center B-cell precursors in two patients with both Hodgkin's disease and non-Hodgkin's lymphoma. *N Engl J Med.* 1999;340:1239–1247.
29. Kuppers R, Roers A, Kanzler H. Molecular single cell studies of normal and transformed lymphocytes. *Cancer Surv.* 1997;30:45–58.
30. Marafioti T, Hummel M, Anagnostopoulos I, et al. Origin of nodular lymphocyte-predominant Hodgkin's disease from a clonal expansion of highly mutated germinal-center B cells. *N Engl J Med.* 1997;337:453–458.
31. Marafioti T, Hummel M, Foss HD, et al. Hodgkin and reed-sternberg cells represent an expansion of a single clone originating from a germinal center B-cell with functional immunoglobulin gene rearrangements but defective immunoglobulin transcription. *Blood.* 2000;95:1443–1450.
32. Braeuninger A, Kuppers R, Strickler JG, et al. Hodgkin and Reed-Sternberg cells in lymphocyte predominant Hodgkin disease represent clonal populations of germinal center-derived tumor B cells. *Proc Natl Acad Sci U S A.* 1997;94:9337–9342.
33. Falini B, Mason DY. Proteins encoded by genes involved in chromosomal alterations in lymphoma and leukemia: clinical value of their detection by immunocytochemistry. *Blood.* 2002;99:409–426.
34. Carbone A, Gloghini A, Gaidano G, et al. Expression status of BCL-6 and syndecan-1 identifies distinct histogenetic subtypes of Hodgkin's disease. *Blood.* 1998;92:2220–2228.
35. Falini B, Bigerna B, Pasqualucci L, et al. Distinctive expression pattern of the BCL-6 protein in nodular lymphocyte predominance Hodgkin's disease. *Blood.* 1996;87:465–471.
36. Muschen M, Rajewsky K, Brauninger A, et al. Rare occurrence of classical Hodgkin's disease as a T cell lymphoma. *J Exp Med.* 2000;191:387–394.
37. Seitz V, Hummel M, Marafioti T, et al. Detection of clonal T-cell receptor gamma-chain gene rearrangements in Reed-Sternberg cells of classic Hodgkin disease. *Blood.* 2000;95:3020–3024.
38. Anonymous. *Cancer Facts & Figures 2007.* Atlanta: American Cancer Society; 2007.
39. Perkins CI, Morris CR, Wright WE, et al. *Cancer Incidence and Mortality in California by Detailed Race/Ethnicity, 1988–1992.* Sacramento, CA: California Department of Health Services Surveillance Section; 1995.
40. Kennedy BJ, Fremgen AM, Menck HR. The National Cancer Data Base report on Hodgkin's disease for 1985–1989 and 1990–1994. *Cancer.* 1998;83:1041–1047.
41. Duggan DB, Petroni GR, Johnson JL, et al. A. Randomized comparison of ABVD and MOPP/ABV hybrid for the treatment of advanced Hodgkin's disease: report of an intergroup trial. *J Clin Oncol.* 2003;21:607–614.
42. Canellos GP, Anderson JR, Propert KJ, et al. Chemotherapy of advanced Hodgkin's disease with MOPP, ABVD, or MOPP alternating with ABVD. *N Engl J Med.* 1992;327:1478–1484.
43. Diehl V, Behringer K. Could BEACOPP be the new standard for the treatment of advanced Hodgkin's lymphoma (HL)? *Cancer Invest.* 2006;24: 713–717.
44. Forsyth PD, Bessell EM, Moloney AJ, et al. Hodgkin's disease in patients older than 70 years of age: a registry-based analysis. *Eur J Cancer.* 1997;33:1638–1642.
45. Eghbali H, Hoerni-Simon G, de Mascarel I, et al. Hodgkin's disease in the elderly. A series of 30 patients aged older than 70 years. *Cancer.* 1984;53:2191–2193.
46. Wedelin C, Bjorkholm M, Biberfeld P, et al. Prognostic factors in Hodgkin's disease with special reference to age. *Cancer.* 1984;53:1202–1208.
47. Landgren O. *Diagnostic and Prognostic Studies in Hodgkin's Lymphoma.* Stockholm: Karolinska Institutet; 2002:54.
48. Westling P. Studies of the prognosis in Hodgkin's disease. *Acta Radiol.* 1965;245 (Suppl):5–125.
49. Landgren O, Algernon C, Axdorph U, et al. Hodgkin's lymphoma in the elderly with special reference to type and intensity of chemotherapy in relation to prognosis. *Haematologica.* 2003;88:438–444.
50. Engert A, Ballova V, Haverkamp H, et al. Hodgkin's lymphoma in elderly patients: a comprehensive retrospective analysis from the German Hodgkin's Study Group. *J Clin Oncol.* 2005;23:5052–5060.
51. Ballova V, Ruffer JU, Haverkamp H, et al. A prospectively randomized trial carried out by the German Hodgkin Study Group (GHSG) for elderly patients with advanced Hodgkin's disease comparing BEACOPP baseline and COPP-ABVD (study HD9elderly). *Ann Oncol.* 2005;16:124–131.

52. Weekes CD, Vose JM, Lynch JC, et al. Hodgkin's disease in the elderly: improved treatment outcome with a doxorubicin-containing regimen. *J Clin Oncol.* 2002;20:1087–1093.
53. Proctor SJ, White J, Jones GL. An international approach to the treatment of Hodgkin's disease in the elderly: launch of the SHIELD study programme. *Eur J Haematol Suppl.* 2005;63–67.
54. Landgren O, Axdorph U, Fears TR, et al. A population-based cohort study on early-stage Hodgkin lymphoma treated with radiotherapy alone: with special reference to older patients. *Ann Oncol.* 2006;17:1290–1295.
55. van Spronsen DJ, Janssen-Heijnen ML, Breed WP, et al. Prevalence of co-morbidity and its relationship to treatment among unselected patients with Hodgkin's disease and non-Hodgkin's lymphoma, 1993–1996. *Ann Hematol.* 1999;78:315–319.
56. Erdkamp FL, Breed WP, Bosch LJ, et al. Hodgkin disease in the elderly. A registry-based analysis. *Cancer.* 1992;70:830–834.
57. Peterson BA, Pajak TF, Cooper MR, et al. Effect of age on therapeutic response and survival in advanced Hodgkin's disease. *Cancer Treat Rep.* 1982;66:889–898.
58. Levis A, Depaoli L, Bertini M, et al. Results of a low aggressivity chemother-apy regimen (CVP/CEB) in elderly Hodgkin's disease patients. *Haematolog-ica.* 1996;81:450–456.
59. Specht L, Nissen NI. Hodgkin's disease and age. *Eur J Haematol.* 1989;43:127–135.
60. Evens AM, Sweetenham JW, Horning SJ. Hodgkin lymphoma in older pa-tients: an uncommon disease in need of study. *Oncology (Williston Park).* 2008;22:1369–1379; discussion 1379, 1385, 1388–1393.
61. Correa P, O'Conor GT. Epidemiologic patterns of Hodgkin's disease. *Int J Cancer.* 1971;8:192–201.
62. Macfarlane GJ, Evstifeeva T, Boyle P, et al. International patterns in the occur-rence of Hodgkin's disease in children and young adult males. *Int J Cancer.* 1995;61:165–169.
63. Aozasa K, Ueda T, Tamai M, et al. Hodgkin's disease in Osaka, Japan (1964–1985). *Eur J Cancer Clin Oncol.* 1986;22:1117–1119.
64. Ng AK, Bernardo MV, Weller E, et al. Second malignancy after Hodgkin disease treated with radiation therapy with or without chemotherapy: long-term risks and risk factors. *Blood.* 2002;100:1989–1996.
65. Dores GM, Metayer C, Curtis RE, et al. Second malignant neoplasms among long-term survivors of Hodgkin's disease: a population-based evaluation over 25 years. *J Clin Oncol.* 2002;20:3484–3494.
66. Ng AK, Bernardo MP, Weller E, et al. Long-term survival and competing causes of death in patients with early-stage Hodgkin's disease treated at age 50 or younger. *J Clin Oncol.* 2002;20:2101–2108.
67. Aleman BM, van den Belt-Dusebout AW, Klokman WJ, et al. Long-term cause-specific mortality of patients treated for Hodgkin's disease. *J Clin On-col.* 2003;21:3431–3439.
68. Hoppe RT. Hodgkin's disease: complications of therapy and excess mortality. *Ann Oncol.* 1997;8(Suppl 1):115–118.
69. Travis LB, Hill DA, Dores GM, et al. Breast cancer following radiother-apy and chemotherapy among young women with Hodgkin disease. *JAMA.* 2003;290:465–475.
70. van Leeuwen FE, Klokman WJ, Stovall M, et al. Roles of radiation dose, chemotherapy, and hormonal factors in breast cancer following Hodgkin's disease. *J Natl Cancer Inst.* 2003;95:971–980.
71. Hill DA, Gilbert E, Dores GM, et al. Breast cancer risk following radio-therapy for Hodgkin lymphoma: modification by other risk factors. *Blood.* 2005;106:3358–3365.
72. Travis LB, Hill D, Dores GM, et al. Cumulative absolute breast cancer risk for young women treated for Hodgkin lymphoma. *J Natl Cancer Inst.* 2005;97:1428–1437.
73. Foss Abrahamsen A, Andersen A, Nome O, et al. Long-term risk of second malignancy after treatment of Hodgkin's disease: the influence of treatment, age and follow-up time. *Ann Oncol.* 2002;13:1786–1791.
74. Aleman BM, van den Belt-Dusebout AW, De Bruin ML, et al. Late car-diotoxicity after treatment for Hodgkin lymphoma. *Blood.* 2007;109:1878–1886.
75. Hjalgrim H, Askling J, Sorensen P, et al. Risk of Hodgkin's disease and other cancers after infectious mononucleosis. *J Natl Cancer Inst.* 2000;92:1522–1528.
76. Lehtinen T, Lumio J, Dillner J, et al. Increased risk of malignant lymphoma in-dicated by elevated Epstein-Barr virus antibodies—a prospective study. *Can-cer Causes Control.* 1993;4:187–193.
77. Mueller N, Mohar A, Evans A, et al. Epstein-Barr virus antibody patterns pre-ceding the diagnosis of non-Hodgkin's lymphoma. *Int J Cancer.* 1991;49:387–393.
78. Mueller NE. Hodgkin's disease. In: Schottenfeld D, Fraumeni JF Jr, eds. *Cancer Epidemiology and Prevention.* New York: Oxford University Press; 1996:893–919.
79. Glaser SL, Lin RJ, Stewart SL, et al. Epstein-Barr virus-associated Hodgkin's disease: epidemiologic characteristics in international data. *Int J Cancer.* 1997;70:375–382.
80. Flavell KJ, Biddulph JP, Powell JE, et al. South Asian ethnicity and material deprivation increase the risk of Epstein-Barr virus infection in childhood Hodgkin's disease. *Br J Cancer.* 2001;85:350–356.
81. Tomita Y, Ohsawa M, Kanno H, et al. Epstein-Barr virus in Hodgkin's disease patients in Japan. *Cancer.* 1996;77:186–192.
82. Alexander FE, Jarrett RF, Lawrence D, et al. Risk factors for Hodgkin's disease by Epstein-Barr virus (EBV) status: prior infection by EBV and other agents. *Br J Cancer.* 2000;82:1117–1121.
83. Sleckman BG, Mauch PM, Ambinder RF, et al. Epstein-Barr virus in Hodgkin's disease: correlation of risk factors and disease characteristics with molecular evidence of viral infection. *Cancer Epidemiol Biomarkers Prev.* 1998;7:1117–1121.
84. Gallagher A, Perry J, Freeland J, et al. Hodgkin's lymphoma and Epstein-Barr virus (EBV): no evidence to support hit-and-run mechanism in cases classified as non-EBV-associated. *Int J Cancer.* 2003;104:624–630.
85. Benharroch D, Shemer-Avni Y, Levy A, et al. New candidate virus in associ-ation with Hodgkin's disease. *Leuk Lymphoma.* 2003;44:605–610.
86. Goedert JJ, Cote TR, Virgo P, et al. Spectrum of AIDS-associated malignant disorders. *Lancet.* 1998;351:1833–1839.
87. Carbone A, Gloghini A. AIDS-related lymphomas: from pathogenesis to pathology. *Br J Haematol.* 2005;130:662–670.
88. Klippel JH. *Primer on the Rheumatic Diseases.* Atlanta: Arthritis Foundation; 2001.
89. Bjornadal L, Lofstrom B, Yin L, et al. Increased cancer incidence in a Swedish cohort of patients with systemic lupus erythematosus. *Scand J Rheumatol.* 2002;31:66–71.
90. Kassan SS, Thomas TL, Moutsopoulos HM, et al. Increased risk of lymphoma in sicca syndrome. *Ann Intern Med.* 1978;89:888–892.
91. Isomaki HA, Hakulinen T, Joutsenlahti U. Excess risk of lymphomas, leukemia and myeloma in patients with rheumatoid arthritis. *J Chronic Dis.* 1978;31:691–696.
92. Mellemkjaer L, Andersen V, Linet MS, et al. Non-Hodgkin's lymphoma and other cancers among a cohort of patients with systemic lupus erythematosus. *Arthritis Rheum.* 1997;40:761–768.
93. Gridley G, McLaughlin JK, Ekbom A, et al. Incidence of cancer among pa-tients with rheumatoid arthritis. *J Natl Cancer Inst.* 1993;85:307–311.
94. Ekstrom K, Hjalgrim H, Brandt L, et al. Risk of malignant lymphomas in patients with rheumatoid arthritis and in their first-degree relatives. *Arthritis Rheum.* 2003;48:963–970.
95. Thomas E, Brewster DH, Black RJ, et al. Risk of malignancy among patients with rheumatic conditions. *Int J Cancer.* 2000;88:497–502.
96. Mellemkjaer L, Alexander F, Olsen JH. Cancer among children of parents with autoimmune diseases. *Br J Cancer.* 2000;82:1353–1357.
97. Hartge P, Wang SS, eds. *Overview of the Etiology and Epidemiology of Lymphoma. Non-Hodgkin's Lymphoma.* Philadelphia: Lippincott Williams & Wilkins, 2004.
98. Landgren O, Kerstann KF, Gridley G, et al. Re: Familial clustering of Hodgkin lymphoma and multiple sclerosis. *J Natl Cancer Inst.* 2005;97:543–544.
99. Smedby KE, Hjalgrim H, Askling J, et al. Autoimmune and chronic inflamma-tory disorders and risk of non-Hodgkin lymphoma by subtype. *J Natl Cancer Inst.* 2006;98:51–60.
100. Engels EA, Cerhan JR, Linet MS, et al. Immune-related condi-tions and immune-modulating medications as risk factors for non-Hodgkin's lymphoma: a case-control study. *Am J Epidemiol.* 2005;162:1153–1161.
101. Zintzaras E, Voulgarelis M, Moutsopoulos HM. The risk of lymphoma development in autoimmune diseases: a meta-analysis. *Arch Intern Med.* 2005;165:2337–2344.
102. Penn I. Neoplastic complications of transplantation. *Semin Respir Infect.* 1993;8:233–239.
103. Haluska FG, Brufsky AM, Canellos GP. The cellular biology of the Reed-Sternberg cell. *Blood.* 1994;84:1005–1019.
104. Garnier JL, Lebranchu Y, Lefrancois N, et al. Hodgkin's disease after renal transplantation. *Transplant Proc.* 1995;27:1785.
105. Goldin LR, McMaster ML, Ter-Minassian M, et al. A genome screen of families at high risk for Hodgkin lymphoma: evidence for a susceptibility gene on chromosome 4. *J Med Genet.* 2005;42:595–601.
106. Cordano P, Lake A, Shield L, et al. Effect of IL-6 promoter polymor-phism on incidence and outcome in Hodgkin's lymphoma. *Br J Haematol.* 2005;128:493–495.
107. Cozen W, Gebregziabher M, Conti DV, et al. Interleukin-6-related genotypes, body mass index, and risk of multiple myeloma and plasmacytoma. *Cancer Epidemiol Biomarkers Prev.* 2006;15:2285–2291.

108. Cozen W, Gill PS, Ingles SA, et al. IL-6 levels and genotype are associated with risk of young adult Hodgkin lymphoma. *Blood.* 2004;103:3216–3221.

109. Glaser SL. Reproductive factors in Hodgkin's disease in women: a review. *Am J Epidemiol.* 1994;139:237–246.

110. Kravdal O, Hansen S. The importance of childbearing for Hodgkin's disease: new evidence from incidence and mortality models. *Int J Epidemiol.* 1996;25:737–743.

111. Kravdal O, Hansen S. Hodgkin's disease: the protective effect of childbearing. *Int J Cancer.* 1993;55:909–914.

112. Swerdlow A, dos Santos Silva I, Doll R. *Cancer Incidence and Mortality in England and Wales: Trends and Risk Factors.* Oxford: Oxford University Press; 2001.

113. McCunney RJ. Hodgkin's disease, work, and the environment. A review. *J Occup Environ Med.* 1999;41:36–46.

114. Grufferman NM. Hodgkin's lymphoma. In: David Schottenfeld J, Joseph F. Fraumeni, eds. *Cancer Epidemiology and Prevention.* New York: Oxford University Press; 2006:872–897.

115. SEER-13: Surveillance, Epidemiology, and End Results (SEER) Program (www.seer.cancer.gov) SEER*Stat Database: Incidence-SEER 13 Regs Limited-Use, Nov 2007 Sub (1973–2005) <Single Ages to 85+, Katrinia/Rita Population Adjustment> -Linked To County Attributes - Total U.S., 1969–2005 Counties, National Cancer Institute, DCCPS, Surveillance Research Program, Cancer Statistics Branch, released April 2008, based on November 2007 submission, 2008.

116. SEER-17: Surveillance, Epidemiology, and End Results (SEER) Program (www.seer.cancer.gov) SEER*Stat Database: Incidence-SEER 17 Regs Limited-Use, Nov 2007 Sub (1973–2005) <Single Ages to 85+, Katrinia/Rita Population Adjustment> -Linked To County Attributes - Total U.S., 1969–2005 Counties, National Cancer Institute, DCCPS, Surveillance Research Program, Cancer Statistics Branch, released April 2008, based on November 2007 submission, 2008.

117. Ferlay J, Bray F, Pisani P, et al. GLOBOCAN 2002, Cancer Incidence, Mortality and Prevalence Worldwide, IARC CancerBase No. 5, version 2.0. Lyon, France, IARC Press, 2004.

# Clinical Manifestations and Natural History of Hodgkin's Lymphoma

Joseph M. Connors

Hodgkin's lymphoma was recognized as a unique illness almost 2 centuries ago. By the early 1900s, detailed descriptions of the typical microscopic appearance allowed confident separation of this type of lymphoma from other diseases causing similar symptoms and lymphadenopathy. Finally, and most importantly in terms of making clear the need for definite identification of the disease, curative treatments, initially with radiation therapy, and later multiagent chemotherapy, became available more than 50 years ago. Thus, Hodgkin's lymphoma has been sufficiently, dependably, and accurately diagnosed that its specific patterns of presentation and clinical behavior are well understood.

It is important to distinguish 2 major variants of Hodgkin's lymphoma, the classic variety including the nodular sclerosing, mixed cellularity, lymphocyte rich and lymphocyte depleted subtypes, and nodular lymphocyte predominant Hodgkin's lymphoma, a rare subtype seen in approximately 5% of cases.[1] Each of these 2 major variants, classic and nodular lymphocyte predominant, has a unique set of presenting symptoms and natural history. An understanding of the typical and unusual ways in which each of these 2 main variants of Hodgkin's lymphoma can present and how the disease spreads throughout the body is essential to their timely diagnosis and initiation of appropriate treatment. In addition, appreciation of the typical patterns of spread and relapse of this lymphoma equips the clinician with the knowledge needed to choose the best and most efficient diagnostic tests to stage the disease correctly and plan a course of treatment that best balances the need to cure this otherwise fatal illness with the need to minimize the impact of late, potentially serious toxicities.

Hodgkin's lymphoma typically, but not exclusively, presents in younger patients, usually between the ages of 20 and 60 years. Patients may feel well but note anatomic changes such as localized lymphadenopathy or they may become ill with constitutional symptoms, such as fever, night sweats, unexplained weight loss or fatigue or nonspecific organ-related symptoms, such as cough, pruritus, or localized bone pain or unexpected laboratory abnormalities, such as anemia, hypoalbuminemia, or an elevated erythrocyte sedimentation rate. Diagnosis may be straightforward, based on the results of a lymph node or bone marrow biopsy, or challenging because of the nonspecific nature of presenting symptoms or laboratory findings. Appreciation of the typical and unusual modes of presentation of the lymphoma is necessary for its timely recognition.

## COMMON SYMPTOMS AND PRESENTING ABNORMALITIES OF CLASSICAL HODGKIN'S LYMPHOMA

Classical Hodgkin's lymphoma almost always causes mass lesions, most typically in centriaxial lymph nodes, but occasionally in other organs, such as the spleen, bone marrow, liver, bone, or lungs. However,

because several of these sites are anatomically deep within the body, indirect evidence of the presence of the lymphoma, such as constitutional symptoms, local organ-specific abnormalities, such as cough or bone pain or incidentally discovered laboratory abnormalities, may precede detection of such mass lesions by physical examination or imaging. Thus, the most common manifestation of Hodgkin's lymphoma, especially in younger patients, is the development of persistent, painless, firm but not hard, supradiaphragmatic lymphadenopathy, usually but not exclusively in the neck or supraclavicular fossa or, less often, axilla (Table 1). However, similar lymphadenopathy may develop within the mediastinum where it does not come to attention until it causes a localizing symptom, such as cough, substernal chest pain, or anterior chest wall swelling. In older patients, retroperitoneal lymphadenopathy may present as an abdominal mass or abdominal or back pain.

Hodgkin's lymphoma typically spreads in a predictable fashion from one set of lymph nodes to adjacent groups, most often starting in supradiaphragmatic nodes (90%) and much less commonly in infradiaphragmatic nodes (10%). Two types of extranodal spread are recognized. Localized extension, presumably by direct invasion or through local lymphatic vessels, may involve any anatomic structure nearby involved lymph nodes, accounting for almost all involvement of the thyroid, pleura, pericardium, perihilar lungs, subcutaneous tissue, skin, epidural tissue, and other similar sites. Such localized contiguous spread is common, especially when the original lymph node involvement is bulky and has a special designation in the staging system applied to Hodgkin's lymphoma.[2,3] For example, involvement localized to neck lymph nodes and the nearby thyroid is designated stage II E. Such localized spread of Hodgkin's lymphoma should be distinguished from more distant spread into extranodal organs, such as, the bone marrow or liver, because such localized extranodal extension does not necessarily imply widespread metastases and measures suitable for the treatment of localized disease, such as radiation, can be curative.

Spread of Hodgkin's lymphoma to distant extranodal organs is almost always preceded by splenic involvement, although the involvement of the spleen may be occult. Such distant extranodal Hodgkin's lymphoma occurs almost exclusively in 4 organs: liver, bone marrow, lung, or bone. Although rare cases of isolated involvement at other extranodal sites, such as skin, brain, gastrointestinal tract, or musculoskeletal tissue have been reported they are quite exceptional and constitute less than 1% of Hodgkin's lymphoma presentations.[1] Even in the presence of confirmed Hodgkin's lymphoma in lymph nodes involvement of such exceptional sites should be accepted as part of the presentation of the Hodgkin's lymphoma only if proven by an appropriate biopsy. Often such associated lesions prove to be due to another neoplasm or infectious disease, not the underlying Hodgkin's lymphoma.

**TABLE 1.** Common and Uncommon Manifestations of Hodgkin's Lymphoma at the Time of Initial Diagnosis

| | |
|---|---:|
| **Common** | |
| Lymphadenopathy | |
|   Supradiaphragmatic | 90% |
|   Infradiaphragmatic | 10% |
| Extranodal disease | |
|   No extranodal extension | 75% |
|   Localized, contiguous with involved lymph nodes | 10% |
|   Disseminated (liver, lung, bone, and bone marrow) | |
|     Classical | 15% |
|     Nodular lymphocyte predominant | 5% |
| B symptoms | 35% |
| **Uncommon** | |
| Pruritus | <5% |
| Pain after alcohol ingestion | <2% |
| **Rare** | <1% |
| Autoimmune | |
|   Hemolytic anemia | |
|   Thrombocytopenia | |
| Paraneoplastic | |
|   Neurologic | |
|     Cerebellar degeneration | |
|     Limbic encephalitis (Ophelia syndrome) | |
|     Subacute myelopathy | |
|     Subacute motor neuropathy | |
|     Guillain-Barre syndrome | |
|     Central pontine myelinolysis | |
|     Diffuse cerebritis | |
|   Renal | |
|     Glomerulonephritis | |
|       Minimal change | |
|       Membranous | |
|       Proliferative | |
|       IgA associated | |
|     Nephrotic syndrome | |

As appropriate for the detection of any new mass lesion, either by physical examination or imaging tests performed to investigate a localizing symptom, such a finding should prompt an appropriate biopsy. It is quite important that such a biopsy consist of either an entire-involved lymph node or a generous excisional biopsy of a deeper mass lesion to provide the pathologist with sufficient material to search for the expected Reed-Sternberg cells and find the typical mixed inflammatory background changes.[4] A definitive diagnosis is a cornerstone of modern oncologic management and should not be compromised by an inadequately small or crushed biopsy.

Manifestations of Hodgkin's lymphoma other than a mass lesion can be divided into localized symptoms, nonspecific constitutional or organ-related symptoms, and laboratory abnormalities. Although not a common cause of such localized symptoms as cough, substernal chest pain, bone pain, or abdominal swelling, Hodgkin's lymphoma should remain on the list of possible explanations until a specific diagnosis is made. An appropriate combination of imaging tests and directed biopsies should provide the needed diagnostic answer. More challenging can be nonspecific constitutional symp-toms, such as fever, night sweats, weight loss, or fatigue. Before the availability of modern imaging techniques, especially fine-detailed computerized tomographic scanning, Hodgkin's lymphoma was appropriately included in any list of differential diagnoses of such non-specific abnormalities. However, currently such scans, occasionally complemented by functional imaging tests such as radionucleotide gallium scanning or positron emission tomography, almost always allow localization of a mass lesion appropriate for biopsy if Hodgkin's lymphoma is present. Similarly, such imaging techniques straight-forwardly assist the assessment of organ-specific symptoms, such as localized pain or cough, quickly identifying appropriate next steps to confirm a diagnosis.

One organ-specific symptom, pruritus, continues to challenge physicians because of its nonspecific nature and the infrequency with which it is caused by Hodgkin's lymphoma. Clinicians, especially family practitioners, primary care internists, and dermatologists, need to remember Hodgkin's lymphoma as a possible cause of intractable itching. Finally, incidentally discovered anemia, thrombocytopenia, neutropenia, lymphopenia, hypoalbuminemia, or elevated erythrocyte sedimentation or similar findings encountered either incidentally or in the assessment of fatigue, unexplained weight loss, fever, night sweats, or other constitutional symptoms may suggest the presence of Hodgkin's lymphoma. Imaging tests followed by an appropriate biopsy or performance of a bone marrow biopsy should provide the additional information necessary to pin down a diagnosis of Hodgkin's lymphoma, if present.

## UNCOMMON SYMPTOMS AND PRESENTING ABNORMALITIES OF CLASSICAL HODGKIN'S LYMPHOMA

Uncommonly, Hodgkin's lymphoma may cause a variety of potentially confusing symptoms or findings. Pain at a site of involved lymph nodes may occur immediately after alcohol ingestion. Although traditionally associated with Hodgkin's lymphoma, such alcohol-related pain is rare (<1%–2% of cases) and not specific, occasionally being caused by other neoplasms or inflammatory diseases such as systemic lupus erythematosis or rheumatoid arthritis.[5] Persistent alcohol-related pain should be investigated with imaging studies focused on the lymph node areas near the pain. If due to Hodgkin's lymphoma, lymphadenopathy should be readily evident.

Although autoimmune hematologic conditions have been reported with Hodgkin's lymphoma in the past, such manifestations are now rare, perhaps in part because such past reports may have been based on mistaken diagnoses of what was actually a non-Hodgkin's lymphoma. Autoimmune hemolytic anemia and thrombocytopenia have been rarely reported with Hodgkin's lymphoma and should be appropriately investigated.[6,7] Most often such conditions are linked to other conditions besides Hodgkin's lymphoma or remain unexplained. Rarely, Hodgkin's lymphoma is found to be present and, if so, appropriate treatment should resolve the autoimmune phenomenon.

Paraneoplastic syndromes have infrequently been reported in association with Hodgkin's lymphoma. Several neurologic manifestations have been described including cerebellar degeneration, which usually presents as a gait abnormality but may involve dysarthria, nystagmus, diplopia, or dysphagia.[8,9] This syndrome seems to be caused by cross-reacting autoantibodies that irreversibly damage nerve fibers within the cerebellum.[10] Arrest of progression and occasional improvement with control of the underlying Hodgkin's lymphoma have been reported.[8] Other uncommon neurologic associations have rarely been reported in association with Hodgkin's lymphoma including limbic encephalitis (also referred to as the Ophelia syndrome),[11] subacute myelopathy,[12] subacute motor neuropathy,[13] Guillain-Barre syndrome,[14] central pontine myelinolysis,[15] and diffuse cerebritis.[16]

The kidneys, although virtually never invaded by metastatic spread of Hodgkin's lymphoma and only occasionally by direct extension, may display paraneoplastic involvement. Glomerulonephritides of various types have been described including minimal change, membranous, proliferative, or IgA-associated glomerulonephritis.[17–22] Clinically, patients may have all or some of the findings of nephrotic syndrome,[23–25] sometimes predating the lymphoma by months to years. The timing of these renal abnormalities is not tightly connected to the lymphoma. They may occur, before, coincident with, after successful treatment of, or at the same time as relapse of the lymphoma.[23–25] In addition, these glomerulonephritides may persist despite control of the lymphoma or regress independently.

Many additional syndromic abnormalities or organ dysfunctions have rarely been reported coincident with Hodgkin's lymphoma including hepatitis, cholangitis, vasculitis, conjunctivitis, uveitis, hypertension, hypercalcemia, hypoglycemia, the syndrome of inappropriate antidiuretic hormone secretion, coagulopathies, and hemophagocytosis.[26] These abnormalities have usually been associated with advanced, often recurrent or neglected, disease and none is diagnostic of Hodgkin's lymphoma. Thus, their presence is not likely to lead to the diagnosis of Hodgkin's lymphoma unless additional findings are present, such as a mass lesion in lymph nodes, spleen, liver, bone, or lungs or an abnormal infiltrate is found in the bone marrow.

Two situations in which Hodgkin's lymphoma is diagnosed deserve special comment because of their unusual modes of presentation. First, Hodgkin's lymphoma coincident with infection due to human immunodeficiency virus (HIV) much more frequently involves extranodal organs and causes coincident B symptoms (night sweats, fever, and weight loss) than ordinary Hodgkin's lymphoma.[27–33] In addition, the extranodal lymphoma may involve unusual organs, such as the central nervous system, musculoskeletal tissue, pleura, or abdominal viscera and may do so in the absence of splenic involvement, both characteristics infrequently encountered with Hodgkin's lymphoma in the absence of HIV infection.[27–30,34,35] This unusually aggressive pattern of metastatic involvement partially explains the poorer response to treatment seen in patients with Hodgkin's lymphoma and HIV infection.[27–30,34,35]

The other situation in which Hodgkin's lymphoma may present atypically is when it affects older patients above the age of 60 to 70 years, which occurs in about 5% of patients.[36–43] In such patients, presentations with systemic symptoms such as weight loss and fatigue are much more common as is subdiaphragmatic involvement. Also, in contrast to younger patients, in which approximately 75% of cases are of the nodular sclerosing subtype, at least 50% of older patients present with the mixed cellularity subtype.[37] This combination of findings associated with advanced age including subdiaphragmatic presentation, which less often presents with an obvious mass that might prompt medical assessment and is therefore harder to detect, prominent constitutional symptoms and mixed cellularity subtype may partially explain the poorer prognosis seen in elderly patients.[36–39]

## CLINICAL MANIFESTATIONS OF NODULAR LYMPHOCYTE PREDOMINANT HODGKIN'S LYMPHOMA

Nodular lymphocyte predominant Hodgkin's lymphoma is seen in approximately 5% of cases of newly diagnosed disease. This variant typically occurs in younger patients with a 2:1 male predominance. More than 80% of cases present with limited stage disease, usually supradiaphragmatic stage I A or II A, or less commonly III A,

with minimal bulk.[44–47] Apparent involvement of extranodal organs, bulky splenic or subdiaphragmatic disease, or constitutional symptoms should prompt additional biopsies, because such findings are unusual in nodular lymphocyte predominant Hodgkin's lymphoma and are often a sign of coincident non-Hodgkin's lymphoma, particularly diffuse large B-cell lymphoma or T-cell rich B-cell lymphoma.[48] Nodular lymphocyte predominant Hodgkin's lymphoma typically has very indolent behavior often persisting as palpable peripheral lymph nodes for months to years before a definite diagnosis is made. It may be preceded or followed by persistent lymphadenopathy due to progressive transformation of germinal centers, a non-neoplastic condition that may prove self-limiting or may be a prodrome to nodular lymphocyte predominant Hodgkin's lymphoma or other lymphocytic neoplasms.[49,50]

## NATURAL HISTORY OF HODGKIN'S LYMPHOMA

Before discovery of reliably curative treatments, Hodgkin's lymphoma was a uniformly fatal illness with patients succumbing to a combination of progressive bulky lymphadenopathy that eventually compromised vital organ function and a wasting syndrome with steadily worsening constitutional symptoms, weight loss, cachexia, inanition, and death. Currently available chemotherapy and radiation treatments cure at least 80% of patients, usually with the first choice of regimen. Thus, fortunately, late manifestations of the disease have become uncommon. However, recurrence does affect a minority of patients. When Hodgkin's lymphoma relapses it typically recurs in sites of previous disease, if those sites were not treated with radiation, or novel sites if the original disease was irradiated. Even if novel sites are involved they are usually in lymph node regions nearby original sites of disease or in the usual extranodal sites, lung, liver, bone, or bone marrow. At recurrence, the histologic subtype most often matches the original diagnosis but a progression to greater numbers of Reed Sternberg cells and a tendency to develop the syncitial variant of nodular sclerosing disease may become evident. Eventually, despite application of the current best available treatments, involvement of vital organs, such as the lungs, liver, and bone marrow, often complicated by systemic infections, marked nutritional compromise and generalized weakness leads to the patient's demise. At autopsy extensive involvement of extranodal organs, including those seldom involved in the earlier stages of the disease, such as the central nervous system, can be documented.

For the clinician, the most important aspect of the later natural history of Hodgkin's lymphoma has to do with the anticipation of relapse, if it is going to occur. Fortunately, most recurrences become evident soon after the completion of primary treatment. Currently, at least half of all recurrences are noted within 1 to 2 years of primary treatment completion and 80% to 90% within 5 years. Patients who remain free of recurrence for more than 10 years rarely develop recurrence and after 15 years the risk of recurrence drops to match the risk of developing the lymphoma independently.[51] Thus, after the first decade of follow-up the most important aspect of continued management is anticipation of late complications of treatment, the majority of which is development of secondary neoplasms.[52–56] Irradiation is the treatment most likely to induce second cancers but chemotherapy, especially if it included alkylating agents such as mechlorethamine or cyclophosphamide, and even the underlying defects that led to the development of Hodgkin's lymphoma in the first place may also play a role. It is important to screen for cancers of the head and neck, thyroid, lung, breast, skin, uterine cervix, pleura (mesothelioma), and soft tissues (sarcoma) and to counsel against exposure to any additive factors such as use of tobacco products. Symptoms suggestive of such second cancers should be promptly evaluated.

**TABLE 2.**   Potential Late Nonneoplastic Complications of Treatment of Hodgkin's Lymphoma With Appropriate Clinical Responses and Preventive Strategies

| Risk/Problem | Incidence/Response |
| --- | --- |
| Dental caries | Neck or oropharyngeal irradiation may cause decreased salivation. Patients should have careful dental care follow-up and should make their dentist aware of the previous irradiation. |
| Hypothyroidism | After external beam irradiation that encompasses the thyroid with doses sufficient to cure Hodgkin's lymphoma at least 50% of patients eventually develop hypothyroidism. All patients whose TSH level becomes elevated should be treated with life-long thyroxine replacement in doses sufficient to suppress thyroid-stimulating hormone (TSH) levels to low normal. This is necessary to correct the hypothyroidism and to assure that the radiation damaged thyroid is not subjected to long-term stimulation by thyroid stimulating hormone, which may increase the risk of thyroid neoplasm. |
| Infertility | ABVD is not known to cause any permanent gonadal toxicity although oligospermia for 1 to 2 yr after treatment is common. Other regimens may cause gonadal damage, especially if alkylating agents or procarbazine was included. Direct or scatter radiation to gonadal tissue also may cause infertility, amenorrhea, or premature menopause but this seldom occurs with the current fields used for the treatment of Hodgkin's lymphoma. Thus, with the current chemotherapy regimens and radiation fields used, most patients will not develop these problems. In general, after treatment, women who continue menstruating are fertile, but men require semen analysis to provide a specific answer. High-dose chemoradiotherapy and hematopoietic stem-cell transplantation almost always cause permanent infertility in both genders although some young women occasionally recover fertility. |
| Impaired immunity to infections | Hodgkin's lymphoma and its treatment can lead to life-long impairment of full immunity to infection. All patients should be given annual influenza immunization and pneumococcal immunization after treatment and again 5 yr later. Patients whose spleen has been irradiated or removed should also be immunized against meningococcal types A and C and *Hemophilus influenza* type B. As for all adults, diphtheria and tetanus immunizations should be kept up to date and appropriate immunizations given to prevent infections such as hepatitis A or B when traveling or if the patient's occupation or activities suggest heightened risk of exposure. |

Optimal follow-up management of a patient with cured Hodgkin's lymphoma also requires an understanding of other late toxicities besides second neoplasms.[57] Table 2 lists the major such late complications and appropriate steps to minimize their negative effects. In an era when most patients are cured correct management of the late infectious, endocrine, reproductive, dental, and other complications of the chemotherapy and radiation required to cure the original lymphoma is integral to ensuring each patient's long-term health.

## CONCLUSIONS

Most cases of Hodgkin's lymphoma present with typical lymphadenopathy detected either incidentally by the patient or by imaging procedures performed for assessment of other conditions or as part of investigation of localized symptoms such as cough or pain. Occasionally, nonspecific constitutional symptoms such as fever or fatigue prompt assessment which, in turn, reveals a mass lesion. The diagnosis is confirmed with an appropriate biopsy. Nowadays, aided by remarkably detailed imaging procedures such as modern computerized tomographic scanning, the clinician usually has little difficulty identifying the site to be biopsied and, thus, the diagnosis of Hodgkin's lymphoma is readily established. Knowledge of the usual pattern of spread of this lymphoma, with its orderly progression through lymph node groups and typical forms of extranodal involvement, facilitates timely diagnosis and informs the choice of procedures necessary to complete staging and plan treatment. Rare manifestations with involvement of unusual sites or presentation with paraneoplastic organ dysfunction can challenge the evaluating physician but a search for mass lesions and an appreciation of these uncommonly encountered findings as potential clues to the presence of Hodgkin's lymphoma eventually prompts appropriate investigation and correct diagnosis of the underlying lymphoma. Finally, an understanding of the usual pattern and timing of relapse and knowledge of the typical types of late toxicity expected after successful eradication of the lymphoma allow the patient's physicians to detect recurrence or secondary complications and devise appropriate management plans.

## REFERENCES

1. Swerdlow SH, Campo E, Harris NL, et al. *WHO Classification of Tumours of Haematopoietic and Lymphoid Tissues.* Lyon, France: International Agency for Research on Cancer; 2008.
2. Carbone PP, Kaplan HS, Musshoff K, et al. Report of the committee on Hodgkin's disease staging classification. *Cancer Res.* 1971;31:1860–1861.
3. Lister TA, Crowther D, Sutcliffe SB, et al. Report of a committee convened to discuss the evaluation and staging of patients with Hodgkin's disease: Cotswolds meeting. *J Clin Oncol.* 1989;7:1630–1636.
4. Hehn ST, Grogan TM, Miller TP. Utility of fine-needle aspiration as a diagnostic technique in lymphoma. *J Clin Oncol.* 2004;22:3046–3052.
5. Bichel J. Is the alcohol-intolerance syndrome in Hodgkin's disease disappearing? *Lancet.* 1972;1:1069.
6. Levine AM, Thornton P, Forman SJ, et al. Positive Coombs test in Hodgkin's disease: significance and implications. *Blood.* 1980;55:607–611.
7. Ozdemir F, Yilmaz M, Akdogan R, et al. Hodgkin's disease and autoimmune hemolytic anemia: a case report. *Med Princ Pract.* 2005;14:205–207.
8. Hammack J, Kotanides H, Rosenblum MK, et al. Paraneoplastic cerebellar degeneration. II. Clinical and immunologic findings in 21 patients with Hodgkin's disease. *Neurology.* 1992;42:1938–1943.
9. Dropcho EJ. Autoimmune central nervous system paraneoplastic disorders: mechanisms, diagnosis, and therapeutic options. *Ann Neurol.* 1995;37(suppl 1):S102–S113.
10. Shams'ili S, Grefkens J, de Leeuw B, et al. Paraneoplastic cerebellar degeneration associated with antineuronal antibodies: analysis of 50 patients. *Brain.* 2003;126:1409–1418.
11. Carr I. The Ophelia syndrome: memory loss in Hodgkin's disease. *Lancet.* 1982;1:844–845.
12. Dansey RD, Hammond-Tooke GD, Lai K, et al. Subacute myelopathy: an unusual paraneoplastic complication of Hodgkin's disease. *Med Pediatr Oncol.* 1988;16:284–286.
13. Schold SC, Cho ES, Somasundaram M, et al. Subacute motor neuronopathy: a remote effect of lymphoma. *Ann Neurol.* 1979;5:271–287.
14. Hughes RA, Britton T, Richards M. Effects of lymphoma on the peripheral nervous system. *J R Soc Med.* 1994;87:526–530.
15. Chintagumpala MM, Mahoney DH Jr, McClain K, et al. Hodgkin's disease associated with central pontine myelinolysis. *Med Pediatr Oncol.* 1993;21:311–314.
16. Epaulard O, Courby S, Pavese P, et al. Paraneoplastic acute diffuse encephalitis revealing Hodgkin's disease. *Leuk Lymphoma.* 2004;45:2509–2512.
17. Bergmann J, Buchheidt D, Waldherr R, et al. IgA nephropathy and hodgkin's disease: a rare coincidence. Case report and literature review. *Am J Kidney Dis.* 2005;45:e16–e19.

18. Dabbs DJ, Striker LM, Mignon F, et al. Glomerular lesions in lymphomas and leukemias. *Am J Med.* 1986;80:63–70.

19. Fer MF, McKinney TD, Richardson RL, et al. Cancer and the kidney: complications of neoplasms. *Am J Med.* 1981;71:704–718.

20. Ma KW, Golbus SM, Kaufman R, et al. Glomerulonephritis with Hodgkin's disease and herpes zoster. *Arch Pathol Lab Med.* 1978;102:527–529.

21. Ronco PM. Paraneoplastic glomerulopathies: new insights into an old entity. *Kidney Int.* 1999;56:355–377.

22. Yum MN, Edwards JL, Kleit S. Glomerular lesions in Hodgkin disease. *Arch Pathol.* 1975;99:645–649.

23. Shapiro CM, Vander Laan BF, Jao W, et al. Nephrotic syndrome in two patients with cured Hodgkin's disease. *Cancer.* 1985;55:1799–1804.

24. Delmez JA, Safdar SH, Kissane JM. The successful treatment of recurrent nephrotic syndrome with the MOPP regimen in a patient with a remote history of Hodgkin's disease. *Am J Kidney Dis.* 1994;23:743–746.

25. Korzets Z, Golan E, Manor Y, et al. Spontaneously remitting minimal change nephropathy preceding a relapse of Hodgkin's disease by 19 months. *Clin Nephrol.* 1992;38:125–127.

26. Bierman PJ, Cavalli F, Armitage J. Unusual syndromes in Hodgkin lymphoma. In: Hoppe RT, Mauch PM, Armitage JO, et al, eds. *Hodgkin Lymphoma.* Philadelphia: Wolters Kluwer; 2007:411–418.

27. Berenguer J, Miralles P, Ribera JM, et al. Characteristics and outcome of AIDS-related Hodgkin lymphoma before and after the introduction of highly active antiretroviral therapy. *J Acquir Immune Defic Syndr.* 2008;47:422–428.

28. Tanaka PY, Pessoa VP Jr, Pracchia LF, et al. Hodgkin lymphoma among patients infected with HIV in post-HAART era. *Clin Lymphoma Myeloma.* 2007;7:364–368.

29. Hentrich M, Maretta L, Chow KU, et al. Highly active antiretroviral therapy (HAART) improves survival in HIV-associated Hodgkin's disease: results of a multicenter study. *Ann Oncol.* 2006;17:914–919.

30. Biggar RJ, Jaffe ES, Goedert JJ, et al. Hodgkin lymphoma and immunodeficiency in persons with HIV/AIDS. *Blood.* 2006;108:3786–3791.

31. Vilchez RA, Finch CJ, Jorgensen JL, et al. The clinical epidemiology of Hodgkin lymphoma in HIV-infected patients in the highly active antiretroviral therapy (HAART) era. *Medicine (Baltimore).* 2003;82:77–81.

32. Re A, Casari S, Cattaneo C, et al. Hodgkin disease developing in patients infected by human immunodeficiency virus results in clinical features and a prognosis similar to those in patients with human immunodeficiency virus-related non-Hodgkin lymphoma. *Cancer.* 2001;92:2739–2745.

33. Powles T, Bower M. HIV-associated Hodgkin's disease. *Int J STD AIDS.* 2000;11:492–494.

34. Xicoy B, Ribera JM, Miralles P, et al. Results of treatment with doxorubicin, bleomycin, vinblastine and dacarbazine and highly active antiretroviral therapy in advanced stage, human immunodeficiency virus-related Hodgkin's lymphoma. *Haematologica.* 2007;92:191–198.

35. Thompson LD, Fisher SI, Chu WS, et al. HIV-associated Hodgkin lymphoma: a clinicopathologic and immunophenotypic study of 45 cases. *Am J Clin Pathol.* 2004;121:727–738.

36. Klimm B, Eich HT, Haverkamp H, et al. Poorer outcome of elderly patients treated with extended-field radiotherapy compared with involved-field radiotherapy after chemotherapy for Hodgkin's lymphoma: an analysis from the German Hodgkin Study Group. *Ann Oncol.* 2007;18:357–363.

37. Klimm B, Diehl V, Engert A. Hodgkin's lymphoma in the elderly: a different disease in patients over 60. *Oncology. (Williston Park)* 2007;21:982–990; discussion 990, 996, 998 passim.

38. Feltl D, Vitek P, Zamecnik J. Hodgkin's lymphoma in the elderly: the results of 10 years of follow-up. *Leuk Lymphoma.* 2006;47:1518–1522.

39. Engert A, Ballova V, Haverkamp H, et al. Hodgkin's lymphoma in elderly patients: a comprehensive retrospective analysis from the German Hodgkin's Study Group. *J Clin Oncol.* 2005;23:5052–5060.

40. Landgren O, Algernon C, Axdorph U, et al. Hodgkin's lymphoma in the elderly with special reference to type and intensity of chemotherapy in relation to prognosis. *Haematologica.* 2003;88:438–444.

41. Kim HK, Silver B, Li S, et al. Hodgkin's disease in elderly patients (> or = 60): clinical outcome and treatment strategies. *Int J Radiat Oncol Biol Phys.* 2003;56:556–560.

42. Stark GL, Wood KM, Jack F, et al. Hodgkin's disease in the elderly: a population-based study. *Br J Haematol.* 2002;119:432–440.

43. Proctor SJ, Rueffer JU, Angus B, et al. Hodgkin's disease in the elderly: current status and future directions. *Ann Oncol.* 2002;13:133–137.

44. Nogova L, Reineke T, Brillant C, et al. Lymphocyte-predominant and classical Hodgkin's lymphoma: a comprehensive analysis from the German Hodgkin Study Group. *J Clin Oncol.* 2008;26:434–439.

45. Anagnostopoulos I, Hansmann ML, Franssila K, et al. European Task Force on Lymphoma project on lymphocyte predominance Hodgkin disease: histologic and immunohistologic analysis of submitted cases reveals 2 types of Hodgkin disease with a nodular growth pattern and abundant lymphocytes. *Blood.* 2000;96:1889–1899.

46. Diehl V, Franklin J, Sextro M, et al. Clinical presentation and treatment of lymphocyte predominance Hodgkin's disease. In: Armitage JO, Diehl V, Hoppe RT, et al, eds. *Hodgkin's Disease.* Philadelphia: Lippincott Williams & Wilkins; 1999:563–582.

47. Bodis S, Kraus MD, Pinkus G, et al. Clinical presentation and outcome in lymphocyte predominant Hodgkin's disease. *J Clin Oncol.* 1997;15:3060–3066.

48. Huang JZ, Weisenburger DD, Vose JM, et al. Diffuse large B-cell lymphoma arising in nodular lymphocyte predominant Hodgkin lymphoma: a report of 21 cases from the Nebraska Lymphoma Study Group. *Leuk Lymphoma.* 2004;45:1551–1557.

49. Osborne BM, Butler JJ. Clinical implications of progressive transformation of germinal centers. *Am J Surg Pathol.* 1984;8:725–733.

50. Poppema S, Kaiserling E, Lennert K. Hodgkin's disease with lymphocytic predominance, nodular type (nodular paragranuloma) and progressively transformed germinal centres—a cytohistological study. *Histopathology.* 1979;3:295–308.

51. Bodis S, Henry-Amar M, Bosq J, et al. Late relapse in early-stage Hodgkin's disease patients enrolled on European Organization for Research and Treatment of Cancer protocols. *J Clin Oncol.* 1993;11:225–232.

52. Connors JM. Hodgkin's lymphoma: the hazards of success. *J Clin Oncol.* 2003;21:3388–3390.

53. Aleman BM, van den Belt-Dusebout AW, Klokman WJ, et al. Long-term cause-specific mortality of patients treated for Hodgkin's disease. *J Clin Oncol.* 2003;21:3431–3439.

54. Henry-Amar M, Somers R. Survival outcome after Hodgkin's disease: a report from the international data base on Hodgkin's disease. *Semin Oncol.* 1990;17:758–768.

55. Henry-Amar M, Hayat M, Meerwaldt JH, et al. Causes of death after therapy for early stage Hodgkin's disease entered on EORTC protocols. EORTC Lymphoma Cooperative Group. *Int J Radiat Oncol Biol Phys.* 1990;19:1155–1157.

56. van Leeuwen FE, Swerdlow SH, Travis LB. Second cancers after treatment of Hodgkin lymphoma. In: Hoppe RT, Mauch PM, Armitage JO, et al, eds. *Hodgkin Lymphoma.* Philadelphia: Wolters Kluwer; 2007:347–370.

57. Vose JM, Constine LS, Sutcliffe SB. Other complications of the treatment of Hodgkin lymphoma. In: Hoppe RT, Mauch PM, Armitage JO, et al, eds. *Hodgkin Lymphoma.* Philadelphia: Wolters Kluwer; 2007:383–392.

# Histopathology of Hodgkin's Lymphoma

Franziska C. Eberle • Haresh Mani • Elaine S. Jaffe

## HISTORICAL BACKGROUND

In 1832, Thomas Hodgkin first reported "On some morbid appearances of the absorbent glands and spleen" describing postmortem findings in 7 patients with enlarged lymph nodes and spleen.[1] Thirty-three years later Wilks[2] confirmed Hodgkin's findings in 15 additional patients and proposed to name the disease "Hodgkin's disease." In 1898 and 1902, the characteristic binucleated and multinucleated cells in Hodgkin's disease were independently described by Carl Sternberg and Dorothy Reed (Fig. 1). She disputed the view of Carl Sternberg, who related the abnormal cellular proliferation to tuberculosis.[3] She made a number of other significant observations, noting an early age peak in children and adolescents, and that the health of the patient was generally excellent before disease onset. She also noted the presence of anergy in patients with Hodgkin's disease.[4] However, neither Reed nor Sternberg recognized the neoplastic nature of the disease. Gall and Mallory[5] established the first modern classification system of lymphoma, based on their studies of 618 cases, which also included Hodgkin's disease. In 1944, Jackson and Parker[6] developed the first classification of Hodgkin's disease which contained 3 subtypes of Hodgkin's disease: paragranuloma, granuloma, and sarcoma (Table 1).

The modern classification of Hodgkin's disease was introduced by Lukes and Butler.[7] Importantly, they recognized the unique features of nodular sclerosis which was former subsumed under the large group of "Hodgkin's granuloma." Recognizing the importance of the inflammatory background, they described lymphocytic and histiocytic (L&H) predominance, and lymphocyte depletion (LD) Hodgkin's lymphomas. L&H Hodgkin's could be nodular or diffuse, and LD was likewise divided into diffuse fibrosis and reticular subtypes. Mixed cellularity remained somewhat of a wastebasket category, for those cases not meeting criteria for one of the other subtypes. In the subsequent Rye conference in New York these 6 subtypes were reduced again to 4 subtypes: lymphocyte predominant, nodular sclerosis, mixed cellularity, and lymphocyte depleted.[8] This classification could be readily used by pathologists with high reproducibility, and correlated well with clinical features, and remained unaltered for almost 3 decades. Based on new phenotypic, genotypic, morphologic, and clinical findings, the Revised European American Lymphoma (REAL) classification in 1994 included Hodgkin's lymphoma as one of the lymphoid neoplasms, and distinguished between 2 major types: nodular lymphocyte predominant Hodgkin's lymphoma (NLPHL) and classical Hodgkin's lymphoma (CHL). CHL was further classified into 4 subtypes: nodular sclerosis CHL (NSCHL), mixed cellularity CHL (MCCHL), lymphocyte-rich CHL (LRCHL), and lymphocyte-depleted CHL (LDCHL).[9] The terminology recommended in the REAL classification was incorporated into the World Health Organization (WHO) classification of tumors of hematopoietic and lymphoid tissues (Table 1), including the substitution of the term Hodgkin's lymphoma for Hodgkin's disease.[10,11]

The original name "Hodgkin's disease" was based on the uncertain status of the disease, infectious or neoplastic, and the uncertain cell of origin. Multiple studies have proven now the neoplastic nature of the Hodgkin's cell and also a B lymphocyte origin in nearly all cases.[12,13] Therefore, the name "Hodgkin's lymphoma" is preferred instead of the term "Hodgkin's disease."

The WHO classification is primarily based on the histopathological and immunophenotypic characteristics of the different Hodgkin's lymphoma subtypes. Findings from molecular analysis and clinical studies from the recent decades confirm the principles of the WHO classification. But at the same time, new epidemiologic and molecular findings suggest that CHL is not a single disease but consists of more than 1 entity with distinct characteristics. Moreover, the CHL subentities NSCHL and MCCHL/LDCHL together with NLPHL form 95% of Hodgkin's lymphoma. Here, we discuss the categories of Hodgkin's lymphoma focusing on NLPHL, NSCHL, and MCCHL/LDCHL.

## CLASSICAL HODGKIN'S LYMPHOMA

Although NLPHL has been identified as an entity distinct from CHL,[14] there is also a greater appreciation today for the differences between NSCHL and the other subtypes, mainly MCCHL/LDCHL and LRCHL.[15] NSCHL affects young adults, is associated with mediastinal involvement, and requires an intact immune system for its development. In addition to histologic differences, its cytokine milieu and background lymphocyte population differ from other subtypes of CHL. The presence of an overlap with primary mediastinal large B-cell lymphoma (PMLBCL) suggests a thymic origin for mediastinal NSCHL. MCCHL and LDCHL represent a spectrum, sharing many features related to incidence, pattern of spread, and association with immunodeficiency.[15] LRCHL, the most recently defined subtype, is perhaps the least well understood, with respect to its epidemiology and cellular origins (Table 2). Epstein-Barr viral (EBV) sequences are found in 20% to 90% of cases of CHL. The incidence of EBV-positivity varies with the age at presentation, the histologic subtype, and epidemiological factors such as geographic distribution or underlying immunodeficiency.[16] EBV-positive CHL is seen most often in the very young or the very old. There has been considerable speculation regarding the variations in the rate of EBV positivity. Can EBV play a hit and run role, or is there another virus linked to CHL pathogenesis?[17-19]

## NODULAR SCLEROSIS CLASSICAL HODGKIN'S LYMPHOMA

Representing approximately 70% of all CHL, and perhaps an even higher proportion in developed countries, NSCHL is the most frequent subtype and its incidence has continued to rise over the past decades.[20] This entity stands apart from other forms of CHL and

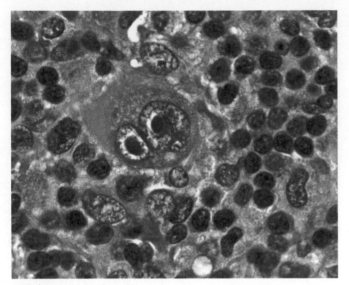

**FIGURE 1.** Classic Reed-Sternberg cell with owl-eye inclusion-like nucleoli. The nucleoli are approximately the same diameter as the background lymphocytes (H&E).

**TABLE 1.** Evolution of Hodgkin's Lymphoma Classification

| Jackson/Parker, 1944 | Lukes/Butler, 1966 | Rye Conference, 1966 | REAL/WHO, 1994/2008 |
|---|---|---|---|
| Paragranuloma | L&H, nodular | LP | NLPHL |
|  | L&H, diffuse |  | LRCHL |
| Granuloma | NS | NS | NSCHL |
|  | MC | MC | MCCHL |
| Sarcoma | LD, diffuse fibrosis | LD | LDCHL |
|  | LD, reticular |  |  |

REAL indicates Revised European American Lymphoma; NS, nodular sclerosis; MC, mixed cellularity.

Hodgkin/Reed Sternberg (HRS) cell is termed a lacunar cell, because the cytoplasmic membrane is often retracted in formalin-fixed tissues (Fig. 2). Compared with classical HRS cells, lacunar cells have smaller nuclei, less prominent nucleoli, and more abundant cytoplasm. Classic HRS cells can also be found but usually are rare in NSCHL. Lacunar cells are found in cellular nodules, containing variable numbers of small lymphocytes. Neutrophils and eosinophils may be abundant, sometimes forming microabscesses within the nodules. The nodules are surrounded by dense collagen bands poor in fibroblasts. HRS cells express interleukin (IL-)13 and fibroblasts from NSCHL type are positive for the IL-13 receptor.[30] The production of transforming growth factor beta by the neoplastic cells also has been implicated in the fibrotic reaction.[31] The fibrosis often begins in the lymph node capsule, with fibrosis invaginating into the lymph node along vascular septa. In contrast to MCCHL and LDCHL, B cells form a higher proportion of the lymphocytic background in NSCHL.[32] In some cases with focal involvement, atypical cells are found within B-cell follicles, consistent with an origin from germinal center B cells.[33,34]

Some morphologic variations of NSCHL exist. The "syncytial variant" of NSCHL is characterized by cohesive sheets of lacunar cells within the nodules. In the "cellular phase" of NSCHL, a nodular growth pattern is present, but concentric fibrous bands are not formed.[35,36] As NSCHL is the most common subtype of CHL in Western countries, and yet differs in its clinical behavior, there have been attempts to grade NSCHL based on the proportion of neoplastic cells. The term "lymphocyte-depleted" (LD) form of NSCHL was coined to describe those cases having a high proportion of HRS cells, often with prominent necrosis.[37] Patients with advanced stage LD-NSCHL had a poorer prognosis and a higher relapse rate than NSCHL without lymphocytic depletion. Interestingly, the adverse prognostic impact of LD-NSCHL was not observed in patients with low-stage disease treated with radiation therapy.[38] A 2-grade system for classification of NSCHL was developed by the British National Lymphoma

NLPHL. NSCHL is more frequent in resource-rich areas and the patient's high socioeconomic status is considered as 1 risk factor.[21,22] The disease affects primarily young adults and is less often observed in the elderly.[23] Interestingly, in contrast to all other forms of CHL and NLPHL, NSCHL demonstrates a female predominance. Association with EBV is rarely reported.[24] Compared with MCCHL and LDCHL, NSCHL shows a different risk factor pattern, suggesting that this entity may not have the same etiology as the other CHL types.[25,26] Gene expression profiling studies have supported the unique aspects of NSCHL, and in addition have identified signatures correlating with the generally good clinical outcome.[27] Prominently expressed genes include those involved in apoptotic induction and cell signaling.

NSCHL also has distinct clinical features. In 80% of patients with NSCHL the mediastinum is involved and 50% of patients with NSCHL present with bulky disease. Involvement of extralymphatic organs or bone marrow is not common. B symptoms occur in approximately 40% of all patients. At time of diagnosis more than 50% of patients have stage II disease.[28,29]

## Histopathology of NSCHL

NSCHL differs from other subtypes in terms of the growth pattern and the characteristics of the neoplastic cells. The characteristic

**TABLE 2.** Major Categories of Hodgkin's Lymphoma

|  | NSCHL | MCCHL and LDCHL | NLPHL |
|---|---|---|---|
| **Risk factors** |  |  |  |
| Socioeconomic status | High | Low | No risk factors |
| HIV infection | Negative | Positive |  |
| Gender predominance | Female | Male | Male |
| Age | Young adults | Children or elderly | Young adults |
| EBV infection | Negative | Positive | Negative |
| Lymphoid tissue involved | Mediastinal, cervical and axial lymph nodes | Generalized disease, lymph nodes and bone marrow | Peripheral and mesenteric lymph nodes, no mediastinal involvement |

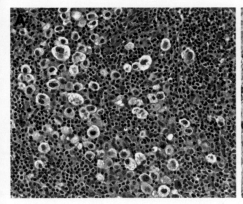
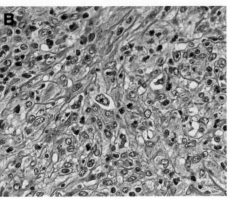

**FIGURE 2.** Nodular sclerosis Hodgkin's lymphoma. A, HRS cells have features of lacunar cells, and cluster within the nodular aggregates (H&E). B, This case is an example of the fibrohistiocytic variant of NSCHL, grade II. Normal lymphocytes are relatively sparse, and histiocytes and eosinophils are abundant (H&E).

Investigation.[39,40] This grading of NSCHL was based on the cellularity of the nodules, the quantity of sclerosis, and the amount and atypia of neoplastic cells. NSCHL was considered grade II if 1 of the 3 following features was fulfilled within the neoplastic nodules: (A) more than 25% with a high proportion of tumor cells and necrosis, (B) more than 80% show a fibrotic or fibrohistiocytic composition, or (C) more than 25% contain numerous large bizarre or anaplastic cells. In the absence of these characteristics, NSCHL was considered grade I. The clinical relevance of grading of NSCHL has not been confirmed in all studies and has remained controversial.[41–43] As therapy has improved, the prognostic significance of grade has diminished.[43] Interestingly, grade seems most relevant in those patients who relapse, with shortened survival seen in those patients relapsing with grade II disease.[42] Variations on the British National Lymphoma Investigation grading system also have been proposed.[44] Grading has not been required by the WHO classification and is considered optional for clinical practice.[43]

A close relationship of NSCHL to PMLBCL and a possible origin from a thymic B cell has been described in recent studies.[45–47] Both entities share several features. The low-affinity immunoglobulin (Ig)E receptor CD23, known to be expressed on thymic B cells and PMLBCL, also is expressed in some cases of NSCHL. A lack of immunoglobulin (Ig) expression and HLA class I antigens is observed in both[48]; and *MAL*, a gene that encodes a protein associated with lipid rafts in T cells and epithelial cells, is expressed in both PMLBCL and some cases of NSCHL with mediastinal involvement.[49,50] Other subtypes of CHL do not express this gene.

The transitional morphology and phenotype of mediastinal gray zone lymphomas (MGZLs) provide further proof of a close relationship between PMLBCL and NSCHL.[11,47] The 2008 WHO classification recognizes a subset of cases in which a distinction between PMLBCL and NSCHL is not possible (Fig. 3). These cases may be designated as "B-cell lymphoma, unclassifiable, with features intermediate between diffuse large B-cell lymphoma and classical Hodgkin's lymphoma." Most but not all of these cases present with mediastinal disease.

Cases with features of MGZLs were most likely included in the past in the category of "Hodgkin's-like" or "Hodgkin's-related" anaplastic large cell lymphoma (ALCL).[51] Because of the strong CD30 expression in both entities, early studies suggested a relationship to ALCL. Today, it is appreciated that they share no biologic relationship, as CHL is of B cell origin and ALCL is of T-cell origin.[52] The optimal therapy for MGZLs is not yet determined.[53,54] However, both chemotherapy and radiation seem required for long-term disease-free survival.[55]

## MIXED CELLULARITY AND LYMPHOCYTE-DEPLETED CLASSICAL HODGKIN'S LYMPHOMA

MCCHL is the second most frequent subtype of all CIIL with a frequency between 10% and 20%, whereas LDCHL is the rarest subtype (<5%) in Western countries.[11] In most developing countries, MCCHL and LDCHL are the predominant CHL subtypes.[56–58] Both entities have overlapping epidemiological, clinical, and biologic features, which clearly differ from NSCHL. In contrast to NSCHL,

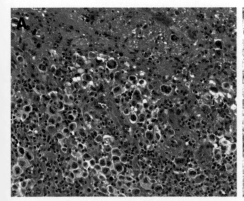
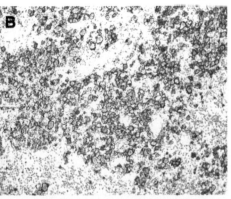

**FIGURE 3.** B-cell lymphoma, unclassifiable, with features intermediate between diffuse large B-cell lymphoma and classical Hodgkin's lymphoma. A, In this example of a "gray zone" lymphoma, the neoplastic cells resemble lacunar cells and are palisaded around an area of necrosis (H&E). B, Immunohistochemical studies showed that the neoplastic cells were strongly CD20-positive and CD15-negative (not shown). This phenotype is atypical for CHL (CD20 immunostain).

low-socioeconomic status seems to be a risk factor for MCCHL and LDCHL.[21] Human immunodeficiency virus (HIV) infection is an additional relevant risk factor for the development of MCCHL or LDCHL, not only in developing countries but also in Western countries.[59–62] A recent study showed that the incidence of Hodgkin's lymphoma is increasing relative to B-immunoblastic lymphomas among HIV-positive patients, as highly active retroviral therapy improves immune function in this cohort.[61]

In contrast to the gender distribution in NSCHL, MCCHL and LDCHL are more common in men than in women. In addition, MCCHL has a bimodal age peak, presenting in both pediatric and elderly patients. LDCHL is primarily a disease of older individuals and associated with greater underlying immune compromise.[63] EBV infection of neoplastic cells is frequently detected in both MCCHL and LDCHL and distinguishes these subtypes from both NSCHL and NLPHL, which are generally EBV negative.[18] In addition to their epidemiologic and pathogenic features, MCCHL and LDCHL also have distinct clinical characteristics. Typically, MCCHL and LDCHL do not involve the thymus gland or mediastinum, which are preferentially involved in NSCHL. In contrast, peripheral lymph nodes and bone marrow are common sites of involvement of MCCHL and LDCHL. B symptoms are frequent. In the past, the histologic subtype was considered a major factor impacting prognosis.[64] Since the development of highly effective therapies, even for patients with advanced stage disease, other factors such as comorbidities including HIV-infection are more important prognostic factors than histologic classification.[65] Nonetheless, histologic subclassification remains relevant, as LDCHL and MCCHL have a worse prognosis compared with other subtypes of CHL.[66]

As NSCHL is subdivided into 2 grades, according to the proportion of tumor cells, MCCHL and LDCHL also may be viewed as 2 grades of a single disease entity.[15] The grading reflects both the proportion of normal lymphocytes within the background and the degree of underlying immunodeficiency in the patient. Subsuming MCCHL and LDCHL into a single entity supports the concept of a 3 disease hypothesis of Hodgkin's lymphoma as already suggested by MacMahon[67] in 1966 (Table 2).

## Histopathology of MCCHL and LDCHL

Morphologically, MCCHL usually shows obliteration of the lymph node architecture. In cases of partial involvement the infiltrate is paracortical, with residual hyperplastic or regressed lymphoid follicles. In contrast to NSCHL, fibrosis if present is fine, fibrillar, and disorganized. Importantly, HRS cells are typical in appearance without lacunar or popcorn variants. As suggested by its name, the background in MCCHL comprises a mixture of different inflammatory cell types including lymphocytes, plasma cells, histiocytes, eosinophils, and neutrophils. The composition of the background can vary from patient to patient. In some cases, a granulomatous reaction may be prominent and may obscure the diagnostic cells.[68]

LDCHL shows a highly variable appearance but is characterized by 1 common feature: relative predominance of HRS cells in relation to the depleted background lymphocytes. Two main patterns of LDCHL were initially described in the Lukes-Butler[69] classification: a reticular/sarcomatous pattern and a diffuse fibrosis pattern. The reticular or sarcomatous variant was characterized by large numbers of HRS cells. This variant is rarely diagnosed today, and many such cases in the past were probably pleomorphic lymphomas of either B or T lineage.[65] Even today the distinction from a pleomorphic B-cell lymphoma may be difficult; such cases are sometimes termed "gray lymphomas," or in the 2008 WHO classification, "B-cell lymphoma, unclassifiable, with features intermediate between diffuse large B-cell

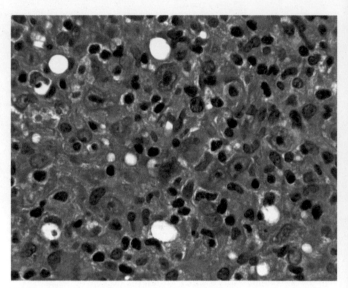

**FIGURE 4.** Lymphocyte-depleted CHL. This uncommon subtype presented in this 90-year-old man with generalized lymphadenopathy. HRS-cells are abundant and the background contains numerous histiocytes (H&E).

lymphoma and classical Hodgkin's lymphoma."[11,70] These tumors often contain Reed-Sternberg-like cells, but differ phenotypically, in that CD20 is more often expressed, and CD15 is negative. Diffuse large B-cell lymphoma of the elderly also may resemble CHL. The neoplastic cells are EBV positive, and show a broad spectrum of cytologic features, including HRS-like cells.[71,72]

The diffuse fibrosis variant is defined as HRS cells embedded in a background of diffuse fibrosis. Fibroblasts can either be increased in number or even absent; recognition of diagnostic HRS cells may be difficult in these cases. Other cases of LDCHL contain abundant histiocytes but relatively few reactive lymphocytes (Fig. 4). This histologic picture may be seen in HIV-associated CHL. LDCHL should be distinguished from NSCHL, grade II, which may contain abundant HRS cells. It is likely that early series contained examples of NSCHL, grade II, miscategorized as LDCHL. LDCHL is the rarest subtype of Hodgkin's lymphoma, and the proportion of cases diagnosed as such has decreased in recent years because of introduction of immunophenotypic and molecular studies and the exclusion of morphologically similar lymphomas.

## LYMPHOCYTE-RICH CLASSICAL HODGKIN'S LYMPHOMA

The most recently identified subtype LRCHL has a rate of approximately 5% of all CHL. In the past, this subtype was often misinterpreted as NLPHL, but with immunophenotypic studies was shown to be a variant of CHL.[9,73] Initially, there was speculation that this might be a variant of NSCHL in "early phase," but in patients with multiple biopsies, the histologic features remained unchanged. The clinical characteristics of LRCHL clearly differ from NSCHL. Patients with LRCHL are predominantly of male gender. The median age is higher than NSCHL and NLPHL.[74,75] Most patients present with peripheral lymphadenopathy, usually stage I or stage II. In contrast to NSCHL, mediastinal involvement is rare. B symptoms are usually absent. The

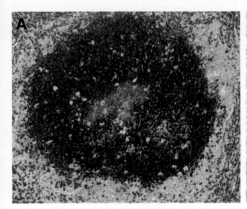

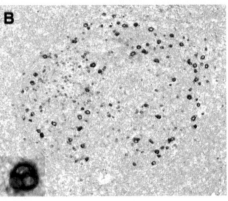

**FIGURE 5.** Lymphocyte-rich CHL. A, HRS cells are found within expanded follicles, mainly at the periphery in the mantle and marginal zone (CD20 immunostain). B, CD30 highlights the HRS cells at the periphery of a B-cell follicle. Inset shows a CD30-positive Reed-Sternberg cell at high power.

tumor cells are usually EBV negative.[76] The prognosis is very good with event-free and overall survival (OS) of 97% at 30 months.

## Histopathology of LRCHL

Most cases of what is now recognized as LRCHL have a nodular growth pattern[73] and were first referred to as follicular Hodgkin's disease.[77] The lymphoid follicles are typically regressed, with the neoplastic cells localized to the far mantle and marginal zones of the follicles (Fig. 5). The individual HRS cells are rosetted by T-cells, so that in immunohistochemical stains the expanded marginal zones have a moth eaten appearance. Other inflammatory cells, including eosinophils and plasma cells, are generally sparse. Cytologically, the HRS cells have the phenotype of CHL; however, their cytologic features are often intermediate between those of lymphocyte predominant (LP) cells and classical HRS cells. They tend to have smaller nucleoli, and less cellular atypia than HRS cells in other forms of CHL. Thus, it is not surprising that these cases were often misdiagnosed as NLPHL before the routine use of immunophenotyping.[73]

A less number of cases of LRCHL have a diffuse growth pattern, with classical HRS cells in a background of mainly small lymphocytes. Cases with these features were probably described first by Lennert and Mohri, who considered them a lymphocyte predominant type of MCCHL.[9,78] The clinical features of this rare variant are not delineated.

### NODULAR LYMPHOCYTE PREDOMINANT HODGKIN'S LYMPHOMA

About 5% of all Hodgkin's lymphomas are classified as NLPHL. This subtype differs from CHL clinically, epidemiologically, and with regard to its immunophenotype and genetics (Table 2).[14] NLPHL is more common in men than in women (3:1).[74] Patients are often young adults between the age of 30 to 50 years, and most often present with peripheral lymphadenopathy without B symptoms. NLPHL is the only subtype in which mesenteric lymph node involvement may be seen. The mediastinum is spared. Association with EBV is rarely seen.[79] The prognosis of NLPHL is good, even in patients who are followed without treatment.[66] Paradoxically, late relapses are not uncommon in NLPHL, but even after relapse the prognosis is good.[74,80]

### Histopathology of NLPHL

NLPHL arises in the follicular environment, and nearly always has a follicular or nodular growth pattern, although over time the process may become diffuse. NLPHL lacks HRS cells. The neoplastic cell of NLPHL was originally termed the L&H cell, after the original description of this form of HL by Lukes et al[7] as "lymphocytic and

histiocytic predominance." These cells have also been referred to as "popcorn" cells, but the WHO classification of 2008 recommended the use of the term "LP cell."[11] In comparison with classical HRS cells, the nucleoli of the LP cells are smaller, multiple, and basophilic. A variety of patterns have been described, but expansion of the follicular structure is nearly always seen.[81]

Progressive transformation of germinal centers (PTGC) is observed in some cases of NLPHL.[82] However, when diagnosed independently, progressive transformation of germinal centers has a low incidence of progression to NLPHL.[83] NLPHL may progress to diffuse large B-cell lymphoma (DLBCL) in about 5% of cases, and in such cases DLBCL and NLPHL are often composite in the same lymph node mass.[84,85] The clinical significance of this form of progression is indeterminate, but some patients still maintain an excellent prognosis.[84,86] Clonal identity between the NLPHL and DLBCL has been shown in most cases studied at the molecular level.[87,88] Another type of histologic progression is to a process histologically indistinguishable from T-cell/histiocyte-rich large B-cell lymphoma.[89] In these cases, the prognosis is often poor, with advanced stage disease and bone marrow involvement. However, cases in which a nodular pattern is maintained, even if T-cell rich, have a better outcome.[90]

### IMMUNOHISTOCHEMISTRY OF HODGKIN'S LYMPHOMA

The diagnosis of Hodgkin's lymphoma is primarily based on the recognition of the typical tumor cells, either HRS cells or LP cells, in the appropriate environment. In addition, the character of the inflammatory background and the surrounding stroma as well as established immunophenotypic and molecular markers help to classify the disease into the various tumor subtypes. A panel of markers is used for immunophenotyping of Hodgkin's lymphoma including B-cell surface markers, transcription factors, and EBV-associated proteins (Table 3).

In nearly all cases of CHL, HRS cells are positive for CD30, a glycoprotein belonging to the tumor necrosis factor receptor superfamily.[91,92] In addition, the majority of HRS cells (85%) also express CD15, the Lewis x carbohydrate adhesion molecule.[93,94] Even though both LP cells and HRS cells are genotypically of B-cell lineage, CD20 and CD79a are only expressed by a minority of CHL cases (10%–40% CD20+).[12,95,96] The wide variation in the proportion of cells expressing CD20 in CHL may be related to changes in antigen retrieval techniques, with a higher proportion of CD20-positive cases seen in recent years. However, overall the B-cell program is lost in most cases of CHL.[96] As noted above, the HRS cells of CHL are positive for EBV most often in MCCHL and LDCHL. EBV is expressed

**TABLE 3.** Immunohistochemical Features of Hodgkin's Lymphoma

|  | LP Cells NLPHL | HRS Cells CHL |
|---|---|---|
| Nonlineage antigens |  |  |
| CD45 | + | − |
| CD30 | − | + |
| CD15 | − | +/− |
| B cell-associated antigens |  |  |
| CD20 | + | −/+ |
| CD79a | + | −/+ |
| J chain | +/− | − |
| IgD | +/− | − |
| B cell-related transcription factors |  |  |
| BOB.1 | + | −/+ |
| OCT 2 | + | −/+ |
| PU.1 | + | − |
| PAX5 | + | + (weak) |
| EBV detection |  |  |
| LMP-1 | − | +/−* |
| EBER | − | +/−* |

*Often positive in MCCHL/LDCHL, usually negative in NSCHL.
+ indicates positive in all cases; +/−, positive in majority of cases; −/+, positive in minority of cases; −, negative in all cases.

with a latency II phenotype and can be detected with immunostains for LMP-1 and EBV in situ hybridization with the EBER probe.[97] Galectin-1 is expressed in CHL but not in NLPHL and seems responsible for mediation of suppression of EBV-specific T-cell immunity.[98]

The phenotype in NLPHL differs in nearly all respects from that of CHL. LP cells are usually negative for both CD15 and CD30.[14] The B-cell markers CD20 and CD79a are positive in nearly all cases of NLPHL. LP cells may express Ig and polypeptides of the light chain fraction (J chain) and Ig are detectable in the majority of cases of NLPHL.[99,100] In addition, the LP cells in a subset of cases of NLPHL express IgD; the IgD-positive cases are most frequent in young males, and often contain nodules relatively rich in T-lymphocytes (Fig. 6).[101] The common leukocyte surface antigen CD45 is detected on LP cells but not on HRS cells.

The B cell-associated transcription factors Pax5, Oct-2, BOB.1, and PU.1 again underscore the B-cell lineage origin of LP cells and

HRS cells but also show specific expression patterns. Pax5, also known as B cell-specific activator protein, is crucial in B-cell lineage commitment and is expressed by LP cells and HRS cells.[102] The other transcription regulating proteins, Oct-2 and BOB.1 that are involved in germinal center formation and Ig production, are expressed by LP cells, but are often negative in CHL.[103] Oct-2 is strongly expressed in normal germinal center cells and more weakly in other B-cell populations. It is also highly expressed in LP cells, and immunostains for Oct-2 are diagnostically useful in cases in which LP cells are sparse (Fig. 6). The unique regulatory protein PU.1 required in the generation of lymphoid and myeloid cells is positive in LP cells but negative in CHL and also in T-cell/histiocyte-rich large B-cell lymphoma (Table 3).[104]

The clinical significance of alterations in the usual phenotype in CHL has been examined in several studies.[95,105,106] A study from the German Hodgkin Study Group found that the absence of CD15 expression and expression of CD20 by the HRS cells were both negative prognostic features.[105] Portlock et al[106] also confirmed an adverse prognostic significance for CD20-positive CHL, with decrease in time to treatment failure and OS in CD20+ cases. However, another study found CD20 to be a positive prognostic factor for both failure-free survival (FFS) and OS.[95] Notably, the clinical impact was lost in patients treated in the more modern era, after 1981. Other immunophenotypic aberrancies also have been observed in CHL. For example, a subset of CHL cases show aberrant T-cell antigen expression, without evidence of T-cell gene rearrangement.[107] CD2, CD3, and CD4 are the most commonly expressed antigens on the surface of the HRS cells.

Although most cases that show a T-cell immunophenotype are also of B-cell origin on molecular analysis,[108] a T-cell origin was suggested in 3 reported cases, based on the presence of T cell receptor gene rearrangements.[109,110] However, conclusive evidence for a T-cell form of CHL is lacking. For one, at the time the 2 reports were published, it was not appreciated that peripheral T-cell lymphomas could express both CD30 and CD15, and mimic CHL at both the phenotypic and morphologic levels.[111] Additionally, cases of pleomorphic T-cell lymphomas after primary cutaneous ALCL, mycosis fungoides, and lymphomatoid papulosis may closely simulate CHL.[112] Much of the biology that we understand regarding CHL is related to its derivation from rescued germinal center B cells.[13] Conceptually, suggesting that the same disease entity may be of T-cell derivation runs counter to the view that lineage is a primary factor in defining disease entities.[9]

The inflammatory background also differs in CHL and NLPHL. NLPHL arises within the follicular environment, and early in the course of disease abundant B cells, generally IgD-positive are

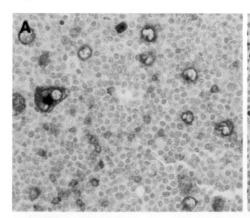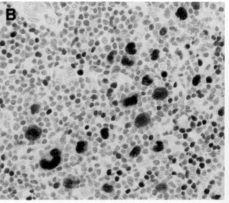

**FIGURE 6.** NLPHL. A, The LP cells in this case were positive for IgD, a finding most frequent in young males (IgD immunostain). B, LP cells stain intensely with OCT-2, which is useful in diagnosis when the atypical cells are sparse. Note the lobulated nuclear contours (OCT-2 immunostain).

present.[113] The individual LP cells are rosetted by T-cells that have the phenotype of intrafollicular T-cells, expressing CD57 and PD-1.[114,115] In contrast, HRS cells in CHL generally are found in a T-cell rich background. The rosetting cells are CD4-positive T-cells that express the costimulatory molecule CD28.[116] The cytokine milieu in CHL may lead to the generation of regulatory T (Treg) cells, positive for CD4, CD25, and CCR4, which may be associated with immune escape.[117,118]

## CONCLUSION

Many years ago MacMahon[67] speculated on the heterogeneity of Hodgkin's disease based on epidemiological observations. He hypothesized that Hodgkin's disease comprised 3 separate disease entities, with differing etiologies. Further studies have supported his hypothesis, and in many respects NLPHL, NSCHL, and MCCHL/LDCHL are distinctive. All cases of Hodgkin's lymphoma are unified by the fact that neoplastic cells are in the minority, and the majority of cells present in the tumor are reactive. However, the various forms of Hodgkin's lymphoma differ in the character of the neoplastic cells and in the inflammatory background. Additional differences in clinical presentation and epidemiology underscored in this review help to define these disease entities. Although it is now accepted that the neoplastic cells are of B-cell lineage, many questions remain concern the etiology of Hodgkin's lymphoma, the downregulation of the B-cell program in CHL, and the basis for the heterogeneity observed clinically and pathologically.

## REFERENCES

1. Hodgkin's T. On some morbid experiences of the absorbent glands and spleen. *Medicochirurgic Trans.* 1832;17:68–97.
2. Wilks S. Cases of enlargement of the lymphatic glands and spleen (or Hodgkin's disease). *Guys Hosp Rep.* 1865;11:56–67.
3. Reed DM. On the pathological changes in Hodgkin's disease, with especial reference to its relation to tuberculosis. *Johns Hopkins Hosp Rep.* 1902;1902:133–196.
4. Dawson PJ. Whatever happened to Dorothy Reed? *Ann Diagn Pathol.* 2003;7:195–203.
5. Gall EA, Mallory TB. Malignant lymphoma: a clinico-pathologic survey of 618 cases. *Am J Pathol.* 1942;18:381–429.
6. Jackson H, Parker F. Hodgkin's disease. II. Pathology. *N Engl J Med.* 1944;231:35–44.
7. Lukes R, Butler J, Hicks E. Natural history of Hodgkin's disease as related to its pathlogical picture. *Cancer.* 1966;19:317–344.
8. Lukes RJ, Craver LF, Hall TC, et al. Report of the nomenclature committee. *Cancer Res.* 1966;26:1311.
9. Harris NL, Jaffe ES, Stein H, et al. A revised European-American classification of lymphoid neoplasms: a proposal from the International Lymphoma Study Group. *Blood.* 1994;84:1361–1392.
10. Jaffe ES, Harris NL, Stein H, et al. *Pathology and Genetics of Tumours of Haematopoietic and Lymphoid Tissues.* Lyon, France: IARC Press; 2001.
11. Swerdlow SH, Campo E, Harris NL, et al. *WHO Classification of Tumours of Haematopoietic and Lymphoid Tissues.* Lyon, France: International Agency for Research on Cancer; 2008.
12. Schmid C, Pan L, Diss T, et al. Expression of B-cell antigens by Hodgkin's and Reed-Sternberg cells. *Am J Pathol.* 1991;139:701–707.
13. Kuppers R, Rajewsky K, Zhao M, et al. Hodgkin's disease: Hodgkin's and Reed Sternberg cells picked from histological sections show clonal immunoglobulin gene rearrangements and appear to be derived from B cells at various stages of development. *Proc Natl Acad Sci USA.* 1994;91:1092–1096.
14. Mason D, Banks P, Chan J, et al. Nodular lymphocyte predominance Hodgkin's disease: a distinct clinico-pathological entity. *Am J Surg Pathol.* 1994;18:528–530.
15. Levy A, Armon Y, Gopas J, et al. Is classicalal Hodgkin's disease indeed a single entity? *Leuk Lymphoma.* 2002;43:1813–1818.
16. Glaser SL, Clarke CA, Darrow LA. Hodgkin's disease etiology and novel viruses: clues from groups exposed to blood products. *Int J Cancer.* 2003;104:796–797.
17. Jarrett RF, MacKenzie J. Epstein-Barr virus and other candidate viruses in the pathogenesis of Hodgkin's disease. *Semin Hematol.* 1999;36:260–269.
18. Armstrong AA, Alexander FE, Cartwright R, et al. Epstein-Barr virus and Hodgkin's disease: further evidence for the three disease hypothesis. *Leukemia.* 1998;12:1272–1276.
19. Delecluse HJ, Marafioti T, Hummel M, et al. Disappearance of the Epstein-Barr virus in a relapse of Hodgkin's disease. *J Pathol.* 1997;182:475–479.
20. Clavel J, Steliarova-Foucher E, Berger C, et al. Hodgkin's disease incidence and survival in European children and adolescents (1978–1997): report from the Automated Cancer Information System project. *Eur J Cancer.* 2006;42:2037–2049.
21. Clarke CA, Glaser SL, Keegan TH, et al. Neighborhood socioeconomic status and Hodgkin's lymphoma incidence in California. *Cancer Epidemiol Biomarkers Prev.* 2005;14:1441–1447.
22. Henderson BE, Dworsky R, Pike MC, et al. Risk factors for nodular sclerosis and other types of Hodgkin's disease. *Cancer Res.* 1979;39:4507–4511.
23. Engert A, Ballova V, Haverkamp H, et al. Hodgkin's lymphoma in elderly patients: a comprehensive retrospective analysis from the German Hodgkin's Study Group. *J Clin Oncol.* 2005;23:5052–5060.
24. Keegan TH, Glaser SL, Clarke CA, et al. Epstein-Barr virus as a marker of survival after Hodgkin's lymphoma: a population-based study. *J Clin Oncol.* 2005;23:7604–7613.
25. Cozen W, Katz J, Mack TM. Risk patterns of Hodgkin's disease in Los Angeles vary by cell type. *Cancer Epidemiol Biomarkers Prev.* 1992;1:261–268.
26. Cozen W, Cerhan JR, Martinez-Maza O, et al. The effect of atopy, childhood crowding, and other immune-related factors on non-Hodgkin's lymphoma risk. *Cancer Causes Control.* 2007;18:821–831.
27. Devilard E, Bertucci F, Trempat P, et al. Gene expression profiling defines molecular subtypes of classicalal Hodgkin's disease. *Oncogene.* 2002;21:3095–3102.
28. Colby T, Hoppe R, Warnke R. Hodgkin's disease: a clinicopathologic study of 659 cases. *Cancer.* 1981;49:1848–1858.
29. Lister TA, Crowther D, Sutcliffe SB, et al. Report of a committee convened to discuss the evaluation and staging of patients with Hodgkin's disease: Cotswolds meeting. *J Clin Oncol.* 1989;7:1630–1636.
30. Ohshima K, Akaiwa M, Umeshita R, et al. Interleukin-13 and interleukin-13 receptor in Hodgkin's disease: possible autocrine mechanism and involvement in fibrosis. *Histopathology.* 2001;38:368–375.
31. Newcom SR, Kadin ME, Ansari AA. Production of transforming growth factor-beta activity by Ki-1 positive lymphoma cells and analysis of its role in the regulation of Ki-1 positive lymphoma growth. *Am J Pathol.* 1988;131:569–577.
32. Pituch-Noworolska A, Drabik G, Kacinska E, et al. Lymphocyte populations in lymph nodes in different histological types of Hodgkin's disease in children. *Acta Haematol.* 2004;112:129–135.
33. Kanzler H, Kuppers R, Hansmann ML, et al. Hodgkin's and Reed-Sternberg cells in Hodgkin's disease represent the outgrowth of a dominant tumor clone derived from (crippled) germinal center B cells. *J Exp Med.* 1996;184:1495–1505.
34. Marafioti T, Hummel M, Foss HD, et al. Hodgkin's and reed-sternberg cells represent an expansion of a single clone originating from a germinal center B-cell with functional immunoglobulin gene rearrangements but defective immunoglobulin transcription. *Blood.* 2000;95:1443–1450.
35. Strickler J, Michie S, Warnke R, et al. The "syncytial variant" of nodular sclerosing Hodgkin's disease. *Am J Surg Pathol.* 1986;10:470–477.
36. Ben-Yehuda-Salz D, Ben-Yehuda A, Polliack A, et al. Syncytial variant of nodular sclerosing Hodgkin's disease. A new clinicopathologic entity. *Cancer.* 1990;65:1167–1172.
37. DeVita VT Jr, Simon RM, Hubbard SM, et al. Curability of advanced Hodgkin's disease with chemotherapy. Long-term follow-up of MOPP-treated patients at the National Cancer Institute. *Ann Intern Med.* 1980;92:587–595.
38. Johnson RE, Zimbler H, Berard CW, et al. Radiotherapy results for nodular sclerosing Hodgkin's disease after clinical staging. *Cancer.* 1977;39:1439–1444.
39. Bennett MH, MacLennan KA, Easterling MJ, et al. The prognostic significance of cellular subtypes in nodular sclerosing Hodgkin's disease: an analysis of 271 non-laparotomised cases (BNLI report no. 22). *Clin Radiol.* 1983;34:497–501.
40. MacLennan K, Bennett M, Tu A, et al. Relationship of histopathologic features to survival and relapse in nodular sclerosing Hodgkin's disease. *Cancer.* 1989;64:1686–1693.
41. Hess J, Bodis S, Pinkus G, et al. Histopathologic grading of nodular sclerosis Hodgkin's disease. Lack of prognostic significance in 254 surgically staged patients. *Cancer.* 1994;74:708–714.
42. Ferry JA, Linggood RM, Convery KM, et al. Hodgkin's disease, nodular sclerosis type. Implications of histologic subclassification. *Cancer.* 1993;71:457–463.

43. Harris NL. Hodgkin's lymphomas: classification, diagnosis, and grading. *Semin Hematol.* 1999;36:220–232.

44. von Wasielewski S, Franklin J, Fischer R, et al. Nodular sclerosing Hodgkin's disease: new grading predicts prognosis in intermediate and advanced stages. *Blood.* 2003;101:4063–4069.

45. Rosenwald A, Wright G, Leroy K, et al. Molecular diagnosis of primary mediastinal B cell lymphoma identifies a clinically favorable subgroup of diffuse large B cell lymphoma related to Hodgkin's lymphoma. *J Exp Med.* 2003;198:851–862.

46. Savage KJ, Monti S, Kutok JL, et al. The molecular signature of mediastinal large B-cell lymphoma differs from that of other diffuse large B-cell lymphomas and shares features with classicalal Hodgkin's lymphoma. *Blood.* 2003;102:3871–3879.

47. Traverse-Glehen A, Pittaluga S, Gaulard P, et al. Mediastinal gray zone lymphoma: the missing link between classical Hodgkin's lymphoma and mediastinal large B-cell lymphoma. *Am J Surg Pathol.* 2005;29:1411–1421.

48. Kanavaros P, Gaulard P, Charlotte F, et al. Discordant expression of immunoglobulin and its associated molecule mb-1/CD79a is frequently found in mediastinal large B-cell lymphomas. *Am J Pathol.* 1995;146:735–741.

49. Copie-Bergman C, Plonquet A, Alonso MA, et al. MAL expression in lymphoid cells: further evidence for MAL as a distinct molecular marker of primary mediastinal large B-cell lymphomas. *Mod Pathol.* 2002;15:1172–1180.

50. Hsi ED, Sup SJ, Alemany C, et al. MAL is expressed in a subset of Hodgkin's lymphoma and identifies a population of patients with poor prognosis. *Am J Clin Pathol.* 2006;125:776–782.

51. Pileri S, Bocchia M, Baroni C, et al. Anaplastic large cell lymphoma (CD30+/Ki-1+): results of a prospective clinicopathologic study of 69 cases. *Br J Haematol.* 1994;86:513–523.

52. Jaffe ES. Anaplastic large cell lymphoma: the shifting sands of diagnostic hematopathology. *Mod Pathol.* 2001;14:219–228.

53. Zinzani PL, Martelli M, Magagnoli M, et al. Anaplastic large cell lymphoma Hodgkin's-like: a randomized trial of ABVD versus MACOP-B with and without radiation therapy. *Blood.* 1998;92:790–794.

54. Cazals-Hatem D, Andre M, Mounier N, et al. Pathologic and clinical features of 77 Hodgkin's lymphoma patients treated in a lymphoma protocol (LNH87): a GELA study. *Am J Surg Pathol.* 2001;25:297–306.

55. Dunleavy D, Pittaluga S, Grant N, et al. Gray zone lymphomas: clinical and histological characteristics and treatment with dose-adjusted EPOCH-R. *Blood.* 2008;112:1228.

56. Zarate-Osorno A, Roman LN, Kingma DW, et al. Hodgkin's disease in Mexico. Prevalence of Epstein-Barr virus sequences and correlations with histologic subtype. *Cancer.* 1995;75:1360–1366.

57. Ambinder RF, Browning PJ, Lorenzana I, et al. Epstein-Barr virus and childhood Hodgkin's disease in Honduras and the United States. *Blood.* 1993;81:462–467.

58. Siddiqui N, Ayub B, Badar F, et al. Hodgkin's lymphoma in Pakistan: a clinico-epidemiological study of 658 cases at a cancer center in Lahore. *Asian Pac J Cancer Prev.* 2006;7:651–655.

59. Clarke CA, Glaser SL. Epidemiologic trends in HIV-associated lymphomas. *Curr Opin Oncol.* 2001;13:354–359.

60. Glaser SL, Clarke CA, Gulley ML, et al. Population-based patterns of human immunodeficiency virus-related Hodgkin's lymphoma in the Greater San Francisco Bay Area, 1988–1998. *Cancer.* 2003;98:300–309.

61. Biggar RJ, Jaffe ES, Goedert JJ, et al. Hodgkin's lymphoma and immunodeficiency in persons with HIV/AIDS. *Blood.* 2006;108:3786–3791.

62. Stein L, Urban MI, O'Connell D, et al. The spectrum of human immunodeficiency virus-associated cancers in a South African black population: results from a case-control study, 1995–2004. *Int J Cancer.* 2008;122:2260–2265.

63. Neiman RS, Rosen PJ, Lukes RJ. Lymphocyte-depletion Hodgkin's disease. A clinicopathological entity. *N Engl J Med.* 1973;288:751–755.

64. Axtell L, Myers M, Thomas L, et al. Prognostic indicators in Hodgkin's disease. *Cancer.* 1972;29:1481–1488.

65. Kant JA, Hubbard SM, Longo DL, et al. The pathologic and clinical heterogeneity of lymphocyte-depleted Hodgkin's disease. *J Clin Oncol.* 1986;4:284–294.

66. Allemani C, Sant M, De Angelis R, et al. Hodgkin's disease survival in Europe and the U.S.: prognostic significance of morphologic groups. *Cancer.* 2006;107:352–360.

67. MacMahon B. Epidemiology of Hodgkin's disease. *Cancer Res.* 1966;26:1189–1201.

68. Kadin ME, Donaldson SS, Dorfman RF. Isolated granulomas in Hodgkin's disease. *N Engl J Med.* 1970;283:859–861.

69. Lukes RJ, Butler JJ. The pathology and nomenclature of Hodgkin's disease. *Cancer Res.* 1966;26:1063–1083.

70. Garcia JF, Mollejo M, Fraga M, et al. Large B-cell lymphoma with Hodgkin's features. *Histopathology.* 2005;47:101–110.

71. Oyama T, Ichimura K, Suzuki R, et al. Senile EBV+ B-cell lymphoproliferative disorders: a clinicopathologic study of 22 patients. *Am J Surg Pathol.* 2003;27:16–26.

72. Park S, Lee J, Ko YH, et al. The impact of Epstein-Barr virus status on clinical outcome in diffuse large B-cell lymphoma. *Blood.* 2007;110:972–978.

73. Anagnostopoulos I, Hansmann ML, Franssila K, et al. European Task Force on Lymphoma project on lymphocyte predominance Hodgkin's disease: histologic and immunohistologic analysis of submitted cases reveals 2 types of Hodgkin's disease with a nodular growth pattern and abundant lymphocytes. *Blood.* 2000;96:1889–1899.

74. Diehl V, Sextro M, Franklin J, et al. Clinical presentation, course, and prognostic factors in lymphocyte- predominant Hodgkin's disease and lymphocyte-rich classicalal Hodgkin's disease: report from the European Task Force on Lymphoma Project on Lymphocyte-Predominant Hodgkin's Disease. *J Clin Oncol.* 1999;17:776–783.

75. Shimabukuro V. Lymphocyte-rich classicalal Hodgkin's lymphoma: clinical presentation and treatment outcome in 100 patients treated within German Hodgkin's Study Group trials (vol 23, pg 5739, 2005). *J Clin Oncol.* 2006;24:2220–2220.

76. Brauninger A. Typing the histogenetic origin of the tumor cells of lymphocyte-rich classicalal Hodgkin's lymphoma in relation to tumor cells of classicalal and lymphocyte-predominance Hodgkin's lymphoma. *Cancer Res.* 2003;63:1644–1651.

77. Ashton-Key M, Thorpe PA, Allen JP, et al. Follicular Hodgkin's disease. *Am J Surg Pathol.* 1995;19:1294–1299.

78. Lennert K, Mohri N. Histologische Klassifizierung und Vorkommen des M. *Hodgkin's Internist.* 1974;15:57–65.

79. Chang K-C, Khen NT, Jones D, et al. Epstein-Barr virus is associated with all histological subtypes of Hodgkin's lymphoma in Vietnamese children with special emphasis on the entity of lymphocyte predominance subtype. *Hum Pathol.* 2005;36:747–755.

80. Regula D, Hoppe R, Weiss L. Nodular and diffuse types of lymphocyte predominance Hodgkin's disease. *N Engl J Med.* 1988;318:214–219.

81. Fan Z, Natkunam Y, Bair E, et al. Characterization of variant patterns of nodular lymphocyte predominant hodgkin lymphoma with immunohistologic and clinical correlation. *Am J Surg Pathol.* 2003;27:1346–1356.

82. Poppema S, Kaiserling E, Lennert K. Nodular paragranuloma and progressively transformed germinal centers: ultrastructural and immunohistochemical findings. *Virchows Arch [B].* 1979;31:211–225.

83. Ferry JA, Zukerberg LR, Harris NL. Florid progressive transformation of germinal centers. A syndrome affecting young men, without early progression to nodular lymphocyte predominance Hodgkin's disease. *Am J Surg Pathol.* 1992;16:252–258.

84. Sundeen JT, Cossman J, Jaffe ES. Lymphocyte predominant Hodgkin's disease, nodular subtype with coexistent "large cell lymphoma." Histological progression or composite malignancy? *Am J Surg Pathol.* 1988;12:599–606.

85. Hansmann M, Stein H, Fellbaum C, et al. Nodular paragranuloma can transform into high-grade malignant lymphoma of B type. *Hum Pathol.* 1989;20:1169–1175.

86. Huang JZ, Weisenburger DD, Vose JM, et al. Diffuse large B-cell lymphoma arising in nodular lymphocyte predominant Hodgkin's lymphoma: a report of 21 cases from the Nebraska Lymphoma Study Group. *Leuk Lymphoma.* 2004;45:1551–1557.

87. Greiner TC, Gascoyne RD, Anderson ME, et al. Nodular lymphocyte-predominant Hodgkin's disease associated with large-cell lymphoma: analysis of Ig gene rearrangements by V-J polymerase chain reaction. *Blood.* 1996;88:657–666.

88. Wickert RS, Weisenburger DD, Tierens A, et al. Clonal relationship between lymphocytic predominance Hodgkin's disease and concurrent or subsequent large-cell lymphoma of B lineage. *Blood.* 1995;86:2312–2320.

89. Rudiger T, Gascoyne RD, Jaffe ES, et al. Workshop on the relationship between nodular lymphocyte predominant Hodgkin's lymphoma and T cell/histiocyte-rich B cell lymphoma. *Ann Oncol.* 2002;13:44–51.

90. Boudova L, Torlakovic E, Delabie J, et al. Nodular lymphocyte predominant Hodgkin's lymphoma with nodules resembling T-cell/histiocyte rich B-cell lymphoma: differential diagnosis between nodular lymphocyte predominant Hodgkin's lymphoma and T-cell/histiocyte rich B-cell lymphoma. *Blood.* 2003;24:24.

91. Stein H, Gerdes J, Schwab U, et al. Identification of Hodgkin's and Sternberg-reed cells as a unique cell type derived from a newly-detected small-cell population. *Int J Cancer.* 1982;30:445–459.

92. Goldbrunner R, Warmuth-Metz M, Tonn JC, et al. Primary Ki-1-positive T-cell lymphoma of the brain–an aggressive subtype of lymphoma: case report and review of the literature. *Surg Neurol.* 1996;46:37–41.

93. Hsu SM, Yang K, Jaffe ES. Phenotypic expression of Hodgkin's and Reed-Sternberg cells in Hodgkin's disease. *Am J Pathol.* 1985;118:209–217.

94. Chittal S, Caveriviere P, Schwarting R, et al. Monoclonal antibodies in the diagnosis of Hodgkin's disease. The search for a rational panel. *Am J Surg Pathol.* 1988;12:9–21.

95. Tzankov A, Krugmann J, Fend F, et al. Prognostic significance of CD20 expression in classicalal Hodgkin's lymphoma: a clinicopathological study of 119 cases. *Clin Cancer Res.* 2003;9:1381–1386.

96. Schwering I, Brauninger A, Klein U, et al. Loss of the B-lineage-specific gene expression program in Hodgkin's and Reed-Sternberg cells of Hodgkin's lymphoma. *Blood.* 2003;101:1505–1512.

97. Weiss LM, Movahed LA, Warnke RA, et al. Detection of Epstein-Barr viral genomes in Reed-Sternberg cells of Hodgkin's disease. *N Engl J Med.* 1989;320:502–506.

98. Gandhi MK, Moll G, Smith C, et al. Galectin-1 mediated suppression of Epstein-Barr virus specific T-cell immunity in classical Hodgkin's lymphoma. *Blood.* 2007;110:1326–1329.

99. Stein H, Hansmann M, Lennert K, et al. Reed-Sternberg and Hodgkin's cells in lymphocyte-predominant Hodgkin's disease of nodular subtype contain J chain. *Am J Clin Pathol.* 1986;86:292–297.

100. Schmid C, Sargent C, Isaacson P. L and H cells of nodular lymphocyte predominant Hodgkin's disease show immunoglobulin light-chain restriction. *Am J Pathol.* 1991;139:1281–1289.

101. Prakash S, Fountaine T, Raffeld M, et al. IgD Positive L&H Cells Identify a Unique Subset of Nodular Lymphocyte Predominant Hodgkin's Lymphoma. *Am J Surg Pathol.* 2006;30:585–592.

102. Foss HD, Reusch R, Demel G, et al. Frequent expression of the B-cell-specific activator protein in Reed-Sternberg cells of classicalal Hodgkin's disease provides further evidence for its B-cell origin. *Blood.* 1999;94:3108–3113.

103. Stein H, Marafioti T, Foss HD, et al. Down-regulation of BOB. 1/OBF. 1 and Oct2 in classicalal Hodgkin's disease but not in lymphocyte predominant Hodgkin's disease correlates with immunoglobulin transcription. *Blood.* 2001;97:496–501.

104. Marafioti T, Mancini C, Ascani S, et al. Leukocyte-specific phosphoprotein-1 and PU. 1: two useful markers for distinguishing T-cell-rich B-cell lymphoma from lymphocyte-predominant Hodgkin's disease. *Haematologica.* 2004;89:957–964.

105. von Wasielewski R, Mengel M, Fischer R, et al. Classical Hodgkin's disease. Clinical impact of the immunophenotype. *Am J Pathol.* 1997;151:1123–1130.

106. Portlock CS, Donnelly GB, Qin J, et al. Adverse prognostic significance of CD20 positive Reed-Sternberg cells in classicalal Hodgkin's disease. *Br J Haematol.* 2004;125:701–708.

107. Tzankov A, Bourgau C, Kaiser A, et al. Rare expression of T-cell markers in classicalal Hodgkin's lymphoma. *Mod Pathol.* 2005;18:1542–1549.

108. Kuppers R, Brauninger A. Reprogramming of the tumour B-cell phenotype in Hodgkin's lymphoma. *Trends Immunol.* 2006;27:203–205.

109. Muschen M, Rajewsky K, Brauninger A, et al. Rare occurrence of classicalal Hodgkin's disease as a T cell lymphoma. *J Exp Med.* 2000;191:387–394.

110. Seitz V, Hummel M, Marafioti T, et al. Detection of clonal T-cell receptor gamma-chain gene rearrangements in Reed-Sternberg cells of classical Hodgkin's disease. *Blood.* 2000;95:3020–3024.

111. Barry TS, Jaffe ES, Sorbara L, et al. Peripheral T-cell lymphomas expressing CD30 and CD15. *Am J Surg Pathol.* 2003;27:1513–1522.

112. Davis T, Morton C, Miller-Cassman R, et al. Hodgkin's disease, lymphomatoid papulosis, and cutaneous T-cell lymphoma derived from a common T-cell clone. *N Engl J Med.* 1992;326:1115–1122.

113. Timmens W, Visser L, Poppema S. Nodular lymphocyte predominance type of Hodgkin's disease is a germinal center lymphoma. *Lab Invest.* 1986;54:457–461.

114. Kamel OW, Gelb AB, Shibuya RB, et al. Leu 7 (CD57) reactivity distinguishes nodular lymphocyte predominance Hodgkin's disease from nodular sclerosing Hodgkin's disease, T-cell-rich B-cell lymphoma and follicular lymphoma. *Am J Pathol.* 1993;142:541–546.

115. Nam-Cha SH, Roncador G, Sanchez-Verde L, et al. PD-1, a follicular T-cell marker useful for recognizing nodular lymphocyte-predominant Hodgkin's lymphoma. *Am J Surg Pathol.* 2008;32:1252–1257.

116. Cossman J, Messineo C, Bagg A. Reed-Sternberg cell: survival in a hostile sea. *Lab Invest.* 1998;78:229–235.

117. Ishida T, Ishii T, Inagaki A, et al. Specific recruitment of CC chemokine receptor 4-positive regulatory T cells in Hodgkin's lymphoma fosters immune privilege. *Cancer Res.* 2006;66:5716–5722.

118. Marshall NA, Christie LE, Munro LR, et al. Immunosuppressive regulatory T cells are abundant in the reactive lymphocytes of Hodgkin's lymphoma. *Blood.* 2004;103:1755–1762.

# Hodgkin's Lymphoma—Patients Assessment and Staging

Mary K. Gospodarowicz

Hodgkin's lymphoma is an important malignant disease. It affects young people, it is highly curable and requires meticulous assessment, treatment, and response evaluation to maximize cure, and minimize treatment-related toxicity. In the past 20 years, advances in chemotherapy and judicious use of combined modality therapy resulted in the improved overall survival of patients with Hodgkin's lymphoma.[1] Currently, more than 80% of younger patients may expect cure.[2] In this review, we will consider the taxonomy of patient assessment, staging, and response evaluation, describe the evolution of staging in Hodgkin's lymphoma, and outline the current procedures used to define disease extent.

The optimal management of any malignant disease requires careful evaluation of the disease, the patient, and available treatment options. This evaluation requires as the first step the confirmation of diagnosis with definition of the specific tumor type and any molecular tumor characteristics. The second step is assessment of disease extent. Disease extent is defined as "stage of disease." The third step is assessment of patient's general health and comorbidities that may impact treatment. Staging, as the estimation of the anatomic disease extent, is therefore only 1 component of patient evaluation and must not be confused with the overall patient assessment.

## TAXONOMY

Disease stage is defined and recorded at the time of initial presentation and diagnosis. It is important as patients with different disease stage at presentation have different prognosis, regardless of the ensuing course of disease. For example, a patient with stage I disease that recurs after treatment will have a better survival than the patient with stage IV disease who recurs. Stage is a form of shorthand language to describe disease extent. For example, in Hodgkin's lymphoma, stage I communicates disease limited to 1 lymph node region, whereas stage III communicates lymph node involvement above and below diaphragm.

In clinical practice, the term "staging" is used at any time disease extent is evaluated during the course of disease. The appropriate term for patient assessment after treatment would be "evaluation of treatment response," and at relapse, "assessment of extent of relapse." Staging (verb) as an activity describes the tests required to determine disease extent. There is also general misunderstanding of "staging" and "prognostic evaluation." Disease stage is only 1 of prognostic characteristics. Prognostic factors may be grouped into tumor related, host or patient related, and environment related.[3,4] Tumor-related factors include "tumor profile" that describes histopathological, molecular, and genetic characteristics, whereas "tumor stage" describes the anatomic disease extent.[3] The prognostic factors should be evaluated in the context of specific treatment intervention and prognosis should be defined with a specific end point in mind. For example, proposed use of chemotherapy with bleomycin and doxorubicin requires

evaluation of pulmonary and cardiac function, whereas proposed use of cisplatin requires evaluation of renal function and hearing.

## Cancer Staging—Principles and Use

Staging of malignant diseases was first proposed in 1920s. It was recognized then that patients with smaller localized cancers survived longer than those with extensive or disseminated disease. They were also cured with surgical resection. Pierre Denoix, father of modern TNM classification noted that the anatomic disease extent is a very powerful predictor of outcome but not the only factor.[5,6] He noted that tumor type, grade, rate of growth, and patients' symptoms were also relevant. Today, many forget that the original intent of staging classification was to describe the anatomic disease extent. Staging classification is therefore a form of language or code to communicate this. For example, in Hodgkin's lymphoma, stage I communicates disease limited to 1 lymph node region, whereas stage III communicates lymph node involvement above and below diaphragm. Knowledge of the anatomic extent of disease is essential to characterize cancer before treatment. Stage is required to develop a treatment plan. The extent of disease is relevant for assessment of outcomes with any form of treatment, although the location of disease is more important when local therapies (surgery and radiotherapy) are used.

The information about stage is used in selecting appropriate diagnostic tests. For example, patients who have advanced stage III and stage IV Hodgkin's lymphoma are recommended to have bone marrow biopsy. Staging is used to select an appropriate treatment plan; all practice guidelines for Hodgkin's lymphoma include stage as one of the decision points for recommending treatment. Staging is necessary to be able to prognosticate and predict the outcome for an individual patient and stage information is used to establish informed consent for treatment.

Stage information is used to assess the outcome of therapeutic intervention in similar groups of patients. We use initial stage and knowledge of the outcome associated with this to select appropriate follow-up monitoring and provide patient and caregiver education. Stage information is also used in research. The analysis of patients' outcomes by stage is used to improve the efficiency of research design and data analysis and enhance the confidence of prediction. We design future studies by identifying subgroups with poor outcomes with current therapies. As all treatments for cancer are associated with some toxicity, stage information is also used to identify groups with excellent outcomes that can benefit from reduced therapy.

## STAGING HODGKIN'S LYMPHOMA

Traditional staging of Hodgkin's lymphoma was based on physical examination and later imaging, which in 1960s and 1970s was with conventional x-rays with contrast (intravenous pyelogram (IVP), inferior vena cava (IVC), and lymphography) or plain tomography.

**TABLE 1.** Cotswold Modification of the Ann Arbor Staging Classification[8]

| | |
|---|---|
| Stage I | Involvement of a single lymph node region of lymphoid structure or involvement of a single extralymphatic site (IE) |
| Stage II | Involvement of 2 or more lymph node regions on the same side of the diaphragm (II) or localized contiguous involvement of only one extranodal organ or site and its regional lymph nodes with or without other lymph node regions on the same side of the diaphragm (IIE) |
| Stage III | Involvement of lymph node regions on both sides of the diaphragm (III), which also may be accompanied by involvement of the spleen (IIIS) or by localized contiguous involvement of only one extranodal organ site (IIIE) or both (IIISE) |
| Stage IV | Disseminated (multifocal) involvement of one or more extranodal organs or tissues, with or without associated lymph node involvement or isolated extralymphatic organ involvement with distant (non-regional) nodal involvement |
| Designations applicable to any stage | |
| A | No symptoms |
| B | Fever (>38°C), night sweats, unexplained loss of >10% body weight in previous 6 mo |
| X | Bulky disease |
| E | Involvement of a single extranodal site that is contiguous or proximal to the known nodal site |

Involvement of hilar nodes on both sides constitutes stage II disease.
Bulky mediastinal disease has been defined as a thoracic ratio of maximum transverse mass diameter greater than or equal to one third of the internal transverse diameter measured at T5/6 intervertebral disc level on chest radiography. Other authors have designated a lymph node mass of 10 cm or more in greatest dimension as bulky disease.
Evidence of invasion of adjacent structures, such as bone, chest wall, or lung is an important consideration, as this may influence management. For example, a mediastinal or hilar mass that invades the adjacent lung is classified as IIE, whereas pulmonary involvement separate from adenopathy represents stage IV disease.

Imaging was used to detect thoracic and abdominal disease, whereas the presence of peripheral lymphadenopathy was determined by careful palpation, which was a highly valued, but known as quite inaccurate clinical skill. Over the past 30 years, modern imaging with computerized tomography (CT) replaced other clinical methods.

Hodgkin's lymphoma was one of the first diseases, where clinical staging and logical progression of the disease was linked to outcomes. The early proposals for staging classification were formalized in 1971 at the Workshop on the Staging of Hodgkin's Disease held in Ann Arbor, MI. The Ann Arbor classification has been formally adopted by the Union Internationale Contre (International Union Against Cancer) Tumor Node Metastasis (UICC TNM) Committee.[7] Today, almost 40 years later, staging classification of Hodgkin's lymphoma remains relevant although imperfect. The last modifications to the Ann Arbor classification were proposed at the Cotswolds meeting in 1998 (Table 1).[8] Although the stage designation is commonly used in practice, detailed descriptors such as "X" for bulky disease are rarely used. The current approach to staging of patients with Hodgkin's lymphoma has evolved over the past 40 years. This gradual evolution was driven by changes in the management and by progress in imaging. There is general paucity of level I evidence to guide staging. To understand the practice today, it is useful to review the history of staging in Hodgkin's lymphoma.[9]

## CLINICAL PRESENTATION AND PATIENT ASSESSMENT

Patients with Hodgkin's lymphoma typically present with asymptomatic lymph node enlargement, most commonly in the neck. However, if peripheral lymph node enlargement is not apparent, patients may present with systemic symptoms such as night sweats or fever. Weight loss is usually associated with advanced disease. Fever, night sweats, and weight loss have prognostic significance in Hodgkin's lymphoma, are known as "systemic" symptoms, and are present in about one third of patients. Pruritus is another relatively common presenting symptom. It used to be associated with adverse outcome, but with modern treatment, it is not. Because intrathoracic presentations are common, cough, and shortness of breath are among other presenting features. Biopsy of enlarged lymph nodes usually is diagnostic.

The clinical assessment starts with confirmation of diagnosis. A careful histopathologic assessment of the biopsy by an experienced pathologist and presence of adequate amount of tissue is paramount. Immunocytochemistry helps to differentiate between Hodgkin's and other types of lymphoma. With modern techniques, the confusion between Hodgkin's lymphoma and non-Hodgkin's lymphoma is less common than in the past.

The modern assessment of the extent of disease in Hodgkin's disease includes careful history, laboratory tests, physical examination, and imaging (Table 2).[10] Patient assessment involves the comprehensive history, specifically enquiring about presence or absence of constitutional "systemic" symptoms including unexplained fever more than 38°C, night sweats, or unintentional weight loss of greater than 10% of body weight. These 3 symptoms are classified as B symptoms and they are used in staging to indicate adverse prognosis. Other lymphoma-related symptoms, such as fatigue, pruritus, and alcohol-induced pain in involved nodal areas, should be noted, although they do not confer adverse prognosis. Laboratory studies should include a complete blood count, lactate dehydrogenase, erythrocyte sedimentation rate, alkaline phosphatase, albumin, and liver

**TABLE 2.** Staging and Assessment of Patients with Newly Diagnosed Hodgkin's Lymphoma

| | |
|---|---|
| History | Presence of systemic symptoms—fever, night sweats, and weight loss |
| | Pruritus and alcohol-related pain |
| | HIV status, cardiac, pulmonary, renal disease, hepatitis B surface antigen, hepatitis B core antibody, and hepatitis C antibody |
| Physical examination | Peripheral lymph node area, lever, and spleen |
| Laboratory tests | Complete blood count, LDH, liver function tests, and ESR |
| Imaging | CT—head and neck, chest, abdomen, and pelvis |
| | PET-CT |
| Bone marrow biopsy | Stages III–IV |
| | B symptoms |

function tests. Bone marrow biopsy is indicated in selected cases of Hodgkin's lymphoma, those with advanced disease or hematologic abnormalities.

In addition, before recommending treatment, clinical assessment should assess fitness of patient to treatment, assess the degree of comorbidities, and state of vital organs. Before starting chemotherapy, the patient should have electrocardiogram (ECG), multigraded acquisition scan (MUGA) scan or echocardiogram, pulmonary function tests, thyroid, and gonadal function tests and, if relevant, semen analysis and sperm storage. None of these tests are relevant to staging per se, but they are essential in assessing the baseline condition of the patient and monitoring treatment toxicity.

The guidelines for staging of Hodgkin's lymphoma call for comprehensive physical examination. Although the physical examination may guide the initial investigations, in all instances, patients presenting with Hodgkin's disease should have full imaging studies including imaging of all major lymph node groups, thorax, and abdomen.

Because staging of Hodgkin's lymphoma evolved over the years, we will consider specific issues in staging Hodgkin's lymphoma and conclude with currently recommended procedures.

## Staging Laparotomy

In 1960s and 1970s, stage I and stage II Hodgkin's lymphoma was managed with radiotherapy alone. Radiotherapy (RT) resulted in almost 100% local control, but was associated with 30% to 50% distant failure, most frequently because of the presence of occult intraabdominal disease. This and limited accuracy of imaging led to the acceptance of surgical staging of Hodgkin's lymphoma. Patients with clinically localized presentations were routinely subjected to laparotomy with splenectomy, and biopsies of the liver and paraaortic lymph nodes. The staging laparotomy in Hodgkin's lymphoma provided valuable information about the patterns of abdominal involvement. Numerous studies consistently revealed clinically occult abdominal disease in 30% to 50% of patients. This occult disease was most commonly found in the spleen. The correlation between clinical factors including the extent of supradiaphragmatic disease, presence of systemic symptoms, elevated erythrocyte sedimentation rate (ESR), age, bulk, and the findings at staging laparotomy led to the development of risk-adjusted management strategies that selectively used combined modality therapy in patients at high risk of occult abdominal disease. With time, improved imaging of the abdomen, increased use of combined modality therapy and the desire to limit the extent of radiotherapy to avoid late toxicity, eliminated the need for staging laparotomy.[9] Randomized studies showed equivalent survival for patients managed with and without staging laparotomy.[11] Although now abandoned, staging laparotomy provided useful information about patterns of disease.[9] Fundamentally, the staging evaluation should meet the needs of clinical patient management. With the availability of improved imaging with CT scanning, the availability of FDG-PET imaging, and the use of combined modality therapy in almost all patients with Hodgkin's disease, staging laparotomy is no longer relevant.

## Bone Marrow Biopsy

Unlike in non-Hodgkin's lymphoma, staging bone marrow biopsy is not required in most of patients with Hodgkin's disease. Numerous studies have documented that the bone marrow involvement in patients with stage I and stage II Hodgkin's lymphoma without unfavorable prognostic factors is extremely rare and false-positive determinations are as frequent as positive.[12,13] Therefore, the bone marrow biopsy should be reserved for patients with stage III and stage IV Hodgkin's lymphoma or those stage I and stage II patients with severe B symptoms or hematologic abnormalities.

## Anatomic Imaging

### Lymphangiogram

In the past, lymphangiography played an important role in the assessment of infradiaphragmatic Hodgkin's lymphoma.[14] The development of lymphangiograms presented a major advance in staging of Hodgkin's lymphoma. The ability to visualize abdominal lymph nodes was useful in staging and response assessment because the contrast remained in situ for a number of months.[15–17] In 1980s, CT gradually replaced lymphangiography with no major effect on the ability to detect intra-abdominal disease.

### Computerized Tomography

Today, full imaging studies in Hodgkin's lymphoma include CT imaging of all lymph node areas, including head and neck, thorax, abdomen, and pelvis.[18] In addition, if extranodal disease is suspected, magnetic resonance imaging is used to assess the extent of soft tissue, spinal canal, or brain involvement. This thorough imaging assessment of the patient serves to define the anatomic disease extent, which is essential for determining the stage. The knowledge of exact disease extent is also very useful in assessing completeness of response to treatment. The obvious limitations of anatomic imaging include inability to visualize microscopic disease, difficulties in interpreting small lymph nodes visualized on CT, and differentiating benign reactive inflammatory infiltrates, fibrosis, etc. from malignant tumor. Lymph nodes under 1 cm in diameter may also represent reactive hyperplasia, but also may harbor Hodgkin's lymphoma. Current convention calls for thoracic and abdominal lymph nodes to be considered as abnormal if they measure more than 10 mm in the short-axis diameter, and the neck, axillary, and inguinal lymph nodes if they measure more than 15 mm in short axis diameter. Clearly, smaller lymph nodes may harbor Hodgkin's lymphoma but many may be reactive.

## Functional Imaging

### Gallium Scintigraphy

CT and conventional x-ray imaging provides anatomic but not functional information. In the past, Gallium scintigraphy was used to define disease extent and response in Hodgkin's and other lymphomas.[19] This originated after the observation that uptake of Gallium-67 citrate was most pronounced in viable tumors. Although used for staging, the major role of Gallium imaging in the last 2 decades was to evaluate the response of tumor to treatment rather than to stage patients. Gallium imaging was found to be poor in detecting small volume disease particularly in the abdomen, where one can find enlarged lymph nodes that are Gallium negative. The absence of Gallium uptake could be interpreted as the absence of disease.

### FDG-PET Imaging

In the past 20 years, the development of PET technology led to extensive investigation of biochemical processes in vivo. PET is a noninvasive, quantitative imaging technique that can visualize biologic processes in vivo. PET has been shown to be superior to [67]Gallium-scintigraphy in lymphoma staging, it is easier to perform, and it delivers a lower radiation dose to the patient.[20–23] With the use of combined PET/CT equipment, disease sites can be defined both based on size criteria and their glucose metabolism.[24] FDG-PET has proven a valuable tool in the management of lymphomas.[25–27] FDG-PET is a useful modality in staging of lymphomas especially when used in conjunction with CT imaging. It is more sensitive than Gallium imaging but in studies comparing staging that includes FDG-PET and staging with modern CT imaging without FDG-PET, the change in the stage is small. In addition, there has been no report suggesting that the outcome of patients staged with and without FDG-PET differs. One should differentiate the role of FDG-PET in the initial staging from the role of FDG-PET in response assessment and guiding further therapy. Several studies have shown FDG-PET to be very sensitive in detecting areas of involvement by Hodgkin's lymphoma. In addition to detecting nodal involvement, FDG-PET is much more sensitive in detecting extranodal involvement, especially in the spleen, bone, and bone marrow. PET in general is able to detect an additional number of Hodgkin's lymphoma sites compared with conventional CT. This usually results in a modification of stage, usually increasing the stage, in about 15% to 20% of patients. Overall, management is changed in 5% to 15% of patients.[28,29] Despite the general use of FDG-PET in staging, most reports include small numbers of patients, often mixing Hodgkin's lymphoma and other lymphomas. One of the largest series is from the prospective study by the Intergruppo Italiano Linfomi.[30] The study included 186 patients from 6 Italian hematological institutions studied between 2002 and 2005. Imaging with FDG-PET was compared with the standard contrast enhanced CT imaging. In this study, overall 910 involved sites were registered with CT and 1090 sites were evaluated with FDG-PET. In this study, the sites seen on FDG-PET were confirmed with another imaging modality (magnetic resonance imaging, ultrasound). As most other studies, the gold standard of biopsy to evaluate discordant site was not used. Overall CT and FDG-PET were concordant in 84% of patients and discordant in 16%. Stage was higher with PET in 14% and lower in 1%. The planned treatment was modified based on PET results in 11 patients. Of patients staged as localized (stage I and stage II), 10 (8%) has stage changed to advanced. Contemporary management of Hodgkin's lymphoma is based on anatomic stage, presence of systemic symptoms, bulky mediastinal disease, ESR, and age. Most patients with Hodgkin's lymphoma receive chemotherapy today. Patients with stage I and stage II disease and no risk factors may receive reduced number of courses of chemotherapy followed by involved field radiotherapy. It would be interesting to see, in how many patients recommended treatment would have been insufficient when CT alone was used to determine disease stage. The current treatment policies have been developed in an era of CT imaging without PET and it is possible that the treatment recommended would compensate for deficiencies in staging. To date, no study to date compared the outcomes of patients staged with and without FDG-PET.

Despite the high sensitivity and specificity, the usefulness of FDG-PET in Hodgkin's lymphoma staging is debated. The increased use of chemotherapy negates the need for the exact definition of anatomic disease extent. However, the trend to minimizing treatment with the use of short chemotherapy and limiting radiotherapy to involved lymph nodes requires precise information on anatomic disease extent. Therefore, in most centers, FDG-PET is recommended as part of staging assessment.

## SUMMARY

Current practice in staging of Hodgkin's lymphoma developed gradually over the past 40 years. Modern imaging made staging laparotomy redundant. Lymphangiograms are no longer performed, and Gallium scintigraphy is rapidly becoming obsolete. There is little argument today that CT imaging is the cornerstone of staging assessment in patients with Hodgkin's lymphoma. The art of physical examination is important, but its limitations are obvious, and therefore imaging should be used not only in the assessment of intrathoracic and intra-abdominal disease, but also to evaluate peripheral lymphadenopathy.

Change takes time, and in number of centers, Gallium scintigraphy continues to be performed, usually because FDG-PET is not approved for staging. However, because FDG-PET has become an essential tool in response assessment, it is a matter of time until all centers will adopt FDG-PET as part of imaging at diagnosis.[31]

It is important to realize that the current guidelines for patient assessment and evaluation have not been prospectively evaluated in the context of modern practice guidelines.[10] Current practice calls for minimizing treatment in patients with stage I and stage II "low risk" presentations. The risk factors include presence of B symptoms, elevated ESR, bulky disease, and age. These "risk factors" in Hodgkin's lymphomas were based on the pattern of failure with radiotherapy alone, in patients evaluated with 1980s imaging techniques, without FDG-PET. The adverse influence of B symptoms on outcomes is still poorly understood, the importance of ESR is questionable. The adverse impact of age is acknowledged but poorly understood. We should ask whether these factors are still relevant in 2009 in the era of chemotherapy and functional imaging.

The earlier review concentrated on the evaluation of patients presenting with newly diagnosed disease. It is important to note that the management of patients with Hodgkin's lymphoma involves a complex algorithms requiring interim assessment of treatment efficacy, overall response evaluation, careful follow-up to detect treatment failure early, and maximize the potential benefit of salvage treatment.[10]

## REFERENCES

1. Tubiana M. Hodgkin's disease: historical perspective and clinical presentation. *Bailleres Clin Haematol.* 1996;9:503–530.
2. Connors JM. State-of-the-art therapeutics: Hodgkin's lymphoma. *J Clin Oncol.* 2005;23:6400–6408.
3. Gospodarowicz MK, O'Sullivan B, Koh E. Prognostic factors: principles and applications. In: Gospodarowicz MK, O'Sullivan B, Sobin L, eds. *Prognostic Factors in Cancer.* 3rd ed. Hoboken, NJ: Wiley; 2006:23–38.
4. Gospodarowicz M, O'Sullivan B. Prognostic factors in cancer. *Semin Surg Oncol.* 2003;21:13–18.
5. Publique MdlS: Nomenclature classification des cancers. *Bulletin de L'Institut National D'Hygiene.* 1950;5:81–84.
6. Gospodarowicz M, Benedet L, Hutter RV, et al. History and international developments in cancer staging. *Cancer Prev Control.* 1998;2:262–268.
7. *TNM Classification of Malignant Tumours.* 6th ed. New York: Wiley-Liss; 2002.
8. Lister TA, Crowther D, Sutcliffe SB, et al. Report of a committee convened to discuss the evaluation and staging of patients with Hodgkin's disease: Cotswolds meeting. *J Clin Oncol.* 1989;7:1630–1636.
9. Carde P, Glatstein E. Role of staging laparotomy in Hodgkin's disease. In: Mauch P, Armitage J, Diehl V, et al, eds. *Hodgkin's Disease.* Philadelphia: Lippincott Williams & Wilkins; 1999:273–293.
10. Hodgkin's Disease/Lymphoma, NCCN Clinical Practice Guidelines in Oncology, 2009.
11. Carde P, Hagenbeek A, Hayat M, et al. Clinical staging versus laparotomy and combined modality with MOPP versus ABVD in early-stage Hodgkin's disease: the H6 twin randomized trials from the European Organization for Research and Treatment of Cancer Lymphoma Cooperative Group. *J Clin Oncol.* 1993;11:2258–2272.
12. Doll DC, Ringenberg QS, Anderson SP, et al. Bone marrow biopsy in the initial staging of Hodgkin's disease. *Med Pediatr Oncol.* 1989;17:1–5.
13. Gupta R, Gospodarowicz M, Lister T. Clinical evaluation and staging of Hodgkin's disease. In: Mauch P, Armitage J, Diehl V, et al, eds. *Hodgkin's Disease.* Philadelphia: Lippincott Williams and Wilkins; 1999:223–240.
14. Mansfield CM, Fabian C, Jones S, et al. Comparison of lymphangiography and computed tomography scanning in evaluating abdominal disease in stages III and IV Hodgkin's disease. A Southwest Oncology Group study. *Cancer.* 1990;66:2295–2299.
15. Rosenberg SA. Lymphography: a great advance, abandoned. *J Clin Oncol.* 2008;26:5662–5663.

16. Castellino RA, Hoppe RT, Blank N, et al. Computed tomography, lymphography, and staging laparotomy: correlations in initial staging of Hodgkin's disease. *AJR Am J Roentgenol.* 1984;143:37–41.

17. Castellino RA, Dunnick NR, Goffinet DR, et al. Predictive value of lymphography for sites of subdiaphragmatic disease encountered at staging laparotomy in newly diagnosed Hodgkin's disease and non-Hodgkin's lymphoma. *J Clin Oncol.* 1983;1:532–536.

18. Vinnicombe SJ, Reznek RH. Computerised tomography in the staging of Hodgkin's disease and non-Hodgkin's lymphoma. *Eur J Nucl Med Mol Imaging.* 2003;30(suppl 1):S42–S55.

19. Even-Sapir E, Israel O. Gallium-67 scintigraphy: a cornerstone in functional imaging of lymphoma. *Eur J Nucl Med Mol Imaging.* 2003;30(suppl 1):S65–S81.

20. Friedberg JW, Fischman A, Neuberg D, et al. FDG-PET is superior to gallium scintigraphy in staging and more sensitive in the follow-up of patients with de novo Hodgkin's lymphoma: a blinded comparison. *Leuk Lymphoma.* 2004;45:85–92.

21. Ha CS, Choe JG, Kong JS, et al. Agreement rates among single photon emission computed tomography using gallium-67, computed axial tomography and lymphangiography for Hodgkin's disease and correlation of image findings with clinical outcome. *Cancer.* 2000;89:1371–1379.

22. Kostakoglu L, Leonard JP, Kuji I, et al. Comparison of fluorine-18 fluorodeoxyglucose positron emission tomography and Ga-67 scintigraphy in evaluation of lymphoma. *Cancer.* 2002;94:879–888.

23. Wirth A, Seymour JF, Hicks RJ, et al. Fluorine-18 fluorodeoxyglucose positron emission tomography, gallium-67 scintigraphy, and conventional staging for Hodgkin's disease and non-Hodgkin's lymphoma. *Am J Med.* 2002;112:262–268.

24. Czernin J, Allen-Auerbach M, Schelbert HR. Improvements in cancer staging with PET/CT: literature-based evidence as of September 2006. *J Nucl Med.* 2007;48(suppl 1):78S–88S.

25. Juweid ME, Stroobants S, Hoekstra OS, et al. Use of positron emission tomography for response assessment of lymphoma: consensus of the Imaging Subcommittee of International Harmonization Project in Lymphoma. *J Clin Oncol.* 2007;25:571–578.

26. Juweid ME. Utility of positron emission tomography (PET) scanning in managing patients with Hodgkin's lymphoma. *Hematology Am Soc Hematol Educ Program.* 2006;259–265:510–511.

27. Juweid ME, Cheson BD. Role of positron emission tomography in lymphoma. *J Clin Oncol.* 2005;23:4577–4580.

28. Hernandez-Maraver D, Hernandez-Navarro F, Gomez-Leon N, et al. Positron emission tomography/computed tomography: diagnostic accuracy in lymphoma. *Br J Haematol.* 2006;135:293–302.

29. Pelosi E, Pregno P, Penna D, et al. Role of whole-body [18F] fluorodeoxyglucose positron emission tomography/computed tomography (FDG-PET/CT) and conventional techniques in the staging of patients with Hodgkin's and aggressive non Hodgkin's lymphoma. *Radiol Med.* 2008;113:578–590.

30. Rigacci L, Vitolo U, Nassi L, et al. Positron emission tomography in the staging of patients with Hodgkin's lymphoma. A prospective multicentric study by the Intergruppo Italiano Linfomi. *Ann Hematol.* 2007;86:897–903.

31. Cheson BD. The International Harmonization Project for response criteria in lymphoma clinical trials. *Hematol Oncol Clin North Am.* 2007;21:841–854.

# Combined Modality Treatment of Hodgkin's Lymphoma

Beate Klimm • Andreas Engert

The first-line treatment of patients with Hodgkin's lymphoma (HL) is tailored according to stage and risk profile at diagnosis. Patients with clinical stages I and II without any risk factor are allocated to the early-stage favorable group, those with risk factors to the early-stage unfavorable group. Patients with stages III and IV disease are assigned to the advanced-stage risk group. The stage is determined according to the Cotswolds staging classification.[1] Besides stage and B symptoms, which include fever, night sweats, and weight loss, most groups have implemented relevant prognostic factors such as larger tumor mass, including bulky disease >10 cm or a large mediastinal tumor $\geq 1/3$ of thoracic diameter. However, there are small differences in the definition of risk factors used and the classification of certain subgroups of HL patients among the different study groups in the Europe and the United States. In the United States, usually patients are either allocated to early or advanced stages. The definitions of treatment groups according to the different study groups in the Europe and the United States are presented in Table 1. All chemotherapy abbreviations mentioned in this article are explained in Table 2.

## TREATMENT OF EARLY-FAVORABLE HL

### Radiotherapy

In the treatment of early stages, extended-field (EF) radiotherapy had been considered standard treatment modality for many years. With this technique, radiation was delivered to all initially involved and adjacent lymph node regions, leading to large irradiation fields compared with the involved-field (IF) radiotherapy, which is restricted to the initially involved lymph node regions only. Together with the successful introduction of MOPP[2] and ABVD[3] chemotherapy for advanced stages in the 1980s, the paradigmatic shift from radiation alone to additional chemotherapy in early stages was accelerated by the realization of long-term toxicity and mortality related to large radiation fields and radiotherapy doses. Longer follow-up of patients who underwent EF-radiotherapy revealed severe late effects as competing causes of death, such as heart failure, pulmonary dysfunction, and secondary malignancies. Furthermore, although complete remission was generally achieved, there was a higher risk of relapsing from the first-line treatment when EF-radiotherapy alone was administered.[4] Two different strategies were explored to prevent these relapses: either applying even more intensive radiotherapy or adding chemotherapy for early-favorable stages to control occult lesions.[5] The latter strategy produced better outcomes and at the same time enabled reduction of radiotherapy to the IF for this risk group.

Thus, radiotherapy alone is almost obsolete, with 1 exception: patients with the first diagnosis of nodular lymphocyte predominant subtype of HL (LPHL) in clinical stage IA without risk factors are usually not included in ongoing trials for classic HL. On the basis of this very favorable prognosis, treatment with 30 Gy IF-radiotherapy

alone is an option for patients with stage IA of this subtype. Although being less toxic, this strategy seems to produce similar responses for LPHL IA patients compared with combined modality treatment.[6] Experimental approaches for these patients focus on the humanized monoclonal anti-CD20 antibody rituximab, which has given impressive results in relapsed LPHL.[7] Compared with IA patients with LPHL, advanced LPHL stages at initial diagnosis have less favorable outcomes and are thus treated according to protocols used for classic HL.[8]

## Chemoradiotherapy and Chemotherapy

Most centers and groups in the Europe and the United States have now accepted combined modality treatment consisting of 2 to 4 cycles of ABVD followed by 30 Gy IF-radiotherapy as the standard of care for early-favorable stage disease. Several randomized studies confirmed the superiority of combined modality treatment over radiotherapy alone. Other trials were conducted to investigate and reduce radiation fields and dose and, likewise, to decrease chemotherapy drug combinations and duration of treatment. The Southwest Oncology Group demonstrated that patients treated with combined modality therapy consisting of 3 cycles of doxorubicin and vinblastine followed by subtotal lymphoid irradiation (STLI) had a markedly superior outcome in terms of freedom from treatment failure (FFTF: 94% vs. 81% at 3 years) than those receiving STLI alone.[9] Another study from Milan revealed that STLI can be effectively replaced by IF-radiotherapy after short duration ABVD chemotherapy, while maintaining a very similar progression-free (97%) and overall survival (OS, 93%) at 5 years.[10] The European Organization for Research and Treatment of Cancer (EORTC) and the Groupe d'Etude des Lymphomes de l'Adulte demonstrated that combined modality with either 6 courses of EBVP (H7F trial) or 3 courses of MOPP/ABV (H8F trial) followed by IF-radiotherapy yielded a significantly better event-free survival (EFS) than achieved by subtotal nodal irradiation alone.[11,12] The aim of their H9F trial was to evaluate a possible dose reduction of radiotherapy (36 Gy or 20 Gy or no radiotherapy) after administering 6 cycles of EBVP. However, the arm without radiotherapy was closed prematurely because of a higher relapse rate than expected.[13] Although EBVP was used instead of ABVD in this setting, the use of chemotherapy alone in early-favorable stages should currently still be regarded as experimental. Another randomized trial for nonbulky, asymptomatic stage I-III HL failed to demonstrate superiority of ABVD + radiotherapy over ABVD alone; however, the total number of patients was small and all patients received 6 cycles of ABVD, even those in clinical stages I and II without risk factors.[14] A combined modality approach was also established in the HD7 trial of the German Hodgkin's Study Group (GHSG). In this trial, 2 cycles of ABVD plus EF-radiotherapy were shown to be superior to

**TABLE 1.** Definition of Treatment Groups of the EORTC/GELA, GHSG, and NCIC/ECOG

| Treatment Group | EORTC/GELA | GHSG | NCIC/ECOG |
|---|---|---|---|
| Early-stage favorable | CS I–II without risk factors (supradiaphragmatic) | CS I–II without risk factors | Standard risk group: favorable CS I–II (without risk factors) |
| Early-stage unfavorable | CS I–II with ≥1 risk factors (supradiaphragmatic) | CS I, CSIIA ≥1 risk factors; CS IIB with C/D but without A/B | Standard risk group: unfavorable CS I–II (at least one risk factor) |
| Advanced stage | CS III–IV | CS IIB with A/B; CS III–IV | High risk group: CS I or II with bulky disease; intraabdominal disease; CS III, IV |
| Risk factors (RF) | A. Large mediastinal mass | A. Large mediastinal mass | A. ≥40 yr |
|  | B. Age ≥50 yr | B. Extranodal disease | B. Not NLPHL or NS histology |
|  | C. Elevated ESR* | C. Elevated ESR* | C. ESR ≥50 mm/h |
|  | D. ≥4 involved regions | D. ≥3 involved areas | D. ≥4 involved nodal regions |

*≥50 mm/h without or ≥30 mm/h with B symptoms.
GJSG, German Hodgkin Lymphoma Study group; EORTC, European Organization for Research and Treatment of Cancer; GELA indicates Groupe d'Etude des Lymphomes de l'Adulte; ECOG, Eastern Cooperative Oncology Group; NCIC, National Cancer Institute of Canada; ESR, erythrocyte sedimentation rate.

EF-radiotherapy alone in terms of FFTF (88% vs. 67% at 7 years). The OS was equal in both arms because of effective salvage treatment.[15]

Further improvement of treatment with respect to the excellent long-term survival rates seems difficult. Thus, strategies to reduce drug dose and toxicity while maintaining efficacy are being pursued. In the subsequent HD10 trial of the GHSG, a possible reduction in chemotherapy from 4 to 2 cycles of ABVD or IF-RT from 30 to 20 Gy was evaluated. In the interim analyses, no significant differences in FFTF and OS were detected between 4 cycles of ABVD and 2 cycles of ABVD or between patients receiving different doses of radiotherapy (30 Gy vs. 20 Gy), but final result have to be awaited.[16] The aim of the current GHSG HD13 trial is to omit the presumably less-effective drugs, bleomycin or dacarbazine, from the ABVD backbone. Patients were thus randomized between 2 cycles of ABVD, ABV, AVD, or AV followed by 30 Gy IF-radiotherapy. However, the arms without dacarbazine (ABV and AV) had to be closed prematurely for safety reason because of more events in these arms. The next trial of the GHSG (HD16) and the current trial of the EORTC (H10F) incorporate positron emission tomography (PET) as a tool, which will hopefully help to evaluate early response to treatment and further reduce chemotherapy or avoid radiation for a part of patients with very good prognosis. A selection of recent and ongoing studies in patients with early-favorable HL is given in Table 3.

## TREATMENT OF EARLY-UNFAVORABLE HL

### From Extended to Involved Field Radiotherapy

Patients with early-unfavorable HL generally qualify for combined modality treatment. However, the ideal chemotherapy and radiation combinations are not yet clearly defined, and there is an ongoing desire to optimize treatment in this risk group. This is further being attempted by reducing radiation doses and field sizes in a similar manner to that for early-favorable stages. Several trials seem to indicate that the reduction of field size does not compromise the efficacy of treatment. Bonadonna et al[10] compared STLI with IF-radiotherapy after 4 cycles of ABVD in patients with early-favorable and unfavorable stages and reported a similar treatment outcome in both arms. In their H8U trial, the EORTC randomized patients between 6 cycles of MOPP/ABV + 36 Gy IF-radiotherapy, 4 cycles of MOPP/ABV + 36 Gy IF-RT, or 4 cycles MOPP/ABV + STLI. There was no difference between arms in terms of response rates, failure-free survival, or OS.[12] The GHSG HD8 trial randomized patients receiving 2 alternating cycles of COPP/ABVD to either extended (arm A) or involved field radiation (arm B). Final results at 5 years did not indicate differences between the 2 arms in terms of FFTF (86% and 84%) and OS (91% and 92%); however, more toxicity was reported in the patients who were treated with EF-radiotherapy.[17] A National Cancer Institute of

**TABLE 2.** Chemotherapy Regimens Used in HL and Their Drug Combinations

| Regimen | Drug Combinations |
|---|---|
| **MOPP** | Mechlorethamine, Oncovin (Vincristine), Procarbazine, Prednisone |
| **COPP** | Cyclophosphamide, Oncovin (Vincristine), Procarbazine, Prednisone |
| **ABVD** | Adriamycin (doxorubicin), Bleomycin, Vinblastine, Dacarbazine |
| **ABV** | Adriamycin (doxorubicin), Bleomycin, Vinblastine |
| **AVD** | Adriamycin (doxorubicin), Vinblastine, Dacarbazine |
| **AV** | Adriamycin (doxorubicin), Vinblastine |
| **EBVP** | Epirubicin, Bleomycin, Vinblastine, Prednisone |
| **VAPEC-B** | Vincristine, Adriamycin (doxorubicin), Prednisolone, Etoposide, Cyclophosphamide, Bleomycin |
| **ChIVPP/EVA** | Chlorambucil, Vinblastine, Procarbazine, Prednisolone, Etoposide, Vincristine, Adriamycin (doxorubicin) |
| **MOPPEBVCAD** | Mechlorethamine, Oncovin (Vincristine), Procarbazine, Prednisone, Epidoxorubicin, Bleomycin, Vinblastine, CCNU (Lomustine), Alkeran, Vindesine |
| **Stanford V** | Mechlorethamine, Adriamycin (doxorubicin), Vinblastine, Vincristine, Bleomycin, Etoposide, Prednisone |
| **BEACOPP** (baseline, escalated or 14) | Bleomycin, Etoposide, Adriamycin (doxorubicin), Cyclophosphamide, Oncovin (vincristine), Procarbazine, Prednisone |

| TABLE 3. Selected Trials for Early-Stage Favorable Hodgkin's Lymphoma | | | | |
|---|---|---|---|---|
| **Trial** | **Therapy Regimen** | **No. Pts.** | **Outcome** | **References** |
| SWOG no. 9133 | A. 3 (Dox.+Vinbl.) + STLI (36–40 Gy) | 165 | 94% (FFTF); 98% (OS) | 9 |
| | B. STLI (36–40 Gy) | 161 | 81% (FFTF); 96% (OS); (3 yr) | |
| Milan 1990–1997 | A. 4 ABVD + STLI | 65 | 97% (FFP); 93% (OS) | 10 |
| | B. 4 ABVD + IF-RT | 68 | 97% (FFP); 93% (OS); (5 yr) | |
| EORTC/GELA H7F | A. 6 EBVP + IF-RT (36 Gy) | 168 | 88% (EFS); 92% (OS) | 11 |
| | B. STNI | 165 | 78% (EFS); 92% (OS); (10 yr) | |
| EORTC/GELA H8F | A. 3 MOPP/ABV + IF-RT (36 Gy) | 270 | 98% (EFS, 5 yr); 97% (OS, 10 yr) | 12 |
| | B. STNI | 272 | 74% (EFS, 5 yr); 92% (OS, 10 yr) | |
| EORTC/GELA H9F | A. 6 EBVP + IF-RT (36 Gy) | 239 | 88% (EFS); 98% (OS) | 13 |
| | B. 6 EBVP + IF-RT (20 Gy) | 209 | 85% (EFS); 100% (OS) | |
| | C. 6 EBVP (no RT) | 130 | 69% (EFS); 98% (OS); (4 yr) closed because of high relapse rate | |
| GHSG HD7 | A. EF-RT 30 Gy (40 Gy IF) | 311 | 67% (FFTF); 92% (OS) | 15 |
| | B. 2 ABVD + EF-RT 30 Gy (40 Gy IF) | 316 | 88% (FFTF); 94% (OS); (7 yr) | |
| GHSG HD10 | A. 4 ABVD + IF-RT (30 Gy) | 847 | Interim anal yr is (2 yr) | 16 |
| | B. 4 ABVD + IF-RT (20 Gy) | | All pts | |
| | C. 2 ABVD + IF-RT (30 Gy) | | 96.6% (FFTF) | |
| | D. 2 ABVD + IF-RT (20 Gy) | | 98.5% (OS) | |
| GHSG HD13 | A. 2 ABVD + IF-RT (30 Gy) | | Ongoing trial | |
| | B. 2 ABV + IF-RT (30 Gy) | | B. and D. closed prematurely for safety reason (many events) | |
| | C. 2 AVD + IF-RT (30 Gy) | | | |
| | D. 2 AV + IF-RT (30 Gy) | | | |

SWOG indicates Southwest Oncology Group: EORTC, European Organization for Research and Treatment of Cancer; GELA, Groupe d'Etude des Lymphomes de l'Adulte; GHSG, German Hodgkin's Lymphoma Study Group; EF/IF-RT, extended/involved-field radiotherapy; STLI, subtotal lymphoid irradiation; STNI, subtotal nodal irradiation; FFTF, Freedom of treatment failure; FFP, freedom from progression; EFS, event-free survival; OS, overall survival.

Canada/Eastern Cooperative Oncology Group trial favored combined modality treatment over ABVD alone in unfavorable nonbulky stage IA/IIA HL.[18] Furthermore, a recent retrospective analysis supports the use of approximately 30 Gy IF-radiotherapy after a good response to ABVD,[19] a strategy that has been adopted in the ongoing GHSG and EORTC trials.

## Optimization of Chemotherapy

In early-unfavorable stages, efforts were made to improve the efficacy of chemotherapy by altering drugs and schedules as well as the number of cycles. In the past, alternation or hybridization of a MOPP-like regimen with ABVD did not produce better outcomes when compared with ABVD alone. Furthermore, studies in advanced-stage HL indicated that ABVD alone is equally effective and less myelotoxic compared with alternating MOPP/ABVD, and both are superior to MOPP alone.[20] Thus, a combined modality treatment consisting of 4 courses of ABVD followed by 30 Gy IF-radiotherapy is considered standard treatment for patients with early-unfavorable HL. Despite the excellent initial remission rates obtained with ABVD and radiotherapy, approximately 15% of patients in early-unfavorable stages relapse within 5 years and about another 5% suffer from primary progressive disease. These outcome rates are rather similar to those in patients in advanced stages when treated with more intensive regimens.

Thus, study groups are currently evaluating different regimens for the early-unfavorable group that were previously pioneered for the treatment of advanced stages. In their ongoing intergroup trial no. 2496, the Eastern Cooperative Oncology Group and Southwest Oncology Group are assessing whether the Stanford V regimen (12 weeks) is superior to 6 cycles of ABVD. In another approach, 4 cycles of ABVD were compared with 4 cycles of BEACOPP-baseline by the EORTC-Groupe d'Etude des Lymphomes de l'Adulte (H9U trial) and by the GHSG (HD11 trial). In addition, 2 EORTC trials analyzed whether 4 cycles of combined modality treatment are equally effective as 6 cycles (EORTC: H8U and H9U trial). In the H9U study, patients were randomly assigned to 6 cycles of ABVD or 4 cycles of ABVD or 4 cycles of BEACOPP-baseline, followed by 30 Gy IF-Radiotherapy in all arms. After a median follow-up of 4 years, no significant difference was observed between the 3 different treatment arms with respect to EFS or OS.[21] Interim results of the GHSG HD11 trial demonstrated very similar rates of FFTF and OS. At 3 years, there was no difference with respect to outcome, either between the ABVD and BEACOPP-baseline arms or between 30 Gy and 20 Gy IF-radiotherapy. Although it should be taken into account that these are relatively early data, currently there is no evidence for changing treatment from 4 to 6 cycles of ABVD or for recommending 4 cycles of BEACOPP-baseline in this group of patients.[22] However, the low FFTF in this risk group led the GHSG to a further intensification of treatment. In the ongoing HD14 trial for early-unfavorable stages, the BEACOPP escalated regimen was introduced, which had shown high efficacy in the treatment of advanced HL.[23] Patients were randomized to receive either 4 cycles of ABVD or 2 cycles of BEACOPP escalated plus 2 cycles of ABVD, both followed by 30 Gy IF-radiotherapy. The latter approach looks very promising at 3 years. In their current EORTC trial H10U, the EORTC incorporates PET and applies a risk-adapted schedule.

**TABLE 4.** Selected Trials for Early-Stage Unfavorable Hodgkin's Lymphoma

| Trial | Therapy Regimen | No. Pts. | Outcome | References |
|---|---|---|---|---|
| EORTC/GELA H8U | A. 6 MOPP/ABV + IF RT (36 Gy) | 336 | 84% (EFS, 5 yr); 88% (OS, 10 yr) | 12 |
| | B. 4 MOPP/ABV + IF RT (36 Gy) | 333 | 88% (EFS, 5 yr); 85% (OS, 10 yr) | |
| | C. 4 MOPP/ABV + STNI | 327 | 87% (EFS, 5 yr); 84% (OS,10 yr) | |
| GHSG HD8 | A. 2 COPP + ABVD + EF RT (30 Gy) + Bulk (10 Gy) | 532 | 86% (FFTF); 91% (OS) | 17 |
| | B. 2 COPP+ABVD + IF RT (30 Gy) + Bulk (10 Gy) | 532 | 84% (FFTF); 92% (OS); (5 yr) | |
| SWOG/ECOG no. 2496 | A. 6 ABVD + IF RT (36 Gy) to bulk (>5 cm) B. 12 wk Stanford V + IF RT (36 Gy) to bulk (>5 cm) | | Ongoing trial | |
| EORTC/GELA H9U | A. 6 ABVD + IF RT | 276 | 91% (EFS); 95% (OS) | 21 |
| | B. 4 ABVD + IF RT | 277 | 87% (EFS); 94% (OS) | |
| | C. 4 BEACOPP bas. + IF RT | 255 | 90% (EFS); 93% (OS); (4 yr) | |
| GHSG HD11 | A. 4 ABVD + IF RT (30 Gy) | 1293 | Interim analysis (3 yr) | 22 |
| | B. 4 ABVD + IF RT (20 Gy) | | All pts | |
| | C. 4 BEACOPP bas. + IF RT (30 Gy) | | 87% (FFTF) | |
| | D. 4 BEACOPP bas. + IF RT (20 Gy) | | 96% (OS) | |
| GHSG HD14 | A. 4 ABVD + IF RT (30 Gy) | | Ongoing trial | |
| | B. 2 BEACOPP esc. + 2 ABVD + IF RT (30 Gy) | | | |

SWOG indicates Southwest Oncology Group; EORTC, European Organization for Research and Treatment of Cancer; GELA, Groupe d'Etude des Lymphomes de l'Adulte; GHSG, German Hodgkin's Lymphoma Study Group; ECOG, Eastern Cooperative Oncology Group; EF/IF-RT, extended/involved-field radiotherapy; STNL, subtotal nodal irradiation; FFTF, Freedom of treatment failure; EFS, event-free survival; OS, overall survival.

Concerning radiotherapy, a new involved-node method leading to even smaller fields is being tested.[24] A selection of recent and ongoing studies in patients with early-unfavorable HL is given in Table 4.

## TREATMENT OF ADVANCED-STAGE HL

### Advent of ABVD Chemotherapy

Before the introduction of combination chemotherapy, more than 95% of patients with advanced HL succumbed to their disease within 5 years. Thus, remission rates in excess of 50% achieved with MOPP were a major breakthrough in oncology. MOPP was successfully used for many years for advanced-stage disease, resulting in long-term remission of nearly 50%.[2,25] The regimen was then replaced by ABVD, after a series of large multicenter trials had proven the superiority of ABVD and alternating MOPP/ABVD over MOPP alone.[26,27] Hybrid regimens such as MOPP/ABV were only equally effective when compared with alternating MOPP/ABVD and even rapidly alternating multidrug regimens such as COPP/ABV/IMEP did not result in better outcome.[28,29] However, more acute toxicity and a higher incidence of leukemia was reported after MOPP/ABV hybrid when compared with ABVD.[25] Therefore, ABVD was regarded the standard regimen against which all new combinations had to be tested. Nevertheless, a long-term follow-up report of 123 patients that had been treated with ABVD for advanced HL revealed a failure free survival of only 47% and an OS of 59% after 14.1 years.[30]

### New Chemotherapy Options

Several groups tried to improve the ABVD results by developing new regimens with additional drugs and by increasing dose intensity and dose density with the support of colony-stimulating factors and modern antibiotics. These new approaches include multidrug regimens such as Stanford V, MOPPEBVCAD, VAPEC-B, ChlVPP/EVA, and BEACOPP variants.[31–36]

Stanford V was developed as a short-duration, reduced-toxicity program and applied weekly over 12 weeks. Consolidating radiotherapy to sites of initial disease was employed. With an estimated 5-year freedom from progression of 89% and OS of 96%, this regimen produced very promising responses. However, the data were generated at a single center.[31] A prospectively randomized multicenter comparison of Stanford V with MOPPEBVCAD and ABVD showed that this regimen was inferior in terms of response rate (76% vs. 89% and 94%) and PFS (73% vs. 85% and 94%) in a multicenter setting. ABVD was still the best choice when it was combined with optional, limited irradiation.[32] These conflicting results might be partially explained by the use of less radiotherapy in the randomized setting and the better treatment quality of single-center reports. The Manchester group developed VAPEC-B, an abbreviated 11-week chemotherapy program and conducted a randomized comparison with the hybrid ChlVPP/EVA. After 5 years, EFS and OS were significantly better with ChlVPP/EVA than with VAPEC-B (EFS: 78 vs. 58%; OS: 89 vs. 79%).[33]

The GHSG HD9 trial compared COPP/ABVD, BEACOPP baseline, and BEACOPP escalated. Results from 1195 randomized patients showed a clear superiority of escalated BEACOPP over BEACOPP-baseline and COPP/ABVD at 5 years.[23] The follow-up data at 10 years confirmed these results: with a median follow-up of 112 months, the FFTF and OS rates were 64% and 75% in the COPP/ABVD group, 70% and 80% in the BEACOPP baseline group, and 82% and 86% in the BEACOPP-escalated group.[34] The subsequent GHSG HD12 trial aimed at deescalating chemotherapy and radiotherapy by comparing 4 courses of BEACOPP-escalated with

**TABLE 5.** Selected Trials for Advanced Hodgkin's Lymphoma

| Trial | Therapy Regimen | No. Pts. | Outcome | Ref. |
|---|---|---|---|---|
| Intergroup Italy | A. ABVD (6 cycles) | 98 | 83% (FFS); 86% (FFP); 90% (OS) | 32 |
| | B. Stanford V (12 wk) | 89 | 67% (FFS); 76% (FFP); 83% (OS) | |
| | C. MEC hybrid (six courses) (+RT initial bulk/ residual mass) | 88 | 85% (FFS); 93% (FFP); 90% (OS) (5 yr) | |
| Intergroup GB and Italy | A. ChlVPP/EVA hybrid (6 cycles) | 144 | 82% (FFP); 78% (EFS); 89% (OS) | 33 |
| | B. VAPEC-B (11 wk) (±RT initial bulk/residual mass) | 138 | 62% (FFP); 58% (EFS); 79% (OS) (5 yr) | |
| GHSG HD9 | A. COPP/ABVD (4 cycles) | 260 | 64% (FFTF); 75% (OS) | 34 |
| | B. BEACOPP baseline (8 cycles) | 469 | 70% (FFTF); 80% (OS) | |
| | C. BEACOPP escalated (8 cycles) | 466 | 82% (FFTF); 86% (OS) (10 yr) | |
| GHSG HD12 | A. 8 BEA esc. | 348 | 4th interim analysis (4 yr) | 35 |
| | B. 8 BEA esc. | 345 | All patients | |
| | C. 4 BEA esc. + 4 BEA baseline | 351 | 88% (8Besc) vs. 86% (4+4) (FFTF) | |
| | D. 4 BEA esc. + 4 BEA baseline (A. + C.: +RT bulk/residual mass) | 352 | 93% (8Besc) vs. 91% (4+4) (OS) | |
| GHSG HD15 | A. 8 BEA esc. | | Trial closed, results awaited | 37 |
| | B. 6 BEA esc. | | Negative predictive value for PET: 94% (12 mo) | |
| | C. 8 BEA-14 | | | |
| | (+RT to PET + residual mass ≥2.5 cm) | | | |
| Intergroup no. 20012 EORTC, … | 8 × ABVD 4 BEA esc. + 4 BEA baseline | | Ongoing trial | |

SWOG indicates Southwest Oncology Group; EORTC, European Organization for Research and Treatment of Cancer; GELA, Groupe d'Etude des Lymphomes de l'Adulte; GHSG, German Hodgkin's Lymphoma Study Group; ECOG, Eastern Cooperative Oncology Group; EF/IF-RT, extended/involved-field radiotherapy; STNI, subtotal nodal irradiation; FFS, failure-free survival; FFP, freedom from progression; FFTF, freedom from treatment failure; EFS, event-free survival; OS, overall survival.

4 courses of escalated and 4 courses of baseline BEACOPP, with or without consolidating radiation to initial bulky and residual disease. In an interim analysis of HD12 at 4 years, there was no significant difference in the FFTF and OS between the different arms so far, but final results are awaited.[35] In the following HD15 trial, patients were randomized between 8 courses of BEACOPP-escalated, 6 courses of BEACOPP-escalated, or 8 courses of BEACOPP-14, which is a time-intensified variant of BEACOPP-baseline.[36] Additional radiotherapy was only applied to residual lesions ≥2.5 cm positive by PET. The chemotherapy question is not yet solved; however, PET demonstrated a high negative predictive value for progression or early relapse for patients with residual disease after the first-line chemotherapy in advanced-stage HL.[37] The question whether escalated BEACOPP is superior to ABVD alone in a randomized setting is currently being evaluated in an intergroup trial initiated by the EORTC (no. 20012). Here, 8 cycles of ABVD are being compared with 4 cycles of BEACOPP-escalated followed by 4 cycles of BEACOPP-baseline. Further intensification of the first-line therapy in high-risk patients by employing high-dose chemotherapy and autologous stem cell transplantation after 4 instead of 8 cycles of ABVD did not improve outcome compared with conventional treatment.[38] A selection of recent and ongoing studies in patients with advanced-stage HL is given in Table 5.

## Role of Consolidating Radiotherapy and PET

The role of consolidating radiotherapy after effective chemotherapy in the treatment of patients with advanced HL is still subject to clinical research. A meta-analysis comparing combined modality approaches and chemotherapy alone reported equal tumor control and even better OS in patients treated with chemotherapy alone.[39] Therefore, randomized trials currently evaluate the impact of radiotherapy after effective chemotherapy for advanced HL. A study conducted by the EORTC indicated that consolidating IF-RT did not result in better outcome in patients who had already achieved a complete remission after 6 to 8 cycles of MOPP/ABV, although radiotherapy may be beneficial to patients with partial remissions.[40] Longer follow-up of the GHSG HD12 trial and the HD15 trial may help to define the role of radiotherapy for residual disease. In the HD15 trial, PET scan was used as a tool to analyze tumor activity in residual masses after chemotherapy. Radiotherapy was only applied to PET-positive residual lesions ≥2.5 cm. The approach led to a substantial lower number of patients receiving radiotherapy than in previous GHSG studies. The method showed a high negative predictive value; thus, consolidation radiotherapy might be omitted in PET-negative patients with residual disease without increasing the risk for progression or early relapse compared with patients in complete remission.[37] In addition, there are data from smaller trials with ABVD suggesting that early PET scan during chemotherapy may discriminate between responders and nonresponders and thus have a potential role for use in response-adapted strategies.[41,42] This approach is currently being investigated in larger randomized GHSG and EORTC studies for advanced-stage HL.

## Elderly HL Patients

Although there is substantial variety in the health status among elderly patients with HL, the age at diagnosis remains an unfavorable risk factor, particularly in patients with advanced stages. In most groups, patients are considered "elderly" if they are older than

60 years. Factors such as more aggressive disease, more frequent diagnosis of advanced stage, comorbidity, poor tolerance of treatment, failure to maintain dose intensity, shorter survival after relapse, and death because of other causes contribute to the poorer outcome of elderly patients. A retrospective analysis of GHSG trials showed that elderly patients have a poorer risk profile, more treatment-associated toxicity, a lower dose-intensity and higher mortality as major factors for poorer outcome.[43] Generally, elderly patients without major comorbidities who are sufficiently fit to tolerate standard therapy have a treatment outcome comparable with that of younger patients. Whenever possible, elderly patients should be treated with a doxorubicin-containing regimen; however, the BEACOPP regimen is too toxic for patients over 60 years.[44] Furthermore, large radiotherapy fields should be avoided.[45] Whether the results of new approaches such as ChlVPP-ABV, ODBEP, PVAG, BACOPP, or VEPEMB would be superior compared with ABVD or equal and less toxic is currently a matter of speculation because of the lack of randomized studies.

## SUMMARY

Currently, combined modality treatment strategies including 2 to 4 cycles of ABVD chemotherapy followed by 30 Gy IF-radiotherapy is the standard treatment for patients with early stages of HL at diagnosis. Patients in the early-favorable risk group achieve an FFTF of more than 90% and an OS of about 95% at 5 years. Patients in the early unfavorable group have an FFTF of about 84% and an OS of 91%.[12,15,17] In many centers 6 to 8 cycles of ABVD plus consolidating radiotherapy to residual disease is still considered the gold standard for patients with advanced-stage HL. The GHSG recommends BEACOPP escalated for patients under the age of 60 because of significant better outcome rates. With ABVD, Stanford V, and MOPPEBVCAD the 5-year failure-free survival rates were 78%, 54%, and 81%. Corresponding 5-year OS rates were 90%, 82%, and 89%.[32] With BEACOPP escalated FFTF and an OS rates of 87% and 91% were observed at 5 years.[23]

With regard to these excellent results, modern treatment strategies aim at further optimizing chemotherapy by simultaneously reducing therapy-induced acute and long-term toxicities. Potential future strategies may use response-adapted therapy approaches guided by early-PET scan and may successfully implement new drugs and experimental strategies in the first-line treatment.

## REFERENCES

1. Lister TA, Crowther D, Sutcliffe SB, et al. Report of a committee convened to discuss the evaluation and staging of patients with Hodgkin's disease: Cotswolds meeting. *J Clin Oncol.* 1989;7:1630–1636.
2. Longo DL, Young RC, Wesley M, et al. Twenty years of MOPP chemotherapy for Hodgkin's disease. *J Clin Oncol.* 1986;4:1295–1306.
3. Bonadonna G, Zucali R, Monfardini S, et al. Combination chemotherapy of Hodgkin's disease with adriamycin, bleomycin, vinblastine, and imidazole carboximide versus MOPP. *Cancer.* 1975;36:252–259.
4. Horwich A, Specht L, Ashley S. Survival analysis of patients with clinical stages I or II Hodgkin's disease who have relapsed after initial treatment with radiotherapy alone. *Eur J Cancer.* 1997;33:848–853.
5. Specht L, Gray RG, Clarke MJ, et al. Influence of more extensive radiotherapy and adjuvant chemotherapy on long-term outcome of early-stage Hodgkin's disease: a meta-analysis of 23 randomized trials involving 3,888 patients. International Hodgkin's Disease Collaborative Group. *J Clin Oncol.* 1998;16:830–843.
6. Nogova L, Reineke T, Eich HT, et al. Extended field radiotherapy, combined modality treatment or involved field radiotherapy for patients with stage IA lymphocyte-predominant Hodgkin's lymphoma: a retrospective analysis from the German Hodgkin's Study Group (GHSG). *Ann Oncol.* 2005;16:1683–1687.
7. Schulz H, Rehwald U, Morschhauser F, et al. Rituximab in relapsed lymphocyte-predominant Hodgkin's lymphoma: long-term results of a phase 2 trial by the German Hodgkin's Lymphoma Study Group (GHSG). *Blood.* 2008;111:109–111.
8. Nogová L, Reineke T, Brillant C, et al. Lymphocyte-predominant and classical Hodgkin's lymphoma: a comprehensive analysis from the German Hodgkin's Study Group. *J Clin Oncol.* 2008;26:434–439.
9. Press OW, LeBlanc M, Lichter AS, et al. Phase III randomized intergroup trial of subtotal lymphoid irradiation versus doxorubicin, vinblastine, and subtotal lymphoid irradiation for stage IA to IIA Hodgkin's disease. *J Clin Oncol.* 2001;19:4238–4244.
10. Bonadonna G, Bonfante V, Viviani S, et al. ABVD plus subtotal nodal versus involved-field radiotherapy in early-stage Hodgkin's disease: long-term results. *J Clin Oncol.* 2004;22:2835–2841.
11. Noordijk EM, Carde P, Dupouy N, et al. Combined-modality therapy for clinical stage I or II Hodgkin's lymphoma: long-term results of the European Organisation for Research and Treatment of Cancer H7 randomized controlled trials. *J Clin Oncol.* 2006;24:3128–3135.
12. Fermé C, Eghbali H, Meerwaldt JH, et al. Chemotherapy plus involved-field radiation in early-stage Hodgkin's disease. *N Engl J Med.* 2007;357:1968–1971.
13. Eghbali H, Brice P, Creemers G-Y, et al. Comparison of Three Radiation Dose Levels after EBVP Regimen in Favorable Supradiaphragmatic Clinical Stages (CS) I-II Hodgkin's Lymphoma (HL): preliminary Results of the EORTC-GELA H9-F Trial. *Blood.* 2005;106:814a.
14. Straus DJ, Portlock CS, Qin J, et al. Results of a prospective randomized clinical trial of doxorubicin, bleomycin, vinblastine, and dacarbazine (ABVD) followed by radiation therapy (RT) versus ABVD alone for stages I, II, and IIIA nonbulky Hodgkin's disease. *Blood.* 2004;104:3483–3489.
15. Engert A, Franklin J, Eich HT, et al. Two cycles of doxorubicin, bleomycin, vinblastine, and dacarbazine plus extended-field radiotherapy is superior to radiotherapy alone in early favorable Hodgkin's lymphoma: final results of the GHSG HD7 trial. *J Clin Oncol.* 2007;25:3495–3502.
16. Engert A, Pluetschow A, Eich HT, et al. Combined Modality Treatment of two or four cycles of ABVD followed by involved field radiotherapy in the treatment of patients with early stage Hodgkin's lymphoma: update interim analysis of the randomised HD10 study of the German Hodgkin's Study Group (GHSG). *Blood.* 2005;106:2673a.
17. Engert A, Schiller P, Josting A, et al. Involved-field radiotherapy is equally effective and less toxic compared with extended-field radiotherapy after four cycles of chemotherapy in patients with early-stage unfavorable Hodgkin's lymphoma: results of the HD8 trial of the German Hodgkin's Lymphoma Study Group. *J Clin Oncol.* 2003;21:3601–3608.
18. Meyer RM, Gospodarowicz MK, Connors JM, et al. Randomized comparison of ABVD chemotherapy with a strategy that includes radiation therapy in patients with limited-stage Hodgkin's lymphoma: National Cancer Institute of Canada Clinical Trials Group and the Eastern Cooperative Oncology Group. *J Clin Oncol.* 2005;23:4634–4642.
19. Vassilakopoulos TP, Angelopoulou MK, Siakantaris MP, et al. Combination chemotherapy plus low-dose involved-field radiotherapy for early clinical stage Hodgkin's lymphoma. *Int J Radiat Oncol Biol Phys.* 2004;59:765–781.
20. Canellos GP, Anderson JR, Propert KJ, et al. Chemotherapy of advanced Hodgkin's disease with MOPP, ABVD, or MOPP alternating with ABVD. *N Engl J Med.* 1992;327:1478–1484.
21. Fermé C, Diviné M, Vranovsky A, et al. Four ABVD and involved-field radiotherapy in unfavorable supradiaphragmatic clinical stages (CS) I-II Hodgkin's Lymphoma (HL): preliminary results of the EORTC-GELA H9-U Trial. *Blood.* 2005;106:813a.
22. Diehl V, Brillant C, Engert A. Recent interim analysis of the HD11 Trial of the GHSG: intensification of chemotherapy and reduction of radiation dose in early unfavorable stage Hodgkin's lymphoma. *Blood.* 2005;106:816a.
23. Diehl V, Franklin J, Pfreundschuh M, et al. Standard and increased-dose BEACOPP chemotherapy compared with COPP-ABVD for advanced Hodgkin's disease. *N Engl J Med.* 2003;348:2386–2395.
24. Girinsky T, van der Maazen R, Specht L, et al. Involved-node radiotherapy (INRT) in patients with early Hodgkin's lymphoma: concepts and guidelines. *Radiother Oncol.* 2006;79:270–277.
25. Bonadonna G, Valagussa P, Santoro A. Alternating non-cross-resistant combination chemotherapy or MOPP in stage IV Hodgkin's disease. A report of 8-year results. *Ann Intern Med.* 1986;104:739–746.
26. Duggan DB, Petroni GR, Johnson JL, et al. Randomized comparison of ABVD and MOPP/ABV hybrid for the treatment of advanced Hodgkin's disease: report of an intergroup trial. *J Clin Oncol.* 2003;21:607–614.
27. Santoro A, Bonadonna G, Valagussa P, et al. Long-term results of combined chemotherapy-radiotherapy approach in Hodgkin's disease: superiority of ABVD plus radiotherapy versus MOPP plus radiotherapy. *J Clin Oncol.* 1987;5:27–37.
28. Connors JM, Klimo P, Adams G, et al. Treatment of advanced Hodgkins disease with chemotherapy—comparison of MOPP/ABV hybrid regimen with

alternating courses of MOPP and ABVD: a report from the National Cancer Institute of Canada Clinical Trials Group. *J Clin Oncol.* 1997;15:1638–1645.

29. Sieber M, Tesch H, Pfistner B, et al. Treatment of advanced Hodgkin's disease with COPP/ABV/IMEP versus COPP/ABVD and consolidating radiotherapy: final results of the German Hodgkin's Lymphoma Study Group HD6 trial. *Ann Oncol.* 2004;15:276–282.

30. Canellos GP, Niedzwiecki D. Long-term follow-up of Hodgkin's disease trial. *N Engl J Med.* 2002;346:1417–1418.

31. Horning SJ, Hoppe RT, Breslin S, et al. Stanford V and radiotherapy for locally extensive and advanced Hodgkin's disease: mature results of a prospective clinical trial. *J Clin Oncol.* 2002;20:630–637.

32. Gobbi PG, Levis A, Chisesi T, et al. ABVD versus modified stanford V versus MOPPEBVCAD with optional and limited radiotherapy in intermediate- and advanced-stage Hodgkin's lymphoma: final results of a multicenter randomized trial by the Intergruppo Italiano Linfomi. *J Clin Oncol.* 2005;23:9198–9207.

33. Radford JA, Rohatiner AZ, Ryder WD, et al. ChlVPP/EVA hybrid versus the weekly VAPEC-B regimen for previously untreated Hodgkin's disease. *J Clin Oncol.* 2002;20:2988–2994.

34. Engert A, Franklin J, Diehl V. Long-Term follow-up of BEACOPP$_{escalated}$ chemotherapy in patients with advanced-stage Hodgkin's lymphoma on behalf of the German Hodgkin's Study Group. *Blood.* 2007;110:211a.

35. Engert A, Franklin J, Mueller R-P, et al. HD12 Randomised Trial comparing 8 dose-escalated cycles of BEACOPP with 4 escalated and 4 baseline cycles in patients with advanced stage Hodgkin's Lymphoma (HL): an analysis of the German Hodgkin's Lymphoma Study Group (GHSG), University of Cologne, D-50924 Cologne, Germany. *Blood.* 2006;108:99a.

36. Sieber M, Bredenfeld H, Josting A, et al. 14-day variant of the bleomycin, etoposide, doxorubicin, cyclophosphamide, vincristine, procarbazine, and prednisone regimen in advanced-stage Hodgkin's lymphoma: results of a pilot study of the German Hodgkin's Lymphoma Study Group. *J Clin Oncol.* 2003;21:1734–1739.

37. Kobe C, Dietlein M, Franklin J, et al. Positron emission tomography has a high negative predictive value for progression or early relapse for patients with residual disease after first-line chemotherapy in advanced-stage Hodgkin's lymphoma. *Blood.* 2008;112:3989–3994.

38. Federico M, Bellei M, Brice P, et al. High-dose therapy and autologous stem-cell transplantation versus conventional therapy for patients with advanced Hodgkin's lymphoma responding to front-line therapy. *J Clin Oncol.* 2003;21:2320–2325.

39. Loeffler M, Brosteanu O, Hasenclever D, et al. Meta-analysis of chemotherapy versus combined modality treatment trials in Hodgkin's disease. International Database on Hodgkin's Disease Overview Study Group. *J Clin Oncol.* 1998;16:818–829.

40. Aleman BM, Raemaekers JM, Tirelli U, et al. Involved-field radiotherapy for advanced Hodgkin's lymphoma. *N Engl J Med.* 2003;348:2396–2406.

41. Hutchings M, Mikhaeel NG, Fields PA, et al. Prognostic value of interim FDG-PET after two or three cycles of chemotherapy in Hodgkin's lymphoma. *Ann Oncol.* 2005;16:1160–1168.

42. Hutchings M, Loft A, Hansen MT, et al. FDG-PET after two cycles of chemotherapy predicts treatment failure and progression-free survival in Hodgkin's lymphoma. *Blood.* 2006;107:52–59.

43. Engert A, Ballova V, Haverkamp H, et al. Hodgkin's lymphoma in elderly patients: a comprehensive retrospective analysis from the German Hodgkin's Study Group. *J Clin Oncol.* 2005;23:5052–5060.

44. Ballova V, Ruffer JU, Haverkamp H, et al. A prospectively randomized trial carried out by the German Hodgkin's Study Group (GHSG) for elderly patients with advanced Hodgkin's disease comparing BEACOPP baseline and COPP-ABVD (study HD9elderly). *Ann Oncol.* 2005;16:124–131.

45. Klimm B, Eich HT, Haverkamp H, et al. Poorer outcome of elderly patients treated with extended-field radiotherapy compared with involved-field radiotherapy after chemotherapy for Hodgkin's lymphoma: an analysis from the German Hodgkin Study Group. *Ann Oncol.* 2007;18:357–363.

# Role of Chemotherapy in Hodgkin's Lymphoma

Pamela Seam • John E. Janik • Dan L. Longo • Vincent T. DeVita, Jr.

There are few success stories in oncology as rewarding or remarkable as the development of curative therapies for Hodgkin's lymphoma (HL). In 1832, in an article entitled "Some Morbid Appearances of the Absorbent Glands and Spleen," Thomas Hodgkin first characterized the lymphadenopathy and splenomegaly associated with HL.[1] Extended-field radiotherapy (EF-RT) became the mainstay of curative therapy until the 1960s when systemic chemotherapy was incorporated into the treatment paradigm to manage disseminated disease. In this article, we will define the relevant features of the staging system in HL, review the landmark chemotherapeutic regimens used to treat both limited and advanced stage classic HL, and finally, discuss the role of 18-fluorodeoxyglucose positron emission tomography (PET) scans in assessing response and minimizing the risk of long-term toxicities. Nodular lymphocyte-predominant HL, regarded as a separate entity under the WHO lymphoma classification, will not be discussed here.

## STAGING AND PROGNOSTIC EVALUATION

The Ann Arbor classification defines 4 clinical and pathologic stages of HL.[2] In 1990, the suffix "X" was incorporated into the classification and indicated the presence of bulky disease, ie, a single mass exceeding 10 cm in largest diameter or a mediastinal mass exceeding one third of the maximum transverse transthoracic diameter on a standard posterior-anterior chest radiograph at the level of T5–T6.[3] In North America, the division of HL into limited stage (stage I–IIA with no areas of bulk) and advanced stage (stage III–IV or stage I–II with B symptoms or areas of bulk) has guided modern treatment strategies. The National Cancer Institute of Canada/Eastern Cooperative Oncology Group (NCIC/ECOG) further distinguishes unfavorable early stage patients as those age $\geq$40, erythrocyte sedimentation rate (ESR) $\geq$50 mm/hr, mixed cellularity or lymphocyte depleted histology, or $\geq$4 sites of disease.[4] The therapeutic implications of these and similar subdivisions used by the European cooperative groups remain unclear.[5,6]

## LIMITED STAGE DISEASE

Given that HL is a radiosensitive disease, EF-RT was the treatment of choice until the late 1980s. Staging laparotomy was frequently performed to confirm that disease was indeed localized. A number of studies demonstrated equivalent or superior long-term disease control in patients receiving chemotherapy alone or combined modality therapy (CMT) versus treatment with radiation therapy alone.[5,7–12] Meta-analyses have solidified these conclusions.[11,12]

Specht et al[11] conducted a meta-analysis in which individual patient data were collected on 1688 patients in 13 studies between 1967 and 1988 using mechlorethamine, vincristine sulfate, procarbazine, and prednisone (MOPP) or a MOPP-like regimen with

radiation therapy versus radiation therapy alone. The addition of chemotherapy to radiotherapy halved the 10-year risk of treatment failure (15.8% vs. 32.7%, $P < 0.00001$), but the effect on overall survival (OS) was not statistically significant. Another analysis of 14 randomized trials performed between 1974 and 1988 and enrolling 1740 patients compared chemotherapy alone with CMT.[12] Among trials in which radiation was added to chemotherapy, the 10-year tumor control rate improved by 11% ($P = 0.0001$) with no improvement in OS ($P = 0.57$). When additional chemotherapy was substituted for radiation in CMT, no difference in tumor control rates ($P = 0.43$) was observed although OS significantly improved for the chemotherapy alone group ($P = 0.045$). The lack of an OS benefit in patients receiving CMT in both meta-analyses highlights the impact of radiation-induced cardiovascular complications and secondary neoplasia.

CMT does produce a superior outcome to radiation therapy alone. A phase III intergroup prospective randomized trial of subtotal lymphoid irradiation (SLI) versus doxorubicin, vinblastine, and SLI for stage IA–IIA disease reported a markedly superior failure-free survival (FFS) rate for patients on the CMT arm (94%) compared with the SLI arm (81%).[10] In another study of stage IA–IIA patients, the freedom from treatment failure (FFTF) at 7 years (88%) was significantly better for the 316 patients who received 2 cycles of doxorubicin, bleomycin, vinblastine, and dacarbazine (ABVD) plus EF-RT versus the 311 patients who received EF-RT alone (67%).[9]

Ferme et al[8] stratified 1538 patients with untreated stage I–II supradiaphragmatic HL into a favorable prognosis group (n = 542) and an unfavorable prognosis group (n = 996).[5] Favorable prognosis patients were randomly assigned to receive 3 cycles of MOPP-ABV plus involved-field radiotherapy (MOPP-doxorubicin, bleomycin, and vinblastine plus IF-RT) or subtotal nodal radiotherapy. Patients with an unfavorable prognosis were randomly assigned to receive 6 or 4 cycles of MOPP-ABV plus IF-RT or 4 cycles of MOPP-ABV plus subtotal nodal radiotherapy. With 92 months of median follow-up, among patients with a favorable prognosis, the 5-year event-free survival (EFS) rate and 10 year OS estimate were 98% and 97%, respectively, for the CMT group and 74% and 92%, respectively, for the radiotherapy alone group. There was no difference in 5-year EFS rates and 10-year OS estimates among the 3 treatment groups in patients with an unfavorable prognosis. The authors concluded that early stage favorable patients should receive chemotherapy plus IF-RT, whereas unfavorable disease patients should receive 4 courses of a doxorubicin containing regimen plus IF-RT. This conclusion ignores the possibility that the outcome might be similar or even improved with the use of chemotherapy alone.

Clinical investigations turned to reducing the size of the radiation field, reducing the radiation dose, limiting the number of cycles of chemotherapy, and using chemotherapy alone. We will focus on the latter 2 approaches, with an emphasis on ABVD and ABVD-like regimens, which are currently the standard of care for stage I–II HL in the United States.[4,7,13–15]

In a phase III trial of 1131 patients with stage I–II favorable disease, Diehl et al[13] randomly assigned patients to 2 or 4 cycles of ABVD followed by IF-RT at either 20 or 30 Gy. The reported FFTF after a median observation time of 2 years was 96.6% with no statistical differences between arms that differed in the number of cycles of chemotherapy or the dose of IF-RT.

In a series of 251 Indian patients, 179 achieved a complete remission (CR) after 6 cycles of ABVD and were further randomized to IF-RT or no further therapy.[14] The 8-year EFS and OS in the chemotherapy-alone arm were 76% and 89%, respectively, as compared with 88% and 100%, respectively, in the chemotherapy plus IF-RT arm.[14] The inclusion of pediatric patients and patients with various stages of disease may have affected the results. Notably, among 99 patients with stage I-II disease, there was no difference in EFS or OS between the 2 arms of the study.

In a study from the Memorial Sloan-Kettering Cancer Center, 152 untreated HL patients with clinical stages IA–IIA, IB–IIB, and IIIA without bulky disease were randomly assigned to 6 cycles of ABVD alone or 6 cycles of ABVD followed by radiation therapy.[15] At 60 months, the freedom from progression (FFP) was 86% for the ABVD plus radiation therapy arm and 81% ($P = 0.61$) for the ABVD arm alone, whereas OS for the 2 arms was 97% and 90%, respectively ($P = 0.08$). The small sample size and the inclusion of patients with B symptoms and IIIA disease may have confounded the results, but they suggest that chemotherapy alone is an acceptable approach for most patients.

Meyer et al[4] conducted a multicenter randomized controlled trial in which 399 patients with nonbulky clinical stage I–IIA HL were stratified into favorable and unfavorable risk cohorts. Patients were randomly assigned to receive either radiotherapy (subtotal nodal radiation for favorable risk or 2 cycles of ABVD followed by subtotal nodal radiation for unfavorable risk) or ABVD as a single modality (4 vs. 6 cycles of ABVD based on radiographic response on CT after 2 cycles of chemotherapy). At a median follow-up of 4.2 years, there was no difference in OS (94% vs. 96%, $P = 0.4$) or EFS (88% vs. 86%, $P = 0.06$) in patients allocated to CMT versus patients allocated to chemotherapy alone. Although the 5 year freedom from disease progression was superior in patients who received radiation therapy ($P = 0.006$), there was a trend toward more deaths due to second cancers and cardiovascular events. The survival of relapsed patients on both arms of the study was more than 70%.

The National Cancer Institute (NCI) reported 25 year follow-up on 136 patients randomized to receive radiation therapy or MOPP chemotherapy.[16] Disease-free survival (DFS) was 61% and 87% for radiation and MOPP, respectively ($P = 0.0034$). OS was 63% and 81% for radiation and MOPP, respectively ($P = 0.048$). Among the patients who remained in CR from chemotherapy, 25-year OS was 93% versus 78% for patients treated with radiation therapy ($P = 0.05$). Secondary malignancies and heart disease accounted for excess deaths among patients in CR previously treated with mantle field radiation therapy. Based on these results and the curative potential of chemotherapy alone in the majority of patients, radiation should be reserved for the 5% to 7% of patients whose disease does not respond to chemotherapy.

## ADVANCED STAGE DISEASE

In 1963, the NCI initiated a pilot study to test MOPP chemotherapy in 43 patients with advanced HL.[17] MOPP was the first regimen capable of prolonging DFS in advanced disease and the first such success in any disseminated solid tumor.[18] Providing the same

therapeutic benefit as MOPP with less hematologic toxicity and lower rates of infertility, ABVD eventually replaced MOPP as the standard of care for advanced HL in the United States.[19] Various combinations of MOPP and ABVD were tested over the next twenty years, but none proved better than ABVD alone. In phase I–II studies, Stanford V (doxorubicin, vinblastine, mechlorethamine, etoposide, vincristine, bleomycin, and prednisone) and bleomycin, etoposide, adriamycin, cyclophosphamide, vincristine, procarbazine, and prednisone (BEACOPP), both administered with radiation therapy, also demonstrated clinical efficacy.[20–22] Phase III trials comparing each of them with ABVD are ongoing.

DeVita et al[23] first reported that MOPP achieved high CR rates (81%), durable CRs (29–42 months), and long-term DFS (47% DFS at 4 years) in stage III–IV patients. At 14 years of follow-up, 157 of 188 treated patients (84%) entered a CR with 101 patients (66%) remaining disease free more than 10 years from the end of treatment.[18]

MOPP, however, caused reversible bone marrow depression, neurotoxicity, and permanent azoospermia in nearly 100% of men.[18,24] Whereas most women age $\leq 26$ years regained normal menses after cessation of therapy, 41% of women age $\geq 26$ became amenorrheic. Nearly all women experienced premature menopause typically in their late 30s. Only one patient in the NCI series developed acute leukemia, but acute leukemia and myelodysplastic syndrome after MOPP or MOPP in combination with radiotherapy were reported elsewhere.[25,26]

To improve treatment outcome, the Milan group developed ABVD "... on an empirical rather than a solid scientific basis ... "[19,27] Less toxic than MOPP, ABVD became the standard of care in advanced HL. In an equivalence trial, 60 patients with untreated stage IIB-IVB HL were randomly assigned to 6 cycles of ABVD versus 6 cycles of MOPP. MOPP (76%) and ABVD (75%) produced the same number of CRs with bone marrow suppression representing the main dose limiting factor. Among 232 previously untreated stage IIB, IIIA, and IIIB patients randomly assigned to receive 3 cycles of MOPP or ABVD followed by radiotherapy, the 7-year FFP (80.8% vs. 62.8%, $P < 0.002$), relapse-free survival (87.7% vs. 77.2%, $P = 0.06$), and OS (77.4% vs. 67.9%, $P = 0.03$) were higher for ABVD than MOPP.[28] There were no significant abnormalities in cardiopulmonary function with either regimen.

To maximize the cure rates achieved with MOPP and ABVD, clinical trials incorporated multiple noncross-resistant agents, and then alternated the component drugs (MOPP/ABVD), sequenced them (MOPP → ABVD), or integrated 7 of 8 drugs into a hybrid therapy (MOPP/ABV).[29–32] Seventy patients with advanced HL, including 16 in first relapse after radiotherapy, were treated with hybrid MOPP/ABV regimen for more than 8 months.[30] IF-RT was given to partial responders. The actuarial OS at 49 months for 54 untreated patients was 90% with no reported drug-induced pulmonary or cardiac toxicity. These results led to a randomized 301 patient study of untreated stage IIIB, IVA, or IVB disease or disease in first relapse after radiotherapy comparing the MOPP/ABV hybrid regimen or MOPP alternating with ABVD.[33] Five-year OS rates and 5-year FFS rates for the 2 regimens were similar. The MOPP/ABV regimen was associated with significantly more episodes of febrile neutropenia (27% vs. 10%, $P = 0.0001$) and stomatitis (7% vs. 1%, $P = 0.01$) versus alternating MOPP/ABVD (10%) ($P = 0.0001$). Although the MOPP/ABV hybrid was as effective as ABVD in an intergroup trial, the incidence of myelodysplastic syndrome and acute leukemia dampened support for the regimen.[34]

In 1992, Cancer and Leukemia Group B reported a landmark trial comparing MOPP alone for 6 to 8 cycles, MOPP alternating with ABVD for 12 cycles, and ABVD alone for 6 to 8 cycles.[35] Lower doses of mechlorethamine and vincristine were used as compared with the original MOPP regimen. In this multicenter study, 361 HL patients with untreated stage III–IV disease or relapsed disease after radiotherapy for localized disease were randomly assigned to receive one of the 3 regimens. CR rates were 67% for MOPP, 82% for ABVD, and 83% for MOPP-ABVD ($P = 0.006$ comparing MOPP with the doxorubicin-containing regimens). At 5 years, FFS rates were 50%, 61%, and 65% for MOPP, ABVD, and MOPP-ABVD, respectively ($P = 0.02$ for the comparison of MOPP with the other regimens). There were no differences in OS at 5 years: 66% for MOPP, 73% for ABVD, and 75% for MOPP-ABVD ($P = 0.28$ comparing MOPP with the doxorubicin-containing regimens). ABVD therapy was clearly as effective as MOPP alternating with ABVD, and both were superior to MOPP alone. Furthermore, ABVD was less myelotoxic than MOPP or MOPP-ABVD with lower rates of severe (18% vs. 47%–53%) and life threatening (3% vs. 21%–28%) neutropenia.

Six percent of patients in the Cancer and Leukemia Group B study did, however, develop severe pulmonary toxicity with 3 patients dying while on therapy.[35] The Stanford V regimen was, therefore, developed to maintain or improve the cure rate seen with ABVD or MOPP-like regimens while minimizing acute and long-term toxicities.[20] Administered over 12 weeks, the 7-drug regimen reduced the cumulative doses of bleomycin, doxorubicin, and nitrogen mustard and omitted procarbazine. Although the first 25 patients received 36 to 44 Gy of mantle irradiation for bulky mediastinal disease, nodular spleens, and persistent nodal disease on CT 2 weeks after the completion of chemotherapy, the protocol was modified to give 36 Gy only to sites of disease 5 cm or greater at diagnosis and macroscopic splenic involvement. With a median follow-up 5.4 years, the 5 year FFP was 89% and OS 96% among 142 patients with stage III–IV or locally extensive mediastinal stage I–II HL.[21] There were no secondary leukemias and no observed cardiopulmonary toxicity, though the follow-up period was short.

In the only published comparison of ABVD, Stanford V, and a MOPP-like regimen, Gobbi et al[36] randomized 355 patients with stage IIB, III, or IV HL to receive 6 cycles of ABVD, 3 cycles of Stanford V, or 6 cycles of MOPP plus epidoxorubicin, bleomycin, vinblastine, lomustine, doxorubicin, and vindesine (MOPPEBVCAD). Among responding patients, 2 sites of previously bulky disease were irradiated 4 to 6 weeks after the end of chemotherapy. With respect to CR rate, 5 year FFS, and 5 year progression free survival (PFS), Stanford V was inferior to ABVD and MOPPEBVCAD with no significant differences in OS among the 3 regimens. Response assessment occurred at different times for patients receiving different regimens (8 and 12 weeks for the first and final assessment in Stanford V patients vs. 16 and 24 weeks for ABVD and MOPPEBVCAD patients), and this difference may have led to inferior results for Stanford V. The initiation of radiotherapy 4 to 6 weeks after the completion of chemotherapy in the Italian study (vs. 2 weeks as written in the original Stanford V protocol) may also have played a role. Finally, radiotherapy being limited to 2 sites of disease in the Stanford V arm and being administered to only 66% of patients in the Italian study (vs. 90% of patients in the original Stanford V study) may have influenced the outcome.

In 1991, the German Hodgkin's Lymphoma Group introduced the regimen BEACOPP.[22] The regimen essentially represented a rearrangement of the COPP/ABVD regimen with shorter treatment duration (24 vs. 32 weeks) and higher dose intensity than COPP/ABVD with increased doses of doxorubicin and cyclophosphamide. Etoposide was included in the regimen, and IF-RT (30 Gy) was given to all sites of initial bulky disease or to residual tumor remaining after chemotherapy. In the pilot study, 29 untreated patients with stage IIB-IV HL received 8 cycles of BEACOPP.[22] The study was later

amended to allow for the inclusion of filgrastim, the restriction of etoposide to the first 3 days of therapy, and a decrease in the dose of doxorubicin to 25 mg/m2 (from 40 mg/m$^2$). Twenty-one patients (72%) received consolidating radiotherapy. At a median follow-up of 40 months, the FFTF rate was 89%. Toxicities were tolerable with grade III/IV neutropenia occurring in 28% of chemotherapy cycles with no treatment-related deaths.

Escalated BEACOPP increased the doses of doxorubicin (from 25 to 35 mg/m$^2$), cyclophosphamide (from 650 to 1200 mg/m$^2$), and etoposide (from 100 to 200 mg/m$^2$).[37] Filgrastim was given to prevent prolonged neutropenia and severe infections. Among 60 stage IIB-IVA patients, the FFTF rate was 90% at 32 months. Seventy-three percent of these patients received radiotherapy to initial bulk lesions and residual disease in addition to 8 cycles of chemotherapy. Although between 71% and 76% of patients developed grade III/IV neutropenia, there was no corresponding rate of grade III/IV infections. Four patients developed secondary malignancies, including 2 leukemias 28 and 35 months after the completion of therapy.

In a prospective study, the German Hodgkin's Lymphoma Group randomly assigned 1201 patients with unfavorable stage IIB, IIIA–IIIB, or IV to receive 8 cycles of COPP-ABVD, BEACOPP, or increased dose BEACOPP, each followed by radiotherapy (30 Gy to sites of initial bulky disease and 40 Gy to any residual tumor).[38] Approximately 70% of patients on all 3 arms received irradiation. The study was terminated at the first interim analysis when it was determined that both BEACOPP groups were superior to COPP-ABVD in terms of the rate of FFTF. The 5-year rate of FFTF was 69% in the COPP-ABVD arm, 76% in the BEACOPP arm, and 87% in the increased-dose BEACOPP arm. Five-year rates of OS were not significantly different between standard dose BEACOPP and escalated dose BEACOPP. There was, however, a statistically significant difference in OS ($P = 0.002$) between the COPP-ABVD group (83%) versus the escalated BEACOPP group (91%). The improvement in FFTF and OS in the escalated BEACOPP group was accompanied by an increased incidence of acute hematologic effects. Ninety percent of patients developed grade 4 neutropenia and 22% patients developed grade 3 or 4 infections. Twenty-two patients developed secondary neoplasms with 14 developing acute leukemias. Thirteen of these patients were in the BEACOPP groups versus one in the COPP-ABVD group. Ten and 9 patients developed solid tumors and second non-HLs, respectively, in the BEACOPP groups. Three and 7 patients developed solid tumors and second NHLs, respectively, in the COPP-ABVD group.

Whether the same improvement in FFTF and OS would have been seen if patients had been randomly assigned to ABVD instead of ABVD-COPP remains unclear.[38] Several factors have prevented the German regimen from gaining acceptance around the world: no data from a randomized phase III trial demonstrate the superiority of BEACOPP over ABVD; BEACOPP is associated with an increased incidence of acute and late toxicities; and the inclusion of radiation therapy in the treatment of patients with advanced disease increases the risks of second cancers and potentially fatal premature heart disease.

## ROLE OF FDG-PET SCANS IN THE MANAGEMENT OF BOTH LIMITED AND ADVANCED STAGE DISEASE

Even as the cure rate for advanced HL approaches 80%, a major concern remains late-onset toxicities including the risk of second malignancies and an increased risk of myocardial infarction or stroke in patients who receive mediastinal radiotherapy and cervical radiation therapy, respectively. The goal of therapy is to maximize therapeutic benefit while minimizing morbidity and mortality. The most frequently used prognostic model in HL is a 7-factor prognostic scoring system, the International Prognostic Score (IPS), that predicts 5-year rates of FFP.[39] By using data collected from 5141 patients treated with chemotherapy for advanced HL, Hasenclever et al identified 7 factors with independent prognostic effects, including albumin <4g/dL, hemoglobin <10.5 g/dL, male sex, age >45 years, stage IV disease, white blood cell count >15000/mm$^3$, and lymphocyte count <600/mm$^3$. Because the IPS relies on fixed pretreatment variables, it neglects possibly the most important prognostic factor, the chemosensitivity of the tumor. Distinguishing between metabolically active lymphoma and residual scar tissue, 18-fluorodeoxyglucose PET may play an important role in the development of a patient response-based treatment strategy.

Hutchings et al[40] prospectively examined the prognostic value of interim 18-fluorodeoxyglucose positron emission tomography (FDG-PET) after 2 cycles of chemotherapy in patients with all stages of HL. Among 16 patients with positive PET scans, 11 patients progressed, and 2 of these patients died. Among 61 patients with negative PET scans, 58 patients were alive and free of disease at a median follow-up of 23 months. The 2-year PFS for PET-positive and PET-negative patients was 96% and 0%, respectively, and in multivariate regression analyses, PET results after 2 cycles of therapy were shown to be a stronger predictor of PFS than clinical stage or extranodal disease.

Gallamini et al[41] further demonstrated the superior prognostic value of midtreatment FDG-PET scans over the IPS. Among 260 patients with newly diagnosed advanced HL who underwent FDG-PET scans after completing 2 cycles of ABVD, the 2-year PFS for patients with positive PET scans was 12.8%. For patients with negative midtreatment PET results, the 2-year PFS was 95%. A multivariate regression analysis was performed and included both the IPS (as a continuous variable) and PET results after 2 cycles of chemotherapy. Only the PET results and stage IV disease had independent prognostic value. The question of whether the midtreatment PET scan should be performed after 2 or after 3 cycles of therapy remains unanswered.

There is only one report in the literature that implements a risk-adapted approach to treating HL.[42] In this study, 108 patients with newly diagnosed HL and adverse prognostic factors received therapy first based on their IPS score and then based on their midtreatment FDG-PET or gallium scan.[39] Patients with an IPS ≤2 received 2 cycles of standard BEACOPP while patients with an IPS ≥3 received 2 cycles of escalated BEACOPP. Patients with a positive interim scan then received 4 cycles of escalated BEACOPP, whereas patients with a negative interim scan received 4 cycles of standard BEACOPP. Among 69 patients with early unfavorable or standard risk disease, 58 received 6 cycles of standard BEACOPP and 10 received 2 cycles of standard BEACOPP followed by 4 cycles of escalated BEACOPP. With a median follow-up of 46 months, the 5-year EFS and OS rates for this group were 84% and 90%, respectively. Among 39 high-risk patients, 31 received 2 cycles of escalated BEACOPP followed by 4 cycles of standard BEACOPP. Only 7 patients received 6 cycles of escalated BEACOPP. With a median follow-up of 49 months, the 5-year EFS and OS rates for this group were 85% and 91%, respectively. The similar EFS and OS rates observed in both risk groups suggest that a risk-adapted treatment plan may be reasonable. To confirm the benefit of more intensive therapy in the setting of a positive midtreatment PET scan, larger prospective clinical trials are needed.

## CONCLUSIONS

The curative potential of combined chemotherapy was first realized with the introduction of MOPP in the 1960s. ABVD has maintained the high-response rate seen with MOPP, minimized some of its toxicities, and substituted others. Because randomized clinical trial data have never proven that CMT is superior to chemotherapy alone, the widespread use of radiation therapy in all stages of disease seems unjustified. As early and late toxicities associated with the use of radiation therapy affect an increasing fraction of long-term survivors, the curative potential of clinical staging and 6 cycles of chemotherapy need to be reexamined. Future clinical investigations should focus on integrating functional imaging with FDG-PET scans into the treatment paradigm as a decision-making tool to identify the small percentage of patients who require more intensive therapy to increase the likelihood of cure.

## REFERENCES

1. Abbondanzo SL. Thomas Hodgkin. *Ann Diagn Pathol.* 2003;7:333–334.
2. Carbone PP, Kaplan SH, Musshoff K, et al. Report of the committee on Hodgkin's disease staging classification. *Cancer Res.* 1971;31:1860–1861.
3. Lister TA, Crowther D, Sutcliffe SB, et al. Report of a committee convened to discuss the evaluation and staging of patients with Hodgkin's disease: Cotswolds meeting. *J Clin Oncol.* 1989;7:1630–1636.
4. Meyer RM, Gospodarowicz MK, Connors JM, et al. Randomized comparison of ABVD chemotherapy with a strategy that includes radiation therapy in patients with limited-stage Hodgkin's lymphoma: National Cancer Institute of Canada Clinical Trials Group and the Eastern Cooperative Oncology Group. *J Clin Oncol.* 2005;23:4634–4642.
5. Noordijk EM, Carde P, Dupouy N, et al. Combined-modality therapy for clinical stage I or II Hodgkin's lymphoma: long-term results of the European Organisation for Research and Treatment of Cancer H7 randomized controlled trials. *J Clin Oncol.* 2006;24:3128–3135.
6. Dühmke E, Franklin J, Pfreundschuh M, et al. Low-dose radiation is sufficient for the noninvolved extended-field treatment in favorable early-stage Hodgkin's disease: long-term results of a randomized trial of radiotherapy alone. *J Clin Oncol.* 2001;19:2905–2914.
7. Longo DL, Glatstein E, Duffey PL, et al. Radiation therapy versus combination chemotherapy in the treatment of early-stage Hodgkin's disease: seven-year results of a prospective randomized trial. *J Clin Oncol.* 1991;9:906–917.
8. Ferme C, Eghbali H, Meerwaldt JH, et al. Chemotherapy plus involved-field radiation in early-stage Hodgkin's disease. *N Engl J Med.* 2007;357:1916–1927.
9. Engert A, Franklin J, Eich HT, et al. Two cycles of doxorubicin, bleomycin, vinblastine, and dacarbazine plus extended-field radiotherapy is superior to radiotherapy alone in early favorable Hodgkin's lymphoma: final results of the GHSG HD7 trial. *J Clin Oncol.* 2007;25:3495–3502.
10. Press OW, LeBlanc M, Lichter AS, et al. Phase III randomized intergroup trial of subtotal lymphoid irradiation versus doxorubicin, vinblastine, and subtotal lymphoid irradiation for stage IA to IIA Hodgkin's disease. *J Clin Oncol.* 2001;19:4238–4244.
11. Specht L, Gray RG, Clarke MJ, et al. Influence of more extensive radiotherapy and adjuvant chemotherapy on long-term outcome of early-stage Hodgkin's disease: a meta-analysis of 23 randomized trials involving 3,888 patients. International Hodgkin's Disease Collaborative Group. *J Clin Oncol.* 1998;16:830–843.
12. Loeffler M, Brosteanu O, Hasenclever D, et al. Meta-analysis of chemotherapy versus combined modality treatment trials in Hodgkin's disease. International Database on Hodgkin's Disease Overview Study Group. *J Clin Oncol.* 1998;16:818–829.
13. Diehl V, Brillant C, Engert A. HD10: investigating reduction of combined modality treatment intensity in early stage Hodgkin's lymphoma. Interim analysis of a randomized trial of the German Hodgkin Study Group (GHSG). *J Clin Oncol.* 2005;23(suppl 1):6506.
14. Laskar S, Gupta T, Vimal S, et al. Consolidation radiation after complete remission in Hodgkin's disease following six cycles of doxorubicin, bleomycin, vinblastine, and dacarbazine chemotherapy: is there a need? *J Clin Oncol.* 2004;22:62–68.
15. Straus DJ, Portlock CS, Qin J, et al. Results of a prospective randomized clinical trial of doxorubicin, bleomycin, vinblastine, and dacarbazine (ABVD) followed by radiation therapy (RT) versus ABVD alone for stages I, II, and IIIA nonbulky Hodgkin disease. *Blood.* 2004;104:3483–3489.
16. Longo D, Glatstein E, Duffey P, et al. A prospective trial of radiation alone vs combination chemotherapy alone for early-stage Hodgkin's disease: implications of 25-year follow-up to current combined modality therapy. *Blood.* 2006;108:98.
17. DeVita VT Jr, Carbone PP. Treatment of Hodgkin's disease. *Med Ann Dist Columbia.* 1967;36:232–234 passim.

18. Longo DL, Young RC, Wesley M, et al. Twenty years of MOPP therapy for Hodgkin's disease. *J Clin Oncol.* 1986;4:1295–1306.
19. Bonadonna G, Zucali R, Monfardini S, et al. Combination chemotherapy of Hodgkin's disease with adriamycin, bleomycin, vinblastine, and imidazole carboxamide versus MOPP. *Cancer.* 1975;36:252–259.
20. Bartlett NL, Rosenberg SA, Hoppe RT, et al. Brief chemotherapy, Stanford V, and adjuvant radiotherapy for bulky or advanced-stage Hodgkin's disease: a preliminary report. *J Clin Oncol.* 1995;13:1080–1088.
21. Horning SJ, Hoppe RT, Breslin S, et al. Stanford V and radiotherapy for locally extensive and advanced Hodgkin's disease: mature results of a prospective clinical trial. *J Clin Oncol.* 2002;20:630–637.
22. Diehl V, Sieber M, Rüffer U, et al. BEACOPP: an intensified chemotherapy regimen in advanced Hodgkin's disease. The German Hodgkin's Lymphoma Study Group. *Ann Oncol.* 1997;8:143–148.
23. Devita VT Jr, Serpick AA, Carbone PP. Combination chemotherapy in the treatment of advanced Hodgkin's disease. *Ann Intern Med.* 1970;73:881–895.
24. Viviani S, Santoro A, Ragni G, et al. Gonadal toxicity after combination chemotherapy for Hodgkin's disease. Comparative results of MOPP vs ABVD. *Eur J Cancer Clin Oncol.* 1985;21:601–605.
25. Valagussa P, Santoro A, Fossati-Bellani F, et al. Second acute leukemia and other malignancies following treatment for Hodgkin's disease. *J Clin Oncol.* 1986;4:830–837.
26. Blayney DW, Longo DL, Young RC, et al. Decreasing risk of leukemia with prolonged follow-up after chemotherapy and radiotherapy for Hodgkin's disease. *N Engl J Med.* 1987;316:710–714.
27. Santoro A, Bonfante V, Bonadonna G. Salvage chemotherapy with ABVD in MOPP-resistant Hodgkin's disease. *Ann Intern Med.* 1982;96:139–143.
28. Santoro A, Bonadonna G, Valagussa P, et al. Long-term results of combined chemotherapy-radiotherapy approach in Hodgkin's disease: superiority of ABVD plus radiotherapy versus MOPP plus radiotherapy. *J Clin Oncol.* 1987;5:27–37.
29. Bonadonna G, Valagussa P, Santoro A. Alternating non-cross-resistant combination chemotherapy or MOPP in stage IV Hodgkin's disease. A report of 8-year results. *Ann Intern Med.* 1986;104:739–746.
30. Klimo P, Connors JM. MOPP/ABV hybrid program: combination chemotherapy based on early introduction of seven effective drugs for advanced Hodgkin's disease. *J Clin Oncol.* 1985;3:1174–1182.
31. Viviani S, Bonadonna G, Santoro A, et al. Alternating versus hybrid MOPP and ABVD combinations in advanced Hodgkin's disease: ten-year results. *J Clin Oncol.* 1996;14:1421–1430.
32. Glick JH, Young ML, Harrington D, et al. MOPP/ABV hybrid chemotherapy for advanced Hodgkin's disease significantly improves failure-free and overall survival: the 8-year results of the intergroup trial. *J Clin Oncol.* 1998;16: 19–26.
33. Connors JM, Klimo P, Adams G, et al. Treatment of advanced Hodgkin's disease with chemotherapy–comparison of MOPP/ABV hybrid regimen with alternating courses of MOPP and ABVD: a report from the National Cancer Institute of Canada clinical trials group. *J Clin Oncol.* 1997;15:1638–1645.
34. Duggan DB, Petroni GR, Johnson JL, et al. Randomized comparison of ABVD and MOPP/ABV hybrid for the treatment of advanced Hodgkin's disease: report of an intergroup trial. *J Clin Oncol.* 2003;21:607–614.
35. Canellos GP, Anderson JR, Propert KJ, et al. Chemotherapy of advanced Hodgkin's disease with MOPP, ABVD, or MOPP alternating with ABVD. *N Engl J Med.* 1992;327:1478–1484.
36. Gobbi PG, Levis A, Chisesi T, et al. ABVD versus modified stanford V versus MOPPEBVCAD with optional and limited radiotherapy in intermediate- and advanced-stage Hodgkin's lymphoma: final results of a multicenter randomized trial by the Intergruppo Italiano Linfomi. *J Clin Oncol.* 2005;23:9198–9207.
37. Tesch H, Diehl V, Lathan B, et al. Moderate dose escalation for advanced stage Hodgkin's disease using the bleomycin, etoposide, adriamycin, cyclophosphamide, vincristine, procarbazine, and prednisone scheme and adjuvant radiotherapy: a study of the German Hodgkin's Lymphoma Study Group. *Blood.* 1998;92:4560–4567.
38. Diehl V, Franklin J, Pfreundschuh M, et al. Standard and increased-dose BEACOPP chemotherapy compared with COPP-ABVD for advanced Hodgkin's disease. *N Engl J Med.* 2003;348:2386–2395.
39. Hasenclever D, Diehl V. A prognostic score for advanced Hodgkin's disease. International Prognostic Factors Project on Advanced Hodgkin's Disease. *N Engl J Med.* 1998;339:1506–1514.
40. Hutchings M, Loft A, Hansen M, et al. FDG-PET after two cycles of chemotherapy predicts treatment failure and progression-free survival in Hodgkin's Lymphoma. *Blood.* 2006;107:52–59.
41. Gallamini A, Hutchings M, Rigacci L, et al. Early interim 2-[$^{18}$F]fluoro-2-deoxy-D-glucose positron emission tomography is prognostically superior to international prognostic score in advanced-stage Hodgkin's lymphoma: a report from a joint Italian-Danish study. *J Clin Oncol.* 2007;25:3746–752.
42. Dann EJ, Bar-Shalom R, Tamir A, et al. Risk-adapted BEACOPP regimen can reduce the cumulative dose of chemotherapy for standard and high-risk Hodgkin's Lymphoma with no impairment of outcome. *Blood.* 2007;109:905–909.

# Role of Radiation Therapy in Hodgkin's Lymphoma

Joachim Yahalom

Radiation is probably the most effective single agent in the curative treatment of Hodgkin's lymphoma (HL). The dramatic effect of ionizing radiation on HL tumors was reported as early as 1901, a short time after Roentgen's discovery of "x-rays." Yet, during the first half of the 20th century, HL remained incurable and responses to radiotherapy were partial or brief due to limitations of antiquated technology of the time and poor clinical application. As x-ray technology and penetration improved in the 1940s and the concept of irradiating beyond the involved area was adopted, patients with early-stage HL could be cured with radiation alone—the only effective curative modality for lymphomas, that was available until the late 1960s.[1]

During the 1960s and 1970s, before the advent of chemotherapy and the use of a dual modality approach, radiation therapy (RT) alone still cured many patients, particularly in early stages. Yet, reliance on RT alone required wide extension of the radiation field and raising the dose to normal tissue tolerance levels ("radical radiotherapy"). Twenty and 30 years later, the long follow-up of the survivors disclosed an unexpected price; the incidence of morbidity and mortality of those patients with HL was significantly higher compared with the normal population. The main complications were secondary tumors (mostly breast and lung cancers).[2] There was also more than expected coronary artery disease associated with the use of radical radiotherapy.

The advent of effective and less-toxic chemotherapy regimens in the late 1970s merged with attempts to secure the cure of larger number of patients; even of those with more advanced disease. This effort translated into using full-dose combined-modality approach with full-dose chemotherapy and extended field radiotherapy. Although this strategy indeed cured more patients, it produced a higher rate of short- and long-term complications. The ensuing reports of survivors' morbidity caused obvious alarm.

The strategic response in the 1990s was to reduce therapy for HL, although hoping to maintain the cure rate. One approach was to keep the concept of combined modality, but reduce significantly the extent of the irradiated volume, decrease the radiation dose, and at the same time also reduce the number of chemotherapy courses. Others considered radiotherapy as the only culprit causing long-term complication, and thus totally eliminated RT from the treatment regimen and consequently relied on more courses or additional combinations of chemotherapy.

These 2 conflicting strategies fostered hot debates and opinionated editorials that naturally confused and distressed new and previously treated patients with HL. Constructively, it also led to the design of several prospectively randomized studies that focused on choice between the 2 approaches described earlier.[3–5]

The advocates of the total exclusion of radiotherapy and substituting it with more chemotherapy made the following arguments:

1. Radiotherapy is the main and possibly the sole cause of the increased long-term morbidity of HL survivors.
2. Reduction in the extent and/or dose is of radiotherapy unlikely to significantly change the risk.
3. A chemotherapy alone strategy will provide an excellent outcome of disease control, that would be at least similar, if not better, than the results obtained with combined modality. If RT is omitted, the decrease in radiation-related late mortality from causes other than HL would probably result in better overall survival (OS) rates.
4. Chemotherapy alone, even if escalated or prolonged, is safe and is unlikely to result in more toxicity.
5. Even if more failures will occur without radiotherapy, salvage with higher dose chemotherapy followed by stem-cell transplantation is simple, well tolerated, and safe.

Those who had reservations about omitting radiotherapy strongly disagreed with the above. They expected disease control rate without RT to decrease and have a negative effect on OS. They also argued that the modern reduction in both extent and dose of radiation that was designed for the setting of combined-modality treatment (as opposed to radiation alone of the past) would markedly reduce or eliminate the radiation-related long-term toxicity. At the same time, the associated reduction in chemotherapy will further enhance the short- and long-term safety profile of the combined therapy program. This approach will also reduce markedly the need for salvage therapy with high-dose therapy and autologous stem-cell transplantation that causes not only physical and psychologic trauma to these young adults and their families, but also increases the risk of short- and long-term serious complications; mostly sterility and secondary leukemia.

## Randomized Studies in Early-Stage HL Comparing Combined-Modality Therapy With Chemotherapy Alone

Several groups tested the hypothesis that chemotherapy alone could provide equivalent disease control to that achieved with combined-modality therapy. The studies from Europe,[6] Asia,[7] and North America[8–10] targeted mostly early-stage favorable and unfavorable patients and were conducted in adults, children or adolescents, or in both. In some the randomization was upfront, in others it was limited to patients who achieved a clear complete response (CR) with chemotherapy. The trials are detailed later and are summarized in Table 1.

### Children Cancer Group (CCG) #5942[10]

The Children Cancer Study Group tested the role of radiation therapy in young patients (<21 years) who attained a CR with risk-adapted chemotherapy (mostly COPP/ABV, 4–6 cycles). They enrolled 829

**TABLE 1.** Randomized Studies that Compared Combined Modality With Chemotherapy Alone

| | Stage | Treatment Arms | EFS or FFP (%) | P | OS | P | Comments |
|---|---|---|---|---|---|---|---|
| CCG 5942 (501 pts) | I–IV (I–II 68%) | COPP/ABV × 4–6 | 85* | 0.02* | 3 yr | NS | No-RT arm closed |
| | | Same + IF 21 Gy | 93* | | | | early (relapses) |
| Mumbai (251 pts) | I–IV (I–II 55%) | ABVD × 6 | 76 | 0.01 | 8 yr | 0.02 | |
| | | ABVD × 6 + IF 30 Gy | 88 | | | | |
| EORTC/GELA H9F (489 pts) | I–II favorable | EBVP × 6 | 69 | 0.001 | 4 yr | NA | No-RT arm closed |
| | | EBVP × 6 + IF 20 Gy | 85 | | | | early (relapses) |
| | | EBVP × 6 + IF 36 Gy | 88 | | | | |
| NCIC/ECOG HD6 (276 pts) | I–II unfavorable, but no B, or bulky | ABVD × 4–6 | 88 | 0.004 | 5 yr | NS | Designed for OS evaluation at 12 yr |
| | | ABVD × 2 + STLI | 95 | | | | |
| MSKCC (152 pts) | I–III A/B nonbulky | ABVD × 6 | 81 | NS | 5 yr | 0.08 | Not powered to detect differences <20% |
| | | ABVD × 6 + EF/IF | 86 | | | | |

*Analyzed as treated.
NA indicates not available; NS, not significant.

patients into the study (68% were early-stage). Five hundred one patients who achieved a CR were then randomized to receive either low-dose (21 Gy)-involved-field radiotherapy (IFRT) or no further treatment. The accrual stopped earlier than planned because of a significantly higher number of relapses on the no-radiotherapy arm.

The 3-year event-free survival (EFS) with an intent-to-treat analysis was 92% for patients randomized to receive RT and 87% for those randomized to no further treatment ($P = 0.057$). Because 30 patients switched their treatment after randomization, an analysis "as treated" was performed and showed a 3-year EFS of 93% for those who received radiation and only 85% for those who were only observed ($P = 0.0024$). At this early analysis, no survival difference was detected.

### The Tata Memorial Hospital Trial[7]

This is a large prospectively randomized study from the main cancer center in Mumbai, India of 251 patients with HL (55% early stage) who received 6 cycles of doxorubicin, bleomycin, vinblastine, and dacarbazine (ABVD) chemotherapy. Of those, only 179 patients (71%) who achieved a CR were randomized to either IFRT of 30 Gy (+10 Gy boost to bulky sites) or to no further therapy.

At a median follow-up of 63 months, the 8-year EFS and OS were significantly better for the patients who received consolidation with IFRT compared with those who received ABVD alone (EFS-88% vs. 76%, $P = 0.01$; OS 100% vs. 89%, $P = 0.002$). Most relapses in the ABVD alone arm were early and systemic, whereas in the ABVD + RT arm, the relapses were late and localized.

### National Cancer Institute of Canada/ECOG Trial HD-6[9]

This intergroup study included 405 patients with nonbulky stage I–II patients. They were randomized to either receive "standard therapy," namely, subtotal nodal irradiation alone for favorable patients and ABVD (2 cycles) followed by subtotal nodal irradiation for unfavorable (B, elevated ESR, ≥3 sites, age ≥40, mixed cellularity (MC) histology) patients, or to the experimental arm that consisted of 6 cycles or 4 cycles (if CR was attained after 2 cycles) of ABVD and no RT.

At a median follow-up of 4.2 years, progression-free survival with ABVD alone was significantly inferior [$P = 0.006$; hazard ratio (HR) = 2.6; 5-year progression-free survival estimates 87% vs. 93%]. At this early point, no survival difference has been detected. Although the "standard" arm that included RT alone for favorable patients is no longer considered the standard of care, the inferior performance

of ABVD alone compared with standard therapy in nonbulky early stage patients cannot be ignored. At a median follow-up of 4 years no OS difference was detected. Originally, the study was statistically designed for a 12-year analysis of survival.

### EORTC/GELA H9[6]

This is a large ongoing trial in favorable early-stage patients with classic HL. All patients received 6 cycles of epirubicin, bleomycin, vinblastine, and prednisone. Only patients who achieved a CR are randomized to either IFRT of 36 Gy, IFRT of 20 Gy, or to no radiation. Because of an excessive number of relapses in no radiation arm, the group closed it early. At the completion of the study, there was no difference between adding consolidation RT of 36 Gy or 20 Gy, but there was a significantly lower failure-free survival at 4 years if no radiation was added (failure-free survival of 87%, 84%, and 69%; $P = 0.001$, respectively). At only 4 years median follow-up, no survival difference was detected.

### Memorial Sloan-Kettering Cancer Center Trial[8]

The Memorial Sloan-Kettering trial included 152 patients with nonbulky early-stage HL. Patients were randomized upfront to either received ABDV X6 alone or ABVD X6 followed by radiotherapy. At 60 months CR duration, freedom from progression, for ABVD + RT versus ABVD alone are 91% versus 87% ($P = 0.61$) and 86% versus 81% ($P = 0.61$), respectively. OS was 97% with ABVD + RT vs. 90% with ABVD alone ($P = 0.08$). Although the differences between the outcome of the 2 treatment groups were not statistically significant, the study was not powered to detect differences between the treatment strategies that were smaller than 20%, because of the small number of patients and events. The superior OS ($P = 0.08$) of the ABVD + RT group is also difficult to explain and is possibly a result of the small size of this trial. The results are summarized in Table 1.

## Effect of Omitting Radiation on Overall Survival

The effect of different treatment approaches used in prospectively randomized studies on OS has always been very difficult to demonstrate in HL. Therefore, disease control and early toxicity considerations often guided the evolution of current treatment strategies.[11] There are multiple factors that explain why superior disease control on one arm of a randomized study does not necessarily translate into a statistically significant survival advantage: patients with HL commonly survive for a long time even with active disease, there are good salvage options; even if salvage fails, the patient could be maintained with disease for several years with single agents or simple RT. In most HL studies, the number of patients and the number of events especially in early-stage disease are small resulting in small differences that rarely meet "statistical significance" sacred criteria. Indeed, advantageous disease control by one treatment may be eventually tempered by its toxicity that will take more time to declare itself; this is relevant to both adding RT or enhancing chemotherapy as an alternative. Finally, most studies are reported early, often without full peer-review and detailed analysis of events and many large cooperative group studies do not have optimal follow-up and information on cause of death. It is thus may be misleading to declare an equality of 2 treatment options because they lack an OS difference and ignore the improved freedom from treatment failure even if significant.

Indeed, with one exception, all studies listed in Table 1 fail to show a significant OS advantage for the combined-modality arm even though the disease control for this approach was significantly better. The median follow-up ranged between 3 and 5 years; the median follow-up in the study showed that survival advantage to adding RT was 8 years.

To overcome the shortfall of small studies statistical power, The Cochrane Hematological Malignancies Group recently performed a meta-analysis of all published prospective randomized comparing combined-modality therapy (CMT) in early-stage HL with chemotherapy alone. They included 5 eligible randomized controlled trials involving 1245 patients. Although the CR rate was similar in patients receiving chemotherapy alone compared with CMT, both tumor control and OS were significantly better in patients receiving CMT. The hazard ratio was 0.40 (95% CI 0.25–0.66) for tumor control and 0.41 (95% CI 0.27–0.60) for OS.[12]

## Transformation From "Radical Radiotherapy" Into Tailored Mini-Radiotherapy: The Effect on Long-Term Complications

In the 1960s and 1970s, when radiotherapy was the primary, and at times the only curative modality for HL, it was used alone or with adjuvant mechlorethamine, vincristine, prednisone, and procarbazine (MOPP) for early and advanced stages. Bulky sites were covered with large radiation field margins, and occasionally even the lungs and the liver were intentionally irradiated. Even for favorable patients, the standard field was total lymphoid irradiation. Its giant size compensated for the lack of good imaging information. The dose was also maximized (the standard dose at Stanford was 44 Gy) and often treatment was given in a technique that delivered even higher doses anteriorly to the heart and breast.[13]

The IFRT that is used now in combined-modality programs is considerably smaller; the radiation is limited to the involved site and is often tailored to include only the reduced postchemotherapy volume.[14] It is estimated that in comparison with total lymphoid irradiation (TLI), the average involved field will reduce the irradiated volume by more than 80%. This is particularly relevant to irradiation of the breast, heart, and lungs. With the old indiscriminate "mantle" field radiotherapy, most of the breast tissue was irradiated. Most breast exposure resulted from the routine irradiation of the axillae and most second breast cancers indeed developed in the outer part of the breast. Yet, approximately, two third of women with early-stage HL do not require radiation of the axillae, and additional protection to the upper and medial aspects of the breast can now be provided by further reducing field size using careful computerized tomographic-based planning that usually allows for smaller mediastinal volumes, particularly after chemotherapy. We can now avoid irradiating the breast in most women and substantially reduce exposure of the heart and lungs.[15]

The large fields of the past limited the radiation technique to simple opposed anterior and posterior fields. The conversion to

smaller and better defined radiation volumes allows the utilization of more conformal radiation therapy, based on better imaging, computerized planning programs, and when indicated, advanced tools such as intensity modulated radiotherapy.[16] Modern breakthroughs in radiotherapy technology that have been implemented recently in HL have already demonstrated better sparing of the heart and coronary arteries. They provide increased accuracy, avoid normal organs, and thus improve the therapeutic ratio.[17]

Recent studies clearly indicate that the risk of secondary solid tumor induction is radiation dose related. This was carefully analyzed for secondary breast and lung cancers as well as for other tumors.[18,19] Although it will take more years of careful follow-up of patients in randomized studies to display the full magnitude of risk tapering by current reduction of radiation field and dose, recent data suggest that this likely to be the case. In a recent Duke University study, 2 groups of patients with early-stage HL were treated with different radiation approaches over the same period. One group received radiotherapy alone, given to extended fields with a median dose of 38 Gy, the second group received chemotherapy followed by involved-field low-dose (median of 25 Gy) radiotherapy. Although 12 patients developed second tumors in the first group and 8 of them died, no second tumors were detected in the second group. The median follow-up was 11.7 and 8.1 years, respectively.[20] Similar observations with an even longer follow-up were made by the Yale group.[21] In the randomized study from Milan, comparing ABVD × 4 followed by subtotal lymphoid irradiation with ABVD × 4 followed by only IFRT, 3 patients developed second cancers after subtotal lymphoid irradiation and no second cancers were detected after IFRT. Median follow-up was 10 years.[22]

The European HL study groups recently introduced an additional reduction in the size of the involved radiation. The reduced size field is tailored to the involved lymph node and not the whole region where they reside as is in IFRT and is thus termed involved node radiotherapy (INRT).[23] Most importantly, for radiotherapy involving the mediastinum or the abdomen, INRT is designed according to the postchemotherapy volume that is often markedly reduced in comparison with the initial volume. Although there is no prospective randomized comparison of INRT with IFRT, a recently retrospective well-controlled comparison of sequential patients with HL treated with only 2 cycles of ABVD followed by either extended-field RT, involved field or further reduction to INRT showed similarly excellent disease control and OS in all RT groups without any difference in in-field or marginal relapse.[24]

## Role of RT

### Special Consideration of Stage, Bulk, and Histologic Type of HL

Most of the discussion on the role of consolidation RT in HL focused on patients with favorable (without bulky disease and/or B symptoms) classic HL and most data from randomized studies is limited to this group of patients. Yet, other groups of patients with HL present other consideration and the data regarding the option of avoiding RT in these patients is limited.

### Lymphocyte-Predominant Hodgkin's Lymphoma

Most (>75%) patients with Lymphocyte-Predominant Hodgkin's Lymphoma (LPHL) present with at an early stage; the disease is commonly limited to one peripheral site (neck, axilla, or groin) and involvement of the mediastinum is extremely rare. The treatment recommendations for LPHL differ markedly from those for classic HL. The American National Comprehensive Cancer Network guidelines, the German Hodgkin's Lymphoma Study Group, and the European Organization for Research and Treatment of Cancer (EORTC) currently recommend involved-field radiation alone as the treatment of choice for early-stage LPHL.[25] It should be emphasized that even if regional radiation fields are selected, the uninvolved mediastinum should not be irradiated, thus avoiding the site most prone for radiation-related short- and long-term side effects. Although there has not been a study that compared extended-field RT (commonly used in the past) with involved field RT, retrospective data suggest that involvedfield is adequate.[26] The radiation dose recommended is between 30 and 36 Gy with an optional additional boost of 4 Gy to a (rare) bulky site.

## Unfavorable Early-Stage HL

Although different study groups slightly use definitions of favorable and unfavorable early stages, all consider bulky disease or B symptoms as unfavorable features. In this category of patients, chemotherapy is not reduced below 4 cycles and adding RT as consolidation is standard of care.

## Advanced-Stage HL

Although the role of consolidation radiotherapy after induction chemotherapy remain controversial, irradiation is often added in patients with advanced stage HL who present with bulky disease or remain in uncertain complete remission after chemotherapy.[27] Retrospective studies have demonstrated that adding low-dose radiotherapy to all initial disease sites after chemotherapy induced complete response decreases the relapse rate by ~25% and significantly improves OS. Interpretation of the impact of radiation in prospective studies has been controversial.[28,29] However, a Southwest Oncology Group randomized study of 278 patients with stage III or IV Hodgkin's disease suggested that the addition of low-dose irradiation to all sites of initial disease after a complete response to mechlorethamine, Oncovin (vincristine), prednisone, bleomycin, Adriamycin (doxorubicin), and procarbazine chemotherapy improves remission duration in patients with advanced-stage disease.[30] An intention-to-treat analysis showed that the advantage of combined-modality therapy was limited to patients with nodular sclerosis. No survival differences were observed. A meta-analysis of several randomized studies demonstrated that the addition of radiotherapy to chemotherapy reduces the rate of relapse but did not show survival benefit for combined modality compared with chemotherapy alone.[31]

Recently, EORTC reported the results of a randomized study that evaluated the role of IFRT in patients with stage III/IV Hodgkin's disease who obtained a CR after MOPP/ABV.[32] Patients received 6 or 8 cycles of MOPP/ABV chemotherapy (number of cycles depended upon the response). Patients who have not obtained a CR (40% of patients) were not randomized to receive chemotherapy and received IFRT. Of the 418 patients who reached a CR 85 patients were not randomized to receive treatment for various reasons. A total of 161 patients were randomized to receive no RT and 172 patients were randomized to receive IFRT. The authors concluded that IFRT does not improve the treatment results in patients with stage III/IV Hodgkin's disease who reached a CR after 6 to 8 courses of MOPP/ABV chemotherapy. The 5-year OS rates were 91% and 85%, respectively ($P = 0.07$). The data indicated that in comparison with chemotherapy alone, there were more cases of leukemia second tumors on the CR combined modality, but surprisingly not in the large group of patients who have not achieved CR with chemotherapy and all received RT. This observation suggests that the increased mortality on the randomized RT arm is a statistical fluke resulting from small number of events. Interestingly, in partial responders after 6 cycles of MOPP/ABV, the addition of IFRT yielded OS and EFS rates that were similar to those obtained in CR to chemotherapy patients. The

EORTC study has several limitations that detract from its applicability to many advanced-stage patients. First, a relatively small fraction of patients were determined to be in CR and thus eligible for randomization on the study. The regimen of MOPP/ABV X 6–8 is toxic and this regimen is no longer used in North America.[33] Second, only few patients with bulky disease were randomized on the EORTC study. Lastly, the claim that added RT caused more secondary malignancies on the combined modality has not been evident in patients with PR receiving even higher doses of RT to multiple areas after MOPP/ABV.

The only randomized study questioning the role of consolidation RT after CR to ABVD X 6 (the most common regimen currently used for advance-stage HL) was performed at Tata Medical Center in India.[7] The study included patients of all stages, but almost half were stages III and IV. A subgroup analysis of the advanced-stage patients showed a statistically significant improvement of both 8-year EFS and 8-year OS with added RT compared with ABVD alone (EFS 78% vs. 59%; $P < 0.03$ and OS 100% vs. 80%; $P < 0.006$).

When advanced-stage HL is treated with the new highly effective and less toxic treatment program of Stanford V, it is imperative to follow the brief chemotherapy program with IFRT to sites originally larger than 5 cm or to a clinically involved spleen.[34] When radiotherapy was fully of partially omitted on this program the results were inferior.[35]

In summary, patients in CR after full-dose chemotherapy program like MOPP/ABV may not need RT consolidation. Yet, patients with bulky disease, incomplete or uncertain CR or patients treated on brief chemotherapy programs will benefit from involved field RT to originally bulky or residual disease.

## RT in Salvage Programs for Refractory and Relapsed HL

High-dose therapy supported by autologous stem-cell transplantation has become a standard salvage treatment for patients who relapsed or remained refractory to chemotherapy or to combined-modality therapy. Many of the patients who enter these programs have not received prior radiotherapy or relapsed at sites outside the original radiation field. These patients could benefit from integrating radiotherapy into the salvage regimen.

Poen et al[36] from Stanford analyzed the efficacy and toxicity of adding cytoreductive (pretransplant; n = 18) or consolidative (posttransplant; n = 6) RT to 24 of 100 patients receiving high-dose therapy. This study showed that most (69%) relapses after autologous stem cell transplantation occurred in sites known to be involved immediately before transplantation. When these sites were irradiated before transplantation, no in-field failures occurred. Although only a trend in favor of IF-RT could be shown for the entire group of transplanted patients, for patients with stages I–III freedom from relapse was significantly improved. Limiting the analysis to patients who received no prior RT also resulted in a significant advantage to IF-RT. Fatal toxicity in this series was not influenced significantly by IF-RT.

At Memorial Sloan-Kettering Cancer Center, we developed a program that integrated RT into the high-dose regimen for salvage of HD. We schedule accelerated hyperfractionated irradiation (b.i.d. fractions of 1.8 Gy each) to start after the completion of reinduction chemotherapy and stem-cell collection and before the high-dose chemotherapy and stem-cell transplantation. Patients who have not been previously irradiated received involved field RT (18 Gy in 5 days) to sites of initially bulky (>5 cm) disease and/or residual clinical abnormalities followed by TLI of 18 Gy (1.8 Gy per fraction, b.i.d.) within an additional 5 days. Patients who had prior RT received only involved-field RT (when feasible) to a maximal dose of 36 Gy.

This treatment strategy has been in place since 1985 with over 350 patients treated thus far. The first generation program demonstrated the feasibility and efficacy of the high-dose combined-modality regimen resulting in an EFS of 47% for the patients receiving TLI followed by cyclophosphamide-etoposide chemotherapy.[37] The recent report of the second generation two-step high-dose chemoradiotherapy program indicated that after a median follow-up of 34 months the intent-to-treat EFS and OS were 58% and 88%, respectively. For patients who underwent transplantation, the EFS was 68%.[38] Treatment-related mortality was 3% with no treatment-related mortality over the last 8 years. The results of this treatment program in refractory patients were similar to those of relapsed patients.[39] Both groups showed favorable EFS and OS compared with most recently reported series. Recent report on quality of life and treatment-related complications of long-tem survivors of the Memorial Sloan-Kettering Cancer Center program disclosed only a small number of late complications and is highly encouraging.[40]

## SUMMARY

Treatment results of favorable early-stage HL (FFTF over 90%) with CMT that includes short-course ABVD and reduced-dose IFRT set a high standard to challenge. At the same time, the trials that attempted to omit radiotherapy in favorable patients who obtained a CR with chemotherapy had thus far inferior outcome for chemotherapy alone. Thus, chemotherapy alone should be given only in the context of a clinical research trial or to highly selected individuals with contraindications to combined modality. Functional imaging may allow the identification of CR patients in whom treatment could possibly be further reduced, but is still experimental. The data available thus far do not support the omission of RT even in PET-negative patients.[41]

## REFERENCES

1. Kaplan HS. Clinical evaluation and radiotherapeutic management of Hodgkin's disease and the malignant lymphomas. *N Engl J Med.* 1968;278:892–899.
2. Boice JD Jr. Second cancer after Hodgkin's disease—the price of success? *J Natl Cancer Inst.* 1993;85:4–5.
3. Longo DL. Hodgkin's disease: the sword of Damocles resheathed. *Blood.* 2004;104:3418.
4. Yahalom J. "Don't throw out the baby with the bathwater"—on optimizing cure and reducing toxicity in Hodgkin's lymphoma. *J Clin Oncol.* 2006;24:544–548.
5. DeVita VT Jr. Hodgkin's disease—clinical trials and travails. *N Engl J Med.* 2003;348:2375–2376.
6. Noordijk E, Thomas J, Ferme C, et al. First results of the EORTC-GELA H9 randomized trials: the H9-F trial (comparing 3 radiation dose levels) and H9-U trial (comparing 3 chemotherapy schemes) in patients with favorable or unfavorable early stage Hodgkin's lymphoma (HL). *J Clin Oncol* 2005;21(suppl 1):Abstract 6506.
7. Laskar S, Gupta T, Vimal S, et al. Consolidation radiation after complete remission in Hodgkin's disease following six cycles of doxorubicin, bleomycin, vinblastine, and dacarbazine chemotherapy: is there a need? *J Clin Oncol.* 2004;22:62–68.
8. Straus DJ, Portlock CS, Qin J, et al. Results of a prospective randomized clinical trial of doxorubicin, bleomycin, vinblastine, and dacarbazine (ABVD) followed by radiation therapy (RT) versus ABVD alone for stages I, II, and IIIA nonbulky Hodgkin's disease. *Blood.* 2004;104:3483–3489.
9. Meyer RM, Gospodarowicz MK, Connors JM, et al. Randomized comparison of ABVD chemotherapy with a strategy that includes radiation therapy in patients with limited-stage Hodgkin's lymphoma: National Cancer Institute of Canada Clinical Trials Group and the Eastern Cooperative Oncology Group. *J Clin Oncol.* 2005;23:4634–4642.
10. Nachman JB, Sposto R, Herzog P, et al. Randomized comparison of low-dose involved-field radiotherapy and no radiotherapy for children with Hodgkin's disease who achieve a complete response to chemotherapy. *J Clin Oncol.* 2002;20:3765–3771.
11. Specht L, Gray RG, Clarke MJ, et al. Influence of more extensive radiotherapy and adjuvant chemotherapy on long-term outcome of early-stage Hodgkin's disease: a meta-analysis of 23 randomized trials involving 3,888 patients. International Hodgkin's Disease Collaborative Group. *J Clin Oncol.* 1998;16:830–843.
12. Rehan F, Brillant C, Schiltz H, et al. Chemotherapy alone versus chemotherapy plus radiotherapy for early stage Hodgkin's lymphoma [abstract]. *Blood.* 2007;110:2320.
13. Kaplan H. The radical radiotherapy of Hodgkin's disease. *Radiology.* 1962;78:553–561.
14. Yahalom J. Changing role and decreasing size: current trends in radiotherapy for Hodgkin's disease. *Curr Oncol Rep.* 2002;4:415–423.
15. Yahalom J. Favorable early-stage Hodgkin's lymphoma. *J Natl Compr Canc Netw.* 2006;4:233–240.
16. Goodman KA, Toner S, Hunt M, et al. Intensity modulated radiation therapy in the treatment of lymphoma involving the mediastinum. *Int J Radiat Oncol Biol Phys.* 2005;62:198–206.
17. Girinsky T, Pichenot C, Beaudre A, et al. Is intensity-modulated radiotherapy better than conventional radiation treatment and three-dimensional conformal radiotherapy for mediastinal masses in patients with Hodgkin's disease, and is there a role for beam orientation optimization and dose constraints assigned to virtual volumes? *Int J Radiat Oncol Biol Phys.* 2006;64:218–226.
18. Travis LB, Gospodarowicz M, Curtis RE, et al. Lung cancer following chemotherapy and radiotherapy for Hodgkin's disease. *J Natl Cancer Inst.* 2002;94:182–192.
19. Travis LB, Hill D, Dores GM, et al. Breast cancer following radiotherapy and chemotherapy among young women with Hodgkin's disease. *JAMA.* 2003;290:465–475.
20. Koontz B, Kirkpatrick J, Clough R, et al. Combined modality therapy versus radiotherapy alone for treatment of early stage Hodgkin's disease: cure versus complications. *J Clin Oncol.* 2006;24:605–611.
21. Salloum E, Doria R, Schubert W, et al. Second solid tumors in patients with Hodgkin's disease cured after radiation or chemotherapy plus adjuvant low-dose radiation. *J Clin Oncol.* 1996;14:2435–2443.
22. Bonadonna G, Bonfante V, Viviani S, et al. ABVD plus subtotal nodal versus involved-field radiotherapy in early-stage Hodgkin's disease: long-term results. *J Clin Oncol.* 2004;22:2835–2841.
23. Girinsky T, van der Maazen R, Specht L, et al. Involved-node radiotherapy (INRT) in patients with early Hodgkin's lymphoma: concepts and guidelines. *Radiother Oncol.* 2006;79:270–277.
24. Campbell BA, Voss N, Pickles T, et al. Involved-nodal radiation therapy as a component of combination therapy for limited-stage Hodgkin's lymphoma: a question of field size. *J Clin Oncol.* 2008;26:5170–5174.
25. Hoppe RT, Advani RH, Ambinder RF, et al. Hodgkin's disease/lymphoma. *J Natl Compr Canc Netw.* 2008;6:594–622.
26. Schlembach PJ, Wilder RB, Jones D, et al. Radiotherapy alone for lymphocyte-predominant Hodgkin's disease. *Cancer J.* 2002;8:377–383.
27. Prosnitz LR, Wu JJ, Yahalom J. The case for adjuvant radiation therapy in advanced Hodgkin's disease. *Cancer Invest.* 1996;14:361–370.
28. Yahalom J, Ryu J, Straus DJ, et al. Impact of adjuvant radiation on the patterns and rate of relapse in advanced-stage Hodgkin's disease treated with alternating chemotherapy combinations. *J Clin Oncol.* 1991;9:2193–2201.
29. Brizel DM, Winer EP, Prosnitz LR, et al. Improved survival in advanced Hodgkin's disease with the use of combined modality therapy [see comments]. *Int J Radiat Oncol Biol Phys.* 1990;19:535–542.
30. Fabian C, Mansfield C, Dahlberg S, et al. Low-dose involved field radiation after chemotherapy in advanced Hodgkin's disease. *Ann Intern Med.* 1994;120:903–912.
31. Loeffler M, Brosteanu O, Hasenclever D, et al. Meta-analysis of chemotherapy versus combined modality treatment trials in Hodgkin's disease. International Database on Hodgkin's Disease Overview Study Group [see comments]. *J Clin Oncol.* 1998;16:818–829.
32. Aleman BM, Raemaekers JM, Tirelli U, et al. Involved-field radiotherapy for advanced Hodgkin's lymphoma. *N Engl J Med.* 2003;348:2396–2406.
33. Duggan DB, Petroni GR, Johnson JL, et al. Randomized comparison of ABVD and MOPP/ABV hybrid for the treatment of advanced Hodgkin's disease: report of an intergroup trial. *J Clin Oncol.* 2003;21:607–614.
34. Horning SJ, Hoppe RT, Breslin S, et al. Stanford V and radiotherapy for locally extensive and advanced Hodgkin's disease: mature results of a prospective clinical trial. *J Clin Oncol.* 2002;20:630–637.
35. Chisesi T, Federico M, Levis A, et al. ABVD versus stanford V versus MEC in unfavourable Hodgkin's lymphoma: results of a randomised trial. *Ann Oncol.* 2002;13(suppl 1):102–106.
36. Poen JC, Hoppe RT, Horning SJ. High-dose therapy and autologous bone marrow transplantation for relapsed/refractory Hodgkin's disease: the impact of involved field radiotherapy on patterns of failure and survival [see comments]. *Int J Radiat Oncol Biol Phys.* 1996;36:3–12.
37. Yahalom J, Gulati SC, Toia M, et al. Accelerated hyperfractionated total-lymphoid irradiation, high-dose chemotherapy, and autologous bone marrow

transplantation for refractory and relapsing patients with Hodgkin's disease. *J Clin Oncol.* 1993;11:1062–1070.

38. Moskowitz CH, Nimer SD, Zelenetz AD, et al. A 2-step comprehensive high-dose chemoradiotherapy second-line program for relapsed and refractory Hodgkin's disease: analysis by intent to treat and development of a prognostic model. *Blood.* 2001;97:616–623.

39. Moskowitz CH, Kewalramani T, Nimer SD, et al. Effectiveness of high dose chemoradiotherapy and autologous stem cell transplantation for patients with biopsy-proven primary refractory Hodgkin's disease. *Br J Haematol.* 2004;124:645–652.

40. Goodman KA, Riedel E, Serrano V, et al. Long-term effects of high-dose chemotherapy and radiation for relapsed and refractory Hodgkin's lymphoma. *J Clin Oncol.* 2008;26:5240–5247.

41. Yahalom J. Omitting radiotherapy after attaining FDG PET-negative status following chemotherapy alone for Hodgkin's lymphoma: a randomized study caveat. *Leuk Lymphoma.* 2007;48:1667–1669.

# Salvage Therapy for Hodgkin's Lymphoma

Fahd Quddus • James O. Armitage

Hodgkin's lymphoma (HL) is a clonal lymphoid malignancy mainly confined to the lymph nodes and the lymphoid organs. HL (previously Hodgkin's disease) affects approximately 7500 new patients annually in the United States.[1] The disease incidence varies considerably and seems to have a bimodal pattern with first peak in the late 20's, and a second peak in patients 55 years and older.[2] The disease is composed of 2 distinct entities: the more common, classic HL, and the rarer nodular lymphocyte predominant HL. Classic HL includes the subgroups, nodular sclerosis, which is the most common type in United States, mixed cellularity, lymphocyte depleted, and lymphocyte rich.

From the period 1960 to 1963, the 5-year survival from HL was 40%. However, with advances in radiation therapy and in combination chemotherapy, from the period 1989 to 1993, the 5-year survival has considerably increased to more than 80%.

## FAILURE TO INITIAL THERAPY

Depending on the initial stage as well as the various prognostic factors, up to 30% of HL patients can be expected to relapse after initial induction of remission.[3] However, the biologic features of HL that contribute to its sensitivity to chemotherapy and radiation therapy during initial treatment can be retained at the time of relapse, thus allowing for durable responses and remissions with second-line (and even third-line) therapeutic measures.

For the purpose of this article, it might be useful to review some of the basic terminologies associated with salvage therapy for HL. "Relapse" itself may be defined as reappearance of disease in sites of prior disease and/or in new sites after an initial complete response to therapy. "Progression" refers to increasing evidence of disease after achieving a partial response, and "refractory disease" refers to a failure to achieve even a partial response.

Despite the high cure rate with initial therapy, in approximately 5% to 10% of patients with HL, the disease is refractory to initial treatment, and 10% to 30% of patients will experience disease relapse after an initial complete response.[4,5] Of note, the majority of the relapses after initial complete response are detected during physical examination or during evaluation of various symptoms rather than routine blood work or imaging.

It is essential to document disease recurrence histologically via a biopsy. Positron emission tomography in combination with computed tomography remains the test of choice for detecting disease activity or relapse post treatment.[6-9] Compared with computed tomography alone, positron emission tomography in combination with computed tomography is better able to distinguish between active tumor and necrosis or fibrosis in residual masses. However, the positive predictive value of positron emission tomography in detecting disease response is only about 65%. As per literature, as much as 40% of so-called positive positron emission tomography scans at the end

of therapy do not recur in the next 5 years of follow-up.[10] Causes of a falsely positive positron emission tomography scan include inflammatory changes postchemotherapy, radiation therapy, rebound thymic hyperplasia, brown fat, inflammation, and infection.[11] In contrast, the negative predictive value of a positron emission tomography is as high as 90%,[7] with the 10% to 20% false negatives likely secondary to possible microscopic disease.

## PROGNOSTIC FACTORS

As the initial treatment strategies for HL become more effective, the various prognostic factors for relapse will possibly change as well. For now, the duration of remission after initial chemotherapy remains the single most important prognostic factor for relapsed HL patients with respect to how well the patients will respond to subsequent salvage therapy. The National Cancer Institute in 1992 updated its experience with long-term follow up of HL patients who had relapsed after initial conventional dose combination chemotherapy.[12] No patient with primary progressive disease survived more than 8 years. In contrast, the 20-year survival rate for patients with early (less than 12 months) and late relapse (more than 12 months) was 11% and 22%, respectively.[12]

The German Hodgkin's Lymphoma Study Group reported on 422 patients with relapsed HL after initial therapy, which included radiation therapy, conventional chemotherapy, and a combination of the 2.[13] The 3 most important prognostic factors for a possible third relapse for these patients included in order of importance: duration of initial remission, stage of disease at relapse, and anemia. It is to be noted that one-third of the included patients underwent hematopoietic stem cell transplantation as salvage therapy.

## TREATMENT

### Radiotherapy

Radiation therapy alone in the setting of disease relapse is now rarely used. Only limited studies have been reported with this particular approach, and the data are supportive of combined modality being superior to radiation alone.[14]

Occasionally, radiation therapy alone can be used with some success in highly selected patient with prolonged period of initial remission, and localized recurrence with no extranodal disease, absence of B symptoms, and the ability of encompassing the entire disease recurrence site within the radiation field.[15-17]

Nodal or involved field radiotherapy is often used in combined-modality salvage of relapse after chemotherapy. Radiation therapy is also frequently added to patients with relapsed disease undergoing high-dose chemotherapy and autologous stem cell transplant, especially to sites of bulky disease. Prospective data showing a benefit of this approach are currently lacking, with concern for added toxicity.

## Conventional Chemotherapy

Until recently, it was standard practice to treat HL patients who relapse after more than 1 year with the same chemotherapy regimen as the one used for initial remission induction. Most commonly used chemotherapy regimens for first-line therapy include doxorubicin, bleomycin, vinblastine, dacarbazine, nitrogen mustard, vincristine, procarbazine, and prednisone (MOPP), or the newer regimens such as Stanford V (nitrogen mustard, doxorubicin, vinblastine, vincristine, bleomycin, etoposide, and prednisone) or bleomycin, etoposide, doxorubicin, cyclophosphamide, vincristine, procarbazine, and prednisone. As such, these patients were able to achieve a second complete remission approximately 80% of the times with a mean survival of about 4 years.[14] Patients who relapsed within a year of disease remission were offered a different chemotherapy regimen avoiding drugs that were used in the first regimen.[18–20] No randomized clinical trial has shown any benefit of one standard salvage chemotherapy regimen over the other to date. However, despite responses, these patients even after achieving a second remission go on to relapse and die of the disease or its complications. Thus, there is currently a shift in practice where almost all eligible patients with relapsed disease are offered high-dose chemotherapy and autologous stem cell transplantation.

Patients ineligible for high-dose chemotherapy and autologous stem cell transplantation can be considered for conventional chemotherapy regimens in combination with radiation therapy if possible. Most such patients can be treated with a first-line conventional chemotherapy regimen that was not used initially.[21–23]

## High-Dose Chemotherapy and Autologous Hematopoietic Stem Cell Transplant

High-dose chemotherapy with autologous hematopoietic stem cell transplantation is the cornerstone of salvage therapy for most relapsed HL patients. It is also considered the standard of care for those who experience progression during remission induction.

The likelihood of attaining a successful second remission is related greatly to the duration of the initial remission.[14] Patients whose initial remission lasted more than 12 months have an impressive 75% to 80% chance of achieving a durable second remission. In contrast, patients whose initial remission lasted less than 12 months have a 40% to 50% chance of a second durable remission. Figures are even more dismal for patients who had progressive disease during induction chemotherapy, with likelihood of attaining a durable remission at only 20%.

In general, the salvage therapy is administered in 2 phases. Initially, a conventional chemotherapy regimen is administered with the hope to reduce the tumor bulk as much as possible. This usually is followed by stem cell mobilization, and subsequent high-dose chemotherapy along with stem cell rescue.

The choice of the conventional chemotherapy regimen used for salvage usually depends on the original chemotherapy regimen used during first remission induction as well as the duration of the initial remission. Patients who have progressed on a certain first-line chemotherapy regimen (ie, doxorubicin, bleomycin, vinblastine, and dacarbazine) may respond better to another chemotherapy regimen, which avoids agents used in the first regimen (ie, MOPP or MOPP-like regimen). A new regimen with novel agents, such as etoposide, methylprednisolone, high-dose cytarabine, and cisplatin, may be more effective.[24] Newer agents such as gemcitabine may also be effective in achieving an adequate reduction in this initial tumor bulk. Ultimately, the goal is to reduce the tumor burden as much as possible, before embarking on the high-dose chemotherapy and autologous stem cell transplant. Patients with the lowest tumor burden before high-dose

chemotherapy and autologous stem cell transplant are most likely to attain a durable second remission.

## Sequential High-Dose Chemotherapy

Keeping in mind the Norton-Simon hypothesis, sequential high-dose chemotherapy regimen offers the highest possible dosing of chemotherapeutic agents in the shortest duration possible.

This dose- and time-intensification approach was initially studied in a phase II multicenter trial by the German Hodgkin's Lymphoma Study Group.[25] Patients included in the study had histologically proven primary progressive or relapsed HL. Treatment consisted of 2 cycles dexamethasone, high-dose cytarabine, and cisplatin; patients with chemosensitive disease received cyclophosphamide followed by peripheral blood stem cell harvest; methotrexate plus vincristine, etoposide and carmustine, etoposide, cytarabine, malphalan plus peripheral blood stem cell transplantation. A total of 102 patients (median age 34 years, range 18–64) were enrolled. The response rate was 80% (72% complete response, 8% partial response). With a median follow-up of 30 months (range 3–61 months), freedom from second failure and overall survival were 59% and 78% for all patients, respectively. Freedom from second failure and overall survival for patients with early relapse were 62% and 81%, for late relapse 65% and 81%; for progressive disease 41% and 48%, and for multiple relapse 39% and 48%, respectively.

Based on the promising results of this study, a prospective randomized European intergroup study was started comparing this intensified regimen with 2 courses of dexamethasone, high-dose cytarabine, and cisplatin followed by carmustine, etoposide, cytarabine, and malphalan. The results of this study (HD-R2 protocol) remain pending at this point.

## Allotransplant

Allogeneic transplant is not routinely considered for HL patients secondary to donor availability as well as the advanced age of many of these patients. In addition, a reduced relapse rate after an allogeneic transplant due to its graft-versus-tumor effect comes at the expense of potentially lethal graft-versus-host toxicity. For patients with HL treated with low-intensity allogeneic transplant, the treatment related mortality at 1 year was approximately 20%, and the 2-year overall survival was approximately 50%.[26] The treatment related mortality was considerably worse for the older age group. Nevertheless, this approach, in particular the nonmyeloablative conditioning regimens, warrants further investigation especially for patients with refractory disease who have failed other therapies.

## New Directions

HL patients who progress after high-dose chemotherapy and autologous stem cell transplantation have few good therapeutic options left, and generally have a poor outcome. In one study, HL patients who failed high-dose chemotherapy and autologous stem cell transplantation, the median time to progression after the next therapy was only 3.8 months, with the median survival after high-dose chemotherapy and autologous stem cell transplantation failure being 26 months.[27]

Of the various novel therapies available, the 2 cytotoxic agents, gemcitabine[28] and vinorelbine[29] seem the most promising. Both agents have shown activity in heavily pretreated HL patients, even though the duration of responses was short. Vinorelbine, a vinca alkaloid, demonstrated activity in patients who were treated in the past with vincristine and vinblastine.[29] Further role of these agents in first and second-line therapies is currently under investigation.

Recent studies also included exploitation of the expression of CD30 on the Reed-Sternberg cells. Antibodies targeting the molecule had shown promise in vitro. Recent trials of SGN-30 (humanized mouse monoclonal antiCD30) and MDX-060 (fully humanized antibody) showed few side effects, however, only limited clinical response was seen.[30,31] Other areas of interest include immunotoxins directed against CD25, as well as immunotherapy with cytotoxic T-cells targeting Ebstein-Barr Virus antigens as well as the Reed-Sternberg cells.

## CONCLUSIONS

Considerable progress has been made in recent years with respect to HL therapy, and its cure rate has significantly increased. Currently, more than 80% of newly diagnosed HL patients are expected to be long-term survivors. Nevertheless, for the subset of patients who relapse or progress after initial therapy, HL remains a challenging disease. Indeed for patients who progress after high-dose chemotherapy and autologous stem cell transplantation (or are ineligible), therapeutic options remain limited, and further new therapies are warranted.

## REFERENCES

1. Jemal A, Murray T, Ward E, et al. Cancer statistics, 2005. *CA Cancer J Clin.* 2005;55:10–30; erratum in *CA Cancer J Clin.* 2005;55:259.
2. Glaser SL, Jarrett RF. The epidemiology of Hodgkin's disease. *Baillieres Clin Haematol.* 1996;9:401–416.
3. Oza AM, Ganesan TS, Leahy M, et al. Pattern of survival in patients with Hodgkin's disease: long follow up in a single center. *Ann Oncol.* 1993;4:385–392.
4. Horning SJ. Hodgkin's disease. In: Cavalli F, Hansen HH, Kaye SB, eds. *Textbook of Medical Oncology.* 2nd ed. London, England: Martin Dunitz; 2000:461–474.
5. Diehl V, Mauch PM, Harris NL. Hodgkin's disease. In: Devita VT Jr, Hellman S, Rosenberg SA, eds. *Cancer: Principles and Practice of Oncology.* vol 2. 6th ed. Philadelphia, PA: Lippincott Williams and Wilkins; 2001:2339–2387.
6. Juweid ME. Utility of positron emission tomography (PET) scanning in managing patients with Hodgkin's lymphoma. *Hematology Am Soc Hematol Educ Program.* 2006;259–265.
7. Cheson BD, Pfistner B, Juweid ME, et al. Revised response criteria for malignant lymphoma. *J Clin Oncol.* 2007;25:579–586.
8. Jerusalem G, Beguin Y, Fassotte MF, et al. Whole-body positron emission tomography using 18F-fluorodeoxyglucose for posttreatment evaluation in Hodgkin's disease and non-Hodgkin's lymphoma has higher diagnostic and prognostic value than classical computed tomography scan imaging. *Blood.* 1999;94:429–433.
9. Hoh CK, Glaspy J, Rosen P, et al. Whole-body FDG-PET imaging for staging of Hodgkin's disease and lymphoma. *J Nucl Med.* 1997;38:343–348.
10. Hutchings A, Loft A, Hansen M, et al. FDG-PET after 2 cycles of chemotherapy predicts treatment failure and progression free survival in Hodgkin's lymphoma. *Blood.* 2005;108:52.
11. Fallanca F, Giovacchini G, Ponzoni M, et al. Cervical thymic hyperplasia after chemotherapy in an adult patient with Hodgkin's lymphoma: a potential cause of false-positivity on [18F]FDG PET/CT scanning. *Br J Haematol.* 2008;140:477.
12. Longo DL, Puffey PL, Young RC, et al. Conventional dose salvage combination chemotherapy in patients relapsing with Hodgkin's disease after combination chemotherapy: the low probability for cure. *J Clin Oncol.* 1992;10:210–218.
13. Josting A, Franklin J, May M, et al. New prognostic score based on treatment outcome of patients with relapsed Hodgkin's lymphoma registered in the database of the German Hodgkin's lymphoma study group. *J Clin Oncol.* 2002;20:221–230.
14. Uematsu M, Tarbell N, Silver B, et al. Wide field radiation therapy with or without chemotherapy for patients with Hodgkin's disease in relapse after initial combination chemotherapy. *Cancer.* 1993;72:207–212.
15. Brada M, Eeles R, Ashley S, et al. Salvage radiotherapy in recurrent Hodgkin's disease. *Ann Oncol.* 1992;3:131–135.
16. Wirth A, Corry J, Laidlaw C, et al. Salvage radiotherapy for Hodgkin's disease following chemotherapy failure. *Int J Radiat Oncol Biol Phys.* 1997;39:599–607.
17. Pezner RD, Lipsett JA, Vora N, et al. Radical radiotherapy as salvage treatment for relapse of Hodgkin's disease initially treated by chemotherapy alone: prognostic significance of the disease-free interval. *Int J Radiat Oncol Biol Phys.* 1994;30:965–970.
18. Pfreundschuh MG, Rueffer U, Lathan B, et al. Dexa-BEAM in patients with Hodgkin's disease refractory to multidrug chemotherapy regimens: a trial of the German Hodgkin's Disease Study Group. *J Clin Oncol.* 1994;12:580–586.
19. Ferme C, Bastion Y, Lepage E, et al. The MINE regimen as intensive salvage chemotherapy for relapsed and refractory Hodgkin's disease. *Ann Oncol.* 1995;6:543–549.
20. Rodriguez J, Rodriquez MA, Fayad L, et al. ASHAP: a regimen for cytoreduction of refractory or recurrent Hodgkin's disease. *Blood.* 1999;93:3632–3636.
21. Bonfante V, Santoro A, Viviani S, et al. Outcome of patients with Hodgkin's disease failing after primary MOPP-ABVD. *J Clin Oncol.* 1997;15:528–534.
22. Bonadonna G, Santoro A, Gianni AM, et al. Primary and salvage chemotherapy in advanced Hodgkin's disease: the Milan Cancer Institute experience. *Ann Oncol* 1991;2(Suppl 1):9–16.
23. Harker WG, Kushlan P, Rosenberg SA. Combination chemotherapy for advanced Hodgkin's disease after failure of MOPP: ABVD and B-CAVe. *Ann Intern Med.* 1984;101:440–446.
24. Aparicio J, Segura A, Garcera S, et al. ESHAP is an active regimen for relapsing Hodgkin's disease. *Ann Oncol.* 1999;10:593–595.
25. Robinson SP, Goldstone AH, Mackinnon S, et al. Chemoresistant or aggressive lymphoma predicts for a poor outcome following reduced intensity allogeneic progenitor cell transplantation: an analysis from the lymphoma working party of the European Group for Blood and Bone Marrow Transplantation. *Blood.* 2002;100:4310–4316.
26. Kewalramani T, Nimer SD, Zelenetz AD, et al. Progressive disease following autologous transplant in patients with chemosensitive relapsed or primary refractory Hodgkin's disease or aggressive non-Hodgkin's lymphoma. *Bone Marrow Transplant.* 2003;32:673–679.
27. Santoro A, Bredenfeld H, Devizzi L, et al. Gemcitabine in the treatment of refractory Hodgkin's disease: results of a multicenter phase II sudy. *J Clin Oncol.* 2000;18:2615 2619.
28. Devizzi L, Santoro A, Bonfante V, et al. Vinorelbine: a new promising drug in Hodgkin's disease. *Leuk Lymphoma.* 1996;22:409–414.
29. Josting A, Rudolph C, Mapara M, et al. Cologne high-dose sequential chemotherapy in relapsed and refractory Hodgkin's lymphoma: results of a large multicenter study of the German Hodgkin's Lymphoma Study Group (GHSG). *Ann Oncol.* 2005;16:116–123.
30. Ansell S, Byrd J, Horwitz S, et al. Phase I/II study of a fully human anti-CD30 monoclonal antibody (MDX-060) in Hodgkin's disease and anaplastic large cell lymphoma. *Blood.* 2003;102 (11, pt 1):181a (abstract 632).
31. Barlett NL, Berstein SH, Leonard JP, et al. Safety, anti-tumor activity and pharmacokinetics of six weekly doses of SGN-30 (anti-CD30 monoclonal antibody) in patients with refractory or recurrent CD30 hematologic malignancies. *Blood.* 2003;102 (11, pt 1):647a (abstract 2390).

# Late Effects of Hodgkin's Disease and Its Treatment

Andrea K. Ng • Peter M. Mauch

Long-term survivors of Hodgkin's lymphoma are at significantly increased risk for a number of late complications, some of which are known to contribute to their excess mortality over time. Several studies have shown that although the cumulative incidence of mortality from Hodgkin's lymphoma plateaus over time, mortality from other causes continues to rise with increasing follow-up time, with second malignancy and cardiac disease being the 2 leading causes of death in these patients.[1–3] A clear understanding of the various late effects of treatment, their timing and associated risk factors can facilitate the development of optimal follow-up plan for long-term survivors, including screening and prevention strategies. Furthermore, recognition of therapy-related complications can guide treatment modification in newly diagnosed patients to minimize future late effects.

## SECOND MALIGNANCY

Since the early 1970s, there has been an accumulation of literature characterizing second malignancies after Hodgkin's lymphoma. Traditionally, second malignancy after Hodgkin's lymphoma had been divided into 3 main categories: leukemia, non-Hodgkin's lymphoma, and solid tumors.

### Leukemia

The increased risk of leukemia was first described in the early 1970s in patients who had been treated for Hodgkin's lymphoma.[4] The risk seemed to be the highest in the first 10 years after treatment. The risk was largely related to the use of alkylating chemotherapy in a dose-related manner.[5,6] Although splenectomy and the addition of large-field radiation therapy to chemotherapy have been postulated as additional risk factors, data are conflicting.[6,7] The prognosis of leukemia after Hodgkin's lymphoma is extremely poor, with a median survival of less than 1 year.[3] With the replacement of mechlorethemine, vincristine, procarbazine, and prednisone (MOPP) by adriamycin, bleomycin, vinblastine, and dacarbazine (ABVD), the risk of leukemia has been substantially reduced. In a recent large, international population-based study by Schonfeld et al,[8] a significant reduction in absolute excess risk of acute myeloid leukemia was found in patients who were treated for Hodgkin's lymphoma after 1985, which is likely explained by changes in chemotherapy over time. However, alkylators are still used in the setting of salvage treatment and are included in some of the modern regimens including bleomycin, etoposide, doxorubicin, cyclophosphamide, procarbazine, and prednisone (BEACOPP) and Stanford V.[9,10] The risk of secondary leukemia may therefore remain even in patients treated in the modern era.

### Non-Hodgkin's Lymphoma

An increased risk of non-Hodgkin's lymphoma after Hodgkin's lymphoma has also been observed.[3,11,12] Its timing and relationship with prior therapy, however, is unclear. Development of non-Hodgkin's lymphoma after Hodgkin's lymphoma may be treatment induced. It could also be part of the natural course of Hodgkin's lymphoma, especially for the lymphocyte predominant subtype, or it may be related to the immunosuppressed status of Hodgkin's lymphoma patients. In a study from the German Hodgkin's Study Group, patients who developed non-Hodgkin's lymphoma within 3 months after completion of Hodgkin's lymphoma therapy had a significantly worse prognosis than patients who developed non-Hodgkin's lymphoma beyond 12 months (2-year OS, 20% versus 42%).[13] Age-adjusted International Prognostic Score also significantly predicted for treatment outcome.

## Solid Tumors

As the number of survivors of Hodgkin's lymphoma increases and with longer follow-up time, solid tumors had emerged as the major subtype of second malignancy, accounting for up to 75% to 80% of all cases of second malignancy.[3,11,12,14,15] Solid tumors typically develop after a long latency of at least 10 years after the initial Hodgkin's lymphoma treatment. In addition, the risk seems to persist as long as beyond 30 years after the initial diagnosis. The most common solid tumors observed in long-term survivors of Hodgkin's lymphoma include breast, lung, and gastrointestinal malignancies.[3,14–16]

Two case-control studies had examined in detail the relationship between radiation dose and the risk of breast cancer after Hodgkin's lymphoma therapy.[16,17] In the study by van Leeuwen et al,[17] the breast cancer risk was significantly increased only after a radiation dose of 38.5 Gy or higher but not at lower doses. In a larger, international case-control study by Travis et al,[16] a radiation dose of >4 Gy to the breast was associated with a 3.2-fold breast cancer risk compared with women who received lower doses of radiation and no alkylating chemotherapy. The risk increased to eightfold for women who received >40 Gy to the breast ($P$ trend $< 0.001$).

A significant radiation dose-response relationship has similarly been shown for the development of lung cancer after Hodgkin's lymphoma. In a case-control study by Travis et al,[18] the increased risk of lung was statistically significant only after exposure to doses of 30 Gy or higher, compared with patients who received <5 Gy to the area of the lung in which cancer developed.

Limited data are available on solid tumor risk after chemotherapy alone. In a British cohort study, which included 1693 patients treated with chemotherapy (largely alkylating chemotherapy) alone, the relative risk of lung cancer after chemotherapy alone was found to be significantly increased at 3.3 compared with the matched-general population.[12] A subsequent case-control study from the same group,[19] and another study by Travis et al,[18] both showed a significant dose-response relationship between cumulative doses of alkylating chemotherapy and lung cancer risk.

Other factors also influence the risk of treatment-related solid tumors after Hodgkin's lymphoma. Young age at mantle irradiation has been consistently shown to be associated with significantly increased risk of breast cancer in women.[3,11,15] Hormonal exposures also seem to play an important role in the development of breast cancer after Hodgkin's lymphoma. Treatment exposure to alkylating chemotherapy and pelvic irradiation with resulting premature menopause had been found to be protective against breast cancer.[16,17] Another well-documented risk factor is tobacco exposure on lung cancer development. In a case-control study by Travis et al,[18] a multiplicative effect of tobacco history on the risk of treatment-related lung cancer was shown. In patients who had received chest irradiation and alkylating chemotherapy, and had a tobacco history, the lung cancer risk was 49-fold higher than patients who had none of the exposures.

## CARDIOVASCULAR DISEASE

The relative risks of cardiac mortality in survivors of Hodgkin's lymphoma have been estimated to range from 2.2 to 7 and the absolute excess risk range from 9.3 to 28/10,000 person-years.[2,3,20–22] A wide spectrum of cardiac complications have been reported in long-term survivors of Hodgkin's lymphoma.[23–27] These include pericardial disease, valvular disease, conduction abnormalities, ventricular dysfunction, and coronary disease.

### Cardiovascular Disease After Mediastinal Irradiation

The relationship between mediastinal irradiation for Hodgkin's lymphoma and long-term risk of fatal cardiovascular complications is well documented.[1,28,29] In addition, the risk seems to be dose related, as demonstrated in the study by Hancock et al,[20] in which cardiac mortality was significantly increased in patients who received more than 30 Gy to the mediastinum, but the increase was not significant in patients who received 30 Gy or less.

In addition to cardiac mortality, data on cardiac morbidity after Hodgkin's lymphoma therapy are also available. In a retrospective study from the University of Florida on 415 patients with history of Hodgkin's lymphoma,[30] 10.4% of patients developed coronary artery disease at a median follow-up of 9 years posttreatment. On multivariable analysis, the only treatment-related risk factor significantly associated with risk of coronary artery disease was the use of a matched mantle and paraaortic field when compared with mantle alone or subdiaphragmatic treatment alone. Aleman et al[31] from the Netherlands reviewed 1474 survivors of Hodgkin's lymphoma younger than 41 years at treatment. At a median follow-up of 18.7 years, the relative risks of myocardial infarction and congestive heart failure were significantly increased at 3.6 and 4.9, respectively. The relative risk of myocardial infarction became significantly elevated after 10 years, and it remained significantly elevated for at least 25 years after treatment. On multivariable analysis, mediastinal radiotherapy was associated with significantly increased risks of valvular disorders, coronary heart disease, and congestive heart failure. Several studies have also shown that traditional cardiac risk factors, including hypertension, hypercholesterolemia, and smoking significantly contribute to the subsequent risk of cardiac disease after Hodgkin's lymphoma therapy.[27,30,32]

### Cardiovascular Disease After Chemotherapy

In recent years, data are available on the relationship between chemotherapy for Hodgkin's lymphoma and risk of cardiac complications. Aviles et al[26] reviewed 399 Hodgkin's lymphoma patients who achieved a complete remission after chemotherapy alone. At a median follow-up of 11.5 years, 20 patients developed congestive heart failure and 19 patients developed myocardial infarction. A total of 21 cardiac deaths were reported. The relative risks of cardiac mortality after ABVD, MBVD (mitoxantrone instead of doxorubicin), and EBVD (epirubicin instead of doxorubicin), compared with the matched normal population, were 46.4, 67.8, and 19.4, respectively.

A British study also demonstrated the independent effect of chemotherapy on risk of cardiac mortality, although the relative risks were less dramatically elevated. This study included 7033 patients with Hodgkin's lymphoma treated from 1967 to 2000.[33] At a mean follow-up of 11.1 years, a total of 166 myocardial infarction deaths were observed. The risk of cardiac mortality was separately analyzed for patients who received chemotherapy with mediastinal irradiation and chemotherapy without mediastinal irradiation. Among patients who were treated with ABVD and mediastinal irradiation, the relative risk of cardiac mortality was significantly elevated at 12.1 ($P = 0.004$). However, patients who received ABVD without mediastinal irradiation were also found to have a significantly elevated relative risk of cardiac mortality of 7.8 ($P = 0.01$). The relative risks of cardiac mortality after treatment with any adriamycin-based chemotherapy with and without mediastinal irradiation were 2.4 ($P = 0.05$) and 3.2 ($P < 0.001$), respectively.

### Screening for Cardiovascular Disease

Because of the well-documented increased risks of cardiac complications in Hodgkin's lymphoma survivors, investigators have described the use of cardiac screening tools in asymptomatic patients. In a prospective study from Stanford University, 294 asymptomatic patients treated with mediastinal irradiation for Hodgkin's lymphoma underwent electrocardiography and echocardiography screening at a median time of 15 years from initial treatment.[23] Significant valvular abnormality, depressed left ventricular fractional shortening, regional wall motion abnormality, decreased left ventricular mass and pericardial thickening, all of which also increased with increasing time from initial irradiation. In the most recent report from the same group, the focus was on coronary disease among participants of the screening trial.[34] During stress testing, 14% developed perfusion defects, impaired wall motion, or both abnormalities. Based on the imaging results, 40 patients (14%) underwent coronary angiography. As a result of the screening, 7 of these asymptomatic patients (2.4%) underwent bypass graft surgery. In addition, 23 patients (8%) subsequently developed coronary events during a median of 6.5 years of follow-up, including 10 cases of acute myocardial infarctions. Of note, the median dose to the mediastinum among patients included in this Stanford screening study was 44 Gy (range, 35–54.6 Gy), which are doses that are considerably higher than those used in current practice.

Adams et al[24] conducted a prospective cardiac screening study along with quality-of-life evaluation on 48 asymptomatic childhood Hodgkin's lymphoma survivors. The median age of the study population at the time of initial therapy was 16.5 years, and the median dose received was 40 Gy. The median follow time was 14.3 years. On echocardiogram, 42% were found to have significant valve defects, 75% had conduction defects, and 22% had echocardiographic changes suggestive of restrictive cardiomyopathy. A significant association between aortic regurgitation and decreased physical component score on the SF-36 was found ($P = 0.01$). A decreased peak myocardial oxygen uptake during exercise ($VO_{2max}$), a predictor of mortality in heart failure, was associated with increased fatigue ($P = 0.02$) and decreased physical component score ($P = 0.00017$). These findings suggest that the late effects of treatment can contribute to quality-of-life impairment and fatigue in long-term Hodgkin's lymphoma survivors.

## OTHER LATE EFFECTS

### Noncoronary Vascular Complications

Emerging data are available on the risk of noncoronary vascular disease as a late complication after Hodgkin's lymphoma therapy. Hull et al[27] reported an actuarial incidence of noncoronary atherosclerotic disease of 2% at 5 years, 3% at 10 years, and 7% at 20 years, respectively, among 415 Hodgkin's lymphoma survivors. The median dose to the low neck was significantly higher in patients who developed subclavian artery stenosis than those who did not (44 Gy and 36 Gy, respectively, $P = 0.002$). Similarly, the median dose to the low neck was 38 Gy among patients who developed carotid artery stenosis and 36 Gy in patients who did not ($P = 0.05$). In addition, hypertension ($P = 0.003$) and diabetes mellitus ($P = 0.001$) were both significant independent factors associated with noncoronary atherosclerotic disease in this population. A report from the Childhood Cancer Survivor Study examined the incidence of stroke in survivors of pediatric Hodgkin's lymphoma.[35] Compared with the siblings, there was a 5.6-fold higher risk of stroke in survivors of Hodgkin's lymphoma who received mantle radiation therapy. The median dose to the mantle field in survivors who developed a stroke was 40 Gy. Unlike the study by Hull et al, hypertension and diabetes mellitus did not significantly increase the risk of stroke, but a smoking history was a significant predictor (OR = 3.37, $P = 0.026$). Currently, the role of screening for noncoronary vascular disease in Hodgkin's lymphoma survivors is unknown. However, it is important to note that modern approaches to Hodgkin's lymphoma therapy use lower radiation doses, smaller fields, and planning techniques that limit dose inhomogeneity and hot spots commonly seen in the neck area with older techniques. It is therefore anticipated that noncoronary vascular complications will be less of a concern in more recently treated patients.

### Thyroid Dysfunction

The most common thyroid abnormality after radiation therapy for Hodgkin's lymphoma is hypothyroidism. In a study by Hancock et al,[36] the actuarial risk of hypothyroidism after radiation therapy for Hodgkin's lymphoma was 47% at 26 years. Other less common thyroid abnormalities observed included Graves' disease, thyroiditis, thyrotoxicosis, thyroid nodules, and thyroid malignancies.

The risk of radiation-related thyroid dysfunction seems to be dose related.[37,38] In a study from the University of Minnesota, the estimated actuarial risk of developing hypothyroidism was 60% at 11 years.[39] In addition, the relative risk of hypothyroidism was estimated to increase by 1.02/Gy. Patients who have received radiation therapy to the neck region for Hodgkin's lymphoma would therefore benefit from thyroid function testing as part of follow-up.

### Sterility

Radiation therapy can induce germinal epithelium depletion in a dose-related manner.[40–43] Decrease in sperm count can be observed after doses as low as 0.15 Gy. A 1-time dose of 0.35 Gy or higher can cause transient azoospermia. The recovery time increases with increasing dose, and doses of 2 Gy or higher to the germinal epithelium can result in permanent azoospermia. At doses of 15 Gy or higher, Leydig cell function can be affected, with potential need for testosterone replacement therapy. In men who are receiving pelvic radiation therapy for Hodgkin's lymphoma, cryopreservation of semen before intiation of therapy should be strongly considered. Adequate testicular shielding can also reduce the risk of permanent azoospermia.

The effect of chemotherapy for Hodgkin's lymphoma on male reproductive function had also been extensively explored. After 6 to 8 cycles of MOPP chemotherapy, 80% to 90% of patients will develop azoospermia.[44] In a recent cohort study conducted by the EORTC, exposure to alkylating chemotherapy was associated with a significantly higher risk of gonadal dysfunction among male patients and longer recovery time of gonadal function.[45] The current standard systemic therapy for Hodgkin's lymphoma, ABVD, can lead to transient azoospermia in about one third of patients, but the majority of patients will have recovery of spermatogenesis after treatment.[44,46] However, the BEACOPP regimen, developed by the German Hodgkin's Study Group for patients with advanced-stage or unfavorable Hodgkin's lymphoma,[9] is associated with an increased risk of sterility. In a recent study on 38 male patients treated with BEACOPP, at baseline, 77% patients had dysspermia. After treatment, 89% patients had azoospermia, 11% had other dysspermia, and no patients had normozoospermia.[47]

Ionizing radiation can cause direct DNA damage to ovarian follicles, leading to follicular atrophy and decreased follicular reserve within the ovary. An ovarian dose of 4 Gy may cause a 30% incidence of sterility in young women but 100% sterility in women over 40 years of age.[43] In women receiving pelvic irradiation for Hodgkin's lymphoma, oophoropexy, which can be achieved laparscopically can reduce the dose delivered to the ovaries and preserve fertility.[48,49]

The effect of chemotherapy on female reproductive function was explored in a cohort study of 518 female survivors of Hodgkin's lymphoma.[50] At a median follow-up of 9.4 years, chemotherapy was associated with a 12.3-fold increased risk of premature menopause compared with radiotherapy alone. A significant dose-response relationship was demonstrated with exposures to alkylating chemotherapy, most notably for procarbazine and cyclophosphamide. In a case-control survey study of female Hodgkin's lymphoma survivors treated with ABVD, no significant subfertility was found.[51] However, the BEACOPP regimen can result in continues amenorrhea in over 50% of women.[14]

## SUMMARY

In view of the increased risk for various late effects after treatment for Hodgkin's lymphoma, patient education regarding the risks, and promoting healthy behavior to reduce modifiable risk factors (eg, sun safety practice, smoking cessation, dietary changes, and weight control) are essential. In addition, early-detection and prevention strategies, especially for the more serious, potentially life-threatening late effects including second malignancies and cardiac disease, should be considered in high-risk patients. These include mammography and breast magnetic resonance imaging screening in women who had received chest irradiation at a young age, and low-dose chest computed tomography screening in survivors with a smoking history and who have received chest irradiation and/or alkylating chemotherapy. Survivors with history of exposures to adriamycin-based chemotherapy or mediastinal irradiation may also benefit from cardiac screening tests, and routine blood pressure and lipid screening. However, the efficacy of these tests, and their optimal timing and frequency, remain to be determined.

It is important to note that most of the documented late effects after Hodgkin's lymphoma therapy are based on patients treated with outdated chemotherapy and radiation fields, doses, and techniques. Modeling data have shown that treatment with limited radiation fields to lower doses can significantly reduce second malignancy risk.[52] Current efforts of additional reduction in radiation field sizes and doses will likely further reduce late complications.[25,53,54] Recent advances in conformal radiation therapy techniques can also effectively limit doses critical normal structures.[55,56] As Hodgkin's lymphoma therapy evolves, it is imperative to continue the long-term follow-up of survivors with careful documentation of late effects associated with new treatments. Understanding the contribution of other modifying factors in the context of modern therapy, including genetic factors, environmental factors, and lifestyle choices may further help guide patient counseling and refine follow-up recommendations.

## REFERENCES

1. Henry-Amar M, Hayat M, Meerwaldt JH, et al. Causes of death after therapy for early stage Hodgkin's disease entered on EORTC protocols. EORTC Lymphoma Cooperative Group. *Int J Radiat Oncol Biol Phys.* 1990;19:1155–1157.
2. Hoppe RT. Hodgkin's disease: complications of therapy and excess mortality. *Ann Oncol.* 1997;8(suppl 1):115–118.
3. Ng AK, Bernardo MP, Weller E, et al. Long-term survival and competing causes of death in patients with early-stage Hodgkin's disease treated at age 50 or younger. *J Clin Oncol.* 2002;20:2101–2108.
4. Arseneau JC, Sponzo RW, Levin DL, et al. Nonlymphomatous malignant tumors complicating Hodgkin's disease. Possible association with intensive therapy. *N Engl J Med.* 1972;287:1119–1122.
5. Kaldor JM, Day NE, Clarke EA, et al. Leukemia following Hodgkin's disease. *N Engl J Med.* 1990;322:7–13.
6. van Leeuwen FE, Chorus AM, van den Belt-Dusebout AW, et al. Leukemia risk following Hodgkin's disease: relation to cumulative dose of alkylating agents, treatment with teniposide combinations, number of episodes of chemotherapy, and bone marrow damage. *J Clin Oncol.* 1994;12:1063–1073.
7. Bonadonna G, Bonfante V, Viviani S, et al. ABVD plus subtotal nodal versus involved-field radiotherapy in early-stage Hodgkin's disease: long-term results. *J Clin Oncol.* 2004;22:2835–2841.
8. Schonfeld SJ, Gilbert ES, Dores GM, et al. Acute myeloid leukemia following Hodgkin lymphoma: a population-based study of 35,511 patients. *J Natl Cancer Inst.* 2006;98:215–218.
9. Diehl V, Franklin J, Pfreundschuh M, et al. Standard and increased-dose BEACOPP chemotherapy compared with COPP-ABVD for advanced Hodgkin's disease. *N Engl J Med.* 2003;348:2386–2395.
10. Horning SJ, Hoppe RT, Breslin S, et al. Stanford V and radiotherapy for locally extensive and advanced Hodgkin's disease: mature results of a prospective clinical trial. *J Clin Oncol.* 2002;20:630–637.
11. van Leeuwen FE, Klokman WJ, Veer MB, et al. Long-term risk of second malignancy in survivors of Hodgkin's disease treated during adolescence or young adulthood. *J Clin Oncol.* 2000;18:487–497.
12. Swerdlow AJ, Barber JA, Hudson GV, et al. Risk of second malignancy after Hodgkin's disease in a collaborative British cohort: the relation to age at treatment. *J Clin Oncol.* 2000;18:498–509.
13. Rueffer U, Josting A, Franklin J, et al. Non-Hodgkin's lymphoma after primary Hodgkin's disease in the German Hodgkin's Lymphoma Study Group: incidence, treatment, and prognosis. *J Clin Oncol.* 2001;19:2026–2032.
14. Behringer K, Breuer K, Reineke T, et al. Secondary amenorrhea after Hodgkin's lymphoma is influenced by age at treatment, stage of disease, chemotherapy regimen, and the use of oral contraceptives during therapy: a report from the German Hodgkin's Lymphoma Study Group. *J Clin Oncol.* 2005;23:7555–7564.
15. Hodgson DC, Gilbert ES, Dores GM, et al. Long-term solid cancer risk among 5-year survivors of Hodgkin's lymphoma. *J Clin Oncol.* 2007;25:1489–1497.
16. Travis LB, Hill DA, Dores GM, et al. Breast cancer following radiotherapy and chemotherapy among young women with Hodgkin disease. *JAMA.* 2003;290:465–475.
17. van Leeuwen FE, Klokman WJ, Stovall M, et al. Roles of radiation dose, chemotherapy, and hormonal factors in breast cancer following Hodgkin's disease. *J Natl Cancer Inst.* 2003;95:971–980.
18. Travis LB, Gospodarowicz M, Curtis RE, et al. Lung cancer following chemotherapy and radiotherapy for Hodgkin's disease. *J Natl Cancer Inst.* 2002;94:182–192.
19. Swerdlow AJ, Schoemaker MJ, Allerton R, et al. Lung cancer after Hodgkin's disease: a nested case-control study of the relation to treatment. *J Clin Oncol.* 2001;19:1610–1618.
20. Hancock SL, Tucker MA, Hoppe RT. Factors affecting late mortality from heart disease after treatment of Hodgkin's disease. *JAMA.* 1993;270:1949–1955.
21. Eriksson F, Gagliardi G, Liedberg A, et al. Long-term cardiac mortality following radiation therapy for Hodgkin's disease: analysis with the relative seriality model. *Radiother Oncol.* 2000;55:153–162.
22. Lee CK, Aeppli D, Nierengarten ME. The need for long-term surveillance for patients treated with curative radiotherapy for Hodgkin's disease: University of Minnesota experience. *Int J Radiat Oncol Biol Phys.* 2000;48:169–179.
23. Heidenreich PA, Hancock SL, Lee BK, et al. Asymptomatic cardiac disease following mediastinal irradiation. *J Am Coll Cardiol.* 2003;42:743–749.
24. Adams MJ, Lipsitz SR, Colan SD, et al. Cardiovascular status in long-term survivors of Hodgkin's disease treated with chest radiotherapy. *J Clin Oncol.* 2004;22:3139–3148.
25. Heidenreich PA, Hancock SL, Vagelos RH, et al. Diastolic dysfunction after mediastinal irradiation. *Am Heart J.* 2005;150:977–982.
26. Aviles A, Neri N, Nambo JM, et al. Late cardiac toxicity secondary to treatment in Hodgkin's disease. A study comparing doxorubicin, epirubicin and mitoxantrone in combined therapy. *Leuk Lymphoma.* 2005;46:1023–1028.
27. Hull MC, Morris CG, Pepine CJ, et al. Valvular dysfunction and carotid, subclavian, and coronary artery disease in survivors of hodgkin lymphoma treated with radiation therapy. *JAMA.* 2003;290:2831–2837.
28. Boivin JF, Hutchison GB, Lubin JH, et al. Coronary artery disease mortality in patients treated for Hodgkin's disease. *Cancer.* 1992;69:1241–1247.
29. Hancock SL, Donaldson SS, Hoppe RT. Cardiac disease following treatment of Hodgkin's disease in children and adolescents. *J Clin Oncol.* 1993;11:1208–1215.
30. Glanzmann C, Kaufmann P, Jenni R, et al. Cardiac risk after mediastinal irradiation for Hodgkin's disease. *Radiother Oncol.* 1998;46:51–62.
31. Aleman BM, van den Belt-Dusebout AW, De Bruin ML, et al. Late cardiotoxicity after treatment for Hodgkin lymphoma. *Blood.* 2007;109:1878–1886.
32. Aleman BM, van den Belt-Dusebout AW, Klokman WJ, et al. Long-term cause-specific mortality of patients treated for Hodgkin's disease. *J Clin Oncol.* 2003; 21:3431–3439.
33. Swerdlow AJ, Higgins CD, Smith P, et al. Myocardial infarction mortality risk after treatment for Hodgkin disease: a collaborative British cohort study. *J Natl Cancer Inst.* 2007;99:206–214.
34. Heidenreich PA, Schnittger I, Strauss HW, et al. Screening for coronary artery disease after mediastinal irradiation for Hodgkin's disease. *J Clin Oncol.* 2007;25:43–49.
35. Bowers DC, McNeil DE, Liu Y, et al. Stroke as a late treatment effect of Hodgkin's Disease: a report from the Childhood Cancer Survivor Study. *J Clin Oncol.* 2005;23:6508–6515.
36. Hancock SL, Cox RS, McDougall IR. Thyroid diseases after treatment of Hodgkin's disease. *N Engl J Med.* 1991;325:599–605.
37. Constine LS, Donaldson SS, McDougall IR, et al. Thyroid dysfunction after radiotherapy in children with Hodgkin's disease. *Cancer.* 1984;53:878–883.
38. Sklar C, Whitton J, Mertens A, et al. Abnormalities of the thyroid in survivors of Hodgkin's disease: data from the Childhood Cancer Survivor Study. *J Clin Endocrinol Metab.* 2000;85:3227–3232.
39. Bhatia S, Ramsay NK, Bantle JP, et al. Thyroid Abnormalities after Therapy for Hodgkin's Disease in Childhood. *Oncologist.* 1996;1:62–67.
40. Clifton DK, Bremner WJ. The effect of testicular x-irradiation on spermatogenesis in man. A comparison with the mouse. *J Androl.* 1983;4:387–392.
41. Lushbaugh CC, Casarett GW. The effects of gonadal irradiation in clinical radiation therapy: a review. *Cancer.* 1976;37:1111–1125.
42. Meistrich ML. Effects of chemotherapy and radiotherapy on spermatogenesis. *Eur Urol.* 1993;23:136–141.
43. Ogilvy-Stuart AL, Shalet SM. Effect of radiation on the human reproductive system. *Environ Health Perspect.* 1993;101(suppl 2):109–116.
44. Anselmo AP, Cartoni C, Bellantuono P, et al. Risk of infertility in patients with Hodgkin's disease treated with ABVD vs MOPP vs ABVD/MOPP. *Haematologica.* 1990;75:155–158.
45. van der Kaaij MA, Heutte N, Le Stang N, et al. Gonadal function in males after chemotherapy for early-stage Hodgkin's lymphoma treated in four subsequent trials by the European Organisation for Research and Treatment of Cancer: EORTC Lymphoma Group and the Groupe d'Etude des Lymphomes de l'Adulte. *J Clin Oncol.* 2007;25:2825–2832.
46. Viviani S, Santoro A, Ragni G, et al. Gonadal toxicity after combination chemotherapy for Hodgkin's disease. Comparative results of MOPP vs ABVD. *Eur J Cancer Clin Oncol.* 1985;21:601–605.
47. Sieniawski M, Reineke T, Nogova L, et al. Fertility in male patients with advanced Hodgkin lymphoma treated with BEACOPP: a report of the German Hodgkin Study Group (GHSG). *Blood.* 2008;111:71–76.
48. Williams RS, Littell RD, Mendenhall NP. Laparoscopic oophoropexy and ovarian function in the treatment of Hodgkin disease. *Cancer.* 1999;86:2138–2142.
49. Williams RS, Mendenhall N. Laparoscopic oophoropexy for preservation of ovarian function before pelvic node irradiation. *Obstet Gynecol.* 1992;80:541–543.
50. De Bruin ML, Huisbrink J, Hauptmann M, et al. Treatment-related risk factors for premature menopause following Hodgkin lymphoma. *Blood.* 2008;111:101–108.
51. Hodgson DC, Pintilie M, Gitterman L, et al. Fertility among female hodgkin lymphoma survivors attempting pregnancy following ABVD chemotherapy. *Hematol Oncol.* 2007;25:11–15.

52. Koh ES, Sun A, Tran TH, et al. Clinical dose-volume histogram analysis in predicting radiation pneumonitis in Hodgkin's lymphoma. *Int J Radiat Oncol Biol Phys.* 2006;66:223–228.

53. Noordijk EM, Thomas J, Fermé C, et al. First results of the EORTC-GELA H9 randomized trials: the H9-F trial (comparing 3 radiation dose levels) and H9-U trial (comparing 3 chemotherapy schemes) in patients with favorable or unfavorable early stage Hodgkin's lymphoma (HL). *J Clin Oncol.* 2005;23:6505a.

54. Girinsky T, van der Maazen R, Specht L, et al. Involved-node radiotherapy (INRT) in patients with early Hodgkin lymphoma: concepts and guidelines. *Radiother Oncol.* 2006;79:270–277.

55. Girinsky T, Ghalibafian M. Radiation treatment in non Hodgkin's lymphomas: present and future directions. *Cancer Radiother.* 2005;9:422–426.

56. Ghalibafian M, Beaudre A, Girinsky T. Heart and coronary artery protection in patients with mediastinal Hodgkin lymphoma treated with intensity-modulated radiotherapy: dose constraints to virtual volumes or to organs at risk? *Radiother Oncol.* 2008;87:82–88.

CHAPTER

# 23

# Peritoneal Surface Malignancies

## A Real Challenge for Surgeons

François Noël Gilly

As far as peritoneal carcinomatosis are concerned, they were regarded as a situation only to be palliated. In the 1980s, some surgeons, in Japan, France and US, decided to develop new therapeutic approaches, combining major surgical resections and intraperitoneal chemohyperthermia. They were first regarded as "dreamers," and almost 20 years were necessary for cytoreductive surgery and hyperthermic intraperitoneal chemotherapy (HIPEC) to be considered as a "gold standard treatment" for colorectal carcinomatosis, pseudomyxoma peritonei, and peritoneal mesothelioma.

In 2009, numerous centers all over the world are dealing with peritoneal surface malignancies, and the new "challenge" is now a surgical one: the first international registration[1] and all the phase II and III trials clearly demonstrated that the completeness of cytoreduction was the key point for the survival results. In other words, we still need more trials to evaluate the real place of HIPEC in this therapeutic strategy, but we already know how important is the surgeon in the treatment of peritoneal surface malignancies.

Another challenge will be the diffusion of the results of the "French speaking network registration on peritoneal surface malignancies treatment": from this large registration (more than 1200 patients treated by cytoreductive surgery and HIPEC), it was strongly demonstrated that the mortality, the morbidity, and the survival results were strongly influenced by the experience of the center. As usual, it is not easy for surgeons to meet a patient and then, to refer him to another surgeon, in another center. However, because of the complexity of cytoreductive surgery and HIPEC, the necessity of a multidisciplinary team, and the specificity of immediate postoperative period, it is an evidence that only experienced centers should go on dealing with such treatment programs.

At least, numerous researches have to been designed: clinical trials with new intra peritoneal drugs, combination of HIPEC with new targeted therapies, new morphologic exams to assess more accurately preoperatively the carcinomatosis extent, and biomolecular screening to select more precise prognostic factors. Twenty years were necessary to come from the "dreamers" to the "evidence." Twenty years will be necessary to go to the final goal: the cure of peritoneal surface malignancies.

## REFERENCE

1. Glehen O, Kwiatkowski F, Sugarbaker PH, et al. Cytoreductive surgery combined with perioperative intraperitoneal chemotherapy for the management of peritoneal carcinomatosis from colorectal cancer. A multi-institutional study of 506 patients. *J Clin Oncol.* 2004;22:3284–3292.

# Progress in the Management of Carcinomatosis

Paul H. Sugarbaker

This special issue of *The Cancer Journal* originated in Lyon, France, November 17 to 19, 2008. This was the 6th Biannual Meeting of the Peritoneal Surface Oncology Group International. The topics for presentation and their authorship were chosen by Olivier Glehen and myself at that time.

It was most appropriate that the biannual meeting in 2008 would be held in France. With the French-speaking consortium that has been engineered Dominique Elias, Francois Gilly, and Olivier Glehen, an effort to optimally manage peritoneal surface malignancy within France has occurred over the last decade that, in my opinion, has reached epic proportion.

The French group has published their own monograph, "*Monographies de L'association Francaise de Chirurgie*" to summarize their accomplishments.[1] Not only has laboratory and clinical research excelled within this French-speaking group but also benefits to patients have been forthcoming. In France, the treatment of colorectal and appendiceal dissemination of cancer to the peritoneal surfaces is treated using cytoreductive surgery (CRS) and heated intraperitoneal chemotherapy (HIPEC) as a standard of care fully funded by the French Health Care System. Not just some but all French people have these treatment modalities available to them. Congratulations to the efforts of Gilly, Glehen, and Elias!

The first meeting of the Peritoneal Surface Oncology Group International was a humble one that occurred in London at The Royal College of Surgeons in 1998. Professor Bill Heald and myself organized this international effort to share thoughts on the prevention and treatment of peritoneal dissemination of gastrointestinal cancer. Approximately 30 speakers and participants were there to enter into the presentations and discussions. Since then, the biannual meeting has become more popular. Figure 1 shows the gradual progression of the interest in peritoneal surface oncology from 1998 through 2008. Over these 10 years, a profound change in the attitudes of oncologists toward peritoneal dissemination of colorectal and appendiceal cancer has occurred. The next meeting will be in Uppsala, Sweden on September 8 to 10, 2010.

The fact that CRS plus HIPEC has reached the level of "standard of care" supported by national guidelines is also presented in the manuscript by Vic J. Verwaal. He presents the long-term experience in the management of colorectal carcinomatosis that started at the Netherlands Cancer Institute under the direction of Frans Zoetmulder and now continues throughout Holland carefully shepherded along by Vic J. Verwaal. The commitment to an optimized nationwide program in the management of carcinomatosis available to all Dutch people is clearly evident in the presentation of Dr. Verwaal.

The program in Spain, Italy, Belgium, Germany, and Scandinavia is strong and rapidly progressing. Perhaps, at this point in time not as well organized as in France and the Netherlands but nevertheless growing on a regular basis.

In the United States, the efforts to develop centers of excellence for the management of peritoneal carcinomatosis have continued to prosper. Pittsburgh, Pennsylvania, Washington, DC, Winston-Salem, North Carolina, Omaha, Nebraska, and Houston, Texas have established centers with experienced surgeons directing the programs. The interest in medical oncologists in referral of colorectal and appendiceal cancer patients with carcinomatosis has increased substantially. The realization that evidence-based medicine supports CRS and HIPEC for carcinomatosis, and that systemic chemotherapy using FOLFOX and Avastin cannot be supported by the literature has led to this "cytoreduction reversal." The wonderful article in the *Journal of Clinical Oncology* by Sanoff et al[2] clearly shows the benefits of oxaliplatin-based chemotherapy for colorectal cancer patients who have objective evidence of their metastatic disease. Unfortunately, with carcinomatosis, there usually is no objective radiologic evidence of disease progression or regression by radiologic studies. To my knowledge, not a single carcinomatosis patient is included in the review of Sanoff et al. There is no evidence that systemic chemotherapy is of benefit to patients with colorectal or appendiceal carcinomatosis.

On the other hand, CRS plus HIPEC has an abundance of data to support its general usage as a standard of care with support from national guidelines. The registry report by Glehen et al, (N = 506) the randomized controlled study reported by Verwaal et al, the French registry of patients (N = 484), the Dutch registry reported in this issue of *The Cancer Journal* by Verwaal (N = 562), the systematic

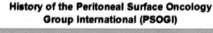

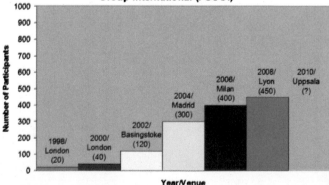

Note: PSOGI in Japanese means clear

**FIGURE 1.** Increasing interest generated in the study of carcinomatosis by the Peritoneal Surface Oncology Group International over a single decade.

review by Yan et al, and approximately 30 phase II studies from single institutions from all over the world all point to CRS plus HIPEC as a standard of care for colorectal and appendiceal malignancy.[3–6] Much has been accomplished, and yet much work needs to be done.

## REFERENCES

1. Elias D, Gilly F, Glehen O. Carcinoses peritoneales d'origine digestive et primitive. Monographies de L'association Francaise de Chirurgie. France: Walters Kluwer; 2008.
2. Sanoff HK, Sargent DJ, Campbell ME, et al. Five-year data and prognostic factor analysis of oxaliplatin and irinotecan combinations for advanced colorectal cancer: N9741. *J Clin Oncol.* 2008;26:5721–5727.
3. Glehen O, Kwiatkowski F, Sugarbaker PH, et al. Cytoreductive surgery combined with perioperative intraperitoneal chemotherapy for the management of peritoneal carcinomatosis from colorectal cancer: a multi-institutional study. *J Clin Oncol.* 2004;22:3284–3292.
4. Verwaal VJ, van Ruth S, de Bree E, et al. Randomized trial of cytoreduction and hyperthermic intraperitoneal chemotherapy versus systemic chemotherapy and palliative surgery in patients with peritoneal carcinomatosis of colorectal cancer. *J Clin Oncol.* 2003;21:3737–3743.
5. Verwaal VJ. Long-term results of cytoreduction and HIPEC followed by systemic chemotherapy. *Cancer J.* 2009;15:212–215.
6. Yan TD, Black D, Savady R, et al. Systematic review on the efficacy of cytoreductive surgery combined with perioperative intraperitoneal chemotherapy for peritoneal carcinomatosis from colorectal carcinoma. *J Clin Oncol.* 2006;24:4011–4019.

# Imaging of Peritoneal Carcinomatosis

Santiago González-Moreno • Luis González-Bayón • Gloria Ortega-Pérez • Concepción González-Hernando

Peritoneal seeding is a well-known mechanism of spread in advanced gastrointestinal and gynecological malignancies, but it may also occur as a manifestation of primary peritoneal neoplasms. The last few decades have witnessed a revolution in the conception and management of peritoneal surface malignancies. We have learnt that prognosis is not uniformly pessimistic for patients with this kind of diseases and that, where only palliative treatments and comfort measures were contemplated, nowadays selected cases may benefit from a radical locoregional approach aiming at long-term disease control.

Imaging studies used routinely in the cancer patient have an important role in the assessment of peritoneal tumor spread, from the initial diagnosis to the evaluation of disease volume and distribution that may help select those patients who will benefit from an aggressive treatment that combines cytoreductive surgery (CRS) with perioperative intraperitoneal chemotherapy (PIC). For this purpose, a close correlation between radiologic and actual surgical findings would be ideal and desirable but reality is that, despite significant technological advances, accuracy of peritoneal neoplastic disease detection by the current imaging studies is not optimal.[1]

Surgical and medical oncologists treating these patients need to be aware of the imaging manifestations of peritoneal carcinomatosis and of the limitations of clinicoradiologic correlation in this scenario. Despite these, dedicated and motivated radiologists can make the most out of the different imaging modalities currently available, offering invaluable information to be incorporated to a therapeutic decision-making process. This article will describe the imaging findings in patients with peritoneal carcinomatosis and their application in clinical practice, focusing in their role in the selection of patients for CRS and PIC.

## DIAGNOSTIC IMAGING OPTIONS IN PERITONEAL CARCINOMATOSIS

### Abdominopelvic Ultrasonography

Abdominopelvic Ultrasonography is often one of the first diagnostic tests in patients with a clinical suspicion of peritoneal carcinomatosis. It is innocuous for the patient because no radiation is delivered. It easily detects peritoneal fluid and may also depict peritoneal implants. However, it is a recognized operator-dependent technique and a careful evaluation of all peritoneal-bearing structures searching for peritoneal disease, which can be time consuming.

### Computed Tomography

Computed tomography (CT) is undoubtedly the most used imaging modality in the evaluation of peritoneal carcinomatosis. It uses x-ray technology. For an adequate yield, administration of intravenous contrast and a large volume of oral contrast are mandatory. Rectal contrast may be used as well for opacification of the large bowel,[2] also allowing for additional individualization of structures in the pelvis. CT scanning technology has significantly evolved over the last few years, arriving to the current state-of-the-art, thin-slice, helical, multidetector machines that offer an improved spatial resolution (a few millimeters) with the possibility of multiplanar (axial, coronal, sagital) or tridimensional reconstructions and a short-image acquisition time. A standard contrast-enhanced CT scan ordered for evaluation of a patient with peritoneal carcinomatosis should include thorax, abdomen, and pelvis. An important advantage to bear in mind is that most clinicians are familiarized with the basic interpretation and reading of CT scan-obtained images.

It has been shown that CT scan accuracy for the detection of peritoneal mucinous lesions varies with their location within the abdomen, being greatest in the gutters, over the free surface of spleen and liver, and less favorable in the pelvis and midabdomen. Tumor nodule size influences sensitivity as well, ranging from 25% for lesions smaller than 0.5 cm to 90% for nodules more than 5 cm in size.[2]

An additional feature influencing the ability of CT to detect peritoneal disease lies in the morphology of the peritoneal lesions. Because CT scan detects variations in shapes and volumes, disease that layers out contouring the shape of normal intraabdominal structures is almost impossible to be depicted, compared with nodular lesions with a defined volume, which are readily demonstrated if their size is above the spatial resolution of the test (Fig. 1).

Of note, de Bree et al[3] report a wide interobserver variability among radiologists in the interpretation of CT scans of patients with peritoneal carcinomatosis of colorectal origin. This variability affects the detection rate of peritoneal disease in general (60% vs. 76%), of small size tumor nodules (9% vs. 24% for lesions smaller than 1 cm), and of lesions on the small bowel and its mesentery, of crucial importance in establishing a surgical indication.

### Magnetic Resonance Imaging

Magnetic resonance imaging (MRI) uses the effect of a strong magnetic field on tissue protons spin motion, resulting in a superior soft tissue contrast compared with CT scan. Intravenous administration of gadolinium has an image-enhancing effect with a dynamic pattern that is characteristic of malignant tissues. Compared with CT scan, MRI acquisition time is somewhat longer and more influenced by respiratory movement artifacts, its spatial resolution is lower, and clinicians find it harder to interpret. It also offers multiplanar and tridimensional reconstructions but, additionally, can obtain differential imaging by manipulation of the signal (T1–T2).

Because peritoneal carcinomatosis lesions sit on soft tissues, it seems logical that it should be an ideal technique to evaluate this disease. Evaluation of peritoneal disease requires fat-suppressed, gadolinium-enhanced, spoiled gradient-echo sequences.[4] Some of the

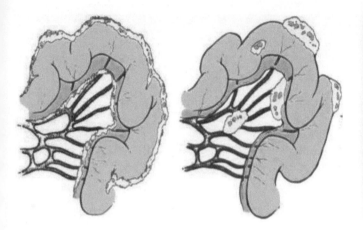

**Layered**                    **Nodular**

**FIGURE 1.** Morphology of peritoneal implants affecting their detection by CT. Layered implants (higher grade, non-mucinous, and invasive lesions) conform the normal shape of abdominal structures and cannot be depicted by CT scan, whereas nodular implants (lower grade, mucinous, and non-invasive lesions) alter that shape making them apparent by this imaging technique. Modified with permission from Paul H. Sugarbaker, MD.

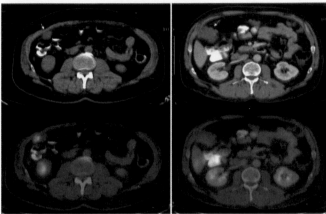

**FIGURE 2.** Peritoneal implants appearance by PET-CT (pointed by arrows) in 2 patients with peritoneal carcinomatosis of colorectal origin. CT scan images are shown above and PET-CT fusion images are shown below. Moderate to high-grade peritoneal lesions may show an increased [18]Fluoro deoxyglucose uptake (left) unless they are mucinous in nature (right). Courtesy of Instituto Tecnológico PET, Madrid, Spain.

aforementioned differences with CT scanning may have contributed to its being less used or less popular for this application, but definitive differential advantages should bring it to a higher rank in peritoneal carcinomatosis evaluation. In a comparative study reported by Low[5] using CT and MRI, the latter showed a significantly improved sensitivity for depicting tumor involving the peritoneum and the intestinal tract. The same author reports on the ability of MRI to depict subtle peritoneal implants, an important feature that constitutes a weakness of CT scanning. Moreover, in patients with moderate to high-volume ascites, it allows for a good evaluation of the parietal or visceral peritoneum covered by fluid, which is not possible with a CT scan.[4]

## [18]Fluoro Deoxyglucose Positron Emission Tomography

[18]Fluoro deoxyglucose positron emission tomography (PET) has revolutionized oncology practice in the last decade. It uses nuclear medicine to provide a metabolic-functional assessment of lesions by measuring the selective uptake of the intravenously administered radiotracer [18]Fluoro deoxyglucose (increased in malignant tissues). Its poor anatomic resolution can be overcome by combining it with a CT scan obtained at the same time (PET-CT) and using image fusion software. The CT scan part of a PET-CT is usually performed without contrast. However, by administering oral and intravenous contrast, we can significantly improve the anatomic resolution and location of malignant lesions pointed out by the PET scan, and thus prevent the patient from having an additional contrast-enhanced CT scan, resulting in patient satisfaction, and cost-efficiency. It is important to know that PET scan may not detect low-grade malignant tumors, and that it can have false-positive results in cases of acute inflammation or active tissue repair, ie, after surgery. Very pertinent to peritoneal carcinomatosis, mucinous tumors do not show activity in PET and therefore are not indicated in these cases (Fig. 2).

## IMAGING CHARACTERIZATION OF PERITONEAL CARCINOMATOSIS

International consensus achieved through a Delphi methodology in Milan in 2006 was unanimous in considering contrast-enhanced, multidetector CT scan of the thorax, abdomen, and pelvis, the procedure of choice in the evaluation of patients for CRS combined with PIC.[6] MRI and PET-CT were considered useful but not fundamental. The assessment of peritoneal disease by CT scan needs to be done in a systematic fashion based on the knowledge of the pathobiology of the disease (histologic grade, biologic aggressiveness, mucinous features, ability to cause distant metastases, or retroperitoneal lymphatic spread) and of the mechanisms of peritoneal spread (peritoneal fluid circulation, "redistribution phenomenon," and gravity distribution) (Table 1).[7]

Free fluid is one of the classic signs of peritoneal carcinomatosis. Ascitic fluid can be seen only in dependent parts like the Douglas pouch if its volume is low or also surrounding the liver, spleen, and filling both gutters if it is more abundant. Free mucus appears hypodense, with a similar distribution and may be interpreted as fluid, although both show differences in attenuation values.

The greater omental fat, in its disposition under the anterolateral parietal peritoneum, can appear stranded or nodular in cases of low to moderate involvement, or conforming a dense omental cake of variable thickness when completely replaced by tumor (Fig. 3). The parietal peritoneum can appear just enhanced by contrast or irregular, thickened, and with associated implants of variable size.

The epigastric region has to be systematically and thoroughly evaluated for its crucial surgical implications, described later (Fig. 4). Structures or areas to be specifically assessed are the lesser omentum (hepatogastric area), the main part of the omental bursa (area between the posterior surface of stomach and the anterior surface of the pancreas), its subpyloric recess[8] (cul-de-sac and most dependent part of the omental bursa), its superior recess (posterior to the caudate process of the liver, between the inferior vena cava and the right diaphragmatic crus), and the liver hylar region.

**TABLE 1.** Elements to Be Assessed in a Systematic Reading of a CT Scan in a Patient With Peritoneal Surface Malignancy Being Evaluated for Cytoreductive Surgery

1. Distant disease sites: liver parenchyma/lungs/pleurae/mediastinum
2. Free fluid or free mucus: presence or absence, volume and distribution
3. Greater omentum
4. Parietal peritoneum (anterior/lateral/pelvic)
5. Right diaphragmatic peritoneum—liver surface
6. Left diaphragmatic peritoneum—splenic surface
7. Epigastrium
   - Lesser omentum (hepato-gastric ligament)
   - Omental bursa
   - Superior recess of omental bursa
   - Subpyloric space
   - Porta hepatis and gallblader
8. Small bowel and small bowel mesentery
9. Large bowel
10. Specific bowel areas
    - Terminal ileum—ileocecal region
    - Rectosigmoid junction
    - Ligament of Treitz—first jejunal loop
11. Pelvis
    - Cul-de-sac of Douglas (relationship with rectum/bladder/uterus)
    - Ovaries (female)
    - Lymphadenopathy (iliac/obturator)
12. Retroperitoneum
    - Lymphadenopathy (paraaortic, paracaval, interaortocaval)
    - Ureters

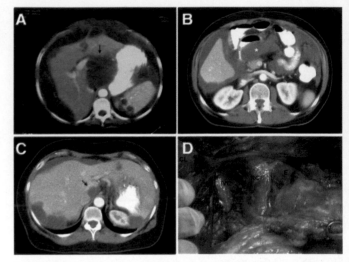

**FIGURE 4.** CT characterization of possible lesions in the epigastric region in mucinous peritoneal carcinomatosis. A, A mucinous mass (arrow) replacing the lesser omentum. B, Mucinous tumor (asterisk) filling the subpyloric space, narrowing the gastric outlet and first duodenal portion. Note the contrast administered per rectum filling the descending colon, anterior to left kidney. In both the cases, a total gastrectomy was needed to clear the tumor. C, CT appearance of a mucinous tumor nodule dwelling in the superior recess of the omental bursa (arrow), with its actual correlation in the surgical field shown to the right (D). The resected tumor can be seen in the right lower corner of the picture, held by a ring forceps, and still attached at its base. Note the classic scalloping of the liver surface by the mucinous tumor in A and C. CL indicates caudate process of liver, reflected up; IVC, inferior vena cava; RC, right diaphragmatic crus; E, esophagus.

Throughout the abdomen and pelvis, mucinous implants can be seen individually or as confluent hypodense lesions. When located between the diaphragmatic peritoneum and the liver or the spleen, the classic "scalloping" of the liver or splenic surfaces can be noticed (Fig. 4).

The appearance of the small bowel and its mesentery needs special attention. Heavy mesenteric involvement causes rigidity and retraction, drawing the bowel loops together against the posterior abdomen, whereas a healthy, elastic small bowel mesentery allows for

a free spread of bowel loops, which in cases with ascites float freely close to the anterior abdominal wall in a "fan-like" configuration (Figs. 5A, B). Yan et al[9] described and classified in 3 categories (classes I, II, and III), the CT appearance of the small bowel and its mesentery in 30 cases of peritoneal mesothelioma. This classification can be extrapolated to other instances of peritoneal carcinomatosis and can be instrumental in surgical decision making and clinical research. A more specific description on bowel and mesenteric CT findings and their influence on surgical planning can be found later. The large bowel may similarly show wall enhancement or increased thickness, associated nodules or masses, or changes in bowel diameter, or in mesenteric fat density. Especial attention should be directed to the ileocecal area, the rectosigmoid colon, and the ligament of Treitz, being preferential areas of involvement in peritoneal carcinomatosis.

The pelvis is a commonly involved area when peritoneal seeding occurs. The Douglas pouch appearance may vary from containing only fluid or mucus to harboring tumor nodules or masses that may secondarily involve by infiltration or just compress the urinary bladder, the rectum, or the uterus. In the female patient, ovaries involved by surface disease (Krukenberg phenomenon) may appear uni- or bilaterally enlarged to a variable size (including massively enlarged ovaries that extend into the lower or mid abdomen) with a mixture of hyper and hypodense areas (Fig. 6).

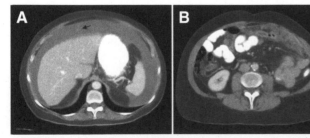

**FIGURE 3.** CT signs of peritoneal carcinomatosis. A, Ascitic fluid surrounding the liver and the spleen may be present and constitutes a classic sign. Note the falciform ligament of the liver as a thin white line (arrow) stretched by the fluid. B, A typical omental cake is apparent mostly in the left hemiabdomen, underneath the abdominal wall.

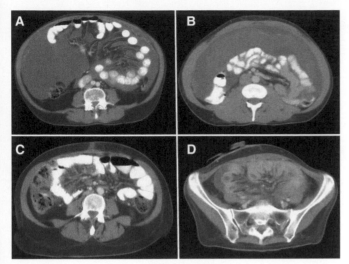

**FIGURE 5.**    CT appearance of the small bowel in peritoneal carcinomatosis. A, Small bowel loops floating in ascitic fluid close to the anterior abdominal wall with a visible, stretched "fan-like" mesentery in a patient with peritoneal mesothelioma (class I of Yan et al[9]). B, Small bowel loops centrally and posteriorly retracted in a patient with signet-ring mucinous peritoneal carcinomatosis of appendiceal origin. Despite the contribution of a pressing omental cake in this configuration, a foreshortened, retracted small bowel mesentery by high-grade disease is to be expected. C, A diseased small bowel mesentery can be noted in this patient with peritoneal carcinomatosis of colorectal origin, expressed by loss of fat clarity, presence of nodularity, and fat stranding (class II of Yan et al[9]). The irregular small bowel surface contour may indicate serosal involvement. D, Enhanced wall thickening of cross-sectioned small bowel loops with loss of the normal architecture and matting along with near obliteration of mesenteric fat (class III of Yan et al[9]) in a patient with peritoneal carcinomatosis of gastric origin.

In gynecologic malignancy, and less frequently in gastrointestinal tumors, pelvic and retroperitoneal lymph node bearing areas (iliac, obturator, paraaortic, para caval, aortocaval) have to be scrutinized in search for lymphadenopathy. Also in the retroperitoneum, ureters need to be assessed for changes in diameter that may indicate urinary obstruction.

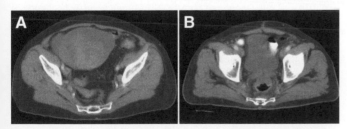

**FIGURE 6.**    CT imaging of the pelvis in mucinous peritoneal carcinomatosis of colorectal origin. A, A female patient with an enlarged 13 cm right ovary (asterisk) replaced by mucinous tumor (Krukenberg phenomenon). B, Pictures a male patient with a mucinous mass (arrow) sitting at the bottom of a low-lying Douglas pouch, infiltrating the anterior rectal wall posteriorly and contacting the seminal vesicles anteriorly; at surgery these were found infiltrated by the tumor as well.

## THE ROLE OF DIAGNOSTIC IMAGING IN THE SELECTION OF PATIENTS FOR CRS AND PIC

CRS combined with PIC has resulted in improved long-term disease control rates in selected patients with peritoneal surface malignancy of various origins, previously considered only for palliative treatment approaches.[10–13] A complete cytoreduction, defined as residual disease volume under 2.5 mm in greatest dimension,[14] is the most important prognostic factor accounting for improved survival in these diseases. Therefore, indications for this procedure revolve around the likelihood to achieve this surgical goal. Generally, peritoneal disease that can be completely resected by a combination of peritonectomy procedures and visceral resections, in a fit patient cleared to undergo major surgery under general anesthesia with no distant disease spread constitute the basis to consider a patient as a candidate for this procedure. Therefore, the role of imaging in the patient selection process is aimed at ruling out extraperitoneal disease involvement, assessing peritoneal disease volume and distribution as a guide for surgical planning, and evaluating possible signs that may preclude the achievement of a complete cytoreduction.

### Evaluation of Extraperitoneal Disease

Distant disease, ie, secondary deposits developed by hematogonous spread or lymphatic dissemination beyond the regional basins, constitutes a contraindication for CRS in a patient with peritoneal carcinomatosis. This includes liver metastases, retroperitoneal lymphadenopathy, and thoracic involvement (lung, pleura, mediastinum). This is the reason why imaging studies performed in a patient under evaluation for CRS and PIC should include the thorax, abdomen, and pelvis. Liver metastases have traditionally been a contraindication, but recent studies have challenged this criterion in the cases of colorectal peritoneal carcinomatosis with a limited number of resectable lesions.[15] Retroperitoneal lymph node involvement (Fig. 7B) can be considered a systemic equivalent of disease in gastrointestinal cancer, whereas in gynecological cancer, it constitutes a more direct, regional form of spread, therefore not a contraindication per se for CRS.

Good quality contrast-enhanced CT scan is routinely used for this purpose. Hepatic, pleural, pulmonary (Fig. 7A), mediastinal, or retroperitoneal (Fig. 7B) involvement are easily identified by this technique if the lesion size falls within the limits of the spatial resolution of this technique. Comparison with previous studies is mandatory. The additional functional information provided by PET or PET-CT scan

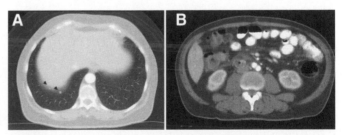

**FIGURE 7.**    Role of CT scan in the assessment of distant disease in peritoneal carcinomatosis of colorectal origin. A, Two small lung metastases (arrowheads) are visible in the right lower lobe not visible by plain chest x-ray film. The complete thoracic CT showed a total of 10 similar lesions distributed in both lungs. The peritoneal disease was considered resectable a priori by CT, but the patient was turned down for CRS. B, Three centimeter retroperitoneal adenopathy (asterisk), PET positive, can be seen in this patient lying anterior to the inferior vena cava and posterior to the caudalmost tip of the third duodenal portion.

can be very useful in cases of doubtful lesions or even in the detection of subtle metastases not depicted by a change in CT morphology, being aware of the limitations of PET. The detection of extraperitoneal disease is currently the main reason for using PET in these patients.

## Evaluation of Peritoneal Disease: Surgical Planning

Peritoneal disease volume, its localization, and distribution are important pieces of information that can influence therapeutic decision making and help in planning a surgical cytoreductive procedure. Quantitative scoring systems such as the peritoneal cancer index[16] that ranges between 0 and 39 are useful tools that can be used for this assessment. For this purpose there is no doubt that CT scan is the current standard that cannot be matched at this time (even less so improved) by PET or PET-CT. In a study correlating the findings of CT, PET-CT, and surgery, the correlation between CT and surgical findings was moderate, whereas that of PET/CT and surgery was low.[17] Underestimation of peritoneal disease extent occurred in 80% of the cases with PET-CT. Therefore, PET or PET-CT scan should not be ordered at the present time with the only aim in mind to evaluate peritoneal disease.

However, one must bear in mind that CT scan underestimates peritoneal disease burden as well in up to 70% of the cases,[17] especially in invasive, nonmucinous tumors (Fig. 8). de Bree et al considered CT scan of limited value in the selection of patients with peritoneal carcinomatosis of colorectal or appendiceal origin for CRS because of interobserver variability. High-peritoneal cancer index at surgical exploration (it has been suggested that over 20 in colorectal cancer and over 10 in gastric cancer) may make a complete cytoreduction unfeasible. Therefore, a peritoneal disease burden already elevated in a CT scan may be an indicator of caution when considering the indication of a cytoreductive procedure. This is not the case in noninvasive processes such as pseudomyxoma peritonei (disseminated peritoneal adenomucinosis), low-grade sarcomatosis, or low-grade or cystic peritoneal mesothelioma, where widespread, voluminous disease can be completely cytoreduced.

Certain findings in a preoperative CT scan will assist the surgeon in the design of a cytoreductive procedure, who in turn will be able to help the patient understand the possible extent of the surgery and prepare for it. Disease around the spleen or in the splenic hylum indicates that a splenectomy is needed, and preoperative vaccinations

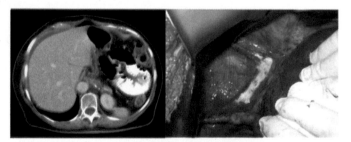

**FIGURE 8.** Underestimation of peritoneal involvement by CT scan in peritoneal carcinomatosis of colorectal origin. CT scan shows a thin rim of perihepatic fluid and an apparently normal, thin, contrast-enhanced right hemidiaphragm. Surgical exploration unexpectedly revealed the pictured whitish plaque of tumor infiltrating the diaphragm in its full thickness (an example of layered disease configuration, as per Fig. 1). Note that this disease location is determined by "gravity distribution," being at the posterior, most dependent portion of the right subphrenic space. An unplanned right partial diaphragmatic resection was required to clear this disease.

for encapsulated bacteria can be provided. Subpyloric space involvement, a large mass in the lesser omentum or in the epigastric region or encasement of the stomach by tumor may indicate the need of a gastric resection, either partial or total. The surgeon's eye should also look for signs of disease in the superior recess of the omental bursa, because it can be easily overlooked and dissection in this area can be challenging. Pelvic and adnexal involvement mark the need for a total abdominal hysterectomy plus bilateral salpingo-oophorectomy, a fact that needs to be specifically addressed with women in child-bearing age. Retroperitoneal tumor implants can be seen in cases that have undergone previous incomplete surgical interventions that have violated the posterior peritoneal lining; in these cases, nodules or masses associated with the ureters and causing proximal ureteral dilatation can be detected. If unilateral, this does not constitute an absolute contraindication for CRS per se, but its detection in preoperative CT scan calls for the availability of expert urological help during the surgical procedure, should this be needed.

## Imaging Indicators of Unresectable Disease

Disease in the small bowel and small bowel mesentery constitutes a sentinel, limiting criterion in the decision-making process involved in CRS. Enough small bowel needs to remain in place to allow for an adequate oral nutrition in the future. Therefore, the evaluation of small bowel loops and their mesentery is a crucial component in the preoperative imaging assessment of a patient with peritoneal carcinomatosis. In a CT scan, this requires maximal luminal filling with contrast. We will look for nodules or masses associated or protruding into the bowel surface, bowel surface irregularities (Fig. 5C), bowel wall thickening (Fig. 5D), changes in bowel diameter, and possible air-fluid levels that may indicate segmental obstruction. The mesenteric fat and the mesenteric vessels contained within need to be carefully assessed as well (Fig. 5C). Diffuse loss of mesenteric fat clarity, mesenteric retraction causing foreshortening, associated nodules or masses (sometimes reported as "mesenteric lymphadenopathy"), and/or loss of the mesenteric vessel normal configuration or architecture are signs of involvement. Experience tells us that even the most sophisticated CT technology usually underestimates actual small bowel involvement revealed at surgical exploration. In a study of 30 cases by Dromain et al, CT scan detected small bowel implants in 26% of the cases, whereas the actual incidence of this type of disease location found at surgery was 83%.

Jacquet et al[18] reported in 1995 that CT signs of segmental bowel obstruction and the presence of tumor nodules over 0.5 cm in the small bowel surface exclusive of the terminal ileum were associated with an 88% chance of arriving to an incomplete cytoreduction, whereas the absence of both features predicted a 92% chance of achieving a complete cytoreduction in patients with mucinous peritoneal carcinomatosis. Similarly, Yan et al[9] described that the presence of an epigastric mass greater than 5 cm in diameter in CT scan and signs of heavy small bowel involvement (referred to as "class III" small bowel configuration) were markers of unresectable disease in patents with diffuse malignant peritoneal mesothelioma, leading to an 100% probability of incomplete cytoreduction when both features were present.

MRI has been reported to be superior to CT scan in the assessment of the intestinal tract and mesenteric involvement, in light of its differential ability to evaluate soft tissue changes[5] Given the limiting nature of diffuse small bowel involvement in a patient candidate for CRS and its underestimation by CT scan, it may be worthwhile using MRI for this purpose in cases of unconfirmed clinical or radiologic suspicion of diffuse small bowel involvement or in patients with a borderline surgical indication.

Disease located in and around the porta hepatis in cases of peritoneal carcinomatosis with invasive clinical and histologic features will preclude the consecution of a complete cytoreduction, and therefore it is a contraindication for the procedure. However, lesions at this location of noninvasive nature such as diffuse peritoneal adenomucinosis or low-grade peritoneal mesothelioma can often be stripped away.

## CONCLUSIONS AND SUMMARY

Limitations of currently available imaging modalities for peritoneal surface malignancy do not allow us to accurately predict whether a complete cytoreduction will be achieved in an individual patient. However, imaging studies provide crucial information that, considered together with other clinical and pathologic features, will help us decide which patient should be offered a surgical exploration with a cytoreductive intent. Close interaction and cooperation between surgical oncologists and radiologists is of utmost importance in this regard. Dedicated, motivated radiologists are required to obtain the most precise and clinically useful readings.

Contrast-enhanced, multidetector CT scan of the thorax, abdomen, and pelvis is the current imaging standard to evaluate these patients for surgery. This study should be obtained within the month before the planned surgical date and not earlier. It offers a reasonable sensitivity for the detection of peritoneal carcinomatosis but an underestimation of peritoneal disease burden, a reasonable detection of extraperitoneal disease, identification of key features that may preclude a complete cytoreduction, and orientation in planning the surgical procedure. Reading of a CT scan in these cases should be done in a systematic fashion.

Gadolimiun-enhanced, fat-suppressed MRI is a good imaging complement to CT scan for the detection of subtle peritoneal, mesenteric, or bowel surface disease, especially in patients with ascites. It may be determinant in cases of dubious CT scan findings. Its integration in peritoneal surface malignancy practices is encouraged but is yet to occur. The role of PET-CT is limited to the detection of extraperitoneal disease, and its role in the evaluation of peritoneal disease extent is marginal.

## REFERENCES

1. Frangioni JV. New technologies for human cancer imaging. *J Clin Oncol.* 2008;26:4012–4021.
2. Archer A, Sugarbaker PH, Jelinek JS. Radiology of peritoneal carcinomatosis. *Cancer Treat Res.* 1996;82:263–288.
3. de Bree E, Koops W, Kröger R, et al. Peritoneal carcinomatosis from colorectal or appendiceal origin: correlation of preoperative CT with intraoperative findings and evaluation of interobserver agreement. *J Surg Oncol.* 2004;86: 64–73.
4. Low RN. Magnetic resonance imaging in the oncology patient: evaluation of the extrahepatic abdomen. *Semin Ultrasound CT MR.* 2005;26:224–236.
5. Low RN. Extrahepatic abdominal imaging in patients with malignancy: comparison of MR imaging and helical CT in 164 Patients. *J Magn Reson Imaging.* 2000;12:269–277.
6. Yan TD, Morris DL, Kusamura S, et al. Preoperative investigations in the management of peritoneal surface malignancy with cytoredutive surgery and perioperative intraperitoneal chemotherapy: expert consensus statement. *J Surg Oncol.* 2008;98:224–227.
7. Sugarbaker PH. Observations concerning cancer spread within the peritoneal cavity and concepts supporting an ordered pathophysiology. *Cancer Treat Res.* 1996;82:79–100.
8. Sugarbaker PH. The subpyloric space; an important surgical and radiologic feature in pseudomyxoma peritonei. *Eur J Surg Oncol.* 2002;28:443–446.
9. Yan TD, Haveric N, Carmignani CP, et al. Abdominal computed tomography scans in the selection of patients with malignant peritoneal mesothelioma for comprehensive treatment with cytoreductive surgery and perioperative intraperitoneal chemotherapy. *Cancer.* 2005;103:839–849.
10. Yan TD, Welch L, Black D, et al. A systematic review on the efficacy of cytoreductive surgery combined with perioperative intraperitoneal chemotherapy for diffuse malignancy peritoneal mesothelioma. *Ann Oncol.* 2007;18:827–834.
11. Yan TD, Black D, Savady R, et al. A systematic review on the efficacy of cytoreductive surgery and perioperative intraperitoneal chemotherapy for pseudomyxoma peritonei. *Ann Surg Oncol.* 2007;14:484–492.
12. Yan TD, Black D, Savady R, et al. Systematic review on the efficacy of cytoreductive surgery combined with perioperative intraperitoneal chemotherapy for peritoneal carcinomatosis from colorectal carcinoma. *J Clin Oncol.* 2006; 24:4011–4019.
13. Yonemura Y, Bando E, Kawamura T, et al. Cytoreduction and intraperitoneal chemotherapy for carcinomatosis from gastric cancer. *Cancer Treat Res.* 2007;134:357–373.
14. González-Moreno S, Kusamura S, Baratti D, et al. Postoperative residual disease evaluation in the locoregional treatment of peritoneal surface malignancy. *J Surg Oncol.* 2008;98:237–241.
15. Elias D, Benizri E, Pocard M, et al. Treatment of synchronous peritoneal carcinomatosis and liver metastases from colorectal cancer. *Eur J Surg Oncol.* 2006;32:632–636.
16. Sugarbaker PH. Management of Peritoneal Surface Malignancy Using Intraperitoneal Chemotherapy and Cytoreductive Surgery: A Manual for Physicians and Nurses. 3rd ed. Grand Rapids, Michigan: The Ludann Company; 1998.
17. Dromain C, Leboulleux S, Auperin A, et al. Staging of peritoneal carcinomatosis: enhanced CT vs. PET/CT. *Abdom Imaging.* 2008;33:87–93.
18. Jacquet P, Jelinek JS, Chang D, et al. Abdominal computed tomographic scan in the selection of patients with mucinous peritoneal carcinomatosis for cytoreductive surgery. *J Am Coll Surg.* 1995;181:530–538.

# Laparoscopy in the Management of Peritoneal Carcinomatosis

Alfredo Garofalo • Mario Valle

The greatest problem in handling a patient affected with peritoneal carcinomatosis is carrying out a correct preoperative assessment of carcinomatosis extent before engaging in an extremely complicated surgical procedure that entails high rates of complications and mortality, even after a simple explorative laparotomy.

From the beginning of our experience, we found it necessary to integrate information deriving from diagnostics of videolaparoscopic staging that resulted in a correct assessment of patients, the peritoneal cancer index (PCI) definition and, above all, the possibility of deciding the feasibility of a complete cytoreduction (CCO) procedure with the aim of bringing patients to a postoperative CCO stage. By using this methodology many patients were excluded from treatment [peritonectomy + hyperthermic intraperineal chemotherapy (HIPEC)] because more than 2/3 of the small intestine was affected or because of extremely high PCI: the patients excluded at the first VLS of stadiation underwent VLS restaging after an average of 6 to 8 cycles of systemic neoadjuvant chemotherapy. A small series of patients affected with neoplastic ascites who did not respond to chemotherapy, in very advanced stages of the disease, were treated with completely videolaparoscopic palliative hyperthermic chemotherapy.

## LAPAROSCOPY IN THE STAGING OF PERITONEAL CARCINOMATOSIS

Before submitting a peritoneal carcinomatosis to peritonectomy with HIPEC, it is necessary to assess the prognosis and feasibility. It is thus fundamental to pre-emptively know the following with accuracy:

- Origin of the tumor,
- PCI,
- Degree of involvement of the small bowel and its mesentery, and
- Number and extension of the organ resection to perform.

Computed tomography scans and magnetic resonance imaging are routinely used in image diagnostics, which allow for a good evaluation of omental cake and show the presence of tumor masses larger than 5 mm, but they do not quantify the extension of the disease in the small bowel and its infiltration into the mesentery. Imaging diagnostics does consent us to exclude approximately 20% of patients with extraregional disease from the procedure. A recent study by Denzen et al[1] demonstrates how a peritoneal carcinomatosis was found in 100% of patients who underwent VLS, whereas an earlier CT showed that only 47.8% were apparently affected ($P < 0.1$) (Fig. 1).

Only recently have studies been performed with 18F-fluorodeoxyglucose-positron emission tomography/CT in the staging of peritoneal carcinomatosis that carry an actual real sensibility of 88%.[2-4]

Peritonectomy with HIPEC has a notable impact on survival only in cases where a complete CC0/1 cytoreduction is performed[5-9]: Morbidity varies from 20% to 30% and mortality from 4% to 8%.[10-14]

This is often found even only with an explorative laparotomy, as is demonstrated by Esquivel et al[15] in his study that reports morbidity from 12% to 23% and mortality from 20% to 36% in advanced neoplasms treated only with laparotomy.

It is thus fundamental to propose peritonectomy with HIPEC only to patients in which a cytoreduction to CC0/1 can realistically be performed with a clear and safe preoperative program. Videolaparoscopic stadiation allows for an evaluation of PCI and of the cytoreduction index with no mortality and with very low morbidity.

## Methods

### Abdominal Cavity Exploration

Once the Hasson trocar was placed, the ascites was completely suctioned out of the peritoneal cavity through the trocar, taking care not to contaminate the wall with ascitic fluid. It was preferable not to position the trocar on the median line or on the umbilicus as there is a high incidence of adhesions both from previous surgery and from tumor masses that may have infiltrated the median line. We preferred to position the trocar in the right or left iliac fossa on the midaxillary line after a clinical evaluation and sonogram of the quadrants. Access to the iliac fossa also allowed for a better view in the presence of an omental cake in the small intestine and the mesentery below, with the possibility to raise the omental cake using the trocar (5 mm) placed in the contralateral iliac fossa (port II). A 30-degree scope was routinely used, and by rotating the scope once inserted, a dissection of adhesions could be performed, therefore reducing viscerolysis to a minimum.

Adhesiolysis was performed at a minimum before the stadiation procedure to avoid the risk of lesion to abdominal organs but nonetheless allowing for a complete evaluation of the cancer index. It was preferable, in the case of tenacious adhesions or neoplastic infiltrations of the median line, to explore the right and left sections separately to avoid viscerolysis and to carry out a second open access to view the contralateral quadrants.

Cytology samples should be taken under direct view. Highly mucinous carcinomatoses sometimes required a 10-mm trocar in port II, so that a larger suction cannula could be used. In peritoneal surface malignancies where the histopathologic findings were unknown or doubtful, it was important to harvest multiple biopsy specimens from the parietal, omental, and pelvic cavity lesions. Diaphragmatic biopsies that can cause perforation and provoke infiltration of the muscular wall should be avoided. In cases where the presence of liver metastases or the involvement of suprahepatic veins was suspected, or in diaphragmatic lesions of more than 2 cm, intraoperative ultrasound imaging through the laparoscope might be useful.

To accomplish the laparoscopic definition of PCI, which is determined on the basis of the distribution and size of the neoplastic nodules, the operating table was moved into at least 4 positions: steep

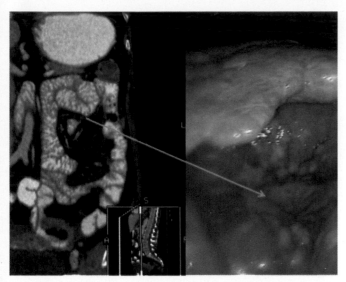

**FIGURE 1.** Peritoneal seeding from colonic cancer: treitz and small bowel mesentery infiltration under omental cake. Negative CT scan PCI: 23. Patient excluded from peritonectomy.

anti-trendelenburg left tilt, steep anti-trendelenburg right tilt, steep Trendelenburg left tilt, and steep Trendelenburg right tilt.[16,17]

## Results

From August 2000 to September 2008, we performed 197 diagnostic VLS procedures in patients with peritoneal surface malignancies (Table 1). The mean time needed for a diagnostic and staging VLS procedure was 30 minutes (range: 15/45 minutes). In one patient with gastric cancer, access to the abdominal cavity was impossible because of thick cancerous adhesions between the small bowel loops and the abdominal wall.

The patient was subjected to midline laparotomy, but the disease was not resectable because of massive involvement of the small intestine loops tightly adherent to the abdominal wall.

In 184 cases, 2 trocars (10 and 5 mm, respectively) were sufficient to carry out the procedure, whereas in 13 cases, it was necessary to add a third 10-mm trocar to gain full view of the abdominal cavity because of neoplastic adhesions located along the midline.

In 70 cases, the peritoneal surface malignancy was due to ovarian tumor, in 40 due to gastric tumor, in 35 due to a recurrent colorectal neoplasm, in 14 due to a pseudomyxoma peritonei, in 10 due to mesothelioma, in 6 due to neoplasm of the uterine cervix, in 6 due to abdominal sarcomatosis, in 5 due to recurrent pancreas neoplasm, in 1 due to peritoneal carcinomatosis to prostate neoplasm, in 1 due to intra-abdominal desmoplastic small round cell tumor, and in 9 due to the carcinomatosis was secondary to a primary breast tumor.

In 4 cases (2%), VLS understaged the carcinomatosis (mesothelioma, gastric cancer, pseudomyxoma, and ovarian cancer) and on laparotomy, massive infiltration of the pancreas was detected in gastric cancer and mesothelioma, which resulted in a CC2 peritonectomy. In the pseudomyxoma and ovarian cancer, the VLS cancer index was less than that confirmed by the PCI determined at surgical exploration, but it was nonetheless possible to carry out a peritonectomy with CC0 cytoreduction.

In 162 (82.2%) cases, advanced carcinomatosis was found with PCI >17. In fact, in 35 cases, PCI was range 0 to 13, in 13 cases 14 to 16, in 48 cases 17 to 23, in 53 cases, 24 to 33, and in 48 cases 34 to 39. Sixty-seven patients were excluded from surgical exploration because of massive infiltration of the small bowel or of its root seen by the VLS.

One hundred forty-one of 197 patients (71.5%) on whom we performed diagnostic VLS procedure had undergone at least 1 prior laparotomy. Ninety-eight (50.7%) patients were treated with a peritonectomy and HIPEC. Four (2%) patients who were not eligible for a peritonectomy because of massive infiltration of the small bowel and occlusion underwent a videolaparoscopic decompressive ileostomy.

As far as morbidity is concerned in videolaparoscopic surgical exploration, we observed 4 (2.08%) complications, of which 2 (1.04%) were intraoperative: one was a perforation of the diaphragm during biopsy, sutured with laparoscopic technique, one early postoperative bleeding treated with a blood transfusion, and 2 (1.04%) were delayed postoperative: infections of the trocar site, which were treated with topical antibiotic therapy. No neoplastic seeding was detected at the trocar sites, and all patients who underwent peritonectomy

**TABLE 1.** Videolaparoscopy in the Stadiation of Peritoneal Carcinomatosis—Personal Experience—2000/2008

| Source Carcinomatosis | Patient | VLS Diagnostic | VLS Unfeasible | Understaging | Trocar Infection | Diaphram Perforation | Intraoperative Bleeding | 2 Trocar | 3 Trocar |
|---|---|---|---|---|---|---|---|---|---|
| Ovary | 70 | 70 | 0 | 1 | 0 | 0 | 0 | 70 | 0 |
| Stomach | 40 | 39 | 1 | 1 | 1 | 1 | 0 | 34 | 6 |
| Colon-rectum | 35 | 35 | 0 | 0 | 1 | 0 | 1 | 33 | 2 |
| Pseudomyxoma | 14 | 14 | 0 | 1 | 0 | 0 | 0 | 14 | 0 |
| Mesothelioma | 10 | 10 | 0 | 1 | 0 | 0 | 0 | 10 | 0 |
| Breast | 9 | 9 | 0 | 0 | 0 | 0 | 0 | 9 | 0 |
| Uterus | 6 | 6 | 0 | 0 | 0 | 0 | 0 | 6 | 0 |
| Sarcoma | 6 | 6 | 0 | 0 | 0 | 0 | 0 | 6 | 0 |
| Pancreas | 5 | 5 | 0 | 0 | 0 | 0 | 0 | 0 | 5 |
| Prostate | 1 | 1 | 0 | 0 | 0 | 0 | 0 | 1 | 0 |
| Intra-abdominal desmoplastic round cell tumor | 1 | 1 | 0 | 0 | 0 | 0 | 0 | 1 | 0 |
| Total | 197 | 196 | 1 | 4 | 2 | 1 | 1 | 184 | 13 |
| % | 100 | 99.49 | 0.51 | 2.03 | 1.02 | 0.51 | 0.51 | 93.40 | 6.60 |

procedures resulted negative to port site metastasis 10 to 40 days from the procedure. We observed no mortality.

## LAPAROSCOPY IN THE TREATMENT OF REFRACTORY ASCITES

The use of laparoscopic assessment of carcinomatosis extent in the restaging of peritoneal carcinomatosis subjected to adjuvant and neoadjuvant chemotherapy has allowed for, on the one hand, the use of a peritonectomy procedure in patients with peritoneal carcinomatosis respondent to neoadjuvant chemotherapy and, on the other hand, a re-evaluation of patients with carcinomatosis that do not respond to systemic chemotherapy. In the nonrespondent group, we observed a group of patients with debilitating ascites who not only failed to respond to systemic chemotherapy but also to any other therapy attempted to diminish the ascites (albumin infusions, diuretics at high dosages repeated paracentesis), which resulted in an extremely negative impact on quality of life. Twenty-eight (14.21%) patients underwent intraperitoneal hyperthermic chemotherapy for the palliation of ascites with a videolaparoscopic technique (Fig. 2).[18–20]

## Methods

A Hasson trocar was placed in the right or left pararectal area through a 1-cm incision taking care not to contaminate the wall with the ascitic fluid. The ascites was completely suctioned out of the peritoneal cavity through the trocar before insufflating with $CO_2$. After placing the 30-degree 5-mm scope under direct vision, a second 5-mm trocar was placed in the iliac fossa contralateral to the scope. If necessary, viscerolysis was performed to free the abdominal cavity of cancerous adhesions. If extended viscerolysis was considered dangerous, it was only pursued to ensure communication between all abdominal quadrants, so that the hyperthermic chemotherapy agent could flow through the inflow tubes and drains to reach all the peritoneal surfaces. Then, 3 additional 5-mm trocars were sequentially placed on the right and left side into the free iliac fossa.

A 5-mm grasper was passed from the peritoneal cavity out through the 5-mm trocar to place closed-suction drains into the pelvic cavity and into the right and left subdiaphragmatic space. These 3 suctioning drains are connected together to provide a single outflow. The 5-mm trocars were removed, and an infusion trocar was placed

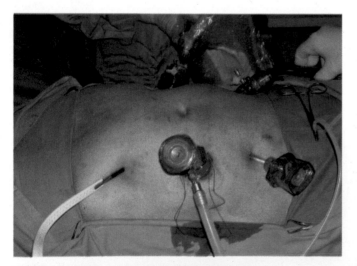

**FIGURE 2.**    Videolaparoscopic HIPEC procedure.

directly through the 10-mm trocar site where the camera had been inserted. To make the peritoneal space watertight, all drains were secured with a purse-string suture to the skin and connected to the perfusion machine, which should be set at an inflow temperature of 43°C to 44°C. An average temperature of 42°C in the whole peritoneal cavity was sought.

The temperature was measured by means of 2 probes. One was at the inflow site and the other at the junction between the 3 outflow drains. The patient's body temperature was monitored by means of 3 probes: at the skin, in the external ear canal, and in the rectum or bladder. The mean duration of laparoscopic preparation was 45 minutes, with a range of 30 to 120 minutes depending on the extent of viscerolysis.

To allow the chemotherapy solution to distribute itself throughout the whole peritoneal surface, the operating table tilt was changed at 15-minute intervals during perfusion as follows: (1) level, (2) trendelenburg + left tilt, (3) trendelenburg + right tilt, (4) level, (5) reverse trendelenburg + left tilt, and (6) reverse trendelenburg + right tilt.

Perfusion lasted 90 minutes after which the chemotherapy agent was recovered and a lavage of 2000 mL of 1.5% dextrose was performed to remove residual chemotherapy. The drains were connected to gravity bags and were removed postoperatively after copious drainage ceased. After removing all drains, the patient was discharged from the hospital.

The hyperthermic intraperitoneal chemotherapy was performed using cisplatin 50 mg/m² and doxorubicin 15 mg/m² for ascites from ovarian cancer, peritoneal mesothelioma, or breast cancer. In ascites from rectal colon and stomach cancer, mitomycin at 12.5 mg/m² was used. The volume of perfusate used was 2000 mL; it consisted of a peritoneal dialysis solution containing 1.5% dextrose. Fresh frozen plasma (1200 mL) was infused during perfusion. Furosemide was administered along with intravenous fluids to maintain a 400-mL/h diuresis.[20]

## Results

Of the 28 patients treated, at the origin of malignant ascites there were 10 cases of gastric cancer, 7 colon cancer, 5 breast lobular cancer, 5 ovarian cancer, and 1 peritoneal mesothelioma. In all cases, we observed a complete disappearance of the ascites within 9 days of laparoscopic perfusion. The average increment on the Karnofsky index postoperative was of 20 points. Even though the treatment is of a palliative nature, the disappearance of the refractory ascites did have an impact on average survival rate, of 152 days (range 21–796). The longest survival times were observed in 3 of 5 cases of breast lobular cancer (807, 736, and 216 days), whereas the shortest survival times were observed in the cases of ascites from gastric cancer. Follow-up ultrasound or CT 1 month after the laparoscopic HIPEC revealed complete resolution of ascites in 26 of the 28 patients, one patient died in the 21st postoperative day free from ascites. In one case, a CT scan 1 year later showed a small, clinically undetectable, ascitic accumulation in the pelvis. In 2 cases of concomitant neoplastic intestinal occlusion, a laparoscopic ileostomy was performed before beginning the hyperthermic intraperitoneal chemotherapy.

In the video-laparoscopic perfusion, for refractory ascites, no intraoperative or postoperative complications and no mortality due to the procedure were observed.[20,21]

## DISCUSSION

### Staging

We began using laparoscopy in the assessment of peritoneal carcinomatosis extent and in the treatment of refractory ascites in 2000, publishing in 2003 the first 48 cases of stadiation and the first 9 cases of closed perfusion.[17]

Objections regarding feasibility tied to the difficulty of trocar positioning in the presence of abdominal wall tumor masses or because of adhesions from previous surgeries, skepticism on the reliability and efficacy of the method in the stadiation phase, fear of neoplastic contamination at the trocar entry sites, and the absence of a curative objective tied to the laparoscopic procedure have been overcome in our experience.

Eight years from our first proposal to use laparoscopy in the staging of peritoneal carcinomatosis, the role of laparoscopic procedure has now become clear, well defined in its indications, technique, and possible applications.

VLS in stadiation allows the following:

- Evaluation of the mesentery (superficial lesions and retractions; Fig. 3),
- Evaluation of lesions on the antimesenteric margin,
- Evaluation of the omental bursa, pelvic cavity, diaphragm, and abdominal wall,
- Evaluation of sectors according to the cancer index, with PCI similar to VLS,
- The possibility of peritoneal washing and biopsies for the typing of the primitive tumor, and
- The predictive evaluation of the cytoreduction index after peritonectomy.

The above-mentioned points give us a certain indication regarding the "feasibility" and "cost/benefit" of a peritonectomy procedure with HIPEC.

Some weak points regarding the use of VLS in stadiation could be tied to the following:

- Evaluation of the thickness of lesions of the diaphragm,
- Evaluation of pancreatic involvement, and
- Necessity of a skilled laparoscopic surgeon, expert in advanced laparoscopy and carcinomatosis.

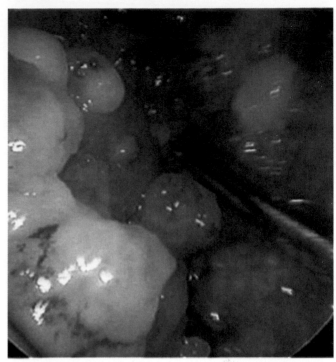

**FIGURE 4.**   Laparoscopic staging of peritoneal carcinomatosis from colonic cancer: PCI: 39. Patient referred to neoadjuvant chemotherapy.

The weak points of the procedure can become points of strength if VLS is coupled with a video-assisted laparoscopic sonogram, which will in turn permit:

- A good evaluation of the thickness of lesions of the diaphragm,
- The qualitative and quantitative evaluation of pancreatic involvement, as well as that of the retrocavity, and
- The evaluation of hepatic metastasis and of their resectability.

The indications for VLS stadiation are as follows:

- Staging of a carcinomatosis already diagnosed via imaging technology (Tc-Rm),
- Staging of a carcinomatosis of dubious origin (biopsy),
- Restaging after neoadjuvant chemotherapy (Figs. 4 and 5),
- Restaging during follow-up in the case of dubious imaging,
- Restaging after adjuvant chemotherapy.

The use of VLS stadiation is not advisable for patients who have already undergone a peritonectomy with the objective of a second look, as the presence of adhesions will not allow for a comprehensive evaluation of the eventual relapse or a good evaluation of all abdominal quadrants. We believe that in the case of dubious relapses in CT scan, the 18F-fluorodeoxyglucose-positron emission tomography/CT can offer further information on the origin and entity of the relapse and of its possible treatment.

## Treatment of Refractory Ascites

Laparoscopic HIPEC may result in deeper penetration of the cancer chemotherapy drug in the peritoneal layers and tumor nodules. In the

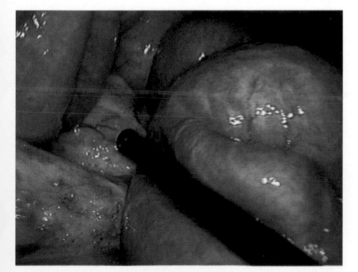

**FIGURE 3.**   Peritoneal seeding from gastric cancer: involvement of the small bowel and its mesentery PCI: 39. Patient excluded from peritonectomy.

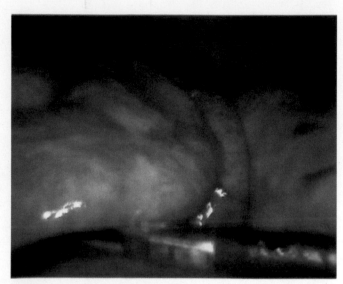

**FIGURE 5.** Same patient from Figure 4 after neoadjuvant chemotherapy: disappearance of the macroscopic lesions, persisting mesentry retraction and infiltration of more than 2/3 of the small bowel. PCI 39. Patient excluded from the procedure.

absence of cytoreductive surgery during these palliative laparoscopic HIPEC procedures, one can assume that the direct cytotoxic effect of this single chemotherapy instillation will be limited. The heated chemotherapy may eradicate viable cancer several cell layers deep on all the peritoneal surfaces. Then, a thin layer of fibrosis may develop on the exposed surfaces. The fibrous layer may direct the cancerous fluid into the capillary bed and thereby into the systemic circulation, causing a resolution of the problematic reaccummulation of ascites.[16,19]

Abdominal sclerosis and induction of dense adhesions are probably the major factor of efficacy of this technique. Ozols et al[19] in their phase I study reported sclerozing peritonitis and subsequent pain at the dose-limiting factor of 18 uM when performing intracavitary chemotherapy with doxorubicin in patients with advanced ovarian cancer. The absence of major complications and treatment-related mortality in our patients suggests that laparoscopic HIPEC is a safe technique.

The treatment is to be considered palliative for ascites that do not respond to therapy and must be performed exclusively on patients that, after VLS stadiation, present a peritoneal carcinomatosis noneligible for peritonectomy with HIPEC according to the PCI, or for extensive evolution of the disease.

The objective of the treatment is to improve on the Karnowsky index, ultimately impacting the patient's quality of life. In patients with PCI <13 affected by peritoneal carcinomatosis from lobular breast cancer, the treatment can be performed even though the carcinomatosis in these cases is the expression of a systemic disease and thus not eligible for peritonectomy surgery with HIPEC.

## CONCLUSIONS

Videolaparoscopy is placed, within a strategy of treatment of peritoneal carcinomatosis, at the beginning of a critical path analysis to classify the patient and provide a correct indication for integrated treatment and, in the end, associated with HIPEC, is an effective palliative instrument for neoplastic refractory ascites.

VLS is safe and reliable, absent of major complications, and mortality. VLS in peritoneal carcinomatosis foresees that the surgeon have experience in advanced videolaparoscopy and in the surgical treatment of carcinomatosis to prevent downstaging and greater complications.

## REFERENCES

1. Denzen U, Hoffmann S, Helmreich-Becker I, et al. Minilaparoscopy in the diagnosis of peritoneal tumor spread: prospective controlled comparison with computed tomography. *Surg Endosc.* 2004;18:1067–1070.
2. Dirisamer A, Schima W, Heinisch M, et al. Detection of histologically proven peritoneal carcinomatosis with fused 18F-FDG-PET/MDCT. *Eur J Radiol.* In press.
3. De Gaetano AM, Calcagni ML, Rufini V, et al. Imaging of peritoneal carcinomatosis with FDG PET-CT: diagnostic patterns, case examples and pitfalls. *Abdom Imaging.* In press.
4. Dromain C, Leboulleux S, Auperin A, et al. Staging of peritoneal carcinomatosis: enhanced CT vs. PET/CT. *Abdom Imaging.* 2008;33:87–93.
5. Glehen O, Kwiatkowski F, Sugarbaker PH, et al. Cytoreductive surgery combined with perioperative intraperitoneal chemotherapy for management of peritoneal carcinomatosis from colorectal cancer: a multi-institutional study. *J Clin Oncol.* 2004;22:3284–3292.
6. Di Giorgio A, Naticchioni E, Biacchi D, et al. Cytoreductive surgery (peritonectomy procedures) combined with hyperthermic intraperitoneal chemotherapy (HIPEC) in the treatment of diffuse peritoneal carcinomatosis from ovarian cancer. *Cancer.* 2008;113:315–325.
7. Rasmussen PC, Laurberg S. New treatment of peritoneal carcinomatosis from colorectal cancer. Cytoreductive surgery and hyperthermic intraperitoneal chemotherapy. *Ugeskr Laeger.* 2007;169:3179–3181.
8. Piso P, Dahlke MH, Ghali N, et al. Multimodality treatment of peritoneal carcinomatosis from colorectal cancer: first results of a new German centre for peritoneal surface malignancies. *Int J Colorectal Dis.* 2007;22:1295–1300.
9. Cavaliere F, Valle M, De Simone M, et al. 120 peritoneal carcinomatoses from colorectal cancer treated with peritonectomy and intra-abdominal chemohyperthermia: a S.I.T.I.L.O. multicentric study. *In Vivo.* 2006;20:747–750.
10. Capone A, Valle M, Proietti F, et al. Petrosillo postoperative infections in cytoreductive surgery with hyperthermic intraperitoneal intraoperative chemotherapy for peritoneal carcinomatosis. *J Surg Oncol.* 2007;96:507–513.
11. Yan TD, Links M, Fransi S, et al. Learning curve for cytoreductive surgery and perioperative intraperitoneal chemotherapy for peritoneal surface malignancy—a journey to becoming a Nationally Funded Peritonectomy Center. *Ann Surg Oncol.* 2007;14:2270–2280.
12. Sugarbaker PH. Reported impact of cytoreductive surgery and hyperthermic intraperitoneal chemotherapy on systemic toxicity. *Ann Surg Oncol.* 2008;15:1800–1801.
13. Yan TD, Black D, Sugarbaker PH, et al. A systematic review and meta-analysis of the randomized controlled trials on adjuvant intraperitoneal chemotherapy for resectable gastric cancer. *Ann Surg Oncol.* 2007;14:2702–2713.
14. Zappa L, Sugarbaker PH. Compartment syndrome of the leg associated with lithotomy position for cytoreductive surgery. *J Surg Oncol.* 2007;96:619–623.
15. Esquivel J, Farinetti A, Sugarbaker PH. Elective surgery in recurrent colon cancer with peritoneal seeding: when to and when not to proceed. *G Chir.* 1999;20:81–86.
16. Valle M, Garofalo A. Laparoscopic staging of peritoneal surface malignancies. *Eur J Surg Oncol.* 2006;32:625–627.
17. Garofalo A, Valle M. Staging videolaparoscopy of peritoneal carcinomatosis. *Tumori.* 2003;89(4 suppl):70–77.
18. Valle M, Garofalo A, Federici O, et al. Laparoscopic intraperitoneal antiblastic hyperthermic chemoperfusion in the treatment of refractory neoplastic ascites. Preliminary results. *Suppl Tumori.* 2005;4:S122–S123.
19. Garofalo A, Valle M, Garcia J, et al. Laparoscopic intraperitoneal hyperthermic chemotherapy for palliation of debilitating malignant ascites. *Eur J Surg Oncol.* 2006;32:682–685.
20. Valle M, Van Der Speeten K, Garofalo A. Laparoscopic hyperthermic intraperitoneal peroperative chemotherapy (HIPEC) in the management of refractory malignant ascites: a multi-institutional retrospective analysis in 52 patients. *J Surg Oncol.* In press.
21. Ozols RF, Young RC, Speyer JL, et al. Phase I study and pharmacological studies of adriamycin administered intraperitoneally to patients with ovarian cancer. *Cancer Res.* 1982;42:4265–4269.

# Morbidity and Mortality with Cytoreductive Surgery and Intraperitoneal Chemotherapy

## The Importance of a Learning Curve

Faheez Mohamed • Brendan J. Moran

Throughout the world, the concept of patient safety is moving to its rightful place as a central pillar of healthcare. A complex interplay of factors leads to good outcomes, and frequently a string of sometimes individually minor errors can culminate in major harm to a patient. The World Health Organization's "Safe Surgery Saves Live" program, launched in June 2008,[1] recently demonstrated a 47% reduction in deaths and 36% reduction in in-hospital complications following implementation of a 19-item "safe surgery checklist."[2] This checklist ensures that all staff involved in the care of the patient are fully aware of the procedure to be performed and that perioperative interventions such as antibiotic and thrombotic prophylaxis are optimized. The mechanism for the observed reduction in deaths reported by the study is unclear, but reflects a renewed interest in elements of surgical practice that can be improved. The surgeon's performance has always been key and the concept of "the learning curve" a favorite of those interested in the introduction of new technologies.[3] Proficiency in a surgical procedure does not come solely from numbers performed and varies widely between individuals.[4]

The modern surgical oncologist requires a range of competencies[5] to provide high-quality care. The traditional apprenticeship model of surgical training is evolving, and as a result there is less acceptance of the "see one, do one, teach one" approach.[6] With less time available for training and increasingly complex technology available, novel approaches are required to impart the knowledge and decision-making skills needed to develop expertise in surgical oncology. For new treatments to become established, an analysis of cost-benefit, efficacy, morbidity, and mortality is essential. The surgical team has a responsibility to ensure morbidity and mortality are minimized. This is fundamental in allowing transition of an experimental treatment to standard of care.[7] The development of the treatment of peritoneal carcinomatosis by cytoreductive surgery (CRS) and hyperthermic intraperitoneal chemotherapy (HIPEC) illustrates the importance of the learning curve. A number of centers around the world now have considerable expertise in the management of peritoneal malignancy providing a useful insight into the factors that influence outcome.

## MORBIDITY AND MORTALITY FOLLOWING CRS AND HIPEC FOR PERITONEAL CARCINOMATOSIS

There have been a number of reports addressing the morbidity and mortality associated with CRS and HIPEC for pseudomyxoma peritonei (PMP)[8] and colonic peritoneal carcinomatosis.[9] Major morbidity involves gastrointestinal tract complications, such as anastomotic leakage, enteric and pancreatic fistulation, cardiopulmonary events, including pneumonia and thromboembolism and intra-abdominal abscesses. A shortcoming of many reports is a nonuniform use of toxicity-reporting criteria.[10] This makes assessment of morbidity and mortality difficult and comparisons between centers less meaningful. Treatment-related morbidity and mortality is related to age, tumor load, extent of CRS, and associated operative factors.[11–16] Many patients have had previous abdominal surgery before definitive cytoreduction, increasing the risk of complications from adhesiolysis and distorted anatomy resulting in a high incidence of small bowel fistulae[14,17] and significant blood loss.[14]

Intraoperative and postoperative hemorrhage has been a major issue in this complex 4 quadrant multiorgan surgery and is often reported as a significant cause for reoperation.[18] A recent personal observation has been that the use of HIPEC for between 30 and 120 minutes facilitates effective hemostasis allowing bleeding vessels to be visualized before abdominal closure with a reduction in the requirement for relaparotomy for bleeding.

Intraperitoneal chemotherapy agents such as oxaliplatin can cause significant hematological toxicity with reports of an increase in postoperative hemorrhage.[19] Neutropenic sepsis is a potentially serious complication usually presenting around day 10 after intraperitoneal mitomycin C, due to bone marrow toxicity.[20] Septic complications may herald or result from neutropenia and require prompt treatment.

Morbidity ranges between 12%[21] and 67.6%[19] in recent studies of CRS and HIPEC for PMP although lack of uniformity in grading morbidity makes comparison difficult. Mortality ranges between 0%[15] and 9%[22] (Table 1). It becomes apparent that early reports from centers had a much higher incidence of morbidity and mortality than more recent updates from the same teams. In Sugarbaker's experience, a mortality rate of 5% and morbidity of 35% reported in 1996[23] were reduced to 1.5% and 27%, respectively, in an update with an expanded series in 1999.[24] A subsequent update has shown a mortality rate of 2% and morbidity of 40%[25] suggesting that this team may have reached the plateau in its learning curve. Similarly, Elias et al[26] reported 36 patients who had complete cytoreduction for PMP over a 7-year period from 1994 to 2001. Five patients died before discharge giving in-hospital mortality of 13.8%. Major morbidity was quoted at 44%. An update in 2008 of 105 patients reported an in-hospital mortality of 7.8% (30 day mortality of 3.8%) and morbidity of 67.6%. Although the mortality rate has almost halved, it is not clear whether morbidity has increased or if the grading of complications has changed.

## THE GLOBAL LEARNING CURVE

Recent reports suggest that the initial high morbidity and mortality seen with CRS and HIPEC decreases with increasing experience.[18,27–29] This is most marked in specialized centers and includes improvements in patient selection, surgical expertise, and postoperative management.[18] This increased information base is culminating in a "global learning curve" reduction of complications (Table 2).

**TABLE 1.**   Morbidity and Mortality of CRS With HIPEC for PMP

| Study | Year | No. Patients | Treatment Modality | Major Morbidity (%) | Mortality (%) |
|---|---|---|---|---|---|
| Witkamp et al[22] | 2001 | 46 | HIPEC (MMC) | 39 | 9 |
| Guner[31] | 2005 | 28 | HIPEC (MMC or Cisplatin) | 36 | 7 |
| Loungnarath et al[15] | 2005 | 27 | HIPEC (MMC or Cisplatin) | 22 | 0 |
| Miner et al[32] | 2005 | 97 | IV/EPIC 5FU (4 patients received HIPEC) | 16 | 4 |
| Sugarbaker et al[25] | 2006 | 356 | HIPEC (MMC) + EPIC (5FU) | 19 | 2 |
| Stewart et al[33] | 2006 | 110 | HIPEC (MMC) | 38 | 6 |
| Yan et al[21] | 2006 | 50 | HIPEC (MMC) + EPIC (5FU) | 12 | 4 |
| Murphy et al[12] | 2007 | 123 | HIPEC (MMC) + EPIC (5FU) | 21 | 5 |
| Smeenk et al[34] | 2007 | 103 | HIPEC (MMC) | 54 | 3 |
| Baratti[35] | 2008 | 95 | HIPEC (MMC and Cisplatin) | 18.7 | 1 |
| Elias et al[19] | 2008 | 105 | HIPEC (MMC/oxaliplatin/irinotecan/induction IV 5FU) | 67.6 | 7.8 |
| Median (range) | | | | 31 (12–67.6) | 4 (0–9) |

NR indicates not reported; MMC, mitomycin C; 5-FU, 5-fluorouracil.

In the United Kingdom, mortality after pediatric cardiac surgery focused attention on approaches to achieving competence in complex surgical procedures. The report "Care in the Operating Theater and the Learning Curve,"[30] discussed that it is understood that outcomes improved with operator experience, but suggested that the learning curve was no longer acceptable although no elaboration of its components was given.

The peritoneal malignancy program was initiated at Basingstoke in 1994, an institution with a documented track record in surgical teaching and high-quality outcomes. Moran[18] analyzed the factors from the Basingstoke experience that influenced the learning curve for CRS and HIPEC primarily for PMP. The initial 100 patients treated were divided into 3 numerically equal groups (33, 33, and 34, respectively), though the whole experience was over a 6-year period that was divided into 3 distinct time intervals (79 months, 16 months, and 9 months). Both major morbidity and mortality fell (Table 2) with increasing experience. Technical failures such as anastomotic leakage and reoperation for bleeding occurred predominantly during the initial experience of CRS and HIPEC. Anastomotic leak rate fell from 12% to 0%, and reoperation for bleeding from 15% to 0% over the 6-year period. Proximal stomal defunctioning is now performed routinely in all patients after anterior resection and restoration of colorectal continuity. Significant intra-abdominal bleeding was detected in 11/100 (11%), and 6/11 required relaparotomy for bleeding, 5 of

whom were in the earliest time period. One of these patients had 4 further laparotomies to evacuate hematoma and control hepatic bleeding. In the initial series, normothermic chemotherapy was used for a short interval. Subsequent meticulous attention to hemostasis aided by the hiatus provided by the time to instill HIPEC has also helped reduce postoperative hemorrhage.

Knowledge of the toxicity of HIPEC and early postoperative intraperitoneal chemotherapy has resulted in a low threshold for dose modification in patients at high risk of perioperative morbidity or mortality. The involvement of at least 2 experienced trained surgeons for CRS with HIPEC is thought to facilitate training, experience, and the management of adverse events. This approach has been effective in attenuating the learning curve. Case selection was the other important element with a smaller proportion of those referred undergoing surgery over time. In total, 61% of those referred underwent surgery in the initial time period, whereas only 37% were operated on in the last period reported.[18]

The review by the team, at The Netherlands Cancer Institute[28] of 323 CRS and HIPEC procedures over a 10.5-year period is illuminating. Again their experience was divided into 3 time periods of between 24 and 36 months to investigate the learning curve for CRS and HIPEC. Peritoneal carcinomatosis was of colonic origin in 184 patients and from PMP in 128 patients. Morbidity was scored according to the National Cancer Institute Common Toxicity Criteria and was regarded as major if grade III (minor surgical intervention such as tube drainage) or IV (major surgical intervention such as relaparotomy). Major morbidity consisted of gastrointestinal complications (31.5%), infections (20.9%), pulmonary complications (12.8%), bone marrow suppression (11.7%), cardiovascular complications (8.4%), and urinary tract complications (8.4%). Overall major morbidity fell from 71% (52/73) between 1996 and 1998 to 34% (44/129) between 2003 and 2006. Perioperative mortality was halved from 8% (6/73) to 4% (5/129) in the same time periods (Table 2). Interestingly, an increase in the number of complete cytoreductions performed was observed after 130 procedures although on multivariable analysis no significant association between treatment period and survival was seen. The authors comment that refining patient selection particularly for colorectal peritoneal carcinomatosis using preoperative imaging helped exclusion of patients unlikely to benefit from CRS and HIPEC and therefore, led to fewer patients with large volume (6 or 7 abdominal regions involved) or unresectable (extensive small bowel) disease being subjected to surgery and its substantial morbidity.

**TABLE 2.**   Major Morbidity and Mortality With Increasing Experience of CRS and HIPEC for Peritoneal Carcinomatosis

| Senior Investigator | % Perioperative Mortality | | |
|---|---|---|---|
|  | Initial | Intermediate | Recent |
| Moran[18] (n = 100)* | 18 (6/33) | 3 (1/33) | 3 (1/33) |
| Zoetmulder coworkers[28] (n = 323)† | 8 (6/73) | 6 (7/121) | 4 (5/129) |
| Morris coworkers[29] (n = 140)‡ | 7 (5/70) | NR | 1 (1/70) |

Initial, intermediate, and recent refer to different time periods within the reported experience.
*Over 6-yr period, reported anastomotic leakage and re-operation for bleeding.
†Over 10.5-yr period.
‡Over 9-yr period. Moderate and severe morbidity figures were reported and have been combined.
NR indicates not reported.

The experience of the Nationally Funded Peritonectomy Center in Sydney, Australia acknowledges the significant financial resources, technical skill, expertise, and experience required to successfully undertake CRS and HIPEC for peritoneal surface malignancy.[29] Results were reported over a period of just under 10 years with 140 consecutive patients undergoing CRS with HIPEC and early postoperative intraperitoneal chemotherapy at the St Georges Hospital in Sydney. Analysis of outcomes was based on comparison of the first 70 patients and the subsequent 70 patients over a 7-year and 2-year period, respectively. Sixty-nine patients had PMP, 40 colorectal peritoneal carcinomatosis, 15 peritoneal mesothelioma, and 16 peritoneal malignancy of other origin. Seventy-three percent (51/70) in the first 7-year period received intraperitoneal chemotherapy compared with 80% (56/70) in the second period. Outcome measures were classed as moderate morbidity requiring an interventional procedure such as radiologic-guided drain insertion, and severe morbidity requiring transfer to intensive care or return to the operating theater. Overall, 61 patients (30 in the initial period and 31 in the subsequent period) suffered moderate morbidity in the form of intra-abdominal collection (n = 44, 31%), pneumothorax (n = 10, 7%), pleural effusion (n = 9, 6%), pancreatic leak (n = 2, 1%), and bile leak (n = 1, 1%) with some patients experiencing more than 1 event. No significant reduction in moderate morbidity over time was reported. Severe morbidity in 28 patients (21 in the initial period and 7 in the subsequent period) included intestinal perforation (n = 10, 7%), postoperative bleeding (n = 9, 6%), fistula (n = 5, 4%), chemotherapy-related neutropenia (n = 5, 4%), acute renal failure requiring dialysis (n = 1, 1%), tracheostomy for prolonged respiratory failure (n = 1, 1%), central line erosion causing pleural effusion requiring thoracotomy (n = 1, 1%), and negative laparotomy for suspected perforation (n = 1, 1%). Again, more than 1 event occurred in some patients. Twenty-seven patients (19%) were readmitted with fistulae (n = 8, 6%), small bowel obstruction (n = 8, 6%), intra-abdominal collection (n = 7, 5%), wound abscess (n = 4, 3%), pancreatic leak (n = 2, 1%), pleural effusion (n = 2, 1%), and pulmonary embolism (n = 1, 1%). Mortality fell from 7% to 1% with 5 deaths in the initial 70 patients and 1 death in the subsequent 70 patients. Causes of death included multiorgan failure, secondary to chemotherapy-related bone marrow suppression in 3 patients on postoperative days 19, 20, and 306. Three patients died of septic shock following peritonitis on postoperative days 7, 15, and 25. The authors comment that they have stopped using intravenous mitomycin C, which has prevented any further cases of neutropenia that were seen during their early experience.

## WHAT CAN THE LEARNING CURVE TEACH US ABOUT CRS AND HIPEC?

All interventional procedures have an inherent risk, and experience undoubtedly diminishes, but can never abolish this. Novel interventions always require careful evaluation, honest audit, and appraisal. For low-volume procedures, multicenter assessment may be required to establish the benefits and risks so that an estimate of risk to benefit can be acquired over time. This is particularly difficult for rare conditions requiring complex, high-risk procedures. The techniques required for optimal management of peritoneal malignancy, namely CRS and HIPEC, serve as a good model in evaluating complex cancer care. Patients, often with advanced metastatic malignancy and a limited life span, undergo a combination of major 4 quadrant abdominal surgery, multivisceral resection, often with several intestinal anastomoses and heated intraperitoneal chemotherapy. The surgical, anesthetic, and nursing techniques required to safely perform macroscopic tumor resection extend across several surgical disciplines including general surgery, hepatobiliary surgery, urology, and gynaecology. Furthermore, the surgery crosses several oncologic subspecialities including colorectal, upper gastrointestinal tract, and gynecologic malignancy.

The practicalities of heated intraperitoneal chemotherapy add another element of complexity to the surgery and undoubtedly add to the morbidity and mortality associated with major gastrointestinal tract surgery. It is likely that chemotherapy increases the risks of anastomotic leakage, in particular, and some have recommended that these risks necessitate defunctioning multiple or low colorectal anastomoses by a proximal stoma.[18] Undoubtedly, presentation and publication of the inherent risks associated with CRS and HIPEC, together with centralization of services and collaboration between units, will be instrumental in reducing morbidity and mortality. The learning curve comprises a combination of surgical and institutional awareness of these issues, a willingness to learn from established units, and an understanding of the infrastructural requirements needed to sustain a service for these complex but eminently treatable conditions.

Team work is essential, and although surgical leadership is crucial, it is recommended that 2 experienced surgeons support each other in the development of the multidisciplinary team required to optimize outcome, minimize risk, and deal with problems as they arise. Rigorous data collection to facilitate service improvement and inform quality assurance is vital for the provision of a high-risk intervention such as CRS with HIPEC. However, with proper patient selection, skilled peritonectomy procedures, standardized perioperative intraperitoneal chemotherapy regimens, and vigilant postoperative care by experienced teams, impressive results can be obtained.[7,16] The modern surgical oncologist must not only master the challenging techniques of CRS, but also understand the rationale, indications, and potential morbidity associated with HIPEC. This is best done in high-volume centers and those wishing to undertake CRS and HIPEC for peritoneal malignancy should be mindful of the learning curve and strive to learn from the mistakes of others. For the full benefits of this treatment strategy to be realized, surgeons have an obligation to minimize morbidity and mortality.

## REFERENCES

1. World Health Organisation: Safe Surgery Saves Lives 2008. Available at: www.who.int/patientsafety/safesurgery/en/.
2. Haynes AB, Weiser TG, Berry WR, et al. A surgical safety checklist to reduce morbidity and mortality in a global population. *N Engl J Med.* 2009;360:491–499.
3. Nizard RS, Porcher R, Ravaud P, et al. Use of the Cusum technique for evaluation of a CT-based navigation system for total knee replacement. *Clin Orthop Relat Res.* 2004:180–188.
4. Dagash H, Chowdhury M, Pierro A. When can I be proficient in laparoscopic surgery? A systematic review of the evidence. *J Pediatr Surg.* 2003;38:720–724.
5. Roach PB, Silverstein JC. Training fellows and core competency: "making quality certain." *J Surg Oncol.* 2009;99:83–84.
6. Pellegrini CA, Warshaw AL, Debas HT. Residency training in surgery in the 21st century: a new paradigm. *Surgery.* 2004;136:953–965.
7. Sugarbaker PH. Clinical research to standard of care: when does the transition occur? *Ann Surg Oncol.* 2003;10:825–826.
8. Yan TD, Black D, Savady R, et al. A systematic review on the efficacy of cytoreductive surgery and perioperative intraperitoneal chemotherapy for pseudomyxoma peritonei. *Ann Surg Oncol.* 2007;14:484–492.
9. Koppe MJ, Boerman OC, Oyen WJ, et al. Peritoneal carcinomatosis of colorectal origin: incidence and current treatment strategies. *Ann Surg.* 2006;243:212–222.
10. Younan R, Kusamura S, Baratti D, et al. Morbidity, toxicity, and mortality classification systems in the local regional treatment of peritoneal surface malignancy. *J Surg Oncol.* 2008;98:253–257.
11. Moran BJ, Mukherjee A, Sexton R. Operability and early outcome in 100 consecutive laparotomies for peritoneal malignancy. *Br J Surg.* 2006;93:100–104.

12. Murphy EM, Sexton R, Moran BJ. Early results of surgery in 123 patients with pseudomyxoma peritonei from a perforated appendiceal neoplasm. *Dis Colon Rectum.* 2007;50:37–42.

13. Butterworth SA, Panton ON, Klaassen DJ, et al. Morbidity and mortality associated with intraperitoneal chemotherapy for Pseudomyxoma peritonei. *Am J Surg.* 2002;183:529–532.

14. Smeenk RM, Verwaal VJ, Zoetmulder FA. Toxicity and mortality of cytoreduction and intraoperative hyperthermic intraperitoneal chemotherapy in pseudomyxoma peritonei–a report of 103 procedures. *Eur J Surg Oncol.* 2006;32: 186–190.

15. Loungnarath R, Causeret S, Bossard N, et al. Cytoreductive surgery with intraperitoneal chemohyperthermia for the treatment of pseudomyxoma peritonei: a prospective study. *Dis Colon Rectum.* 2005;48:1372–1379.

16. Glehen O, Osinsky D, Cotte E, et al. Intraperitoneal chemohyperthermia using a closed abdominal procedure and cytoreductive surgery for the treatment of peritoneal carcinomatosis: morbidity and mortality analysis of 216 consecutive procedures. *Ann Surg Oncol.* 2003;10:863–869.

17. Sugarbaker PH, Ronnett BM, Archer A, et al. Pseudomyxoma peritonei syndrome. *Adv Surg.* 1996;30:233–280.

18. Moran BJ. Decision-making and technical factors account for the learning curve in complex surgery. *J Public Health (Oxf).* 2006;28:375–378.

19. Elias D, Honore C, Ciuchendea R, et al. Peritoneal pseudomyxoma: results of a systematic policy of complete cytoreductive surgery and hyperthermic intraperitoneal chemotherapy. *Br J Surg.* 2008;95:1164–1171.

20. Verwaal VJ, van Tinteren H, Ruth SV, et al. Toxicity of cytoreductive surgery and hyperthermic intra-peritoneal chemotherapy. *J Surg Oncol.* 2004;85: 61–67.

21. Yan TD, Links M, Xu ZY, et al. Cytoreductive surgery and perioperative intraperitoneal chemotherapy for pseudomyxoma peritonei from appendiceal mucinous neoplasms. *Br J Surg.* 2006;93:1270–1276.

22. Witkamp AJ, de Bree E, Kaag MM, et al. Extensive surgical cytoreduction and intraoperative hyperthermic intraperitoneal chemotherapy in patients with pseudomyxoma peritonei. *Br J Surg.* 2001;88:458–463.

23. Jacquet P, Stephens AD, Averbach AM, et al. Analysis of morbidity and mortality in 60 patients with peritoneal carcinomatosis treated by cytoreductive surgery and heated intraoperative intraperitoneal chemotherapy. *Cancer.* 1996;77:2622–2629.

24. Stephens AD, Alderman R, Chang D, et al. Morbidity and mortality analysis of 200 treatments with cytoreductive surgery and hyperthermic intraoperative intraperitoneal chemotherapy using the coliseum technique. *Ann Surg Oncol.* 1999;6:790–796.

25. Sugarbaker PH, Alderman R, Edwards G, et al. Prospective morbidity and mortality assessment of cytoreductive surgery plus perioperative intraperitoneal chemotherapy to treat peritoneal dissemination of appendiceal mucinous malignancy. *Ann Surg Oncol.* 2006;13:635–644.

26. Elias D, Laurent S, Antoun S, et al. [Pseudomyxoma peritonei treated with complete resection and immediate intraperitoneal chemotherapy]. *Gastroenterol Clin Biol.* 2003;27:407–412.

27. Cavaliere F, Valle M, De Rosa B, et al. [Peritonectomy and chemohyperthermia in the treatment of peritoneal carcinomatosis: learning curve]. *Suppl Tumori.* 2005;4:S119–S121.

28. Smeenk RM, Verwaal VJ, Zoetmulder FA. Learning curve of combined modality treatment in peritoneal surface disease. *Br J Surg.* 2007;94:1408–1414.

29. Yan TD, Links M, Fransi S, et al. Learning curve for cytoreductive surgery and perioperative intraperitoneal chemotherapy for peritoneal surface malignancy–a journey to becoming a Nationally Funded Peritonectomy Center. *Ann Surg Oncol.* 2007;14:2270–2280.

30. The Bristol Royal Infirmary Inquiry: Care in the Operating Theatre and the Learning Curve. Available at: www.bristol-inquiry.org.uk.

31. Guner Z, Schmidt U, Dahlke MH, et al. Cytoreductive surgery and intraperitoneal chemotherapy for pseudomyxoma peritonei. *Int J Colorectal Dis.* 2005;20:155–160.

32. Miner TJ, Shia J, Jaques DP, et al. Long-term survival following treatment of pseudomyxoma peritonei: an analysis of surgical therapy. *Ann Surg.* 2005;241:300–308.

33. Stewart JH IV, Shen P, Russell GB, et al. Appendiceal neoplasms with peritoneal dissemination: outcomes after cytoreductive surgery and intraperitoneal hyperthermic chemotherapy. *Ann Surg Oncol.* 2006;13:624–634.

34. Smeenk RM, Verwaal VJ, Antonini N, et al. Survival analysis of pseudomyxoma peritonei patients treated by cytoreductive surgery and hyperthermic intraperitoneal chemotherapy. *Ann Surg.* 2007;245:104–109.

35. Baratti D, Kusamura S, Nonaka D, et al. Pseudomyxoma peritonei: clinical pathological and biological prognostic factors in patients treated with cytoreductive surgery and hyperthermic intraperitoneal chemotherapy (HIPEC). *Ann Surg Oncol.* 2008;15:526–534.

# Cytoreductive Surgery Plus Intraperitoneal Chemohyperthermia in Patients with Colorectal Cancer at High Risk for Local-Regional Recurrence

Jeremie H. Lefevre • Dominique M. Elias

Colorectal cancer (CCR) remains the third commonest cause of cancer death in Western Europe and North America.[1] During the course of the disease, the onset of peritoneal carcinomatosis (PC) is considered a terminal condition, and patients are often treated palliatively.[2] The larger studies investigating the prognosis of isolated PC treated with chemotherapy included between 50 and 392 patients and resulted in a median survival duration of 5.2 to 12.6 months.[3–6] However, with complete cytoreductive surgery (CCRS) and hyperthermic intraperitoneal chemotherapy (HIPEC), the overall 5-year survival rate ranges from 22% to 49% in patients with colorectal PC.[3,7–9]

This review focuses on the concept of early repeated combined treatment: the "second-look" approach. The aim is to treat patients with PC at an early asymptomatic stage with CCRS + HIPEC. The 2 justifications for this early and systematic second look are that CCRS + HIPEC yield lower morbidity and better survival results when the extent of peritoneal disease is minimal.

After defining the second-look concept and a historical review, we will present this approach for 3 different types of patients: patients at high risk of developing PC after resection of the primary tumor, patients having already undergone CCRS + HIPEC, and patients presenting carcinoembryonic antigen (CEA) elevation or a positive positron emission tomography (PET).

## THE SECOND-LOOK CONCEPT

The second-look concept was first used by Wangensteen[10] in 1948. The principles are based on the systematic use of planned reoperation in asymptomatic patients with malignant disease who are theoretically at risk for developing recurrent or metastatic disease despite initial curative surgery. They used an interval of 6 months between resection of the primary and the second look.[11] The definition of high-risk patients and this arbitrary interval were far from optimal nor indeed was the efficacy of treatment (with surgery alone). This old approach had to be revisited in the light of recent progress.

## HIGH-RISK PATIENTS AFTER RESECTION OF THE PRIMARY TUMOR

### Preliminary Works

In the preliminary works (1940) by the team in the Department of Surgery in Minnesota, high-risk patients were defined as having involved nodes at histologic analysis.[11] This team developed the second-look program performing a systematic laparotomy every 6 months. Whenever recurrent disease was found, it was removed. Patients underwent further reoperations until no residual cancer was found. Among 234 asymptomatic patients with a previously resected

abdominal (colonic, rectal, gastric, or ovarian) cancer with invaded lymph nodes, 51% had residual disease diagnosed during one of the 338 second-look procedures meaning that half of the cohort underwent exploratory laparotomy. The mortality rate was 6.8%, and only 10% of patients who were found to have residual cancer during the second-look procedure were converted to a negative status.[11] Moreover, in the subgroup with colonic cancer (n = 91), peritoneal seeding was initially confined to the region of the primary lesion but subsequently spread to the entire abdomen and pelvis.[12] Progress was, therefore, definitely required for better selection of patients and more efficient treatment.

### Better Selection of Patients After Resection of the Primary Tumor

The selection of patients who may benefit from a second-look approach is now easier in light of the different series in the literature in which some subgroups of high-risk patients have been defined: patients exhibiting limited synchronous PC with the primary tumor, with synchronous ovarian metastases, with a perforated primary tumor, and an initial emergency presentation with blood loss or obstruction.[1,13–18] Many studies have reported contradictory results concerning the predictivity of developing PC when tumor cells are found in systematic peritoneal washings during resection of the primary, so this method is usually considered not sufficiently reliable.[19] Guidelines, therefore, do not recommend systematic peritoneal washing.

### The Second-Look Approach in the Area of CCRS + HIPEC: The Institut Gustave Roussy Experience

Since 1948, adjuvant therapies have completely modified the prognosis of patients with N+ CCR or liver metastasis or both. Nowadays, with modern systemic oxaliplatin-containing and irinotecan-containing chemotherapy, patients with isolated resectable PC can achieve a median survival of 24 months.[20] However, only CCRS + HIPEC is able to prolong median survival to roughly 63 months with a 5-year survival rate of 51%[20] in very selected patients. Throughout the published series of CCRS + HIPEC, the morbidity of the procedure seemed to be much lower and survival results were higher when the extent of peritoneal disease was limited. This argued in favor of using CCRS + HIPEC as early as possible in the natural history of PC. However, diagnosing PC at an early stage is impossible, both clinically (no symptoms) and radiologically (no signs), and in most cases, biologic modifications are not contributive. The only way to diagnose minimal PC early is to systematically perform laparotomy. The second-look concept, therefore, gained momentum because CCRS + HIPEC were performed earlier to remove limited peritoneal seeding, and this combined procedure proved to be far more efficient with less morbidity.[3,8,21–23]

To our knowledge, the only study to have reported results on the second-look approach with the use of CCRS + HIPEC came from our department.[24] This series included 29 patients during a 7-year period. Patients presented with macroscopically proven PC at initial surgery (minimal PC which was resected), patients with ovarian metastasis, and patients with a perforated tumor (spontaneous or inadvertent intraoperative perforation) at initial surgery were considered for second-look surgery, which was to be performed in asymptomatic patients. Thus, a new surgical exploration for reversal of a stoma, abnormalities on computed tomography (CT) scan, tumor marker elevation, or for clinical symptoms are not included in the definition of a second-look procedure as expounded in this article.

The principles of the procedure have already been described.[24] After surgical resection of the primary tumor, these "high-risk PC" patients commonly received adjuvant oxaliplatin-based or irinotecan-based chemotherapy regimens for 6 months. Six months later, if the complete workup was negative (no clinical symptoms nor any CT scan abnormality or blood tumor marker elevation), second-look surgery was proposed to the patients and was performed during the following month.

A median xyphopubic incision was systematically used, and the abdominal cavity was completely explored. Only a laparotomy with complete and systematic exploration of the abdominal cavity is able to detect early stage PC. The entire abdominal cavity cannot be explored and palpated extensively during laparoscopy, which does not allow one to reopen all previous dissection planes, and is, therefore, not indicated. Surgical exploration is often difficult. In our series of second-look surgical procedures, the mean operating time for exploratory laparotomies was 295 minutes.[24] If PC was discovered, the mean number of involved peritoneal areas and the mean peritoneal score for the extent of peritoneal seeding (Sugarbaker's score which can range from 1 to 39) was calculated.[23] After exploration, 3 options were defined as follows:

1. Patients with macroscopic PC, confirmed at frozen section analysis, underwent CCRS + HIPEC. Macroscopically detectable peritoneal disease had to be completely resected before administering HIPEC.
2. If there was no macroscopic PC, HIPEC was only performed in patients whose synchronous PC was resected with the primary tumor.

For the remaining patients, HIPEC was not performed. As usual in our institute, HIPEC was administered with oxaliplatin (300 mg/m$^2$) and irinotecan (200 mg/m$^2$) in 2 L/m$^2$ of dextrose, more than 30 minutes at 43° (gradient: 42°C–45°C) using the Coliseum technique. Before HIPEC, patients received systemic leucovorin (20 mg/m$^2$) and 5-fluorouracil (400 mg/m$^2$), resulting in the administration of a tritherapy.

## Results of Second-Look Surgery for High-Risk Patients With Colorectal Cancer

PC was observed in 16 patients (55%), and CCRS + HIPEC were performed. These patients had mild PC with a low peritoneal index (mean 10.2) compared with series treating symptomatic PC. Six patients with no PC at the second-look procedure were submitted to HIPEC because they had PC at the time of the first surgery, and finally only 7 (24%) had an exploratory laparotomy.

Concerning complications, no postoperative mortality was observed, and the morbidity rate was 38%. The mean hospital stay

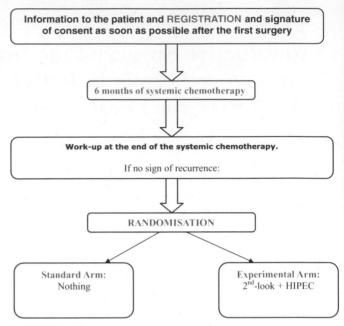

**FIGURE 1.**  Design of the trial.

was 16.4 days (7–24 days). Severe morbidity (grade III and IV) was observed in only 14% of the patients. Compared with series of symptomatic PC with severe morbidity (23%–40%), these results confirm that when PC is diagnosed and treated earlier, lower morbidity is observed.[22,25,26]

This systematic second-look surgery at 12 months found macroscopic PC in 62% of the patients with PC (resected) at initial surgery, in 75% of the patients who initially had ovarian metastases, and in 33% of patients with a perforated primary at initial surgery. Interestingly, among the 7 patients who did not receive HIPEC at second-look surgery (because no macroscopic PC was discovered), 3 subsequently developed PC. With a short follow-up of 27 months (6–96 months), long-term survival is not available, but the early results of this new approach are encouraging: 8 of 16 patients treated with CCRS + HIPEC are free of disease, 4 relapsed in the peritoneum, and 4 developed isolated visceral metastases.

We are in the process of submitting to the Ministry of Health, a randomized multicentric trial comparing simple follow-up to exploratory laparotomy plus "systematic" HIPEC in colorectal patients initially treated with surgery and adjuvant chemotherapy who have a high risk of developing PC (Fig. 1).

## HIGH-RISK PATIENTS BECAUSE THEY WERE ALREADY TREATED WITH CCRS + HIPEC

Some series have reported the use of second-look surgery after CCRS + HIPEC for patients with a mucinous appendiceal neoplasm.[27,28] In these studies, 98 patients underwent a second-look procedure and 45 patients had 3 or more surgeries. Second-look surgery was systematic (ie, true second look) for 29 patients (30%), and performed for abnormal clinical, radiologic, or biologic findings in the other patients. The majority of patients (n = 58, 59%) had the first second-look surgery within a year after the initial procedure. The 5-year overall survival rate was higher compared with that of patients who did not undergo reoperation, and prolonged survival in patients with 3 or more reoperations was significantly associated with complete cytoreduction.

The same procedures have been undertaken for PC of colorectal origin. In a series of 86 patients who underwent CCRS + HIPEC, 18 developed signs and symptoms of recurrent colon or rectal cancer in the absence of extra-abdominal dissemination, so further surgery was considered of possible benefit.[29] This indication for CCRS + HIPEC is totally different from the early described second-look procedure where patients were asymptomatic without any clinical sign of recurrence. In this series of 18 symptomatic patients, second-look surgery was successful if the patient had complete cytoreduction at the time of definitive treatment for PC ($P = 0.04$). Patients, in whom cytoreduction was incomplete at the time of initial treatment, did not benefit from the second-look procedure. This result confirms that patients should not undergo HIPEC unless cytoreduction is complete.[8,20,30] Moreover, the completeness of cytoreduction proved to be an important prognostic indicator at the time of second-look surgery. Patients who had CC0 or CC1 cytoreduction at the time of the second-look procedure were statistically significantly more likely to have prolonged 1-year ($P = 0.047$) and 2-year ($P = 0.066$) survivals.[29]

To our knowledge, no study has assessed the results of systematic second-look surgery after CCRS + HIPEC for PC of colorectal origin. Before proposing this systematic second-look procedure, you need to answer the following 3 questions:

1. If a first combined CCRS + HIPEC procedure has failed to cure PC, is a repeated procedure indicated to treat recurrent PC, and if so, should the drugs be modified?
2. How to define high-risk patients likely to redevelop isolated PC?
3. What should be the cost-efficiency results for the society?

## OTHER SELECTION TOOLS FOR HIGH-RISK PATIENTS WHO MAY BENEFIT FROM CCRS + HIPEC

Faced with these interesting results, one might question the value of this second-look approach for patients who present with isolated CEA elevation or isolated uptake on the PET scan during follow-up after previous resection of a CCR. In these cases, second-look surgery is not systematically proposed for asymptomatic patients but for abnormal biologic or imaging findings.

### Isolated CEA Elevation

After surgical resection, CEA usually declines progressively and normalizes within 4 to 6 weeks.[31,32] Elevation may be secondary to a local or distant recurrence of the cancer. As was the case for the first second-look surgery for asymptomatic patients, some old data are available concerning CEA elevation and repeated surgery. Wanebo et al[33] reported that among a cohort of 358 patients operated between 1970 and 1976 for CCR, 16 were reoperated on for significant CEA elevation without any other sign of recurrence. Liver metastases were found in 6 patients and a local recurrence in 6. Two patients had a negative exploration and the remaining 2 patients had lung metastases. Among the 16 patients, 6 (42.8%) underwent a curative resection. In another larger study by Martin et al,[34] 146 patients were operated on for CEA elevation with no radiologic sign of extra-abdominal spread. In these patients, 139 (95%) had recurrences, and 81 (58%) of these lesions were resectable for potential cure. In this interesting study, no details were provided on the discovery of PC, but it is likely that patients with unresectable disease had at least some PC. Given the proven efficacy of CCRS + HIPEC, the rate of curative second-look surgery should be higher.

A recent review provides other arguments for the rationale of second-look surgery when faced with CEA elevation.[35] Approximately 75% of all recurrences give rise to an increase in CEA.[36] Compared with a regular clinical evaluation and other tests such as liver function tests, other serum markers, and CT scan examination, CEA monitoring is more effective in detecting early evidence of recurrent disease than any other single entity.[37–39] Serum CEA levels may rise before the development of cancer-related symptoms with a median lead time of 4.5 to 8 months.[34,40,41] A meta-analysis of 7 nonrandomized trials showed a 9% improvement in 5-year survival for patients whose CEA levels were followed-up postoperatively.[42,43]

However, in the majority of the studies, the recurrences were located on the liver, and few data are available on the rate of PC discovered through CEA elevation. CEA is most sensitive for hepatic or retroperitoneal metastases and less sensitive for local, peritoneal, or pulmonary involvement.[41] Even if the discovery of hepatic metastases does not prohibit the use of HIPEC,[44,45] the number of patients who would benefit from CRRS + HIPEC will probably be low. Moreover, some authors argue that the cost of monitoring is as high as that of the rate of negative second-look procedures.[41,46] Moertel et al[41] reported the results of 1217 patients with resected colon cancer, among whom 1017 had postoperative CEA monitoring. Among those patients, 417 developed a recurrence from CCR. Fifty-nine percent of these patients had CEA elevation (>5 ng/mL) before the discovery of the recurrence, but 16% of 600 patients without a tumor recurrence exhibited false-positive CEA elevation. Finally, approximately 2.9% of patients with CEA elevation were alive and disease free for more than 1 year after salvage surgery. A similar proportion (2%) of patients without CEA monitoring, were also alive and disease free more than 1 year after surgery.

Finally, the concept of second-look surgery with CCRS + HIPEC in case of resectable PC for asymptomatic patients with CEA elevation has yet to be validated and further studies are warranted.

### Isolated Uptake on PET Scan

Conventional imaging modalities like CT scan exhibit high-diagnostic sensitivity, but it is difficult to distinguish between postoperative scars and relapse.[47] In contrast, the use of fluor-18-deoxyglucose-PET with a high diagnostic value in the detection of recurrent colorectal carcinoma may be a valuable tool for identifying patients likely to benefit from a second-look approach. A recent meta-analysis on the sensitivity and specificity of this modality included 27 published studies.[47] PET was found to be an accurate technique for detecting pelvic metastasis or local regional recurrence, with a sensitivity comprised between 70% and 100% and a specificity of 85% to 100%. In contrast, when PC is present, it strongly underestimates the real extent of this disease, as we previously showed.[48]

Its major role is to rule out extra-abdominal disease, which may preclude CCRS + HIPEC. Finally, the detection of isolated peritoneal uptake on fluor-18-deoxyglucose-PET, during follow-up, could be a valuable indication for proposing a laparotomy aimed at ultimately performing a CCRS + HIPEC, but there are no data concerning this point.

## CONCLUSIONS

This review has highlighted the efficiency of second-look surgery associated with CCRS + HIPEC in selected high-risk patients after resection of their primary. This procedure is less morbid and more efficient than classic CCRS + HIPEC, because of the early detection of asymptomatic, burgeoning PC. Further studies are needed to validate our preliminary results in a randomized fashion in larger cohorts.

## ACKNOWLEDGMENTS

*The authors thank Lorna Saint Ange for editing.*

## REFERENCES

1. McArdle CS, McMillan DC, Hole DJ. The impact of blood loss, obstruction and perforation on survival in patients undergoing curative resection for colon cancer. *Br J Surg.* 2006;93:483–488.
2. Koppe MJ, Boerman OC, Oyen WJ, et al. Peritoneal carcinomatosis of colorectal origin: incidence and current treatment strategies. *Ann Surg.* 2006;243:212–222.
3. Verwaal VJ, van Ruth S, de Bree E, et al. Randomized trial of cytoreduction and hyperthermic intraperitoneal chemotherapy versus systemic chemotherapy and palliative surgery in patients with peritoneal carcinomatosis of colorectal cancer. *J Clin Oncol.* 2003;21:3737–3743.
4. Jayne DG, Fook S, Loi C, et al. Peritoneal carcinomatosis from colorectal cancer. *Br J Surg.* 2002;89:1545–1550.
5. Sadeghi B, Arvieux C, Glehen O, et al. Peritoneal carcinomatosis from nongynecologic malignancies: results of the EVOCAPE 1 multicentric prospective study. *Cancer.* 2000;88:358–363.
6. Chu DZ, Lang NP, Thompson C, et al. Peritoneal carcinomatosis in nongynecologic malignancy. A prospective study of prognostic factors. *Cancer.* 1989;63:364–367.
7. Elias D, Blot F, El Otmany A, et al. Curative treatment of peritoneal carcinomatosis arising from colorectal cancer by complete resection and intraperitoneal chemotherapy. *Cancer.* 2001;92:71–76.
8. Glehen O, Kwiatkowski F, Sugarbaker PH, et al. Cytoreductive surgery combined with perioperative intraperitoneal chemotherapy for the management of peritoneal carcinomatosis from colorectal cancer: a multi-institutional study. *J Clin Oncol.* 2004;22:3284–3292.
9. Yan TD, Black D, Savady R, et al. Systematic review on the efficacy of cytoreductive surgery combined with perioperative intraperitoneal chemotherapy for peritoneal carcinomatosis from colorectal carcinoma. *J Clin Oncol.* 2006;24:4011–4019.
10. Wangensteen OH. Cancer of the colon and rectum; with special reference to earlier recognition of alimentary tract malignancy; secondary delayed re-entry of the abdomen in patients exhibiting lymph node involvement; subtotal primary excision of the colon; operation in obstruction. *Wis Med J.* 1949;48:591–597.
11. Gilbertsen VA, Wangensteen OH. A summary of thirteen years' experience with the second look program. *Surg Gynecol Obstet.* 1962;114:438–442.
12. Gunderson LL, Sosin H, Levitt S. Extrapelvic colon—areas of failure in a reoperation series: implications for adjuvant therapy. *Int J Radiat Oncol Biol Phys.* 1985;11:731–741.
13. Zoetmulder FA. Cancer cell seeding during abdominal surgery: experimental studies. *Cancer Treat Res.* 1996;82:155–161.
14. Sweitzer KL, Nathanson SD, Nelson LT, et al. Irrigation does not dislodge or destroy tumor cells adherent to the tumor bed. *J Surg Oncol.* 1993;53:184–190.
15. Jacquet P, Elias D, Sugarbaker PH. [Tumor implantation in cicatrization sites following surgery for digestive cancers.] *J Chir (Paris).* 1996;133:175–182.
16. Willett C, Tepper JE, Cohen A, et al. Obstructive and perforative colonic carcinoma: patterns of failure. *J Clin Oncol.* 1985;3:379–384.
17. Slanetz CA Jr. The effect of inadvertent intraoperative perforation on survival and recurrence in colorectal cancer. *Dis Colon Rectum.* 1984;27:792–797.
18. Jestin P, Nilsson J, Heurgren M, et al. Emergency surgery for colonic cancer in a defined population. *Br J Surg.* 2005;92:94–100.
19. Yang SH, Lin JK, Lai CR, et al. Risk factors for peritoneal dissemination of colorectal cancer. *J Surg Oncol.* 2004;87:167–173.
20. Elias D, Lefevre JH, Chevalier J, et al. Complete cytoreductive surgery plus intraperitoneal chemohyperthermia with oxaliplatin for peritoneal carcinomatosis of colorectal origin. *J Clin Oncol.* 2009;27:681–685.
21. Verwaal VJ, van Ruth S, Witkamp A, et al. Long-term survival of peritoneal carcinomatosis of colorectal origin. *Ann Surg Oncol.* 2005;12:65–71.
22. Elias D, Raynard B, Farkhondeh F, et al. Peritoneal carcinomatosis of colorectal origin. *Gastroenterol Clin Biol.* 2006;30:1200–1204.
23. Sugarbaker PH, Schellinx ME, Chang D, et al. Peritoneal carcinomatosis from adenocarcinoma of the colon. *World J Surg.* 1996;20:585–591; discussion 592.
24. Elias D, Goere D, Di Pietrantonio D, et al. Results of systematic second-look surgery in patients at high risk of developing colorectal peritoneal carcinomatosis. *Ann Surg.* 2008;247:445–450.
25. Shen P, Hawksworth J, Lovato J, et al. Cytoreductive surgery and intraperitoneal hyperthermic chemotherapy with mitomycin C for peritoneal carcinomatosis from nonappendiceal colorectal carcinoma. *Ann Surg Oncol.* 2004;11:178–186.
26. Glehen O, Cotte E, Schreiber V, et al. Intraperitoneal chemohyperthermia and attempted cytoreductive surgery in patients with peritoneal carcinomatosis of colorectal origin. *Br J Surg.* 2004;91:747–754.
27. Esquivel J, Sugarbaker PH. Second-look surgery in patients with peritoneal dissemination from appendiceal malignancy: analysis of prognostic factors in 98 patients. *Ann Surg.* 2001;234:198–205.
28. Mohamed F, Chang D, Sugarbaker PH. Third look surgery and beyond for appendiceal malignancy with peritoneal dissemination. *J Surg Oncol.* 2003;83:5–12; discussion 12–13.
29. Portilla AG, Sugarbaker PH, Chang D. Second-look surgery after cytoreduction and intraperitoneal chemotherapy for peritoneal carcinomatosis from colorectal cancer: analysis of prognostic features. *World J Surg.* 1999;23:23–29.
30. Elias D, Sideris L, Pocard M, et al. Efficacy of intraperitoneal chemohyperthermia with oxaliplatin in colorectal peritoneal carcinomatosis. Preliminary results in 24 patients. *Ann Oncol.* 2004;15:781–785.
31. Nakamura T, Tabuchi Y, Nakae S, et al. Serum carcinoembryonic antigen levels and proliferating cell nuclear antigen labeling index for patients with colorectal carcinoma. Correlation with tumor progression and survival. *Cancer.* 1996;77(8 Suppl):1741–1746.
32. Fletcher RH. Carcinoembryonic antigen. *Ann Intern Med.* 1986;104:66–73.
33. Wanebo JH, Stearns M, Schwartz MK. Use of CEA as an indicator of early recurrence and as a guide to a selected second-look procedure in patients with colorectal cancer. *Ann Surg.* 1978;188:481–493.
34. Martin EW Jr, Minton JP, Carey LC. CEA-directed second-look surgery in the asymptomatic patient after primary resection of colorectal carcinoma. *Ann Surg.* 1985;202:310–317.
35. Goldstein MJ, Mitchell EP. Carcinoembryonic antigen in the staging and follow-up of patients with colorectal cancer. *Cancer Invest.* 2005;23:338–351.
36. Mayer RJ, Garnick MB, Steele GD Jr, et al. Carcinoembryonic antigen (CEA) as a monitor of chemotherapy in disseminated colorectal cancer. *Cancer.* 1978;42(3 Suppl):1428–1433.
37. Hall NR, Finan PJ, Stephenson BM, et al. The role of CA-242 and CEA in surveillance following curative resection for colorectal cancer. *Br J Cancer.* 1994;70:549–553.
38. Sugarbaker PH, Gianola FJ, Dwyer A, et al. A simplified plan for follow-up of patients with colon and rectal cancer supported by prospective studies of laboratory and radiologic test results. *Surgery.* 1987;102:79–87.
39. Rocklin MS, Senagore AJ, Talbott TM. Role of carcinoembryonic antigen and liver function tests in the detection of recurrent colorectal carcinoma. *Dis Colon Rectum.* 1991;34:794–797.
40. McCall JL, Black RB, Rich CA, et al. The value of serum carcinoembryonic antigen in predicting recurrent disease following curative resection of colorectal cancer. *Dis Colon Rectum.* 1994;37:875–881.
41. Moertel CG, Fleming TR, Macdonald JS, et al. An evaluation of the carcinoembryonic antigen (CEA) test for monitoring patients with resected colon cancer. *JAMA.* 1993;270:943–947.
42. Bruinvels DJ, Stiggelbout AM, Kievit J, et al. Follow-up of patients with colorectal cancer. A meta-analysis. *Ann Surg.* 1994;219:174–182.
43. Berman JM, Cheung RJ, Weinberg DS. Surveillance after colorectal cancer resection. *Lancet.* 2000;355:395–399.
44. Elias D, Benizri E, Pocard M, et al. Treatment of synchronous peritoneal carcinomatosis and liver metastases from colorectal cancer. *Eur J Surg Oncol.* 2006;32:632–636.
45. Kianmanesh R, Scaringi S, Sabate JM, et al. Iterative cytoreductive surgery associated with hyperthermic intraperitoneal chemotherapy for treatment of peritoneal carcinomatosis of colorectal origin with or without liver metastases. *Ann Surg.* 2007;245:597–603.
46. Staab HJ, Anderer FA, Stumpf E, et al. Eighty-four potential second-look operations based on sequential carcinoembryonic antigen determinations and clinical investigations in patients with recurrent gastrointestinal cancer. *Am J Surg.* 1985;149:198–204.
47. Zhang C, Chen Y, Xue H, et al. Diagnostic value of FDG-PET in recurrent colorectal carcinoma: a meta-analysis. *Int J Cancer.* 2009;124:167–173.
48. Dromain C, Leboulleux S, Auperin A, et al. Staging of peritoneal carcinomatosis: enhanced CT vs. PET/CT. *Abdom Imaging.* 2008;33:87–93.

# Surgical Techniques in Visceral Resection and Peritonectomy Procedures

Philip Bao • David Bartlett

Current surgical management of the peritoneal surface malignancies can be performed with curative intent, and potential long-term survival when a strategy of cytoreductive surgery with peritoneal chemoperfusion is used for select patients and cancers. Controversies regarding the administration of peritoneal chemotherapy (technique, hyperthermia, agent of choice, and timing) will likely remain unresolved because of its nonuniform practice across different centers and the difficulty generating valid clinical trial data addressing best methods, but there is little disagreement that, at minimum, adequate cytoreduction is critical to successful outcome. The rationale for visceral resection and peritonectomy is to remove all macroscopic tumors that may cause symptoms, such as obstruction and ascites, while creating an optimal environment for tumor cell exposure to perfusate. If appropriate cytoreduction cannot be achieved, most centers would not proceed with hyperthermic intraperitoneal chemoperfusion (HIPEC).

## IMPORTANCE OF COMPLETE CYTOREDUCTION

Slightly different terminology exists to describe the completeness of cytoreduction achieved during surgery, but the cytoreduction is considered adequate if either no macroscopic tumor remains (R0) or if only nodules less than approximately 2.5 mm (R1) remain to allow tumor penetration of intraperitoneal chemotherapy.[1-4] Larger gross residual tumor nodules are classified as R2 debulkings and are insufficient. Numerous studies stratify survival analyses on the basis of this surgical endpoint, and the completeness of cytoreduction serves as a major prognostic factor for outcome in treating pseudomyxoma peritonei, sarcomatosis, malignant peritoneal mesothelioma, and gastrointestinal carcinomatosis of different origins.[5-10] Median survival after inadequate cytoreduction, despite additional chemoperfusion, seems little different from that observed with palliative treatments only.[11] In addition, that disease recurrence most frequently occurs in the peritoneal cavity supports the importance of the local-regional control to which cytoreduction contributes.[12] Finally, in the setting of recurrence, cytoreduction and HIPEC procedures can be repeated with some survival benefit.[13]

## MORBIDITY AND MORTALITY OF AGGRESSIVE CYTOREDUCTION

However, the aggressive cytoreductive surgery is not without significant morbidity and mortality, ranging from 20% to 50% and 2% to 12%, respectively, in some series.[8,14-18] Multivisceral resections, multiple anastomoses, and patient population often malnourished from cancer, and prior systemic therapies each increase the potential for perioperative complications. Median operative blood loss is reported to be several liters, and hospital stays average about 2 weeks. It is difficult to distinguish the relative contributions of cytoreduction versus chemoperfusion to perioperative morbidity, but certainly the most common complications are surgical, and many require procedural interventions—anastomotic leak, fistula, and abscess—as opposed to hematologic toxicity attributable to chemotherapy. In particular, reports of anastomotic leak rates range from 6% to 18%. The frequency of complications, as would be expected with most complex surgical procedures, is proportional to operative time and blood loss. Although one study has suggested that multivisceral resection alone is not necessarily associated with increased morbidity, reoperative rates, and poor survival,[19] this patient population requires careful postoperative monitoring for early detection of complications.

Clearly, the extent of adequate cytoreduction depends on the extent of carcinomatosis, and thus prudent surgical judgment to proceed is required on initial exploration of the abdominal cavity because preoperative imaging usually underestimates what will be found. Even with the complete cytoreduction, extensive colorectal carcinomatosis with a Peritoneal Carcinomatosis Index greater than 20 may carry poor prognosis.[20] Thus when considering cytoreductive surgery, the twin principles of appropriate patient selection and meticulous surgical technique, as in all surgery, should be observed.

## TECHNIQUES IN VISCERAL RESECTION AND PERITONECTOMY

The techniques of visceral resection and peritonectomy follow logically from the oncologic goals of cytoreduction and the need to minimize perioperative morbidity. Certainly, many organs, such as the spleen, can be safely removed, but functional bowel length should be preserved where possible. Tumor histology and patterns of peritoneal spread will also influence the extent of cytoreduction indicated, with malignant mesothelioma requiring more radical peritonectomy due to diffuse involvement of the peritoneum, as opposed to colon cancer where resection of visible tumor may just require limited resections.[21] Debulking and HIPEC procedures easily last upward of 6 to 10 hours, thus, due diligence should be given to patient positioning and padding; maintenance of normothermia; deep vein thrombosis prophylaxis with sequential compression devices and subcutaneous heparin; and appropriately timed preoperative antibiotics redosed if necessary during the case.

Sugarbaker[22] provides detailed technical descriptions of visceral and parietal peritonectomy to clear the diaphragms, omentum, lesser sac, major viscera, and pelvis of tumor burden. Above all, systematic exploration of all compartments and subsequent clearance of the peritoneal cavity is necessary to identify sites of disease and achieve optimal cytoreduction. The goal of the complete cytoreduction needs to be weighed against the potential morbidity of each aspect of the procedure performed and the potential alteration of the patient's quality of life. These issues also need to be assessed in the context of the biology of the tumor being treated.

Effective cytoreduction requires many specialized tools to enhance visibility and exposure, minimize blood loss, and limit the duration of the procedure. A versatile self-retaining retractor (eg, Thompson Retractor, Thompson Surgical Instruments, Inc., Traverse City, MI) is required to free the assistants' hands, and surgical headlights improve visibility throughout the peritoneal cavity. For hemostasis, we use electrocautery and argon beam coagulator. As the length of the procedure may influence morbidity and mortality, any instruments that can be safely used to expedite the case should be considered. We use automatic clips, coagulating dissectors (eg, LigaSure, Valleylab, Boulder, CO), and vascular, bowel, and skin stapling devices. The case should proceed in a uniform and a standard fashion, so that the routine is comfortable and nothing is left unattended. The following is a detailed description of the procedure in the order that we prefer.

## LAPAROSCOPIC EXPLORATION TO ASSESS RESECTABILITY

Our goal is to perform laparotomy only on patients who can be resected completely of all gross disease. Thus, laparoscopy may be performed to assess R0 resectability before formally opening the abdomen. It can rule out some patients and get them back onto systemic chemotherapy quickly. If safe laparoscopic access cannot be attained quickly, then the surgeon should proceed expeditiously with laparotomy.

By using the computed tomography scan as a guide, a safe location for the trocar should be planned first. We use an open cutdown technique in these cases, as the risk of an inadvertent enterotomy is high with its attendant costs of a leak or fistula. The abdomen is explored using 2 or 3 ports. Given the long case ahead, we try to complete laparoscopic assessment within 15 minutes. If a complete cytoreduction seems feasible, we then convert to an open procedure. Once opened, the peritoneal cavity is assessed again, and for those patients in whom at least an R1 resection can be performed, we will proceed, but if an R2 resection is the best that can be achieved then the procedure is terminated.

## INCISION

Maximizing visualization mandates using a long-midline excision from xiphoid to pubis. The patient has often had a prior laparotomy, and consideration should be made for complete resection of the abdominal scar and the umbilicus, especially when an umbilical hernia is present or palpable tumor is present in the abdominal wall. Entering the abdomen can often be challenging as patients with significant carcinomatosis will often have intestine cemented to the anterior abdominal wall, especially at the midline scar. In this circumstance, the peritoneum and even the posterior rectus fascia should be left on the intestine and the abdomen entered more laterally. Attempts to separate intestine from the anterior abdominal wall through tumor nodules will lead to serosal tears and full-thickness bowel injuries, which just increase operative time and postoperative complications.

In patients with bulky peritoneal carcinomatosis, the better decision may be to not enter the peritoneum directly but rather to stay in the subperitoneal plane and perform the anterior abdominal wall peritonectomy before entering the abdomen. This plane can be dissected to the pericolic gutters on both sides before formally entering the abdomen laterally. This completes the anterior wall peritonectomy in a safe and efficient manner.

## ANTERIOR ABDOMINAL WALL AND FALCIFORM LIGAMENT

Once the abdomen is open, the anterior abdominal wall is inspected and all gross disease removed. In general, electrocautery at high temperatures can resect nodules rapidly with minimal blood loss. For areas of the anterior abdominal wall that are diffusely involved, formal peritoneal stripping is performed. This can be performed before opening the abdomen as described earlier or the peritoneum can be pulled down from the posterior fascia at the midline, creating a dissection plane to the pericolic gutters on both sides, up to the diaphragm superiorly and down to the bladder inferiorly. We use empty sponge clamps or ring forceps to grasp the peritoneum and maintain a broad base, using blunt and electrocautery dissection to complete the anterior wall peritonectomy in a relatively short time. The falciform and round ligaments are taken down and resected completely in all patients. This will help retraction of the abdominal wall and also aid the flow of perfusate during HIPEC. The falciform is divided to the suprahepatic vena cava superiorly and then separated from the liver capsule to the umbilical fissure at the branch point of the liver segments 4B and 3 portal pedicles.

## LYSIS OF ADHESIONS

Once the anterior abdominal wall is dissected, the self-retaining retractor is assembled for maximum exposure of the abdominal cavity (Fig. 1). A complete lysis of adhesions is then performed. Care must be taken to avoid serosal injuries to the bowel, and areas matted with tumor involvement or scar can be marked for resection. We prefer not to commit to any bowel resection until full exploration has been performed. During the complete lysis of adhesions, the assessment of the extent of disease continues, and a determination is made whether to proceed with attempted cytoreduction and HIPEC versus changing the goals of the procedure to palliating impending sites of obstruction and other problems.

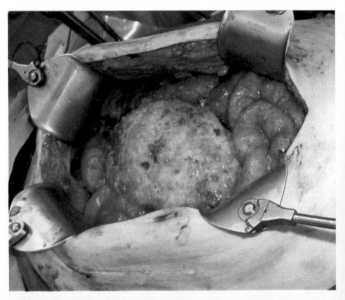

**FIGURE 1.**  Optimal exposure with a self-retaining retractor and incision from xiphoid to pubis. The head of the patient is to the left.

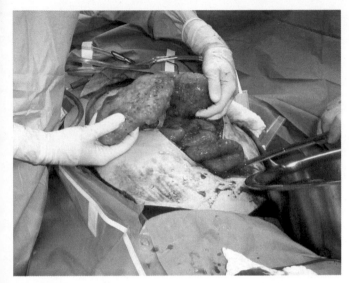

**FIGURE 2.**   A large omental cake of tumor involvement.

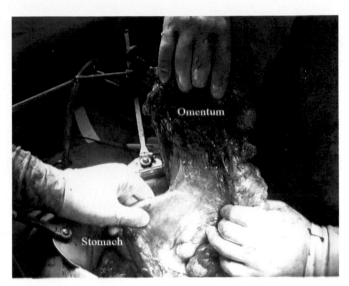

**FIGURE 4.**   The greater omentum resected from the greater curve of the stomach.

## GREATER OMENTECTOMY

After lysis of adhesions, a greater omentectomy is performed. This is standard both to remove a common site of tumor implantation and to facilitate fluid circulation during chemoperfusion (Fig. 2). The omentum should be lifted and taken off the transverse colon sharply, avoiding injury to the transverse colon that can lead to late perforations and fistulas (Fig. 3). If the omentum is fixed with tumor to the transverse colon, it must be decided whether the complete transverse colon should be resected or small areas of serosa taken to achieve complete cytoreduction. The rest of the abdomen should be assessed for resectability, as it would make no sense to perform a transverse colectomy to clear 1- to 2-mm residual deposits with gross tumor left on the superior vena cava or the base of the bladder. Sometimes it is necessary to cut through the tumor, lifting the omentum off the trans-

verse colon, so that no bridges are burned before complete inspection of the peritoneal cavity.

The omentum is also taken off the greater curvature of the stomach (Fig. 4). If it is involved with bulky tumor, the gastroepiploic arcade is typically not preserved, but if the omentum is free of disease, then attempts should be made to preserve this gastric vascular supply. This will allow some flexibility for subsequent procedures during the case that may further compromise blood flow to the stomach.

## SPLENECTOMY

As the omentum is dissected from the greater curvature of the stomach, the decision for splenectomy is made. The spleen is often involved with peritoneal carcinomatosis either by the extension of omental disease into the splenic hilum or by the extension of subdiaphragmatic peritoneal disease over the splenic capsule. The splenic capsule itself may have significant direct tumor involvement. The spleen is usually taken en bloc with the greater omentum (Fig. 5). Care should be taken to carefully dissect tumor from the pancreas as pancreatic leaks can be a significant cause of morbidity with these procedures. The spleen is mobilized from its peritoneal attachments and lifted up to expose the splenic artery and the vein, which can best be approached posteriorly away from the peritoneum and the omentum. We use vascular staplers to divide the splenic vessels. The soft tissue is dissected directly off the pancreas, and the spleen and omentum removed together. In cases where the tumor is invading the tail of the pancreas, a distal pancreatectomy can be performed en bloc with the omentectomy and the splenectomy as well. We generally divide the splenic vessels first with a vascular stapler and then the pancreas with another staple load, oversewing the staple line with interrupted, overlapping figure-of-eight sutures to assure control of the pancreatic duct. In addition, a drain is usually left at the end of the case to monitor for pancreatic leak.

## LEFT HEMI-DIAPHRAGM PERITONECTOMY

After splenectomy, the retractors are in an ideal location to complete the left diaphragm peritonectomy. The peritoneum is incised anteriorly over a long distance. It is then grasped with the sponge

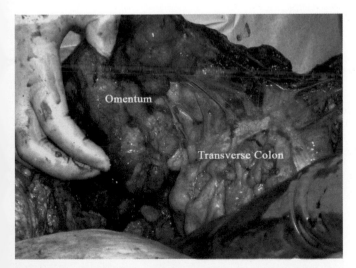

**FIGURE 3.**   Carcinomatosis of the greater omentum along the transverse colon.

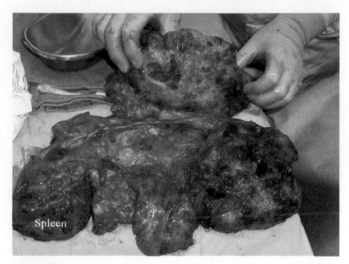

**FIGURE 5.** En bloc greater omentectomy and splenectomy.

clamps, and a combination of blunt and sharp dissection with electrocautery is used to peel the peritoneum off the diaphragm. In cases of minimal peritoneal involvement, isolated resection of nodules can be performed, but diffuse disease requires formal peritonectomy. The integrity of the diaphragm should be protected as any full-thickness injury will lead to contamination of the chest cavity. Regardless of whether the diaphragm is injured, a pleural effusion may result requiring postoperative drainage. Although we do not routinely place prophylactic chest tubes for this purpose, this has been described and should be considered for larger diaphragmatic defects before repair. The left hemidiaphragm peritonectomy is usually one of the easier procedures. It is often less involved with tumor than the right hemidiaphragm, and there are certainly fewer structures of concern in this compartment. Peritonectomy should be taken over to the esophageal hiatus medially and then the peritoneum severed. We usually come back to dissect the right hemidiaphragm and tissue overlying the pericardium later during the case.

## SMALL INTESTINE

At this point, the entirety of the small intestine is run from the ligament of Treitz to the cecum. There are often tumor nodules at the ligament of Treitz, and these are resected as well as any other tumor along the way. Both sides of the mesentery are inspected and tumor excised with electrocautery. Tumor involving the serosa of the bowel is generally left intact until the entire small bowel is assessed. It is advisable to avoid making numerous full-thickness injuries to the small bowel to remove serosal tumor deposits as the risk of leak and fistulization will increase dramatically. Rather, the goal should be to remove large segments of bowel in continuity that are diffusely involved with tumor. Small nodules on the serosa may need to be left behind if the extent of the involvement is significant. Tumor nodules from colon cancer often will invade along the mesentery where the blood supply enters the small intestine, and this can be especially problematic to resect without full-thickness injury to the bowel. Once the small bowel has been inspected completely without committing to any resection, a decision is made to perform resections while leaving adequate bowel length for normal nutritional function and minimizing the number of anastomoses. Our goal is to maintain at least 200 cm of small intestine; however, we will accept as little as 120 cm if this achieves a

complete cytoreduction. The surgeon must consider whether adequate colon will be left behind for fluid absorption and whether a gastrectomy and gastrojejunostomy will be required, which would further limit the functional residual intestine. Leaving 100 cm of small intestine combined with an ileostomy and a gastrojejunostomy will likely commit the patient to lifetime parenteral nutrition. Once it is decided how much of the small intestine can be safely removed, the bowel can be divided with a stapler, and the mesentery resected with the LigaSure device. As much of the mesentery as possible is left to minimize the risk of ischemia to other parts of the intestine. This can be, especially, critical when a minimal amount of intestine remains. The anastomosis of resected bowel is then deferred until after HIPEC.

## LARGE INTESTINE

The large intestine is then traced and inspected. The transverse colon will have been assessed previously at the time of the omentectomy. The cecum is often involved with tumor around the mesoappendix, and an appendectomy should be performed if it is still in place. The abdominal wall peritonectomy should have been carried down to the pericolic gutters and any residual tumors should be taken off the right and left colon. As with the small intestine, no decisions should be made regarding resection until the entire colon and rectum have been assessed. The transverse colic mesentery needs to be inspected carefully and tumor resected. The appendices epiploica of the sigmoid colon are often involved and should likewise be excised. Because of gravity tumor often involves the pelvic peritoneum and invades into the anterior rectum and posterior bladder. The need for low anterior resection is evaluated in the context of what residual bowel exists for reconnection and the need for diverting loop ileostomy.

## PELVIC PERITONECTOMY

The pelvic peritonectomy is probably the most challenging procedure. Care must be taken not to injure the ureters, the iliac vessels, the male vas deferens, the bladder, and the rectum. The pelvic peritoneum is least likely to be bluntly dissected, and so in general, a sharp dissection is required. The peritoneum is again incised using a long incision anteriorly. A flap of peritoneum is then grasped with the sponge clamps and taken off the lateral pelvic walls and bladder (Fig. 6). The peritoneum is then incised at the pelvic inlet posteriorly and

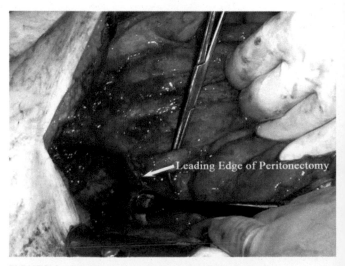

**FIGURE 6.** Peritonectomy along the right pelvis.

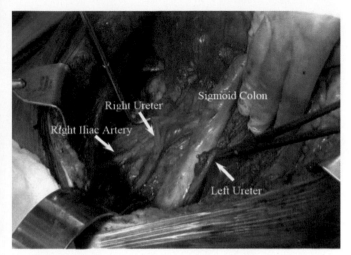

**FIGURE 7.** Completed pelvic peritonectomy with identification and preservation of the iliac vessels and ureters.

lifted to identify the bilateral iliac vessels and ureters early (Fig. 7). Each ureter is traced to its insertion in the bladder, lifting the peritoneum off and the different planes of peritoneum brought together to complete the peritonectomy. Although it is ideal to take the entire pelvic peritoneum en bloc, this is rarely successful or necessary. The advantage of taking a large section is that it enhances the ability to bluntly dissect the peritoneum. The most important aspect though is not to injure any of the pelvic structures.

Male patients should be warned of potential impotence. During pelvic peritonectomy, the gonadal blood supply can be compromised leading to testicular atrophy. The vas deferens may also be involved and killed, in which case the patient may have a dry ejaculate. Temporary bladder dysfunction may also occur, and the patient should be aware of these issues before debulking. In general, the iliac vessels are not invaded from carcinomatosis. However occasionally in advanced cases, the adventitia of the vessels may be stripped in an attempt to dissect tumor from these areas. Vessels must be inspected and reinforced as appropriate to prevent pseudoaneurysm formation.

## BLADDER AND URETERS

The base of the bladder and anterior rectum are often invaded by peritoneal tumor at the base of the cul de sac. Committing to a resection of the rectum in this location usually commits the patient to a diverting ileostomy, and therefore care should be taken to avoid full-thickness injury of the rectum if possible. Likewise, a bladder injury in this location might compromise the urethral orifice or lead to difficult leaks and urinary fistulas. Disease extensively infiltrating the bladder in this location may limit the ability to perform a complete peritonectomy and cytoreduction. A cystectomy with ileal conduit would generally be considered too high risk in the context of carcinomatosis and HIPEC; however, limited bladder dome involvement can be resected and reconstructed if necessary.

Because of the superficial location of the ureters under the peritoneum, it is a common site of involvement with tumor-related obstruction or an inability to excise tumor without injuring the ureters. Usually, the ureter is involved deeper than the pelvis, and significant palliation and avoidance of chronic stents can be achieved by resecting the ureteral involvement and reimplanting the ureter.

## UTERUS AND OVARIES

For female patients, the uterus, the tubes, and the ovaries are often involved with carcinomatosis. The ovaries should be taken out routinely regardless of gross involvement as the ovaries are at high risk and most of patients are not of childbearing potential. Likewise, the fallopian tubes and the broad ligament should be taken without hesitation, and this can be performed simply and quickly. The uterus, if there is a deep invasion of carcinomatosis, is also removed. This often will be at the deep cul de sac where thick invasion of the cervix or vagina will be found necessitating a total hysterectomy. However, if the uterus has limited involvement the individual nodules themselves can be excised quite safely. Any procedure that leads to a suture line such as at the vaginal cuff can potentially increase the morbidity of the procedure; therefore if the uterus does not need to be removed, it should be left in situ.

## RECTUM

If the tumor invades the rectum, a low anterior resection must be performed, this can be performed en bloc with the pelvic peritonectomy. The sigmoid colon should be divided as far distally as possible to allow for a tension-free reconstruction. The rectum and its mesentery should be completely mobilized, lifted up, and the rectum divided below the level of tumor involvement. As this form of tumor never involves the anal sphincters, sphincter preservation can always be achieved. In general, we will use a diverting ileostomy to protect any low rectal anastomoses. Depending on the degree of small bowel and colon left, low rectal anastomoses can result in poor quality of life, and this should be considered in the context of the patient's disease and chances of long-term palliation or cure. In some patients, protecting these anastomoses with a diverting loop colostomy is preferable, so that if the patient decides not to have it reversed, they are not then left with a potentially high-output ileostomy. Because low anterior resection is frequently required, patient positioning should be anticipated. One option is to place all patients in the lithotomy position at the beginning of the case. We prefer to use a split leg table for improved patient safety and apply an end-to-end anastomosis (EEA) stapler through the anus.

## LESSER OMENTECTOMY

The lesser omentum should be excised routinely. This is another frequent site of tumor involvement, and its removal enhances distribution of the perfusate throughout the lesser sac. Care must be taken to preserve the left gastric artery, although if involved with tumor, it can also be taken. We have been impressed that the stomach is able to tolerate extensive perigastric dissection, including the sacrifice of all named blood vessels and the vagus nerve. We have not performed pyloromyotomies or pyloroplasties routinely because of the increased leak risk from these suture lines, and fortunately, we have not had any patients with significant long-term problems of gastric emptying. The lesser omentum should be taken all the way to the caudate lobe and the obliterated ligamentum venosum. This is an area frequently involved by tumor and should be resected completely.

## STOMACH

The stomach is often involved with tumor especially in cases of extensive carcinomatosis. Tumor commonly involves the antrum, extending to the first portion of the duodenum and around the porta hepatis. Both lesser and greater curves are also occasionally involved by extension of bulky tumor within the lesser or greater omentum, respectively. Performing a total gastrectomy and esophagojejunal anastomosis in the context of HIPEC with the other complex procedures being performed simultaneously greatly increases the risk of surgery and affects the quality of life postoperatively. Therefore, it is our practice to avoid a total gastrectomy whenever possible. We do our best to strip tumor from the stomach, repairing serosal defects when feasible. Occasionally with invasive disease, an antrectomy is required. We hold to the philosophy of taking as little of the stomach as necessary and reconstructing with a loop gastrojejunostomy, which is likely safest as it requires one less anastomosis compared with a roux reconstruction. The consequences of delayed gastric emptying with a normal stomach need to be weighed against the risk of a gastrojejunostomy and a gastric staple line. It is a decision that needs to be made in the operating room in the context of what other disease is being left behind, the quality of the tissues, the nutritional status of the patient, and the total number of anastomoses after complete cytoreduction. Gastrojejunostomy will also contribute to a short gut syndrome when extensive small bowel resection is required. The combination of gastrojejunostomy and loop ileostomy leads to an increased risk of dehydration in the perioperative period, and this can affect long-term quality of life. If a gastrectomy is required, the gastrojejunostomy should be performed as close to the ligament of Treitz as possible to maximize the absorption of the small intestine.

## PORTA HEPATIS

The flow of peritoneal fluid into the lesser sac leaves tumor deposits on the posterior aspect of the porta hepatis around the foramen of Winslow, which can lead to early bile duct obstruction. In general, we take an aggressive approach at the porta hepatis. One must be prepared to spend time with careful dissection, placing loops individually around the proper hepatic artery, the portal vein, and the common bile duct. Dissection of all soft tissues is carried posteriorly as far as possible into the liver. We do not routinely perform a cholecystectomy unless the gallbladder is directly involved or exposure of the porta hepatis requires it, and this is only in 10% to 20% of cases. Major injury to the common bile duct must be avoided as a bile duct reconstruction in the setting of carcinomatosis, malnutrition, and HIPEC would be a high risk. Blood loss can also be significant from small posterior branches off the portal vein. The right gastric artery may be the only intact named blood supply to the stomach, and its preservation must be considered in some cases. Direct invasion into the portal vein, bile duct, or hepatic artery would prohibit R0 resection in most cases.

## RIGHT HEMIDIAPHRAGM PERITONECTOMY

After the porta hepatic, the right hemidiaphragm is dissected. The liver must first be mobilized from its peritoneal attachments. The triangular ligaments are divided across the liver surface. The inferior peritoneal attachments should also be divided close to the liver, and the liver should be completely mobilized so that it can be rotated medially. This can sometimes be quite difficult with extensive carcinomatosis, and parenchymal lacerations or capsular tears may result in insidious bleeding. It is important at this point in the case to be sure that the patient is still warm and not coagulopathic. In general, tears and lacerations can be controlled with pressure, cautery, and patience. Once the liver is mobilized and rotated medially, a long-linear incision is made in the peritoneum beginning anteriorly and moving laterally. The peritoneal sheet is then grasped with multiple sponge clamps, and a combination of blunt and sharp dissection is used to strip the peritoneum off the diaphragm (Fig. 8). It is best to continue this as a single large layer as this enhances the ability to bluntly dissect the layer from the diaphragm.

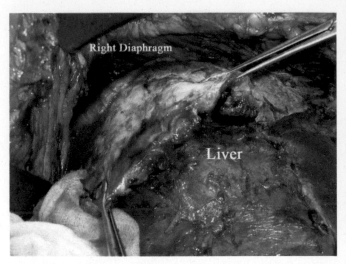

**FIGURE 8.**    Right hemidiaphragm peritonectomy. Full-thickness injury to the diaphragm must be avoided, and the liver capsule also stripped of disease.

Special care should be taken along the central tendon of the diaphragm. At this site, the plane between the peritoneum and the diaphragm is less well developed and is often fused. Small holes in the diaphragm should be expeditiously repaired before any significant contamination into the pleural cavity can occur. Rents in the diaphragm are closed using figure-of-eight sutures around the defect with the last suture tied down during a Valsalva breath. Most cases can be performed without the need for a chest tube. The peritonectomy is then continued all the way posteriorly to the retrohepatic vena cava and superiorly and medially to the suprahepatic vena cava. It is important to visualize the vena cava before beginning the peritonectomy to avoid inadvertent injury to the cava or right hepatic vein. Although it is satisfying to take the entire peritoneum as a single sheet, we find that as the specimen gets larger it may become more manageable to amputate the peritoneum and continue the peritonectomy with a second sheet posteriorly. Any bleeding phrenic veins should be oversewn completely. We have found that simple electrocautery of these vessels is inadequate, with instances of postoperative hemorrhage likely due to movement of the diaphragm.

## PERIHEPATIC DISSECTION

Tumor will often attach to crevices of the liver including the umbilical fissure, the areas in the hilum, and the liver capsule, the left side of the retrohepatic vena cava, and the area between the caudate lobe and segment 4. All of these areas should be inspected carefully. Nodules should be resected carefully, avoiding blood loss from the adrenal gland, vena cava, and other major vessels wherever possible. The capsule of the liver can be stripped where necessary. We find that 10% to 20% of the liver capsule is usually involved, and bleeding from the liver can be controlled with electrocautery or the argon beam coagulator, as long as the patient is not coagulopathic. We will occasionally ablate tumor on the liver capsule when extensive stripping of the capsule is not feasible. As described earlier, the falciform and round ligaments are common sites for tumor involvement, and this may extend down into the umbilical fissure. The liver overlying the portal triad in the umbilical fissure should be divided for better access to tumor in this area. The tumor should then be stripped off the portal triad, avoiding injury to the vessels or bile duct. The left hepatic artery can sometimes be quite small and should be identified and preserved before extensive stripping in this area.

## RECONSTRUCTION

After the HIPEC procedure, we reopen the abdomen and perform any reconstructions. We have found it safer to perform anastomoses after HIPEC because of the potentially damaging affects of the chemotherapy and the physical agitation of the abdominal cavity during the perfusion. The high-flow rates and temperatures stress anastomotic closures and seem to increase the leak rate in our hands. Although impairment of anastomotic healing has been demonstrated with intraperitoneal mitomycin,[23] there is also concern that joining the edematous bowel often observed after perfusion is likewise risky. However, no study evidence clearly supports one sequence over another.[21] Regardless, standard surgical practices to reduce tension and ensure adequate blood supply to the anastomosis in question should be observed always. This is particularly true for pelvic anastomoses associated with anterior resection or proctectomy and esophageal or proximal gastric anastomoses.

The small and large intestines are surveyed carefully, oversewing all serosal defects. Small serosal defects may be tolerated in the setting of cytoreduction and HIPEC, but consideration must be given to the potential for prolonged postoperative ileus and significant bowel distention. The development of a fistula is a major complication that will greatly impair the patient's recovery.

We perform the anastomoses in a standard fashion using staplers. In an effort to reduce bowel complications, we oversew the staple lines with a simple running layer of absorbable suture. Alternatively, these staple lines may be inverted with seromuscular Lembert sutures. Protecting anastomoses with diverting or defunctionalizing ostomies is also an important consideration given the high morbidity of a leak. We routinely perform diverting loop ileostomy in the setting of a low pelvic anastomosis, and all patients are counseled on this possibility preoperatively. Proximal anastomoses associated with total or near-total gastrectomy are also at high risk for complications because of extensive dissection and disruption of the vasculature as well as a functional distal obstruction from the prolonged postoperative ileus frequently seen after these procedures. In this instance, a diverting jejunostomy has been proposed to facilitate distal decompression.[24]

## GASTROSTOMY, JEJUNOSTOMY, AND DRAINS

We prefer not to place a gastrostomy tube or feeding jejunostomy tube because of the risk of complications. Our overall philosophy is to minimize the number of bowel injuries and suture lines. The addition of a simple gastrostomy tube or a jejunostomy after aggressive cytoreduction and HIPEC may increase the risk of postoperative leaks and bowel obstruction. It should be noted that the limit to enteral feeding is usually prolonged ileus and not a decrease in appetite; therefore, early tube feeds will not be tolerated.

Also, the use of postoperative drains is an individual preference for surgeons. Patients will likely develop a reactive ascites in the early postoperative period, which would lead to copious drainage from any peritoneal drains left behind. Although most of the randomized trials have demonstrated no advantage to drains, it remains the normal practice for most surgeons. We have limited our drain use to pancreatic resections and ureteral implantation or anastomoses.

## CLOSURE

Before closure, the entire peritoneal cavity should be carefully inspected for bleeding. It is important that the patient at this point is not coagulopathic. The number of dissected planes is often quite significant, and bleeding needs to be controlled carefully throughout the abdomen.

The most frequent complications are seen at the abdominal incision. This may be due to a higher risk of infection from the duration of surgery and tissue trauma as well as poor overall tissue health and impairments of healing related to HIPEC and nutritional status. As with all other aspects of the procedure, the closure of the abdominal fascia and skin needs to be performed carefully. In addition to early postoperative wound complications, the incidence of ventral hernia formation is also quite high. We have changed from using absorbable suture to a running closure with nonabsorbable polypropylene, which seems to reduce this risk.

The intense adhesion formation after cytoreduction and HIPEC can result in a challenging ileostomy takedown procedure. We use an antiadhesion barrier around the bowel just below the abdominal wall to ease ostomy reversal. Takedown of the stoma can be performed as early as 6 to 8 weeks later. The stoma itself can be matured after skin closure or simply opened at bedside the next day with little functional consequence.

## MINIMALLY INVASIVE CYTOREDUCTION AND HIPEC

In patients at high risk for laparotomy, the possibility of a minimally invasive debulking or cytoreductive surgery and HIPEC have been described. We do not prefer this technique because of the difficulty in carefully assessing the entire abdominal cavity, although in selective cases with patient factors for high morbidity and minimal peritoneal disease, this may be worth considering. The omentectomy should be completed, and then a careful inspection with isolated resection of all nodules performed laparoscopically, just as when open. In cases where the omentum is bulky and will require an incision for removal, a hand port may be added. The hand port has the advantage of allowing better exploration of the abdomen by tactile sensation. Also, the perfusion cannulas can be easily placed through the port. Again, this should be considered in only highly selected cases.

## CONCLUSIONS

In summary, a technically complete yet safe cytoreduction to complement intraperitoneal chemoperfusion is the goal of surgical management for peritoneal surface malignancies. Adherence to principles of good surgical technique is expected to reduce perioperative morbidity and mortality, whereas attention to oncologic principles, accounting for tumor natural history and biology, should maximize long-term outcomes. The cytoreductive surgery and the intraperitoneal chemoperfusion are marathon procedures that benefit from a team approach involving anesthetists, critical care specialists, and surgeons.

## REFERENCES

1. Sugarbaker PH. Management of peritoneal-surface malignancy: the surgeon's role. *Langenbecks Arch Surg.* 1999;384:576–587.
2. Verwaal VJ, van Ruth S, de Bree E, et al. Randomized trial of cytoreduction and hyperthermic intraperitoneal chemotherapy versus systemic chemotherapy and palliative surgery in patients with peritoneal carcinomatosis of colorectal cancer. *J Clin Oncol.* 2003;21:3737–3743.
3. Dedrick RL, Myers CE, Bungay PM, et al. Pharmacokinetic rationale for peritoneal drug administration in the treatment of ovarian cancer. *Cancer Treat Rep.* 1978;62:1–11.
4. Jones RB, Myers CE, Guarino AM, et al. High volume intraperitoneal chemotherapy ("belly bath") for ovarian cancer. Pharmacologic basis and early results. *Cancer Chemother Pharmacol.* 1978;1:161–166.

5. Baratti D, Kusamura S, Nonaka D, et al. Pseudomyxoma peritonei: clinical pathological and biological prognostic factors in patients treated with cytoreductive surgery and hyperthermic intraperitoneal chemotherapy (HIPEC). *Ann Surg Oncol.* 2008;15:526–534.

6. Glehen O, Kwiatkowski F, Sugarbaker PH, et al. Cytoreductive surgery combined with perioperative intraperitoneal chemotherapy for the management of peritoneal carcinomatosis from colorectal cancer: a multi-institutional study. *J Clin Oncol.* 2004;22:3284–3292.

7. Glehen O, Schreiber V, Cotte E, et al. Cytoreductive surgery and intraperitoneal chemohyperthermia for peritoneal carcinomatosis arising from gastric cancer. *Arch Surg.* 2004;139:20–26.

8. Shen P, Hawksworth J, Lovato J, et al. Cytoreductive surgery and intraperitoneal hyperthermic chemotherapy with mitomycin C for peritoneal carcinomatosis from nonappendiceal colorectal carcinoma. *Ann Surg Oncol.* 2004;11:178–186.

9. Brigand C, Monneuse O, Mohamed F, et al. Peritoneal mesothelioma treated by cytoreductive surgery and intraperitoneal hyperthermic chemotherapy: results of a prospective study. *Ann Surg Oncol.* 2006;13:405–412.

10. Rossi CR, Deraco M, De Simone M, et al. Hyperthermic intraperitoneal intraoperative chemotherapy after cytoreductive surgery for the treatment of abdominal sarcomatosis: clinical outcome and prognostic factors in 60 consecutive patients. *Cancer.* 2004;100:1943–1950.

11. Sadeghi B, Arvieux C, Glehen O, et al. Peritoneal carcinomatosis from nongynecologic malignancies: results of the EVOCAPE 1 multicentric prospective study. *Cancer.* 2000;88:358–363.

12. Bijelic L, Yan TD, Sugarbaker PH. Treatment failure following complete cytoreductive surgery and perioperative intraperitoneal chemotherapy for peritoneal dissemination from colorectal or appendiceal mucinous neoplasms. *J Surg Oncol.* 2008;98:295–299.

13. Yan TD, Bijelic L, Sugarbaker PH. Critical analysis of treatment failure after complete cytoreductive surgery and perioperative intraperitoneal chemotherapy for peritoneal dissemination from appendiceal mucinous neoplasms. *Ann Surg Oncol.* 2007;14:2289–2299.

14. Gusani NJ, Cho SW, Colovos C, et al. Aggressive surgical management of peritoneal carcinomatosis with low mortality in a high-volume tertiary cancer center. *Ann Surg Oncol.* 2008;15:754–763.

15. Smeenk RM, Verwaal VJ, Zoetmulder FA. Toxicity and mortality of cytoreduction and intraoperative hyperthermic intraperitoneal chemotherapy in pseudomyxoma peritonei—a report of 103 procedures. *Eur J Surg Oncol.* 2006;32:186–190.

16. Stephens AD, Alderman R, Chang D, et al. Morbidity and mortality analysis of 200 treatments with cytoreductive surgery and hyperthermic intraoperative intraperitoneal chemotherapy using the coliseum technique. *Ann Surg Oncol.* 1999;6:790–796.

17. Verwaal VJ, van Tinteren H, Ruth SV, et al. Toxicity of cytoreductive surgery and hyperthermic intra-peritoneal chemotherapy. *J Surg Oncol.* 2004;85:61–67.

18. Kusamura S, Younan R, Baratti D, et al. Cytoreductive surgery followed by intraperitoneal hyperthermic perfusion: analysis of morbidity and mortality in 209 peritoneal surface malignancies treated with closed abdomen technique. *Cancer.* 2006;106:1144–1153.

19. Franko J, Gusani NJ, Holtzman MP, et al. Multivisceral resection does not affect morbidity and survival after cytoreductive surgery and chemoperfusion for carcinomatosis from colorectal cancer. *Ann Surg Oncol.* 2008;15:3065–3072.

20. da Silva RG, Sugarbaker PH. Analysis of prognostic factors in seventy patients having a complete cytoreduction plus perioperative intraperitoneal chemotherapy for carcinomatosis from colorectal cancer. *J Am Coll Surg.* 2006;203:878–886.

21. Kusamura S, O'Dwyer ST, Baratti D, et al. Technical aspects of cytoreductive surgery. *J Surg Oncol.* 2008;98:232–236.

22. Sugarbaker PH. Peritonectomy procedures. *Ann Surg.* 1995;221:29–42.

23. Fumagalli U, Trabucchi E, Soligo M, et al. Effects of intraperitoneal chemotherapy on anastomotic healing in the rat. *J Surg Res.* 1991;50:82–87.

24. Sugarbaker PH. Cytoreduction including total gastrectomy for pseudomyxoma peritonei. *Br J Surg.* 2002;89:208–212.

# Long-Term Results of Cytoreduction and HIPEC Followed by Systemic Chemotherapy

Vic J. Verwaal

Peritoneal carcinomatosis has been treated by the cytoreductive plus hyperthermic intraperitoneal chemotherapy (HIPEC) procedure for the last 20 years. In the early years of this treatment, it was debated whether the good results were related to patient selection or positive effects of the combined treatment. It was also questioned whether the long-term quality of life benefits were balanced with the efforts for both patients and resources. As a result of continued clinical and laboratory research in the beginning of the 21st century in The Netherlands, the HIPEC procedure became an established treatment for peritoneal carcinomatosis of colorectal origin and pseudomyxoma peritonei. Nowadays, the indication for the HIPEC procedure is extended to other peritoneal surface malignancies such as peritoneal mesothelioma and ovarian cancer. Currently, these other malignancies are treated with the HIPEC procedure in trial protocols.

In the early days of this complex treatment, there were still many shortcomings in the technique and patient management. Now, as a result of many conferences, international workshops and side by side intraoperative teaching, this treatment has been brought to a high level of care. Standardized protocols are available that allow for greater availability of the benefits. Also, there has been a shift in patient selection. In the 1990s, the HIPEC procedure was offered to patients who were at the end stage of their disease having been previously treated with multiple lines of systemic chemotherapy. Today more patients receive the HIPEC procedure upfront. Nowadays, a discussion on prophylactic treatment with the HIPEC procedure for T4 carcinomas is to prevent the progression of carcinomatosis.

## DUTCH ORGANIZATION

The first randomized trial on the HIPEC procedure was conducted in The Netherlands. Perhaps it is not surprising that after the early results of this trial became available in 2003, the waiting list soon go out of hand. To overcome the extremely long-waiting list, new HIPEC centers were setup throughout the country. All the new centers were trained by the "founding" center, The Netherlands Cancer Institute. This training included side by side intraoperative teaching in the new centers. Meanwhile, a national group was founded to discuss HIPEC matters both on patient level and on organizational level.

Currently, the results of the procedures and the adverse outcomes are presented biannually in the Dutch HIPEC group meeting. Also discussed are possible new indications and new trials. The group also provides a base for any new center to start. As a result of proper training and education, new centers can start at a high level of knowledge and performance. In this way, the learning curve has been greatly reduced. The results of the HIPEC procedure of the Dutch groups are presented in Figure 1. In France, a similar organization was set up, and the results were reported by the peritoneal surface workshop meeting in Lyon, France in 2008.

## DATA ON LONG-TERM RESULTS OF CYTOREDUCTION AND HIPEC

Long-term results of cytoreduction followed by HIPEC were published in 2005. The first publication of long-term results had a median follow-up of 46 months.[1] In this publication, there was a median survival of 42.9 months for those patients who underwent a complete cytoreduction. This publication shows the results of the patients treated in the early days of the HIPEC era. The interpretation of the results of this publication was difficult because of possible selection bias and nonstandardized technique.

In 2003, the randomized trial comparing standard chemotherapy with cytoreduction followed by HIPEC and adjuvant therapy was published.[2] In this publication of a prospective randomized trial, the group of patients treated by the HIPEC procedure were not preselected. This study showed that cytoreduction followed by HIPEC had a significant better survival than systemic chemotherapy alone. In the intention to treat analysis, the results of the study showed median survival of 12.5 months in the standard arm and 22.3 months in the experimental arm.

This study was updated in 2008.[3] This update was based on the original 105 patients. The randomized trial protocol stated that patients who progressed should be treated with the best available at that time. As such, patients randomized to the standard treatment who had an intra-abdominal recurrence were offered treatment with the HIPEC procedure after the randomized trial was published in 2003.

To overcome a cross-over problem from the standard arm to the HIPEC arm, the patients were censored at the moment of the cross over. Although this may have presented a major issue in data evaluation, it was only the case in 2 patients.

In the update of the original trial, the follow-up was complete in all patients until August 2007. At that moment, there was a median follow-up of 94 months (range from 72 to 115 months). In Figure 2, the Kaplan-Meier survival curve is shown. Patients of the standard arm had a median survival of 12.6 months. The median survival of patients from the experimental arm was 22.2 months. This difference was significant with a $P$ value of 0.028. The 6-year survival was only 5% in the standard arm and 20% in the experimental arm. It is still important to bear in mind that this analysis was by intention to treat.

Figure 3 shows details of the survival in the experimental arm. From this graph, it is obvious that the requirement for success is the completeness of the cytoreduction. The 5-year survival rate in those patients who had a complete cytoreduction was 45%. In those patients in whom the attempt for a complete cytoreduction was fruitless, the survival was still very poor. The median survival was less than 1 year.

In the randomized trial, bias from patient selection was ruled out by randomizing all patients referred for peritoneal carcinomatosis of colorectal origin. At that time, there was little data to support

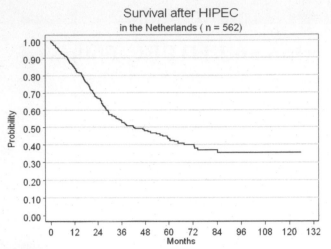

**FIGURE 1.**    Dutch multicenter data showing the survival of patients with colorectal carcinomatosis treated by cytoreductive surgery plus heated intraperitoneal chemotherapy.

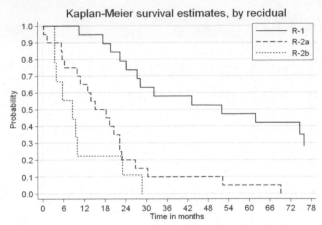

**FIGURE 3.**    Kaplan-Meier survival estimates by residual in patients with colorectal carcinomatosis R-1 = no remaining macroscopic tumor, R-2a = residual tumor smaller than 2.5 mm, and R-2b = residual tumors greater than 2.5 mm (modified form *Ann Surg Oncol.* 2008;15:2426–2432).

any rational patient selection. After the randomized trial, important selection criteria became available. Data on prognostic factors pointed out the patients most likely to benefit.[4,5] Data on toxicity pointed to be considered ineligible for treatment.[6,7] All the publications taken together summarized all options available for these patients. In this way, eligible for this extensive treatment became standardized.[8]

## DATA REGARDING THE LEARNING CURVE

The learning curve of cytoreduction followed by HIPEC has been extensively studied.[9] In the publication by Smeenk et al, an increase of the median survival was seen from a survival probability at 24 months increased from 59.7% in 1996–1998 to 61.9% in 1999–2002 and 71.7% in 2003–2006. The survival rate at 24 months was 49.0% for peritoneal carcinomatosis and 83.1% for pseudomyxoma peritonei.

Besides the effect on survival, there has been also a decrease in toxicity. Not only the toxicity itself decreased but also the outcome of complications improved.[10] It is important to emphasize that the learning curve of an institute reflects not only the capability of that institute but also the world's knowledge at that moment on a disease or its treatment. The lack of general knowledge of peritoneal carcinomatosis and the HIPEC procedure in the 1990s led to slow learning curves. Now that we understand the disease and its treatment more completely and now that education programs are available for institutes introducing this treatment, learning curves will be much shorter. This phenomenon is called the "world learning curve."

Accepting the possibility that the learning curve has now come to its maximum, and knowing that the results for those patients treated on the slope of the learning curve had a 5-year survival of 45%, one can predict that the median survival of those patients treated today will be beyond 5 year.

## LONG-TERM RESULTS OF ALTERNATIVES

Stage IV colorectal cancer is general described as any metastasized colorectal cancer. Peritoneal carcinomatosis is one of the different subcategories of stage IV colorectal cancer. In general, Medical Oncologists treat all stage IV colorectal cancers subcategories on the same protocols. The results of the medical treatment show a median survival of 1 to 2 years. Large randomized trials show even better results with the newest agents.[11]

It is important to realize that the inclusion criteria for the randomized trials is "measurable disease." Peritoneal carcinomatosis is typically not seen on computed tomography (CT) scans, and therefore not seen as a measurable disease.[12] For that reason, medical oncologic studies mainly include patients with CT measurable liver metastasis and not with immeasurable peritoneal carcinomatosis patients. In most of the chemotherapy trials on treatment of stage IV, colorectal cancer patients with peritoneal carcinomatosis are "deselected."

Figure 4 shows the different form of stage IV colorectal cancer. It displays a typical CT scan of a liver metastasis on the left upper picture (Fig. 4A), beneath it is an intraoperative picture of the same liver shown (Fig. 4B). On the right side an intraoperative picture

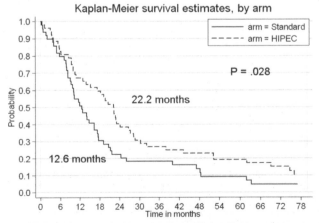

**FIGURE 2.**    Kaplan-Meier survival estimates, by arm in patients with colorectal carcinomatosis (modified from *Ann Surg Oncol.* 2008;15:2426–2432).

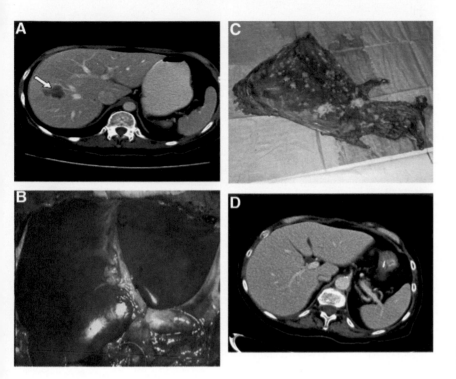

**FIGURE 4.**   A–D, Different forms of colorectal cancer.

of peritoneal carcinomatosis is shown (Fig. 4C), with beneath it the CT scan of the same area (Fig. 4D). The difference in intraoperative observations and CT findings are obvious.

Peritoneal carcinomatosis often presents itself with multiple colon obstructions. This reduces the patient's tolerance of chemotherapy. Folprecht et al[13] performed a study on effectiveness of chemotherapy in patients affected with peritoneal carcinomatosis; they reported

that they had a diminished response. Newer studies indicate differences in gen progressions between liver metastasis and peritoneal metastasis. These data are still preliminary, but they reflect differences in tumor biology between liver metastasis and peritoneal carcinomatosis. For these reasons, the results of the treatment of stage IV colorectal cancer in studies containing mainly liver metastasis cannot be transferred to peritoneal carcinomatosis. In my opinion, there

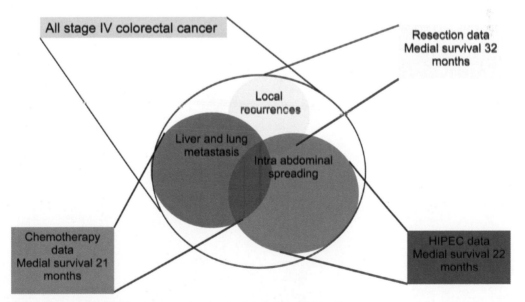

**FIGURE 5.**   Summary of the results of treatment subgroups of stage IV colorectal cancer.

are no reliable data available on the long-term results of the medical treatment of peritoneal carcinomatosis.

## QUALITY OF LIFE STUDIES

The HIPEC procedure is a complex treatment and can come with serious complications. It is often discussed whether the HIPEC procedure is worthwhile in perspective of quality of life. There are only a few data available on this issue. McQuellon et al[14] studied this topic extensively. He found in 109 patients, interviewed between 3.1 to 8.0 years after treatment, that 10 patients (62.5%) had a very good to excellent health status. Furthermore, he found no limitations on moderate activity were reported in 94% of the patients.

One must realize that, alongside the favorable quality of life results, there is the misery of those patients who failed the treatment. Verwaal et al studied in his thesis, the quality of life of patients treated for peritoneal carcinomatosis of colorectal origin. He found that there was a decreased quality of life shortly after the procedure. In the long run, he found that the quality of life was mostly related to the presence of recurrences of disease and not to the treatment.

## GUIDELINES

The international guidelines for the HIPEC procedure were considered in the consensus meeting in Milano in 2006. The guidelines included eligibility, workup, and treatment details. These guidelines are based on scientific evidence and formulated by an international panel of experts. The guidelines have been published; based on this evidence, cytoreduction followed by HIPEC is incorporated in many national guidelines for treatment.[15]

## CONCLUSIONS

Based on this data, and lack of other data, cytoreduction followed by HIPEC should be considered for colorectal peritoneal carcinomatosis in those patients who fit to undergo major surgery. Long-term survival with acceptable quality of life can be achieved in select patients. Selection of the patients is still a critical issue. Unfortunately, there are limited data available for peritoneal carcinomatosis patients treated with systemic chemotherapy and recommendations for the use of systemic chemotherapy in these patients are not available. Figure 5 shows a summary of the results of treatment of 4 subgroups of stage IV colorectal cancer.

## REFERENCES

1. Verwaal VJ, van RS, Witkamp A, et al. Long-term survival of peritoneal carcinomatosis of colorectal origin. *Ann Surg Oncol.* 2005;12:65–71.
2. Verwaal VJ, van RS, de BE, et al. Randomized trial of cytoreduction and hyperthermic intraperitoneal chemotherapy versus systemic chemotherapy and palliative surgery in patients with peritoneal carcinomatosis of colorectal cancer. *J Clin Oncol.* 2003;21:3737–3743.
3. Verwaal VJ, Bruin S, Boot H, et al. 8-year follow-up of randomized trial: cytoreduction and hyperthermic intraperitoneal chemotherapy versus systemic chemotherapy in patients with peritoneal carcinomatosis of colorectal cancer. *Ann Surg Oncol.* 2008;15:2426–2432.
4. Glockzin G, Schlitt HJ, Piso P. Peritoneal carcinomatosis: patients selection, perioperative complications and quality of life related to cytoreductive surgery and hyperthermic intraperitoneal chemotherapy. *World J Surg Oncol.* 2009; 7:5.
5. Verwaal VJ, van Tinteren H, van Ruth S, et al. Predicting the survival of patients with peritoneal carcinomatosis of colorectal origin treated by aggressive cytoreduction and hyperthermic intraperitoneal chemotherapy. *Br J Surg.* 2004;91:739–746.
6. Verwaal VJ, van Tinteren H, Ruth SV, et al. Toxicity of cytoreductive surgery and hyperthermic intra-peritoneal chemotherapy. *J Surg Oncol.* 2004;85:61–67.
7. Younan R, Kusamura S, Baratti D, et al. Morbidity, toxicity, and mortality classification systems in the local regional treatment of peritoneal surface malignancy. *J Surg Oncol.* 2008;98:253–257.
8. Verwaal VJ, Kusamura S, Baratti D, et al. The eligibility for local-regional treatment of peritoneal surface malignancy. *J Surg Oncol.* 2008;98:220–223.
9. Smeenk RM, Verwaal VJ, Zoetmulder FA. Learning curve of combined modality treatment in peritoneal surface disease. *Br J Surg.* 2007;94:1408–1414.
10. Moran BJ, Mukherjee A, Sexton R. Operability and early outcome in 100 consecutive laparotomies for peritoneal malignancy. *Br J Surg.* 2006;93:100–104.
11. Sanoff HK, Sargent DJ, Campbell ME, et al. Five-year data and prognostic factor analysis of oxaliplatin and irinotecan combinations for advanced colorectal cancer: N9741. *J Clin Oncol.* 2008;26:5721–5727.
12. de Bree E, Koops W, Kroger R, et al. Preoperative computed tomography and selection of patients with colorectal peritoneal carcinomatosis for cytoreductive surgery and hyperthermic intraperitoneal chemotherapy. *Eur J Surg Oncol.* 2006;32:65–71.
13. Folprecht G, Kohne CH, Lutz MP. Systemic chemotherapy in patients with peritoneal carcinomatosis from colorectal cancer. *Cancer Treat Res.* 2007;134:425–440.
14. McQuellon RP, Loggie BW, Lehman AB, et al. Long-term survivorship and quality of life after cytoreductive surgery plus intraperitoneal hyperthermic chemotherapy for peritoneal carcinomatosis. *Ann Surg Oncol.* 2003;10:155–162.
15. Esquivel J, Sticca R, Sugarbaker P, et al. Cytoreductive surgery and hyperthermic intraperitoneal chemotherapy in the management of peritoneal surface malignancies of colonic origin: a consensus statement. Society of Surgical Oncology. *Ann Surg Oncol.* 2007;14:128–133.

# Pharmacokinetics and Pharmacodynamics of Perioperative Cancer Chemotherapy in Peritoneal Surface Malignancy

Kurt Van der Speeten • Oswald A. Stuart • Paul H. Sugarbaker

The peritoneal surface remains an important failure site for patients with gastrointestinal and gynecologic malignancies. Tumor cells may exfoliate from the primary tumor into the peritoneal cavity preoperatively due to transserosal growth.[1] Alternatively, at the time of surgery, tumor cells can be dispersed from transected lymph or blood vessels or by manipulation of the primary tumor. Once malignant cells are free inside the peritoneal cavity, they become trapped at sites of trauma where fibrin accumulations and blood clots will secure them and enhance their growth.[2,3]

Eventually, this will result in the development of clinical peritoneal carcinomatosis (PC). The reported incidence in literature varies widely. For example, in a review of 2756 patients by Jayne et al, they reported the incidence of PC at the time of initial surgery to be 7.7%.[4] A review of colonic cancer patients who had recurrences suggests that peritoneal seeding occurred in 25% to 35% of patients.[5]

## NATURAL HISTORY

In the past, oncologists have assumed that PC is equal to distant metastases and as such they regarded it as an incurable component of the intra-abdominal malignancy. Chu et al[6] were the first to investigate the impact of PC upon survival. In 100 patients with biopsy-proven PC, they reported a mean survival of 8.5 months in colorectal cancer patients, 2.4 months in pancreatic cancer patients, and 2.2 months in gastric cancer patients. The European prospective multicenter trial EVOCAPE 1 (Evolution of PC 1) reported remarkably similar results in nongynecologic malignancy patients with PC who received 5-fluorouracil based systemic chemotherapy.[7] In 2002, Jayne et al[4] reported a median survival of 7 months in colorectal cancer patients who had synchronous peritoneal implants. Some reliable data on this topic come from the control arm of the phase III trial by Verwaal et al.[8] A recent update from this trial revealed a median disease-specific survival of 12.6 months in patients with PC from colorectal cancer who received 5-fluorouracil-leucovorin-based systemic chemotherapy.[9] More recent systemic chemotherapy protocols based on the use of oxaliplatin, irinotecan, and biologic agents have improved survival in colorectal cancer patients with PC. Elias et al[10] reported a 23.9-months median survival in 48 colorectal cancer patients with small volume carcinomatosis who were treated with systemic chemotherapy containing oxaliplatin or irinotecan. No long-time survivors were reported in these series.

## REVISED HYPOTHESIS REGARDING PERITONEAL CARCINOMATOSIS

During the last 2 decades, novel therapeutic approaches have emerged for PC patients. These treatments are based on a revised hypothesis that considers PC as a local-regional disease warranting a local-regional therapeutic approach. These treatment modalities combine cytoreductive surgery and perioperative chemotherapy. An aggressive surgical approach combining visceral resections and peritonectomy procedures should address the macroscopic disease, whereas, perioperative intraperitoneal chemotherapy is aimed at residual microscopic disease.[11] The perioperative intraperitoneal chemotherapy includes hyperthermic intraperitoneal perioperative chemotherapy (HIPEC) or early postoperative intraperitoneal chemotherapy or both. Elias et al[12] in 2002 first reported the clinical use of intraoperative intravenous 5-fluorouracil and leucovorin in conjunction with oxaliplatin-based hyperthermic intraperitoneal perioperative chemotherapy. Most recent protocols advocate this bidirectional (simultaneous intraperitoneal and intravenous chemotherapy) intraoperative chemohyperthermia.

## CLINICAL RESULTS IN TREATING PERITONEAL CARCINOMATOSIS

Spratt et al[13] reported, for the first time in 1980, the use of heated triethylenethio-phosphoramide (thiotepa) in a patient with pseudomyxoma peritonei. Since then one randomized control trial and several phase II studies have explored the peroperative intraperitoneal route of drug delivery.[8,9,14–21] In an update on their phase III trial, Verwaal et al[9] reported a 45% 5-year survival in colorectal PC patients receiving optimal cytoreduction and HIPEC with mitomycin C followed by systemic chemotherapy. Elias et al[21] recently analyzed the results of combined cytoreductive surgery and perioperative chemotherapy in 1290 patients with PC from a variety of primary malignancies. At 5 years, 37% of these patients were still alive. These encouraging clinical results are in strong contrast with historical control groups and patients treated with systemic chemotherapy.

Although further clinical data from phase II and III trials supporting this combined treatment protocols are necessary, an optimalization of the wide variety of different perioperative cancer chemotherapy protocols used in these treatment regimens is equally important. To this date, a clear understanding of the pharmacology of perioperative chemotherapy is still lacking. It is possible that increased safety and important treatment improvements may originate from analyzing the pharmacological data. This review aims to clarify the pharmacokinetic and pharmacodynamic data currently available regarding the intraperitoneal delivery of cancer chemotherapy agents in patients with PC.

## PHARMACOKINETIC PRINCIPLES OF PERIOPERATIVE CHEMOTHERAPY

Because the intraperitoneal route of delivering chemotherapy is logistically less convenient and technologically more challenging than conventional intravenous chemotherapy, the case needs to be made for the pharmacokinetic advantage of intraperitoneal chemotherapy.

## The Peritoneal Plasma Barrier

In 1941, Baron[22] described in detail the ultrastructure of the peritoneum in man. The peritoneum consists of a monolayer of mesothelial cells supported by a basement membrane and 5 layers of connective tissue, which account for a total thickness of 90 $\mu$m. The connective tissue layers include interstitial cells and a matrix of collagen, hyaluron, and proteoglycans. The cellular component consists of fibroblasts, pericytes, parenchymal cells, and blood capillaries.

Contrary to intuitive thinking it is not the mesothelial lining, which is the main transport barrier. Flessner et al[23] demonstrated in a rodent model that neither removal of the stagnant fluid layer on the mesothelium nor removal of the mesothelial lining influenced the mass transfer coefficient over the barrier. Human studies in patients undergoing partial or total peritonectomy showed that the clearance of mitomycin C was not significantly changed by the removal of the mesothelium.[24] Basic research suggests that rather the blood capillary wall and the surrounding interstitium are the principal barriers for transport from the peritoneal space to the plasma.[25] Fluid enters the vascular compartment by diffusion from the peritoneal compartment or by absorption through the peritoneal lymphatic stomata, which are concentrated on the diaphragmic surface.[26,27] Diffusion of fluid through the parietal peritoneum generally results in flow to the plasma compartment. Drainage through the visceral peritoneum covering the surfaces of liver, spleen, stomach, small and large bowel, and mesentery is into the portal venous blood.[28]

## Dedrick Diffusion Model

The pharmacokinetic rationale of perioperative intraperitoneal cancer chemotherapy is based on the dose intensification provided by the peritoneal plasma barrier. On the basis of peritoneal dialysis research, Dedrick et al[29] in 1978 concluded that the peritoneal permeability of a number of hydrophilic anticancer drugs may be considerably less than the plasma clearance of that same drug. The peritoneal clearance is inversely proportional to the square root of its molecular weight. This results in a significantly higher concentration in the peritoneal cavity when compared with the plasma after intraperitoneal administration.[30,31] A simplified mathematical diffusion model considers the plasma to be a single compartment separated by an effective membrane from another single compartment, the peritoneal cavity (Fig. 1). This results in the following equation:

$$\text{Rate of mass transfer} = PA(C_P - C_B).$$

Where PA = permeability area (PA = effective contact area x permeability), $C_P$ = concentration in peritoneal cavity, and $C_B$ = concentration in the blood.[32] This simple conceptual model indicates the importance of the effective contact area. Although the equation permits calculation of the pharmacokinetic advantage, the model does not tell anything about the specific penetration of the cancer chemotherapy drug into the tissue or tumor nodule.[33] Also, it does not predict the value of the effective contact area. It simply describes the transfer between 2 compartments.

## Pharmacokinetic Variables

### Dose

A wide variety of drug doses have been used in these perioperative cancer chemotherapy treatment protocols. Most groups use a drug dose based on calculated body surface area (mg/m$^2$) although Rubin et al[34] demonstrated that there is an imperfect and gender-biased correlation between actual peritoneal surface area and calcu-

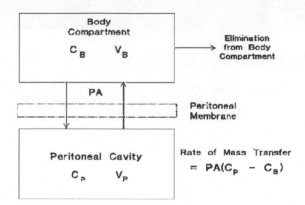

**FIGURE 1.** Traditional two-compartment model of peritoneal transport in which transfer of a drug from the peritoneal cavity to the blood occurs across the "peritoneal membrane." The permeability-area product (PA) governs this transfer and can be calculated by measuring the rate of drug disappearance from the cavity and dividing by the overall concentration difference between the peritoneal cavity and the blood (or plasma). $C_B$, the free drug concentration in the blood (or plasma); $V_B$, volume of distribution of the drug in the body; $C_P$, the free drug concentration in the peritoneal fluid; $V_p$, volume of the peritoneal cavity. (Adapted from Dedrick RL, Flessner MF. Pharmacokinetic problems in peritoneal drug administration: tissue penetration and surface exposure. *J Natl Cancer Inst.* 1997;89:480–487).

lated body surface area. Body surface area is an accurate predictor of drug metabolism, and in this regard is a useful predictor of systemic toxicity. A significant number of institutions use a closed method for intraoperative hyperthermic chemotherapy. They calculate the dose of cancer chemotherapy per liter from the body surface area. A large volume of this cancer chemotherapy solution (usually 6 L) is placed in a reservoir. In this method, the amount of chemotherapy solution is placed within the peritoneal space and thus, the amount of drug in contact with the peritoneal surface is determined by the amount of distention (between 2 and 6 L) of the abdominal cavity during the HIPEC procedure. This may result in a variable permeability area and unpredictable systemic exposure.

### Volume

Following the above-mentioned equation, the rate of mass transfer over the peritoneal-plasma membrane will improve with an increasing effective contact area. A large volume of artificial ascites can increase the contact surface of the chemotherapy solution with the peritoneum. Keshaviah et al[35] demonstrated a linear rise in mass transfer in 10 patients who were dialyzed with different volumes ranging from 0.5 to 3 L. Elias et al[36] confirmed these findings in PC patients where constant concentrations of oxalipatin (410 mg/m$^2$) were administered intraperitoneally in volumes of 2 and 2.5 L/m$^2$. Platinum intraperitoneal maximal concentrations decreased with 20% in the 2.5 L/m$^2$ group. Similarly, Sugarbaker et al[37] reported a slower clearance of chemotherapy when a constant dose was administered intraperitoneally in larger volumes.

A consistent drug dose and consistent volume of chemotherapy solution, both based on the body surface area, may be the most effective method of obtaining a predictable systemic toxicity and exposure of the tumor nodules to the cancer chemotherapy.

## Duration

The literature reports a wide variety of durations of intraperitoneal chemotherapy protocols ranging from 30 to 120 minutes. The dose-response curves and their dependency on exposure time have been mathematically modeled by Gardner.[38] According to his model, a plateau in tumor cell kill will be reached, after which a prolonged exposure time offers no further cytotoxic advantage. Theoretically, the most advantageous exposure time for cytotoxic effects in PC patients should be carefully weighed against the systemic exposure and bone marrow toxicity. The duration of perioperative chemotherapy regimens should be pharmacology driven and not arbitrary.

## Carrier Solution

The choice of carrier solution to deliver the cancer chemotherapy drug is not pharmacokinetically neutral. Hypotonic, isotonic, and hypertonic solutions were explored with both low and high molecular weight chemotherapy molecules. The ideal carrier solution should provide the following: enhanced exposure of the peritoneal surface, prolonged high intraperitoneal volume, slow clearance from the peritoneal cavity, and absence of adverse effects to peritoneal membranes.[39] This is especially important in the setting of early postoperative intraperitoneal chemotherapy where maintenance of a high dwell volume of chemotherapy solution over a prolonged time period improves the distribution of the drug and the effectiveness of the treatment.[40] Mohamed et al[41] showed that a isotonic high molecular weight dextrose solution will prolong the intraperitoneal retention of the artificial ascites. Several in vitro and animal studies suggested a pharmacokinetic advantage of hypotonic carrier solutions in a HIPEC setting.[42,43] Elias et al[44] studied the pharmacokinetics of heated oxaliplatin with increasingly hypotonic carrier solutions in colorectal PC patients. They reported no significant differences in absorption and intratumoral oxaplatin but a very high incidence of unexplained postoperative bleeding (50%) and unusually severe trombocytopenia in patients treated with hypotonic carrier solutions. Further clarification of the safety and efficacy of hypotonic carrier solutions is required before their use can be recommended.

## Pressure

Dedrick et al[45] postulated that the penetration distance is equal to the square root of the ratio of the tissue diffusivity and the rate constant for drug removal from the tissue $(D/k)^{1/2}$. Unpublished observations by Flessner et al[23] in a rat model showed a doubling of the extracellular space in the anterior abdominal wall of rats when the pressure of intra-abdominal peritoneal dialysis solution was raised from 0 to 4 cm $H_2O$. An increased effective tissue diffusivity was postulated.

Several reports in animal models confirm the increased accumulation and antitumor effect of intraperitoneal cisplatin, oxaliplatin, and doxorubicin when the abdominal pressure is raised.[46–49] The useful application of this increased intra-abdominal pressure is limited by its respiratory and hemodynamic tolerance. At this time, the only useful clinical application is in palliating refractory malignant ascites in PC patients by laparoscopic HIPEC at 12 to 15 mm Hg.[50–52]

# PHARMACODYNAMIC PRINCIPLES OF PERIOPERATIVE CHEMOTHERAPY

Pharmacokinetics explores what the body does to the cancer chemotherapy drug, whereas pharmacodynamics explores what the drug does to the body. The efficacy of intraperitoneal cancer chemotherapy protocols is governed as much by nonpharmacokinetic variables (tumor nodule size, density, vascularity, interstitial fluid pressure, and binding) as by the above-mentioned pharmacokinetic variables.

## TUMOR NODULE AS PHARMACOLOGIC ENDPOINT

Figure 2 shows a conceptual model combining pharmacokinetic and pharmacodynamic variables with the tumor nodule as the pharmacologic end point.

In vitro experiments with multicellular models showed that direct tissue penetration of most cytotoxic agents is very limited (usually less than 1 mm).[53] Los et al[54,55] reported similar limited penetration of 1 to 2 mm after intraperitoneal cisplatinum administration in an animal model. Further support for these experimental data comes from clinical studies reporting completeness of cytoreduction as the most significant prognostic factor for disease-free survival and overall

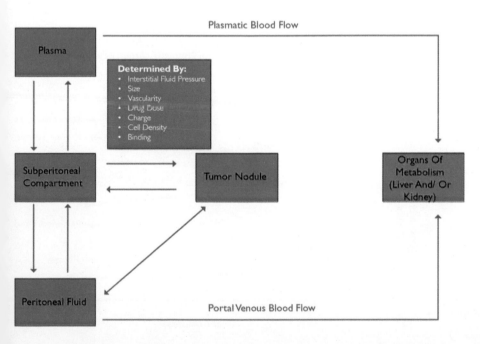

**FIGURE 2.** Conceptual model of 5-fluorouracil distribution and metabolism during bidirectional intraoperative chemotherapy.

survival in patients with PC.[8,14,21,56,57] For example, in a recent multicentric review of 523 colorectal PC patients, multivariate analysis showed that the risk of death increased by 39% when going from CCR-0 to CCR-1.[21]

## TEMPERATURE

Adding hyperthermia to intraperitoneal chemotherapy may increase the tumor response to cancer chemotherapy by several mechanisms. First, heat alone has a direct antitumor effect. Mild hyperthermia more than 41° induces selective cytotoxicity of malignant cells by several mechanisms: impaired DNA repair, protein denaturation, and inhibition of oxidative metabolism in the microenvironment of malignant cells leading to increased acidity, lysosomal activation, and increased apoptotic cell death.[58-60] Thermal tolerance can be induced in this setting by up-regulation of heat shock proteins.[61] This may limit the importance of a direct antitumor effect of heat. Second, applying mild hyperthermia augments the cytotoxic effects of some chemotherapeutic agents. Synergy between heat and cancer chemotherapy drugs may arise from multiple events such as heat damage to ABC transporters (drug accumulation), intracellular drug detoxification pathways, and to repair mechanisms of drug-induced DNA adducts.[62] Such augmented effects were postulated for doxorubicin,[63] platinum complexes,[64,65] mitomycin C,[65] melphalan,[66] docetaxel, irinotecan, and gemcitabine.[67]

Third, experimental data suggest that hyperthermia may increase the penetration depth of the cancer chemotherapy solution into tissues and tumor nodules. Jacquet et al[68] reported that tissue penetration of doxorubicin was significantly enhanced when the cancer chemotherapy solution was administered intraperitoneally at 43°C. In addition, hyperthermia did not affect the pharmacokinetic advantages of intraperitoneal doxorubicin with low plasma and distant tissue levels.

## CYTOTOXIC DRUGS USED WITH PERIOPERATIVE CHEMOTHERAPY

### Doxorubicin

Doxorubicin ($C_{27}H_{29}NO_{11}$) or hydroxyldaunorubicin (adriamycin) is an anthracycline antibiotic. Historically, it has been categorized as a DNA-intercalating drug but experimental work suggests that interaction of doxorubicin with the cell surface membrane rather than its intracellular uptake is an essential first step for doxorubicin cytotoxity.[69,70] Because of its wide in vitro and in vivo activity against a broad range of malignancies, its slow clearance from the peritoneal compartment because of the high molecular weight of the hydrochloride salt (579, 99 d), its favorable area under the curve ratio of intraperitoneal to intravenous concentration times of 230, and the absence of risk for dose-limiting cardiotoxicity when used intraperitoneally; doxorubicin was considered a potential beneficial agent for perioperative intraperitoneal delivery. This was supported by both experimental and clinical pharmacokinetic data.[68,71-75] Figure 3 shows the pharmacologic profile of intraperitoneally administered doxorubicin.[75] The consistent finding of doxorubicin sequestration in tumor nodules raises questions about the possible underlying mechanism. Simple diffusion forces as proposed by Dedrick and Flessner are not enough to explain the phenomenon. In the absence of experimental data supporting active transport of cancer chemotherapy drugs over membranes, the authors postulate active binding to the cell membrane as a possible mechanism. Levels of cytotoxic drugs in tumor nodules cannot be predicted by measuring drug concentrations in peritoneal fluid and plasma. The sequestration phenomenon of doxorubicin in tumor nodules is a constant one in its presence regardless the underlying pathology or subtype. A consequence is that the cancer chemotherapy levels measured in the tumor nodules may be far more important than considered in the past.

### Mitomycin C

Mitomycin C is an alkylating antibiotic, which has been used extensively in intraperitoneal cancer chemotherapy treatment protocols in appendiceal and colorectal PC patients. In vitro data suggest thermal enhancement of mitomycin C.[65] A remarkable difference in drug dosimetry between different groups of investigators is reported. Van Ruth et al[76] at the Dutch Cancer Institute reported a dose-finding study. Their data suggest that a dose of 35 mg/m² resulted in the highest peritoneal/plasma AUC ratio with acceptable toxicity. To maintain the concentration throughout the 90 minutes perfusion time, the dose was divided in 3 fractions: 50% at the start, 25% after 30 minutes, and 25% at 60 minutes. Jacquet et al[77] reported a mean AUC ratio of 23.5 when using a dose of 12.9 ± 3.8 mg/m². The toxicity profile of mitomycin C, including anastomotic dehiscence and impaired wound healing, has been well characterized.[78-80] Sugarbaker et al[80] in a clinical series of 356 procedures reported 19% grade IV events

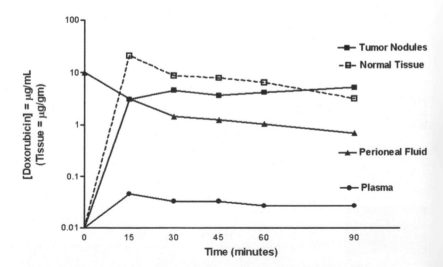

**FIGURE 3.** Pharmacologic profile of intraoperative intracavitary doxorubicin.

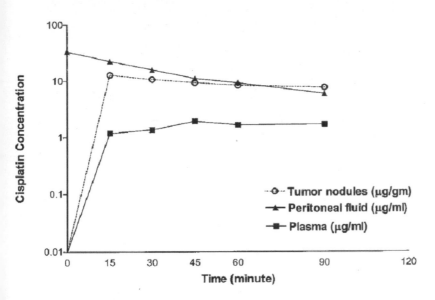

**FIGURE 4.** Pharmacologic profile of intraoperative intracavitary cisplatin.

requiring an urgent intervention. Of these grade IV events, 28% were hematological and 26% gastrointestinal.

## Cisplatin

Cisplatin (cis-diamminedichloroplatinum-III, CDDP) causes apoptotic cell death by formation of DNA adducts.[81] It has been well studied in the setting of adjuvant intraperitoneal chemotherapy of residual small volume ovarian cancer. Three randomized trials showed a significant survival benefit.[82–84] Combined with cytoreductive surgery and hyperthermia, cisplatin has been used for intracavitary therapy for ovarian cancer, gastric cancer, and peritoneal mesothelioma. Urano et al[85] showed an excellent in vitro an in vivo thermal augmentation of cisplatin. Figure 4 shows the pharmacologic profile of cisplatin during intraperitoneal chemotherapy. In contrast to the doxorubicin data, the intratumoral concentrations of cisplatin reflect the intraperitoneal concentrations. The penetration of cisplatin into tumor nodules was studied by several groups. Los et al[86] for the first time described intratumoral distribution of cisplatin after intraperitoneal administration and suggested that the advantage over intraperitoneal versus intravenous administration was maximal in the first 1.5 mm. Van der Vaart et al[87] investigated the cisplatin-induced DNA adduct formation and could measure this 3 to 5 mm into the tumor tissue.

## Oxaliplatin

Oxaliplatin [oxalato-1,2-diaminocyclohexane-platinum(II)] is a third generation platinum complex with a similar cytotoxic mechanism as cisplatinum. In contrast with cisplatin, it has a proven activity in colorectal and appendiceal malignancies. Its clinical use in PC patients as a component of bidirectional intraoperative chemotherapy has been pioneered by Elias et al.[36] In a dose escalation and pharmacokinetic study, they showed that 460 mg/m² of oxaliplatin in 2 L/m² of chemotherapy solution more than 30 minutes was well tolerated.[12] The low area under the curve ratio is compensated by the rapid absorption of the drug into the tissue. They report a median survival of 63 months and a 5-year survival rate of 51% with this approach.[10] In contrast to cisplatin and mitomycin, oxaliplatin is not stable in chloride-containing solutions and can only be administered in dextrose 5%.[88] This may result in serious electrolyte disturbances and hyperglycemia during the intracavitary therapy.[89]

## Carboplatin

Carboplatin [(1,1-cyclobutanedicarboxylato)platinum(II)] is a higher molecular weight platinum compound than cisplatin, which at the present time is mostly used in normothermic intraperitoneal chemotherapy protocols in patients with advanced ovarian cancer. Cjezka et al[90] in a clinical study with normothermic carboplatin reported a relative bioavailability (calculated as AUC-values), which was at least 6 times higher in the intraperitoneal fluid than in the serum for 48 hours. Los et al[55] compared carboplatin and cisplatin after intraperitoneal administration in a rat model of PC. Their data demonstrate that despite a clear pharmacokinetic advantage of carboplatin over cisplatin, its capacity to penetrate into peritoneal cancer nodules and tumor cells is far lower than that of cisplatin. These data limit its clinical application.

## Irinotecan (CPT-11)

Irinotecan is a topoisomerase-I inhibitor. Irinotecan itself has little if any cytotxic activity and can only exert its anticancer activity through its metabolite SN-38. This metabolization takes place in the liver by carboxylesterase. Several side pathways and degradation processes have been described.[91] This has several consequences. First, patients with Gilbert syndrome should not receive irinotecan as they lack the enzymes necessary for degradation of the drug.[92] Second, pharmacokinetics is very different in animal models and humans.

Irinotecan has a very high molecular weight (677 d) and was considered a pharmacokinetic advantageous molecule for intraperitoneal administration. Guichard et al[93] reported high CPT-11 and SN-38 AUCs and low clearances from the peritoneal cavity after intracavitary administration in mice. Contrasting human pharmacokinetic data were reported by Maruyama et al.[94,95] They showed in both malignant ascites patients and gastric or colonic PC patients that little or no CPT-11 was converted intraperitoneally to SN-38 after intraperitoneal administration. Despite this lack of pharmacologic understanding for its cytotoxic activity, Maruyama et al[96] and other authors report excellent growth inhibition in animal models of PC.[97,98] Elias et al[99] performed most of the clinical work with intraperitoneal irinotecan. In a phase-I study, they combined intraperitoneal oxaliplatin with escalating doses of irinotecan during HIPEC. At 400 mg/m², they reported a tissue concentration that was 16 to 23 times higher than that

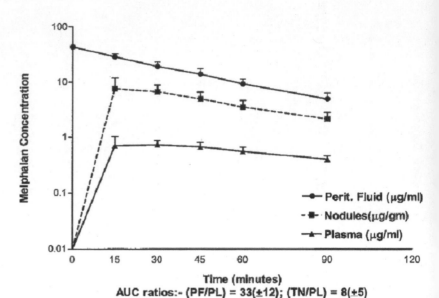

**FIGURE 5.** Pharmacologic profile of intraoperative intracavitary melphalan.

of unbathed tissues. This, however, came at the price of 58% grade 3 to 4 hematological toxicity.

## Melphalan

Melphalan (L-phenylalanine mustard) is a chemotherapy drug belonging to the class of nitrogen mustard alkylating agents. Alberts et al[100] were the first to investigate the pharmacokinetics of intraperitoneal melphalan. Melphalan systemic absorption from the peritoneal cavity averaged only 39% of the administered dose. Urano et al[85] showed a remarkable heat augmentation of melphalan. Glehen et al[101] investigated the effect of hyperthermia on the pharmacokinetics of intraperitoneal melphalan in a rat model. Hyperthermia decreased the AUC of peritoneal fluid without increasing the plasma AUC. Intra-abdominal tissue concentrations were markedly elevated compared with normothermic controls. Figure 5 shows the pharmacologic profile of melphalan during intraoperative intraperitoneal administration. Sugarbaker et al[102] in a pharmacokinetic and phase-II study of intraoperative intraperitoneal melphalan showed that 90% of the cancer chemotherapy drug was absorbed during the 90-minutes procedure with a 30 times higher exposure at the peritoneal surface than in the blood. Concentrations in tumor nodules were 10 times higher than concentrations in the blood. This favorable pharmacokinetic profile and tissue distributions combined with cytotoxic activity against a wide range of malignancies makes melphalan an excellent salvage drug for intraperitoneal treatment protocols.

## Gemcitabine

Gemcitabine (2′,2′-difluorodeoxycitidine) is a pyrimidine analogue with a wide range of in vitro cytotoxic activity, particularly against pancreatic cancer. It has some advantageous pharmacokinetic characteristics for intracavitary administration. Pestiau et al[103] investigated the pharmacokinetics and tissue distribution of intraperitoneal gemcitabine in a rat model. The AUC ratio (intraperitoneal/intravenous) after intraperitoneal administration was $26.8 \pm 5.8$. Hyperthermic administration resulted in increased tissue concentrations. Several investigators explored the use of normothermic intraperitoneal gemcitabine in advanced cancer outside the setting of cytoreductive surgery.[104–106]

Resected advanced pancreatic cancer with high risk of recurrence in the operative field is a potential indication for intraoperative intraperitoneal administration of heated gemcitabine in an adjuvant setting.

## Taxanes

The taxanes paclitaxel and docetaxel represent one of the most interesting new classes of cancer chemotherapy drugs. The taxanes stabilize the microtubule against depolymerization, thereby disrupting normal microtubule dynamics.[107] They exert cytotoxic activity against a broad range of tumors. Because of their high molecular weight, these molecules have a remarkable high AUC ratio of respectively 853 and 861.[108] This translates itself into a clear pharmacokinetic advantage for intraperitoneal administration.[109] The data regarding possible thermal augmentation of taxanes are conflicting.[110–113] Taxanes have been used in a neoadjuvant intraperitoneal setting as well as intraoperatively and postoperatively.[82,83,114–116]

## BIDIRECTIONAL INTRAOPERATIVE CHEMOTHERAPY

By combining intraoperative intravenous and intraoperative intraperitoneal cancer chemotherapy a bidirectional diffusion gradient is created through the intermediate tissue layer, which contains the cancer nodules. This offers opportunities for optimizing cancer chemotherapy delivery to the target peritoneal tumor nodules. Elias and Sideris[36] first reported the clinical use of intraoperative intravenous 5-fluorouracil and leucovorin in conjunction with oxaliplatin-based hyperthermic intraperitoneal perioperative chemotherapy. This was based on earlier in vitro and in vivo studies suggesting a synergistic effect of oxaliplatin and 5-fluorouracil.[117,118]

Figure 6 shows the concentrations of 5-fluorouracil in tumor nodules harvested from 9 patients during the bidirectional (intraperitoneal doxorubicin and mitomycin C plus intravenous 5-fluorouracil) intraoperative chemotherapy treatment. Although the 5-fluorouracil is administered as a normothermic intravenous solution, it penetrates rapidly into the heated tumor nodules. Normothermic administered 5-fluorouracil becomes subject to the augmentation of mild hyperthermia of the subperitoneal compartment. By modulating the timing

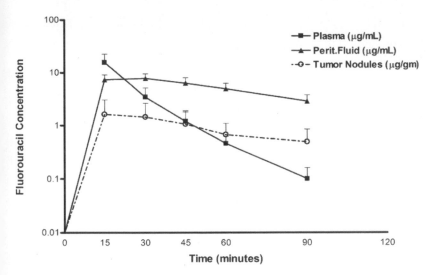

**FIGURE 6.** 5-Fluorouracil concentrations in plasma, peritoneal fluid and tumor nodules after intravenous administration during hyperthermic intraperitoneal chemotherapy procedure.

of intravenous chemotherapy, we can achieve heat targeting to the peritoneal membrane and the tumor nodules contained in it. Timing of intravenous chemotherapy emerges as an important new variable in cancer chemotherapy as it directly influences the pharmacokinetics and pharmacodynamics of the cancer chemotherapy drug.

## INDIVIDUAL DRUG SENSITIVITY OF TUMORS

The efficacy of perioperative cancer chemotherapy protocols is governed not only by the above-mentioned pharmacokinetic and non-pharmacokinetic variables. Ultimately, individual drug sensitivity of a tumor to cancer chemotherapy may be equally important. There is solid evidence supporting a tumor-specific heterogeneous activity of cytotoxic drugs in cell cultures of different tumors.[119,120] Mahteme et al[121] confirmed the same heterogeneous cytotoxic response of cytotoxic drugs in PC samples in a variety of tumors. To date, however, there are no prospective data supporting an improved clinical outcome from drug selection based on in vitro drug sensitivity testing.

## CONCLUSION

In the last 2 decades, perioperative cancer chemotherapy protocols have emerged for the treatment of PC patients. This has resulted in remarkable clinical successes in contrast with prior failures. Now that the concept is proven, time has come to further improve the treatment protocols. This improvement should be driven by further pharmacokinetic and pharmacodynamic research. Our recent data support the importance of the tumor nodule as the most meaningful pharmacologic end point. A similar pharmacokinetic advantage of different cancer chemotherapy drugs (expressed as AUC ratio) can result in very different concentrations in tumor nodules. Timing of perioperative intravenous chemotherapy may substantially influence the pharmacokinetics.

## REFERENCES

1. Sheperd NA, Baxter KJ, Love SB. The prognostic importance of peritoneal involvement in colonic cancer: a prospective evaluation. *Gastroenterology.* 1997;112:1096–1102.
2. Sugarbaker PH. Successful management of microscopic residual disease in large bowel cancer. *Cancer Chemother Pharmacol.* 1999;43(Suppl):S15–S25.
3. Oosterling SJ, Van der Bij GJ, Van Egmond M, et al. Surgical trauma and peritoneal recurrence of colorectal carcinoma. *Eur J Surg Oncol.* 2005;31: 29–37.
4. Jayne DG, Fook S, Loi C, et al. Peritoneal carcinomatosis from colorectal cancer. *Br J Surg.* 2002;89:1545–1550.
5. Brodsky JT, Cohen AM. Peritoneal seeding following potentially curative resection of colonic carcinoma: implications for adjuvant therapy. *Dis Colon Rectum.* 1991;34:723–727.
6. Chu DZ, Lang NP, Thompson C, et al. Peritoneal carcinomatosis in nongynecologic malignancy. A prospective study of prognostic factors. *Cancer.* 1989;63:364–367.
7. Sadeghi B, Arvieux C, Glehen O, et al. Peritoneal carcinomatosis from non-gynecologic malignancies: results of the EVOCAPE 1 multicentric prospective study. *Cancer.* 2000;88:358–363.
8. Verwaal VJ, Van Ruth S, De Bree E, et al. Randomized trial of cytoreduction and hyperthermic intraperitoneal chemotherapy versus systemic chemotherapy and palliative surgery in patients with peritoneal carcinomatosis of colorectal cancer. *J Clin Oncol.* 2003;21:3737–3743.
9. Verwaal VJ, Bruin S, Boot H, et al. 8-year follow-up of randomized trail: cytoreduction and hyperthermic intraperitoneal chemotherapy versus systemic chemotherapy in patients with peritoneal carcinomatosis of colorectal cancer. *Ann Surg Oncol.* 2008;15:2426–2432.
10. Elias D, Lefevre JH, Chevalier J, et al. Complete cytoreductive surgery plus intraperitoneal chemohyperthermia with oxaliplatin for peritoneal carcinomatosis of colorectal origin. *J Clin Oncol.* 2009;27:681–685.
11. Sugarbaker PH. Peritonectomy procedures. *Surg Oncol Clin N Am.* 2003;12: 703–727.
12. Elias D, Bonnay M, Puizillou JM, et al. Heated intra-operative intraperitoneal oxaliplatin after complete resection of peritoneal carcinomatosis: pharmacokinetics and tissue distribution. *Ann Oncol.* 2002;13:267–272.
13. Spratt JS, Adcock RA, Muskovin M, et al. Clinical delivery system for intraperitoneal hyperthermic chemotherapy. *Cancer Res.* 1980;40:256–260.
14. Glehen O, Kwiatkowski F, Sugarbaker PH, et al. Cytoreductive surgery combined with perioperative intraperitoneal chemotherapy for the management of peritoneal carcinomatosis from colorectal cancer: a multi institutional study. *J Clin Oncol.* 2004;22:3284–3292.
15. Glehen O, Mithieux F, Osinsky D, et al. Surgery combined with peritonectomy procedures and intraperitoneal chemohyperthermia in abdominal cancers with peritoneal carcinomatosis: a phase II study. *J Clin Oncol.* 2003;21:799–806.
16. Yan TD, Black D, Sugarbaker PH, et al. A systematic review and meta-analysis of the randomized controlled trials on adjuvant intraperitoneal chemotherapy for respectable gastric cancer. *Ann Surg Oncol.* 2007;14:2702–2713.
17. Bijelic L, Jonson A, Sugarbaker PH. Systematic review of cytoreductive surgery and heated intraoperative intraperitoneal chemotherapy for treatment of peritoneal carcinomatosis in primary and recurrent ovarian cancer. *Ann Oncol.* 2007;18:1943–1950.
18. Yan TD, Welch L, Black D, et al. A systematic review of the efficacy of cytoreductive surgery combined with perioperative intraperitoneal chemotherapy for diffuse malignancy peritoneal mesothelioma. *Ann Oncol.* 2007;18:827–834.
19. Yan TD, Black D, Savady R, et al. A systematic review on the efficacy of cytoreductive surgery and perioperative intraperitoneal chemotherapy for pseudomyxoma peritonei. *Ann Surg Oncol.* 2007;14:484–492.
20. Yan TD, Black D, Savady R, et al. Systematic review on the efficacy of cytoreductive surgery combined with perioperative intraperitoneal chemotherapy

for peritoneal carcinomatosis from colorectal carcinoma. *J Clin Oncol.* 2006;24:4011–4019.

21. Elias D, Glehen O, Gilly F. Carcinose péritonéales d'origine digestive et primitive. Rapport du 110 éme congrès Ages de l'AFC. Arnette: Wolters Kluwer France; 2008.

22. Baron MA. Structure of the intestinal peritoneum in man. *Am J Anat.* 1941;69:439–497.

23. Flessner MF, Henegar J, Bigler S, et al. Is the peritoneum a significant transport barrier in peritoneal dialysis? *Perit Dial Int.* 2003;23:542–549.

24. De Lima Vazquez V, Stuart OA, Mohamed F, et al. Extent of parietal peritonectomy does not change intraperitoneal chemotherapy pharmacokinetics. *Cancer Chemother Pharmacol.* 2003;52:108–112.

25. Stelin G, Rippe B. A phenomenological interpretation of the variation in dialysate volume with dwell time in CAPD. *Kidney Int.* 1990;38:465–472.

26. Bettendorf U. Lymph flow mechanism of the subperitoneal diaphragmatic lymphatics. *Lymphology.* 1978;11:111–116.

27. Bettendorf U. Electronmicroscopic studies on the peritoneal resorption of intraperitoneally injected latex particles via the diaphragmatic lymphatics. *Lymphology.* 1979;12:66–70.

28. Katz MH, Barone RM. The rationale of perioperative intraperitoneal chemotherapy in the treatment of peritoneal surface malignancies. *Surg Oncol Clin N Am.* 2003;12:673–688.

29. Dedrick RL, Myers CE, Bungay PM, et al. Pharmacokinetic rationale for peritoneal drug administration in the treatment of ovarian cancer. *Cancer Treat Rep.* 1978;62:1–11.

30. Dedrick RL. Theoretical and experimental bases of intraperitoneal chemotherapy. *Semin Oncol.* 1985;12(3 Suppl 4):1–6.

31. Flessner MF, Fenstermacher JD, Dedrick RL, et al. A distributed model of peritoneal-plasma transport: tissue concentration gradients. *Am J Physiol.* 1985;248:F425–F435.

32. Flessner MF. The transport barrier in intraperitoneal therapy. *Am J Physiol Renal Physiol.* 2005;288:433–442.

33. Flessner MF. Intraperitoneal drug therapy: physical and biological principles. *Cancer Treat Res.* 2007;134:131–152.

34. Rubin J, Clawson M, Planch A, et al. Measurements of peritoneal surface area in man and rat. *Am J Med Sci.* 1988;295:453–458.

35. Keshaviah P, Emerson PF, Vonesh EF, et al. Relationship between body size, fill volume and mass transfer area coefficient in peritoneal dialysis. *J Am Soc Nephrol.* 1994;4:1820–1826.

36. Elias DM, Sideris L. Pharmacokinetics of heated intraoperative intraperitoneal oxaliplatin after complete resection of peritoneal carcinomatosis. *Surg Oncol Clin N Am.* 2003;12:755–769.

37. Sugarbaker PH, Stuart OA, Carmignani CP. Pharmacokinetic changes induced by the volume of chemotherapy solution in patients treated with hyperthermic intraperitoneal mitomycin C. *Cancer Chemother Pharmacol.* 2006;57:703–708.

38. Gardner SN. A mechanistic, predictive model of dose-response curves for cell cycle phase-specific and—non-specific drugs. *Cancer Res.* 2000;60:1417–1425.

39. Mohamed F, Sugarbaker PH. Carrier solutions for intraperitoneal chemotherapy. *Surg Oncol Clin N Am.* 2003;12:813–824.

40. Pestieau SR, Schnake KJ, Stuart OA, et al. Impact of carrier solutions on the pharmacokinetics of intraperitoneal chemotherapy. *Cancer Chemother Pharmacol.* 2001;47:269–276.

41. Mohamed F, Marchettini P, Stuart OA, et al. Pharmacokinetics and tissue distribution of intraperitoneal paclitaxel with different carrier solutions. *Cancer Chemother Pharmacol.* 2003;52:405–410.

42. Kondo A, Maeta M, Oka A, et al. Hypotonic intraperitoneal cisplatin chemotherapy for peritoneal carcinomatosis in mice. *Br J Cancer.* 1996;73:1166–1170.

43. Tsujitani S, Oka A, Kondo A, et al. Administration in a hypotonic solution is preferable to dose escalation in intraperitoneal cisplatin chemotherapy for peritoneal carcinomatosis in rats. *Oncology.* 1999;57:77–82.

44. Elias D, Otmany A, Bonnay M, et al. Human pharmacokinetic study of heated intraperitoneal oxaliplatin in increasingly hypotonic solutions after complete resection of peritoneal carcinomatosis. *Oncology.* 2002;63:346–352.

45. Dedrick RL, Flessner MF. Pharmacokinetic problems in peritoneal drug administration: tissue penetration and surface exposure. *J Natl Cancer Inst.* 1997;89:480–487.

46. Esquis P, Consolo D, Magnin G, et al. High intraabdominal pressure enhances the penetration and antitumor effect of intraperitoneal cisplatin on experimental carcinomatosis. *Ann Surg.* 2006;244:106–112.

47. Jacquet P, Stuart OA, Chang D, et al. Effect of intra-abdominal pressure on pharmacokinetics and tissue distribution of doxorubicin after intraperitoneal administration. *Anticancer Drugs.* 1996;7:596–603.

48. Gesson-Paute A, Ferron G, Thomas F, et al. Pharmacokinetics of oxaliplatin during open versus laparoscopically assisted heated intraoperative chemotherapy (HIPEC): an experimental study. *Ann Surg Oncol.* 2008;15:339–344.

49. Thomas F, Ferron G, Gesson-Paute A, et al. Increased tissue diffusion of oxaliplatin during laparoscopically assisted versus open heated intraoperative intraperitoneal chemotherapy (HIPEC). *Ann Surg Oncol.* 2008;15:3623–3624.

50. Garofalo A, Valle M, Garcia J, et al. Laparoscopic intraperitoneal hyperthermic chemotherapy for palliation of debilitating malignant ascites. *Eur J Surg Oncol.* 2006;32:682–685.

51. Facchiano E, Scaringi S, Kianmanesh R, et al. Laparoscopic hyperthermic intraperitoneal chemotherapy (HIPEC) for the treatment of malignant ascites secondary to unresectable peritoneal carcinomatosis from advanced gastric cancer. *Eur J Surg Oncol.* 2007;34:154–158.

52. Patriti A, Cavazzoni E, Graziosi L, et al. Successful palliation of malignant ascites from peritoneal mesothelioma by laparoscopic intraperitoneal hyperthermic chemotherapy. *Surg Laparosc Endosc Percutan Tech.* 2008;18:426–428.

53. Tannock IF, Lee CM, Tunggal JK, et al. Limited penetration of anticancer drugs through tumor tissue: a potential cause of resistance of solid tumors to chemotherapy. *Clin Cancer Res.* 2002;8:878–884.

54. Los G, Mutsaers PH, Lenglet WJ, et al. Platinum distribution in intraperitoneal tumors after intraperitoneal cisplatin treatment. *Cancer Chemother Pharmacol.* 1990;25:389–394.

55. Los G, Verdegaal EM, Mutsaers PH, et al. Penetration of carboplatin and cisplatin into rat peritoneal tumor nodules after intraperitoneal chemotherapy. *Cancer Chemother Pharmacol.* 1991;28:159–165.

56. Smeenk RM, Verwaal VJ, Antonini N, et al. Survival analysis of pseudomyxoma peritonei patients treated by cytoreductive surgery and hyperthermic intraperitoneal chemotherapy. *Ann Surg.* 2007;245:104–109.

57. Sugarbaker PH, Chang D, Koslowe P. Prognostic features for peritoneal carcinomatosis in colorectal and appendiceal cancer patients when treated by cytoreductive surgery and intraperitoneal chemotherapy. *Cancer Treat Res.* 1996;81:89–104.

58. Sticca RP, Dach BW. Rationale for hyperthermia with intraoperative intraperitoneal chemotherapy agents. *Surg Oncol Clin N Am.* 2003;12:689–701.

59. Dahl O, Dalene R, Schem BC, et al. Status of clinical hyperthermia. *Acta Oncol.* 1999;38:863–873.

60. Sugarbaker PH. Laboratory and clinical basis for hyperthermia as a component of intracavitary chemotherapy. *Int J Hyperthermia.* 2007;23:431–442.

61. Lepock JR. How do cells respond to their thermal environment? *Int J Hyperthermia.* 2005;21:681–687.

62. Kampinga HH. Cell biological effects of hyperthermia alone or combined with radiation or drugs: a short introduction to newcomers in the field. *Int J Hyperthermia.* 2006;22:191–196.

63. Hahn GM, Braun J, Har-Kedar I. Thermochemotherapy: synergism between hyperthermia (42–43°) and adriamycin (or bleomycin) in mammalian cell inactivation. *Proc Nat Acad Sci.* 1975;72:937–940.

64. Kusumoto T, Holden SA, Teicher BA. Hyperthermia and platinum complexes: time between treatments and synergy in vitro and in vivo. *Int J Hyperthermia.* 1995;11:575–586.

65. Barlogie B, Corry PM, Drewinko B. In vitro thermochemotherapy of human colon cancer cells with cis-dichlorodiammineplatinum(II) and Mitomycin C. *Cancer Res.* 1980;40:1165–1168.

66. Urano M, Ling CC. Thermal enhancement of melphalan and oxaliplatin cytology in vitro. *Int J Hyperthermia.* 2002;18:307–315.

67. Mohamed F, Marchettini P, Stuart OA, et al. Thermal enhancement of new chemotherapeutic agents at moderate hyperthermia. *Ann Surg Oncol.* 2003;10:463–468.

68. Jacquet P, Averbach AM, Stuart OA, et al. Hyperthermic intraperitoneal doxorubicin: pharmacokinetics, metabolism and tissue distribution in a rat model. *Cancer Chemother Pharmacol.* 1998;41:147–154.

69. Tritton TR. Cell surface actions of adriamycin. *Pharmac Ther.* 1991;49:293–309.

70. Lane P, Vichi P, Bain DL, et al. Temperature dependence studies of adriamycin uptake and cytotoxocity. *Cancer Res.* 1987;47:4038–4042.

71. Johansen PB. Doxorubicin pharmacokinetics after intravenous and intraperitoneal administration in the nude mouse. *Cancer Chemother Pharmacol.* 1981;5:267–270.

72. Ozols RF, Grotzinger KR, Fisher RI, et al. Kinetic characterization and response to chemotherapy in a transplantable murine ovarian cancer. *Cancer Res.* 1979;39:3202–3208.

73. Ozols RF, Locker GY, Doroshow JH, et al. Pharmacokinetics and tissue penetration in murine ovarian cancer. *Cancer Res.* 1979;39:3209–3214.

74. Ozols RF, Young RC, Speyer JL, et al. Phase I and pharmacological studies of adriamycin administered intraperitoneally to patients with ovarian cancer. *Cancer Res.* 1982;42:4265–4269.

75. Van der Speeten K, Stuart OA, Mahteme H, et al. A pharmacologic analysis of intraoperative intracavitary cancer chemotherapy with doxorubicin. *Cancer Chemother Pharmacol.* 2008;63:799–805.

76. Van Ruth S, Verwaal VJ, Zoetmulder FA. Pharmacokinetics of intraperitoneal mitomycin C. *Surg Oncol Clin N Am.* 2003;12:771–780.

77. Jacquet P, Averbach A, Stephens AD, et al. Heated intraoperative intraperitoneal mitomycin C and early postoperative intraperitoneal 5-fluorouracil: pharmacokinetic studies. *Oncology.* 1998;55:130–138.

78. Smeenk RM, Verwaal VJ, Zoetmulder FA. Toxicity and mortality of cytoreduction and intraoperative hyperthermic intraperitoneal chemotherapy in pseudomyxoma peritonei. A report of 103 procedures. *Eur J Surg Oncol.* 2006;32:186–190.

79. Glehen O, Osinsky D, Cotte E, et al. Intraperitoneal chemohyperthermia using a closed abdominal procedure and cytoreductive surgery for the treatment of peritoneal carcinomatosis: morbidity and mortality analysis of 216 consecutive procedures. *Ann Surg Oncol.* 2003;10:863–869.

80. Sugarbaker PH, Alderman R, Edwards G, et al. Prospective morbidity and mortality assessment of cytoreductive surgery plus perioperative intraperitoneal chemotherapy to treat peritoneal dissemination of appendiceal mucinous malignancy. *Ann Surg Oncol.* 2006;13:635–644.

81. Cepeda V, Fuertes MA, Castilla J, et al. Biochemical mechanisms of cisplatin cytotoxicity. *Anticancer Agents Med Chem.* 2007;7:3–18.

82. Armstrong DK, Bundy B, Wenzel L, et al. Intraperitoneal cisplatin and paclitaxel in ovarian cancer. *N Engl J Med.* 2006;354:34–43.

83. Markman M, Bundy BN, Alberts DS, et al. Phase III trial of standard-dose intravenous cisplatin plus paclitaxel versus moderately high-dose carboplatin followed by intravenous paclitaxel and intraperitoneal cisplatin in small-volume stage III ovarian carcinoma: an intergroup study of the Gynecologic Oncology Group, Southwestern Oncology Group, and Eastern Cooperative Oncology Group. *J Clin Oncol.* 2001;19:1001–1007.

84. Alberts DS, Liu PY, Hannigan EV, et al. Intraperitoneal cisplatin plus intravenous cyclophosphamide versus intravenous cisplatin plus intravenous cyclophosphamide for stage III ovarian cancer. *N Engl J Med.* 1996;335:1950–1955.

85. Urano M, Kuroda M, Nishimura Y. For the clinical application of thermochemotherapy given at mild temperatures. *Int J Hyperthermia.* 1999;15:79–107.

86. Los G, Mutsaers PH, Van der Vijgh WJ, et al. Direct diffusion of cis-diamminedichloroplatinum(II) in intraperitoneal rat tumors after intraperitoneal chemotherapy: a comparison with systemic chemotherapy. *Cancer Res.* 1989;49:3380–3384.

87. Van der Vaart PJ, van der Vange N, Zoetmulder FA, et al. Intraperitoneal cisplatin with regional hyperthermia in advanced ovarian cancer: pharmacokinetics and cisplatin-DNA adduct formation in patients and ovarian cancer cell lines. *Eur J Cancer.* 1998;34:148–154.

88. Jerremalm E, Hedeland M, Wallin I, et al. Oxaliplatin degradation in the presence of chloride: identification and cytotoxicity of the monochloro monooxalato complex. *Pharm Res.* 2004;21:891–894.

89. De Somer F, Ceelen W, Delanghe J, et al. Severe hyponatremia, hyperglycemia and hyperlactatemia are associated with intraoperative hyperthermic intraperitoneal chemoperfusion with oxaliplatin. *Perit Dial Int.* 2008;28:61–66.

90. Czejka M, Jäger W, Schüller J, et al. Pharmacokinetics of carboplatin after intraperitoneal administration. *Arch Pharm (Weinheim).* 1991;324:183–184.

91. Mathijssen RH, van Alphen RJ, Verweij J, et al. Clinical pharmacology and metabolism of irinotecan (CPT-11). *Clin Cancer Res.* 2001;7:2182–2194.

92. Wasserman E, Myara A, Lokiec F, et al. Severe CPT-11 toxicity in patients with Gilbert's syndrome: two case reports. *Ann Oncol.* 1997;8:1049–1051.

93. Guichard S, Chatelut E, Lochon I, et al. Comparison of the pharmacokinetics and efficacy of irinotecan after administration by the intravenous versus intraperitoneal route in mice. *Cancer Chemother Pharmacol.* 1998;42:165–170.

94. Maruyama M, Toukairin Y, Baba H, et al. Experimental study on CPT-11 intraperitoneal chemotherapy. Metabolism of CPT-11 in malignant ascites. *Gan To Kagaku Ryoho.* 2000;27:1858–1860.

95. Maruyama M, Toukairin Y, Baba H, et al. Pharmacokinetic study of the intraperitoneal administration of CPT-11 for patients with peritoneal seedings of gastric and colonic cancers. *Gan To Kagaku Ryoho.* 2000;28:1505–1507.

96. Maruyama M, Nagahama T, Yuassa Y. Intraperitoneal versus intravenous CPT-11 for peritoneal seeding and liver metastasis. *Anticancer Res.* 1999;19:4187–4191.

97. Choi SH, Tsuchida Y, Yang HW. Oral versus intraperitoneal administration of irinotecan in the treatment of nude mice. *Cancer Lett.* 1998;124:15–21.

98. Hribaschek A, Kuhn R, Pross M, et al. Intraperitoneal versus intravenous CPT-11 given intra- and postoperatively for peritoneal carcinomatosis in a rat model. *Surg Today.* 2006;36:57–62.

99. Elias D, Matsuhisa T, Sideris L, et al. Heated intra-operative intraperitoneal oxaliplatin plus irinotecan after complete resection of peritoneal carcinomatosis: pharmacokinetics, tissue distribution and tolerance. *Ann Oncol.* 2004;15:1558–1565.

100. Alberts DS, Chen HS, Chang SY, et al. The disposition of intraperitoneal bleomycin, melphalan, and vinblastine in cancer patients. *Recent Results Cancer Res.* 1980;74:293–299.

101. Glehen O, Stuart OA, Mohamed F, et al. Hyperthermia modifies pharmacokinetics and tissue distribution of intraperitoneal melphalan in a rat model. *Cancer Chemother Pharmacol.* 2004;54:79–84.

102. Sugarbaker PH, Stuart OA. Pharmacokinetic and phase II study of heated intraoperative intraperitoneal melphalan. *Cancer Chemother Pharmacol.* 2007;59:151–155.

103. Pestiau SR, Stuart OA, Chang D, et al. Pharmacokinetics of intraperitoneal gemcitabine in a rat model. *Tumori.* 1998;84:706–711.

104. Sabbatini P, Aghajanian C, Leitao M, et al. Intraperitoneal Cisplatin with intraperitoneal gemcitabine in patients with epithelial ovarian cancer: results of a phase I/II trial. *Clin Cancer Res.* 2004;10:2962–2967.

105. Morgan RJ Jr., Synold TW, Bixin X, et al. Phase I trial of intraperitoneal gemcitabine in the treatment of advanced malignancies primarily confined to the peritoneal cavity. *Clin Cancer Res.* 2007;13:1232–1237.

106. Gamblin TC, Egorin MJ, Zuhowski EG, et al. Intraperitoneal gemcitabine pharmacokinetics: a pilot and pharmacokinetic study in patients with advanced adenocarcinoma of the pancreas. *Cancer Chemother Pharmacol.* 2008;62:647–653.

107. Ceelen WP, Pahlman L, Mahteme H. Pharmacodynamic aspects of intraperitoneal cytotoxic therapy. *Cancer Treat Res.* 2007;134:195–214.

108. Sugarbaker PH, Mora JT, Carmignani P, et al. Update on chemotherapuetic agents utilized for perioperative intraperitoneal chemotherapy. *Oncologist.* 2005;10:112–122.

109. Mohamef F, Sugarbaker PH. Intraperitoneal taxanes. *Surg Oncol Clin N Am.* 2003;12:825–833.

110. Rietbroek RC, Katschinski DM, Reijers MHE, et al. Lack of thermal enhancement for taxanes in vitro. *Int J Hyperthermia.* 1997;13:525–533.

111. Schrump DS, Zhai SP, Nguyen DM, et al. Pharmacokinetics of paclitaxel administered by hyperthermic retrograde isolated lung perfusion techniques. *J Thorac Cardiovasc Surg.* 2002;123:686–694.

112. Cividalli A, Cruciani G, Livdi E, et al. Hyperthermia enhances the response of paclitaxel and radiation in a mouse adenocarcinoma. *Int J Radiat Oncol Biol Phys.* 1999;44:407–412.

113. Mohamed F, Stuart OA, Glehen O, et al. Docetaxel and hyperthermia: factors that modify thermal enhancement. *J Surg Oncol.* 2004;88:14–20.

114. Yonemura Y, Bandou E, Sawa T, et al. Neoadjuvant treatment of gastric cancer with peritoneal dissemination. *Eur J Surg Oncol.* 2006;32:661–665.

115. De Bree E, Rosing H, Beijnen JH, et al. Pharmacokinetic study of docetaxel in intraoperative hyperthermic i.p. chemotherapy for ovarian cancer. *Anticancer Drugs.* 2003;14:103–110.

116. De Bree E, Rosing H, Filis D, et al. Cytoreductive surgery and intraoperative hyperthermic intraperitoneal chemotherapy with paclitaxel: a clinical and pharmacokinetic study. *Ann Surg Oncol.* 2008;15:1183–1192.

117. Mathé G, Kidani Y, Segiguchi M, et al. Oxalato-platinum or 1-OHP, a third generation platinum complex: an experimental and clinical appraisal and preliminary comparison with cisplatinum and carboplatinum. *Biomed Pharmacother.* 1989;43:237–250.

118. de Gramont A, Tournigand C, Louvet C, et al. [Oxaliplatin, folonic acid and 5-fluorouracil (folfox) in pretreated patients with metastatic advanced cancer. The GERCOD]. *Rev Med Interne.* 1997;18:769–775.

119. Nygren P, Fridborg H, Csoka K, et al. Detection of tumor-specific cytotoxic drug activity in vitro using the fluorometric microculture cytotoxicity assay and primary cultures of tumor cells from patients. *Int J Cancer.* 1994;56:715–720.

120. Larsson R, Kristensen J, Sandberg C, et al. Laboratory determination of chemotherapeutic drug resistance in tumor cells from patients with leukemia, using a fluorometric microculture cytotoxicity assay (FMCA). *Int J Cancer.* 1992;50:177–185.

121. Mahteme H, von Heideman A, Grundmark B, et al. Heterogeneous activity of cytotoxic drugs in patient samples of peritoneal carcinomatosis. *Eur J Surg Oncol.* 2008;34:547–552.

# Epithelial Appendiceal Neoplasms

Paul H. Sugarbaker

## PRIMARY APPENDICEAL NEOPLASM

### Mucocele of the Appendix

The appendix has no known contribution to gastrointestinal function. Therefore, it is removed as an incidental organ in many surgical procedures within the abdomen or pelvis. On study of the mucosa of the appendix, it is obvious that this structure contains many goblet cells, and consequently, its exocrine production of mucus is copious. The density of these goblet cells is far greater within the epithelium of the appendix than within the colon. If any important function of the appendix does exist, perhaps its role in mucus production and lubrication of the fecal contents within the right colon should be mentioned.

With this mucus-producing epithelial lining, it is not surprising that a majority of the epithelial tumors of the appendix are mucinous. Also, it is not surprising that most appendiceal tumors begin as a mucocele (Fig. 1). The mucocele of the appendix may be symptomatic versus asymptomatic, small (less than 5 cm) versus large, neoplastic versus benign, and unruptured versus ruptured. The precise incidence of a mucocele of the appendix over the lifespan of a human is not known. However, because a mucocele is so frequently encountered, it must be quite common. Fortunately, a great majority of mucoceles removed with appendectomy are benign.

When a mucocele is encountered, it is extremely important to determine whether the wall of that structure is intact or has been

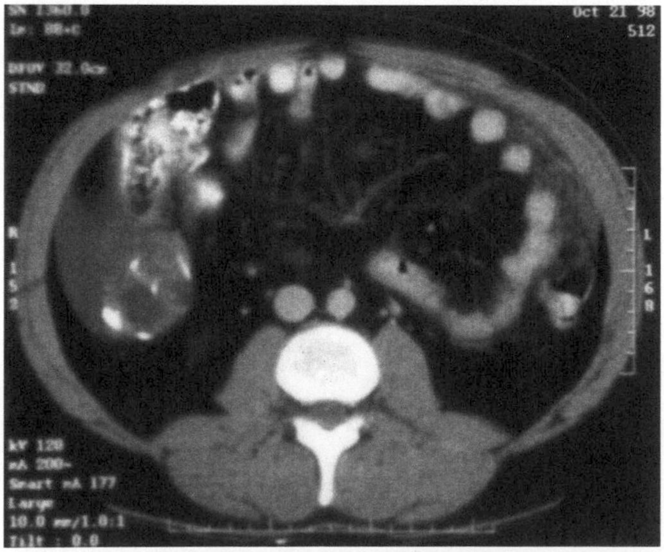

**FIGURE 1.** Mucocele of the appendix as seen on abdominal CT.

breached. A gross assessment of the appendix either by open surgery or by laparoscopic surgery is essential. Also, proper surgical management of the mucocele is essential; rupture of a neoplastic mucocele by a traumatic appendectomy can be considered an iatrogenic surgical disaster.[1]

Important data regarding the management of the mucocele of the appendix were provided by Misdraji et al[2] at the Massachusetts General Hospital. In 49 low-grade mucinous neoplasms, those with disease confined to the appendix behaved as benign disease, and no recurrence was seen with a six-year follow-up. The same low-grade tumor with extra-appendiceal spread had only a 45% 5-year survival. They concluded that an unruptured mucocele that contained low-grade cancer was a benign process, and it should be treated by simple appendectomy. In contrast, low-grade mucinous tumors (benign appearing histology), when there was access to the free peritoneal cavity, were often lethal.

Unfortunately, gross examination of the appendix at the time of appendectomy and an assessment of the size of the mucocele cannot tell the surgeon if it is benign or malignant.[2] The prudent surgical approach is to regard every mucocele of the appendix as malignant. This means that special care in the resection of an appendiceal mucocele must occur to avoid trauma and possible rupture of the appendix as it is removed. Often, this means conversion of a laparoscopic appendectomy to an open laparotomy.

Not only the appendiceal mucocele must be removed intact by a gentle surgical technique but also the peritoneal spaces surrounding the appendix must be carefully inspected. Any fluid or mucus in the vicinity must be recovered and sent for cytologic examination. Aspiration of fluid from beneath the right liver within the right retrohepatic space is indicated; also aspiration of fluid from the pelvis is essential. Careful observation of both the right and left ovary looking for cystic tumors may establish the Krukenberg Syndrome.[3] If these spaces and tissues are adequately sampled, the patient's subsequent treatment can be more knowledgeably planned.

A large number of patients with a neoplastic mucocele will have epithelial cells present in mucus outside of the appendix. In this situation, the criteria for diagnosis of the pseudomyxoma peritonei syndrome have been established.[4] Of course, if tumor nodules outside of the appendix exist, these must be biopsied to confirm intracoelomic disseminated disease.

### Mucinous Appendiceal Neoplasms Versus Intestinal Type

For colon cancer, approximately 10% of patients will have a mucinous histologic type of adenocarcinoma. In contrast, approximately 90% of appendiceal epithelial cancers are of a mucinous histologic type, and the intestinal type of disease (nonmucinous) is unusual. When the intestinal type of disease occurs, it is usually from an appendiceal

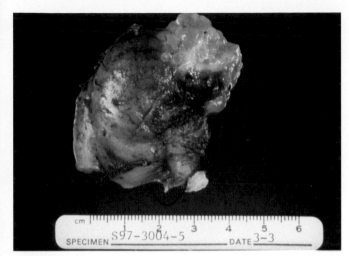

**FIGURE 2.** Ruptured appendiceal mucinous neoplasm with pathology of diffuse peritoneal adenomucinosis. Mucus-containing malignant cells extruded into the free peritoneal cavity from the end of the appendix. The entire appendix and mesoappendix were removed to sample the appendiceal lymph nodes.

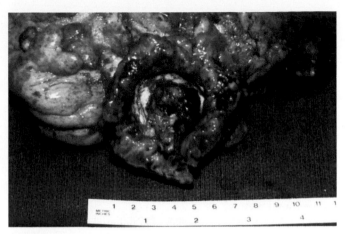

**FIGURE 4.** Ruptured appendiceal mucinous neoplasm with pathology of peritoneal mucinous carcinoma. The appendix has been destroyed by the invasive cancer.

malignancy at the orifice of the appendix, and the initial cancer dissemination is to lymph nodes. Uniformly, epithelial malignancies that exist along the lumen of the appendix or at its tip are of a mucinous histologic type; the initial cancer dissemination is through the wall of the appendix into the peritoneal space (Fig. 2).

## Gross and Histologic Types of Mucinous Appendiceal Neoplasms

A breakthrough in the management of mucinous appendiceal neoplasms came with the recognition that a broad spectrum of aggressiveness exists within mucinous appendiceal neoplasms. The histologic types were classified by Ronnett et al[5] from the extent of cel-

lular atypia of the epithelial cells and the architecture of these cells within the peritoneal cancer deposits. The least aggressive mucinous tumors present as a ruptured mucocele and were classified as diffuse peritoneal adenomucinosis (Fig. 3). Histologically, adenomucinosis was characterized by multifocal mucinous tumors adherent to but not invading into visceral or parietal peritoneal surfaces. Microscopically, the peritoneal lesions contain scant histologically benign appearing mucinous epithelium within abundant extracellular mucus. An intense hyalinizing fibrotic reaction that separates the pools of mucin was another important histologic feature. The need to distinguish secondary involvement of the ovaries by a perforated mucinous appendiceal tumor from mucinous borderline tumors of the ovary has been established previously.[6]

Peritoneal mucinous adenocarcinoma was characterized by invasive appendiceal and peritoneal lesions (Fig. 4). The histology shows abundant epithelium with glandular or signet ring cell morphology with sufficient architectural complexity and cytologic atypia to warrant a diagnosis of mucinous adenocarcinoma (Fig. 5).

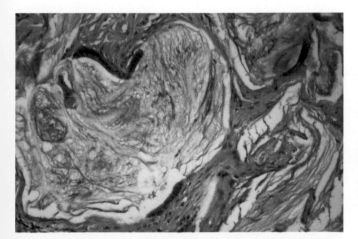

**FIGURE 3.** Peritoneal lesions of disseminated peritoneal adenomucinous showed simple mucinous epithelial strips with abundant extracellular mucin. Bland epithelium had no cytologic atypia or mitosis (hematoxylin and eosin, ×400).

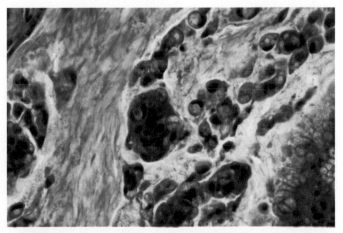

**FIGURE 5.** Peritoneal lesion of mucinous carcinomatosis showed the invasion of tumor cells with cytologic atypia. Signet ring cells are numerous (hematoxylin and eosin, ×500).

Mucinous adenocarcinomas could be further separated into 3 grades by evaluating the epithelial content of the tumor to more completely describe a histologic progression of aggressive cancer behavior. Well-differentiated mucinous adenocarcinoma was composed predominantly of single tubular glands. The tumor cells were well polarized similar to epithelium of an adenoma. Atypia of the tumor cells was remarkable, and an invasive component was identified. Moderately differentiated mucinous adenocarcinoma showed characteristics between well-differentiated and poorly differentiated adenocarcinoma. It was composed of solid sheets of malignant cells admixed with glandular formations. The polarity of the tumor cells was minimal or absent. Poorly differentiated adenocarcinoma was composed of highly irregular glandular structures or lacked glandular differentiation. The polarity of the cancer cells had disappeared completely. Often, signet ring cells were present.[7]

An intermediate type of appendiceal mucinous tumor was described by Ronnett et al.[5] In the intermediate or hybrid type of tumor, the predominant histologic features were those of adenomucinosis; however, focal areas (lower than 5% of the field of view) were of mucinous adenocarcinoma (Fig. 6). Exhaustive study of the clinical material available from many different foci of peritoneal carcinomatosis may be necessary to establish an intermediate histologic type.

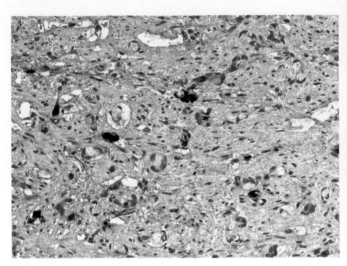

**FIGURE 7.**   Adenocarcinoid shows an admixture of small uniform glands and single infiltrating tumor cells that resemble goblet cells. Some fields of view show copious mucus. Many cells are stained by neuroendocrine immunostain, chromogranin (×200).

## The Adenocarcinoid Histologic Type

As the name implies, adenocarcinoid tumors of the appendix possess a dual morphology showing both carcinoid and mucinous adenocarcinoma components.[8] The carcinoid component is positive for neuroendocrine immunostains including synaptophysin, chromogranin, and neurospecific enolase (Fig. 7).

## Surgical Management of the Primary Appendiceal Neoplasm

Although solid clinical information is lacking, epithelial neoplasms of the appendix more than 2 cm in diameter have traditionally been managed by right colon resection. The rationale for prophylactic right colectomy was the resection of occult lymph nodal metastases within the ileocolic lymphatic system. Gonzalez-Moreno et al[9] addressed this surgical tradition by analyzing clinical data on 501 patients with epithelial malignancy of the appendix. All patients had peritoneal seeding at the time of referral and were treated in a uniform manner by cytoreductive surgery and perioperative intraperitoneal chemotherapy. The surgical procedure was appendectomy in 198 patients, right colectomy in 280 patients, and no colectomy in 23 patients. Patients with a right colectomy did not have a survival advantage. Varisco et al[10] performed a retrospective chart review and meta-analysis for adenocarcinoid of the appendix. Their data supported the use of appendectomy alone in localized cases of adenocarcinoid of the appendix provided there was no cecal involvement, and the tumor's histology was of low grade. Gonzalez-Moreno et al, in his review, determined that the incidence of lymph node metastases was 4.2% with the mucinous appendiceal malignancies. It was statistically significantly higher with the intestinal type adenocarcinomas of the appendix (66.7%). Surprisingly, the presence of lymph node metastases had no influence on prognosis ($P = 0.155$). These authors suggested that this new information on appendiceal mucinous neoplasms indicated a more selective approach to the use of right colectomy in the management of mucinous appendiceal tumors. Routine right colon resection can only be recommended with an intestinal type of appendiceal cancer.

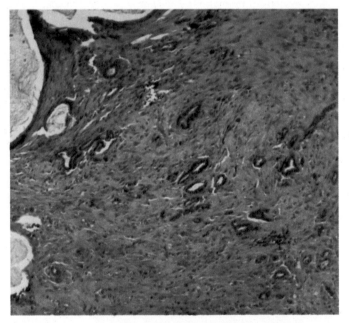

**FIGURE 6.**   The hybrid type of appendiceal mucinous tumor predominantly demonstrated features of disseminated peritoneal adenomucinosis (right upper corner). However, as shown in the center of the photomicrograph, if sufficient tissue was examined, focal areas of well-differentiated adenocarcinoma are identified (hematoxylin and eosin, ×80). In this patient, 15 slides showed disseminated peritoneal adenomucinosis, and in 1 of these, foci of mucinous adenocarcinoma were identified. The cystic foci seen in this figure adjacent to areas of adenocarcinoma are not likely to be dilated glands of carcinoma. They represent the predominant histologic pattern of diffuse peritoneal adenomucinosis seen in this patient.

The current approach recommended by Sugarbaker and coworkers uses the sentinel node concept developed by Morton and colleagues to help decide if right colectomy is necessary with an appendiceal tumor.[11] At the time of appendectomy or with a reoperation, the appendiceal lymph nodes are dissected away from the posterior aspect of the cecum. Approximately 4 nodes lie in and along the appendiceal artery. This en-bloc resection of the appendiceal lymph nodes is then submitted to the pathologist for a cryostat section. If gross and microscopic examinations of these sentinel appendiceal lymph nodes are negative, prophylactic right colectomy is not indicated.

Also, a positive margin on the base of the appendix should not be used as an indication for a right colectomy. Caecectomy can be used to obtain a negative margin of excision and can save the right colon and ileocecal valve function for the patient.

## Second-Look Surgery in Patients With Appendiceal Mucinous Neoplasms

Recently, a new approach to the management of mucinous appendiceal neoplasms, a proactive approach, has evolved. Now, patients with a perforated mucocele of the appendix are carefully evaluated and then selectively brought back to the operating room.

If the evaluation of the specimens obtained at the time of appendectomy shows the presence of mucinous peritoneal carcinomatosis, the treatment recommended by this author is straightforward. The patient needs cytoreductive surgery and hyperthermic intraperitoneal chemotherapy for a long-term survival.[12] However, frequently a dilemma exists after the resection of a mucocele in which the wall of the appendix has been perforated but no diagnosis of peritoneal surface malignancy can be established. In this situation, the author's recommendation for management is as follows: If the appendiceal specimen with perforation shows adenomucinosis, follow-up with computed tomography (CT) scans on a 6 monthly basis for 5 years is recommended. With follow-up, if pseudomyxoma peritonei is detected clinically, its progression should be sufficiently indolent to allow a curative approach to the disease process. In contrast, if the appendiceal tumor shows mucinous adenocarcinoma in the appendix specimen, a second-look surgery should be recommended. This should be an open laparotomy with wide exposure of the abdomen and pelvis, so that complete exploratory laparotomy can be performed. The undersurface of the diaphragms and the omental bursa must be visualized. The ligament of Treitz and the left paracolic sulcus are important. Of course, the rectovesical or rectouterine space must be inspected to its most inferior aspect. The small bowel should be visualized from the ligament of Treitz to the ileocecal valve.

In patients in whom progressive mucinous adenocarcinoma is documented, cytoreductive surgery to remove all evidence of mucinous adenocarcinoma is necessary. Also, greater and lesser omentectomy and sampling of the appendiceal lymph nodes must occur. If these lymph nodes are positive, right colectomy is indicated. The patient is treated with hyperthermic intraperitoneal chemotherapy to eradicate the nonvisible cellular component of the disease.

If recurrent mucinous adenocarcinoma cannot be established, then the patient undergoes a sampling of the appendiceal lymph nodes, greater and lesser omentectomy, and treatment with hyperthermic intraperitoneal chemotherapy. This approach is seen as a prophylaxis against subclinical disease developing at a later time. The timing for the second look is recommended at approximately 6 months after the appendectomy.

This selective second look is designed to prevent the rapid progression of a mucinous adenocarcinoma that may not be recognized by CT and tumor marker surveillance. Treatment of mucinous adenocarcinoma with an extensive pseudomyxoma peritonei carries with it a reduced prognosis and a greater morbidity and mortality. In contrast, the treatment of small volume mucinous adenocarcinoma is associated with an improved prognosis.

## PERITONEAL DISSEMINATION OF MUCINOUS APPENDICEAL NEOPLASMS

### Intracoelomic Dissemination

The characteristic distribution of a mucinous appendiceal neoplasm throughout the abdomen and pelvis constitutes a distinct feature of this disease process.[13,14] The unique pattern of dissemination with small bowel sparing was the original observation that led to the cytoreductive approach to this disease process.

When the appendix bursts from internal pressure from the mucus-producing neoplasm, mucus and mucinous tumor cells are released into the free peritoneal cavity. Because of the slippery fluid, these cells do not adhere in the area proximal to the perforated appendix. Rather, by physical principles of fluid dynamics, they follow the flow of peritoneal fluid. The fluid rises out of the pelvis along the right paracolic sulcus and moves around the abdomen in a clockwise direction. Large volumes of fluid are absorbed through the open lymphatic lacunae on the undersurface of the right hemidiaphragm, and tumor cells are drawn to these sites of fluid resorption. The falciform ligament diverts nonabsorbed fluid down to the lower abdomen. Further fluid is removed by the open lymph pores on the greater omentum. Tumor becomes entrapped within the greater omentum and leads to the "omental cake" formation. This large accumulation of mucinous tumor within the greater and lesser omentum is the hallmark of the pseudomyxoma peritonei syndrome. Tumor cells also become entrapped in the left paracolic sulcus, especially where the sigmoid colon is attached to the left lateral pelvic sidewall. Fluid and tumor cells cascade into the pelvis and are entrapped within the cul-de-sac by gravity. The ovaries, right and left on a monthly basis, present a "sticky surface" for tumor-cell implantation.[3] Also, hormonal factors may cause extremely rapid progression of the disease once it becomes implanted within the ovarian stroma.

The small bowel, because of its continuous peristalsis, is relatively uninvolved with the mucinous tumor implants. The cul-de-sac created by the ligament of Treitz is a prominent site for accumulation of tumor cells. Also, the terminal ileum has an increased density of pores for fluid accumulation. The volume of disease in and around the terminal ileum and ascending colon may be considerably greater than that which occurs along the course of the majority of the small bowel and small bowel mesentery.

This characteristic distribution of mucinous neoplasms of the appendix, both adenomucinosis and peritoneal mucinous carcinoma, creates the clinical picture called pseudomyxoma peritonei. If the clinical entity referred to as pseudomyxoma peritonei is caused by a low-grade appendiceal mucinous neoplasm, it is called the pseudomyxoma peritonei syndrome.[4]

The signs and symptoms of this disease are determined by the patterns of peritoneal dissemination of the mucinous tumor cells. Esquivel and Sugarbaker[15] studied, in a retrospective review, the clinical characteristics of 217 patients with the diagnosis of pseudomyxoma peritonei syndrome. The results of their study are shown in Table 1. The most common initial symptom in men and women combined was appendicitis. However, in none of these patients did the appendicitis occur as a first event in the dissemination of the disease. All patients presenting with appendicitis had moderate to large volume dissemination of the mucinous tumor around the abdomen and pelvis. Apparently, the primary tumor had leaked mucin and mucinous cancer cells on many occasions before the episode of appendicitis. The second

**TABLE 1.**   Clinical Presentation of 217 Patients With Pseudomyxoma Peritonei Syndrome

|  | No. Patients | Men | Women |
|---|---|---|---|
| Appendicitis | 58 (27) | 36 (34) | 22 (20) |
| Increased abdominal girth | 49 (23) | 28 (27) | 21 (19) |
| Ovarian mass | 44 (20) | — | 44 (39) |
| Hernia | 30 (14) | 26 (25) | 4 (4) |
| Ascites | 9 (4) | 5 (5) | 4 (4) |
| Abdominal pain | 8 (4) | 5 (5) | 3 (3) |
| Other | 19 (9) | 5 (5) | 14 (12) |
|    Total | 217 (100) | 105 (48) | 112 (52) |

Values in parentheses are percentages.
Used with permission from *Br J Surg.* 2000;87:1414–1418.

**TABLE 2.**   Visceral Resections and Peritonectomy Procedures That May Be Required for Complete Cytoreduction

| Cytoreduction | |
|---|---|
| **Visceral Resections** | **Peritonectomy Procedures** |
| Resection of prior abdominal incisions | Anterior parietal peritonectomy |
| Greater omentectomy ± splenectomy | Left upper quadrant peritonectomy |
| Rectosigmoid colon resection | Pelvic peritonectomy |
| Hysterectomy and oophorectomy | Right upper quadrant peritonectomy |
| Cholecystectomy | Lesser omentectomy with stripping of the omental bursa |

most common symptom for men and third most common symptom for women were increasing abdominal girth as a result of progressive mucinous ascites. This "jelly belly" often progressed to enormous size before patients recognized the expanding abdomen (Fig. 8). For women, the most common symptom was an ovarian mass. This phenomenon is very similar in it pathobiology to the Krukenberg syndrome; in this syndrome, gastric cancer cells move via the coelomic space to the ovary. In pseudomyxoma peritonei, the mucinous tumor cells move from the appendix to the ovary. The fourth most common presentation in both men and women was a new onset hernia that was filled by a mucoid fluid. Approximately one third of the hernias were right inguinal hernia, one third left inguinal hernia, and another third umbilical hernias.

## Management of Appendiceal Mucinous Neoplasms With Peritoneal Dissemination

Current standard of care for patients with appendiceal mucinous neoplasms requires a "comprehensive management plan." First, the patient undergoes cytoreductive surgery. This is a combination of visceral resections and peritonectomy procedures. After all visible evidence of tumor has been surgically removed, an attempt to eradicate microscopic disease and small tumor nodules occurs using a hyperthermic intraperitoneal chemotherapy treatment.

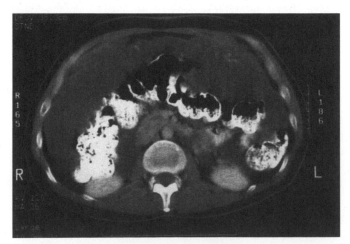

**FIGURE 8.**   CT on a patient presenting with a large "omental cake" and a large volume of mucinous ascites.

The cytoreductive surgery involves a series of visceral resections and peritonectomy procedures.[16] The various combinations of surgical procedures are listed in Table 2. It should be emphasized that no organ or peritoneal surfaces resected unless there is a visible tumor layered out on this structure. Oftentimes, with adenomucinosis, the mucinous tumor is noninvasive and can be wiped away from the involved visceral or parietal peritoneum; in this situation, the organ or peritoneal surface is not resected.

Very often the visceral resections are performed in combination with peritonectomy procedures. For example, the old abdominal incision proceeds just before the complete anterior parietal peritonectomy. The left upper quadrant peritonectomy is performed before greater omentectomy and splenectomy, so that these structures are elevated out of the left upper quadrant and can be removed under direct vision. The pelvic peritonectomy is begun before resection of the rectosigmoid colon, the uterus, and the ovaries. The pelvic peritoneum, rectosigmoid colon, and uterus are removed en bloc and submitted as a single specimen to the pathologist. The right upper quadrant peritonectomy precedes the cholecystectomy. The cholecystectomy becomes the anatomic lead-in to the lesser omentectomy with stripping of the omental bursa. These procedures have been diagrammed and described in several prior publications.[17]

There are multiple different chemotherapy regimens used to eradicate residual tumor nodules and free tumor cells within the peritoneal cavity. Over the past 20 years, an evolution of intraperitoneal treatments has occurred at the Washington Cancer Institute. Currently, the regimen in use is hyperthermic intraperitoneal doxorubicin and mitomycin C plus systemic 5-fluorouracil hyperthermic intraperitoneal chemotherapy plus 5-fluorouracil (HIPEC-plus). The standardized order for HIPEC-plus is given in Table 3. As shown in Figure 9, an open method for chemotherapy administration that allows for manual distribution of the heat and chemotherapy solution is used.[18]

## OUTCOMES OF THE TREATMENT OF APPENDICEAL EPITHELIAL NEOPLASM USING QUANTITATIVE PROGNOSTIC INDICATORS AT THE WASHINGTON CANCER INSTITUTE

To understand the outcomes of treatment, one must establish quantitative prognostic indicators by which to evaluate these treatment strategies. These quantitative prognostic indicators serve as guidelines in the selection of patients for treatments to maximize benefits of therapy and to exclude patients who have little or no likelihood for improvement.[19] They are of great utility in high-risk and costly

**TABLE 3.** Physicians Orders for Bidirectional Intraoperative Chemotherapy (HIPEC-PLUS 5-FU)

1. Add mitomycin C _____ mg to 2 L of 1.5% dextrose peritoneal dialysis solution.
2. Add doxorubicin _____ mg to the same 2 L of 1.5% dextrose peritoneal dialysis solution.
3. Dose of mitomycin C and for doxorubicin is 15 mg/m$^2$ for each chemotherapy agent.
4. Add _____ mg 5-fluorouracil (400 mg/m$^2$ for women and 600 mg/m$^2$ for men) and leucovorin _____ mg (20 mg/m$^2$) to separate bags of 250 mL normal saline. Begin rapid IV infusion of both drugs simultaneous with IP chemotherapy.
5. Send all the above to operating room _____ at _____ o'clock for 90-min treatment.

HIPEC-Plus 5-Fu, hyperthermic intraperitoneal chemotherapy plus 5-fluorouracil.

management protocols to prevent patients who are unlikely to benefit from entering into these treatments. Requirements of a useful quantitative prognostic indicator include reproducibility, prediction of morbidity and mortality, and prediction of survivorship. The goal is to establish management protocols and patient selection criteria, which will standardize the decision-making process for multiple institutions. Collaborative studies between institutions are greatly facilitated when standardized clinical tools for patient management of peritoneal surface malignancy are available. The data presented in the following paragraphs are extracted from a database of 802 patients having surgery for peritoneal dissemination of an appendiceal epithelial neoplasm.

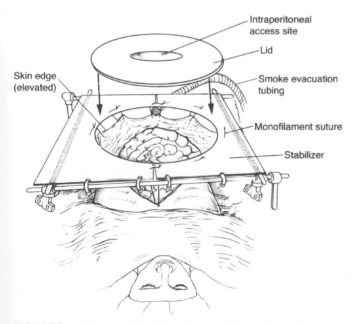

**FIGURE 9.** Apparatus for hyperthermic intraperitoneal chemotherapy administered by an open technique that attempts to achieve uniform distribution of heat and chemotherapy solution. After assembling the apparatus, it is covered by surgical drapes with a cruciate hole for access.

*Labels in figure:* Intraperitoneal access site; Lid; Smoke evacuation tubing; Monofilament suture; Stabilizer; Skin edge (elevated)

## Histopathology as a Quantitative Prognostic Indicator

As discussed earlier in this article, mucinous appendiceal neoplasms have a broad spectrum of biologic aggressiveness. Adenomucinosis describes a noninvasive peritoneal surface malignancy that may become widely dissemination on peritoneal surfaces. In contrast, peritoneal mucinous carcinoma may show the same propensity for widespread intraperitoneal dissemination that is facilitated by large quantities of mucus, but this histopathology shows invasion into surrounding structures. Also, an intermediate type of disease exists in which 95% or more of the fields of view show adenomucinosis, but areas of mucinous adenocarcinoma exist.[5] In the histologic assessment of prognosis, the intermediate type is included with the mucinous carcinoma group.

The survival of patients with mucinous appendiceal neoplasm, when treated in a uniform fashion using cytoreductive surgery and perioperative intraperitoneal chemotherapy, is profoundly affected by the patient's histologic type. Figure 10 shows the survival of patients treated at the Washington Cancer Institute by histopathology. The top portion of Figure 10 includes all patients with a complete and an incomplete cytoreductions that are in the database. The bottom graph is limited to patients who have had a complete cytoreduction. The impact of histopathology on survival persists with complete cytoreduction.

## Peritoneal Cancer Index

Unlike other carcinomatosis assessments, the peritoneal cancer index (PCI) is determined at the time of surgical exploration of the abdomen and pelvis.[19] The PCI is determined according to the diagram and instructions presented in Figure 11.

For mucinous appendiceal neoplasms that show the adenomucinosis histology, the PCI is of value in determining prognosis. As shown in the top portion of Figure 12, this noninvasive malignancy has an excellent prognosis, 94% at 20 years, if the PCI is less than 20. However, if it can be completely removed although the extent of tumor is great, the survival is 64% at 20 years. When the appendiceal mucinous neoplasm has an invasive component, as in the mucinous carcinomatosis histology, the PCI continues to show a statistically significant effect on the survival (bottom portion of Fig. 12).

These data establish a new standard of care for appendiceal mucinous neoplasms. The traditional "watch and wait policy" with "serial debulking procedures" should be of only historical interest. The definitive cytoreduction with perioperative intraperitoneal chemotherapy used in a proactive manner early in the course of this disease provides the highest likelihood of long-term survival. The top portion of Figure 12 shows that this is true for the noninvasive malignancies, and the bottom portion of Figure 12 establishes it for mucinous adenocarcinoma.

## Peritoneum as the First Line of Defense

A majority of oncologists accept the fact that the optimal treatment with a highest rate of cure, the greatest preservation of function, and the lowest morbidity and mortality is an optimal initial treatment. In treating carcinomatosis, this fact has been documented. The peritoneum is the first line of defense in carcinomatosis.[20] If extensive prior surgery with cancer cells present within the peritoneal space is performed, then these cancer cells will implant at surgical resection sites and deep to the peritoneum. Surgery in which there is disregard for the peritoneum as the first line of defense in carcinomatosis will jeopardize subsequent attempts to achieve an optimal cytoreduction. Cancer progression deep to the peritoneal surfaces, especially disease embedded within scar tissue, is difficult or impossible to remove by peritonectomy or to eradicate by intraperitoneal chemotherapy.

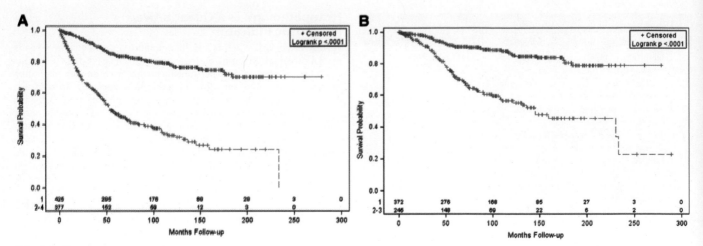

**FIGURE 10.**    Peritoneal surface malignancy of appendiceal origin. Survival by histopathology of patients treated at Washington Cancer Institute. A, Includes all patients. The blue line (N = 425) indicates patients with adenomucinosis. The red line (N = 377) indicates patients with mucinous adenocarcinoma and includes patients with intermediate type histology. B, Limited to patients with a complete cytoreduction. There were 372 adenomucinosis patients (blue line) and 245 patients (red line) with mucinous adenocarcinoma.

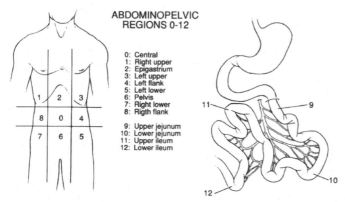

**FIGURE 11.**    Peritoneal cancer index (PCI). Two transverse planes and 2 sagittal planes divide the abdomen into 9 regions. The upper transverse plane is located at the lowest aspect of the costal margin, and the lower transverse plane is placed at the anterior superior iliac spine. The sagittal planes divide the abdomen into 3 equal sectors. The lines define the 9 regions, which are numbered in a clockwise direction with 0 at the umbilicus and 1 defining the space beneath the right hemidiaphragm. Regions 9 to 12 divide the small bowel into upper and lower jejunum and upper and lower ileum. Lesion size score is determined after complete lysis of all adhesions and the complete inspection of all parietal and visceral peritoneal surfaces. It refers to the greatest diameter of tumor implants that are distributed on the peritoneal surfaces. Primary tumors or localized recurrences at the primary site that can be removed definitively are excluded from the lesion size assessment. If there is confluence of disease matting abdominal or pelvic structures together, this is automatically scored as lesion size 3 even if it is a thin confluence of cancerous implants.

## Prior Surgical Score

Prior surgical score (PSS) quantitates the extent of surgery that was performed before definitive cytoreductive surgery and hyperthermic intraperitoneal chemotherapy.[19] The assessment uses a diagram similar to that for the PCI but excludes abdominopelvic regions 9 to 12. The PSS is a summation of the abdominopelvic regions 0 to 8 that have been traumatized by a prior surgery or by the additive effects of several prior surgeries. For a PSS of 0, only a biopsy was performed before definitive comprehensive management; PSS 1 indicates one region with prior surgery; PSS 2 indicates 2 to 5 regions previously dissected; PSS 3 indicates that 5 or more regions were dissected previously. This is equivalent to a prior attempt at complete cytoreduction but in the absence of perioperative intraperitoneal chemotherapy. The top of Figure 13 shows the statistically significant ($P = 0.0005$) impact of PSS on the survival of patients with adenomucinosis. The bottom of Figure 13 shows the lack of significance of PSS on survival of patients with mucinous carcinoma.

The data on PSS and nonaggressive mucinous appendiceal malignancies establishes the adverse effects of prior right colectomy and prior hysterectomy in this patient population. Respect for the peritoneum as a first line of defense is a reality in dealing with this disease.[20] The only definitive surgical interventions that can be supported in the light of this data are definitive cytoreduction with perioperative chemotherapy as the first major intervention in this group of patients.

## Completeness of Cytoreduction

The completeness of cytoreduction score (CC score) functions as a major quantitative prognostic indicator for patients with mucinous appendiceal neoplasms. It is an assessment performed after the cytoreductive surgery is complete. Figure 14 demonstrates the CC score for mucinous appendiceal neoplasms.[19] A complete cytoreduction is defined as CC 0 or CC 1. The tumor nodules with a mucinous appendiceal neoplasm are thought to be well penetrated by the intracavitary chemotherapy, which is always used as part of the comprehensive management plan. Therefore, tumor eradication can be predicted by

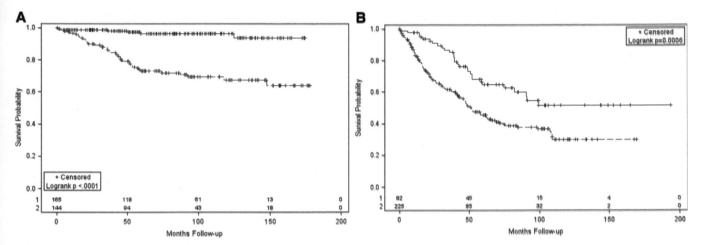

**FIGURE 12.**   Survival by peritoneal cancer index (PCI) for mucinous appendiceal neoplasms. A, Adenomucinous patients with PCI 1 to 20 (blue line, N = 165) versus 21 to 39 (red line, N = 144). B, Mucinous carcinoma patients with PCI 1–20 (blue line, N = 82) versus 21–39 (red line, N = 225).

removal of all tumors down to nodules less than 2.5 cm in diameter. In contrast, hard, fibrotic, nonmucinous intestinal type cancer nodules are poorly penetrated by chemotherapy solution. Only cytoreduction down to no visible evidence of disease would be expected to result in long-term survival with a tumor nodule not well penetrated by the intracavitary chemotherapy.

Also, some cancers may be remarkably more responsive to chemotherapy than to others. This is the situation with a majority of primary ovarian cancers. Their complete response to perioperative chemotherapy is frequently seen even though tumor nodules within the CC 1 or CC 2 category remain after cytoreduction. A bidirectional chemotherapy (intraperitoneal combined with intravenous) used in the operating room may achieve a complete response in these patients despite the presence of visible disease after cytoreduction.

The survival of patients with mucinous appendiceal neoplasms by CC score is shown in Figure 15. This quantitative prognostic in-

dicator has profound predictive value in patients with appendiceal cancer.

## Survival by Presence Versus Absence of Lymph Node Involvement

Lymph node metastases are unusual in patients with appendiceal mucinous neoplasms. They are seen only in patients with peritoneal mucinous carcinoma. Figure 16 shows the survival of these patients by the presence of regional lymph nodes versus their absence. There was a marginally significant reduced survival with positive lymph nodes.

## Survival by an Interpretive Assessment of Small Bowel Regions

In these patients, a minimally or moderately invasive mucinous tumor is widely disseminated within the abdomen and pelvis. By using parietal peritonectomy procedures, disease beneath the right and

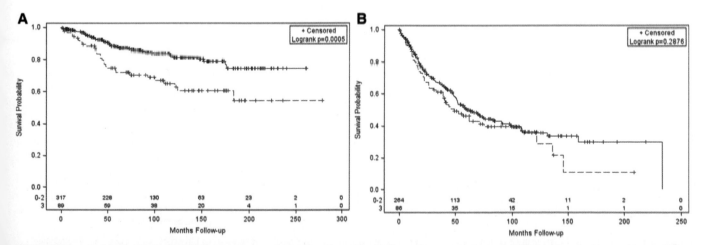

**FIGURE 13.**   Survival of patients with mucinous appendiceal neoplasms by prior surgical score (PSS). A, Survival in patients with adenomucinosis of PSS 0 to 2 (blue line, N = 317) versus PSS of 3 (red line, N = 89). B, PSS does not have a significant impact on survival of mucinous peritoneal carcinomatosis patients. PSS 0 to 2 (blue line, N = 264) versus PSS of 3 (red line, N = 86).

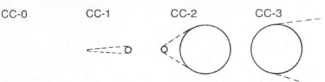

## COMPLETENESS OF CYTOREDUCTION AFTER SURGERY (CC SCORE)

CC-0          CC-1          CC-2          CC-3

No disease    Present→0.25cm   0.25cm → 2.5cm   >2.5cm

**FIGURE 14.**   Completeness of cytoreduction score. A CC-0 is apparent when there is no peritoneal seeding visualized within the operative field. CC-1 indicates nodules persisting after cytoreduction less than 2.5 cm. CC-2 has nodules between 2.5 and 5 cm, whereas a CC-3 indicates nodules greater than 5 cm or a confluence of unresectable tumor nodule at any site within the abdomen or pelvis.

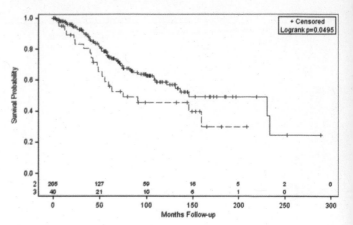

**FIGURE 16.**   Survival of patients with mucinous appendiceal neoplasms by the absence of disease in regional lymph nodes (blue line, N = 205) versus its presence (red line, N = 40).

left hemidiaphragm, in the paracolic sulcus, and in the pelvis can be definitively resected. However, disease on small bowel and small bowel mesentery cannot be adequately removed by peritonectomy. Consequently, disease at this anatomic site can result in an incomplete cytoreduction. Data from the CC score establishes that incomplete cytoreduction in these patients is accompanied by a greatly reduced prognosis.

The CT scan performed with optimal intravenous and oral contrast can identify patients who have small bowel compartmentalization versus diffuse involvement of the small bowel.[21] Figure 8 shows a CT scan where a large volume of adenomucinosis surrounds a compartmentalized small bowel with normal contours and no apparent digestive dysfunction. This patient would have a high likelihood of complete cytoreduction. In contrast, the CT in Figure 17 shows diffuse infiltration of the small bowel regions by mucinous tumor. This patient has a small or even absent likelihood of complete cytoreduction. Although this radiologic prognostic indicator has been well described

and can be completely used to predict complete cytoreduction, survival data to support it have not been published. Frequently, the diffuse involvement of small bowel regions by mucinous tumor is seen in patients who have had one or more attempts at cytoreduction without complete removal of tumor and without the use of intraperitoneal chemotherapy.

## Morbidity and Mortality

Sugarbaker et al[22] performed a prospective assessment of the morbidity and mortality on 356 procedures in patients who had an appendiceal mucinous neoplasm. All of these patients had cytoreductive surgery with peritonectomy procedures plus heated intraoperative intraperitoneal chemotherapy. The total 30-day in-hospital mortality was 2%. Nineteen percent of the procedures were accompanied by at least 1 grade IV adverse event (Fig. 18). Eleven percent of patients required a return to the operating room (Fig. 19). The mortality

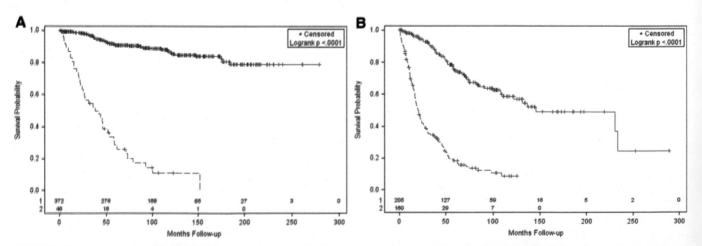

**FIGURE 15.**   Survival of patients with mucinous appendiceal neoplasms by completeness of cytoreduction score. A, Shows adenomucinosis patients; the blue line (N = 372) indicates patients with complete cytoreduction, and the red line (N = 46) indicates incomplete cytoreduction. B, The impact of complete versus incomplete cytoreduction for mucinous carcinoma patients. The blue line indicates complete cytoreduction (N = 205), and the red line indicates incomplete cytoreduction (N = 160).

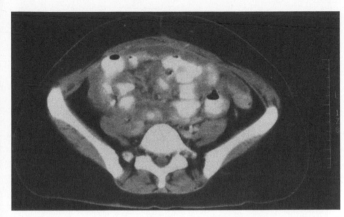

**FIGURE 17.** CT of the abdomen of a patient with appendiceal mucinous neoplasm that shows infiltration of the small bowel regions with tumor. This patient has a small or even absent likelihood of complete cytoreduction.

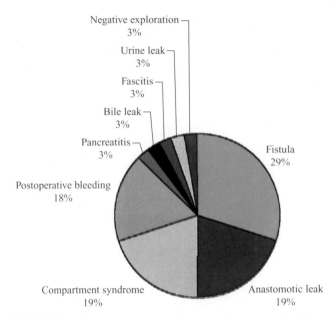

**FIGURE 19.** Cause for return to the operating room in 40 procedures (11.2%). The predominant cause for each reoperative procedure is listed. (Reprinted with permission from *Ann Surg Oncol.* 2006;13:635–644.)

of 2% and the overall grade IV morbidity of 19% in these patients were thought to be acceptable in the light of modern standards for the management of patients with complex gastrointestinal cancer.

Yan et al,[23] in their systematic review of the efficacy of cytoreductive surgery and perioperative intraperitoneal chemotherapy to treat mucinous appendiceal neoplasms, surveyed the most recent

updates from 10 institutions. This morbidity or mortality assessment involved 718 patients from 8 different institutions. Two institutions did not have morbidity or mortality data available. The overall morbidity rate varied from 33% to 56%. The overall mortality ranged from 0% to 18%.

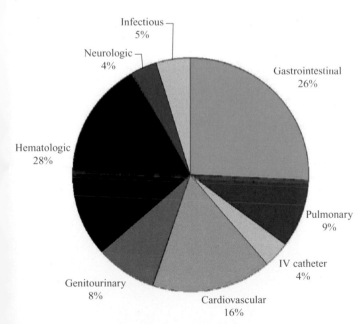

**FIGURE 18.** Grade IV adverse events occurred in 67 (19%) of 356 procedures. Because some procedures had more than a single adverse event, there were a total of 80 grade IV adverse events. The incidence of these 80 adverse events is shown. (Reprinted with permission from *Ann Surg Oncol.* 2006;13:635–644.)

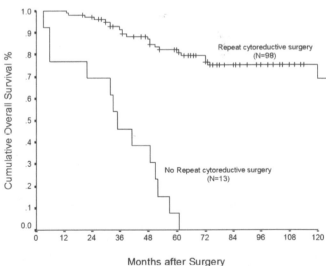

**FIGURE 20.** Survival of 111 patients who developed disease progression after initial cytoreductive surgery (CRS) and perioperative intraperitoneal chemotherapy (PIC) for peritoneal dissemination from appendiceal mucinous neoplasms, stratified by repeat CRS (*P* < 0.001). (Reprinted with permission from *Ann Surg Oncol.* 2007;14:484–492.)

## Follow-Up and Reoperative Procedures After Comprehensive Management

After definitive treatment, these patients with mucinous appendiceal neoplasm are followed up carefully with CEA and CA 19-9 tumor markers and CT scan of chest, abdomen, and pelvis. The CEA and CA 19-9 tumor markers, when used together, are an excellent tool for surveillance of these patients.[24] Also, the follow-up is complemented by the CT scan performed on a 6-monthly basis. The goal of this follow-up plan is to detect recurrence in a timely fashion, so that additional treatments can be initiated.

Yan et al[25] studied reoperative surgery in patients with both adenomucinosis and peritoneal mucinous adenocarcinoma. In those, 111 of 402 patients (28%) developed progressive disease. Ninety-eight patients had a repeat cytoreductive surgery with intraperitoneal chemotherapy and 13 did not. The survival of patients who were considered poor candidates for a repeat cytoreductive effort versus those patients who had a second cytoreduction is shown in Figure 20. By these data, one is led to think that careful follow-up and reoperation if patients can again be made disease-free is the appropriate treatment strategy for this group of patients.

## REFERENCES

1. Dhage-Ivatury S, Sugarbaker PH. Update on the surgical approach to mucocele of the appendix. *J Am Coll Surg.* 2006;202:680–684.
2. Misdraji J, Yantiss RK, Graeme-Cook FM, et al. Appendiceal mucinous neoplasms: a clinicopathologic analysis of 107 cases. *Am J Surg Pathol.* 2003;27:1089–1103.
3. Sugarbaker PH, Averbach AM. Krukenberg syndrome as a natural manifestation of tumor cell entrapment. In: Sugarbaker PH, ed. *Peritoneal Carcinomatosis: Principles of Management.* Boston, MA: Kluwer; 1996:63–191.
4. Sugarbaker PH, Ronnett BM, Archer A, et al. Pseudomyxoma peritonei syndrome. *Adv Surg.* 1996;30:233–280.
5. Ronnett BM, Shmookler BM, Sugarbaker PH, et al. Pseudomyxoma peritonei: new concepts in diagnosis, origin, nomenclature, relationship to mucinous borderline (low malignant potential) tumors of the ovary. In: Fechner RE, Rosen PP, eds. *Anatomic Pathology.* ASCP Press: Chicago; 1997:197–226.
6. Ronnett BM, Kurman RJ, Shmookler BM, et al. The morphologic spectrum of ovarian metastases of appendiceal adenocarcinomas: a clinicopathologic and immunohistochemical analysis of tumors often misinterpreted as primary ovarian tumors or metastatic tumors from other gastrointestinal sites. *Am J Surg Pathol.* 1997;21:1144–1155.
7. Yan H, Pestieau SR, Shmookler BM, et al. Histopathologic analysis in 46 patients with pseudomyxoma peritonei syndrome: failure versus success with a second-look operation. *Mod Pathol.* 2001;14:164–171.
8. Mahteme H, Sugarbaker PH. Treatment of peritoneal carcinomatosis from adenocarcinoid of appendiceal origin. *Br J Surg.* 2004;91:1168–1173.
9. Gonzalez-Moreno S, Sugarbaker PH. Right hemicolectomy does not confer a survival advantage in patients with mucinous carcinoma of the appendix and peritoneal seeding. *Br J Surg.* 2004;91:304–311.
10. Varisco B, McAlvin B, Dias J, et al. Adenocarcinoid of the appendix: is right hemicolectomy necessary? A meta-analysis of retrospective chart reviews. *Am Surg.* 2004;70:593–599.
11. Morton DL, Thompson JF, Essner R, et al. Validation of the accuracy of intraoperative lymphatic mapping and sentinel lymphadenectomy for early-stage melanoma: a multicenter trial. Multicenter Selective Lymphadenectomy Trial Group. *Ann Surg.* 1999;230:453–463.
12. Sugarbaker PH. New standard of care for appendiceal epithelial neoplasms and pseudomyxoma peritonei syndrome? *Lancet Oncol.* 2006;7:69–76.
13. Sugarbaker PH. Pseudomyxoma peritonei: a cancer whose biology is characterized by a redistribution phenomenon. *Ann Surg.* 1994;219:109–111.
14. Carmignani CP, Sugarbaker TA, Bromley CM, et al. Intraperitoneal cancer dissemination: mechanisms of the patterns of spread. *Cancer Metastasis Rev.* 2003;22:465–472.
15. Esquivel J, Sugarbaker PH. Clinical presentation of the pseudomyxoma peritonei syndrome. *Br J Surg.* 2000;87:1414–1418.
16. Sugarbaker P. Peritonectomy procedures. *Ann Surg.* 1995;221:29–42.
17. Sugarbaker PH. Peritonectomy procedures. *Surg Oncol Clin N Am.* 2003;12:703–727.
18. Sugarbaker PH. An instrument to provide containment of intraoperative intraperitoneal chemotherapy with optimized distribution. *J Surg Oncol.* 2005;92:142–146.
19. Jacquet P, Sugarbaker PH. Current methodologies for clinical assessment of patients with peritoneal carcinomatosis. *J Exp Clin Cancer Res.* 1996; 15:49–58.
20. Sugarbaker PH. Peritoneum as the first line of defense in carcinomatosis. *J Surg Oncol.* 2007;95:93–96.
21. Jacquet P, Jelinek JS, Chang D, et al. Abdominal computed tomographic scan in the selection of patients with mucinous peritoneal carcinomatosis for cytoreductive surgery. *J Am Coll Surg.* 1995;181:530–538.
22. Sugarbaker P, Alderman R, Edwards G, et al. Prospective morbidity and mortality assessment of cytoreductive surgery plus perioperative intraperitoneal chemotherapy to treat peritoneal dissemination of appendiceal mucinous malignancy. *Ann Surg Oncol.* 2006;13:635–644.
23. Yan TD, Black D, Savady R, et al. A systematic review on the efficacy of cytoreductive surgery and perioperative intraperitoneal chemotherapy for pseudomyxoma peritonei. *Ann Surg Oncol.* 2007;14:484–492.
24. Carmignani CP, Hampton R, Sugarbaker CE, et al. Utility of CEA and CA 19–9 tumor markers in diagnosis and prognostic assessment of mucinous epithelial cancers of the appendix. *J Surg Oncol.* 2004;87:162–166.
25. Yan TD, Bijelic L, Sugarbaker PH. Critical analysis of treatment failure after complete cytoreductive surgery and perioperative intraperitoneal chemotherapy for peritoneal dissemination from appendiceal mucinous neoplasms. *Ann Surg Oncol.* 2007;14:2289–2299.

# Patient Selection for a Curative Approach to Carcinomatosis

Pompiliu Piso • Gabriel Glockzin • Phillip von Breitenbuch • Talal Sulaiman • Felix Popp • Marc Dahlke
• Jesus Esquivel • Hans Juergen Schlitt

Many patients with gastrointestinal malignancies experience a peritoneal dissemination as a part of the natural history of their disease. Of all patients with colorectal cancer (CRC), up to 25% will be diagnosed with peritoneal carcinomatosis during the course of their disease, with or without associated liver or other distant metastases.[1] These patients have a poor prognosis. However, this has changed over the last decades. Just before the era of systemic and targeted chemotherapy for colon cancer, natural history of patients with peritoneal carcinomatosis arising from colon cancer presented in the European multicenter EVOCAPE I study a median survival of 5.2 months (n = 118).[2] Even though there are no studies investigating systemic treatment modalities for patients with isolated peritoneal dissemination, the survival times of patients with metastatic colon cancer have improved dramatically.[3] Sugarbaker et al[4] and Glehen and Gilly introduced cytoreductive surgery (CRS) and hyperthermic intraperitoneal chemotherapy (HIPEC) as a new therapeutic option for selected patients with peritoneal carcinomatosis more than 20 years ago. Feasibility, efficacy, and safety of CRS and HIPEC have been investigated in numerous clinical trials and many peritoneal surface malignancies treatment centers were established in the United States, Europe, and Japan. There are 2 prospective randomized controlled trials, 1 nonrandomized comparative study, and numerous observational studies regarding clinical and oncologic outcome of patients with peritoneal carcinomatosis arising from CRC. The survival probability at 5 years can be in selected patients as high as 40% with a median survival of more than 40 months.[5-8]

Therefore, a paradigm shift may take place in the treatment of selected patients with peritoneal carcinomatosis arising from CRC, similar to the treatment of liver metastases.[9] Even in the absence of a prospective randomized trial, surgery has become standard of care for patients with resectable liver metastases. In fact, the prognosis of these 2 different patient groups is rather similar, provided a complete cytoreduction was achieved. CRS and HIPEC cannot be offered to every patient with peritoneal carcinomatosis. However, patients should be systematically evaluated for this treatment. There is some evidence suggesting that at least 3% of all patients with CRC can be treated successfully with a positive impact on their prognosis.[10] The selection process is a very difficult one and will be discussed in detail in this article.

## CYTOREDUCTIVE SURGERY AND HYPERTHERMIC INTRAPERITONEAL CHEMOTHERAPY

CRS consists of numerous surgical procedures depending on the extent of peritoneal tumor manifestation. Surgery may include parietal and visceral peritonectomy, greater omentectomy, splenectomy, cholecystectomy, resection of liver capsule, small bowel resection, colonic and rectal resection, gastrectomy, lesser omentectomy, pancreatic resection, hysterectomy, oophorectomy, and urinary bladder

resection.[11] The aim of CRS is to obtain complete macroscopic cytoreduction (CC-0/1) as a precondition for the application of HIPEC. The residual disease is classified intraoperatively using the completeness of cytoreduction (CCR) score. CCR-0 indicates no visible residual tumor and CC-1 residual tumor nodules ≤2.5 mm. CC-2 and CC-3 indicate residual tumor nodules between 2.5 mm and 2.5 cm and >2.5 cm, respectively.[12]

In case of CCR-0/1, CRS is followed by HIPEC. HIPEC can be performed in open or closed abdomen technique. For the performance of HIPEC, a special roller pump is necessary to circulate the perfusate via several catheters placed into the peritoneal cavity. The intraperitoneal temperature is usually 41°C to 43°C. Several drugs can be used for CRC: cisplatinum, mitomycin C, oxaliplatin, and irinotecan.[13-16]

## TOOLS FOR APPROPRIATE SELECTION

Selecting patients with peritoneal carcinomatosis arising from colorectal malignancies is part of the learning curve for multimodality treatment consisting of CRS and HIPEC.[17,18] The surgeon's experience will play an important role in the decision making. Several criteria will help the surgeon to find a personalized treatment strategy and to finally decide, if further information is necessary (Table 1). These criteria will be described here.

During the clinical examination, the surgeon will have to look for the performance status, comorbidity, signs of ascites, palpable tumor, or intestinal obstruction. If the patients had been already operated elsewhere, the operation reports/notes with precise description of the findings (in particular distribution, size, and localization of all nodules) have to be available. If necessary, the first surgeon has to be contacted, in particular to find out details like small bowel involvement, micronodular disease, etc. The histology has to be clearly defined and specify the grade of differentiation, the presence of lymph node metastases, and, in case of peritoneal disseminated adenomucinosis, to exclude adenocarcinoma. On computed tomography (CT) scans, positron emission tomography-CT or magnetic resonance imaging, the surgeon should try to quantify the tumor volume, for example, by peritoneal cancer index (PCI), and to assess the possible extent of resection and the probability of CCR-0/1.[19] However, Koh et al[20] have shown that preoperative CT-PCI does not correlate with the intraoperative PCI.

With all this information, interdisciplinary decision on further treatment (involving surgical oncologists, gastroenterologists, and medical oncologists) can be taken. For marginal cases, a second opinion from a referral center for peritoneal surface malignancies can help, being often lower.

The probability of complete cytoreduction has to be proven again during laparotomy. At this stage, a realistic PCI can be calculated and the small bowel can be explored in all its length. If CCR-0/1 seems achievable, the procedure will be completed, provided there

**TABLE 1.** Factors to Influence the Decision Making

Tumor-specific factors
  Primary tumor
  Histology with grading
  Extra-abdominal disease
  Liver metastases
  Paraortic lymph node metastases
  Peritoneal cancer index
  Small bowel involvement
  Involvement of the hepatogastric ligament
  Biliary/ureteral obstruction
  Response to previous chemotherapy
Other factors
  Peformance status
  Comorbidities
  Learning curve
  Informed consent
  Predictable postoperative quality of life
  Tumor board decision
Useful additional tools for selection (case dependent)
  Positron emission tomography scan/PET-CT
  Diagnostic laparoscopy

are an adequate small bowel length and gastrointestinal reconstruction possibilities.

## Performance Status and Comorbidities

As CRS and HIPEC represent an aggressive treatment strategy with an operation going on over 6 to 10 hours or more, the patients' general condition plays a crucial role, reflecting not only possible intraoperative but also postoperative complications. The performance status can be quantified by different scores. These are mainly the Eastern Cooperative Oncology Group Performance Status (2 or less) and the Karnofsky Index (75% or more).[21]

Some factors can be optimized preoperatively by training and conditioning, for example, in specialized fitness or rehabilitation centers. Immunonutrition may play an important role here, as there is some evidence that it lowers morbidity rates after multivisceral resections.[22]

Others factors are influenced by the presence of associated diseases. Cardiovascular, renal, or pulmonary comorbidity will influence the decision making, and if malfunctions cannot be corrected, CRS and HIPEC may be contraindicated. The presence of other malignancies will also have an impact on the decision to treat peritoneal carcinomatosis if their prognosis is worse than that of the peritoneal malignancy.

For some groups, age >75 years represents a relative contraindication for CRS and HIPEC; however, most of the centers will agree that age alone should not be an impediment for this multimodality treatment strategy. There is some experience with CRS and HIPEC in pediatric patients. A German group has published long-term survival data in a 12-year-old boy with a peritoneal carcinomatosis arising from a colon cancer.[23]

## Primary Tumor

The tumor site of the primary tumor is an important selection criteria, as the prognosis is different. Basically, patients with an appendix cancer have a better prognosis than those with colon cancer. This could have been demonstrated by the prospective randomized trial of The Netherlands Cancer Institute, published in 2003 and 2008.[5,7] On the other hand, patients with colon cancer have a better prognosis than those with rectal cancer. In fact, there are just a few data on this issue, suggesting that there is no 5-year survivor among patients with rectal cancer and peritoneal carcinomatosis.[24]

The histology of the tumor may also play an important role as we know that patients with well differentiated carcinomas will have a better prognosis than those with poorly differentiated.[25] A special situation is the signet cell carcinoma, often associated with a very poor prognosis, for many authors a relative contraindication for extended cytoreduction, although in some cases with low tumor volume and no other metastases, the indication may be evaluated.

The presence of the lymph node metastases at the primary site is also one factor to be taken into consideration for the decision making.[26,27] A high number of lymph node metastases suggests a high recurrence rate, in particular, of disseminated disease. During the consensus meeting in Milan 2006 (5th International Workshop on Peritoneal Surface Malignancies), 50% of all experts considered a combination of 3 cycles of best available systemic therapy followed by CRS and HIPEC and the same systemic therapy of the best strategy for patients with positive lymph node metastases.[28]

Appendiceal malignacy with disseminated peritoneal adenomucinosis represents a separate entity, as the tumor biology is completely different. Nonruptured mucinous adenoma is seldom diagnosed, if the rupture occurs, disseminated peritoneal adenomucinosis will be the consequence (Fig. 1). If only serial debulking is performed, best series showed a 10-years survival rate of 70%; however, no patients survived longer than 20 years.[29] Opposed to that best results for CRS and HIPEC demonstrated 20-years survival probabilities of 70%.[30] This has to be considered when evaluating elderly patients with an increased morbidity and possible quality of life (QoL) impairment after extended surgery.

## Response to Prior Treatments

Many patients with CRC and peritoneal carcinomatosis receive palliative treatment with systemic chemotherapy. In the United States,

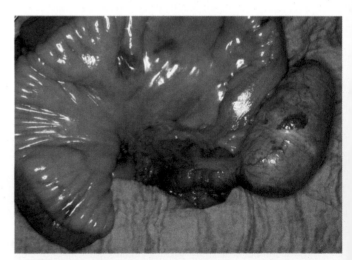

**FIGURE 1.** Appendix mucocele, just before rupturing. Appendectomy could prevent a disseminated peritoneal adenomucinosis in this patient.

most patients have failed every possible combination of cytotoxic biologic agents and often present with a debilitated body and depleted bone marrow.[28] However, if there are signs (eg, according to the response evaluation criteria in solid tumors) suggesting a response to chemotherapy, this will positively influence the prognosis after CRS and HIPEC. This and the length of the tumor-free interval give us a clue regarding the biologic aggressiveness of the tumor and will influence the decision making.[1,26] Progressive disease under systemic chemotherapy will negatively influence (together with other factors) the decision to perform CRS and HIPEC or not. However, this might be different for high-grade mucinous tumors, as we know that they rarely respond to systemic treatments.

## Recurrent Disease

Even after complete cytoreduction, patients with high PCI and high-grade tumor are at risk to be diagnosed with recurrent peritoneal disease. If the disease is located at more than 1 site and the free interval was less than 6 months, no long-term survival can be achieved by redo surgery with HIPEC. However, if the recurrence is limited to 1 site and had occurred later than 6 months after treatment, re-CRS and HIPEC may improve the survival of these patients, with the same prognosis as anticipated after the primary intervention. These patients should be at any rate evaluated for multimodality treatment consisting of CRS and HIPEC.[31]

Some recent data suggest that for patients with primary colon cancer with carcinomatosis or high risk for carcinomatosis (eg, positive peritoneal cytology or perforation of the primary tumor or limited peritoneal seeding), second-look surgery may play a role.[32] Because peritoneal carcinomatosis is difficult to be visualized in CT scan, second-look surgery may improve the rate of detection at early stages. Elias et al[33] published a 55% early detection rate after second-look surgery at 1 year.

## Extra-Abdominal Metastases

The presence of extra-abdominal metastases will limit the survival of patients with peritoneal carcinomatosis and influence their prognosis.[34] Mostly is that the case for lung metastases, mediastinal lymph node metastases, bone metastases, or brain metastases. The biology of these tumor locations will not be influenced by the locoregional abdominal treatment. As these metastases occur because of invasion of blood or lymphatic vessels, they are regarded as systemic cancer dissemination, localized pleural affection may be different as it is caused either by direct diaphragmatic tumor penetration or by intraoperative contamination during diaphragmatic resection. There are some reports on simultaneous pleurectomy in patients with appendiceal malignancies; however, it is associated with a high morbidity and poor prognosis.[35]

## Liver Metastases

The presence of liver metastases is a sign of hematogenous dissemination of the primary tumor. For many groups, this will be contraindication for extended parietal and visceral peritonectomy as it will not influence the prognoses of these patients. However, if we regard the prognosis of patients with limited number of liver metastases treated by surgery and systemic immunochemotherapy, their 5-year survival probability will be at least 40%. Therefore, it will not limit the prognosis of selected patients with peritoneal carcinomatosis, if the peritoneal disease can be treated successfully. This is why, in particular, French centers do treat patients with up to 3 small, peripheric localized, and resectable liver metastases and limited peritoneal carcinomatosis.[36] The long-term results in these patients are not different to those of patients without liver metastases. During the consensus meeting in Milan

2006 (5th International Workshop on Peritoneal Surface Malignancies), 66% of all experts considered the presence of liver metastases not to be an exclusion criteria for CRS and HIPEC.[28]

## Paraaotic Lymph Node Metastases

As for liver metastases, the presence of paraaortic lymph node metastases is a sign of dissemination outside of peritoneal cavity suggesting an aggressive tumor biology. Patients with high number of metastatic lymph nodes at site of the primary tumor are at risk to develop paraaortic lymph node metastases.[26,27] If this occurs, there is an increased risk to be diagnosed with mediastinal paraaortic lymph node metastases. This can be demonstrated by PET-CT scan. However, opposed to liver metastases, this issue has not been addressed in any trial until now. Therefore, it is difficult to interpret the value of this selection criterion alone.

## Biliary and Ureteral Obstruction

If a biliary or ureteral obstruction or both can be diagnosed by ultrasound or CT scan, it is mostly a sign of direct penetration beyond the peritoneal barrier, into the retroperitoneum or into the hilar structures of the liver and can be regarded as surgically not resectable.[27,34] However, external compression because of large tumor masses with secondary obstruction should not be regarded as a contraindication, as the resection of these masses, in particular in patients with pseudomyxoma peritonei, is possible without segmental ureteral or bile duct resection.

## Small Bowel Involvement

A noninvolved small bowel offers best chances of complete cytoreduction (Fig. 2). If the small bowel mesentery has evidence of gross disease with several segmental sites of partial obstruction, there is no surgical option to remove all affected sites. An extended removal of the small bowel will not only cause a short bowel syndrome but also a recurrence within short time, often less than 3 months. Even evidence of intestinal obstruction at more than 1 site, for example, in CT scan, should exclude these patients from CRS and HIPEC protocols.[28,34,37]

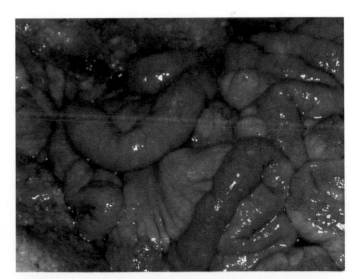

**FIGURE 2.** Complete macroscopic cytoreduction probable: no small bowel involvement underneath the omental cake in a patient with mucinous adneocarcinoma of the ascending colon.

## Gastro-Hepatic Ligament

If the lesser omentum is affected and a tumor nodule with a diameter of more than 5 cm can be visualized in CT scans, the probability of removal of left gastric artery is very high. During omentectomy, the right and left gastroepiloic vessels have to be resected. If, as often the case, a splenectomy has to be performed, the blood supply of the whole stomach is possible only because of preserved left gastric vessels. If a large tumor mass in the gastrohepatic ligament (including the left gastric vessels) has to be removed, a total gastrectomy has also to be completed.[34] This will impair the QoL extremely, in particular if a total colectomy has also to be performed and should be done only in patients having less aggressive histology and biologic behavior, in whom a complete cytoreduction can be achieved.

## Quantification of the Tumor Volume

To be able to analyze the impact of the tumor volume on patients prognosis, several scores have been developed, for example, PCI (Washington Cancer Institute), Gilly staging system (Lyon), P-score (Japanese Research Society for Gastric Cancer), or simplified PCI (The Netherlands Cancer Institute). The most frequently used score is the PCI (Fig. 3).[12] The abdomen is divided into 9 regions and the small bowel into 4: each assigned a lesion-size (LS) score of 0 to 3 that would be representative of the largest implant visualized. LS-0 denotes the absence of implants, LS-1 indicates implants <0.25 cm, LS-2 between 0.25 and 5 cm, and LS-3 >5 cm or a confluence of disease. These figures amount to a final numerical score of 0 to 39. There is some evidence suggesting that patients with a PCI >20 will not benefit from CRS and HIPEC. The main reason is the fact, that no long-term survivors (>5 years postoperatively) have been published. However, during the consensus meeting in Milan 2006 (5th International Workshop on Peritoneal Surface Malignancies), 33% of all experts considered a PCI of more than 20 not to be an absolute exclusion criteria for CRS and HIPEC.[28] The tumor volume may not play the same role for pseudomyxoma peritonei patients with low grade and noninvasive mucinous tumor masses. PCI >20 will not influence the prognosis, as long as a complete cytoreduction can be achieved (Fig. 4).[38]

## Postoperative Quality of Life

Short-term QoL is practically determined by the postoperative morbidity. This is after CRS and HIPEC relatively high but comparable with other major gastrointestinal surgery. Morbidity rates after CRS and HIPEC range from 25% to 41%.[26,39,40]

Despite relatively high morbidity rates and consecutive initial impairment of QoL, several studies could show an improvement of QoL after CRS and HIPEC in long-term survivors. McQuellon et al reported an initial decrease of physical, functional, and well-being scores with an increase relative to baseline levels during follow-up at 3, 6, and 12 months. One year after surgery, 74% of the patients resumed >50% of their normal activities.[41]

The same group has then analyzed the QoL in long-term survivors (>3 years). Seventeen patients have been included in this study. Ten of them described their health as excellent or very good. No limitations on moderate activity were reported in 94% of cases. An improved functional well being, physical well being, and global QoL could be demonstrated. The authors concluded that long-term survival with good QoL is possible in selected patients after CRS and HIPEC.[42]

In another publication, McQuellon et al had analyzed the health outcomes after CRS and HIPEC for patients with disseminated peritoneal cancer of appendiceal origin. Fifty-eight patients had been included in this study. Emotional well being improved during the study period, whereas physical well being and physical functioning declined at 3 months and then improved to near baseline levels at 6 and 12 months. By 1 year, nearly 85% of study participants reported having normal activity or having few symptoms.[43]

Schmidt et al evaluated QoL after CRS and HIPEC in 67 patients with peritoneal carcinomatosis using the EORTC QLQ-C30

## Peritoneal Cancer Index

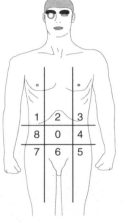

| Regions | Lesion Size | Lesion Size Score |
|---|---|---|
| 0   Central | _____ | LS 0   No tumor seen |
| 1   Right Upper | _____ | LS1   Tumor up to 0.5 cm |
| 2   Epigastrium | _____ | LS2   Tumor up to 5.0 cm |
| 3   Left Upper | _____ | LS3   Tumor > 5.0 cm or confluence |
| 4   Left Flank | _____ | |
| 5   Left Lower | _____ | |
| 6   Pelvis | _____ | |
| 7   Right Lower | _____ | |
| 8   Right Flank | _____ | |
| 9   Upper Jejunum | _____ | |
| 10 Lower Jejunum | _____ | |
| 11 Upper Ileum | _____ | |
| 12 Lower Ileum | _____ | |

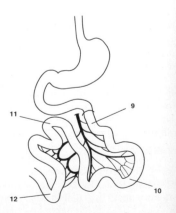

**FIGURE 3.**   Peritoneal cancer index helps to quantify the tumor volume.

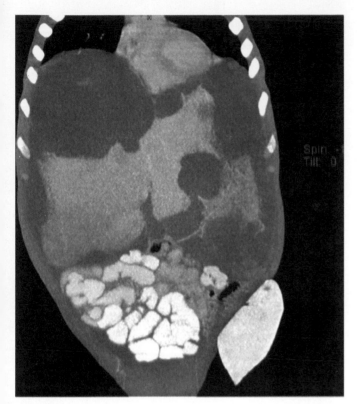

**FIGURE 4.** High PCI in patients with pseudomyxoma is not predictable for complete cytoreduction. The small bowel was not involved in this patient.

questionnaire. The mean score for global health status of long-term survivors was decreased compared with the control population showing particularly an impairment of role and social functioning.[44]

## Informed Consent

Different parts of the treatment have to be discussed with the patient in detail, referring in particular to the probabilities of different organ resections (in particular combinations like total gastrectomy and colectomy), ostomies, postoperative morbidity, QoL, and risk of recurrence. The patient has to evaluate these facts and balance them against possible improvement of his prognosis, giving the patient realistic figures on expected outcome. At this point, patient's motivation will influence the decision to perform CRS and HIPEC. Patient's motivation is important at this stage and it will influence the whole postoperative course.

## DECISION MAKING

### Consensus Statement of the Peritoneal Surface Oncology Group

The Peritoneal Surface Malignancy Group defined 8 clinical and radiologic variables that increase the probability of CCR in patients with peritoneal carcinomatosis of colonic origin: (1) Eastern Cooperative Oncology Group performance status ≤2, (2) no evidence of extra-abdominal disease, (3) up to 3 small, resectable parenchymal hepatic metastases, (4) no evidence of biliary obstruction, (5) no evidence of ureteral obstruction, (6) no evidence of intestinal obstruction at more than 1 site, (7) small bowel involvement: no evidence of gross disease in the mesentery with several segmental sites of partial obstruction, and (8) small volume disease in gastro-hepatic ligament.[34]

As presented, many selection criteria have to be assessed for each patient to be able to decide, if surgery should be undertaken

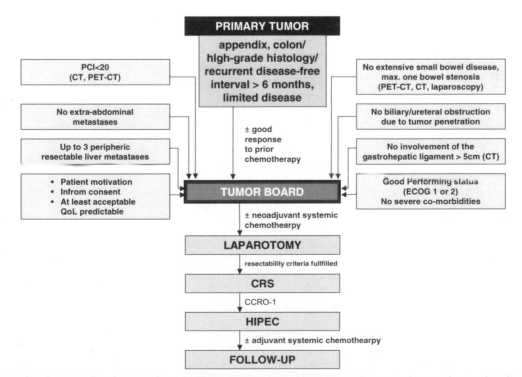

**FIGURE 5.** Algorithm for patient selection, for a curative approach to carcinomatosis arising from colorectal malignancies.

with the aim of CRS and HIPEC (Fig. 5). All these factors have to be discussed interdisciplinary and with the patient to formulate an individualized treatment option. It is difficult to decide on the relative importance of each criteria. As far as we know, completeness of cytoreduction, tumor volume (expressed by PCI), and histology are essential, in many multivariate analysis independent prognostic factors.[45] There are some attempts to formulate scores to describe the disease severity. Pelz et al described a 3-point scale including symptoms, extent of peritoneal dissemination (PCI), and primary tumor histology. The disease severity was expressed by 4 severity scores; advanced disease was an independent predictor of adverse outcome on multivariate analysis.[25]

It is important to create awareness in the medical community regarding the possibility to treat selected patients with peritoneal carcinomatosis and the selection criteria. This would increase the rate of early referrals and the percentage of evaluated patients. It would also result in a lower PCI with higher rates of complete cytoreduction. Because these are the main factors to influence patients' prognosis, the benefit in terms of survival length will be substantial. For patients with peritoneal carcinomatosis arising from appendiceal and colon cancer selected according to the described criteria, CRS and HIPEC will improve prognosis and should be considered standard of care.[46]

## REFERENCES

1. Koppe MJ, Boermann OC, Oyen JG, et al. Peritoneal carcinomatosis of colorectal origin: incidence and current treatment strategies. *Ann Surg.* 2006;243:212–222.
2. Sadeghi B, Arvieux C, Glehen O, et al. Peritoneal carcinomatosis from nongynecologic malignancies: results of the EVOCAPE 1 multicentric prospective study. *Cancer.* 2000;88:358–363.
3. Van Cutsem E, Geboes K. The multidisciplinary management of gastrointestinal cancer. The integration of cytotoxics and biologicals in the treatment of metastatic colorectal cancer. *Best Pract Clin Gastroenterol.* 2007;21:1089–1108.
4. Sugarbaker PH, Cunliffe WJ, Belliveau J, et al. Rationale for integrating early postoperative intraperitoneal chemotherapy into the surgical treatment of gastrointestinal cancer. *Semin Oncol.* 1989;16:83–97.
5. Verwaal VJ, van Ruth S, de Bree E, et al. Randomized trial of cytoreduction and hyperthermic intraperitoneal chemotherapy versus systemic chemotherapy and palliative surgery in patients with peritoneal carcinomatosis of colorectal cancer. *J Clin Oncol.* 2003;21:3737–3743.
6. Verwaal VJ, Bruin S, Boot H, et al. 8-year follow-up of randomized trial: cytoreduction and hyperthermic intraperitoneal chemotherapy versus systemic chemotherapy in patients with peritoneal carcinomatosis of colorectal cancer. *Ann Surg Oncol.* 2008;15:2426–2432.
7. Elias D, Delperro JR, Sideris L, et al. Treatment of peritoneal carcinomatosis from colorectal cancer: impact of complete cytoreductive surgery and difficulties in conducting randomized trials. *Ann Surg Oncol.* 2004;11:518–521.
8. Mahteme H, Hansson J, Berglund A, et al. Improved survival in patients with peritoneal metastases from colorectal cancer: a preliminary study. *Br J Cancer.* 2004;90:403–407.
9. Shen P, Thai K, Stewart JH, et al. Peritoneal surface disease from colorectal cancer: comparison with the hepatic metastases surgical paradigm in optimally resected patients. *Ann Surg Oncol.* 2008;15:3422–3432.
10. Moran BJ, Meade B, Murphy E. Hyperthermic intraperitoneal chemotherapy and cytoreductive surgery for peritoneal carcinomatosis of colorectal origin: a novel treatment strategy with promising results in selected patients. *Colorectal Dis.* 2006;8:544–550.
11. Sugarbaker PH. Peritonectomy procedures. *Ann Surg.* 1995;221:29–42.
12. Jacquet P, Sugarbaker PH. Clinical research methodologies in diagnosis and staging of patients with peritoneal carcinomatosis. *Cancer Treat Res.* 1996;82:359–374.
13. Glehen O, Gilly FN. Quantitative prognostic indicators of peritoneal surface malignancy: carcinomatosis, sarcomatosis, and peritoneal mesothelioma. *Surg Oncol Clin N Am.* 2003;12:649–671.
14. Sugarbaker PH. Laboratory and clinical basis for hyperthermia as a component of intracavitary chemotherapy. *Int J Hyperthermia.* 2007;23:431–442.
15. Glehen O, Cotte E, Kusamura S, et al. Hyperthermic intraperitoneal chemotherapy: nomenclature and modalities of perfusion. *J Surg Oncol.* 2008;98:242–246.
16. Elias D, Benizri E, Dipietrantonio D, et al. Comparison of two kinds of intraperitoneal chemotherapy following complete cytoreductive surgery of colorectal peritoneal carcinomatosis. *Ann Surg Oncol.* 2006;14:509–514.
17. Moran BJ. Decision-making and technical factors account for the learning curve in complex surgery. *J Public Health.* 2006;28:375–378.
18. Smeek RM, Verwaal VJ, Zoetmulder FA. Learning curve of combined modality treatment in peritoneal surface disease. *Br J Surg.* 2007;94:1408–1414.
19. Yan TD, Morris DL, Shigeki K, et al. Preoperative investigations in the management of peritoneal surface malignancy with cytoreductive surgery and perioperative intraperitoneal chemotherapy: expert consensus statement. *J Surg Oncol.* 2008;98:224–227.
20. Koh JL, Yan TD, Glenn D, et al. Evaluation of preoperative computed tomography in estimating peritoneal cancer index in colorectal peritoneal carcinomatosis. *Ann Surg Oncol.* 2009;16:327–333.
21. Reuter NP, Macgregor JM, Woodall CE, et al. Preoperative performance status predicts outcome following heated intraperitoneal chemotherapy. *Am J Surg.* 2008;196:909–913.
22. Waitzberg DL, Saito H, Plank, et al. Postsurgical infections are reduced with specialized nutrition support. *World J Surg.* 2006;30:1592–1604.
23. Reingruber B, Boetcher MI, Klein P, et al. Hyperthermic intraperitoneal chemoperfusion is an option for treatment of peritoneal carcinomatosis in children. *J Pediatr Surg.* 2007;42:17–21.
24. Da Silva G, Cabanas J, Sugarbaker PH. Limited survival in the treatment of carcinomatosis from rectal cancer. *Dis Colon Rectum.* 2005;48:2258–2263.
25. Pelz JO, Stojadinovic A, Nissan A, et al. Evaluation of a peritoneal surface disease severity score in patients with colon cancer with peritoneal carcinomatosis. *J Surg Oncol.* 2009;99:9–15.
26. Glehen O, Kwiatkowski F, Sugarbaker PH, et al. Cytoreductive surgery combined with perioperative intraperitoneal chemotherapy for the management of peritoneal carcinomatosis from colorectal cancer: a multi-institutional study. *J Clin Oncol.* 2004;22:3284–3292.
27. Verwaal V, Kusamura S, Baratti D, et al. The eligibility for loco-regional treatment of peritoneal surface malignancy. *J Surg Oncol.* 2008;98:220–223.
28. Esquivel J, Elias D, Baratti D, et al. Consensus statement on locoregional treatment of colorectal cancer with peritoneal dissemination. *J Surg Oncol.* 2008;98:263–267.
29. Culliford AT, Brooks AD, Sharma S, et al. Surgical debulking and intraperitoneal chemotherapy for established peritoneal metastases from colon and appendix cancer. *Ann Surg Oncol.* 2001;8:787–795.
30. Sugarbaker PH. New standard of care for appendiceal epithelial neoplasms and pseudomyxoma peritonei syndrome? *Lancet Oncol.* 2006;7:69–76.
31. Bijelic L, Yan TD, Sugarbaker PH. Treatment failure following complete cytoreductive surgery and perioperative intraperitoneal chemotherapy for peritoneal dissemination from colorectal or appendiceal mucinous neoplasms. *J Surg Oncol.* 2008;98:295–299.
32. Sugarbaker PH. Comprehensive management of disseminated colorectal cancer. *Ann Surg Oncol.* 2008;15:3327–3330.
33. Elias D, Goere D, Di Pietrantonio D, et al. Results of systematic second-look surgery in patients at high risk of developing colorectal peritoneal carcinomatosis. *Ann Surg.* 2008;247:445–450.
34. Esquivel J, Sticca R, Sugarbaker P, et al. Cytoreductive surgery and hyperthermic intraperitoneal chemotherapy in the management of peritoneal surface malignancies of colonic origin: a consensus statement. Society of Surgical Oncology. *Ann Surg Oncol.* 2007;14:128–133.
35. Pestieau SR, Esquivel J, Sugarbaker PH. Pleural extension of mucinous tumor in patients with pseudomyxoma peritonei syndrome. *Ann Surg Oncol.* 2000;7:199–203.
36. Elias D, Benizri E, Pocard M, et al. Treatment of synchronous peritoneal carcinomatosis and liver metastases from colorectal cancer. *Eur J Surg Oncol.* 2006;32:632–636.
37. Glockzin G, Ghali N, Lang SA, et al. Peritoneal carcinomatosis. Surgical treatment, including hyperthermic intraperitoneal chemotherapy. *Chirurg.* 2007;78:1102–1106.
38. Moran B, Baratti D, Yan TD, et al. Consensus statement on the loco-regional treatment of appendiceal mucinous neoplasms with peritoneal dissemination (pseudomyxoma peritonei). *J Surg Oncol.* 2008;98:277–282.
39. Shen P, Hawksworth J, Lovato J, et al. Cytoreductive surgery and intraperitoneal hyperthermic chemotherapy with mitomycin C for peritoneal carcinomatosis from nonappendiceal colorectal carcinoma. *Ann Surg Oncol.* 2004;11:178–186.
40. Hansson J, Graf W, Pahlman L, et al. Postoperative adverse events and long-term survival after cytoreductive surgery and intraperitoneal chemotherapy. *Eur J Surg Oncol.* 2009;35:202–208.
41. McQuellon RP, Loggie BW, Fleming RA, et al. Quality of life after intraperitoneal hyperthermic chemotherapy (IPHC) for peritoneal carcinomatosis. *Eur J Surg Oncol.* 2001;27:65–73.

42. McQuellon RP, Loggie BW, Lehman AB, et al. Long-term survivorship and quality of life after cytoreductive surgery plus intraperitoneal hyperthermic chemotherapy for peritoneal carcinomatosis. *Ann Surg Oncol.* 2003;10:155–162.

43. McQuellon RP, Danhauer SC, Russell GB, et al. Monitoring health outcomes following cytoreductive surgery plus intraperitoneal hyperthermic chemotherapy for peritoneal carcinomatosis. *Ann Surg Oncol.* 2007;14:1105–1113.

44. Schmidt U, Dahlke MH, Klempnauer J, et al. Perioperative morbidity and quality of life in long-term survivors following cytoreductive surgery and hyperthermic intraperitoneal chemotherapy. *Eur J Surg Oncol.* 2005;31:53–58.

45. Yan TD, Black D, Savady R, et al. Systematic review on the efficacy of cytoreductive surgery combined with perioperative intraperitoneal chemotherapy for peritoneal carcinomatosis from colorectal cancer. *J Clin Oncol.* 2006;24:4011–4019.

46. Yan TD, Morris DL. Cytoreductive surgery and perioperative intraperitoneal chemotherapy for isolated colorectal peritoneal carcinomatosis: experimental therapy or standard of care? *Ann Surg.* 2008;248:829–835.

# Management of Peritoneal Carcinomatosis From Colorectal Cancer

## Current State of Practice

Eddy Cotte • Guillaume Passot • Faheez Mohamed • Delphine Vaudoyer • François Noël Gilly • Olivier Glehen

In the past, carcinomatosis from colorectal cancer has been regarded as a terminal disease; most oncologists have regarded it as a condition only to be palliated. In the 1980s, a renewed interest in peritoneal surface malignancies developed through new multimodal therapeutic approaches. Publications regarding previously unexplored treatment options, such as peritonectomy procedures,[1] hyperthermic intraperitoneal chemotherapy (HIPEC),[2,3] and early postoperative intraperitoneal chemotherapy,[4] have appeared. Promising results were reported by groups using the combination of a comprehensive cytoreductive surgery to treat macroscopic disease with perioperative intraperitoneal chemotherapy to treat microscopic disease.[5–7] It is the only plan that has shown curative results for carcinomatosis in phase II studies, international registries, and one phase III trials.[7–12] Although these data were viewed with great skepticism for many years, it seems impossible to ignore today that a significant proportion of patients with colorectal carcinomatosis are long-term survivors. The traditional view that discovery of colorectal carcinomatosis was the beginning of the end is no longer tenable. Novel protocols and guidelines need to be developed and validated when colorectal carcinomatosis is discovered on preoperative exams, intraoperatively, or during follow-up. This evidence to support this will be reviewed, and the results of systemic chemotherapy compared with combined treatment (cytoreductive surgery with perioperative intraperitoneal chemotherapy) for the management of colorectal carcinomatosis.

## NATURAL HISTORY AND PALLIATIVE TREATMENT OF COLORECTAL CARCINOMATOSIS

In colorectal cancer, despite advances in the early detection of the primary tumor, carcinomatosis is detected in approximately 10% of patients at the time of primary cancer resection.[13,14] The mechanisms causing carcinomatosis are multifactoral and include hematogenous metastasis,[15] peritoneal dissemination of free cancer cells because of serosal involvement of the primary tumor,[16] implantation of free cancer cells due to the presence of adherence molecules,[17] and presence of cancer cells in lymph fluid or venous blood retained within the peritoneal cavity.

Prospective studies to document the clinical features and natural history of carcinomatosis from colorectal cancer remain limited. Data come from 3 prominent studies in the literature. The first study by Chu et al[13] prospectively followed up 45 patients and observed an overall median survival of 6 months. A decade later, in a French multicentric prospective study of 370 patients including 118 patients with colorectal carcinomatosis, the median survival was 5.2 months for colorectal cancer patients.[18] Jayne et al[14] published a retrospective analysis of 3019 patients with colorectal cancer. Thirteen percent of patients were identified with peritoneal carcinomatosis, and the median survival of patients with synchronous disease was 7 months.

Since the development of new systemic chemotherapy protocols using irinotecan, oxaliplatinum, and targeted therapy, the prognosis of metastatic colorectal cancer has been improved, with median survival reaching 24 months.[19–21] These more recent studies include a significant number of patients with liver or lung metastasis (measurable disease) with specific mention of peritoneal carcinomatosis in less than 5% of cases. Peritoneal carcinomatosis represents a metastatic evolution of colorectal cancers but its development, natural history, and response to systemic chemotherapy differ from liver or lung metastases, as demonstrated in several studies.[22,23] Elias et al[24] reported a median survival of 23.9 months for 48 patients with isolated and limited colorectal carcinomatosis treated with modern systemic chemotherapy. For patients with colorectal carcinomatosis, based on current evidence, palliative systemic chemotherapy achieves median survival of between 7 and 24 months. In these patients, long-term survival is rarely, if ever achieved.

## THE RATIONALE FOR A LOCOREGIONAL TREATMENT

### Cytoreductive Surgery and Peritonectomy Procedures

Reducing tumor volume has always been considered an important factor in achieving tumor response to chemotherapy. Cytoreductive surgery attempts to remove all macroscopic disease with extensive visceral resections and peritonectomy procedures, stripping involved portions of the peritoneum. Types of procedure for cytoreductive surgery and peritonectomy have been extensively described by Sugarbaker.[1] When tumor involves visceral peritoneal surfaces, organ resections (splenectomy, large bowel, or small bowel resection) are needed. When tumor involves parietal peritoneal surfaces, parietal peritonectomy or stripping of the peritoneum is required (Figs. 1 and 2). Although large portions of stomach or large bowel can be killed without serious consequences in terms of nutrition, only limited portions of small bowel can be resected. Frequently, implants on small bowel surfaces are the major limitation to complete or sufficient cytoreduction. The combination of both cytoreductive surgery and peritonectomy procedures with HIPEC could act as a "dose intensification device" improving results, with the goal of complete eradication of disease with a single procedure.[5] It is well known that the penetration of intraperitoneal chemotherapy into peritoneal carcinomatosis nodules is limited between 2 and 5 mm, even when combined with heat.[25] Thus, the goal of cytoreductive surgery for curative intent is to achieve maximum reduction of tumor volume.

### Hyperthermic Intraperitoneal Chemotherapy

Intraperitoneal administration of anticancer drugs has many pharmacokinetic advantages and gives high response rates within the

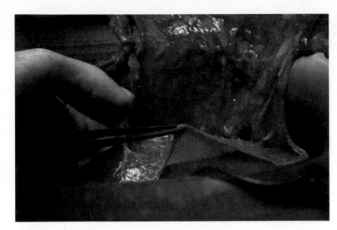

**FIGURE 1.** Peroperative view of stripping of Glisson's capsule involved by mucinous malignant nodules.

abdomen, because the "peritoneal plasma barrier" provides dose-intensive therapy. High concentrations of anticancer drug may be in direct contact with tumor cells, with reduced systemic concentrations and lower systemic toxicity.[2] The direct cytotoxicity of heat has been demonstrated in vitro at 42.5°C.[26] Hyperthermia at 42°C has been shown to enhance the antitumor effects of agents, such as oxaliplatin, mitomycin C, doxorubicin, irinotecan, or cisplatin, by augmenting cytotoxicity or increasing the penetration of drugs into tissue or both.[27–30] This concept of thermal enhancement of drugs with hyperthermia lead to the development of a new local-regional treatment: HIPEC.

## CYTOREDUCTIVE SURGERY COMBINED WITH PERIOPERATIVE INTRAPERITONEAL CHEMOTHERAPY

### Survival Results

The survival results reported by many authors in prospective or retrospective studies demonstrate the importance of residual tumor volume

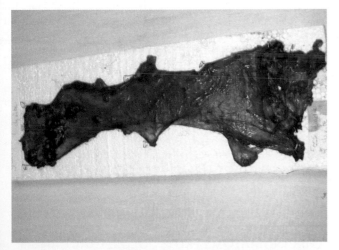

**FIGURE 2.** Specimen of complete parietal peritonectomy of right gutter.

after cytoreductive surgery (Table 1). All phase II studies reported median survival of more than 2 years for patients treated with complete macroscopic cytoreductive surgery or with residual tumor nodules less than 2.5 mm after cytoreduction. The more recent studies reported 5 year survival rates of more than 50%. In 2 large multicenter registries including more than 500 patients, all patients treated by the combination of complete cytoreductive surgery with perioperative intraperitoneal chemotherapy reported median survival of more than 30 months and 5-year survival of more than 30%.[10,31] Moreover, the long-term results of the randomized Dutch trial comparing HIPEC with mitomycin C and cytoreductive surgery to intravenous chemotherapy alone (5-fluorouracil, leucovorin) for the treatment of carcinomatosis from colorectal origin were recently reported.[32] The benefit of this combined procedure was clearly demonstrated (2-year survival rate of 43% in the HIPEC group versus 16% in the control: $P = 0.014$), and the trial was stopped for ethical reasons.[7] This benefit was confirmed by long-term results with a 5-year survival rate of 45% for patients treated in the experimental arm.

Two other interesting studies were recently conducted. The first was published by Shen et al.[33] They compared their experience with cytoreductive surgery and HIPEC for colorectal carcinomatosis with liver resection for hepatic metastasis. No significant difference was found in overall survival, morbidity, and mortality rates between patients in both groups. The second was reported by Elias et al.[24] They compared long-term survival of patients with isolated and resectable peritoneal carcinomatosis in comparable groups of patients treated with systemic chemotherapy or by cytoreductive surgery plus HIPEC. Although modern systemic chemotherapy may lead to a long median survival of 24 months, results were still significantly in favor of the combined treatment with a median survival of 63 months and a 5-year survival of 51%.

The combination of cytoreductive surgery with HIPEC had clearly demonstrated its survival benefit for the treatment of carefully selected patients with resectable colorectal carcinomatosis. The exact role of HIPEC needs clarification and evaluation into phase III trials. Would the combination of complete cytoreductive surgery with modern systemic chemotherapy produce similar results to the same regimen plus HIPEC? No evidence is available in the literature, and the only trial attempting to answer the question was stopped because of difficulties in patient recruitment.[34]

### Morbidity and Mortality Results

The combination of cytoreductive surgery with HIPEC is a complex procedure that exposes patients to high but acceptable morbidity and mortality rates, ranging from 16% to 65% and 0% to 16%, respectively.[35] The main morbidity cytoreductive surgery combined with HIPEC is from complications of surgery: anastomotic leakages, intraperitoneal sepsis, or abscesses. The principal morbidity from HIPEC is hematological toxicity, which is reported to occur in 8% to 31% of cases. Multivariate analyses in large studies showed that the independent factors influencing morbidity were duration of surgery, extent of carcinomatosis, the number of anastomoses performed, and incomplete cytoreductive surgery.[36–39]

When cytoreductive surgery and HIPEC were performed in institutions with an experience of more than 200 procedures, morbidity and mortality rates were 24% and 3%, respectively.[36–39] The combination of extensive surgery and intraperitoneal chemotherapy needs to be performed in specialized centers involved in the management of peritoneal surface malignancies. Surgeons must be competent in the visceral and parietal peritonectomy procedures that are required for the treatment of carcinomatosis. In addition, the surgeon and team

**TABLE 1.** Survival of Patients With Colorectal Carcinomatosis Treated by Cytoreductive Surgery Combined With Perioperative Intraperitoneal Chemotherapy

| Series | Year | Nb | Median Survival (mo) | 2-yr Survival (%) | 3-yr Survival (%) | 5-yr Survival (%) |
|---|---|---|---|---|---|---|
| Pestieau et al[9] | 2000 | 104 | — | — | — | — |
| CC-0 ou 1 | | 44 | 24 | — | — | 30 |
| Culliford et al[53] | 2001 | 64 | 34 | | — | 28 |
| Elias et al[8] | 2001 | 64 | 36 | 54,7 | — | 18,4 |
| Pilati et al[54] | 2003 | 34 | 18 | 31 | — | — |
| Matherne et al[55] | 2004 | 18 | 32 | 60 | — | 28 |
| Verwaal et al[56] | 2004 | 102 | 20 | — | — | — |
| CC-0 | | 50 | 39 | — | | — |
| Glehen et al[12] | 2004 | 53 | 13 | 32 | — | 11 |
| CC-0 | | 23 | 33 | 54 | — | 22 |
| Glehen et al[10] | 2004 | 506 | 19 | — | 39 | 19 |
| CC-0 | | 271 | 32 | — | 47 | 31 |
| Verwaal et al[57] | 2005 | 117 | 22 | 28 | — | 19 |
| Rodrigo et al[58] | 2006 | 70 | 33 | — | 44 | 32 |
| Cavaliere et al[42] | 2006 | 120 | — | — | 33,5 | — |
| Rouers et al[59] | 2006 | 21 | 34 | — | — | 36,6 |
| Kianmanesh et al[45] | 2007 | 43 | 38 | 72 | — | — |
| Shen et al[33] | 2008 | 121 | 34 | — | 48 | 26 |
| Elias et al[24] | 2008 | 48 | 63 | 81 | — | 51 |
| Verwaal et al[32] | 2008 | 117 | 22 | — | — | 45 |
| Yan et al[15] | 2008 | 50 | 29 | — | 39 | — |

CC-0 indicates complete cytoreductive surgery; CC-1, residual tumor nodules of less than 2.5 mm.

must possess knowledge of chemotherapeutic agents and their toxicity during the perioperative period.

## Indications and Contraindications

Results of large multicenter studies have identified several prognostic factors, which can be used to refine selection of patients who can benefit from the combination of cytoreductive surgery with HIPEC.[10,31] A consensus for these indications has been established within peritoneal surface malignancy treatment centers[40,41] but has not been validated by large prospective studies.

This combined management seems to be reserved for patients less than 70 years (physiologic age less than 65) with no cardio-respiratory or renal failure, with Eastern Cooperative Oncology Group performance status of 2 or less, especially when extensive cytoreductive surgery has to be combined with HIPEC, with a high risk of postoperative complications.

HIPEC is indicated when carcinomatosis is amenable to effective cytoreductive surgery allowing either a macroscopic complete resection, or a small residual tumor volume, with residual cancer nodules less than 2.5 mm. In all series, completeness of cytoreductive surgery represents the most important prognostic factor.[10,15,42] Median survival of more than 30 months was seen only in patients treated with complete cytoreductive surgery. Some clinical and radiographic variables have been associated with an increased chance of achieving a complete removal of all tumor during cytoreductive surgery: no evidence of extra-abdominal disease, up to 3 small resectable parenchymal liver metastases, no evidence of biliary, ureteric, or intestinal obstruction at more than one site, no evidence of gross disease in the mesentery or several segmental sites of partial obstruction, and small volume disease in the gastro-hepatic ligament.[40]

The extent of carcinomatosis represents the second most important prognostic factor. It was the most important factor in the most recent multicenter trial, which included more than 80% of patients treated with complete cytoreductive surgery.[31] Several classifications have been used to quantify carcinomatosis extent. Peritoneal Cancer Index of Sugarbaker was chosen by an expert panel to be a useful quantitative prognostic tools.[43] Some authors consider that cytoreductive surgery plus HIPEC is contraindicated in patients with a Peritoneal Cancer Index (PCI) >20.[44]

In cases of carcinomatosis synchronous with the primary tumor, a comparative retrospective study suggested that patients should be treated with cytoreductive surgery followed by HIPEC at the time of primary tumor removal.[9] This management plan avoids the theoretical risk of cancer dissemination through sites of peritonectomy and resection. Prospective studies are needed to confirm these findings.

Extra-abdominal metastases or massive retroperitoneal lymph node involvement are also an absolute contraindication. An aggressive local-regional treatment cannot be envisaged with noncontrolled systemic disease. Multiple liver metastases are also a classic contraindication for this combined therapeutic approach. However, trials have reported that when liver metastasis number 3 or less and are chemosensitive, they can be resected at the time of cytoreductive surgery for peritoneal disease with no adverse impact on outcome.[12,31,45,46]

## RECOMMENDATIONS FOR THE MANAGEMENT OF PATIENTS WITH A DIAGNOSIS OF PERITONEAL CARCINOMATOSIS FROM COLORECTAL CANCER

On the basis of published evidence, cytoreductive surgery with HIPEC is most beneficial in young patients (physiological age less than

## CARCINOMATOSIS EXTENT - EVALUATION

### Peritoneal Cancer Index (PCI) de Sugarbaker

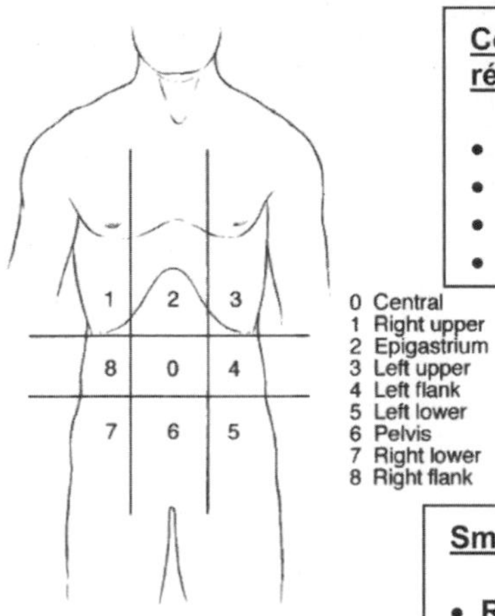

**Cotation by région :**

- **0** : no lesion
- **1** : L ≤ 0.5 cm
- **2** : 0.5 < L ≤ 5 cm
- **3** : L > 5 cm

0  Central
1  Right upper
2  Epigastrium
3  Left upper
4  Left flank
5  Left lower
6  Pelvis
7  Right lower
8  Right flank

**Small intestin :**

- **R9** : proximal jejunum
- **R10** : distal jejunum
- **R11** : proximal ileon
- **R12** : distal ileon

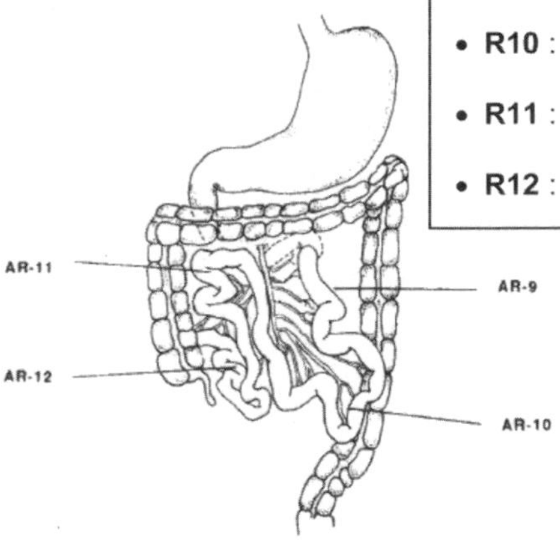

AR-11
AR-12
AR-9
AR-10

| | Before surgery | After surgery |
|---|---|---|
| Region 0 | | |
| Region 1 | | |
| Region 2 | | |
| Region 3 | | |
| Region 4 | | |
| Region 5 | | |
| Region 6 | | |
| Region 7 | | |
| Region 8 | | |
| Region 9 | | |
| Region 10 | | |
| Region 11 | | |
| Region 12 | | |
| Total | | |

### Gilly's classification

| | Before surgery | After surgery |
|---|---|---|
| • **Stage 0** : no lesion (positive cytology)<br>• **Stage 1** : Malignant granulations less than 5 mm in diameter, localized in one part of the abdomen<br>• **Stage 2** : Malignant granulations less than 5 mm in diameter, diffuse to the whole abdomen<br>• **Stage 3** : Localized or diffuse malignant granulations 5 mm to 2 cm in diameter<br>• **Stage 4** : Localized or diffuse large malignant masses (more than 2 cm in diameter) | | |

**FIGURE 3.** Quantitative prognostic evaluation of peritoneal carcinomatosis.

65 years), with low volume disease treated, in specialized centers, involved in the management of peritoneal surface malignancies.[31,40]

All surgeons and medical oncologist who discover peritoneal carcinomatosis from colorectal cancer before, during, or after surgery should consider this therapeutic plan with the intent of cure, especially in young patients with limited disease. Explorative laparotomy with no description of the distribution or extent of carcinomatosis should be avoided. The peroperative discovery of carcinomatosis should describe sites of tumor that may jeopardize the chance of complete cytoreductive surgery: involvement of the porta hepatis or extensive small bowel and mesenteric involvement.[31,47] Many quantitative intraoperative classifications have been described to help assessment from the detailed PCI to the more simple, the classification of Gilly[43] (Fig. 3). The accuracy of assessment of disease extent is crucial in optimizing treatment and avoiding inappropriate referral to specialized centers. Imaging studies at present do not give us the quality of information that the surgeon's intraoperative eye can provide.[48–50]

Respect for the peritoneum is essential.[51] Extensive peritonectomy procedures without perioperative intraperitoneal chemotherapy should be avoided when a potentially curative procedure is possible. Removal of peritoneal surfaces without immediate intraperitoneal chemotherapy will allow tumor cells to become implanted within deeper layers of the abdomen resulting in ureteric and biliary obstruction. This may jeopardize the chance of future curative procedure combining complete cytoreductive surgery with HIPEC and substantially increase the risk of morbidity.

Regarding perioperative intraperitoneal chemotherapy, HIPEC is the treatment of choice for the majority of experts.[41] The addition of heat to intraperitoneal chemotherapy seems to improve survival.[4] Early postoperative intraperitoneal chemotherapy may increase postoperative complications.[10,31] No consensus has been reached on the optimal technology for HIPEC.[52] Oxaliplatinum and mitomycin C are the anticancer drugs that are recommended in combination with hyperthermia for the treatment of colorectal carcinomatosis.[31,40,41] The use of irinotecan or drugs combinations is still under evaluation.[27]

## CONCLUSIONS

In 2009, potential cure of peritoneal carcinomatosis from colorectal cancer is a realistic goal in selected patients. Surgical treatment of peritoneal carcinomatosis should be regarded in the same way as other metastasis sites (liver or lung). On the discovery of peritoneal carcinomatosis, surgeons and oncologists have the responsibility to consider the suitability of their patients for cytoreductive surgery with HIPEC. The evidence suggests that this treatment option can no longer be ignored. Treatment should be centralized in experienced peritoneal surface malignancy centers to limit the toxicity and maximize the survival.

## REFERENCES

1. Sugarbaker PH. Peritonectomy procedures. *Ann Surg.* 1995;221:29–42.
2. Glehen O, Mohamed F, Gilly FN. Peritoneal carcinomatosis from digestive tract cancer: new management by cytoreductive surgery and intraperitoneal chemohyperthermia. *Lancet Oncol.* 2004;5:219–228.
3. Sugarbaker PH. New standard of care for appendiceal epithelial neoplasms and pseudomyxoma peritonei syndrome? *Lancet Oncol.* 2006;7:69–76.
4. Elias D, Benizri E, Di Pietrantonio D, et al. Comparison of two kinds of intraperitoneal chemotherapy following complete cytoreductive surgery of colorectal peritoneal carcinomatosis. *Ann Surg Oncol.* 2007;14:509–514.
5. Glehen O, Mithieux F, Osinsky D, et al. Surgery combined with peritonectomy procedures and intraperitoneal chemohyperthermia in abdominal cancers with peritoneal carcinomatosis: a phase II study. *J Clin Oncol.* 2003;21:799–806.
6. Piso P, Dahlke MH, Loss M, et al. Cytoreductive surgery and hyperthermic intraperitoneal chemotherapy in peritoneal carcinomatosis from ovarian cancer. *World J Surg Oncol.* 2004;2:21.
7. Verwaal VJ, van Ruth S, de Bree E, et al. Randomized trial of cytoreduction and hyperthermic intraperitoneal chemotherapy versus systemic chemotherapy and palliative surgery in patients with peritoneal carcinomatosis of colorectal cancer. *J Clin Oncol.* 2003;21:3737–3743.
8. Elias D, Blot F, El Otmany A, et al. Curative treatment of peritoneal carcinomatosis arising from colorectal cancer by complete resection and intraperitoneal chemotherapy. *Cancer.* 2001;92:71–76.
9. Pestieau SR, Sugarbaker PH. Treatment of primary colon cancer with peritoneal carcinomatosis: comparison of concomitant vs. delayed management. *Dis Colon Rectum.* 2000;43:1341–1346; discussion 7–8.
10. Glehen O KF, Sugarbaker PH, Elias D, et al. Cytoreductive surgery combined whith perioperative intraperitoneal chemotherapy for the management of peritoneal carcinomatosis from colorectal cancer: a multi-institutional study. *J Clin Oncol.* 2004;22:3284–3292.
11. Yan TD, Sim J, Morris DL. Selection of patients with colorectal peritoneal carcinomatosis for cytoreductive surgery and perioperative intraperitoneal chemotherapy. *Ann Surg Oncol.* 2007;14:1807–1817.
12. Glehen O, Cotte E, Schreiber V, et al. Intraperitoneal chemohyperthermia and attempted cytoreductive surgery in patients with peritoneal carcinomatosis of colorectal origin. *Br J Surg.* 2004;91:747–754.
13. Chu DZ, Lang NP, Thompson C, et al. Peritoneal carcinomatosis in nongynecologic malignancy. A prospective study of prognostic factors. *Cancer.* 1989;63:364–367.
14. Jayne DG, Fook S, Loi C, et al. Peritoneal carcinomatosis from colorectal cancer. *Br J Surg.* 2002;89:1545–1550.
15. Yan TD, Morris DL. Cytoreductive surgery and perioperative intraperitoneal chemotherapy for isolated colorectal peritoneal carcinomatosis: experimental therapy or standard of care? *Ann Surg.* 2008;248:829–835.
16. Iitsuka Y, Kaneshima S, Tanida O, et al. Intraperitoneal free cancer cells and their viability in gastric cancer. *Cancer.* 1979;44:1476–1480.
17. Sugarbaker PH. Intraperitoneal chemotherapy and cytoreductive surgery for the prevention and treatment of peritoneal carcinomatosis and sarcomatosis. *Semin Surg Oncol.* 1998;14:254–261.
18. Sadeghi B, Arvieux C, Glehen O, et al. Peritoneal carcinomatosis from nongynecologic malignancies: results of the EVOCAPE 1 multicentric prospective study. *Cancer.* 2000;88:358–363.
19. Folprecht G, Lutz MP, Schoffski P, et al. Cetuximab and irinotecan/5-fluorouracil/folinic acid is a safe combination for the first-line treatment of patients with epidermal growth factor receptor expressing metastatic colorectal carcinoma. *Ann Oncol.* 2006;17:450–456.
20. Hurwitz H, Fehrenbacher L, Novotny W, et al. Bevacizumab plus irinotecan, fluorouracil, and leucovorin for metastatic colorectal cancer. *N Engl J Med.* 2004;350:2335–2342.
21. Goldberg RM, Sargent DJ, Morton RF, et al. Randomized controlled trial of reduced-dose bolus fluorouracil plus leucovorin and irinotecan or infused fluorouracil plus leucovorin and oxaliplatin in patients with previously untreated metastatic colorectal cancer: a North American Intergroup Trial. *J Clin Oncol.* 2006;24:3347–3353.
22. Folprecht G, Kohne CH, Lutz MP. Systemic chemotherapy in patients with peritoneal carcinomatosis from colorectal cancer. *Cancer Treat Res.* 2007;134:425–440.
23. Kohne CH, Cunningham D, Di CF, et al. Clinical determinants of survival in patients with 5-fluorouracil-based treatment for metastatic colorectal cancer: results of a multivariate analysis of 3825 patients. *Ann Oncol.* 2002;13:308–317.
24. Elias D, Lefevre JH, Chevalier J, et al. Complete cytoreductive surgery plus intraperitoneal chemohyperthermia with oxaliplatin for peritoneal carcinomatosis of colorectal origin. *J Clin Oncol.* 2009;27:681–685.
25. van Ruth S, Verwaal VJ, Hart AA, et al. Heat penetration in locally applied hyperthermia in the abdomen during intra-operative hyperthermic intraperitoneal chemotherapy. *Anticancer Res.* 2003;23:1501–1508.
26. Crile G Jr. The effects of heat and radiation on cancers implanted on the feet of mice. *Cancer Res.* 1963;23:372–380.
27. Elias D, Raynard B, Bonnay M, et al. Heated intra-operative intraperitoneal oxaliplatin alone and in combination with intraperitoneal irinotecan: pharmacologic studies. *Eur J Surg Oncol.* 2006;32:607–613.
28. Le Page S, Kwiatkowski F, Paulin C, et al. In vitro thermochemotherapy of colon cancer cell lines with irinotecan alone and combined with mitomycin C. *Hepatogastroenterology.* 2006;53:693–697.
29. Van der Speeten K, Stuart OA, Mahteme H, et al. A pharmacologic analysis of intraoperative intracavitary cancer chemotherapy with doxorubicin. *Cancer Chemother Pharmacol.* 2009;63:799–805.
30. Sugarbaker PH. Getting chemotherapy into the cancerous tissue. *Ann Surg Oncol.* 2008;15:3320; author reply 3321.

31. Elias D, Gilly FN, Glehen O. Carcinoses péritonéales d'origine digestive et primitive. Arnette ed. Paris: Association Française de Chirurgie; 2008.

32. Verwaal VJ, Bruin S, Boot H, et al. 8-year follow-up of randomized trial: cytoreduction and hyperthermic intraperitoneal chemotherapy versus systemic chemotherapy in patients with peritoneal carcinomatosis of colorectal cancer. *Ann Surg Oncol.* 2008;15:2426–2432.

33. Shen P, Thai K, Stewart JH, et al. Peritoneal surface disease from colorectal cancer: comparison with the hepatic metastases surgical paradigm in optimally resected patients. *Ann Surg Oncol.* 2008;15:3422–3432.

34. Elias D, Delperro JR, Sideris L, et al. Treatment of peritoneal carcinomatosis from colorectal cancer: impact of complete cytoreductive surgery and difficulties in conducting randomized trials. *Ann Surg Oncol.* 2004;11:518–521.

35. Younan R, Kusamura S, Baratti D, et al. Morbidity, toxicity, and mortality classification systems in the local regional treatment of peritoneal surface malignancy. *J Surg Oncol.* 2008;98:253–257.

36. Glehen O, Osinsky D, Cotte E, et al. Intraperitoneal chemohyperthermia using a closed abdominal procedure and cytoreductive surgery for the treatment of peritoneal carcinomatosis: morbidity and mortality analysis of 216 consecutive procedures. *Ann Surg Oncol.* 2003;10:863–869.

37. Kusamura S, Younan R, Baratti D, et al. Cytoreductive surgery followed by intraperitoneal hyperthermic perfusion: analysis of morbidity and mortality in 209 peritoneal surface malignancies treated with closed abdomen technique. *Cancer.* 2006;106:1144–1153.

38. Sugarbaker PH, Alderman R, Edwards G, et al. Prospective morbidity and mortality assessment of cytoreductive surgery plus perioperative intraperitoneal chemotherapy to treat peritoneal dissemination of appendiceal mucinous malignancy. *Ann Surg Oncol.* 2006;13:635–644.

39. Levine EA, Stewart JH IV, Russell GB, et al. Cytoreductive surgery and intraperitoneal hyperthermic chemotherapy for peritoneal surface malignancy: experience with 501 procedures. *J Am Coll Surg.* 2007;204:943–953; discussion 53–55.

40. Esquivel J, Elias D, Baratti D, et al. Consensus statement on the loco regional treatment of colorectal cancer with peritoneal dissemination. *J Surg Oncol.* 2008;98:263–267.

41. Esquivel J, Sticca R, Sugarbaker P, et al. Cytoreductive surgery and hyperthermic intraperitoneal chemotherapy in the management of peritoneal surface malignancies of colonic origin: a consensus statement. *Ann Surg Oncol.* 2007;14:128–133.

42. Cavaliere F, Valle M, De Simone M, et al. 120 peritoneal carcinomatoses from colorectal cancer treated with peritonectomy and intra-abdominal chemohyperthermia: a S.I.T.I.L.O. multicentric study. *In Vivo.* 2006;20:747–750.

43. Portilla AG, Shigeki K, Dario B, et al. The intraoperative staging systems in the management of peritoneal surface malignancy. *J Surg Oncol.* 2008;98:228–231.

44. Sugarbaker PH. Successful management of microscopic residual disease in large bowel cancer. *Cancer Chemother Pharmacol.* 1999;43(Suppl):S15–S25.

45. Kianmanesh R, Scaringi S, Sabate JM, et al. Iterative cytoreductive surgery associated with hyperthermic intraperitoneal chemotherapy for treatment of peritoneal carcinomatosis of colorectal origin with or without liver metastases. *Ann Surg.* 2007;245:597–603.

46. Elias D, Benizri E, Pocard M, et al. Treatment of synchronous peritoneal carcinomatosis and liver metastases from colorectal cancer. *Eur J Surg Oncol.* 2006;32:632–636.

47. Bereder JM, Classe JM, Ducreux M, et al. Accord d'experts sur le compte rendu opératoire minimal descriptif d'une carcinose péritonéale. *J Chir (Paris).* 2007;144:463.

48. Cotton F, Pellet O, Gilly FN, et al. MRI evaluation of bulky tumor masses in the mesentery and bladder involvement in peritoneal carcinomatosis. *Eur J Surg Oncol.* 2006;32:1212–1216.

49. Hinshaw JL, Pickhardt PJ. Imaging of primary malignant tumors of peritoneal and retroperitoneal origin. *Cancer Treat Res.* 2008;143:281–297.

50. Chi DS, Ramirez PT, Teitcher JB, et al. Prospective study of the correlation between postoperative computed tomography scan and primary surgeon assessment in patients with advanced ovarian, tubal, and peritoneal carcinoma reported to have undergone primary surgical cytoreduction to residual disease 1 cm or less. *J Clin Oncol.* 2007;25:4946–4951.

51. Elias D, Goere D. Respectons le péritoine! C'est notre première ligne de défense contre la carcinose. *J Chir (Paris).* 2007;144:275–276.

52. Glehen O, Cotte E, Kusamura S, et al. Hyperthermic intraperitoneal chemotherapy: nomenclature and modalities of perfusion. *J Surg Oncol.* 2008;98:242–246.

53. Culliford AT IV, Brooks AD, Sharma S, et al. Surgical debulking and intraperitoneal chemotherapy for established peritoneal metastases from colon and appendix cancer. *Ann Surg Oncol.* 2001;8:787–795.

54. Pilati P, Mocellin S, Rossi CR, et al. Cytoreductive surgery combined with hyperthermic intraperitoneal intraoperative chemotherapy for peritoneal carcinomatosis arising from colon adenocarcinoma. *Ann Surg Oncol.* 2003;10:508–513.

55. Mahteme H, Hansson J, Berglund A, et al. Improved survival in patients with peritoneal metastases from colorectal cancer: a preliminary study. *Br J Cancer.* 2004;90:403–407.

56. Verwaal VJ, van Tinteren H, van Ruth S, et al. Predicting the survival of patients with peritoneal carcinomatosis of colorectal origin treated by aggressive cytoreduction and hyperthermic intraperitoneal chemotherapy. *Br J Surg.* 2004;91:739–746.

57. Verwaal VJ, van Ruth S, Witkamp A, et al. Long-term survival of peritoneal carcinomatosis of colorectal origin. *Ann Surg Oncol.* 2005;12:65–71.

58. da Silva RG, Sugarbaker PH. Analysis of prognostic factors in seventy patients having a complete cytoreduction plus perioperative intraperitoneal chemotherapy for carcinomatosis from colorectal cancer. *J Am Coll Surg.* 2006;203:878–886.

59. Rouers A, Laurent S, Detroz B, et al. Cytoreductive surgery and hyperthermic intraperitoneal chemotherapy for colorectal peritoneal carcinomatosis: higher complication rate for oxaliplatin compared to Mitomycin C. *Acta Chir Belg.* 2006;106:302–306.

# Technology of Hyperthermic Intraperitoneal Chemotherapy in the United States, Europe, China, Japan, and Korea

Jesus Esquivel

Significant advances have been made recently in the field of cytotoxic chemotherapy and biologic agents in the management of unresectable metastatic gastrointestinal cancers with hematogenous or lymphatic dissemination or both. The earliest success with the surgical management of metastatic disease was complete resection of locally recurrent colon and rectal cancer. Next, the resection of liver metastases from the same disease was shown to be of benefit in a selected group of patients. Isolated peritoneal metastases are a common site of recurrence after potentially curative resections of colorectal and appendiceal cancers and also account for significant morbidity and mortality in this group of patients. Extension of the concept of complete surgical eradication of macroscopic metastatic disease to bring about long-term survival to patients with peritoneal surface malignancies secondary to gastrointestinal cancers is being done with an ever-increasing frequency and is being combined with hyperthermic intraperitoneal chemotherapy (HIPEC) to target residual microscopic disease. Better surgical techniques that include peritonectomy procedures, standardized methods to deliver intraoperative intraperitoneal hyperthermic chemotherapy and better patient selection criteria, have resulted in a significant improvement in survival and in morbidity and mortality of the surgical management of this particular group of cancer patients.[1,2] The most recent report by Dr. Dominique Elias on the outcome of patients with limited carcinomatosis who underwent a complete cytoreductive surgery followed with HIPEC using oxaliplatin showed an unprecedented 63-month median survival and a 51% 5-year survival rate.[3] However, there has never been a prospective randomized trial designed and completed to evaluate the impact of the addition of HIPEC after having a complete cytoreductive surgery. The rationale for adding HIPEC to target microscopic residual disease has been well established. Because of the peritoneal-plasma barrier, intraperitoneal administration of chemotherapy results in intraperitoneal levels that are 20 to 1000 times higher than plasma levels, Figure 1. In the operating room, intraoperative intraperitoneal hyperthermic chemotherapy is used. The large volume of chemotherapy solution required to administer HIPEC removes tissue debris and blood products from the abdominal cavity to minimize fibrin entrapment of cancer cells. The chemotherapy not only directly destroys tumor cells, but also eliminates viable platelets, neutrophils, and monocytes from the peritoneal cavity. This diminishes the promotion of tumor growth associated with the wound healing process.

Heat is part of the optimizing process and is used to bring as much dose intensity to the abdominal and pelvic surfaces as is possible. Hyperthermia with intraperitoneal chemotherapy has several advantages. First, heat by itself has more toxicity for cancerous tissue than for normal tissue. This predominant effect on cancer increases as the vascularity of the malignancy decreases. Second, hyperthermia increases the penetration of chemotherapy into tissues. As tissues soften in response to heat, the elevated interstitial pressure of a tumor mass may decrease and allow improved drug penetration. Third, and probably most important, heat increases the cytotoxicity of selected chemotherapy agents. This synergism occurs only at the interface of heat and body tissue at the peritoneal surface.[4]

It has been 30 years since the first HIPEC was delivered by Spratt et al[5] in 1979 at the University of Louisville to a male patient with pseudomyxoma peritonei. During these 3 decades, there have been significant changes on how to deliver the heated perfusate, which drugs and concentrations to use, how long should the perfusion be, and how hot should the temperature be. In recent years, there has also been an explosion in the number of devices in the market available to carry out the intraoperative perfusion of hyperthermic chemotherapy. However, despite the wider acceptance to combine extensive cytoreductive surgery with intraoperative intraperitoneal heated chemotherapy, the specifics of the HIPEC administration continue to lack uniformity. The most recent consensus statement issued by the Peritoneal Surface Oncology Group International after the 2006 meeting in Milan concluded that the debate on the best method to deliver HIPEC is still open, and as a group, we declared that there is no sufficient evidence in the literature confirming the superiority of one technique over the other in terms of outcome, morbidity, and safety to the personnel in the operating room.[6]

The purpose of this chapter is to review the most common methods to deliver HIPEC from the technical standpoint, describing their advantages and disadvantages. We will also review the most common regimens combining chemotherapy and heat in the treatment of several peritoneal surface malignancies.

## MODALITIES OF PERFUSION

To maximize the advantage of the synergistic effect of chemotherapy and hyperthermia, several HIPEC delivering devices that allowed intraoperative perfusion of the peritoneal cavity with heated chemotherapy have been developed. Basically, they all are capable of delivering constant hyperthermia by a closed continuous circuit, with a pump, a heater, a heat exchanger, and real-time temperature monitoring. Despite the increasing numbers and designs of newer machines, most institutions become familiar with one machine and learn to troubleshoot that particular device. This allows for standardization of the delivery of HIPEC at each institution. To avoid systemic hyperthermia during the perfusion, core temperatures are kept at around 35°C before initiating HIPEC. Precooling can be obtained by using cooling blankets and other devices, but for the most part limiting the use of body warming during the cytoreductive phase of the procedure will bring

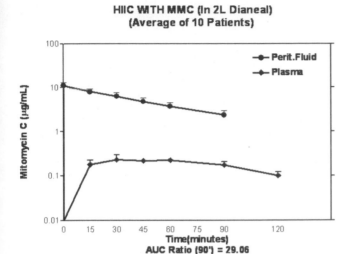

**FIGURE 1.**   Concentration of mitomycin C in plasma versus peritoneal fluid.

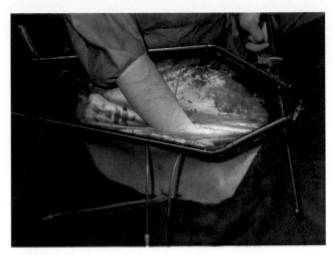

**FIGURE 2.**   Open "colisuem" technique for HIPEC.

the temperature to the desired range. During the actual perfusion, temperature probes are placed at different sites of the circuit and the intraperitoneal cavity: heat generator, heat exchanger, inflow and outflow catheters and some centers add temperature probes to the liver and bladder. During the Milan consensus, it was agreed that the desirable intra-abdominal temperature range that needs to be maintained during HIPEC should be between 41.5°C and 43°C. This temperature is usually accomplished by an inflow temperature between 46°C and 48°C.[6]

## OPEN ABDOMEN "COLISEUM TECHNIQUE"

The open abdominal technique of delivering the intraperitoneal hyperthermic chemotherapy at the time of surgery has also been referred as the coliseum technique.[7] After the cancer resection is complete, a Tenckhoff catheter and closed suction drains are placed through the abdominal wall and made watertight with a purse-string suture at the skin. Temperature probes are secured to the skin edge. By using a long running no. 2 monofilament suture, the skin edges are secured to the self-retaining Thompson retractor. A plastic sheet is incorporated into these sutures to create a covering for the abdominal cavity. A slit in the plastic cover is made to allow the surgeon's double-gloved hand access to the abdomen and pelvis (Fig. 2). During the 90 minutes of perfusion, all the anatomic structures within the peritoneal cavity are uniformly exposed to heat and to chemotherapy. The surgeon gently but continuously manipulates all viscera to keep adherence of peritoneal surfaces to a minimum. Roller pumps force the chemotherapy solution into the abdomen through the Tenckhoff catheter and pull it out through the 4 drains. A heat exchanger keeps the fluid being infused at 44°C to 46°C, so that the intraperitoneal fluid is maintained at 42°C to 43°C. The smoke evacuator is used to pull air from beneath the plastic cover through activated charcoal, preventing potential contamination (by chemotherapy aerosols) of air in the operating room.

After the intraoperative perfusion is complete, the abdomen is suctioned dry of fluid. The abdomen is then reopened, retractors repositioned, and reconstructive surgery is performed. It should be re-emphasized that no suture lines are constructed until after the chemotherapy perfusion is complete. One exception to this rule is closure of the vaginal cuff to prevent leakage of intraperitoneal chemotherapy solution.

## ADVANTAGES OF THE OPEN COLISEUM TECHNIQUE

Having access to the entire abdomen and pelvis during the intraperitoneal perfusion allows the surgeon not only to ensure an adequate treatment with heat and chemotherapy of every abdomino-pelvic region but also prevents excessive heating of normal tissue that can exacerbate postoperative ileus and increase the incidence of postoperative perforation or fistula formation. In addition, the open method provides an access to sample the perfusate and measure concentrations of the chemotherapeutic solution. It is also possible to sample tumor nodules throughout the 90 or 120 minutes and then determine the concentration of the chemotherapeutic agent in the tumor nodules. Another advantage is that in the event that there is bleeding during the intraperitoneal perfusion, the volume in the abdomen can be decreased quite rapidly by decreasing the rate of the inflow and keeping more fluid in the reservoir. This maneuver will assist in identifying and controlling the bleeding site.[8]

## POTENTIAL DISADVANTAGES

Having an open abdomen during the intraperitoneal hyperthermic chemotherapeutic perfusion leads to heat dissipation and makes it harder to achieve a uniform hyperthermia throughout the entire 90 to 120 minutes, particularly if higher temperatures are desired.

Another disadvantage when compared with the closed method is the potential exposure of the operating room personnel to the chemotherapeutic agents. Because the surgeon is required to manipulate the viscera, increased potential exists also for contact exposure. The heated chemotherapy can aerosolize, creating a potential inhalational exposure. Sugarbaker and coworkers[9] evaluated the safety of the operating room personnel. Urine from members of the operating team was assayed for chemotherapy levels. Air was sampled proximal to the operative field, and levels were measured. Finally, sterile gloves commonly used in the operating room were examined for permeability to chemotherapy. All assessments of potential exposures were found to be in compliance with established safety standards. Thus, the theoretical risk of exposure of the operating team to chemotherapy during the open coliseum technique has not been substantiated.

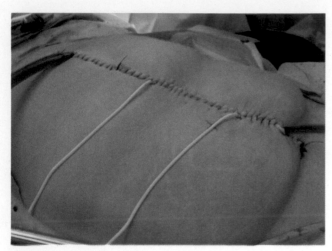

**FIGURE 3.**    Closed abdomen technique for HIPEC.

## CLOSED ABDOMEN TECHNIQUE

The closed abdominal technique is gaining popularity in the United States, but continues to be used less often than the coliseum technique in Europe, Japan, China and Korea. Typically, after the cytoreduction is completed, 1 or 2 inflow catheters and 2 outflow catheters are placed.[8] The outflow catheters are placed in dependent positions such as the pelvis and under the right hemidiaphragm. Temperature probes are placed in the abdomen proximal to and remote from the catheter tips to monitor inflow and outflow temperatures. After temporary closure of the skin, the preheated peritoneal dialysis solution is allowed to fill the peritoneal cavity. Usually, 2 to 3 L are required to distend the cavity and achieve a flow rare of approximately 1500 mL/min (Fig. 3). The abdominal cavity is manually agitated externally during the perfusion period to promote uniform distribution of the heated chemotherapy perfusate. After completion of the perfusion, the abdomen is reopened, the perfusate is evacuated, and disposed of it in the proper fashion, and the abdominal cavity is irrigated with 2 to 3 L of saline to wash away any residual chemotherapy.

## ADVANTAGES OF THE CLOSED TECHNIQUE

The principal advantage of the closed technique is that the potential for environmental contamination with chemotherapy agents is greatly reduced over the open method, and there is also less opportunity for heat loss anteriorly, allowing the appropriate intraperitoneal temperature to be reached faster and maintained more easily. By closing the skin while leaving the fascia open, better flow and distribution of the perfusate is achieved. In some centers, the HIPEC procedure is performed after completion of the entire surgical phase, with inflow and outflow tubes inserted through the abdominal wall before the final closure of the laparotomy incision. At the completion of the perfusion, the tubing is removed, and anesthesia can be reversed. This modification of the closed method saves the need for reopening of the abdomen; however, many surgeons will prefer to do the gastrointestinal reconstructions after the hyperthermic chemotherapeutic perfusion.

## POTENTIAL DISADVANTAGES

The main disadvantage of the closed technique is the lack of uniform distribution of the heated intraperitoneal chemotherapy, which theoretically could result in significant morbidity. When methylene blue was instilled with the closed technique, uneven distribution was observed by Sugarbaker and coworkers.[9] Elias et al[10] observed poor thermal distribution during the closed method by the use of 6 thermal probes placed in different positions. Inadequate circulation of the heated intraperitoneal chemotherapy can lead to accumulation of both, heat and chemotherapy in dependent parts of the abdomen. This undesirable pooling may result in increase systemic absorption and can instigate foci of hyperthermic injury that can contribute to postoperative ileus, bowel perforation, and fistula formation.

## PERITONEAL CAVITY EXPANDER

To expand the volume of the peritoneal cavity and facilitate the distribution of the perfusate, Fujimura et al[11] developed a technique of using a peritoneal cavity expander. The expander is composed of a cylinder made of acrylic that contains inflow and outflow catheters that are secured over the wound. The cylinder fills with the perfusate as it is instilled into the peritoneal cavity, allowing the small bowel to float freely. This technique has been used in Japan and South Korea. Disadvantages were reported by Elias et al,[10] who found oozing around the wound and tumor recurrences inside the parietal wound that had not been treated because of the presence of the expander.

## LAPAROSCOPIC TECHNIQUE

The palliative role of HIPEC in patients with intractable ascites has been recognized and published extensively.[12,13] Recently, a group of French investigators reported on the increased tissue diffusion of oxaliplatin during laparoscopically assisted versus open heated intraoperative intraperitoneal chemotherapy in an animal study.[14] The use of the laparoscopic route to perform cytoreductive surgery to palliate metastatic disease to the ovaries,[15] to completely remove primary ovarian carcinomas with limited peritoneal dissemination,[16] and to do staged HIPEC in patients that had an open cytoreductive surgery[17] has also been reported. Our group has reported on a patient with peritoneal mesothelioma who underwent a laparoscopic cytoreduction with HIPEC. In this case, the inflow catheters were placed through the trocar incisions, and the outflow catheters were placed trough the mini-laparotomy incision that was required to remove the specimen from the greater omentectomy (Fig. 4).

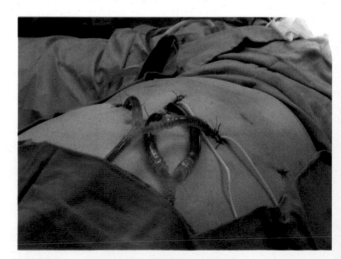

**FIGURE 4.**    Laparoscopic HIPEC technique.

**TABLE 1.** Comparison of HIPEC Technique in Patients With Appendix Cancer

| Institution | Method | Drugs | Dosage | Timing | Outflow Temperature, °C | Duration, min |
|---|---|---|---|---|---|---|
| **United States** | | | | | | |
| Washington Hospital Center | Open | IP MMC | 15 mg/m$^2$ | All at time 0 | 41 | 90 |
| | | IP Dox | 15 mg/m$^2$ | | | |
| | | IV 5FU | 400 mg/m$^2$ | | | |
| | | IV Leu | 20 mg/m$^2$ | | | |
| Wake Forest University | Closed | MMC | 40 mg | 30 mg at time 0 | 40 | 120 |
| St Agnes Hospital | Closed | MMC | 40 mg | 30 mg at time 0 | 42 | 90 |
| | | | | 10 mg at 45 min | | |
| University California, San Diego | Closed | MMC | 10 mg/L perfusate up to 60 mg | 2/3 at time 0 | 41–42 | 60 |
| | | | | 1/3 at 45 min | | |
| **Germany** | | | | | | |
| Regensburg University | Closed | MMC | 20 mg/m$^2$ | All at time 0 | 41–42 | 60 |
| **Spain** | | | | | | |
| MD Anderson España | Open | MMC | 10 mg/m$^2$ (female) | All at time 0 | 42 | 90 |
| | | | 12.5 mg/m$^2$ (male) | | | |
| **Sweden** | | | | | | |
| Uppsala University | Open | IP Oxali | 460 mg/m$^2$ | All at time 0 | 41 | 30 |
| | | IV 5-FU | | 1 h before | | |
| **United Kingdom** | | | | | | |
| Basingstoke | Open | MMC | 15 mg/m$^2$ | All at time 0 | 42 | 60 |
| **Switzerland** | | | | | | |
| Kantonsspital St Gallen | Open | MMC | 25 mg/m$^2$ | 1/3 every 30 min | 42 | 90 |
| **Japan** | | | | | | |
| Kusatu General Hospital | Open | MMC + CDDP | 20 mg | All at time 0 | 42 | 60 |
| Kishiwada Tokushukai and Ikeda Hospital | | | 100 mg | | | |
| **France** | | | | | | |
| Institut Gustave Roussy | Open | Oxali | 460 mg/m$^2$ | At 43 min | 43 | 30 |
| | | IV 5-FU | | | | |
| Centre Hospitalier Lyon Sud | Closed | MMC + CDDP | 20 mg/m$^2$ | All at time 0 | 42 | 90 |
| | | | 20 mg/m$^2$ | | | |

MMC indicates mitomycin C; Dox, doxorubicin; Leu, leucovorin; Oxali, oxaliplatin; CDDP, cisplatinum.

## DISCUSSION

Over the last 2 decades, there have been significant improvements in the care of patients with peritoneal surface malignancies. The unprecedented 63-month median survival on 48 patients with complete cytoreduction of their metastatic disease to the peritoneum from colon cancer recently reported by Elias et al[3] is a testament to the fact that peritoneal carcinomatosis can be treated with curative intent in a selected group of patients. The current treatment modality of choice seems to be the combination of a complete cytoreduction and the administration of HIPEC at the time of surgery. However, nobody knows for sure what the added benefit of HIPEC is after having had a complete cytoreduction, and it is very difficult with the current literature to separate its impact from the added benefits of better surgical techniques, better selection criteria that is based on understanding the biologic behavior of some peritoneal surface malignancies, and improvements in systemic therapy. Most of the cytoreductive surgeon's community believes that the strategy of treatment requires both, cytoreduction and HIPEC. Meanwhile, a large component of the medical oncology community and the insurance companies continue to challenge the role of HIPEC stating that it is associated with too high of

a complication rate, and its benefit has never been proven. As part of this manuscript, I requested information regarding not only the technique used to deliver HIPEC from different centers around the world but also asked them to provide data regarding the drugs and dosages that are being used, when are the drugs given, how hot is the chemotherapeutic perfusion, and for how long is it carried out. Table 1 is the summary of the HIPEC that is being used for patients with appendix cancer. An analysis of the data from these 12 hospitals demonstrates that there is not any kind of consensus on which method is best. Four different drugs are being used for the same purpose: eliminate microscopic residual disease; however, the dose of even the most commonly used drug, mitomycin C, varies significantly among institutions. Regarding heat, there are fewer variations regarding how hot it should be (41°C–42°C), but the range on how long should the HIPEC be continued goes from 30 minutes by some centers to 120 minutes by others. The same can be said about the HIPEC treatment for colon and gastric cancer with peritoneal dissemination (Tables 2–3). Although it seems that our better understanding of the biologic behavior of peritoneal dissemination in addition to the strong pharmacological rationale for HIPEC supports this procedure from

**TABLE 2.** Comparison of HIPEC Technique in Patients With Colon Cancer

| Institution | Method | Drugs | Dosage | Timing | Outflow Temperature, °C | Duration, min |
|---|---|---|---|---|---|---|
| United States | | | | | | |
|   Washington Hospital Center | Open | IP MMC | 15 mg/m$^2$ | All at time 0 | 41 | 90 |
| | | IP Dox | 15 mg/m$^2$ | | | |
| | | IV 5FU | 400 mg/m$^2$ | | | |
| | | IV Leu | 20 mg/m$^2$ | | | |
|   Wake Forest University | Closed | MMC | 40 mg | 30 mg at time 0 | 40 | 120 |
|   St Agnes Hospital | Closed | MMC | 40 mg | 30 mg at time 0 | 42 | 90 |
| | | | | 10 mg at 45 min | | |
|   University California, San Diego | Closed | MMC | 10 mg/L perfusate up to 60 mg | 2/3 at time 0 | 41–42 | 60 |
| | | | | 1/3 at 45 min | | |
| Germany | | | | | | |
|   Regensburg University | Closed | MMC | 20 mg/m$^2$ | All at time 0 | 41–42 | 60 |
| | | Dox | 15 mg/m$^2$ | | | |
| | | Oxali | 300 mg/m$^2$ | | | |
| Spain | | | | | | |
|   MD Anderson España | Open | Oxali | 460 mg/m$^2$ | All at time 0 | 43 | 30 |
| Sweden | | | | | | |
|   Uppsala University | Open | IP Oxali | 460 mg/m$^2$ | All at time 0 | 41 | 30 |
| | | IV 5-FU | | 1 h before | | |
| United Kingdom | | | | | | |
|   Basingstoke | Open | MMC | 15 mg/m$^2$ | All at time 0 | 42 | 60 |
| Switzerland | | | | | | |
|   Kantonsspital St Gallen | Open | MMC | 25 mg/m$^2$ | 1/3 every 30 min | 42 | 90 |
| France | | | | | | |
|   Institut Gustave Roussy | Open | Oxali | 460 mg/m$^2$ | At 43 min | 43 | 30 |
| | | IV 5-FU | | | | |
|   Centre Hospitalier Lyon Sud | Closed | MMC | 20–40 mg/m$^2$ | All at time 0 | 42 | 90 |

MMC indicates mitomycin C; Dox, doxorubicin; Leu, leucovorin; Oxali, oxaliplatin.

**TABLE 3.** Comparison of HIPEC Technique in Patients With Gastric Cancer

| Institution | Method | Drugs | Dosage | Timing | Outflow Temperature, °C | Duration, min |
|---|---|---|---|---|---|---|
| Germany | | | | | | |
|   Regensburg University | Closed | CDDP + Dox | 75 mg/m$^2$ | All at time 0 | 41–42 | 60 |
| | | | 15 mg/m$^2$ | | | |
| Japan | | | | | | |
|   Kusatu General Hospital | Open | MMC + CDDP | 20 mg | All at time 0 | 42 | 60 |
|   Kishiwada Tokushukai and Ikeda Hospitals | | | 100 mg | | | |
| China | | | | | | |
|   Jilin Tumor Hospital | Closed | 5FU | 750 mg/L | n/a | 41 | 60 |
| | | CDDP | 20 mg/L | | | |
| | | MMC | 10 mg/L | | | |
| Korea | | | | | | |
|   Asian Medical Center | Semi-open | MMC | 6 mg | Every 10 min × 5 | 42 | 60 |
| | | CDDP | 60 mg | | | |
| | | Etoposide | 30 mg | | | |
|   Kyungpook National University Hospital | Open | MMC | 10 mg/m$^2$ | All at time 0 | 42 | 60 |
| France | | | | | | |
|   Centre Hospitalier Lyon Sud | Closed | MMC | 20–40 mg/m$^2$ | All at time 0 | 42 | 90 |

CDDP indicates cisplatinum; Dox, doxorubicin; MMC, mitomycin C.

a scientific standpoint, it is going to be very difficult to make decisions regarding clinical trials because there are too many variables. This situation is similar to the use of intraperitoneal chemotherapy in ovarian cancer. With data from 3 prospective randomized studies, the National Cancer Institute of the United States issued a clinical alert urging physicians to consider intraperitoneal chemotherapy in optimally debulked ovarian cancer patients but could not recommend a particular regimen because of the frequent dose adjustments in the trials. So, unless medical and surgical oncologists work together to design protocols that will be powered enough to demonstrate the real benefit of adding HIPEC, the current situation will be slightly improved in terms of the number of HIPEC cases that are performed. At the present time, less than 1% of patients with colon cancer and peritoneal dissemination undergo cytoreductive surgery and HIPEC in the United States, which is also a testament that HIPEC continues to be a frequently questioned and controversial procedure.

## REFERENCES

1. Sugarbaker PH. Peritonectomy procedures. *Ann Surg.* 1995;221:29–42.
2. Verwaal VJ, Bruin S, Boot H, et al. 8-Year follow-up of randomized trial: cytoreduction and hyperthermic intraperitoneal chemotherapy versus systemic chemotherapy in patients with peritoneal carcinomatosis of colorectal cancer. *Ann Surg Oncol.* 2008;15:2426–2432.
3. Elias D, Lefevre JH, Chevalier J, et al. Complete cytoreductive surgery plus intraperitoneal chemohyperthermia with oxaliplatin for peritoneal carcinomatosis of colorectal origin. *J Clin Oncol.* 2008;27:1–8.
4. Sugarbaker PH. Management of peritoneal surface malignancy. Preface. *Surg Oncol Clin N Am.* 2003;12:xxi–xxiv.
5. Spratt JS, Adcock RA, Muskovin M, et al. Clinical delivery system for intraperitoneal hyperthermic chemotherapy. *Cancer Res.* 1980;40:256–260.
6. Glehen O, Cotte E, Kusamura S, et al. Hyperthermic intraperitoneal chemotherapy: nomenclature and modalities of perfusion. *J Surg Oncol.* 2008;98:242–246.
7. Sugarbaker PH, Yu W, Yonemura Y. Gastrectomy, peritonectomy and perioperative intraperitoneal chemotherapy: the evolution of treatment strategies for advanced gastric cancer. *Semin Surg Oncol.* 2003;21:233–248.
8. Esquivel J, Sugarbaker PH, Helm W. *Intraperitoneal Cancer Therapy.* New Jersey: Humana Press; 2007:163–177.
9. Stephens AD, Alderman R, Chang D, et al. Morbidity and mortality of 200 treatments with cytoreductive surgery and hyperthermic intraperitoneal chemotherapy using the coliseum technique. *Ann Surg Oncol.* 1999;6:790–796.
10. Elias D, Antoun S, Goharin A, et al. Research on the best chemohyperthermia technique of treatment of peritoneal carcinomatosis after complete resection. *Int J Surg Invest.* 2000;1:431–439.
11. Fujimura T, Yonemura Y, Fushida S, et al. Continuous hyperthermic peritoneal perfusion for the treatment of peritoneal dissemination in gastric cancers and subsequent second-look operation. *Cancer.* 1990;65:65–71.
12. Facchiano E, Scaringi S, Kianmanesh R, et al. Laparoscopic hyperthermic intraperitoneal chemotherapy (HIPEC) for the treatment of malignant ascites secondary to unresectable peritoneal carcinomatosis from advanced gastric cancer. *Eur J Surg Oncol.* 2007;34:154–158.
13. Patriti A, Cavazzoni E, Graziosi L, et al. Successful palliation of malignant ascites from peritoneal mesothelioma by laparoscopic intraperitoneal hyperthermic chemotherapy. *Surg Laparosc Endosc Percutan Tech.* 2008;18:426–428.
14. Thomas F, Ferron G, Gesson-Paute A, et al. Increased tissue diffusion of oxaliplatin during laparoscopically assisted versus open heated intraoperative intraperitoneal chemotherapy (HIPEC). *Ann Surg Oncol.* 2008;15:3623–3624.
15. Van Dam P, Van Dam L, Verkinderen P, et al. Robotic-assisted laparoscopic cytoreductive surgery for lobular carcinoma of the breast metastatic to the ovaries. *J Min Inv Gyn.* 2003;14:746–749.
16. He YL, Zhang LY, Peng DX. Laparoscopic cytoreductive surgery for ovarian carcinoma: report of 4 cases. *Di Yi Jun Yi Da Xue Xue Bao.* 2004;24:479–480.
17. Knutsen A, Sielaff TD, Greeno E, et al. Staged laparoscopic infusion of hyperthermic intraperitoneal chemotherapy after cytoreductive surgery. *J Gastro Surg.* 2006;10:1038–1043.

# Particle Therapy in All Its Parts

Benjamin Movsas  •  Theodore S. Lawrence

"Technology presumes there's just one way to do things and there never is"—Robert M. Pirsig

Although particle therapy for cancer is certainly not new, there has recently been tremendous interest and energy to develop multiple particle therapy centers over the last few years. However, much controversy swirls around the topic of particle therapy. Is it actually better than current state-of-the-art radiation with photons? What evidence-based medicine is available to document such claims? What are the key differences between the 2 main forms of particle therapy: protons and carbon ions? How should the concern regarding cost effectiveness be addressed? Perhaps there's one issue that everyone can agree upon. Building a particle therapy center to treat cancer patients is a massive enterprise. In this special issue of *The Cancer Journal*, our goal is to address the fundamental issues that one should consider regarding particle therapy.

To this end, we have invited leading experts in particle therapy from around the world. This issue begins with Drs. Blakely and Chang explaining the underlying biology of charged particles. This article introduces the key theoretical concepts of particle therapy compared with photons: the potential for improved dose distributions (described later) that apply to both carbon and proton beams and, in the case of carbon, an improved biologic effectiveness. A carbon beam can kill hypoxic cells, which exist in the center of a tumor and may be the cause of treatment failure after photon radiation, as effectively as well-oxygenated cells. The next article by Dr. Lomax reviews the physical interactions that take place when particles impinge on tissue. This article discusses how protons and carbon have the potential to produce "better" dose distributions than photons. "Better" has 2 strict definitions in radiation oncology: (1) for the same tumor dose, there can be less normal tissue dose or (2) for the same normal tissue dose, there can more tumor dose. Once these basic issues have been described, Drs. Flanz and Smith next walk us through the detailed technological aspects of proton therapy. These excellent articles set up the clinical question: what is the evidence that charged particles have delivered the potential that the physics and biology have suggested? In other words, are these better dose distributions producing measurable clinical improvement?

The next 4 articles focus on the clinical experience thus far using particle therapy. We are pleased that leading clinical experts have

shared their knowledge and summarized the clinical data available. Dr. Merchant focuses on pediatric indications. The chief goal in the application of particle therapy in pediatrics is to maintain tumor dose while decreasing late normal tissue injury (eg, neurocognitive function) and the potential risk of second cancers. In particular, as the risk of second malignancies increases with time and the majority of children are cured, the potential benefits of decreasing the dose to normal tissue would seem to be the greatest. Although pediatric tumors are one of the least controversial applications for charged particle therapy, it is worth noting that radiation is playing a decreasing role in the treatment of pediatric cancers (for instance, a recent study questions its role in childhood acute lymphoblastic leukemia[1]) and the doses of radiation administered are decreasing as well. Thus, it would seem that 2 or 3 facilities could reasonably treat all of the children in the United States.

As the great majority of patients who have received particle therapy have been treated for prostate cancer, we asked for a separate article to be devoted to the role of protons in treating prostate cancer by Drs. Efstathiou, Trofimov, and Zietman. Unfortunately, there is currently no clinical evidence that protons can achieve either higher dose to the tumor or lower dose to the critical normal structures than state of the art photon therapy. These authors discuss the need for a randomized trial to assess this question. Dr. Schulz-Ertner reviews the clinical experience in adults with particle beams, which consists chiefly of retrospective reviews and phase II trials, in a fair but overall positive light. For the sake of balance, we asked Dr. Brada to also review the current clinical experience in his fair but overall negative light. All of these experts have worked hard to provide us with an evidence-based perspective, but, in the absence of randomized trials, the interpretation of the evidence can lead to different conclusions!

Although the emphasis in the United States has been on proton therapy, both Japanese and German investigators have established carbon beam facilities, which, as described above, have distinct potential advantages over protons. Drs. Weber and Kraft provide a thoughtful review comparing and contrasting protons versus carbon ions. In the last article, perhaps the most challenging issue is addressed by Drs. Steinberg and Konski: what are the cost utility issues for particle therapy? If protons cost the same as photons, the ratio of "heat to light" in our discussions would be greatly altered. However, the enormous costs of the current facilities ($150 million for protons and $250 million for carbon) and the current favorable reimbursement for prostate cancer have driven a business model that may not select the patients most likely to benefit from this strategy.

To date, as might be expected, essentially all particle centers have been developed by individual institutions. However, as Pirsig suggests, is there really only "one way" to accomplish this technological goal? For such a massive enterprise, it would seem that a regional or national consortium approach might be best able to integrate the clinical, academic, physics, administrative and financial resources so that patients most likely to benefit from particle therapy could be treated in prospective trials that would determine the role of particle therapy technology. In this way, the whole of radiation oncology could produce future treatments that are greater than the sum of our individual parts or "particles."

## REFERENCE

1. Pui CH, Campana D, Pei D, et al. Treating childhood acute lymphoblastic leukemia without cranial irradiation. *N Engl J Med*. 2009;360:2730–2741.

# Biology of Charged Particles

Eleanor A. Blakely • Polly Y. Chang

## HISTORICAL BACKGROUND

Marie Curie's original observation of different types of radiation tracks streaking through her simple "cloud chamber" revealed that the contrails of $\alpha$ particles were straighter and thicker than the much thinner and tortuous path of $\beta$-emitting radiation contrails.[1] The dose absorbing events in these 2 kinds of radiation tracks have different biologic consequences even at the same level of total dose due to spatial differences in the distribution of the energy absorption. Enhanced biologic damage from clustered damage of $\alpha$ particles was recognized early on as a potential therapeutic tool; however, the short range of penetration of the $\alpha$ particle from radioisotopes was limiting.

The invention of the cyclotron by Ernest O. Lawrence in 1930 for which he was awarded a Nobel prize in 1939 changed the world in many ways, but the opportunity it provided to produce beams of neutrons and particles at increasing higher energies allowed these new radiation modalities to penetrate the cells, tissues, and to depths of the human body. Ernest and his brother John Lawrence, who was a physician, established the Donner Biomedical Laboratory that has now become the Life Sciences Division at the Lawrence Berkeley National Laboratory, Berkeley, California. Ernest placed strong emphasis on the medical use of his cyclotrons, and John developed the Donner Laboratory's medical use of radioisotopes and radiation for the diagnosis and treatment of diseases, in imaging and in safety, for which he became known as the "Father of Nuclear Medicine."

Robert Wilson's suggestion that the Bragg peak of beams of atomic nuclei[2] would be useful for radiotherapy generated worldwide interest in trying to understand the basis for the enhanced biologic effects of dense particle tracks, and it earned him the title of "Father of Hadron Therapy." The word "hadron" comes from the Greek "hadros" meaning "robust." A hadron is any elementary subatomic particle that interacts strongly with other particles.[3] Many elementary particles do not occur under normal circumstances in nature but can be created and detected during energetic collisions of particles produced in a particle accelerator. Atomic constituents include electrons, protons, and neutrons, as well as photons, neutrinos and muons, and some other exotic particles. Protons and neutrons are made up of quarks. "Particle" is a misnomer, however, because the dynamics of particles are governed by quantum mechanics, and therefore exhibit wave-particle duality. All particles and their interactions can almost completely be described by a quantum field theory called the "standard model."[4] There are 40 species of elementary particles in the standard model (24 fermions, 12 vector bosons, and 4 scalar bosons). These particle species can combine to form composite particles, accounting for the hundreds of other species of particles discovered since the 1960s. Photons are bosons. In nature, quarks are always found bound together in groups called hadrons because of a phenomenon known as color confinement.

Hadrons are divided into baryons (protons, neutrons: each made of 3 quarks), and mesons are made of a quark and an antiquark. Carbon ions are composite baryons, and for this reason technically not hadrons, but have been incorrectly included in the popular description of hadron therapy.[3]

Cornelius Tobias pioneered the biomedical applications of accelerated hadron beams with the first biologic experiments using protons performed in 1948, followed by first human exposures to accelerated protons and $\alpha$ particles in 1955. Between 1956 and until the closure of the 184-in cyclotron in 1986, 1500 patients were recruited and treated in the Hadron Therapy Clinical Trials with protons or helium ions at Berkeley using the Irradiation Stereotaxic apparatus for humans, a unique early device that allowed precision placement of the patient for particle radiotherapy.

Early biologic studies in the United States,[5–13] Sweden,[14–18] and in the former Soviet Union[19,20] mapped the changing biologic effects of protons, deuterons, and helium ions at high energies as they emerged from the beam vacuum pipe, until reaching their stopping lowest energy in material, usually with their maximum effect in the Bragg ionization peak. Desirable dose profiles with these low atomic number (Z) beams were used in clinical studies in the United States (Berkeley, Boston), Sweden (Uppsala), Japan (Chiba), and former Soviet Union to treat primarily pituitary and radiotherapy patients.

The heavy ion linear accelerator at Berkeley became a source of "heavy" ions (particles with higher atomic number than the "light" beams of protons or helium ions) for cell biology studies.[21] On the basis of information obtained from this work, Tobias and Todd[22] first suggested the therapeutic use of heavier ions, which was further developed by Tobias et al[23,24] and Tobias.[25] For this reason, some consider Tobias the "Father of Heavy-Ion Therapy." Within the same year, research at 2 US accelerators (the Princeton synchrotron[26] and the Berkeley BEVATRON[27]) demonstrated that large synchrotrons designed for proton acceleration were suitable for accelerating nitrogen and heavier nuclei. The Berkeley BEVALAC complex was created in 1975 by using the heavy ion linear accelerator as an injector to the BEVATRON[28] in another building just below it on the hillside overlooking the campus of the University of California, Berkeley. Tobias and Tobias[29] chronicled the story of this machine in the book he wrote with his wife Ida entitled *People and Particles*.

The BEVALAC became an international biophysical laboratory where a cadre of distinguished visiting scientists joined the Berkeley Laboratory staff of radiation physicists, treatment planners, chemists, biologists, and clinicians involved in the ongoing research program funded by the US Department of Energy and the National Institutes of Health with an ultimate goal of clinical radiotherapy comparing treatment outcomes using helium ions, with those using charged particles of higher atomic number, including carbon ions in May 1977, neon in November 1977, argon in March 1979, and silicon beams in November 1982. Dr. Joseph R. Castro led these phase I and II trials with Dr. Theodore L. Phillips, both from the University of California, San Francisco, Department of Radiation Oncology. The National Aeronautics and Space Administration also supported relevant work estimating radiation risk due to occupational exposure to charged particles in space flight. A significant portion of the early scientific justification for the safe and successful evaluations of radiation risks, and the rationale developed for the use of high-energy charged particles for cancer therapy were generated at the BEVALAC. In addition, the facility provided a unique opportunity for the early pioneers in this field to train and to gain experience with high-energy charged particle beams.

An international set of accelerators on 4 continents (North America, Asia, Europe, and Africa) have successfully continued the quest started in Berkeley to use charged particles for cancer radiotherapy, and a new cadre of scientists and clinicians have emerged with many recent major contributions to the field that are summarized in this article. There have been many leaders demonstrating the success of proton radiotherapy after the treatment of the first proton patient in Berkeley in the mid 1950s. The Uppsala accelerators in Sweden, the Harvard Cyclotron in Boston, MA, the Dubna, ITEP, and St. Petersburg facilities in Russia, the Chiba and Tsukuba accelerators in Japan, the Clatterbridge machine in England, the Paul Scherrer Institute in Switzerland, the Loma Linda University Medical Center in Loma Linda, CA, the Louvain-la-Neuve in Belgium, and the Francis H. Burr Proton Therapy Center at Massachusetts General Hospital were early leaders demonstrating the success of proton radiotherapy. They have been joined by US proton centers in Davis (CA), Boston (MA), Bloomington (IN), Houston (TX), and Jacksonville (FL), and proton facilities in Vancouver (Canada), Nice and Orsay (France), Berlin (Germany), Catania (Italy), Tsuraga City and Shiuoka (Japan), Ilsan (Korea), and Wanjie (China). Proton therapy facilities are also under construction in PSI, Villigen (Switzerland), Philadelphia, Pennsylvania and Western Chicago, IL, Essen (Germany), Taipei (Taiwan), Oklahoma City (Oklahoma), Hampton (Virginia), Protvino (Russia), and Ruzomberok (Slovak Republic). Proton machines are being planned in Trento (Italy), Faure (South Africa), Koeln (Germany), Beijing (China), and Uppsala (Sweden).

Important clinical success in treating large numbers of specific tumor sites with carbon ions began in Chiba, Japan in 1994 led by Dr. Hirohiko Tsujii for the first time in a clinical setting with a dedicated heavy-ion accelerator for medical purposes as a part of a national 10-year strategy for cancer control. Dr. Gerhard Kraft spearheaded the use of the first European carbon ion treatment at the physics laboratory Gesellschaft fur Schwerionenforschung in Darmstadt, Germany, under the clinical direction of Prof. Dr. Jurgen Debus of Heidelberg, who will soon be operating the newly built Heidelberg Ion Therapy accelerator in a clinical setting in Heidelberg. These 2 carbon ion programs have each established significant milestones documenting careful clinical success with carbon treatments in specific tumor sites and in continuing to develop the potentials of carbon beam delivery. New dual proton and carbon therapy facilities have also been operating in Hyogo (Japan) since 2002 and are currently being built in Pavia (Italy), Marburg (Germany), Kiel (Germany), and Gunma (Japan), and are also planned in Wiener Neustadt (Austria). There are no high-energy heavy particle accelerators for radiotherapy in the North American continent, although several groups have plans under consideration. The following sections of this article describe the biophysical rationale that led to interest in particles for therapy.

## PARTICLE BEAM CHOICES FOR RADIOTHERAPY

### Depth-Dose Ionization Profiles

The BEVALAC was used to accelerate the beams from protons to uranium up to energies (E) of up to 1 GeV/atomic mass unit (amu). Early investigations at this accelerator complex addressed the question of which beam would provide the maximum effectiveness at depth, without risk of radiation damage to surrounding normal tissues? The linear energy transfer (LET) value representing the optimal ionization density, or quality of the radiation per unit track length, was thought to be near 100 keV/$\mu$m from $\alpha$ particle studies. This guided the early focus on beams of carbon up to argon at energies of each in the range from 300 to 800 MeV/amu that would be useful to cover tumor locations in the depth of a human body. Higher energies are required for the heavier ion beams to achieve the same depth-dose profile of lighter ion beams. However, peak-to-plateau dose ratios decline at higher energies, and LET values are changing with the increasing mixture of LET values from the fragmentation of primary heavy ions into particles of lower atomic number and concomitant lower effective LET values.

When primary particles fragment, the resulting secondary particles of lower atomic number have a longer range of penetration and produce a pure dose beyond the Bragg peak that is the result of the fragmentation events. Secondary fragments have lower LET values than the primary beam, and thus dilute the total effective LET of the beam. The contribution of fragmentation dose in also increased in the "tail" region beyond the Bragg peak from particle beams of increasing atomic number. An instrument called a BERKLET developed by Llacer et al[30,31] was used to measure LET and residual energy of particles allowing for the identification of the particle's charge as a function of depth of beam penetration, and allowing for comparisons with theoretical models of beam physics. Radiobiological measurements completed in correlative studies with the BERKLET confirmed that the relative biologic effectiveness (RBE) of primary ions decreased with increasing additional fragmentation dose. For many clinical applications, the narrow diameter ion beams need to be modulated to cover a larger diameter field. Several methods, such as scattering foils, ridged filters and propellors, wobbler magnets, spot or raster scanning are used to achieve the larger radiation fields, and to shape the beam that can contribute fragmentation dose to varying degrees,[32-34] which broadens the range of particle Z and E. Also the LET value is not sufficient to characterize track structure, because ions of different atomic number at the same LET can have very different track structures. Both particles E and Z are needed to define beam quality.

Some of the individual Bragg curves for heavy ion beams that were investigated for their biologic effectiveness are presented in Figure 1. The range of LET values represented by these beams are depicted graphically in Figure 2. Figure 2 depicts the dose average LET values for 570 MeV/amu argon, 530 MeV/amu silicon, 425 MeV/amu neon, and 400 MeV/anu carbon from the entrance plateau of the Bragg curve through the stopping Bragg peak. With increasing atomic number, the range of LET values in the stopping Bragg peak regions shifted to a greater prevalence of LET values between 100 keV/$\mu$m and 1000 keV/$\mu$m. However, quite significantly, the LET value of the entrance plateau region also shifted to the right, resulting in an LET of nearly 100 keV/$\mu$m in the plateau of the argon ion beams, which contributed to a loss of one of the main clinical advantages of the peak-to-plateau dose ratio in the Bragg ionization curve. Biologic effects of argon ions in the distal edge of the Bragg peak decreased, because LET values were beyond the maximum for biologic effectiveness. It is for this reason that heavier ion beams are considered not clinically useful.

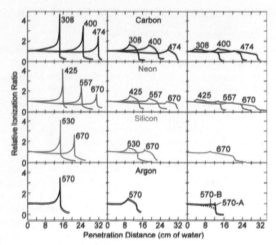

**FIGURE 1.** Bragg peaks of carbon, neon, silicon, and argon at various indicated initial energies of extraction. Unmodified beams (left panel), and spread out Bragg Peaks of 4-cm (middle panel) and 10-cm width (right panel) are presented. Adapted from Ref. 40, with permission from Elsevier.

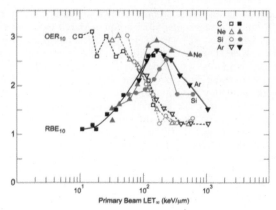

**FIGURE 3.** Variation of OER as a function of LET measured at various points in SOBPs of carbon, neon, silicon, and argon ions (courtesy of E. Blakely).

## RBE and OER Values

Measurements were made of the RBE of the different beams for various endpoints compared with x- or $\gamma$-rays as defined by the International Commission on Radiation Units and Measurements (ICRU 1986). The quality factor RBE in radiation protection, based on the ICRU Report 40[35] and most recently by the International Atomic Energy Agency (IAEA)/ICRP,[36] is the ratio of the absorbed doses of 2 radiations (usually a standard radiation vs. a test radiation) required to produce the same biologic effect. There are several textbooks[37–39] and book chapters[40,41] that have carefully summarized the decades of effort invested in measuring detailed RBE values in particle beams.

Each particle beam of a specific atomic number can be represented by a family of RBE values that changes dependent on the absorbed dose, the reference absolute dose calibration method, the range of particle energies, and the biologic system and end point used to determine the RBE. In fact the maximum effectiveness for each beam can be vastly different at the same LET. The maximum RBE for irradiated cultured human fibroblasts at 10% survival for carbon, neon, silicon, and argon ion beams as a function of LET is shown in Figure 3. RBE values usually increase at lower doses or higher survival due to differences in the shape of the low-LET radiation response at low dose. The RBE values increase from nearly 1.0 for carbon ions at 10 to 20 keV/$\mu$m to nearly 3.0 for neon ions at 150 keV/$\mu$m, but the data are fitted by individual curves for each ion. The maximum RBE for protons (not shown) lies below the LET for the maximum helium ion ($\alpha$ particle) RBE.[42]

The oxygen enhancement ratio (OER) is also plotted in Figure 3. The OER is a parameter that is determined from the ratio of doses under hypoxia versus full oxic conditions that yield the same level of a biologic effect such as cell killing. Prior work demonstrated that tumors were resistant to radiation effects if they outgrew their vascular supply and became necrotic or hypoxic, and that this dependence on oxygen was reduced for charged particles at high-LET.

**FIGURE 2.** Upper panel: Bragg ionization curves studied for 570 MeV/amu argon, 530 MeV/amu silicon, 425 MeV/amu neon, and 400 MeV/amu carbon beams (pristine, 4- and 10-cm extended Bragg peaks). The short thick line below each curve designates the location of the entrance plateau, the longer thick line represents the Bragg peak region, and the dotted line between them represents the ionization region between the plateau and peak. Lower panel: calculated dose-averaged LET$^\infty$ values for pristine and extended Bragg peaks of each ion beam described above. The initial short thick line on the LET$^\infty$ axis represents the LET value calculated for the plateau region of each beam. The longer thick line corresponds to the LET values across the Bragg peak region designated above. The dotted line signifies LET values for the region between the plateau and the peak. Adapted from Ref. 40, with permission from Elsevier.

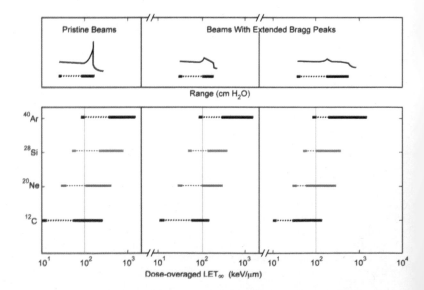

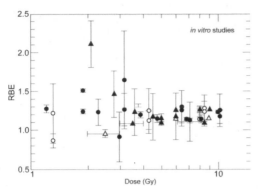

**FIGURE 4.**   Experimental proton RBE values (relative to $^{60}$CO) as a function of dose or fraction for cell inactivation measured in vitro in the center of a SOBP. Closed symbols show measurements using Chinese Hamster cell lines; open symbols stand for other cell lines. Circles represent RBEs for <100-MeV beans and triangles for >100-Me beams. Reprinted from Ref. 44, with permission from Elsevier.

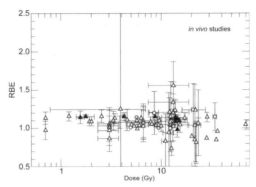

**FIGURE 5.**   Experimental proton RBE values (relative to $^{60}$CO) as a function of dose or fraction measured in vivo in the center of a SOBP. Closed symbols show RBE values for jejunal crypt cells, open symbols stand for RBEs for all other tissues. Circles represent RBEs for <100-MeV beams and triangles for >100-MeV beams. Reprinted from Ref. 44, with permission from Elsevier.

Recent evidence indicates that many additional molecular and cellular changes over and above reductions in OER are associated with high LET effects, as will be described later in this article. As Figure 3 demonstrates, the OER value declines with increasing LET until it is nearly 1.0 at LET values around 200 to 300 keV/$\mu$m.

A major issue in making radiobiological measurements supporting assessment of clinical beams is what biologic model is the best to use in the laboratory to measure beam effectiveness, and another is how can one integrate information one may have from the numerous diverse biologic systems into clinically relevant parameters that can be folded into a robust treatment planning system for pertinent beam delivery options to effectively target the diverse array of tumor tissues in a target area while maximally sparing the normal tissue in the vicinity. Decisions on these matters are impacting new proton and carbon facilities being planned or built and have in some cases slowed the development of internationally adopted treatment protocols.[43]

Paganetti et al[44,45] reviewed the published experimentally determined proton RBE values to evaluate the current clinical use of a generic proton RBE of 1.0 or 1.1. Figure 4 from Paganetti et al summarizes published in vitro RBE value for Chinese hamster cell inactivation measured in the center of a proton spread out Bragg peak (SOBP) and plotted as a function of dose per fraction for proton beams <100 MeV and for >100 MeV beams. The data are widely variable due to the diversity of technical protocols and biologic systems. Figure 5 summarizes the proton RBE values for in vivo jejunal crypt cell survival as a function of dose or fraction in the center of a SOBP. Both of these figures illustrate the magnitude of variability in proton RBE reported with 0.86 to 2.1 (mean of 1.22 and a standard error of 0.02) from the in vitro analysis and with 0.73 to 1.55 (mean of 1.10 and a lower standard error of 0.01) for the in vivo analysis. Figure 6 summarizes the RBEs for cell survival in monoenergetic low energy proton beams of <8.7 MeV as a function of energy and dose per fraction. These low energy beams were produced in physics laboratories, but illustrate the higher proton RBE values of up to 3.7 reported at doses of >1 Gy with a nearly stopping 0.72 MeV proton beam.

The consensus from these analyses and other excellent reviews[38,46,47] is that the RBE for protons of 65 to 250 MeV beams shows a modest increase with depth in the SOBP, and a clear rise in

effective dose at the distal edge of the Bragg peak. In vivo experiments report a slightly lower RBE than reported in vitro. The clinical implications of these results have indicated that the use of an RBE of 1.1 is "reasonable," with no recordable complication in many years of proton treatments with this RBE value, but it is not ideal in situations where critical structures, such as spinal cord, are located immediately behind the target volume.[47] A proton RBE of 1.0 is used for 150 to 250 MeV beams in Tsukuba (Japan) and Uppsala (Sweden), whereas a proton RBE of 1.1 is used at Massachusetts General Hospital, Loma Linda University, Paul Scherrer Institut (Switzerland), Orsay (France), and Faure (South Africa).

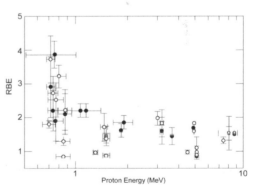

**FIGURE 6.**   Experimental proton RBE values (track segment measurements; relative to $^{60}$Co) as a function of dose or fraction (upper figure) and energy (lower figure) for cell inactivation measured in vitro for near monoenergetic protons (<10 MeV/amu (16m 17, 28, 29, 41–46); 12 and 31 MeV (41); 222 MeV (28)). RBE values based on the ratios of values (zero dose interpolations) are not included. In the upper figure, closed circles show RBEs for proton energies >1 MeV and open circles show RBEs for proton energies <1 MeV. In the lower figure, closed circles show RBEs for doses >4 Gy and open circles show RBEs for doses <4 Gy. Reprinted from Ref. 44, with permission from Elsevier.

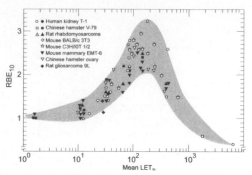

**FIGURE 7.** Aerobic $RBE_{10}$ versus mean $LET^{\infty}$ for monoenergetic and extended Bragg peak data using mammalian cell survival data measured in vitro. The results are compiled from 8 different cell systems.[93–93j] Solid symbols, $RBE_{10}$ in plateau and distal spiral ridge filter peak; open symbols, $RBE_{10}$ in plateau and peak (no spiral ridge filters). Adapted from Ref. 40, with permission from Elsevier.

Paganetti[48] parameterized a relation between proton RBE, dose homogeneity in the cell nucleus, and induction rates for different lesion types using a track structure model and the lethal lesion/potentially lethal lesion model of Curtis.[49] Formalisms such as these provide a framework for a mechanistic interpretation of RBE values. Dicello[50] has described the absorption characteristics of photons, protons, and heavy ions in the tissue that contribute to the major differences in the microdosimetry of these radiation modalities. Endo et al[51] (2007) have published an outstanding description of the more complex microdosimetric evaluation of secondary particles produced by 290 MeV/amu ions. Endo et al reported that the modeling based on a biologic response function as a lineal energy, indicates that the RBE of carbon ions had a maximum of 4.5 at the Bragg peak, then decreases rapidly, with the RBE of fragments around the stopping carbon ions being dominated by boron particles.

Differences in RBE for heavier ion beams due to technical and biologic differences can also be quite variable. Figure 7 provides an indication of the magnitude of some of the variability of the RBE measurements acquired with an array of biologic systems and beam geometries using heavier ion beams at the Berkeley BEVALAC. Recent published work with carbon ions, however, indicates many ongoing collaborative programs and information sharing between international institutions are in progress to validate any differences in beam and dose specifications due to delivery options and RBE parameters,

and to determine whether there is any impact on clinical outcome.[52] Isoeffective doses and RBEs for cell survival measured with cultured human salivary gland (HSG) cells (Table 1) and murine gut crypt survival after single doses (Table 2) and fractionated doses (Table 3) in 6-cm spread out Carbon 290 MeV/amu Bragg Peaks at Gesellschaft fur Schwerionenforschung in Germany and at the National Institute of Radiologic Sciences in Japan, indicates that the carbon beams at these 2 institutes are biologically identical within ±15% for in vitro data and ±3% for an in vivo end point after single and daily fractionated irradiations. Care was taken in these studies to make comparisons under identical beam energies and physical geometries of exposure with an identical biologic system. The reason for the 15% difference between carbon ion effects at each institute is not known.

Each clinical particle therapy program must indeed confirm RBE levels with their own accelerator-specific parameters before commissioning of an accelerator. However, it must be recognized that radiation oncologists do not simply use the RBE measurements taken from the laboratory to prescribe particle doses for patients. As the most recent technical report by IAEA/ICRU[36] points out, the application of the RBE concept in radiation therapy is a complex function of clearly defined RBE measurements made with biologic systems within various regions or depths of the ion beam, a consideration of any dose fractionation, and the dose distribution in the tumor as well as nearby critical normal tissues, and folds in a factor based on past personal clinical experience and information reported from other treatment centers. This fact has contributed to the current emphasis of using a theoretical approach to execute treatment planning that is based on historical summaries of clinical and radiobiological measurements, beam delivery methods, and transport codes to describe the physics within the stopping particle beams. These topics will be considered again later in this article.

## Biologically Effective Dose

The biologically effective dose (BED) is a concept that folds together the particle physical depth dose and the enhanced biologic effectiveness that the dosimeter cannot measure. To compare the overall biologic effectiveness of beams of equivalent depth over realistic extended Bragg peaks, range filters were designed to extend the effective Bragg peak region by accumulating the stopping particles over the broader dimensions required in radiotherapy. The goal was to give a region of isoeffective cell killing several folds wider than the stopping width of a pristine Bragg peak. There are several parameters to consider in this task, including the beam characteristics of energy deposition and fragmentation, and the model for cell inactivation that is used to predict the low-dose response in the mixed LET radiation fields, the specific available cell line sensitivities selected for the

### TABLE 1.    Isoeffective Doses and RBEs of 6-cm SOBP for HSG Cell Kill

| Position Within the SOBP | Isoeffective Dose (Gy)* | | RBE | | RBE Ratio (GSI/NIRS) |
| --- | --- | --- | --- | --- | --- |
| | GSI | NIRS | GSI | NIRS | |
| Proximal | 3.66 ± 0.17 | 3.47 ± 0.19 | 1.53 ± 0.13 | 1.61 ± 0.15 | 0.95 ± 0.12 |
| Middle | 3.22 ± 0.12 | 3.44 ± 0.44 | 1.74 ± 0.14 | 1.63 ± 0.24 | 1.07 ± 0.18 |
| Distal | 2.43 ± 0.11 | 2.55 ± 0.12 | 2.30 ± 0.20 | 2.19 ± 0.19 | 1.05 ± 0.13 |
| Distal end | 2.31 ± 0.11 | 2.37 ± 0.14 | 2.42 ± 0.21 | 2.36 ± 0.22 | 1.03 ± 0.13 |
| Cobalt-60 $\gamma$ rays | 5.59 ± 0.42 | | | | |

Values are mean ± SD.
*$D_{10}$ (dose required to reduce surviving fraction down to 10%).
GSI, Gesellschaft fuř Schwerionenforschung; NIRS, National Institute of Radiological Sciences.
Adapted from Ref. 52, with permission from Elsevier.

**TABLE 2.** Isoeffective Doses and RBEs of 6-cm SOBP for Gut Crypt Survivals After Single Doses

| Position Within the SOBP | Isoeffective Dose (Gy)* | | RBE | | RBE Ratio (GSI/NIRS) |
| --- | --- | --- | --- | --- | --- |
| | GSI | NIRS | GSI | NIRS | |
| Proximal | $10.27 \pm 0.20$ | $10.32 \pm 0.14$ | $1.47 \pm 0.03$ | $1.44 \pm 0.02$ | $1.00 \pm 0.02$ |
| Middle | $9.10 \pm 0.23$ | $9.45 \pm 0.08$ | $1.63 \pm 0.04$ | $1.57 \pm 0.02$ | $1.04 \pm 0.08$ |
| Distal | $8.27 \pm 0.10$ | $8.25 \pm 0.17$ | $1.80 \pm 0.02$ | $1.80 \pm 0.03$ | $1.00 \pm 0.02$ |
| Cobalt-60 $\gamma$ rays | $14.86 \pm 0.08$ | | | | |

Values are mean $\pm$ SD.
*$D_{10}$ (dose required to reduce the number of crypts per circumferences to 10).
GSI, Gesellschaft für Schwerionenforschung; NIRS, National Institute of Radiological Sciences.
Adapted from Ref. 52, with permission from Elsevier.

modeling and their RBE-LET dependence, and the dose level desired for the isoeffective region.

Range filters used at the BEVALAC were designed by Lyman.[54] The filter designs were based on physical beam parameters and available biologic data at the time. As cellular information accumulated with the initial filter design, the information was used to design better filters. The physical dose profile in the extended beams was less at the distal edge to compensate for the enhanced effectiveness of the stopping ions and achieve isoeffectiveness across the extended peak. A representative biologic dose-response profile was developed, and several filters of a newer spiral design were tooled to extend Bragg peaks to a width of 4 or 10 cm. In some cases, different particle beams required different filters to achieve isoeffective killing across the extended peak. In certain other cases, the physical and biologic properties of beams seemed to be similar enough to use the same filter for isoeffectiveness.

To demonstrate the isoeffectiveness of the available filters using single cell line (human T-1 fibroblast), the repair-misrepair model for cellular inactivation[55] was used to fit heavy-ion survival data by least-squares regression and to calculate aerobic RBE values at the 50% survival level (estimated to be approximately the daily dose fraction administered). The repair-misrepair model was selected, because it yields a fit to cell survival data that is representative of fits made with other available models. This model also has other characteristics useful for analytical interpretation.

The $RBE_{50}$ values for the ranges studied were multiplied by the measured physical dose at each range studied. The resultant normalized BED has been plotted over each of 6 Bragg curves of physical dose in Figure 8. The same 4- and 10-cm spiral ridge filters were used for each beam studied. The data for the 4-cm carbon and neon beams show fairly good success in attaining uniformity of aerobic cell killing across the peak. However, the corresponding OER values plotted be-

low each Bragg curve and the corresponding hypoxic BED values (not shown) demonstrated that it is not possible to design filters to simultaneously achieve isoeffectiveness for both aerobic and hypoxic cells. The BED and physical dose plots for the longer ranged 400 MeV/amu carbon beam with the 10-cm spiral ridge filter are depicted in the upper right panel of Figure 8. There is quite a bit of scatter in the replicate estimates of $RBE_{50}$ in the proximal and midpeak regions and less scatter in the distal position, however, the filter design of physical dose seems to slightly overcompensate for effective dose in the distal peak. More physical dose in the distal end of the extended peak is needed for isoeffectiveness across the full range of the peak. The OER value for this long-range carbon beam is rather high, averaging about 2.5 to 2.6 over the 10-cm width, but ranging from $2.8 \pm 0.2$ in the proximal peak to $1.0 \pm 0.2$ in the distal peak.

The BED and physical doses for the 557 MeV/amu neon beam with the 10-cm spiral ridge filter are plotted in the middle right panel of Figure 8. Notice that data from 2 replicate monolayer experiments show proximal and midpeak scatter for neon too; however, the isoeffect is somewhat flatter across the 10 cm of the extended peak. The OER values across the peak of this beam average about 2.1 to 2.3 and ranged from $2.3 \pm 0.2$ in the proximal peak to $1.6 \pm 0.1$ in the distal peak.

The lower left of Figure 8 presents the 570 MeV/amu argon OER values and physical and BED as a function of range. This beam is different from the others, because it shows that for the 4-cm filter design, the BED is quite similar to the physical dose, except that it is slightly less effective in the distal end of the peak. However, the normalized peak-to-plateau dose ratio is still quite advantageous (>1.5) in a narrower region straddling the physical proximal peak. This beam is also unique because of its extremely low OER, which averages about 1.4 across the entire width of the extended peak, including the preproximal and distal regions.

**TABLE 3.** Isoeffective Doses and RBEs of 6-cm SOBP for Gut Crypt Survivals After Fractionated Doses

| Position Within the SOBP | Isoeffective Dose (Gy)* | | RBE | | RBE Ratio (GSI/NIRS) |
| --- | --- | --- | --- | --- | --- |
| | GSI | NIRS | GSI | NIRS | |
| Proximal | $13.30 \pm 0.41$ | $13.70 \pm 0.54$ | $1.71 \pm 0.05$ | $1.66 \pm 0.07$ | $1.03 \pm 0.05$ |
| Middle | $11.68 \pm 0.15$ | $12.24 \pm 0.37$ | $1.95 \pm 0.03$ | $1.86 \pm 0.06$ | $1.05 \pm 0.04$ |
| Distal | $10.14 \pm 0.20$ | $9.89 \pm 0.17$ | $2.24 \pm 0.04$ | $2.30 \pm 0.3$ | $1.98 \pm 0.02$ |
| Cobalt-60 $\gamma$ rays | $22.75 \pm 0.19$ | | | | |

Values are mean $\pm$ SD.
*$D_{10}$ (dose required to reduce the number of crypts per circumferences to 30).
GSI, Gesellschaft für Schwerionenforschung; NIRS, National Institute of Radiological Sciences.
Adapted from Ref. 52, with permission from Elsevier.

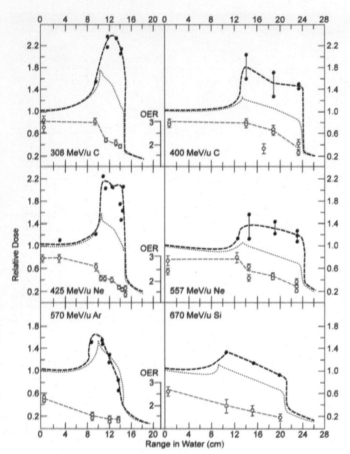

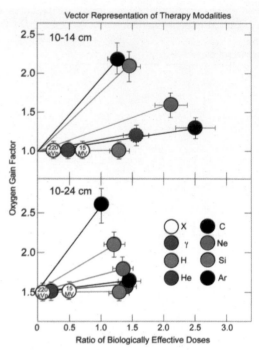

**FIGURE 8.** Physical Bragg ionization curves (dotted line) and biologically effective dose normalized to 1.0 at the beam entrance (●) and OER (○) as a function of range for heavy-ion beams with 4-cm extended Bragg peaks and a total depth of 14 cm, and with 10-cm extended Bragg peaks and a total depth of 21 to 24 cm. The biologic measurements of RBE and OER were made at the 50% survival levels. Adapted from Ref. 40, with permission from Elsevier.

**FIGURE 9.** Vector representation of low LET and high LET particle therapy modalities for treatment of a small, shallow field (upper panel), and a large, deep field (lower panel). Adapted from Ref. 40, with permission from Elsevier.

The lower right panel of Figure 8 presents data for a 670 MeV/amu silicon beam with a 10-cm filter. The results are similar to the 557 MeV/amu neon beam above except that the OER is generally lower than neon and closer to the values obtained with argon ions.

The 4-cm filter design seems to be adequate for the carbon and neon beams, but not for the argon beam. The BED distribution can be optimized for the argon beam by using a spiral ridge filter design with a much less sloped physical dose. The 10-cm filter design seems to slightly overcompensate for biologic killing at this level of biologically effect in the distal peak of the 400 MeV/amu carbon, 557 MeV/amu neon, and 670 MeV/amu silicon ion beams. The use of dual parallel-opposed fields with these extended beams can compensate for some of the lack of isoeffectiveness by smoothing the mixed LET field over the entire extended peak region.

## Comparison of the Beams

Evaluation of the therapeutic advantages of particle beams as described earlier, led to a comparison of each of the beams with other

available therapy modalities. By using the criterion of the oxygen gain factor (OGF), which is the ratio of the OER obtained with the reference low LET radiation source to the OER obtained with the high LET test beam, as an indicator of the high LET advantage, and the ratio of the peak to plateau BED values for cellular survival end points in vitro, a vector representation was constructed to compare the following radiations: low LET sources (γ- and x-rays), protons, helium, carbon, neon, silicon, and argon ion beams. These plots presented in Figure 9 were made to describe the treatment of 2 targets: a 10 × 10-cm field, 4-cm deep at 12-cm average tissue depth (upper panel), and a 10 × 10-cm field at 19-cm average tissue depth (lower panel). Particle beams were used with initial energies that yield approximately 14 cm (upper panel) or 21 to 24 cm (lower panel) for each particle species.

The most therapeutically advantageous positions on the figure are located closer to the upper right quadrant. For the smaller, more shallow target volume (upper panel of Fig. 9), it seems that 308 MeV/amu carbon is superior in the ratio of BED, with 425 MeV/amu neon, 530 MeV/amu silicon, and 570 MeV/amu argon falling off to BED ratios that are similar to protons. Conversely, argon (570 MeV/amu) and silicon (530 MeV/amu) have the best OGF advantages, with neon and carbon showing successively less OGF advantage. Helium ions and protons show an enhanced BED ratio but are most similar to the low LET radiations with respect to OGF, which results in their intermediate placement in the vector plot.

For larger, deeper tumor (lower panel of Fig. 9), the relative placement of each of the therapy modalities is altered, except for the location of the 187 MeV/amu proton and 225 MeV/amu helium data. At this range, the effects of 400 MeV/amu carbon and helium beams are quite similar. The 557 MeV/amu neon beam has a somewhat greater OGF advantage. The low LET modalities have deteriorated considerably in their effective dose ratio. The argon data (estimated for a 700 MeV/amu beam) and the 670 MeV/amu silicon data clearly have an advantageous OGF value even at the greater depth. A similar vector analysis was constructed by Raju[38] to compare radiotherapy modalities with somewhat similar conclusions.

Based on this comparison, the best BED ratio for situations corresponding to therapy needs can be obtained with accelerated carbon beams. All other heavy beams tested, as well as pions, are markedly better than the effective depth-dose ratios achievable with neutrons, x-rays, or γ-rays. A significant depression of the OER at the various depths required for therapy has been achieved with silicon and argon beams, which still retained advantageous BED ratios. The depression of the oxygen effect with silicon or argon ion beams is greater than that achievable with neutrons or pions, or with heavy ions of lower atomic number.

After the completion of this comparison, a significant validation of the results presented earlier was published by the Japanese and later the German programs, before the initiation of systematic and comprehensive clinical trials in each country with carbon ions.[56-62] It should be noted, however, that the Japanese program initially chose to adapt the Berkeley Laboratory approach to charged particle radiotherapy with beam delivery with passive particle beam delivery with fixed ridge filters, whereas the German program opted for active beam delivery with 3D scanned beams. In addition, the 2 programs selected different tumor sites to begin their treatments: the Japanese program treating a wide assortment of tumor sites, whereas the German program initially focused on head and neck tumors.

## PARTICLE TRACK STRUCTURE

Track structure is the spatial and temporal organization of atomic and molecular events that results from the interaction of charged particles with matter. In an accelerator, individual charged particles stripped of their electrons can be produced as ion beams at energies of several hundred MeV/amu having a range sufficient to penetrate a human body. At high energy, the tracks created by the ions in film emulsion reveal a dense, tight cross-sectional "core" caused largely by glancing collisions, and a "penumbra," which is due to energetic knock-on collisions. In contrast, at the stopping low energy range of the track, the cross-sectional track structure is limited to a tight core of ionization.[63] Chatterjee et al[64] have calculated the yield of different chemical species for aqueous systems in the core and penumbra, and the subsequent diffusion of free radical density distributions modifying the track structure with time. Different chemical species produced by the physical absorption of energy in aqueous materials results in biochemical changes in the absorbing material, such as DNA.[65]

Track structure models describe the relationship between the spatial distribution of energy deposition in the form of locations of ionization and excitation and the geometric structure of target molecules. Some of these theoretical models, such as the MOCA14[66,67] and PITS[68] codes, consider the stochastics of ion tracks in evaluating frequency distributions, but have been limited to dealing with maximum energies of 5 MeV/nucleon and have not been extended to high atomic number (Z) and energy (E) ions. A deterministic model of frequency distributions for total energy deposited in small volumes similar to DNA molecules from high energy ions of interest for cancer therapy and other applications has been developed.[69] This model predicts that at high energies, the lateral extension of an ion's track, denoted as the track width, will extend to several hundred micrometers or even a few millimeters due to δ-ray transport.

The concept of dose is significantly different for charged particles compared with conventional radiations due to enhanced biologic

effectiveness at high LET. One charged particle track depending on the particle atomic number and energy can deposit extremely high energy in a very small, discrete path along its track. This nonhomogeneous nature of particle radiations is in contrast with more homogenous photon radiation fields. This distribution of energy absorption feature of particles leads to clustered biologic damage.[70] Particle doses are, therefore, frequently expressed in terms of particle fluence (particle number per unit area per unit of time). Dose is a general term. More often the term "effective dose" is used. Dose fractionation reduces the effects of low-LET radiation, but it is less effective after high-LET radiation, and in some cases, an increased dose effect was observed with dose fractionation.[71] RBE values increase as the particle dose increases. However, a significant hypersensitivity at very low doses (<0.1 Gy) of 100 MeV/amu carbon ions has been reported with V79-4 Chinese hamster cells.[72] The implications of this hypersensitivity to the edge of carbon-ion treatment fields where the dose decreases significantly are currently unknown.

## Biophysical Modeling and Treatment Planning

Modeling of particle beam physics, biophysical responses, patient parameters including tumor and organ motion, beam delivery controls, and treatment planning are underway at most, if not all medical particle accelerators, using novel and some commercially available approaches. The importance of computer-assisted control of beam doses to patient tumors cannot be emphasized enough, because it is integral to patient safety and interinstitutional comparisons of patient outcome. Recent work to evaluate the clinical spatial resolution achievable with protons and heavier charged particles have suggested some reconsiderations may be appropriate due to inherent physical uncertainties.[73] Uncertainties in particle radiobiology are also an issue, and an area requiring intense further effort to optimize current empirical strategies for the future of individualized beam delivery. Lyman[54] used a linear-quadratic cell survival-based model to predict the biologically equivalent particle dose in concert with a beam model based on a computer program (BRAGG), that is used to calculate a Bragg curve of a heavy charged-particle beam. The Japanese program also used survival data for the spread out carbon Bragg peaks[57,74] calculated from the empirical data fitted by a linear-quadratic model with the parameters α and β for HSG tumor cells irradiated by monoenergetic carbon-ion beams[56] using an equation for mixed-beam radiation based on the theory of dual radiation action.[75,76] Recent microdosimetric measurements made with a spherical-walled tissue-equivalent proportional counter at various depths in a plastic phantom have been compared with the HSG survival data for photons, protons, helium, carbon, neon, silicon, and iron ions.[77] The estimated α terms of the linear-quadratic model with a fixed β value reproduced the experimental results for cell irradiation for ion beams with LETs of less than 450 keV/μm, except in the region near the distal peak.

The German carbon ion program developed a novel local effect model (LEM) to convolute the nonhomogenous dose distribution in the particle track with the nonlinear photon dose effect curve.[78] With this procedure, the effects of the particle can be calculated on the basis of the photon dose effect curve. The main biologic parameter of the calculation is the shape (shoulder) of the photon dose effect curve, eg, the α/β ratio. The LEM calculations yield good agreement with experimental data and show that large RBE values are correlated to small α/β values and vice versa. A series of incremental improvements have been added to the LEM.[79-86]

## LATE TISSUE EFFECTS

It is impossible in this short review to cover comprehensively the several decades of additional proton and carbon radiobiology studies over and above RBE and OER that have been published (e.g., see Failla memorial lecture by C.A. Tobias[86a]). This includes studies in differences in molecular damage to DNA, cell cycle effects, dose fractionation/repair, increased sensitivity of radioresistant cell lines, and enhanced cell transformation. For example, results from some of these studies have led to implementation of hypofractionation with carbon ions.

Dosimetry studies on external beam radiation treatment with respect to second cancer induction have been comprehensively reviewed.[87] However, the data for induction of cancer in humans by protons or heavy ions is insufficient for the estimation of cancer risks.[87a] Because of this important issue of clinical concern for particle radiotherapy, we briefly describe here 3 normal tissues that have been studied in the laboratory to evaluate tissue effects with particles, skin, harderian gland, and mammary gland.

## Skin

Decades of clinical experience with skin responses to conventional radiotherapy have led to a significant understanding of radiation-induced skin damage and the need for dose sparing for cosmesis. Recent irradiation studies with full-thickness human skin biopsy specimens obtained from cosmetic surgery have irradiated specimens with low doses of x-rays down to 10 mGy[88] demonstrated that molecular changes were associated with the radiation response of skin. Gene expression changes in 5 core regulatory genes were assessed by real-time radiotherapy polymerase chain reaction (PCR) on human skin biopsies, and the results showed that low doses of radiation can produce changes in gene expression, although time- and dose-response relationships may be complex.

There are several concepts regarding early skin changes due to particle radiation exposures in space that have relevance for clinical radiotherapy with ion beams. It is anticipated that spacecraft shielding will prevent erythema and desquamation; however, subclinical changes could predispose an individual to delayed wound healing. Mouse skin studies with low doses of iron ion beams investigating effects on laminin immunoreactivity have shown[89] that 1 hour after exposure to 1 GeV/amu iron ions over the dose range of 0.03 to 1.6 Gy, neither the visual appearance nor the mean pixel intensity of laminin in the basement membrane was altered compared with sham-irradiated tissue. However, the mean pixel intensity of laminin immmunoreactivity using several different antibodies was significantly decreased in epidermal basement membrane at 48 and 96 hours after exposure to 0.8 Gy of iron ions. In contrast, collagen type IV, another component of the basement membrane, was unaffected. These studies demonstrate quantitatively that densely ionizing radiation elicits changes in skin microenvironments distinct from those induced by sparsely ionizing radiation.

There is a significant literature on the early skin reactions of rodents to single and fractionated doses of various individual charged particle beams because of its importance in preclinical studies for heavy charged particle radiotherapy.[90–94] Skin RBE values for single dose fractions were 1.3 for helium peak ions, 1.5 for carbon peak ions, 1.7 for neon peak ions, and 1.9 for argon ions Human skin reactions were also scored in pilot studies with helium, carbon, or neon ions[95] and compared with an earlier analysis of RBE relative to dose per fraction.[96] The results indicated that skin reactions to stopping 400 MeV/amu neon ions were comparable with fission neutron skin reactions for human, rat, pig, and mouse skin.

Particle beam induction of rat skin tumors has been investigated.[97–100] Results from studies examining the induction of malignant and benign skin tumors at 1 year after exposure to 56Fe, 20Ne, or 40Ar show that differences in tumor yield as a function of

dose and time is dependent on the particle beam used. The effect of the 250 ppm dietary vitamin A-acetate on tumor induction was equivalent to lowering the 56Fe LET effect to approximately that of neon ions. The antioxidant vitamins served as a countermeasure to the tumor induction, and this result is consistent with reports of vitamin mitigation of both UV-[101] and radiation-induced cataract.[102] The yield of skin fibromas as a function of time for a single 3 Gy fraction of 56Fe ion radiation versus 4 fractions of the same radiation, and total absorbed dose delivered over a 10 days interval (a minimum of 2 days between fractions) has also shown that there are no significant differences in the single or fractionated dose regimen.

## Harderian Gland

For a long time, the murine Harderian gland model and the rat skin[97] provided the only experimental animal radiation-induced tumor data in vivo available allowing a comparison of the effects of different particle beams. The Harderian gland lies behind the murine eye, but it is not present in humans.[103] reported RBE values of ~30 for induction of Harderian gland tumors by argon and iron ion beams, and lower RBE values with radiation beams of lower LET[104] extended the study to include protons, niobium, and lanthanum ions, as well as iron, neon and helium ions and 60Co photons, extending the LET values up to 953 keV/$\mu$m. The results indicated that the RBE-LET relationship did indeed reach a plateau at ~100 to 200 keV/$\mu$m, and unlike the data for cell killing and mutations, did not decrease steeply at higher-LET values. An analysis of the Harderian tumor data using particle fluence rather than dose allowed a calculation of a risk coefficient that is a monotonic function of LET for the particles studied.[105] It was suggested that fluence-based risk coefficients for estimating the risk of cancer from exposure to radiations in space be used. This concept of a risk cross section or risk per particle fluence was further examined by Curtis who derived human cancer risk cross sections for low-LET radiation from the data with this approach from the atomic-bomb survivors.[106] Both the fluence-based and microdosimetry event-based methodologies provide a way of dealing with the major objection to the conventional system: using LET alone as a universal physical descriptor of the radiation field to determine the biologic effect. The fluence-based system allows for different values of the risk cross section for different particle types that have the same LET. This work led to National Council for Radiation Protection and Measurements Report No. 137,[107] which compared the conventional method of estimating risk from a mixed radiation field of high- and low-LET components with fluence- and event-related methodologies, using risk cross section and a specific quality function. The result of the analysis where each of the approaches was applied to the same idealized shielding situation in space revealed that under the specified conditions, the differences in the risk calculated by each method was less than a factor of two. In this National Council for Radiation Protection and Measurements Report, it was concluded that when more fluence-based data are available and dosimetric techniques are refined, then the approach should be revisited, but at this time, radiation risk estimates and radiation protection for work in space should continue to be based on the concepts of absorbed dose, quality factor, and dose equivalent.

## Mammary Gland

The risk of mammary carcinomas in a Sprague-Dawley rat model irradiated whole body with energetic iron ions, photons, or iron ions and photons at 60 days of age and followed to death in a series of 3 studies have been investigated by Dicello et al.[108] The animals were continuously monitored for all disease and effects from the radiations and major tissues and tumors were archived. In the second part of the study reported separately, half of all animals were given Tamoxifen to investigate the potential of this drug that is known to reduce the risk of mammary carcinomas. Results from the first completed study illustrates cumulative excess lifetime incidence of mammary tumors (both adenocarcinomas and benign fibroadenomas) as function of dose for photon-, proton- and iron-irradiated rats. The data suggest that iron ions are more efficient in inducing mammary tumors at lower doses in a nearly linear response up to 0.5 Gy with decreasing effects at higher doses and reaching a maximum value nearly the same as that observed for animals irradiated with photons or protons. The curves for all 3 irradiated populations level at ~30% excess incidence but in a different dose-dependent manner. Because of the high natural incidence of breast cancer in this animal model, the reduced slope of higher doses for iron-irradiated animals is associated with the reduced population at risk, and the increased risk of other lethal diseases was noted. Protons (250 MeV) were also apparently more effective than $^{60}$Co $\gamma$-rays.

## Second Primary Malignancies

With increasing efficacy in oncological treatments resulting in increased number of long-term survivors, follow-up on second primary malignancies (SPM) and treatments is emerging as a main concern in radiotherapy and chemotherapy. Factors that contribute to SPM include age at exposure, tissue or organ specificity, dose, dose per fraction, dose rate. In a recent review, Tubiana[109] not only analyzed and interpreted results obtained from patients after their initial treatments but also evaluated whether SPMs could be prevented either by improving the dose distribution in normal tissues or by reducing the dose per fraction and the dose rate. Similar studies with protons or carbon ions need to be completed to address these issues.

## AREAS OF CURRENT RESEARCH

## Investigating Molecular Mechanisms of Action

Although particle therapy has demonstrated advantages when compared with the more traditional radiotherapy modalities, the mechanisms underlying this increased efficacy are still not clearly understood. Tumor cells can die by several mechanisms that global RBE measurements for cell inactivation do not delineate. Modes of death such as apoptosis, mitotic catastrophe,[110] autophagy,[111] or necrotic death are now emerging as prevalent to different degrees in various tumors. High-grade gliomas (HGG) have a poor outcome; however, it was recently demonstrated that the main response of HGG to therapy is autophagic death, despite the fact that autophagy is defective in HGG.[112] There may well be a LET-dependence for the underlying gene expression that leads to each of these various modes of death. The molecular basis of high-LET charged particle radiotherapy is definitely emerging to reveal some striking differences with the molecular basis of conventional radiotherapies. Summarized below are mechanistic studies on normal and tumor human cells in vitro, and work ongoing in murine systems in vivo.

## In Vitro Normal Human Cells

The regulation of protein expression of 2 cell cycle regulators, TP53 and CDKN1A (p21/CIP1/WAF1), in normal human fibroblasts after exposure to x-rays and carbon, xenon, bismuth, and uranium ions in normal human fibroblasts over a period of up to 24 hours after radiation exposure showed transient dose- and LET-dependent accumulation of TP53 protein. Conversely, CDKN1A levels increased and peaked at 3 to 6 hours after exposure with persisting level of this protein at 24 hours strongly dependent on the dose and the LET for x-rays and carbon ions. No further increase in CDKN1A expression was

observed at very high LET.[113] Further, strikingly similar patterns of protein clusters were generated for p21, PCNA, H2AX, and MRE11B (hMre11) in the normal fibroblasts after exposure low energy bismuth to carbon ions covering a spectrum of LETs ranging from about 300 to 13,600 keV/$\mu$m. These results suggest that additional factors, including chromatin compaction, may pay a role in the clustering of proteins in response to particle radiation exposure.[114]

Molecular changes in normal cultured differentiating human lens epithelial cells exposed to high-energy accelerated iron-ion beams as well as to protons and x-rays showed that transcription and translation of *CDKN1A* are both temporally regulated after a single 4-Gy radiation doses. Furthermore, qualitative differences in the distribution of CDKN1A immunofluorescence signals after exposure to x-rays, protons or iron ions, suggesting that LET effects likely play a role in the misregulation of gene function in these cells.[115]

## In Vitro Human Cancer Cell Line Studies

A mutation in the *TP53* is associated with radioresistance in many cancer cell lines. Iwadate et al[116] performed experiments using 2 human glioma cell lines expressing wild-type *TP53* (U-87 and U-138) and 2 expressing mutant *TP53* (U-251 and U-373), and compared the effectiveness of 290 MeV/amu carbon ions and x-rays. He found that the carbon radiation was more cytotoxic against glioma cells than x-rays. The effects of the carbon beams were not dependent on the *TP53* status but were reduced by G1 arrest, which was independent of the *p21* expression. The expression of *BAX* remained unchanged in all 4 cell lines. These results indicated that high LET carbon ions can induce cell death in glioma cells more effectively than x-rays, and that other than *p53*-dependent apoptosis may participate in the cytotoxicity of carbon ions.

Comparisons have been made between human glioma cell lines with normal human fibroblasts to determine the different modes of cell inactivation after either $\gamma$-ray or 20, 40, or 80 keV/$\mu$m carbon ion irradiation.[117] Tsuboi et al in 2007 defined radiation cell death as apoptosis (type I cell death), autophagic (type II cell death), or necrosis (type III cell death).[117] Carbon ions reduced the reproductive potency of all glioma cells in an LET-dependent way to identical levels despite their different $\gamma$-ray radiosensitivities. A *p53*-wild-type glioma cell line (U87MG) demonstrated a higher yield of apoptosis than other cell lines, whereas fibroblasts hardly displayed any cell death, indicating senescence-like growth arrest even after high-LET irradiation. A *p53*-mutant tumor cell line (TK1) demonstrated very low yield of cell death with prominent G2/M arrest. Results of radiosensitivity differ according to what mode of cell inactivation is selected. Although fibroblasts depend on G1 block after ionizing radiation, G2/M blocks may play crucial roles in the radioresistance of *p53*-mutant glioma cells.

Bcl-2 is an antiapoptotic protein that is frequently overexpressed in 30% to 50% of tumors, and overexpression is associated with radioresistance. To determine whether overexpression of Bcl-2 in tumor cells contributes to the radioresistance in human cancers, Hamada et al[118] constructed a Bcl-2-overexpressing HeLa cell and compared the sensitivity of these cells compared with the control neo cells with low LET $\gamma$-rays and high LET helium, and 2 different energies of both carbon and neon ions. Their results provide evidence that particle radiation at the appropriate LET enhances the apoptotic response while prolonging G2/M arrest, resulting in reducing the survival of radioresistant tumors that overexpress Bcl-2. By using human hepatoma SMMC-7721 cells, Ma et al[119] demonstrated that apoptosis rate is correlated with the expression of STAT-3, a signal transducer and activator of transcription, in these cells after either x-ray or C-ions.

PCR-loss of heterozygosity analysis of 6 highly informative microsatellite markers on chromosome 17 from 4 head and neck cancer cell lines after x-ray and carbon ion exposure showed characteristic differences between the DNA structural damage after the x-rays or carbon ions. Most of the x-ray damage occurred in the target region on one of the homologous chromosomes, whereas carbon ion beams caused deletions of the counterparts in both homologous chromosomes.[120]

Several gene expression studies using the Affymetrix Gene chip analysis have compared changes in gene expression in a number of different tumor oral squamous cancer cell lines (OSCC) after either x-rays or SOBP 290 MeV/n carbon ions (LET = 78 keV/$\mu$m). Among 98 genes with significantly altered gene expression levels after irradiation, the validated up-regulation of *SPHK1* was identified to be dose-responsive and temporally responsive to carbon ion, but to a much lesser extent to x-rays.[121] *SPHK1* is a kinase that modulates cell growth and controls of proliferation. *SPHK1* is overexpressed in a variety of solid tumors, including breast, stomach, ovary, kidney, and lung, compared with normal tissues in the same individual. In chemotherapy, up-regulation of *SPHK1/S1P* pathway plays a crucial role in the resistance of prostate cancer cells, whereas inhibition of *SPHK1* triggers apoptosis of cancer cells. The question of how significant up-regulation of *SPHK1* after carbon ions is when compared with x-rays or how it alters the radiosensitivity of the OSCC remains to be answered.

Additional studies comparing alterations of gene expression querying over 18,400 transcripts and variants in OSCC samples after 1, 4, or 7 Gy of 290 MeV/amu carbon or 400 MeV/n neon identified 84 genes that were uniquely differentially expressed after heavy ions but not substantially altered by x-ray.[122] Network and gene ontology analysis using the ingenuity pathway analysis software revealed that 60 of the 84 candidate genes were mapped to 4 functional genetic networks that included genes associated with cell death, cell cycle, cancer, and transforming growth factor (TGF)-$\beta$ signaling. Quantitative PCR validation of 5 selected genes, 3 associated with TGF-$\beta$ signaling pathway (TGF-$\beta$ receptor 2, E3 ubiquitin ligase, bone morphogenic protein 7) and 2 associated with cell cycle: G1/S checkpoint regulation (Cyclin D1 and E2F transcription factor 3) showed that, indeed, the altered expression of these genes were specific only to carbon and neon ions but were not affected after x-rays.

Differential gene array analysis of 6 human malignant melanoma cell lines after carbon ion exposure using a single color microarray (CodeLink Human Whole Genome Bioarraym, GE Healthcare Biosciences Corp) identified 22 genes that were uniquely responsive to carbon ions in all 6 cell lines.[123] Of these, 19 were temporally down-regulated between 1 and 3 hours after radiation and consists of genes that are related to cell cycle progression, cell proliferation, cell death, and cell communication. In contrast, up-regulated genes are found to respond to both carbon and x-ray and include many tumor protein p53 target genes. These findings suggest that the suppression of cell cycle-related genes with the prolongation of G2/M arrest may contribute to the sensitivity of melanoma cell lines to carbon beams, and that radiation-induced *p53*-related genes may play contribute to cellular sensitivity to both C-ions and x-rays.

### Murine In Vivo Studies

Several studies using murine tumor models addressed the impact of tumor microenvironment on alterations in gene expression profiles. Imadome et al[124] reported that the level of expression of stress-responsive and cell-communication genes was up-regulated in 4 mouse tumors (NR-S1, SCCVII, NFSa and 8520) transplanted into the hind limb of C3H/HeNrs mice after a single C-ion exposure. C-ion ir-

radiation resulted in significant changes in expression of genes known to be related to radiation-induced tumor regression. Gene Ontology results further showed that the main genes categories associated with C-ion responses included stress responses to endogenous stimulus or defense response or death, cell communication, and cell cycle genes. Stress-related molecules, such as *Cdkn1a* and *Mgmt*, are involved in cell fate signal transduction pathways and are known to play a role in DNA repair, cell cycle, and death. Another stress responsive gene (eg, *Polk*), that is a member of the DNA polymerase family, has been shown to be involved in the translation of different types of DNA damage. *MAP-kinase* and *Fas*-associated death domain genes (*MADD* and *FADD*) are adaptor proteins in cell death signaling. All together, such up-regulated expression of these genes suggests that C-ions induced abundant unrepaired damage and could potentially affect cell fate. In addition, up-regulated expression of proinflammatory genes such as the *Ikbke/IKKi/IKKe*, a key integrator of signaling induced by proinflammatory stimuli and a functional coordinator between C/EBP and NFkb pathways, other immune-related genes, such as interleukins and chemokines, and *ICAM1*, adhesion molecule associated with the activation of cytotoxic T-lymphocytes suggest increased immunogenicity of tumors. These findings were supported by histologic evaluation of tumor slices indicating abundant infiltration of inflammatory cells after exposure to C-ions.

The novel proangiogenic factor Ephrin-A1 has been reported to contribute to radioresistance to C-ions and $\gamma$-rays in murine tumors.[125] By using the single color oligo microarray system with 44,000 mouse sequences, differential gene expression from tumors derived from irradiated animals previously transplanted with either the NR-S1 or SCCVII squamous cell carcinoma cells. Parallel tumor growth delay measurements postirradiation indicated that tumors derived from NR-S1 are resistant to both $\gamma$-rays and C-ion beam. Four genes, *ephrin A1 (Efna1)*, *small proline-rich protein 1A (Sprr1a)*, *SLIT-ROBO Rho GTPase activating protein 3 (Srgap3)*, and *RIKEN 2 day neonate thymus thymic cells cDNA clone E430023D08 3′ (Xrra1)* were differential expressed in NR-S1 and SCCVII tumors after irradiation. Immunohistochemical analysis of tissue sections confirmed that *Ephrin-A1* was not expressed in either tumor before irradiation but stained strongly positive in NR-S1 cells 1 day after C-ions but not in SCCVII cells, along with significant increase in microvascular density and up-regulation of vascular endothelial growth factor expression, suggesting that radiation-induced changes in gene expression related to angiogenesis have the potential of modulating the tumor microenvironment, thereby affecting responsiveness to radiation treatment.

### Microbeams

Charged particle microbeam facilities are operating, and new ones are being built to investigate a number of unanswered scientific questions, most notably centered on nontargeted effects of radiation. The classic paradigm in radiation biology asserts that all radiation effects on living materials are due to the direct action of radiation on living tissue, and it assumes the validity of linear extrapolation of high dose effects to predict the effects at lower doses. Microbeams are powerful tools because they allow the discrete targeting of dose and identification of untargeted regions in 2-dimensional or 3-dimensional biologic model systems as a function of dose and with the use of various forms of microscopy, allow a reinspection with time after exposure to elucidate mechanisms. The x-ray and charged particle microbeams have confirmed novel nontargeted effects in bystander cells deduced from other less direct methods and have confirmed adaptive responses to high dose in systems preirradiated with low doses of radiation.[126–129] Currently, there is experimental agreement for cell cycle effects in heavy ion bystander cells, demonstrating transient inhibition of the cell cycle progression as reflected by the induction of cell cycle inhibiting proteins, and an enhancement of apoptosis and reduction of clonogenic survival in human and rodent bystander cells. However, conflicting evidence exists in normal cell studies with regard to the induction of DNA or cytogenetic damage in heavy ion bystander cells[130] (http://www.njp.org/). Overall, the most significant finding supported by the majority of the heavy ion studies available to date is that in contrast to many direct effects, bystander cells do not seem to be enhanced with increasing LET.[130] The observation that there is not an increased RBE for bystander effects at high LET could be important to clinical situations with charged particles.

## SUMMARY

The early radiobiology of accelerated charged particles from protons up to argon ions that have been under consideration for clinical applications clearly demonstrated that the enhanced biologic effects exceeded the advantageous depth-physical dose profile of the Bragg peak. The biologic effects of the dense high-LET particle tracks traversing DNA, cells, and tissues at the end of their range yielded both quantitative and qualitative differences compared with radiation effects from low-LET x-ray and $\gamma$-rays. Testing particle radiations with greater atomic numbers and concomitant increasingly higher LET in the stopping distal Bragg peak demonstrated that the biologic effectiveness reached a maximum and then declined, suggesting that ion beams heavier than carbon or neon were less optimal.

During this time of emerging particle radiobiology, the technical landscape in radiation oncology was also evolving with 3D-conformal treatment clearly becoming the accepted goal, and patient imaging methods increasing resolution capabilities. The complex issues of individual patient tumor geometries and locations near critical tissues in the human body has led to an appropriate current use of protons or helium ions for some clinical treatments where precision and critical structures may be involved, especially in pediatric cases, whereas carbon ions are recognized as the best choice for other clinical situations, notably radioresistant tumors. This article briefly reviews the radiobiological history behind the consideration of various charged particles for radiotherapy.

With the advent of fluorescent microscopy and highly specific antibodies, imaging of particle radiobiological effects on cells have elucidated new information regarding underlying mechanisms of damage and repair in the early time course after particle exposures. Particle microbeams are evaluating low dose effects adjacent to high dose profiles. New genomic and proteomic tools have revealed specific gene and protein networks associated with low- or high-LET radiation effects. Beam scanning capabilities have heightened the need for computer control of beam energies, particle fluence, and precise tissue-specific radiobiological responses. Continued research is still needed for improvements in theoretical models of beam physics, delivery options, and biologic parameters of acute and late tissue response as these will also be essential to future institutional comparisons of patient outcome.

## REFERENCES

1. Rutherford E, Chadwick J, and Ellis CD. *Radiations From Radioactive Substances.* Cambridge: University Press; 1930.
2. Hall E. Protons for radiotherapy: a 1946 proposal. *Lancet Oncol.* 2009;10:196.
3. Welsh JS. Basics of particle therapy: introduction to hadrons. *Am J Clin Oncol.* 2008;31:493–495.
4. Weinburg S. A model of leptons. *Phys Rev Lett.* 1967;19:1264–1266.
5. Ashikawa JK, Sondhaus CA, Tobias CA, et al. Acute effects of high-energy protons and alpha particles in mice. *Radiat Res.* 1967;7:312–324.
6. Hall EJ, Kellerer AM, Rossi HH, et al. The relative biological effectiveness of 160 MeV protons. II. Biological data and their interpretation in terms of microdosimetry. *Int J Radiat Oncol Biol Phys.* 1978;4:1009–1013.
7. Raju MR, Amols HI, Bain E, et al. A heavy particle comparative study. Part III: OER and RBE. *Br J Radiol.* 1978;51:712–719.
8. Raju MR, Amols HI, Dicello JF, et al. A heavy particle comparative study. Part I: depth-dose distributions. *Br J Radiol.* 1978;51:699–703.
9. Raju MR, Bain E, Carpenter SG, et al. A heavy particle comparative study. Part II: cell survival versus depth. *Br J Radiol.* 1978;51:704–711.
10. Raju MR, Carpenter SG. A heavy particle comparative study. Part IV: acute and late reactions. *Br J Radiol.* 1978;51:720–727.
11. Robertson JB, Williams JR, Schmidt RA, et al. Radiobiological studies of a high-energy modulated proton beam utilizing cultured mammalian cells. *Cancer.* 1975;35:1664–1677.
12. Tepper J, Verhey L, Goitein M, et al. In vivo determinations of RBE in a high energy modulated proton beam using normal tissue reactions and fractionated dose schedules. *Int J Radiat Oncol Biol Phys.* 1977;2:1115–1122.
13. Tobias CA, Anger HO, Lawrence JH. Radiological use of high energy deuterons and alpha particles. *Am J Roentgenol Radium Ther Nucl Med.* 1952;67:1–27.
14. Falkmer S, Larsson B, Stenson S. Effects of single dose proton irradiation of normal skin and Vx2 carcinoma in rabbit ears: a comparative investigation with protons and roentgen rays. *Acta radiol.* 1959;52:217–234.
15. Larsson B. Blood vessel changes following local irradiation of the brain with high-energy protons. *Acta Soc Med Ups.* 1960;65:51–71.
16. Larsson B, Graffman S, Jung B. Fixation of carbon-11 in the cells of proton-irradiated blood. *Nature.* 1965;207:543–544.
17. Stenson S. Weight change and mortality of rats after abdominal proton and roentgen irradiation. A comparative investigation. *Acta Radiol Ther Phys Biol.* 1969;8:423–432.
18. Stenson S. Effects of proton and roentgen radiation on the rectum of the rat. *Acta Radiol Ther Phys Biol.* 1969;8:263–278.
19. Ueno Y, Grigoriev YG. The RBE of protons with energy greater than 126 MeV. *Br J Radiol.* 1969;42:475.
20. Wainson AA, Lomanov MF, Shmakova NL, et al. The RBE of accelerated protons in different parts of the Bragg curve. *Br J Radiol.* 1972;45:525–529.
21. Sayeg JA, Birge AC, Beam CA, et al. The effects of accelerated carbon nuclei and other radiations on the survival of haploid yeast. II. Biological experiments. *Radiat Res.* 1959;10:449–461.
22. Tobias CA, Todd PW. Heavy charged particles in cancer therapy. *Natl Cancer Inst Monogr.* 1967;24:1–21.
23. Tobias CA, Lyman JT, Chatterjee A, et al. Radiological physics characteristics of the extracted heavy ion beams of the bevatron. *Science.* 1971;174:1131–1134.
24. Tobias CA, Lyman JT, Lawrence JH. Some considerations of physical and biological factors in radiotherapy with high-LET radiations including heavy particles, pi mesons, and fast neutrons. *Prog At Med.* 1971;3:167–218.
25. Tobias CA. Pretherapeutic investigations with accelerated heavy ions. *Radiology.* 1973;108:145–158.
26. White MG, Isaila M, Prelec K, et al. Acceleration of nitrogen ions to 7.4 Gev in the Princeton Particle accelerator. *Science.* 1971;174:1121–1123.
27. Grunder HA, Hartsough WD, Lofgren EJ. Acceleration of heavy ions at the Bevatron. *Science.* 1971;174:1128–1129.
28. Ghiorso A, Grunder H, Hartsough W, et al. The bevalac: an economical facility for very high energetic heavy particle research. *IEEE Trans Nucl Sci NS.* 1973;20:155.
29. Tobias CA, Tobias I. *People and Particles.* San Francisco: San Francisco Press Inc.; 1997.
30. Llacer J, Schmidt JB, Tobias CA. Characterization of fragmented heavy-ion beams using a three-stage telescope detector: detector configuration and instrumentation. *Med Phys.* 1990;17:158–162.
31. Llacer J, Schmidt JB, Tobias CA. Characterization of fragmented heavy-ion beams using a three-stage telescope detector: measurements of 670-MeV/amu 20Ne beams. *Med Phys.* 1990;17:151–157.
32. Castro JR, Petti PL, Daftari IK, et al. Clinical gain from improved beam delivery systems. *Radiat Environ Biophys.* 1992;31:233–240.
33. Ludewigt B. Beam spreading methods. In: Linz U, Chapman J, Hall E, eds. *Ion Beams in Tumor Therapy.* Weinbheim, Germany: Chapman and Hall; 1995.
34. Renner TR, Chu WT. Wobbler facility for biomedical experiments. *Med Phys.* 1987;14:825–834.
35. ICRU. *International Commission on Radiation Units and Measurements.* North Carolina: Oxford University Press; 1986.
36. IAEA/ICRU. *Relative Biological Effectiveness in Ion Beam Therapy.* 2008; TRS 461.

37. Linz U, ed. *Ion Beams in Tumor Therapy.* Weinheim: Chapman and Hall; 1995.
38. Raju MR. *Heavy-Particle Radiotherapy.* New York: Academic Press; 1980.
39. Skarsgard L, ed. *Pion and Heavy Ion Radiotherapy.* Amsterdam: Elsevier Biomedical; 1983.
40. Blakely EA, Ngo FQH, Curtis SB, et al. Heavy-ion radiobiology: cellular studies. *Adv Radiat Biol.* 1984;11:195–389.
41. Leith JT, Ainsworth J, Alpen E. Heavy ion radiobiology: normal tissue studies. *Adv Radiat Biol.* 1983;10:191.
42. Belli M, Cera F, Cherubini R, et al. Inactivation and mutation induction in V79 cells by low energy protons: re-evaluation of the results at the LNL facility. *Int J Radiat Biol.* 1993;63:331–337.
43. Wambersie A, Hendry JH, Andreo P, et al. The RBE issues in ion-beam therapy: conclusions of a joint IAEA/ICRU working group regarding quantities and units. *Radiat Prot Dosimetry.* 2006;122:463–470.
44. Paganetti H, Niemierko A, Ancukiewicz M, et al. Relative biological effectiveness (RBE) values for proton beam therapy. *Int J Radiat Oncol Biol Phys.* 2002;53:407–421.
45. Paganetti H. Significance and implementation of RBE variations in proton beam therapy. *Technol Cancer Res Treat.* 2003;2:413 426.
46. Gerweck LE, Kozin SV. Relative biological effectiveness of proton beams in clinical therapy. *Radiother Oncol.* 1999;50:135–142.
47. Tilly N, Johansson J, Isacsson U, et al. The influence of RBE variations in a clinical proton treatment plan for a hypopharynx cancer. *Phys Med Biol.* 2005;50:2765–2777.
48. Paganetti H. Interpretation of proton relative biological effectiveness using lesion induction, lesion repair, and cellular dose distribution. *Med Phys.* 2005;32:2548–2556.
49. Curtis SB. Lethal and potentially lethal lesions induced by radiation—a unified repair model. *Radiat Res.* 1986;106:252–270.
50. Dicello JF. Absorption characteristics of protons and photons in tissue. *Technol Cancer Res Treat.* 2007;6(4 Suppl):25–29.
51. Endo S, Takada M, Onizuka Y, et al. Microdosimetric evaluation of secondary particles in a phantom produced by carbon 290 MeV/nucleon ions at HIMAC. *J Radiat Res (Tokyo).* 2007;48:397–406.
52. Uzawa A, Ando K, Koike S, et al. Comparison of biological effectiveness of carbon-ion beams in Japan and Germany. *Int J Radiat Oncol Biol Phys.* 2009;73:1545–1551.
53. Deleted in proof.
54. Lyman JT. Computer modeling of heavy charged-particle beams. In: LD Skarsgard, ed. *Pion and Heavy Ion Radiotherapy: Preclinical and Clinical Studies.* Amsterdam: Elsevier; 1983:139–148.
55. Tobias CA, Blakely EA, Ngo FQH, et al. The repair-misrepair model of cell survival. In: Meyn RE, Withers HR, eds. *Radiation Biology and Cancer.* New York: Raven; 1980:195–230.
56. Furusawa Y, Fukutsu K, Aoki M, et al. Inactivation of aerobic and hypoxic cells from three different cell lines by accelerated (3)He-, (12)C- and (20)Ne-ion beams. *Radiat Res.* 2000;154:485–496.
57. Kanai T, Endo M, Minohara S, et al. Biophysical characteristics of HIMAC clinical irradiation system for heavy-ion radiation therapy. *Int J Radiat Oncol Biol Phys.* 1999;44:201–210.
58. Kraft G. Tumor therapy with heavy charged particles. *Prog Particle Nuclear Phys.* 2000;45:S473–S544.
59. Kraft G, Scholz M, Bechthold U. Tumor therapy and track structure. *Radiat Environ Biophys.* 1999;38:229–237.
60. Weyrather WK, Debus J. Particle beams for cancer therapy. *Clin Oncol.* 2003;15:S23–S28.
61. Weyrather WK, Kraft G. RBE of carbon ions: experimental data and the strategy of RBE calculation for treatment planning. *Radiother Oncol.* 2004;73(Suppl 2):S161–S169.
62. Weyrather WK, Ritter S, Scholz M, et al. RBE for carbon track-segment irradiation in cell lines of differing repair capacity. *Int J Radiat Biol.* 1999;75:1357–1364.
63. Tobias CA, et al. Tracks in Condensed Systems. Proceedings Sixth International Congress of Radiation Research. In: 6th International Congress of Radiation Research. Tokyo, Japan: Japanese Association for Radaition Research; 1979.
64. Chatterjee A, Maccabee HD, Tobias CA. Radial cutoff LET and radial cutoff dose calculations for heavy charged particles in water. *Radiat Res.* 1973;54:479–494.
65. Chatterjee A, Holly WR. Computer simulation of initial events in the biochemical mechanisms of DNA damage. *Adv Radiat Biol.* 1993;17:181–226.
66. Wilson W, Toburen LH, Miller JH, et al. Cross sections used in proton track simulations. In: Workshop on Electronic and Ionic Collision Cross Sections needed in the modeling of Radiation Interactions with Matter. Argonne, IL: Argonne National Laboratory; 1984.

67. Charlton DE, Goodhead DT, Wilson WE, et al. Energy deposition in cylindrical volumes; 1) protons energy 0.3–4.0 < V, 2) Alpha particle energy 1.0 MeV to 20.0 MeV. In: Monograph 85/1. Chilton, UK: MRC Radiobiology Unit; 1985.
68. Wilson WE, Miller JH, Nikjpoo H. PITTS: a code for positive ion track structure. In: Varma MN, Chatterjee A, eds.*Computational Approaches in Molecular Biology—Monte Carlo Methods.* New York: Plenum Press; 1993.
69. Cucinotta FA, Nikjoo H, Goodhead DT. Model for radial dependence of frequency distributions for energy imparted in nanometer volumes from HZE particles. *Radiat Res.* 2000;153:459–468.
70. Chatterjee A, Holley WR. Biochemical mechanisms and clusters of damage for high-LET radiation. *Adv Space Res.* 1992;12:33–43.
71. Ngo FQH. Effects on mammalian cells of fractionated heavy-ion doses. In: L. Skarsgard, ed. *Pion and Heavy-Ion Radiotherapy: Preclinical and Clinical Studies.* New York: Elsevier Science Publishing; 1982.
72. Bohrnsen G, Weber KJ, Scholz M. Measurement of biological effects of high-energy carbon ions at low doses using a semi-automated cell detection system. *Int J Radiat Biol.* 2002;78:259–266.
73. Andreo P. On the clinical spatial resolution achievable with protons and heavier charged particle radiotherapy beams. *Phys Med Biol.* 2009;54:N205–N215.
74. Kanai T, Furusawa Y, Fukutsu K, et al. Irradiation of mixed beam and design of spread-out Bragg peak for heavy-ion radiotherapy. *Radiat Res.* 1997;147:78–85.
75. Kellerer AM, Rossi HH. A generalized formation of dual radiation action. *Radiat Res.* 1978;75:471–488.
76. Zaider M, Rossi HH. The synergistic effects of different radiations. *Radiat Res.* 1980;83:732–739.
77. Kase Y, Kanai T, Matsumoto Y, et al. Microdosimetric measurements and estimation of human cell survival for heavy-ion beams. *Radiat Res.* 2006;166:629–638.
78. Scholz M, Kraft G. The physical and radiobiological basis of the local effect model: a response to the commentary by R. Katz. *Radiat Res.* 2004;161:612–620.
79. Combs SE, Bohl J, Elsässer T, et al. Radiobiological evaluation and correlation with the local effect model (LEM) of carbon ion radiation therapy and temozolomide in glioblastoma cell lines. *Int J Radiat Oncol Biol Phys.* 2009;85:126–137.
80. Elsasser T, Kramer M, Scholz M. Accuracy of the local effect model for the prediction of biologic effects of carbon ion beams in vitro and in vivo. *Int J Radiat Oncol Biol Phys.* 2008;71:866–872.
81. Elsasser T, Scholz M. Cluster effects within the local effect model. *Radiat Res.* 2007;167:319–329.
82. Gemmel A, Hasch B, Ellerbrock M, et al. Biological dose optimization with multiple ion fields. *Phys Med Biol.* 2008;53:6991–7012.
83. Kase Y, Kanai T, Matsufuji N, et al. Biophysical calculation of cell survival probabilities using amorphous track structure models for heavy-ion irradiation. *Phys Med Biol.* 2008;53:37–59.
84. Kramer M, et al. Treatment planning for scanned ion beams. *Radiother Oncol.* 2004;73:S80–S85.
85. Kramer M, Scholz M. Rapid calculation of biological effects in ion radiotherapy. *Phys Med Biol.* 2006;51:1959–1970.
86. Scholz M, Matsufuji N, Kanai T. Test of the local effect model using clinical data: tumour control probability for lung tumours after treatment with carbon ion beams. *Radiat Prot Dosimetry.* 2006;122:478–479.
86a. Tobias CM. Failla Memorial Lecture: the future of heavy ion science in biology and medicine. *Radiat Res.* 1985;103:1–33.
87. Xu XG, Bednarz B, Paganetti H. A review of dosimetry studies on external-beam radiation treatment with respect to second cancer induction. *Phys Med Biol.* 2008;53:R193–R241.
87a. National Council for Radiation Protection and Measurements. *Information Needed to Make Radiation Protection Recommendations for Space Missions Beyond Low-Earth Orbit.* Report # 153. Bethesda, MD: National Council for Radiation Protection and Measurements; 2006.
88. Goldberg Z, Schwietert CW, Lehnert B, et al. Effects of low-dose ionizing radiation on gene expression in human skin biopsies. *Int J Radiat Oncol Biol Phys.* 2004;58:567–574.
89. Costes S, Streuli CH, Barcellos-Hoff MH. Quantitative image analysis of laminin immunoreactivity in skin basement membrane irradiated with 1 GeV/nucleon iron particles. *Radiat Res.* 2000;154:389–397.
90. Leith JT, Lewinsky BS, Schilling WA. Modification of the response of mouse skin to x-irradiation by bleomycin treatment. *Radiat Res.* 1975;61:100–109.
91. Leith JT, McDonald M, Howard J. Residual skin damage in rats 1 year after exposure to X rays or accelerated heavy ions. *Radiat Res.* 1982;89:209–213.
92. Leith JT, Powers-Risius P, Woodruff KH, et al. Response of the skin of hamsters to fractionated irradiation with X rays or accelerated carbon ions. *Radiat Res.* 1981;88:565–576.

93. Leith JT, Lewinsky BS, Schilling WA. Comparison of skin responses of mice after single or fractionated exposure to cyclotron-accelerated helium ions and 230 kv x-irradiation. *Radiat Res.* 1975;62:195–215.

93a. Blakely EA, Tobias CA, Ngo FQH, et al. Comparison of helium and heavy ion beams for therapy based on cellular radiobiological data. *Int J Radiat Oncol Biol Phys.* 1978;4(suppl 2):93–94. Abstract.

93b. Blakely EA, Tobias CA, Yang TCH, et al. Inactivation of human kidney cells by high-energy monoenergetic heavy-ion beams. *Radiat Res.* 1979;80:122–160.

93c. Blakely EA, Tobias CA, Ngo FQH, et al. In: Pirruccecllo MC, Tobias CA, eds. *Biological and Medical Research With Accelerated Heavy Ions at the Bevalac.* Lawrence Berkeley Laboratory, LBL 11220; 1980:73–86.

93d. Lucke-Huhle C, Blakely EA, Chang PY, et al. Drastic G2 arrest in mammalian cells after irradiation with heavy-ion beams. *Radiat Res.* 1979;79:97–112.

93e. Ngo FQH, Blakely EA, Tobias CA. Sequential exposures of mammalian cells to low- and high-LET radiations: I: lethal effects following x-ray and neon-ion irradiation. *Radiat Res.* 1981;87:59–78.

93f. Roots R, Yang TC, Craise L, et al. Rejoining capacity of DNA breaks induced by accelerated carbon and neon ions in the spread Bragg peak. *Int J Radiat Biol.* 1980;38:203–210.

93g. Chapman JD, Blakely EA, Smith KC, et al. Radiobiological characterization of the inactivating events produced in mammalian cells by helium and heavy ions. *Int J Radiat Oncol Biol Phys.* 1977;3:97–102.

93h. Curtis SB, Schilling WA, Tenforde TS, et al. Survival of oxygenated and hypoxic tumor cells in the extended-peak regions of heavy charged-particle beams. *Radiat Res.* 1982;90:292–309.

93i. Yang TCH, Blakely EA, Chatterjee A, et al. Response of cultured mammalian cells to accelerated krypton particles. *Life Sci Space Res.* 1977;87:511–520.

93j. Goldstein LS, Phillips TL, Ross GY. Biological effects of accelerated heavy ions: II: fractionated irradiation of intestinal crypt cells. *Radiat Res.* 1981;86:529–541.

94. Leith JT, Woodruff KH, Howard J, Lyman JT, et al. Early and late effects of accelerated charged particles on normal tissues. *Int J Radiat Oncol Biol Phys.* 1977;3:103–108.

95. Blakely E, Castro JR. Assessment of acute and late effects to high-LET radiation. Proceedings of National Institute of Radiological Sciences: International Seminar on the Application of Heavy Ion accelerator to Radiation Therapy of Cancer, nirs-m-103/himac-008. National Institute of Radiological Research, Chiba, Japan, 1994:149–157.

96. Field SB. An historical survey of radiobiology and radiotherapy with fast neutrons. *Curr Top Radiat Res.* 1976;11:1–86.

97. Burns FJ, Albert RE. Dose response for skin tumors induced by single and split doses of argon ions. In: Pirruccello MC, Tobias CA, eds. *Biological and Medical Research with Accelerated Heavy Ions.* Berkeley, CA: Lawrence Berkeley Laboratory, LBL11220; 1980.

98. Burns FJ, et al. High-LET radiation-induced malignant and benign tumors in rat skin. In: Suzuki M, ed. *Risk Evaluation of Cosmic-Ray Exposure in Long-Term Nammed Space Mission.* Tokyo: Kodansha Scientific Ltd.; 1999:109–119.

99. Burns FJ, Zhao P, Xu G, et al. Fibroma induction in rat skin following single or multiple doses of 1.0 GeV/nucleon 56Fe ions from the Brookhaven Alternating Gradient Synchrotron (AGS). *Phys Med.* 2001;17(Suppl 1):194–195.

100. Heimbach RD, Burns FJ, Albert RE. An evaluation by alpha-particle Bragg peak radiation of the critical depth in the rat skin for tumor induction. *Radiat Res.* 1969;39:332–344.

101. Ayala MN, Soderberg PG. Vitamin E can protect against ultraviolet radiation induced cataract in albino rats. *Ophthalmic Res.* 2004;36:264–269.

102. Karslioglu I, Ertekin MV, Koçer I, et al. Protective role of intramuscularly administered vitamin E on the levels of lipid peroxidation and the activities of antioxidant enzymes in the lens of rats made cataractous with gamma-irradiation. *Eur J Ophthalmol.* 2004;14:478–485.

103. Fry RJ, Powers-Risius P, Alpen EL, et al. High-LET radiation carcinogenesis. *Adv Space Res.* 1983;3:241–248.

104. Alpen EL, Powers-Risius P, Curtis SB, et al. Fluence-based relative biological effectiveness for charged particle carcinogenesis in mouse Harderian gland. *Adv Space Res.* 1994;14:573–581.

105. Curtis SB, Townsend LW, Wilson JW, et al. Fluence-related risk coefficients using the Harderian gland data as an example. *Adv Space Res.* 1992;12:407–416.

106. Curtis SB, Nealy JE, Wilson JW. Risk cross sections and their application to risk estimation in the galactic cosmic-ray environment. *Radiat Res.* 1995;141:57–65.

107. NCRP, Fluence-Based and Microdosimetric Event-based Methods for Radiation Protection in Space, in NCRP Report # 137. National Council for Radiation Protection and Measurements: Bethesda, MD, 2001.

108. Dicello JF, Christian A, Cucinotta FA, et al. In vivo mammary tumourigenesis in the Sprague-Dawley rat and microdosimetric correlates. *Phys Med Biol.* 2004;49:3817–3830.

109. Tubiana M. Can we reduce the incidence of second primary malignancies occurring after radiotherapy? A critical review. *Radiother Oncol.* 2009;91:4–15; discussion 1–3.

110. Ianzini F, Mackey M, Mitotic catastophe. In: Gewirtz DA, Holt SE, Grant S, eds. *Apoptosis, Senescence and Cancer.* 2nd ed. Totowa, New Jersey: Humana Press; 2007:73–91.

111. Mizushima N, Levine B, Cuervo AM, et al. Autophagy fights disease through cellular self-digestion. *Nature.* 2008;451:1069–1075.

112. Pirtoli L, Cevenini G, Tini P, et al. The prognostic role of beclin 1 protein expression in high-grade gliomas. *Autophagy.*

113. Fournier C, Wiese C, Taucher-Scholz G. Accumulation of the cell cycle regulators TP53 and CDKN1A (p21) in human fibroblasts after exposure to low- and high-LET radiation. *Radiat Res.* 2004;161:675–684.

114. Jakob B, Scholz M, Taucher-Scholz G. Biological imaging of heavy charged-particle tracks. *Radiat Res.* 2003;159:676–684.

115. Chang PY, Bjornstad KA, Rosen CJ, et al. Effects of iron ions, protons and X rays on human lens cell differentiation. *Radiat Res.* 2005;164(4 Pt 2):531–539.

116. Iwadate Y, Mizoe J, Osaka Y, et al. High linear energy transfer carbon radiation effectively kills cultured glioma cells with either mutant or wild-type p53. *Int J Radiat Oncol Biol Phys.* 2001;50:803–808.

117. Tsuboi K, Moritake T, Tsuchida Y, et al. Cell cycle checkpoint and apoptosis induction in glioblastoma cells and fibroblasts irradiated with carbon beam. *J Radiat Res (Tokyo).* 2007;48:317–325.

118. Hamada N, Hara T, Omura-Minamisawa M, et al. Energetic heavy ions overcome tumor radioresistance caused by overexpression of Bcl-2. *Radiother Oncol.* 2008;89:231–236.

119. Ma J, Ye L, Da M, et al. Heavy ion irradiation increases apoptosis and STAT-3 expression, led to the cells arrested at G2/M phase in human hepatoma SMMC-7721 cells. *Mol Cell Biochem.* 2009;328:17–23.

120. Yamamoto N, Ikeda C, Yakushiji T, et al. Genetic effects of X-ray and carbon ion irradiation in head and neck carcinoma cell lines. *Bull Tokyo Dent Coll.* 2007;48:177–185.

121. Higo M, Uzawa K, Kawata T, et al. Enhancement of SPHK1 in vitro by carbon ion irradiation in oral squamous cell carcinoma. *Int J Radiat Oncol Biol Phys.* 2006;65:867–875.

122. Fushimi K, Uzawa K, Ishigami T, et al. Susceptible genes and molecular pathways related to heavy ion irradiation in oral squamous cell carcinoma cells. *Radiother Oncol.* 2008;89:237–244.

123. Matsumoto Y, Iwakawa M, Furusawa Y, et al. Gene expression analysis in human malignant melanoma cell lines exposed to carbon beams. *Int J Radiat Biol.* 2008;84:299–314.

124. Imadome K, Iwakawa M, Nojiri K, et al. Upregulation of stress-response genes with cell cycle arrest induced by carbon ion irradiation in multiple murine tumors models. *Cancer Biol Ther.* 2008;7:208–217.

125. Nojiri K, Iwakawa M, Ichikawa Y, et al. The proangiogenic factor ephrin-A1 is up-regulated in radioresistant murine tumor by irradiation. *Exp Biol Med (Maywood)* 2009;234:112–122.

126. Bigelow A, Garty G, Funayama T, et al. Expanding the question-answering potential of single-cell microbeams at RARAF, USA. *J Radiat Res (Tokyo).* 2009;50(Suppl A):A21–A28.

127. Gerardi S. Ionizing radiation microbeam facilities for radiobiological studies in Europe. *J Radiat Res (Tokyo).* 2009;50(Suppl A):A13–A20.

128. Matsumoto H, Tomita M, Otsuka K, et al. A new paradigm in radioadaptive response developing from microbeam research. *J Radiat Res (Tokyo).* 2009;50(Suppl A):A67–A79.

129. Prise KM, Schettino G, Vojnovic B, et al. Microbeam studies of the bystander response. *J Radiat Res (Tokyo).* 2009;50(Suppl A):A1–A6.

130. Voss KO, Fournier C, Taucher-Scholz G. Heavy ion microprobes: a unique tool for bystander research and other radiobiological applications. *New J Phys.* 2008;10:075011.

# Charged Particle Therapy

## The Physics of Interaction

Antony J. Lomax

The principle of radiation therapy is relatively simple. Radiation applied to the patient deposits energy through the ionization of atoms, and this deposited energy damages and ultimately sterilizes cells. The exact mechanism is, however, complex and rather indirect. For instance, the overwhelming majority of energy is deposited as heat, raising the temperature of the irradiated medium by only a tiny amount (a few microKelvin), with no negative consequences for the cells. Occasionally, the ionized atoms can also produce free radicals, highly reactive chemical products, which can directly damage the irradiated cells. Despite this, the principle of radiotherapy remains simple. The higher the delivered energy to the tissue—referred to as dose in radiotherapy—the higher is the probability that the tissue will be terminally damaged. Of course, this principle applies to both tumors and normal tissues, and the art of radiotherapy is, therefore, to concentrate the dose in the tumor while sparing the surrounding normal tissues as much as possible. Thus, any radiation type that can localize the deposited dose within a well-defined volume should bring advantages for radiotherapy.

Charged particles exhibit exactly such a characteristic. As an example, Figure 1 shows the so-called depth-dose curve for protons. This shows how the deposited energy (dose) changes as a function of penetration of a proton beam through water. The horizontal axis shows this penetration in centimeters. This curve is typical for charged particles, with a shallow plateau dose on entrance to the medium increasing slowly at first and then rapidly, ultimately resulting in a sharply defined maximum of high dose in the so-called Bragg peak. Beyond this, the dose even more rapidly drops to almost zero within a few millimeters. The Bragg peak characteristics of protons were recognized as being particularly attractive for radiotherapy by Wilson[1] in 1946, when he published his seminal paper on the possibilities of using protons to combat cancer. After this, the first patients were treated with protons in 1954 at Berkeley, followed shortly afterward by the use of heavier charged particles that were investigated clinically at the same facility.[2]

Development was slow during the next 40 years or so, with proton therapy (and particle therapy generally) mainly being restricted to research facilities. However, it was probably with the opening of the first hospital-based proton facility at Loma Linda in California in 1991 that particle therapy at last was shown to be a viable radiotherapy technique that could make it from research to clinical application. At the time of writing, the Loma Linda facility was treating more than 140 patients a day on its 3 proton treatment rooms, showing the potential feasibility of high throughput, hospital-based particle therapy facilities. Based on this experience, the promising initial clinical results, and the clearly improved dose distributions resulting from particle therapy, it is currently experiencing a boom period, with an unprecedented number of new, hospital-based facilities being built and proposed throughout the world.

In this article, we will review the most important properties of charged particles and the characteristics of their interactions with materials, both in the homogenous and in the inhomogenous cases. The aim is to provide a basic knowledge of such interactions, so that the lay reader can understand how high-energy particle beams can be generated and modulated into useable radiotherapeutic beams and to highlight some of the consequences of these interactions on particle therapy when applied to in vivo biologic systems, such as the human patient. For simplicity, in this article, we will concentrate on proton therapy. However, most of the physical effects and interactions described here are also similar for heavier charged particles.

## ENERGY LOSS AND DEPOSITED DOSE

When protons pass through a medium, for example water, they experience Coulomb interactions with the orbiting electrons of the atoms in the medium—that is the opposite charges of the protons and the electrons release electrons from the atomic shells, ionizing the atom and setting free the electron. This causes an "avalanche" effect because the freed electron can also go on to ionize other neighboring atoms. In the process, the protons lose energy, albeit a very small amount, simply because the mass of the proton is more than that of the electron (protons are about 1800 times heavier than electrons). Nevertheless, depending on the density of the material through which the protons are traversing, they may interact with many thousands or millions of electrons per cm of medium they traverse. However, this process is not linear. The rate of change of energy as a function of traversed material (mathematically referred to as $dE/dX$) is given by the Bethe-Bloch formula as follows:

$$\frac{1}{\rho}\frac{dE}{dX} = k \cdot \frac{Z}{A} \cdot \left(\frac{z}{\beta}\right)^2 \cdot \left[13.8 + \ln\left(\frac{\beta^2}{1-\beta^2}\right) - \beta^2 - \ln(I)\right]$$

(1)

Although not a trivial formula, there are just a few characteristics of this that are important to note. First, the deposited energy (and therefore the deposited dose) is dependent on the density of the material ($\rho$) and on its chemical composition (the ratio of atomic number to atomic weight, $Z/A$). More importantly, at least from the point of view of the depth-dose curve shown in Figure 1, the deposited energy is inversely proportional to the square of the velocity of the particle ($\beta$). Thus, when the particle has high velocity, the particle delivers less dose, whereas as the velocity decreases, the particle deposits more and more dose. Relating this to the depth-dose curve shown in Figure 1, on entering the medium (from the left in the figure), the protons have highest energy and therefore the highest velocity. As they traverse the medium, they interact with the orbiting electrons as discussed earlier, and they lose energy (and therefore velocity) and deposit increasingly more dose. Toward the end of their range, where they have the lowest energy and velocity, because of the dependence

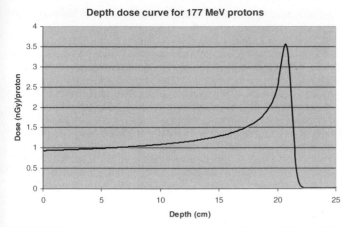

**FIGURE 1.** An example depth-dose curve (in water) for a 177-MeV, Quasi-monoenergetic proton beam. Because of the characteristics of proton energy loss, this demonstrates a sharp "Bragg peak" at a well-defined range (in this case at about 21 cm).

of the deposited dose on the inverse of the square of their velocity, the deposited dose rises rapidly, resulting in the characteristic Bragg peak seen at the distal end of the curve. Beyond this peak, the protons have no energy left, and therefore the dose rapidly drops to zero. From the physics point of view, the deposited energy is referred to in terms of the amount of energy deposited per unit mass and has the units of Joules per kilogram (J/kg). For convenience, however, in radiotherapy, the deposited energy is referred to as "dose" and takes the units of the Gray (Gy), where 1 Gy equals 1 J/kg. Typical prescription doses to a tumor are between 30 and 80 Gy, generally uniformly deposited over the whole tumor volume and delivered in small daily "fractions" of 1.8 to 2.0 Gy per day, a process unsurprisingly known as "Fractionation."

## THE RANGE AND THE SHAPE OF THE BRAGG PEAK

The position of the Bragg peak in depth is simply related to the initial energy (velocity) of the protons. The higher the energy, the deeper the Bragg peak in the medium. This relationship, although again not linear, is a simple, monotonic function from which it is easy to predict the Bragg peak depth exactly if the initial energy of the protons is known, together with the chemical and physical characteristics of the medium to which it is applied. Figure 2 shows a plot of range against initial energy for protons in water. For radiotherapy purposes, initial proton energies between 70 (for eye irradiations) and up to 230 to 250 MeV are used, relating to the maximum Bragg peak ranges of 32 to 38 cm in water.

This Bragg peak behavior is characteristic of all charged particles, either to a lesser or to a greater amount, with the sharpness and relative height of the Bragg peak increasing as the mass of the particle increases. Indeed, the Bragg peak was first discovered for decay products of radium by Bragg and Kleeman[3,4] in Adelaide, Australia, at the beginning of the twentieth century.

However, there is a little more to the story of the Bragg peak. Two other important effects determine its shape and dictate that the "simple" formula shown above could never be fitted to even the most basic of experimental measurements of a proton depth-dose curve. The first is due to interactions of the protons with atomic nuclei of which more in the following sections. The second is the effect of the energy spectrum of the incident protons and of an effect known as range straggling.

Of these, the effect of the energy spectrum is perhaps the most easily explained. It is impossible for any source of accelerated protons to produce perfectly monoenergetic beams—that is a stream of protons in which every proton has exactly the same energy. In practice, such proton beams will exhibit a spread of energies, typically of the order of 1% of the initial energy of the beam. Therefore, although these can still be considered to be quite monoenergetic in nature, there is an inevitable spreading of the Bragg peak, with protons with lower energies having a slightly lower range and those with higher energies stopping somewhat deeper. The net effect is to spread, or widen, the pristine Bragg peak that would result from perfectly monoenergetic

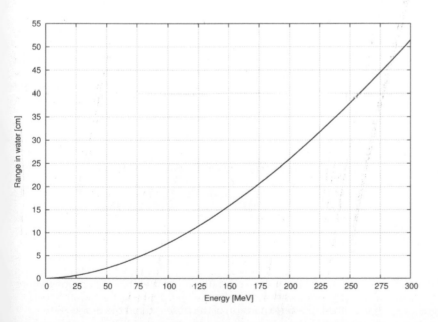

**FIGURE 2.** Energy-range plot for protons in water. This shows the depth of the Bragg peak as a function of initial proton energy. Typically, most proton facilities operate with maximum proton energies of between 230 and 250 MeV, providing maximum ranges of 32 to 38 cm in water.

beams. Range straggling, on the other hand, is an effect that will even spread out monoenergetic beams. Simply put, range straggling occurs because energy loss interactions of the protons with orbiting electrons are governed by statistics, with each proton losing a varying amount of energy with each interaction. Once again, the more interactions a proton undergoes, the more energy it will lose, and the smaller its residual range in the medium, whereas a proton that undergoes fewer interactions will clearly have a slightly higher residual range. Thus, range straggling will also blur even a perfectly monoenergetic beam, broadening the Bragg peak somewhat. As a rule of thumb, range straggling will also smear out the Bragg peak by about 1% of the Bragg peak's range.

## NUCLEAR INTERACTIONS AND THEIR EFFECTS

In addition to protons interacting with orbiting electrons (by far the most common interaction), protons will occasionally also interact with atomic nuclei in 1 of 3 ways: coulomb interactions similar to that with electrons, more of which will be described in the next section, and elastic and inelastic nuclear interactions.

Elastic and inelastic interactions with atomic nuclei are rather complex processes. Suffice it to say, however, that both involve protons impinging directly with the nuclei, from which they are either elastically deflected (the nuclei remains intact) or the proton disturbs the nucleus sufficiently that fragments of the nuclei are knocked out (inelastic collisions). Both have important consequences on the incident protons and on the nuclei themselves. The first, and probably most significant, is that protons are essentially "lost" from the beam at the rate of about 1% per cm of penetration. Thus, for a beam with a range of 20 cm, about 20% of the protons will be lost to nuclear interactions by the time the depth of the Bragg peak is reached. This has important consequences on the shape of the measured Bragg peak, over and above that already described in the previous section. This loss of proton "fluence" essentially suppresses the Bragg peak somewhat to that expected from energy loss alone, simply because the number of protons reaching the Bragg peak is lower than that entering the medium.

Second, as a result of inelastic nuclear interactions, secondary neutrons are produced. This has been a source of some worry for proton therapy in the last few years because neutrons are supposed to be highly efficient at damaging tissue in relation to other radiation qualities (see next section and the concept of "relative biologic effectiveness [RBE]"). Consequently, a number of articles have been published recently, attempting to assess the neutron component of therapeutic proton beams and their potential biologic effect [5–7 and references therein].

Finally, short-lived radioisotopes, such as O-15 and C-11, can be produced. Although these are of very small yields, the fact that these are positron emitters has been exploited to "image" the result of proton (and carbon ion) irradiations after delivery by imaging the patient directly after treatment in a conventional positron emission tomography scanner.[8,9]

In summary, the characteristics of the depth-dose curve measured for a quasi monoenergetic Bragg peak (c.f. Fig. 1) is dependent on 4 main factors: energy loss through coulomb interactions with orbiting electrons, the initial energy spectrum, range straggling, and proton fluence loss due to nuclear interactions. Of these, only the energy spectrum is a parameter that can be manipulated by an experimenter or therapist. The other 3 are determined solely by the laws of physics.

## LATERAL SCATTER AND BEAM DIVERGENCE

Up to now, we have considered the interactions of protons in a 1-dimensional sense—that is in the form of a depth-dose curve. But now, we must consider what is actually being plotted in this curve and extend our discussion to the other spatial dimensions.

Consider again Figure 1. This actually shows what can be called the integral depth-dose curve for protons of 177 MeV. By this, we mean that the dose displayed on the vertical axis is the total dose delivered at all points of an infinite plane, oriented orthogonally to the beam direction, at each depth. In practice, such a curve is obtained either by measuring the dose with a small volume detector as a function of depth in a broad beam or by using a very wide area detector (typically of 8–10 cm diameter) when measuring a narrow "pencil beam" of protons. For the second example, a wide detector is used, so as to collect all the deposited energy ±4 to 5 cm around the central axis of the pencil beam. That such a wide detector is necessary to collect the total dose at a given dose is due to the lateral scattering of protons. That is, the inevitable divergence of a perfectly parallel proton beam is due to interactions in the medium. A typical cross-sectional plot through such a pencil beam is shown in Figure 3. On entering the medium, the beam has a certain width but widens slowly as it penetrates the medium. Similarly, to the energy loss curve, the beam widens ("diverges") only slowly to begin with, but in the region of the Bragg peak, this scattering becomes more pronounced, resulting in a rather bulbous shape in and around the Bragg peak.

Such scattering is due to 3 processes. The first is related to the energy loss described in The Range and the Shape of the Bragg Peak section. When interacting with orbiting electrons, the protons not only lose a small amount of energy but also divert slightly from their path. In practice, however, because of the huge difference in weight between protons and electrons, this effect is so small that it can effectively be ignored. Thus, the main component of scattering comes from 2 other processes related to the nuclear interactions described earlier.

Coulomb interactions with nuclei are, in principle, similar to the interactions of the Coulomb interactions with electrons. As protons and nuclei are both positively charged, the protons experience a repulsive force from the nuclei and are thus deflected from their path. However, in contrast to the case when they interact with orbiting electrons, nuclei are much heavier and can deflect the protons by much greater amounts. As with the Coulomb interactions with electrons, protons undergo many thousands of such interactions per cm and hence this effect is known as "multiple Coulomb scattering (MCS)." It is the predominant process by which the primary protons of an incident beam are deflected. As stated by Goitein,[10] in his excellent book, the contribution to beam width at the Bragg peak is approximately 2% of the range of the Bragg peak in water, and the broadening can be well represented by a Gaussian function. Thus, for a Bragg peak deposited at 20 cm in water, the additional lateral broadening due to MCS would be about 4 mm $\sigma$ (the full width at half maximum width

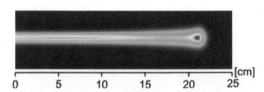

**FIGURE 3.** A cross-section through a narrow proton pencil beam of 177 MeV protons, showing the effects of multiple Coulomb scattering on the beam. The beam direction is from left to right. Increased scattering at the end of the range (where the protons have their lowest energy) is clearly manifested as the bulbous expansion of the dose around the Bragg peak.

of a Gaussian profile is 2.35 times the sigma—so this would result in a full width at half maximum of about 1 cm because of scattering alone).

A smaller, but nevertheless important, effect is the effect of elastic and inelastic collisions on the lateral penumbra of protons. Both effects result in either larger deflections of the primary protons (elastic) or the production of secondary protons with wide angular divergence (inelastic), together with heavier fragments. Such events occur much more rarely than Coulomb interactions with the nuclei, and thus produce a long, but low-magnitude "tail" of dose on top of the almost purely Gaussian form resulting from the MCS process (Pedroni et al[11]). As shown in the work of Pedroni et al, although the magnitude of this halo is small (typically only a few percent of the dose in the primary proton beam), it is a large enough effect to be seen in routine dosimetric measurements (particularly for small fields) and in particularly complex dose distributions, and thus should be taken into account whenever possible.

## LINEAR ENERGY TRANSFER AND RBE

We now move away from the physics-based interactions and look more into the biologic effects of proton interactions. We have already introduced the concept of $dE/dX$ and energy loss in The Range and the Shape of the Bragg Peak section, and have seen that, in the Bragg peak region, the rate of deposition of energy reaches a maximum. One can therefore think of the concept of energy deposition density, more correctly termed "linear energy transfer" (LET). This is the amount of energy (KeV) deposited per micrometer. The LET is very closely related to $dE/dX$ and the higher the $dE/dX$, the higher the LET. Thus, in the Bragg peak region, there is a higher LET than in the plateau area, or a higher ionization density. This increased density of ionizations also effects the ability of the radiation to damage cells and leads to a higher relative biological effectiveness (RBE). Simply put, the higher the RBE, the higher the effectiveness of the radiation to damage tissue in relation to a specified reference irradiation. As our knowledge of radiation and its biologic effect is based on x-ray and mega-voltage photon irradiations, the reference irradiation is taken to be that of 1.17 and 1.33 MeV photons resulting from Co-60 decays. Put more formally, the RBE can be expressed as follows:

$$RBE_{protons} = \frac{D_\alpha^{isoeffect}}{D_{protons}^{isoeffect}}$$

where D ($\alpha$, isoeffect) is the dose required to obtain a given effect (say 50% cell death for cells in vitro) for photon (Co-60) irradiation and D (protons, isoeffect) is the dose of proton irradiation required to achieve the same isoeffect. From equation 2, it is clear that a RBE $>$ 1 implies that, for the same applied dose (Gy or J/kg) of protons and the reference irradiation, protons will have an increased biologic effect.

Although the concept of RBE is very simple, it is a complex problem because, in practice, the RBE is dependent on many parameters, including end-point (isoeffect), dose, cell/tissue type, and the micro- and macroenvironment of the irradiated tissues. Thus, it is very likely that RBE values measured in vitro will be different to those measured in vivo. However, it is generally true that, as LET increases, RBE increases and thus the RBE in the Bragg peak of a proton beam will be somewhat higher than that in the plateau.

Many results of in vitro measurements for the RBE of protons have been published, and all clearly show an increased RBE in the Bragg peak, and particularly in the distal fall-off region, where the LET is highest. It is outside the scope of this article to summarize these results, but suffice it to say that the RBE has variously been measured to be between 2 and 4 for very low proton energies (in the extreme

distal tail of the Bragg peak curve), but a more modest 0.9 to 2.1 in the plateau, with an average value of over all studies of ~1.2. Interestingly, however, when such measurements have been made in vivo, the RBE values tend to be somewhat lower, with values between 0.7 and 1.6 (mean ~1.1) in the plateau region. For an excellent review of the RBE data for proton beam irradiations see the article by Paganetti et al.[12]

In summary, although quite high RBE values have been measured in vivo for protons, and there is a clear increase of RBE in the Bragg peak, the currently accepted method of dealing with RBE for proton therapy is to assume a global RBE of 1.1. That is, when prescribing a dose to a tumor, typically about 10% less physical dose (Gy or J/kg) will be delivered as would be delivered for a comparable photon irradiation. Although this is a rather coarse method, it has the advantage of simplicity and transparency, and of the 50,000 or so patients treated with protons in the last 40 years, there is no clinical evidence to suggest that this approach may be wrong. Nevertheless, the strong evidence of an increased RBE in the Bragg peak cannot, and should not, be ignored, and when designing proton treatments, it is generally judicious to try to avoid using highly weighted Bragg peaks, which impinge on critical normal structures in case the biologic effectiveness is indeed increased in these areas.

Although it is outside the scope of this article to go into detail for the RBE of heavier charged particles, such as C-12, nevertheless, some comments should be made. Indeed, it is from the point of view of RBE that proton and heavy ion therapy differ significantly, not only from the basic theory of RBE but also in the magnitude of the effect. Whereas a global value of 1.1 for proton therapy, although not strictly correct, has been shown clinically to be a reasonable solution, this is not the case for carbon ions, where the RBE varies from somewhat higher than 1 in the plateau to RBEs of 3 to 4 in the Bragg peak. With such large differences, it is imperative that this effect is incorporated into the planning of such treatments, such that the physical depth-dose curve is modified to obtain a homogenous biologically effective dose across the tumor. In summary, although it seems that one can work safely and effectively with a global RBE of 1.1 for protons, this is not the case with heavier ions, and a considerable knowledge of the underlying radio biology is necessary to effectively and safely use such particles for therapy.

## THE EFFECTS OF DENSITY HETEROGENEITIES

Until now, we have concerned ourselves with the effects of protons in homogenous materials or tissues, both from the physical characteristics of proton interactions and from the possible differences in biologic effectiveness as a result of increased ionization densities in the Bragg peak region. Clearly, however, outside of the laboratory or quality assurance phantom, proton therapy is being applied to patients who are anything but homogenous. External beam radiotherapy, whether it is with photons, electron, or protons, must inevitably pass through many different parts of a patient's anatomy to reach the tumor, and these can have very different densities and chemical compositions. Such density heterogeneities can have profound effects on the pristine proton beams thus far considered.

In the first instance, the effect of differing tissues on the range of protons must be considered. As we discussed in The Range and the Shape of the Bragg Peak section earlier, protons lose energy through many interactions with orbiting electrons, and the rate of energy loss is dependent on the density of the material and (to a lesser extent) on the chemical composition. Thus, protons will lose more energy as they traverse 1 cm of bone than they will traverse 1 cm of water, or significantly less when traversing 1 cm of air. This effectiveness of a material to induce energy loss on protons is known as the "stopping

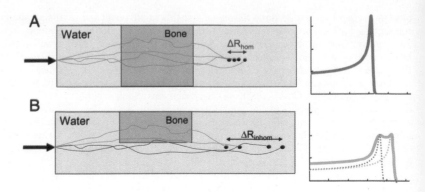

**FIGURE 4.** A schematic representation of the effect of density heterogeneities on a pencil beam of protons. When such a beam traverses a bone-soft tissue interface, then the protons can effectively take different paths through the heterogeneities, leading to different energy losses and a degradation of the Bragg peak.

power" of the material. To accurately determine where in a patient (or inhomogenous phantom) the Bragg peak will be deposited, it is necessary to know the stopping powers of the tissues through which the beam is passing. In practice, this can be conveniently determined from x-ray computer tomographic (CT) data, which can be considered to be a rather quantitative method for imaging (electron) density (Schneider et al[13]). Although the transformation from CT data to proton stopping power is unfortunately not a one-to-one relationship (different materials with the same CT value can have different stopping powers and

vice versa), it is possible to generate quite accurate conversion tables, which are specific for biologic tissues and can provide CT-derived stopping powers for biologic tissues with an accuracy of 1% to 2% (Schaffner and Pedroni[14]).

The issue is complicated, however, when tissue densities or stopping powers vary orthogonally to the beam direction. That is, the beam passes along interfaces between tissues with different stopping powers. Such a case is schematically shown in Figure 4. A narrow proton pencil beam enters the phantom from the left-hand side and

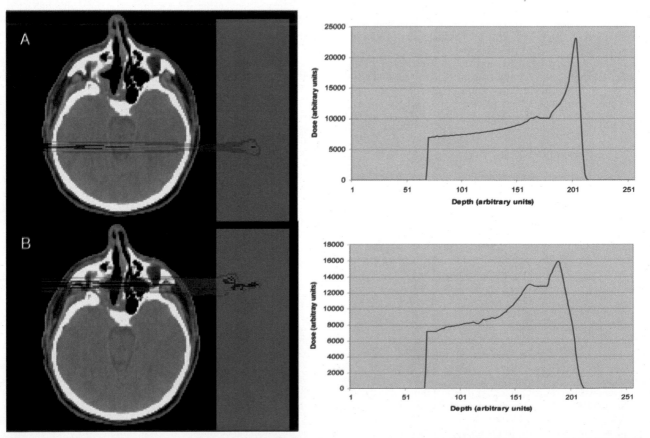

**FIGURE 5.** The effect of real density heterogeneities on a proton pencil beam. A, The pencil beam passes through a relatively homogenous region, and the Bragg peak is preserved (right-hand plot). B, When passing through a more heterogeneous region, the Bragg peak is badly degraded.

then passes along a density heterogeneity, which is centered on the central axis of the beam. What will be the effect on the Bragg peak of the incident proton pencil beam? This is shown in an extremely simplified form in Figure 4b. In this figure, representative proton tracks have been drawn to show the paths of individual protons as they pass through the phantom. As discussed in Nuclear Interactions and Their Effects section, the different protons undergo different MCS events, with some being scattered into the denser region, and others being scattered away. Clearly, those protons scattered into the dense region will then experience more interactions than those passing through the lower density region (because of the higher density region having a higher stopping power) and will thus lose more energy. On exiting the dense region, they will have generally lower residual energy than those protons that have predominantly passed through the lower density region and will therefore have a lower residual range. The net effect of this (at least for this very simplified case) is that the resultant Bragg peak (if measured distal to the heterogeneity) will essentially split into 2 separate Bragg peaks. Thus, our pristine and sharp Bragg peak of Figure 1 becomes badly degraded and broadened by the presence of the density heterogeneity. In practice of course, there will be a smoothing between these 2 "Bragg peak," simply because many protons will also be scattered in and out of the density heterogeneity, thus blurring out the difference between the 2 peaks. However, the net effect will be similar. Density heterogeneities can significantly spread out (or blur) the Bragg peak.

This effect was dramatically demonstrated in the early 1980s by the Boston group, both theoretically (using Monte Carlo-based calculations) and with measurements through a water-filled human skull.[15,16] Figure 5 shows the effect of Bragg peak degradation for a proton pencil beam calculated through the skull base region of a patient's CT data set. The applied beam was a 177-MeV beam similar to that shown in Figure 1, calculated to pass totally through the skull base region and stop in a simulated detector on exit from the patient. The resultant integral "Bragg peak," calculated by integrating all deposited dose in the planes perpendicular to the pencil beam direction in the simulated detector, is shown in Figure 5b. The effects of the bone-air and bone-brain interfaces in the skull base on the Bragg peak are clearly seen because the Bragg peak is badly degraded in comparison with the pristine peak shown in Figures 1 and 5a.

Density heterogeneities then have a profound effect on proton beams, and in almost every region of a patient, such heterogeneities are unavoidable (except with the possible exceptions of irradiations of the eye and in the upper cranium). Thus, the use of CT data (from which stopping power for tissues can be derived) and accurate dose calculation models (which to a greater or lesser extent can approximate the effects of such heterogeneities on the applied proton beam) are an essential prerequisite for proton therapy. Indeed, it is no coincidence that the indications for proton therapy only started expanding from the late 1970s and early 1980s, at the time when x-ray CT scanners were first becoming clinically available. Without such data, it is impossible to accurately calculate the deposited dose in a patient.

Density heterogeneities are an issue of some worry for practitioners of proton therapy. However, an awareness of the problems, and a range of techniques for dealing with these issues, can ensure that these problems can largely be overcome. As a testimony to this, one needs only to look at one of the success stories of clinical proton therapy—the irradiation of skull base chordomas and chondrosarcomas. These are tumors that occur in one of the most heterogeneous areas of the body, with many bone-soft tissue and even bone-air interfaces, all of which can significantly affect the applied proton beam in ways described earlier. Tumor control rates between 60% and 80% for such cases, however, pay testimony to the effectiveness of proton therapy in this region and to the planning and delivery strategies developed to deal with these effects.[17-19]

## SUMMARY

Being relatively heavy charged particles, the interactions of protons with tissue are quite different to those of photons. These differences are directly responsible for the rather attractive characteristic of protons—the well-defined maximum range and sharply defined Bragg peak. In this article, we have tried to outline the main physics principles underlying this well-known curve and to hint at some of the more deep lying, but nevertheless important, processes that govern the interaction of protons with tissues. To summarize these as succinctly as possible, Table 1 provides a quick reference to the characteristics of a proton beam and the underlying physical process that determine this.

**TABLE 1.** Summary of the Main Characteristics of Proton Interactions and Their Dependencies or Consequences

| Characteristic/Effect | Dependencies/Consequences |
|---|---|
| Bragg peak shape | Energy loss through Coulomb Interactions with orbiting electrons. As the deposited energy is inversely proportional to the square of the velocity of the protons, most energy is deposited in a sharp Bragg peak at the end of the range |
| Bragg peak range | Dependent on the initial energy of the protons and the density of the material through which the protons pass |
| Bragg peak width | Dependent on the energy spectrum of initial beam and range straggling (1% of range of Bragg peak) |
| Proton fluence reduction | Results from proton interactions with nuclei |
| | Reduces with range at a rate of roughly 1%/cm and tends to surpress the Bragg peak c.f. the pure energy loss curve. |
| Lateral beam width | Dependent on initial width of beam and multiple Coulomb scattering (MCS) in tissue |
| | Contributions from MCS can be estimated to be roughly 2% of the range of the proton beam |
| Nuclear interactions | Primary cause of proton fluence loss |
| | Result in wider deflections of protons and production of secondary particles (neutrons, secondary protons, heavier by-products) |
| Density heterogeneities | Inevitably degrade (spread-out) the Bragg peak and will effect overall proton range |
| RBE | Indicates the additional biological effect resulting from high ionization densities (LET) in the Bragg peak |
| | Will increase towards and beyond the Bragg peak region and can vary between 1.0 and 2.0 |
| | In practice, a global value of 1.1 is taken by all proton facilities currently |

In summary, it is impossible to understand how proton beams can be modulated, and how and why proton treatments are designed and delivered the way they are, without understanding some of the underlying principles of proton interactions with matter. This article hopefully provides necessary background and basic knowledge to understand a little more that how particle therapy works.

## ACKNOWLEDGMENTS

*The authors thank Uwe Schneider and Sairos Safai for proof reading this article, and Sairos Safai and Silvan Zenklusen for providing Figures 2 and 3, respectively.*

## REFERENCES

1. Wilson RR. Radiological use of fast protons. *Radiology.* 1946;47:487–491.
2. http://ptcog.web.psi.ch/Archive/Patientstatistics-update02Mar2009.pdf.
3. Bragg WH, Kleeman R. On the ionization curve of radium. *Philos Mag.* 1904;S.6:726–738.
4. Bragg WH, Kleeman R. On the alpha particles of radium, and their loss of range in passing through various atoms and molecules. *Philos Mag.* 1905;S.6:318–340.
5. Hall EJ. Intensity-modulated radiation therapy, protons, and the risk of second cancers. *Int J Radiat Oncol Biol Phys.* 2006;65:1–7.
6. Paganetti H, Bortfeld T, Delaney TF. Neutron dose in proton radiation therapy: in regard to Eric J. Hall (Int J Radiat Oncol Biol Phys 2006;65:1–7). *Int J Radiat Oncol Biol Phys.* 2006;66:1594–1595; author reply 1595.
7. Gottschalk B. Neutron dose in scattered and scanned proton beams: in regard to Eric J. Hall (Int J Radiat Oncol Biol Phys 2006;65:1–7). *Int J Radiat Oncol Biol Phys.* 2006;66:1594; author reply 1595.
8. Parodi K, Paganetti H, Shih HA, et al. Patient study of in vivo verification of beam delivery and range, using positron emission tomography and computed tomography imaging after proton therapy. *Int J Radiat Oncol Biol Phys.* 2007;68:920–934.
9. Knopf A, Parodi K, Paganetti H, et al. Quantitative assessment of the physical potential of proton beam range verification with PET/CT. *Phys Med Biol.* 2008;53:4137–4151.
10. Goitein M. *Radiation Oncology—A Physicist's-Eye View.* New York: Springer Science+Business Media; 2008.
11. Pedroni E, Scheib S, Böhringer T, et al. Experimental characterization and physical modelling of the dose distribution of scanned proton pencil beams *Phys Med Biol.* 2005;50:541–561.
12. Paganetti H, Niemierko A, Ancukiewicz M, et al. Relative biological effectiveness (RBE) values for proton beam therapy. *Int J Radiat Oncol Biol Phys.* 2002;53:407–421.
13. Schneider U, Pedroni E, Lomax AJ. On the calibration of CT-Hounsfield units for radiotherapy treatment planning. *Phys Med Biol.* 1996;41:111–124.
14. Schaffner B, Pedroni E. The precision of proton range calculations in proton radiotherapy treatment planning: experimental verification of the relation between CT-HU and proton stopping power *Phys Med Biol.* 1998;43:1579 1592.
15. Goitein M, Sisterson JM. The influence of thick inhomogeneities on charged particle beams. *Radiat Res.* 1978;74:217–230.
16. Urie M, Goitein M, Holley WR, et al. Degradation of the Bragg peak due to inhomogeneities. *Phys Med Biol.* 1986;31:1–15.
17. Hug EB, Loredo LN, Slater JD, et al. Proton radiation therapy for chordomas and chondrosarcomas of the skull base. *J Neurosurg.* 1999;91:432–439.
18. Noel G, Feuvret L, Calugaru V, et al. Chordomas of the base of the skull and upper cervical spine. One hundred patients irradiated by a 3D conformal technique combining photon and proton beams. *Acta Oncol.* 2005;44:700–708.
19. Ares C, Hug EB, Lomax AJ, et al. Effectiveness and safety of spot scanning proton radiation therapy for chordomas and chondrosarcomas of the skull base: first long-term report. *Int J Radiat Oncol Biol Phys.* In press.

# Technology for Proton Therapy

Jacob Flanz • Alfred Smith

A proton therapy facility is composed of hardware and software technologies and clinical components that interact in an integrated fashion to provide safe, accurate, and efficient treatments to cancer patients. To fulfill its mission and accomplish its goals, a modern proton therapy system should contain technologies that have been tested and proven to be safe, robust, and reliable; however, an upgrade path should be provided for the implementation of new developments that advance the field of proton therapy without undue cost or interference with the operations of the overall facility.

The major technology components of a proton therapy system include:

- Beam production systems
- Beam transport systems
- Treatment delivery systems
- Patient support and treatment set up systems
- Treatment control and safety systems
- Data management systems
- Treatment planning systems
- Imaging systems
- System interfaces and information technology networks

Figure 1 shows a typical layout for technologies on the treatment floor of a multiroom proton therapy facility.

Different combinations of the technologies comprising the components listed earlier can create different treatment beam properties; therefore, it is important to know what factors in a system can affect the delivered treatment. Clinical beam parameters such as dose rate and range (penetration in the patient) are related to the beam current and energy; thus, ensuring that the correct dose distribution is delivered to patient places constraints on the accelerator technology. For that reason, it is important to understand the relationships between technology and clinical requirements.

## Beam Production Systems

Proton therapy can require beam penetrations as deep as 37 cm in water equivalent material and as shallow as the skin. Depending on the chosen treatment delivery technology (such as scattered or scanned beams), these requirements have translated, for practical implementation, into proton energies ranging from 70 to 230–250 million electron volts (MeV) to treat tumors in a wide range of patients and tumor sites. Dose rates ranging from 0.5 to 10 Gy/min for average target volumes have been used.

The beam production system generates a beam of desired energy, current, and size and includes the proton accelerator and sometimes an associated energy selection system. Accelerators that have thus far reliably produced high energies in clinical environments include cyclotrons and synchrotrons. Both accelerators are capable of providing high levels of sustained, reliable beam uptime. (If an overall system uptime of >95% is desired, this can translate into a reliability factor of >98% for the accelerator.) Additionally, it is important to consider the beam time structure produced by the accelerator, because this will play a role in the determination of the beam spreading system that can be used.

### Cyclotrons

The charged particle beam path in a simple cyclotron is shown in Figure 2. Two magnetic dipoles are positioned with a gap between them, and an electric field is created in the gap. The beam is injected into gap at the center of the cyclotron and accelerated by the electric field each time it crosses the gap. When the beam leaves the electric field region, it enters the magnetic field region and is bent 180 degrees, then reenters the electric field region at the correct time to be accelerated in the opposite direction. As the charged particle energy increases, so does the radius of the path of the particle. When the energy is sufficient the particle is extracted from the cyclotron. In the case of a cyclotron whose beam extraction energy is constant, the beam is then directed to an energy degrader and selection system.

The electric field goes through 1 cycle (or multiple) for each particle revolution—this is the "cyclotron frequency" of the RF accelerating voltage. The angular frequency of the oscillating electric field is given by $\omega = qB/m$, where $q$ is proton charge, $B$ is magnetic field strength, and $m$ is proton mass. The effects of relativistic mass cause the proton to get progressively more out of step with the accelerating voltage as its velocity increases (the relativistic mass is given by $m_r = m_o/sqrt(1 - v^2/c^2)$, where $m_o$ is the invariant or rest mass, $v$ is the proton velocity, and $c$ is speed of light). Note that as the velocity increases, the relativistic mass increases. The accelerating RF voltage and the protons will get out of synchronization (and limit the maximum energy) unless the frequency of the RF field decreases or the magnetic field increases.

The "synchrocyclotron" and the "isochronous cyclotron" were developed to address this problem. The synchrocyclotron varies the frequency of the accelerating voltage to track the relativistic effects. The accelerator at the Harvard Cyclotron Laboratory was a synchrocyclotron, which used a rotating condenser to vary the RF angular frequency. One effect of this scheme is that only protons that arrive at the accelerating gaps at the right time are accelerated—this creates a pulsed time structure in the extracted proton beam. Because the accelerating frequency is variable in a synchrocyclotron, it is no longer necessary to use high-accelerating voltages such as was used in cyclotrons.

In the isochronous cyclotron, the magnetic field increases to compensate for the relativistic mass effects. The extracted proton beam is constant and not pulsed or bunched.

The C230 isochronous cyclotron built by ion beam applications for proton therapy was constructed for the proton facility at the

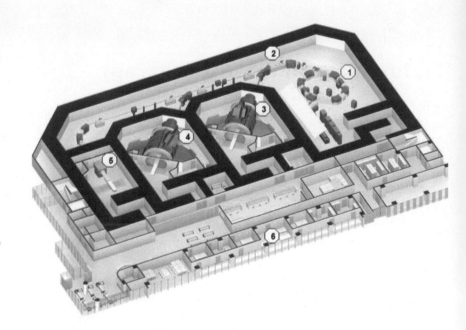

**FIGURE 1.** A typical layout for technologies on the treatment floor of a multiroom proton therapy facility. The items include (1) the beam production system, (2) the beam transport system, (3) and (4) rotating gantries beam delivery systems, (5) a fixed horizontal beam delivery system, and (6) support spaces.

Massachusetts General Hospital; it became operational in 1997.[1] The C230 operates at room temperature, accelerates protons to 230 MeV, and can extract proton beams with currents as high as 300 nA. The overall weight of the iron core and the copper coils is 220 tons, and it has a footprint of 4 m diameter. The C230 opens at the center, which allows for maintenance.

Recently, superconducting technology has been applied to cyclotrons making it possible to significantly reduce their size. Superconducting synchrocyclotrons can be small enough to be installed on an isocentric gantry and rotated about the patient. The Comet cyclotron built by Varian/Accel is a superconducting accelerator weighing only 80 tons.[2] The current carrying coils are in a superconducting cryostat, which allow high currents to be reached. Consequently, an intense magnetic field can be achieved, which allows for proton acceleration up to 250 MeV. The beam properties are largely the same as the room temperature cyclotron. Still River Systems have obtained a patent on a superconducting synchrocyclotron, which is reported to weigh 20 tons; this accelerator will be mounted on a gantry, making it possible to have a single room proton therapy system.[3]

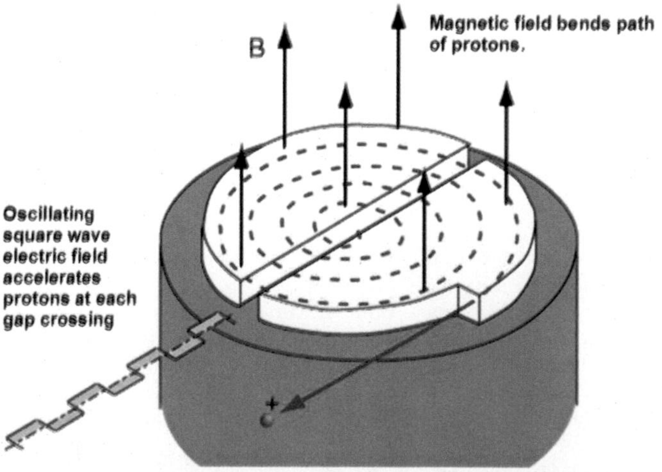

### Synchrotrons

Synchrotrons are circular ring devices where protons travel in vacuum pipes under the influence of magnets that are positioned around the circumference of the circle. Acceleration is achieved by the application of RF fields in an accelerating cavity located in the ring. The magnetic fields must be increased synchronously with the acceleration to keep the particles constrained in the constant radius path. A variety of beam focusing schemes can be used to constrain the beam size, which will affect the size and expense of the magnetic elements controlling the beam. One effect of this acceleration process is that there is an injection and acceleration time period with no beam produced. The beam is then extracted either quickly (rapid cycling)[4] or in a slow controlled way, resulting in a pulsed beam with a time period (variable or fixed) that depends on the synchrotron design. The extracted beam can in some implementations be coordinated with patient motion.

The overall size of the proton synchrotron is determined both by the strength of the magnetic field and by the combination of elements used in the ring. For hospital-based room temperature synchrotrons, the energy ranges from 270 to 330 MeV. As opposed to some cyclotrons that can extract the beam only at the highest accelerated energy, synchrotrons can extract a different energy with each extracted pulse or in some cases modify the extracted beam energy during a pulse.

The Hitachi, Ltd., synchrotron such as the one installed in the University of Texas M. D. Anderson proton therapy facility is shown schematically in Figure 3.[5] The first hospital-based implementation of this synchrotron was at the Tsukuba University Proton Therapy Center in Japan. Concepts for smaller synchrotrons have been developed such as those used for the system developed by ProTom International.

### Accelerator Development

New concepts are being considered for proton accelerators used for cancer therapy; some of these new developments are discussed here. The design of new accelerators has been focused on reducing the size

**Magnetic field bends path of protons.**

B

**Oscillating square wave electric field accelerates protons at each gap crossing**

+

**FIGURE 2.** A representation of the bottom half components in a cyclotron including the charged particle beam path (in red).

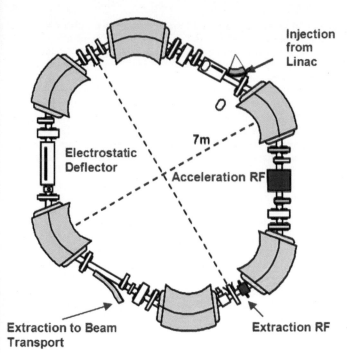

**FIGURE 3.** A schematic of the components of the Hitachi, Ltd., synchrotron installed in the University of Texas M. D. Anderson Proton Therapy Center, also showing the beam injection and extraction regions.

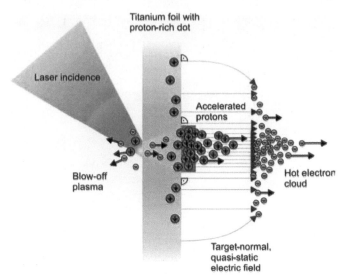

**FIGURE 4.** A representation of the laser induced proton beam acceleration mechanism showing the incident laser beam, and the resulting charge polarization, which induces the accelerating field. Reprinted from *Nature*. 2006;439:445–448, with permission from Lippincott Williams & Wilkins.

and cost of the accelerator or adding functionality to enhance clinical operations. Some of these designs use nonstandard acceleration schemes and some are hybrid concepts of proven methods.

### CycLINAC

A CycLINAC uses a cyclotron as an injector to an RF linear accelerator.[6] This reduces the size and the complexity of both the cyclotron and the LINAC. This system offers the advantage that it can use the "electronic" aspects of a LINAC to control the beam energy and current on a pulse to pulse basis, which increases the flexibility of a "cyclotron only" system, which produces a constant beam energy. In addition, it would be possible to use the cyclotron for positron emission tomography isotope production, thus increasing the functionality of the facility.

### Fixed Focusing Alternating Gradient Accelerators

Fixed focusing alternating gradient accelerators merge aspects of cyclotrons and synchrotrons.[7] This system is comprised of a ring of magnets like a synchrotron, however, instead of the magnetic field ramping with the increasing particle energy during acceleration, the magnet system is designed to accommodate a large range of beam energies as in a synchrotron, and the fields are fixed as in a cyclotron. Work is being conducted to determine whether fixed focusing alternating gradients can be developed for particle therapy.

### *High-Gradient Linear Accelerator*

One concept currently under investigation is that of a high gradient electrostatic or dielectric wall accelerator accelerator.[8] New dielectrics are capable of holding off very high voltages without arcing and gradients over 100 MeV/m may be achieved. This system will use pulsed DC Voltage, as opposed to a large and complex RF system

needed for a LINAC. Such accelerators could produce a short-pulsed beam of clinically useful energy, with pulse by pulse control of beam energy, size and intensity, and could be mounted on a gantry. A dielectric wall accelerator for proton therapy is currently being developed by the Lawrence Livermore Laboratory in collaboration with TomoTherapy.

### *Laser Particle Acceleration*

Results from experiments have indicated that it is possible to create a very large electric field by using an intense laser pulse (intensity $\sim 10^{20}$ W/cm$^2$) to knock out electrons from a thin target.[9] The resulting charge polarization can result in an electric field of TV/m that accelerates protons out of the target. Using this concept, (see Fig. 4) beam energies in the range of several tens of MeV have been reached. This suggests that therapeutic beam energies could be produced using thin targets. Proton beams produced by laser acceleration have a broad energy spectrum and magnetic spectrometry must be used to select a narrow energy band required for therapy beams. This process throws away a large percentage of protons in the beam, although it may be possible to use this to create spread-out Bragg peak (SOBP) fields. Recent tests have shown that, by concentrating the proton source at the center of the electric field axis, the energy spectrum can be improved. There are many challenges in producing high-energy beams with the required clinical characteristics using laser acceleration.

## Beam Transport Systems

Beam transport systems consist of a series of bending (dipole) magnets and focusing (quadrupole) magnets that direct the beam to the treatment rooms. This is certainly required in multiroom facilities served by a single accelerator and may be useful in a single room facility. During transport, the proton beam is contained within a vacuum tube (large enough to contain the beam without losses) running through the magnet cores. At the appropriate junction in the beam transport line, a bending magnet switches the beam to the treatment room scheduled for beam.

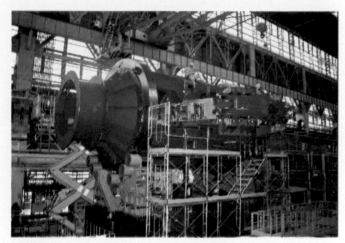

**FIGURE 5.** The Hitachi, Ltd., 360 degrees rotating gantry structure (red) including the mounted beam transport elements (pink).

When the proton beam enters a treatment room, it is transported to the treatment nozzle near the patient through another series of bending and focusing magnets. There are 2 types of beam lines in treatment rooms: isocentric gantries and fixed (usually horizontal) beam lines. In isocentric gantry rooms, a gantry structure supports the beam line including large bending magnets that cause the beam to be bent in one direction and then in the opposite direction so that the beam enters the treatment nozzle in a path perpendicular to the original beam direction to the gantry isocenter, where the patient is located. The gantries, along with their magnets and counterweights, using present technology, typically weigh 120 to 190 tons. The rotating diameter of an isocentric gantry is typically 10 m or larger, some smaller diameter (compact) gantries exist; however, depending upon the design they weigh even more. The entire gantry structure can be rotated in space around the patient treatment enclosure such that the beam exiting the treatment nozzle can be directed to the patient from any angle within a 360-degree gantry rotation or in some cases in a more limited range. The largest isocentric gantries, because of their size, require a large shielded vault approximately 3 stories high. Figure 5 shows a Hitachi, Ltd. isocentric gantry on the factory floor assembled for testing before shipment. Three of these gantries were installed in the University of Texas M. D. Anderson Proton Therapy Center.

In fixed-beam treatment rooms, the beam is directed to the treatment nozzle through an array of magnets that are fixed in space and do not rotate around the patient. The patient is rotated and translated in space with a robotic patient positioner to enable the beam to enter the patient from various angles. Fixed-beam rooms require about one-third the space as gantry rooms therefore the shielded volume is much smaller. Fixed-beam rooms can be used for a variety of treatment sites, although a full study of its applicability for a variety of tumor sites has not been done.

## Beam Delivery Systems

The primary goal of external beam radiotherapy is to deliver the prescribed dose distribution to an irregularly shaped target volume located at depth within a patient. In proton therapy, a small (a few millimeters in diameter) pencil beam entering the treatment delivery nozzle from the beam transport system must be spread and shaped in 3 dimensions (or 4) so that the delivered high dose distribution conforms to the target volume. There are 2 techniques for spreading and shaping a proton beam for delivery of highly conformal treatments: beam scattering and scanning. These are discussed here.

The scattering technique uses scattering devices in the treatment delivery nozzle (usually a double scatterering system for large fields and single scatterer for small [eg, radiosurgery] fields) to spread the beam laterally and a range modulator wheel or ridge filter[10] to create a spread out Bragg peak (SOBP) in the target volume. Using the latter, the scattering system is truly passive since there are no moving parts during a treatment. However, the term passive scattering, has been used for any scattering system, even in the case of a range modulator wheel, which is a dynamic component that can even include a modulated beam current to obtain a uniform longitudinal dose distribution. Between the nozzle exit and the patient surface, a treatment field-specific aperture is used to shape the field laterally to conform to the maximum beams eye view extent of the target volume and a range compensator is used to correct for patient surface irregularities, density heterogeneities in the beam path, and changes in the shape of the distal target volume surface. The size of the SOBP is chosen to cover the greatest extent in depth of the target volume. The SOBP size is constant over the entire target volume: therefore, in general, there is some pull back of the high dose region into normal tissues proximal to the target volume. Because multiple treatment fields are usually used, each directed from a different angle, this high-dose pull back into normal tissue is not additive over all fields. Figure 6 shows how an SOPB can be obtained from a superposition of several Bragg peaks that have been shifted in range and given variable weights to obtain a uniform dose in the high dose region.

The second type of beam delivery uses beam scanning techniques (often called pencil beam scanning).

In beam scanning techniques, there are 2 different methods of magnetically moving the beam throughout the target volume:

- Dose driven scanning—The pencil beam is positioned at a location in the target volume and stays there until the desired dose at that location is reached. The beam is then cut off (or not), the magnet current is adjusted to position the beam at a new location, and the beam is turned on. This sequence is repeated as the beam is moved through multiple target positions. This method is sometimes called discrete spot scanning.
- Time driven scanning—The pencil beam is positioned at a location and either stays there for a given time or is moved continuously with a speed that is synchronized with the accelerator beam current output. The beam is not cut off as it moves from position to position. This method is called line, segment, raster, or continuous scanning and it also contains, as a subset, a form of what is called spot scanning.

In both the aforementioned techniques, the energy changes required for achieving the desired longitudinal dose distribution (not necessarily an SOBP) can be accomplished with energy changes from the accelerator for synchrotrons or energy changes made in the energy selection system for cyclotrons. In either case, energy absorbers in the treatment nozzle are often used in conjunction with the aforementioned methods.

In current practice, scanned proton beams have been used to deliver 3 general types of treatments:

1. SOBP fields—Scanning magnets can be use to scan a pattern that forms large uniform fields in the treatment nozzle. In this manner, large, uniform fields can be produced without the use of

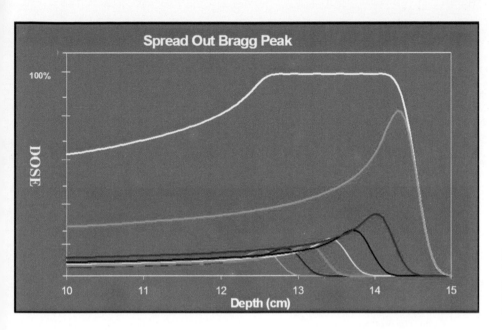

**FIGURE 6.** A plot showing how individual Bragg peaks of different ranges and doses can be added up to produce an SOBP, which is uniform in the desired depth range.

physical scattering devices with their related loss of protons and production of secondary neutrons. Using this scanning method, the SOBP is formed by use of energy changes as described above. This method, often called uniform beam scanning, requires the use of treatment specific apertures and range compensators to shape the treatment beam to the target volume in the same manner as in passive scattering techniques.

2. Single field uniform dose—Scanning beams can produce a highly conformal uniform dose distribution in the target volume with a single field delivery without the use of a patient specific aperture or compensator. The dose distribution within each range layer in the target volume can be highly nonuniform to achieve this effect, but the resulting total dose distribution can be uniform and conformal. This effect is unique with charged particle beams and cannot be achieved with uncharged particles.

3. Nonuniform, single field dose distribution—Scanning beams can be used to deliver treatment plans calculated by optimization techniques analogous to the treatment planning techniques used for intensity modulated x-ray treatments. Optimization for scanned-beam proton treatment plans can lead to multiple optimized beams where each treatment field is nonuniform in dose delivery but the summed dose distribution of all treatment fields results in a uniform, conformal dose in the target volume.

It is important to note that even for a uniform field delivery with a scanned beam, it may be necessary to deliver a different dose to different parts of the target to optimize the dose distribution and the penumbra. Thus, in effect, a nonuniform dose delivery, or in the case of time-driven scanning, intensity modulation is required for uniform overall dose distribution. This is different from the situation using uncharged particles, thus the term intensity modulation is not a useful description for charged particle therapy.

## Patient Positioning Systems

During treatments, patients are supported and positioned in the treatment beam by a device that has 6 degrees of freedom—3 translations and 3 rotations. In isocentric gantry treatment rooms, the combination of the gantry rotation and couch motion provides great flexibility in delivering multiple beams, each from a different direction (angle), to optimize the treatment. Recently, robots have been adapted to particle therapy applications—robots can be used for holding and positioning imaging systems or used to replace traditional patient couches in treatment rooms. Accuracy and reproducibility, which are different concepts are both important in the specification of these systems.

Each treatment room also contains lasers and imaging devices (x-ray tubes and image receptors). The lasers are used for initial patient set up (to get the patient close to the treatment position) and the imaging systems provide orthogonal images of the patients internal anatomy that, when compared with digitally reconstructed images calculated by the treatment planning system, are used to reposition the patient relative to the treatment beam exactly as required by the treatment plan, ie, in same position used for the computed tomography scans that are used in treatment planning.

It may be useful, with modern technology, to consider whether the patient should be moved to the beam or whether the beam can be moved to the patient. This can potentially lead to new positioning and immobilization solutions for initial setup and for management of patient/organ motion.[11] To improve efficiency and increase patient throughput, some believe it may be helpful to have patient set up rooms outside the treatment rooms where patients can be immobilized and positioned for treatment by use of imaging devices in the set up room. If pediatric patients are treated, anesthesia can also be started in the set up room. After the set up procedure has been completed, the patient can be transported to the treatment room and transferred to the treatment support device by use of a robotic transfer. After the treatment has been given, the patient is offloaded onto the transport system and taken back to the treatment set up room. Such systems make it possible to reduce the average time required to treat patients in the treatment room.

## Treatment Control and Safety Systems

Modern proton therapy systems have an overall control system that enables integration of the operations of the various proton therapy components. The control system can schedule the beam for particular treatment rooms, select the appropriate beam energy and beam delivery parameters, coordinate the motion of gantries, nozzles, couches, etc., and monitor the treatment process to ensure that the treatment is delivered accurately and according to the treatment prescription. Although all these functions are necessary, they need not all be tightly coupled depending on the system design.

The treatment safety system ensures that all aspects of the treatment process are carried out safely and provides safety for patients, employees, and the equipment itself. Critical safety elements, which can lead to injury to patients or a mistreatment, are protected through a system of redundant interlocks that ensure that there can be no single point of safety failure; and a detailed-failure mode analysis is used to determine an appropriate set of independent systems for ensuring the safety of critical systems or operations.

## Facility Integration

Modern proton therapy facilities should be fully integrated with respect to the various internal technology or clinical components and with other hospital functions. In this respect, proton therapy facilities should be as integrated as modern conventional radiation therapy departments. All functions of the proton therapy facility including imaging, treatment planning, data management and electronic charting, machine shop, patient treatment positioning, and treatment control should be compliant with DICOM RT/ION standards. The proton facility should also be integrated with all hospital functions such as diagnostic imaging, billing, scheduling, pathology, and medical labs. Full technology integration is necessary for safe and efficient operation of the proton facility.

## CONCLUSIONS

We have described the technologies typically found in a modern proton therapy facility. We have not described treatment planning or data management systems because they are very similar to their conventional counterparts, although the techniques for charged beam

planning optimization are still being developed. There are other technologies that have not been discussed, because they have not been implemented in but a very few situations. Such technologies include cone beam imaging in treatment rooms, multileaf collimators, and methods for reducing errors in scanned beam treatments when organ motion is present. We have not described or shown technologies for all vendors that manufacture and sell proton therapy systems; however, we have described typical technologies and have attempted to cover the breadth of technologies found in proton therapy facilities.

### REFERENCES

1. Flanz J, Durlacher S, Goitein M, et al. Overview of the MGH-Northeast proton therapy center plans and progress. *Nucl Instrum Methods Phys Res B.* 1995;99:830–834.
2. Geisler A, Baumgarten C, Hobl A, et al. Status report of the ACCEL 250 MeV medical cyclotron. In: *Proceedings of the 17th International Conference on Cyclotrons and Their Applications.* Tokyo, Japan: Particle Accelerator Society of Japan; 2004:178–182.
3. Matthews J. Accelerators shrink to meet growing demand for proton therapy. *Physics Today.* March 2009:22.
4. Peggs S, Barton D, Beebe-Wang J, et al. The rapid cycling medical synchrotron, RCMS. In: *Proceedings of EPAC.* Paris, France: 2002:2754–2756.
5. Hiramoto K, Umezawaa M, Saito K, et al. The synchrotron and its related technology for ion beam therapy. *Nucl Instrum Methods Phys Res B.* 2007;261: 786–790.
6. Amaldi U, Berra P, Braccini S, et al. The CycLINAC: an accelerator for diagnostics and hadrontherapy. In: *PTCOG Meeting.* Paris, France: 2004.
7. Collot J, Mori Y, Mandrillon P, Meot F, Edgecock R. The rise of the FFAG. *CERN Courier.* 2008;48:21–28.
8. Sampayan S, Caporaso G, Carder B, et al. High gradient insulator technology for the dielectric wall accelerator. In: *Particle Accelerator Conference.* Dallas, Texas: 1995. UCRL-JC-119411.
9. Faure J, Glinec Y, Pukhov A, et al. A laser-plasma accelerator producing monoenergetic electron beams. *Nature.* 2004;431:541–544.
10. Kostjuchenko V, Nichiporov D, Luckjashin V. A compact ridge filter for spread out Bragg peak production in pulsed proton clinical beams. *Med Phys.* 2001;28:1427–1430.
11. Langen KM, Jones DTL. Organ motion and its management. *Int J Radiat Oncol.* 2001;50:265–278.

# Proton Beam Therapy in Pediatric Oncology

Thomas E. Merchant

Proton beam therapy (PBT) is the future of pediatric radiotherapy. It will be used to increase the cure rates for pediatric cancer and eliminate many of the acute, early, and late effects of treatment. Cure rates will increase when investigators are able to exploit the physical characteristics of the proton beam to increase radiation dose to critical subregions of the targeted volume or by therapeutic intent when patients are referred for definitive irradiation in lieu of less successful alternatives. PBT will increase the likelihood for some patients that therapeutic doses will be administered as caregivers have increased confidence in radiotherapy for children and fewer fears of treatment effects. Side effects of radiotherapy will be eliminated for many and reduced for others who receive PBT because of the reduced dose to normal tissues. The increased conformity anticipated with newer proton delivery methods, including spot scanning, will magnify the differences between protons and photons. Side effects will also be reduced as target volume margins continue to shrink for the most common brain and solid tumors and by environment of care. The latter refers to improved methods of immobilization and verification that are requisite for proton therapy as well as an increase in expertise in all aspects of care. The increased availability and awareness of proton therapy will congregate pediatric patients to proton centers of excellence to increase experience in targeting and normal tissue avoidance.

Despite the heralded advantages, there remain a number of relevant concerns about the current state of PBT for children. These include the lack of clinical experience and known uncertainties in proton physics related to treatment planning systems and radiobiological effects. The statement that only a small number of patients have been treated using protons is unquestionable given information available in the peer-reviewed literature. The small number of patients impacts the amount of follow-up and late effects data. Negative patient selection plagues interpretation of the early outcomes for many of the pediatric series. Most series are replete with incurable cases or those that experts would agree benefit marginally. There has been a lack of optimization afforded to patients treated with proton therapy. Patients referred from a distance to the very limited number of proton centers may not receive integrated care—has surgery or chemotherapy been optimally provided for these children? Furthermore, current protocols for proton therapy include significant variability in target volume definitions, dose prescription, and normal tissue dose constraints. Many protocols do not adhere to the International Commission on Radiation Units and Measurements Reports 50, 62, and 78 definitions for the targeted volumes[1-3] and most do not explicitly include internal and set-up margins. Proton therapy targets may be larger than photon targets for certain tumors because of available protocols. There has been a lack of uniformity in immobilization and verification procedures among proton centers and some are lacking state of the art image guided therapy. A good example is that none of the active proton centers in the US currently has in-room cone beam computed tomography available for children; cone beam computed tomography is now widely available for children treated using photons. Some centers use kilovoltage imaging with fiducial markers, others do not implant these markers and rely on boney anatomy. How does this impact treatment?

In the United States in 2009, proton therapy is available for children at 5 treatment centers located in Boston, Massachusetts, Houston, Texas, Loma Linda, California, Bloomington, Indiana, and Jacksonville, Florida. These centers are located in or near US urbanized areas with the respective rankings of 7 (Boston), 10 (Houston), 25 (Riverside-San Bernadino, CA), 33 (Indianapolis), and 43 (Jacksonville). In order of anticipated completion date, newer centers (urbanized center ranking in parenthesis) are under construction in Oklahoma City, Oklahoma (49), Philadelphia, Pennsylvania (4), Hampton, Virginia (Virginia Beach, VA; 27), and Warrenville, Illinois (near Chicago, IL; 3).[4]

Pediatric patients will be referred for proton therapy based on perceived benefit unlike patients with base of skull of tumors (chordoma and chondrosarcoma),[5] ocular tumors (uveal melanoma),[6] and prostate cancer[7] for which the indications are more established. The advantages for pediatric patients have been generalized and nearly limited to central nervous system (CNS) tumors and those with head and neck sarcomas; however, despite the lack of data and clear indications, this group has the most to gain from a reduction in side effects. The use of proton therapy is in evolution. Current delivery methods are evolving. Passive scattering beams are the current mode of therapy. Passive scanning has been Food Drug Administration cleared in the United States since 2006 and is currently available at some centers but has yet to be used routinely for children and is not a significant fundamental gain over passive scattering. Although several centers have treated a handful of patients, at the time of this writing, active magnetic scanning remains in development in the US and is only available at the Paul Scherrer Institute in Villigen, Switzerland.

Since the time that the hospital-based high-energy cyclotron and rotational gantry for proton beam delivery has been commercially available, investigators have worked with industry to further the advancement of hardware and software to improve proton therapy.

Newer beam line detection systems may increase the speed of proton therapy, newer verification systems including robotic treatment couches; digital imaging positioning systems and post-treatment dosimetry using positron emission tomography will enhance treatment precision and advances in immobilization, verification and the use of anesthesia will improve throughput and efficacy of treating pediatric patients. Considering magnetic scanning and the advancements in hardware, software, and treatment methods and their expected impact on normal tissue dose and target conformity, will data acquired before the use of these systems be of limited value when attempting to show the advantage of protons over photons?

The clinical concept of radiation therapy is to deliver dose to the tumor and spare normal tissue. This concept embodies the central theme for pediatric radiotherapy and drives the development of new methods and innovations. Using present photon methods, increasing conformity is tied to increasing the low-dose volume and the pediatric radiation oncologist is limited in their ability to break current dose barriers. Further, radiation insensitive tumors require very high doses and are unapproachable using photon therapy. PBT is heralded as the next logical step in radiation therapy for children because it may be used to reduce dose to normal tissues while increasing conformity of the high-dose volume—there are likely to be fewer acute and long-term side effects as a result. Proton therapy may be used to reduce combined modality reactions, which are common as combined modality therapy is often used in the pediatric patient. Dose reductions are physically achieved by lowering collateral irradiation. Absent lateral or distant beam scatter and increase conformity of the high-dose volume under certain conditions will reduce the risk of side effects including secondary tumors and cancers. Although PBT is considered, the means for future dose escalation in radiotherapy because it may be easier to deliver higher doses, selectively irradiate portions of the tumor, treat tumors described as radio-insensitive, or increase systemic therapy, these possibilities rank second in importance to normal tissue reduction in the pediatric patient.

One of the common statements made by the naysayer of advanced treatment technology is that with current advances in oncology, radiotherapy for children will soon be a thing of the past. The counterpoint is that the indications for radiotherapy in children are actually increasing for patients with brain and solid tumors. Indeed, radiotherapy questions are a major focus of clinical trials in the US pediatric cooperative groups, which seek to optimize radiation dose and volume. Younger children are routinely irradiated because of the well-defined role of radiotherapy or to improve on past results when radiotherapy was excluded or delayed in treatment regimens. The latter is due to advancements in technology. With the exception of leukemia, selected carcinomas, extracranial germ cell tumors, and hepatic tumors, radiation therapy is indicated for children with brain tumors, Hodgkin disease, bone and soft tissue tumors, neuroblastoma, and renal and ocular tumors. Appropriate protocols currently include the use of proton therapy, which is sanctioned by the cancer therapy evaluation program of the US national cancer institute. Another common statement is that there is no evidence that reducing the volume of irradiation is clinically beneficial. Dose and outcome correlations have been established in models developed to study cognitive effects in brain tumors patients such as ependymoma and medulloblastoma.[8,9] Endocrine effects are directly correlated with dose to the hypothalamus.[10] And flat and long bone growth are known to be directly correlated with radiation dose and volume in pediatric sarcomas.[11]

## Pediatric Solid Tumors

PBT may be indicated for the treatment of retinoblastoma. Although fewer than a 100 cases of retinoblastoma have been treated using PBT during the past 40 years in the US, it has been shown dosimetrically that focal treatment of the retina alone or treatment of the entire optic globe may be advantageously performed using protons to spare ocular and extraocular structures in this vulnerable and young patient population.[12] Although bone and soft tissue sarcomas may appear at any site in the pediatric patient and head and neck sarcomas appear uniquely suitable for proton therapy, even the patient with a large pelvic or extremity sarcoma may have an advantageous reduction in dose to normal tissue dose and an improved ability to preserve growth and development[13,14] (Fig. 1). In the era of dose escalation for patients with residual neuroblastoma, proton therapy may be used to spare renal parenchyma and other critical structures (Fig. 2). Although neuroblastoma is the most common extracranial pediatric solid tumor, much work will have to be done to deploy protons for this abdominal and occasionally thoracic tumor because of tissue heterogeneity and the potentially problems of organ motion. Unresectable or incompletely resected osteosarcoma with a high risk for local failure may benefit from the dose escalation possibilities of proton therapy (Fig. 3). Common sites in the head and neck in axial skeleton regions are those for which proton therapy might be indicated. The treatment of nasopharyngeal cancer, one of the few pediatric cancers also seen in adults, has been shown in comparative dosimetry studies to benefit from the use of protons instead of photons. The potential sparing of the parotid glands and spinal cord show substantial advantages in selected cases (Fig. 4).

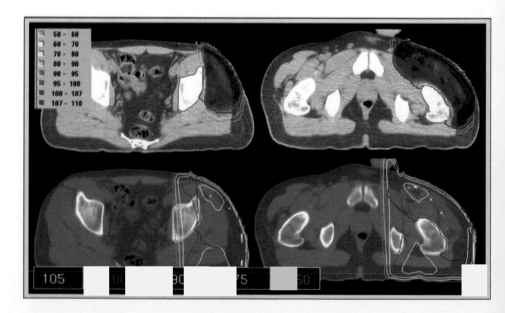

**FIGURE 1.**  Proton (upper images) and photon (lower images) dose distributions generated on axial computed tomography images for a child with Ewing sarcoma. The $D_{50}$ of the ipsilateral femur is 2.69 Gy for PBT compared with 54.25 Gy for photon irradiation.

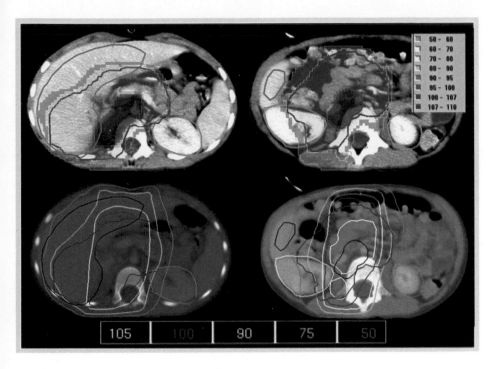

**FIGURE 2.** Proton (upper images) and photon (lower images) dose distributions generated on axial computed tomography images for a child with abdominal neuroblastoma arising from the right adrenal gland. The $D_{50}$ of the ipsilateral kidney is comparable for the 2 treatment modalities; however, the $D_{50}$ of the left kidney is 0.06 Gy for PBT compared with 9.60 Gy for photon irradiation.

## Hodgkin Disease

With an unlimited resource, one might consider research and development of proton therapy for Hodgkin disease. Reductions in dose to heart, lungs, and breasts are significant. The late effects, commonly observed in these patients, may be substantially reduced (Fig. 5).

## CNS Tumors

For pediatric patients with CNS tumors, proton therapy research opportunities are abundant based on photon benchmark outcomes for children with localized brain tumors. These opportunities include the study of cognitive, endocrine and neurologic effects in ependymoma,

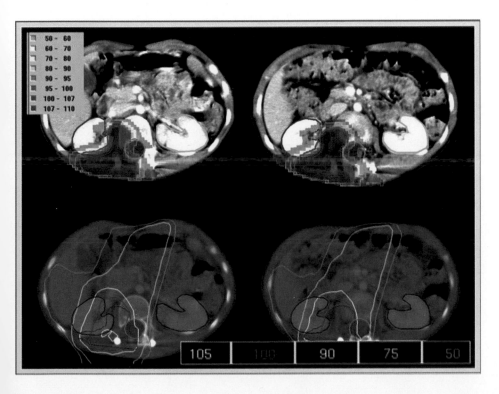

**FIGURE 3.** Proton (upper images) and photon (lower images) dose distributions generated on axial computed tomography images for a child with right paraspinal osteosarcoma. The $D_{50}$ of the contralateral kidney is comparably low for the 2 treatment modalities; however, the $D_{50}$ of the right kidney is 20.28 Gy for PBT compared with a dose limiting 49.61 Gy for photon irradiation. Similarly, the $D_{50}$ of the spinal cord is 25.9 Gy for the proton plan compared with the dose limiting 55.8 Gy for the photon plan, which was developed to administer 60 Gy to the target.

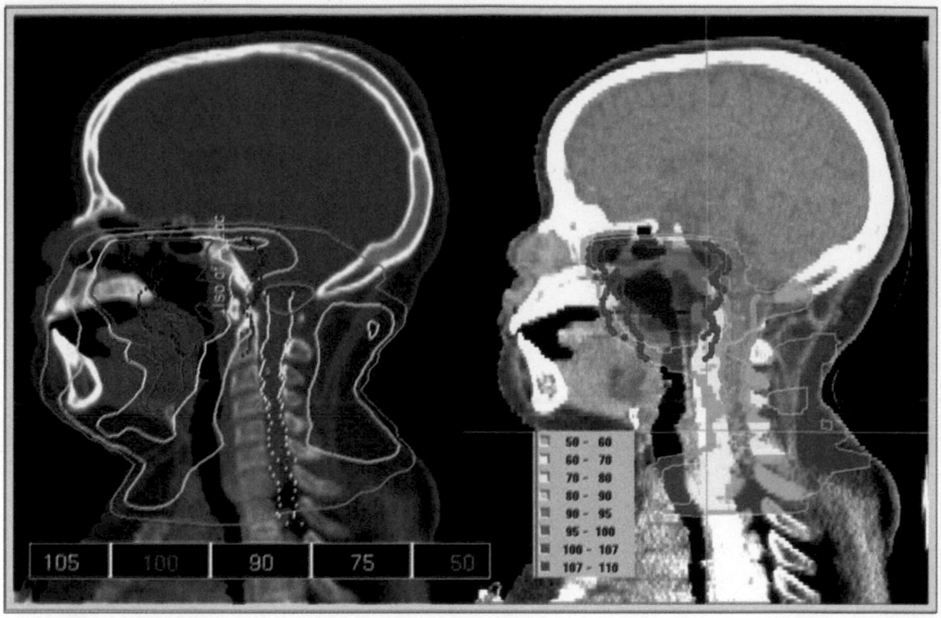

**FIGURE 4.** Proton (right) and photon (left) dose distributions generated on sagittally reconstructed computed tomography images for a child with nasopharynx cancer. The $V_{25Gy}$ of the bilateral parotid glands was 35% for the left parotid and 65% for the right parotid for PBT compared with 98% for the left parotid and 100% for the right parotid for photon irradiation.

low grade glioma, craniopharyngioma, and medulloblastoma. The objective of current research should be to identify the extent of CNS effects for which proton therapy might be able to improve outcomes.

In the study of radiation-related CNS effects in children, it is important to consider that some patients do not experience side effects and that not all side effects are attributable to radiation therapy. For some patients, it may not matter how radiotherapy is administered. However, this is probably not the case for most patients, especially the very young. Advances such as proton therapy are required for those at risk. There are a number of contributing clinical and host factors, and it is important to understand the critical combinations of dose and volume and competing risks. For example, high-dose volumes contribute the greatest effects, whereas low-dose volumes may be contributory but their effect may be an order of magnitude lower in relevant models. The competing risk of tumor recurrence may exceed the incidence of vasculopathy, secondary tumor formation, or other adverse events.

## Ependymoma

Although our recent report that included comparative dosimetric planning of photons and protons for ependymoma[15] did not show substantial differences between these modalities, with further investigation using newer models, it seems that this patient cohort may be ideally suited for study and would be an excellent group to contrast with medulloblastoma or supratentorial primitive neuroectodermal tumors treated with craniospinal irradiation.[16] Patients with ependymoma have a high rate of survivorship, and annually there are nearly 300 children under the age of 19 years in the US who develop this tumor.[17] Postoperative radiation therapy is the standard of care for ependymoma in the US and high doses are often administered to focal regions of the brain, pushing limits of normal tissue tolerance.[18]

Based on our cognitive outcome data published in 2004[19] and despite showing that the average child will have preserved IQ after radiation therapy, including the vulnerable child under the age of 3, dose effects models predict for lower IQ and reading scores for an important proportion of children.[8,20] We recently found that read-

ing scores decline in a statistically significant manner after radiation therapy and that the decline is greatest for the youngest children and those with supratentorial tumor location.[20] We have found significant effects for low-, intermediate-, and high-dose volumes on IQ and reading scores after treatment. In considering future research, it will be important for investigators using protons to consider the contribution of hydrocephalus—patients who have decreasing ventricle size after radiation therapy tend to have an improvement in IQ scores—and hormone deficiencies. Although the risk of hormone deficiency remains low in these children, those who present with growth hormone deficiency or who do not seek therapy for radiation induced hormone deficiency tend to have lower levels of cognitive function.

In summary, patients with ependymoma define a vulnerable population because of their young age, their survivorship is increasing and they are an excellent comparison group for children with medulloblastoma—the most common malignant brain tumor in children. Demonstrating an improvement in psychology scores after proton therapy may be a challenge that is further enhanced by planned reductions in the clinical target volume margin from 10 to 5 mm. Evaluating reading scores after radiation therapy seems to be an important opportunity and investigators should consider the clinical factors of age and tumor location as well as hydrocephalus[21] and growth hormone deficiency. Investigators also should consider stratifying supratentorial and infratentorial tumors. Although not discussed, the incidence of hearing loss, already low with photons, may be eliminated or further reduced with protons[22] (Fig. 6).

## Low-Grade Glioma

Low-grade glioma represents a unique opportunity to study proton therapy in children and modeling suggests a benefit when using protons compared with photons.[15] Survivorship is high and there is a variety of cognitive domains that are affected by irradiation. Although IQ is largely preserved, there are problems in academic achievement affecting reading and spelling and problem and adaptive behavior. Age is a major factor in the study of cognitive effects in children with low-grade glioma. Age can affect baseline scores as well as change

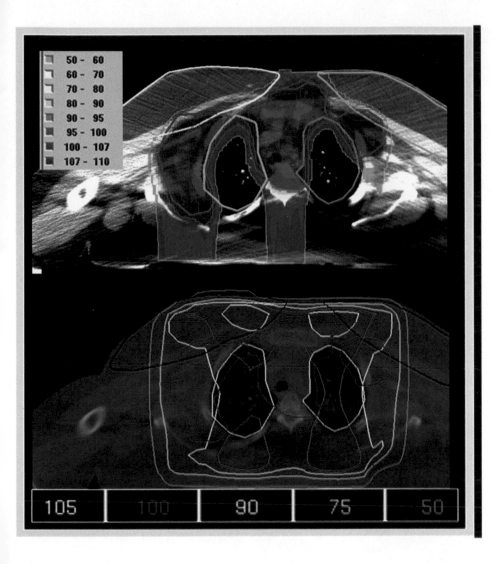

**FIGURE 5.** Proton (upper) and photon (lower) dose distributions generated on axial reconstructed computed tomography images for a child with Hodgkin disease. The dose to the bilateral breasts was <0.2% of the prescribed dose using protons compared with 3% to 6% for PBT. The differences in the mean dose to the heart were 12% of the prescribed dose for the proton plan compared with 98% for the photon plan.

over time. We recently modeled the affect of age and radiation dose on IQ as a function of time after treatment. The model was statistically significant and showed that the affect of age was more than a magnitude greater than the affect of radiation dose.[23] The study also demonstrated the influence of NF-1 and other factors. Confirming these findings in children treated with protons will require considerable effort. Although the hypothalamus is unlikely to be spared in children with central or optic pathway tumors treated with protons, we have shown that despite high-dose irradiation to the hypothalamus, not all children will develop endocrine deficiencies. This finding implies host differences in normal tissue radiosensitivity and genetic predictors of radiation effects should be sought for these and other patients.

In summary, patients with low-grade glioma are relatively young, often pretreated with chemotherapy and the rate of survivorship is high. Most irradiated patients have optic pathway tumors, and there is substantial variability in the targeted volume (Fig. 7). From a psychology standpoint, outcomes using photons is a challenge for protons especially as the clinical target volume margin has been reduced to 5 mm. Age overwhelms the effect of radiation dose in photon models but this must be confirmed using protons. There are a number of conditions to consider including age and NF-1 status, and inves-

tigators must stratify these patients by tumor location: central versus cerebellum. There is a very high rate of pre-existing endocrine deficiency; however, not all patients will develop hormone deficiencies suggesting that host biology should be considered in models of radiation dose and effect. The effect of chemotherapy in the assessment of radiotherapy-related treatment effects other than hearing loss has yet to be considered.

## Craniopharyngioma

Craniopharyngioma represents a group of children with significant pre- and post-treatment morbidity. In our recent report, we showed some of the differences between large and small intracranial structures. Recent models using IQ, radiation dose volume, and age demonstrate potential benefits of protons over photons[15] (Fig. 8).

Investigators at the Institute Gustave Roussy have expended considerable effort to study the effects of proton therapy on these children.[24]

## Medulloblastoma

Conventional therapy for medulloblastoma involving children over the age of 3 years at the time of diagnosis has traditionally

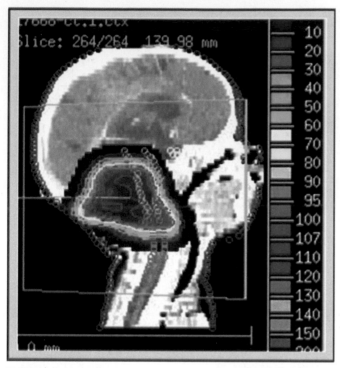

**FIGURE 6.** Proton dose distributions generated on sagittal computed tomography image for a child with ependymoma.

included surgery followed by craniospinal irradiation. The addition of chemotherapy as an adjunct to radiotherapy is recent and has been used to lower the craniospinal dose for standard-risk patients and increase disease control for high-risk patients.[25] Traditional doses of craniospinal irradiation to 36 Gy followed by anatomic posterior fossa treatment to 54 Gy have resulted in rate of decline in IQ of 3.9 points per year.[26] These declines are not surprising given the doses and overall irradiated volume of normal tissue. Efforts to reduce cognitive dysfunction through the use of lower craniospinal doses and combination chemotherapy have not shown a benefit.[27] This is not surprising when one views the curve of volume versus dose for the total brain comparing 36 Gy with 23.4 Gy craniospinal irradiation and full posterior fossa irradiation to 54 Gy.[25] Only doses in the intermediate range are reduced and for a limited volume of normal tissue. Omitting posterior fossa irradiation and confining the boost treatment after craniospinal to the tumor bed with a limited margin results in significant dose volume reductions. This has been accomplished in a series of prospective trials at St. Jude Children's Research Hospital.[28] A similar study using a different chemotherapy regimen is now ongoing in the Children's Oncology Group. Future strategies in the treatment of medulloblastoma with radiotherapy include craniospinal irradiation to dose levels of 18 or 23.4 Gy, based on risk factor considerations, following by treatment of the primary site alone using clinical target volume margins between 5 and 10 mm. Age is a major factor when considering cognitive outcomes for children with medulloblastoma treated with radiotherapy. Patients older than 7 years with average risk medulloblastoma who receive 23.4 Gy craniospinal irradiation typically do not have a decline of IQ. Younger patients treated with the same regimen have a decline in IQ that would be clinical significant within the first 5 years after treatment. Younger patients who require higher doses based on risk

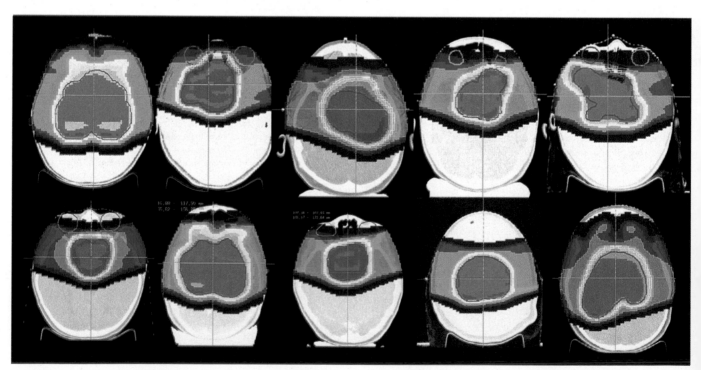

**FIGURE 7.** Proton dose distributions generated on axial computed tomography images for 10 children with optic pathway glioma.

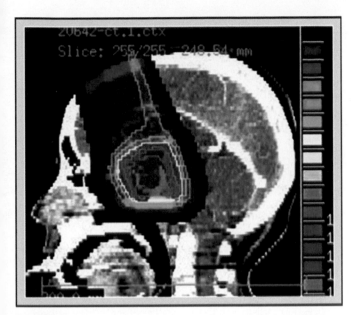

**FIGURE 8.**  Proton dose distributions generated on sagittal computed tomography image for a child with craniopharyngioma.

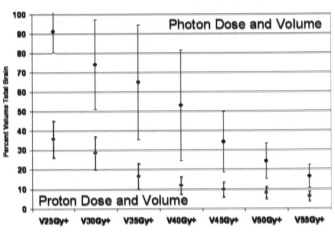

**FIGURE 9.**  Critical combinations of radiation dose and treatment volume based on photon irradiation of medulloblastoma. The photon data represent values that would result in a statistically significant decline in IQ based on follow-up data (unpublished) from Ref. 9. Proton data for the same dose intervals was generated from a similar group of patients to show that the acquired data for proton patients will be substantially different than data acquired for photon patients and less likely to result in a decline in cognition.

have the greatest decline after treatment—the average patient would approach the deficient range (IQ <85) within 3 years after treatment. Older children with high-risk medulloblastoma treated with the high-dose craniospinal irradiation also have a clinically significant fall off in IQ during the first 5 years of follow-up.[29]

Regional differences in the effects of radiation dose on normal brain have been demonstrated for children with medulloblastoma, although the volume that receives the highest dose has the greatest impact on outcome.[9] All dose intervals contribute to decline in IQ suggesting that efforts to reduce craniospinal dose, dose to the primary site, and collateral irradiation to normal tissue, when combined, should reduce side effects and take priority in the treatment of these patients. The same holds true for children age <3 years with medulloblastoma. The clinical target volume margins have been reduced from 10 to 5 mm. As the craniospinal doses are lowered for older children and the clinical target volume margins are further reduced for all, a physical plateau in our ability to reduce dose to normal tissue will be achieved with photons despite the use of intensity modulated radiation therapy in its most conformal form. Our recent article on comparative dosimetry demonstrated some of the differences for small and large intracranial structures and the typical dose volume reductions that might be achieved.[15] Although the differences in the graphs of volume and dose do not appear to be particularly large for total brain and temporal lobe structures, as an example, the difference in decline of IQ as a function of time after radiation therapy was shown to be statistically significant based on a dose effects model that included age and mean dose.

Our recent work in this area has discovered critical dose and volume combinations for photon dose and volume. We have been able to plot the percent volume of the total brain against the volume and dose combination would result in a clinically significant effect. Similar patients treated with protons would have significantly smaller volumes treated to the same dose thus marking a potential benefit for proton irradiation over photons (Fig. 9).

Similar to other patients groups included in this report, medulloblastoma comprises a group of children that include the young and vulnerable[30] where the side effects of irradiation and survivorship are high. From a psychology standpoint, further target volume reductions and changes in photon therapy are unlikely to improve functional outcomes. Clinical target volume margins are being reduced from 10 to 5 mm in current and future trials. There seems to be a modeled benefit for protons, despite the burden of the craniospinal dose. Age is a dominant clinical factor and most domains are affected. Considering endocrine effects, it may be difficult to show an advantage if the craniospinal dose is greater than 18 Gy because the incidence of growth hormone deficiency seems to be consistent above levels of 18 to 20 Gy.

## CONCLUSIONS

Within a decade, nearly all children with potentially curative localized brain and solid tumors will be treated with protons therapy. Pediatric oncologists will be compelled to refer patients for treatment using protons because of the potential reduced side effects and for more precise treatment. The indications for PBT will increase according to treatment capacity. The technology demands for more precise localization of treatment in pediatric radiation oncology will be driven by PBT. Current hypotheses in pediatric clinical trials favor the use of proton beam to achieve their specific aims. Clinical protocols in national consortia have optimized the use of conformal radiation therapy in children with all types of tumors attempting to maximize the dose to the tumor and limit those to normal tissues. Further gains using x-rays are unlikely.

In 1990, the first dedicated US clinical center for proton therapy became available for routine treatment of cancer primarily adult patients. Once safety was been established for adults, the use of proton therapy in pediatric patients began to increase. Today radiation oncology programs are emerging that focus successfully on the pediatric population. Children are very sensitive to the effects of irradiation and appear to be some of the best candidates for proton therapy. Pediatric patients have the most to gain from advancements in radiotherapy including PBT because reductions in the acute and late effects of therapy are one of the top priorities in clinical trial designs. The increased availability of proton centers linked to academic centers of excellence has the potential to congregate pediatric oncology and pediatric radiation oncology patients in those centers. Protons are superiors to photons comparing the conformity of radiation dose to the targeted volume and in reducing dose to normal tissues. The advantages of protons in conformal irradiation dose to the target volume and reducing dose to normal tissues may be exploited to reduce the toxicity of radiation alone or when combined with conventional or experimental chemotherapy. Proton beam irradiation also allows for an increase of radiation dose and local tumor control is the primary issue in preventing treatment failure. A number of investigators have used software to compare normal tissues dose distributions of intensity modulated protons versus those of intensity modulated photons using cases common in the pediatric practice. This includes brain, musculoskeletal, and solid tumors. The differences have been found to be clinically significant and capable of reducing side effects and improving functional outcomes. Because toxicity reduction has been a primary objective for many of the cooperative clinical groups' clinical trials, the use of proton beam alone or in conjunction with other treatments has the potential to measurably reduce treatment related effects for future efforts to intensify therapy. The precision of proton therapy to increase the dose to subvolumes of the tumor or tumor bed complements the risk-based treatment strategies developed worldwide. The increased precision of proton therapy may also be used to exploit the potential benefits of functional or metabolic imaging. Although the indications for proton therapy have not been established for all pediatric tumor types, stages of disease or clinical conditions including patient age, there is consensus that these patients have the most to gain from this modality.

## REFERENCES

1. ICRU Report 50. *Prescribing, Recording and Reporting Photon Beam Therapy.* Washington DC: International Commission on Radiation Units and Measurements; 1992.
2. ICRU Report 62. *Prescribing, Recording and Reporting Photon Beam Therapy (Supplement to ICRO Report 50).* Washington DC: International Commission on Radiation Units and Measurements; 1999.
3. ICRU Report 78. *Prescribing, Recording and Reporting Proton-Beam Therapy.* Washington DC: International Commission on Radiation Units and Measurements; 2007.
4. http://www.demographia.com/db-ua2000pop.htm.
5. Hug EB, Sweeney RA, Nurre PM, et al. Proton radiotherapy in management of pediatric base of skull tumors. *Int J Radiat Oncol Biol Phys.* 2002;52:1017–1024.
6. Dendale R, Lumbroso-Le Rouic L, Noel G, et al. Proton beam radiotherapy for uveal melanoma: results of Curie Institut-Orsay proton therapy center (ICPO). *Int J Radiat Oncol Biol Phys.* 2006;65:780–787.
7. Slater JD, Rossi CJ Jr, Yonemoto LT, et al. Proton therapy for prostate cancer: the initial Loma Linda University experience. *Int J Radiat Oncol Biol Phys.* 2004;59:348–352.
8. Merchant TE, Kiehna EN, Li C, et al. Radiation dosimetry predicts IQ after conformal radiation therapy in pediatric patients with localized ependymoma. *Int J Radiat Oncol Biol Phys.* 2005;63:1546–1554.
9. Merchant TE, Kiehna EN, Li C, et al. Modeling radiation dosimetry to predict cognitive outcomes in pediatric patients with CNS embryonal tumors including medulloblastoma. *Int J Radiat Oncol Biol Phys.* 2006;65:210–221.
10. Merchant TE, Goloubeva O, Pritchard DL, et al. Radiation dose-volume effects on growth hormone secretion. *Int J Radiat Oncol Biol Phys.* 2002;52:1264–1270.
11. Krasin MJ, Xiong A, Wu S, et al. The effects of external beam irradiation on the growth of flat bones in children: modeling a dose-volume effect. *Int J Radiation Oncology Biol Phys.* 2005;62:1458–1463.
12. Krengli M, Hug EB, Adams JA, et al. Proton radiation therapy for retinoblastoma: comparison of various intraocular tumor locations and beam arrangements. *Int J Radiat Oncol Biol Phys.* 2005;61:583–593.
13. Kozak KR, Adams J, Krejcarek SJ, et al. A dosimetric comparison of proton and intensity-modulated photon radiotherapy for pediatric parameningeal rhabdomyosarcomas. *Int J Radiat Oncol Biol Phys.* 2009;74:179–186.
14. Lee CT, Bilton SD, Famiglietti RM, et al. Treatment planning with protons for pediatric retinoblastoma, medulloblastoma, and pelvic sarcoma: how do protons compare with other conformal techniques? *Int J Radiat Oncol Biol Phys.* 2005;63:362–372.
15. Merchant TE, Hua CH, Shukla H, et al. Proton versus photon radiotherapy for common pediatric brain tumors: comparison of models of dose characteristics and their relationship to cognitive function. *Pediatr Blood Cancer.* 2008;51:110–117.
16. MacDonald SM, Safai S, Trofimov A, et al. Proton radiotherapy for childhood ependymoma: initial clinical outcomes and dose comparisons. *Int J Radiat Oncol Biol Phys.* 2008;71:979–986.
17. CBTRUS. *Statistical Report: Primary Brain Tumors in the United States, 1995–1999.* Hinsdale, IL: Central Brain Tumor Registry of the United States; 2002.
18. Mulhern RK, Merchant TE, Gajjar A, et al. Late neurocognitive sequelae among survivors of pediatric brain tumors. *Lancet Oncol.* 2004;5:399–408.
19. Merchant TE, Mulhern RK, Krasin MJ, et al. Preliminary results from a phase II trial of conformal radiation therapy and the evaluation of radiation-related CNS effects for pediatric patients with localized ependymoma. *J Clin Oncol.* 2004;22:3156–3162.
20. Conklin HM, Li C, Xiong X, et al. Predicting change in academic abilities after conformal radiation therapy for localized ependymoma. *J Clin Oncol.* 2008;26:3965–3970.
21. Merchant TE, Lee H, Zhu J, et al. The effects of hydrocephalus on intelligence quotient in children with localized infratentorial ependymoma before and after focal radiation therapy. *J Neurosurg.* 2004;101(2 suppl):159–168.
22. Hua C, Bass JK, Khan RB, et al. Hearing loss after radiotherapy for pediatric brain tumors: effect of cochlea dose. *Int J Radiat Oncol Biol Phys.* 2008;72:892–899.
23. Merchant TE, Conklin HM, Wu S, et al. Late effects of conformal radiation therapy for pediatric patients with low-grade glioma: prospective evaluation of cognitive, endocrine and hearing deficits. *J Clin Oncol.* In press.
24. Habrand JL, Saran F, Alapetite C, et al. Radiation therapy in the management of craniopharyngioma: current concepts and future developments. *J Pediatr Endocrinol Metab.* 2006;19(suppl 1):389–394.
25. Merchant TE. Central nervous system tumors in children. In: Gunderson L, Tepper J, eds. *Clinical Radiation Oncology.* 2nd ed. Philadelphia, PA: Elsevier; 2007:1575–1591.
26. Walter AW, Mulhern RK, Gajjar A, et al. Survival and neurodevelopmental outcome of young children with medulloblastoma at St Jude Children's Research Hospital. *J Clin Oncol.* 1999;17:3720–3728.
27. Ris MD, Packer R, Goldwein J, et al. Intellectual outcome after reduced-dose radiation therapy plus adjuvant chemotherapy for medulloblastoma: a Children's Cancer Group study. *J Clin Oncol.* 2001;19:3470–3476.
28. Merchant TE, Kun LE, Krasin MJ, et al. A multi-institution prospective trial of reduced-dose craniospinal irradiation (23.4 Gy) followed by conformal posterior fossa (36 Gy) and primary site irradiation (55.8 Gy) and dose-intensive chemotherapy for average-risk medulloblastoma. *Int J Radiat Oncol Biol Phys.* 2008;70:782–787.
29. Mulhern RK, Palmer SL, Merchant TE, et al. Neurocognitive consequences of risk-adapted therapy for childhood medulloblastoma. *J Clin Oncol.* 2005;23:5511–5519.
30. Newhauser WD, Fontenot JD, Mahajan A, et al. The risk of developing a second cancer after receiving craniospinal proton irradiation. *Phys Med Biol.* 2009;54:2277–2291.

# The Clinical Experience With Particle Therapy in Adults

Daniela Schulz-Ertner

The main reason for using charged particle beams in radiation therapy is their favorable depth-dose profile, characterized by an increased energy deposition with a sharp maximum at the end of the particle's path, the so-called Bragg Peak. The location of the Bragg peak is determined by the energy of the particles. Favorable dose distributions with steeper dose gradients at the tumor margins when compared with photon beams can thus be achieved, and particles are therefore expected to allow for dose escalation within the target volume and reduction of radiation-induced toxicity.

The relative biologic effectiveness (RBE) of particle beams increases with increasing linear energy transfer (LET). For clinical applications of proton radiotherapy (RT), multiplication of the absorbed dose with the factor 1.1 is the standard procedure leading to the biologic effective proton dose quantified in terms of Cobalt Gray equivalents (GyE). This is possible because the radiobiological properties of protons do not differ substantially from those of photons. By using high-LET beams like carbon ions, the RBE is elevated within the Bragg Peak region, and local RBE values might show a wide range depending on different parameters such as particle type and energy, dose, the cell type and the biologic endpoint looked at.[1] These factors need to be addressed during the treatment planning process for carbon ion radiation therapy.[2] For conventional RT with photons, the oxygenation of the irradiated tissue is known to be a dose-modifying factor, but using carbon ion RT, the oxygen enhancement ratio is reduced in the maximum of the RBE. High-LET beams are therefore assumed to offer biologic advantages in the treatment of tumors with low radioresponsiveness against photon RT and in tumors with hypoxic regions. Furthermore, the therapeutic ratio of carbon ion RT might be further increased by the use of short-course fractionation schemes, enabling a reduction of overall treatment time without increasing toxicity.[3] Secondary cancer induction after carbon ion RT, however, is controversially discussed. There exist only very few experimental data,[4,5] but no long-term clinical data.

Most of the particle therapy facilities in operation use passive beam delivery methods. At this time, only 2 facilities, the Paul Scherrer Institute in Villigen, Switzerland and the Gesellschaft für Schwerionenforschung (GSI) in Darmstadt, Germany, rely on active beam delivery, which allows better sparing of normal tissues, but it is more sensitive to intrafractional target movements. For both, passive and active beam delivery techniques, reproducible immobilization and positioning with high accuracy is mandatory. Rigid immobilization during treatment, stereotactic target localization, and image guidance with pretreatment correction of interfractional setup deviations are used at many centers.

This article reviews the clinical experience with particle therapy in adult patients available so far. Prostate cancer is covered in a separate contribution.

## CNS TUMORS

There are 2 clinical trials available on particle therapy in malignant gliomas. Fitzek et al investigated 23 patients with glioblastoma multiforme treated within a prospective dose escalation trial with a combination of protons and photons using target doses of 90 GyE. Actuarial overall survival rates were 34% and 18% at 2 and 3 years, respectively. In 7 patients, histology after RT revealed radionecrosis. In one patient, a tumor recurrence could be confirmed after RT within the region treated with 90 GyE.[6] Mizoe et al enrolled 48 patients with anaplastic astrocytoma (n = 16) and glioblastoma multiforme (n = 32) in a clinical phase I/II trial of combined photon and carbon ion RT. All patients received concurrent chemotherapy with nimustine hydrochloride (ACNU). Treatment involved photon RT with 50 Gy delivered within 5 weeks in conventional fractionation, followed by 8 fractions of carbon ion RT up to total carbon ion doses between 16.8 and 24.8 GyE. The median survival time was 35 months for anaplastic gliomas and 17 months for glioblastoma multiforme,[7] which seems even better than the median survival time of 14.6 months reported for combined radiochemotherapy with temozolomide in the glioblastoma multiforme patients in the most recent European Organization for Research and Treatment of Cancer (EORTC) trial.[8]

A main shortcoming of both the trials is the fact that no simultaneous application of temozolomide has been performed. Experimental data hint at a possible advantage of a combination of carbon ion RT and temozolomide in comparison with photons plus temozolomide in the glioma cell lines.[9]

Proton RT was investigated prospectively by Fitzek et al in 20 patients with World Health Organization (WHO) grade II and III glioma as well. They treated patients with WHO grade II gliomas with 68.2 GyE; and patients with WHO grade III gliomas received 79.7 GyE. Five-year overall survival was 71% for WHO grade II tumors and 23% for WHO grade III tumors. In this series, a high rate of radionecrosis was observed.[10]

The results of the dose escalation trials with protons and carbon ions show that dose escalation alone will not overcome therapy resistance of glioblastoma multiforme or low-grade gliomas. Furthermore, the limits of radiation therapy with respect to toxicity to normal brain tissue became evident. Future investigations will, therefore, need to focus on multidisciplinary therapy approaches.

## UVEAL MELANOMA

Radiation therapy aims at local tumor control and eye retention. Episcleral plaque brachytherapy was found to be superior to surgery especially in the treatment of medium-sized choroidal melanomas in a randomized Collaborative Ocular Melanoma Study[11] and in a retrospective nonrandomized comparative trial.[12] In a prospective randomized phase III trial, helium ion radiation therapy improved local

**TABLE 1.** Particle Therapy of Uveal Melanomas

| References | Institute | Patients | RT | 5y-LC (%) |
|---|---|---|---|---|
| Egger et al[14] | PSI, Switzerland | 2645 | Protons | 99 |
| Courdi et al[15] | Nice, France | 538 | Protons, 57.2 GyE | 89 |
| Dendale et al[16] | CPO, France | 1406 | Protons, 60 GyE | 96 |
| Desjardins et al[17] | Paris, France | 1272 | Protons | 96 |
| Hocht et al[18] | Berlin, Germany | 245 | Protons, 60 GyE | 95.5 |
| Damato et al[19] | Clatterbridge, UK | 349 | Protons | 97 |
| Tsuji et al[20] | NIRS, Japan | 59 | Carbon ions | 97.4* |

*3y-LC.
PSI indicates Paul Scherrer Institute; CPO, Centre de Protontherapie d'Orsay; LC, local control; NIRS, National Institute of Radiological Sciences; RT, radiotherapy.

control and eye retention rates when compared with brachytherapy with $^{125}$I plaques in medium to large tumors of the posterior segment and in tumors close to the optic nerve. In this trial, however, a higher rate of anterior segment complications was reported after ion beam irradiation.[13] Later on, research focused on proton therapy at several proton facilities. Proton RT yields 5-year local control rates in the range of 96% and eye retention rates between 75% and 92% (Table 1). A target dose of 60 GyE in 4 fractions is the most commonly used treatment scheme. Eye enucleations due to radiation-induced complications, such as neovascular glaucomas, are reported in about 6% of the patients.

Carbon ion RT has been delivered in a phase I/II dose escalation trial in 59 patients with locally advanced or unfavorably located choroidal melanomas. A local control rate of 97.4% was achieved at 3 years.[20] The cumulative neovascular glaucoma rate was, however, relatively high with 42.6% at 3 years in this trial. The most important risk factors for neovascular glaucoma were found to be the volume treated to doses higher than 50 GyE and inclusion of the optic disc.[21,22]

Based on the results obtained in the aforementioned trials, particle therapy with protons is currently considered the best alternative to surgery for uveal melanomas that can not be covered with a sufficient dose using episcleral plaque brachytherapy. Proton RT is well established at a number of specialized centers, and the local control rates are uniquely well more than 90% at 5 years. Results of carbon

ion RT are encouraging, but further investigation is needed aiming at the reduction of RT-induced toxicity.

## SKULL BASE TUMORS

After incomplete resection of skull base chordomas and chondrosarcomas, adjuvant high dose RT is recommended. There exists a dose-response relationship for chordomas, explaining the favorable results after particle therapy with protons and carbon ions when compared with photon treatment.[23] Colli and Al-Mefty analyzed retrospectively protons versus photons in a nonrandomized trial and found that chordoma patients treated with protons had a significantly higher local control probability. The 4-year local control probability was 90% for patients treated with protons versus 19% for patients treated with photons.[24] High local control rates after proton RT were also found by others (Table 2). Carbon ion RT yielded similar control rates in patients with skull base chordomas. At GSI, cumulative local control and overall survival rates at 5 years were 70% and 86%, respectively. Severe late toxicity was observed in less than 5% of the patients, whereas overall treatment time could be significantly reduced to 3 weeks.[23] At the National Institute of Radiologic Sciences (NIRS), 25 patients with chordoma of the skull base and cervical spine have been treated with carbon ion RT. A local control rate of 88% at 3 years was observed.[3] A randomized trial comparing protons and carbon ions in the treatment of chordomas is not yet available.

Particle therapy also yielded high local control rates in chondrosarcomas of the skull base. For this indication, the advantage of particles over photons is less clear because high-dose precision photon RT has been shown to achieve comparably high local control rates.[31] Nevertheless, there exist only few data on high-dose photon RT in chondrosarcomas, whereas the experience with particle therapy is based on several patient series with much higher patient numbers. After proton and carbon ion RT, 5-year local control rates between 75% and 100% have been reported (Table 3).

The indication of proton RT in skull base tumors other than chordoma and chondrosarcoma is debatable. There exists limited experience with proton RT in the treatment of acoustic neuromas, pituitary gland tumors, and meningiomas. At the MGH in Boston, MA, 88 patients with vestibular schwannoma were treated with 12 GyE of proton radiosurgery. The 5-year local control was 93.6%, and the 5-year normal facial and trigeminal nerve function rates were 91.1% and 89.4%, respectively.[35] Bush et al[36] report a local control rate of 100% in 31 schwannoma patients using fractionated proton RT at Loma Linda University Medical Center, CA. At Loma Linda University

**TABLE 2.** Particle Therapy of Skull Base Chordomas

| References | Institute | Patients | RT | 5y-LC (%) |
|---|---|---|---|---|
| Colli and Al-Mefty[24] | Sao Paulo, Brazil | 53 | Protons vs. photons | 90.9 vs. 19.4* |
| Noel et al[25] | CPO, France | 100 | Photons + protons, 67 GyE | 53.8* |
| Weber et al[26] | PSI, Switzerland | 18 | Protons, 74 GyE | 87.5† |
| Igaki et al[27] | Tsukuba, Japan | 13 | Protons + photons, 72 GyE | 46 |
| Castro et al[28] | LBL, USA | 53 | Helium/neon ions, 65 GyE | 63 |
| Hug et al[29] | LLUMC, USA | 33 | Protons, 70.7 GyE | 59 |
| Terahara et al[30] | MGH, USA | 115 | Protons, 68.9 GyE | 59 |
| Schulz-Ertner et al[23] | GSI, Germany | 96 | Carbon ions, 60–70 GyE | 70 |
| Tsujii et al[3] | NIRS, Japan | 25 | Carbon ions, 48–60.8 GyE | 88† |

*4y-LC.
†3y-LC.
PSI indicates Paul Scherrer Institute; LLUMC, Loma Lina University Medical Center; CPO, Centre de Protontherapie d'Orsay; MGH, Massachusetts General Hospital Boston; LBL, Lawrence Berkeley Laboratory; GSI, Gesellschaft für Schwerionenforschung; LC, local control; OS, overall survival; RT, radiotherapy; NIRS, National Institute of Radiologic Sciences.

**TABLE 3.** Particle Therapy of Skull Base Chondrosarcoma

| References | Institute | Patients | RT | 5y-LC (%) |
|---|---|---|---|---|
| Weber et al[26] | PSI | 11 | proton RT, 68 GyE | 100* |
| Hug et al[29] | LLUMC | 25 | proton RT, 70.7 GyE | 75 |
| Rosenberg et al[32] | MGH | 200 | protons + photons, 72.1 GyE | 98† |
| Castro et al[28] | LBL | 27 | helium and neon ions, 65 GyE | 78 |
| Noel et al[32] | CPO | 18 | protons + photons, 67 GyE | 85* |
| Schulz-Ertner et al[33] | GSI | 54 | carbon ions, 60 GyE (BED 75 GyE) | 89.8‡ |

*3y-LC.
†Patients without macroscopic tumor residuals included.
‡4y-LC.
PSI indicates Paul Scherrer Institute; LLUMC, Loma Lina University Medical Center; CPO, Centre de Protontherapie d'Orsay; MGH, Massachusetts General Hospital Boston; LBL, Lawrence Berkeley Laboratory; GSI, Gesellschaft für Schwerionenforschung; LC, local control; RT, radiotherapy.

Medical Center, 47 patients with pituitary adenoma were treated with proton RT, and the local control was obtained in 44 of these patients. Less than 10% of the patients developed severe late effects.[37] For meningiomas, the local control rates between 87.5% and 100% have been reported after proton RT.[38–42] Follow-up is less than 5 years in most of these series, patient numbers are small and reported severe toxicity rates are about 5% to 10%.

For most of these indications, however, excellent treatment results with control rates between 90% and 100%, and the toxicity rates of less than 5% have also been reported after precision photon RT.

A possible advantage of particle therapy, however, remains for atypical and malignant meningiomas, where dose escalation improved local control rates in comparison with photon RT.[43] Further evaluation of particle therapy in this subgroup of skull base meningiomas, taking into consideration the pathologic criteria, is needed to determine the benefit of dose escalation.

## HEAD AND NECK TUMORS

Thornton et al investigated proton therapy as a boost treatment in combination with photon RT in 32 patients with paranasal tumors within a clinical phase I/II. The majority of the patients included in the study were diagnosed with squamous cell carcinomas. Patients with adenocarcinomas and adenoid cystic carcinomas were eligible for the trial as well, whereas patients with lymph node metastases and distant metastases were excluded. The local control rate at 3 years was 89%.[44] In the meanwhile, modern photon intensity-modulated radiation therapy (IMRT) has been shown to allow for dose escalation within the macroscopic tumor as well using an integrated boost concept. It is questionable whether the small difference in the quality of achieved dose distributions of proton and modern photon IMRT translates into a clinical benefit.

Carbon ion radiation therapy was evaluated in a dose escalation study in 36 patients with locally advanced head and neck tumors at NIRS, Japan. Patients were treated with tumor doses between 52.8 and 70.2 GyE. Mizoe et al reported a 5-year local control rate of 75%. Most favorable results were obtained in the adenoid cystic carcinoma and malignant melanoma patients. In adenoid cystic carcinoma and melanoma, the local control rates of 90% and 100%, respectively, have been achieved. Despite the assumption of a radiobiological advantage of carbon ion RT in hypoxic tumors, results in squamous cell carcinomas were disappointing with a local control rate of 34%.[45] One of the main reasons is assumed to be the omission of simultaneous chemotherapy in this trial. In ongoing trials, further investigating carbon ion RT in locally advanced head and neck tumors, concurrent chemotherapy is given.

Carbon ion RT has been investigated even more extensively in locally advanced malignant salivary gland tumors, such as adenoid cystic carcinomas, because a randomized Radiation Therapy Oncology Group/Medical Research Council (RTOG/MRC) trial had shown a significant improvement of the 10-year locoregional control rate with the use of high-LET neutrons when compared with photon RT.[46] A major drawback in the use of neutrons was the relatively high rate of severe late effects, which was estimated to be 10.6% in a metaanalysis of 570 patients with adenoid cystic carcinoma treated at different European neutron facilities.[47]

Most recently, Pommier et al[48] published data of 23 patients with locally advanced adenoid cystic carcinoma treated with protons at the MGH in Boston. Locoregional control was 93%. At GSI, a clinical phase I/II trial investigated combined photon IMRT and a carbon ion boost in the treatment of locally advanced adenoid cystic carcinomas. Locoregional control rates were better than locoregional control rates observed in a historical series of patients treated with photon IMRT alone. The difference was not statistically significant at

**TABLE 4.** Particle Therapy in Locally Advanced Head and Neck Tumors and Malignant Salivary Gland Tumors

| References | Institute | Patients | Tumor Characteristics | RT | 5y-LC (%) |
|---|---|---|---|---|---|
| Slater et al[50] | LLUMC | 29 | SCC oropharynx | Photons + protons, 75.9 GyE | 84 |
| Tokuuye et al[51] | Tsukuba | 33 | Head and neck | Photons + protons, 76 GyE | 74 |
| Mizoe et al[45] | NIRS | 36 | Head and neck | Carbon ions, 48.6–70.2 GyE | 100 MM 50 ACC 34 SCC |
| Pommier et al[48] | MGH | 23 | Locally advanced ACC | Photons + protons, 75.9 GyE | 93 |
| Schulz-Ertner et al[49] | GSI | 63 | Locally advanced ACC | Photons + carbon ions, 72 GyE | 77.5* |
| | | | | Photon IMRT, 66 Gy | 24.6* |
| Tsujii et al[3] | NIRS | 64 | Locally advanced ACC | Carbon ions, 57.6 GyE | 82† |

*4y-LC.
†3y-LC.
SCC indicates squamous cell carcinoma; MM, malignant melanoma; ACC, adenoid cystic carcinoma; LLUMC, Loma Lina University Medical Center; NIRS, National Institute of Radiologic Sciences; MGH, Massachusetts General Hospital Boston; GSI, Gesellschaft für Schwerionenforschung; LC, local control; RT, radiotherapy; IMRT, intensity-modulated radiation therapy.

**TABLE 5.** Particle Therapy in Stage I NSCLC

| References | Institute | Patients | RT | 5y-LC (%) | 5y-OS (%) |
|---|---|---|---|---|---|
| Miyamoto et al[55] | NIRS | 50 | Carbon ions, 72 GyE, 9 fractions | 94.7 | 50<br>IA: 55.2<br>IB: 42.9 |
| Miyamoto et al[56] | NIRS | 79 | Carbon ions<br>Stage IA: 52.8 GyE, 4 fractions<br>Stage IB: 60 GyE, 4 fractions | 90 | 45<br>IA: 62<br>IB: 25 |
| Shioyama et al[54] | Tsukuba | 51 | Proton RT, 76 GyE | IA: 89<br>IB: 39 | IA: 70<br>IB: 16 |
| Nihei et al[57] | NCCHE | 37 | Proton RT, 70–94 GyE, 20 fractions | 80[2] | 84[3] |

*2y-LC.
†2y-OS.
NCCHE indicates National Cancer Center Hospital East; LC, local control; OS, overall survival; RT, radiotherapy; NIRS, National Institute of Radiologic Sciences; NSCLC, nonsmall-cell lung cancer.

the time of the last analysis.[49] The results of proton and carbon ion RT in tumors of the head and neck region are summarized in Table 4.

## LUNG CANCER

Primary photon RT is considered in medically inoperable patients. Dose escalation within the target volume is assumed to improve local control probability. Most recently, modern photon RT, such as stereotactic single dose irradiation and hypofractionated stereotactic irradiation with photons, has yielded respectable results in stage I-II NSCLC with local control rates between 67.9% and 92% at 2 years.[52,53] After proton RT, 5-year in-field control rates of 89% and 39% were observed in stage IA and stage IB NSCLC, respectively. Overall survival rates were 70% and 16%.[54] Similar results were found in other proton trials (Table 5). In parallel, carbon ion radiation therapy has been investigated in the NSCLC patients. A common dose fractionation scheme for carbon ion RT in stage I NSCLC has been 72 GyE given in 9 fractions. The 5-year local control rate was 94.7%. By using this hypofractionated fractionation scheme, grade 3 pneumonitis occurred in less than 5% of all patients.[55] The same authors could show that a fractionation scheme of 4 fractions within 1 week is also feasible in stage I NSCLC with respect to radiation-induced toxicity.[56] Single dose irradiation with carbon ion RT is currently investigated at the NIRS. Furthermore, respiratory gating and image-guided RT are being integrated into modern photon RT and particle therapy and will most likely allow for further sparing of normal lung tissue in the future.

## HEPATOCELLULAR CARCINOMA

Particle therapy allows better sparing of normal liver parenchyma from high doses of RT when compared with photon RT. Published data are available from retrospective and prospective phase I/II trials only (Table 6). Hashimoto et al treated 225 patients with hepatocellular carcinoma with proton RT at Tsukuba, Japan. Local control and overall survival rates were 87.8% and 55.6%, respectively, at 5 years. Coexisting liver cirrhosis influenced overall survival.[58] Overall, carbon ion RT yielded local control and overall survival rates comparable with proton RT.[62]

## TUMORS OF THE BONE AND SOFT TISSUE SARCOMAS

Protons are used at most of the proton facilities to treat paraspinal tumors, because a steep dose gradient between the tumors and the

myelon can be achieved allowing for dose escalation especially in chordomas, chondrosarcomas, and osteosarcomas. Results after proton and carbon ion RT in extracranial chordoma, chondrosarcoma, and osteosarcoma are inhomogeneous, and patient numbers included in prospective and retrospective series are small (Table 7).

Furthermore, there exist only few data on particle therapy in soft tissue sarcomas. Kamada et al evaluated carbon ion RT in a clinical phase I/II trial in 57 patients with locally advanced sarcomas of the bone and soft tissues. Patients with bone tumors, mainly osteosarcomas, chondrosarcomas, and chordomas, were treated at the NIRS using target doses between 52.8 and 73.6 GyE in 16 fractions. Local control and overall survival rates were 73% and 46%, respectively, at 3 years. Remarkable results were observed in a subgroup of 15 patients with inoperable osteosarcoma, where 11 of 15 patients have been locally controlled.[67] In a retrospective analysis of 30 sacral chordoma patients treated with carbon ion RT alone at NIRS, Imai et al[66] found a high local control rate of 96%. Local control rates after irradiation of spinal and sacral chordomas with protons and other charged particles reported by other centers are somewhat lower (Table 7), but this might be due to different definitions used for the analysis of local and distal failures.

## OTHER TUMORS

Sugahara et al[68] treated 46 patients with esophageal carcinoma with proton RT and observed a 5-year local control rate of 83% in selected

**TABLE 6.** Particle Therapy in Liver Tumors

| References | Institute | Patients | RT | LC (%) | 2y-OS (%) |
|---|---|---|---|---|---|
| Bush et al[59] | LLUMC | 34 | Proton RT | 75 | 55 |
| Hata et al[60] | Tsukuba | 21 | Proton RT | 93 | 62 |
| Kawashima et al[61] | Chiba | 30 | Proton RT | 96 | 66 |
| Kato et al[62] | NIRS | 24 | Carbon ion RT | 81 | 50 |
| Tsujii et al[3] | NIRS | 44 | Carbon ion RT, 52.8 GyE, 4 fractions | 95* | 58* |

*3y-OS.
LLUMC indicates Loma Lina University Medical Center; NIRS, National Institute of Radiologic Sciences; LC, local control; OS, overall survival; RT, radiotherapy.

**TABLE 7.** Particle Therapy in Paraspinal and Sacral Tumors

| References | Institute | Patients | Tumor Type | RT | 5y-LC (%) |
|---|---|---|---|---|---|
| Rutz et al[63] | PSI | 26 | Chordoma | Protons, 70.5–73.2 GyE | 77 |
| Tsujii et al[3] | NIRS | 69 | Chordoma | Carbon ions, 70.4 GyE | 98* |
| Schoenthaler et al[64] | LBL | 14 | Chordoma | He and Ne ion RT | 55 |
| Hug et al[65] | MGH | 47 | Osteogenic, chondrogenic | Photons + protons 55.3–82 GyE | 100 CS |
| | | | | | 53 CH |
| | | | | | 59 OS |
| | | | | | 76 others |
| Imai et al[66] | NIRS | 30 | Chordoma | Carbon ions, 52.8–73.6 GyE | 96 |
| Kamada et al[67] | NIRS | 57 | Osteogenic, chondrogenic, soft tissue sarcoma | Carbon ions, 52.8–73.6 GyE | 73* |

*3y-LC.

PSI indicates Paul Scherrer Institute; MGH, Massachusetts General Hospital Boston; LBL, Lawrence Berkeley Laboratory; NIRS, National Institute of Radiologic Sciences; LC, local control; CS, chondrosarcoma; CH, chondroma; OS, osteosarcoma.

patients with early stage tumors. First results of carbon ion RT in patients with pancreatic cancer have been published by Tsujii et al. In a phase I/II dose escalation trial, 22 patients with resectable pancreatic cancer were treated preoperatively with carbon ion RT doses between 44.8 and 48.0 GyE given in 16 fractions within 4 weeks. Three-year overall survival was 23.8%.[3]

Carbon ion RT in primary stage I-IV renal cell carcinoma was investigated by Nomiya et al. Ten patients (7 patients with stage I and 3 patients with stage IV tumors) were included in the trial and were treated with a median total dose of 72 GyE in 16 fractions within 4 weeks. The 5-year local control and overall survival rates were 100% and 74%, respectively. One patient developed grade 4 skin toxicity; no other severe radiation-induced toxicities occurred.[69]

The effectiveness of carbon ion RT has been investigated in 30 patients with stage IIIB and 14 patients with stage IVA carcinoma of the uterine cervix at the NIRS. Patients were treated with carbon ion RT doses between 52.8 and 72 GyE in a first dose searching study. In a subsequent phase I/II trial, the pelvic dose was fixed to 44.8 GyE, and an additional boost dose between 24 and 28 GyE was applied to the cervical tumor, resulting in a cumulative dose of 68.8 to 72.8 GyE. The 5-year local control rates for patients in the first and second phase I/II trials were 45% and 79%, respectively. Even patients with large stage IVA tumors showed a high local control rate of 69%. A major problem was the relatively high rate of severe gastrointestinal late effects necessitating surgery in 8 of 44 patients.[70] Further evaluation with higher patient numbers is required to prove effectiveness of carbon ion RT in these tumor types.

## FUTURE PERSPECTIVES

Although proton RT offers potential benefits in a number of pediatric malignancies by minimizing the risk for secondary malignancies, evidence for the advantage of proton RT in adult patients for most tumor entities does not yet exist. Nevertheless, the lack of clinical phase III trials comparing protons with modern photon RT should not lead to the conclusion that proton RT does not have advantages. Prospective trials provide evidence that proton RT is the treatment of choice for uveal melanomas not manageable with brachytherapy. High effectiveness of proton RT has also been demonstrated for specific skull base tumors, such as chordomas and chondrosarcomas, in nonrandomized trials with large patient numbers. Similar results have been achieved with carbon ion RT in these tumors. Carbon ion RT was furthermore found to be effective in nonsquamous cell head and neck tumors and locally advanced adenoid cystic carcinomas.

The role of proton RT and carbon ion RT in the treatment of early stage lung cancer, hepatocellular carcinoma, primary paraspinal tumors, and gastrointestinal tumors remains to be further defined,

because similar treatment results have been reported with advanced photon RT techniques.

Before particle therapy can be transferred to clinical routine, the proof of its superiority over photon RT in prospective randomized trials would be desirable. However, phase III trials are difficult to perform, because most of the particle therapy centers are still physics-based facilities. They do not provide daily CT-based target localization techniques nor do they use tumor tracking methods to overcome the problems of intrafractional target movements.

## REFERENCES

1. Scholz M, Kellerer AM, Kraft-Weyrather W, et al. Computation of cell survival in heavy ion beams for therapy: the model and its approximation. *Rad Environ Biophysics.* 1997;36:59–66.
2. Krämer M, Jäkel O, Haberer T, et al. Treatment planning for heavy ion radiotherapy: physical beam model and dose optimization. *Phys Med Biol.* 2000;45:3299–3317.
3. Tsujii H, Mizoe J, Kamada T, et al. Clinical results of carbon ion radiotherapy at NIRS. *J Radiat Res.* 2007;48(Suppl):A1–A13.
4. Ando K, Koike S, Oohira C, et al. Tumor induction in mice locally irradiated with carbon ions: retrospective analysis. *J Radiat Res (Tokyo).* 2005;46:185–190.
5. Bettega D, Calzolari P, Hessel P, et al. Neoplastic transformation induced by carbon ions. *Int J Radiat Oncol Biol Phys.* 2009;73:861–868.
6. Fitzek MM, Thornton AF, Rabinov JD, et al. Accelerated fractionated proton/photon irradiation to 90 cobalt gray equivalent for glioblastoma multiforme: results of a phase II prospective trial. *J Neurosurg.* 1999;91:251–260.
7. Mizoe JE, Tsujii H, Hasegawa A, et al. Phase I/II clinical trial of carbon ion radiotherapy for malignant gliomas: combined X-ray radiotherapy, chemotherapy, and carbon ion radiotherapy. *Int J Radiat Oncol Biol Phys.* 2007;69:390–396.
8. Stupp R, Mason WP, van den Bent MJ, et al. Radiotherapy plus concomitant and adjuvant temozolomide for glioblastoma. *N Engl J Med.* 2005;352:987–996.
9. Combs SE, Dohl J, Elsässer T, et al. Radiobiological evaluation and correlation with the local effects model (LEM) of carbon ion radiation therapy and temozolomide in glioblastoma cell lines. *Int J Radiat Biol.* 2009;85:126–137.
10. Fitzek MM, Thornton AF, Harsh G IV, et al. Dose-escalation with proton/photon irradiation for Daumas-Duport lower-grade glioma: results of an institutional phase I/II trial. *Int J Radiat Oncol Biol Phys.* 2001;51:131–137.
11. Jampol LM, Moy CS, Murray TG, et al. The COMS randomized trial of iodine 125 brachytherapy for choroidal melanoma. IV. Local treatment failure and enucleation in the first 5 years after brachytherapy. COMS report no. 19. *Ophthalmology.* 2002;109:2197–2206.
12. Augsburger JJ, Correa ZM, Freire J, et al. Long-term survival in choroidal and ciliary body melanoma after enucleation versus plaque radiation therapy. *Ophthalmology.* 1998;105:1670–1678.
13. Char DH, Quivey JM, Castrop JR, et al. Helium ions versus iodine 125 brachytherapy in the management of uveal melanoma. A prospective, randomized, dynamically balanced trial. *Ophthalmology.* 1993;100:1547–1554.
14. Egger E, Zografos L, Schalenbourg A, et al. Eye retention after proton beam radiotherapy for uveal melanoma. *Int J Radiat Oncol Biol Phys.* 2003;55:867–880.
15. Courdi A, Caujolle JP, Grange JD, et al. Results of proton therapy of uveal melanomas treated in Nice. *Int J Radiat Oncol Biol Phys.* 1999;45:5–11.

16. Dendale R, Lumbroso-Le Rouic L, Noel G, et al. Proton beam radiotherapy for uveal melanoma: results of Curie Institut-Orsay proton therapy center (ICPO). *Int J Radiat Oncol Biol Phys.* 2006;65:780–787.

17. Desjardins L, Lumbroso L, Levy C, et al. Treatment of uveal melanoma with iodine 125 plaques or proton beam therapy: indications and comparison of local recurrence rates. *J Fr Ophtalmol.* 2003;26:269–276.

18. Hocht S, Bechrakis NE, Nausner M, et al. Proton therapy of uveal melanomas in Berlin. 5 years of experience at the Hahn-Meitner Institute. *Strahlenther Onkol.* 2004;180:419–424.

19. Damato B, Kacperek A, Chopra M, et al. Proton beam radiotherapy of choroidal melanoma: the Liverpool-Clatterbridge experience. *Int J Radiat Oncol Biol Phys.* 2005;62:1405–1411.

20. Tsuji H, Ishikawa H, Yanagi T, et al. Carbon-ion radiotherapy for locally advanced or unfavourably located choroidal melanoma: a phase I/II dose-escalation study. *Int J Radiat Oncol Biol Phys.* 2007;67:857–862.

21. Hirasawa N, Tsuji H, Ishikawa H, et al. Risk factors for neovascular glaucoma after carbon ion radiotherapy of choroidal melanoma using dose-volume histogram analysis. *Int J Radiat Oncol Biol Phys.* 2007;67:538–543.

22. Tsujii H, Mizoe J, Kamada T, et al. Overview of clinical experiences on carbon ion radiotherapy at NIRS. *Radiother Oncol.* 2004;73(Suppl 2):41–49.

23. Schulz-Ertner D, Karger CP, Feuerhake A, et al. Effectiveness of carbon ion radiotherapy in the treatment of skull-base chordomas. *Int J Radiat Oncol Biol Phys.* 2007;68:449–457.

24. Colli BO, Al-Mefty O. Chordomas of the craniocervical junction. Follow-up review and prognostic factors. *J Neurosurg.* 2001;95:933–943.

25. Noel G, Feuvret L, Calugaru V, et al. Chordomas of the base of the skull and upper cervical spine. One hundred patients irradiated by a 3D conformal technique combining photon and proton beams. *Acta Oncologica.* 2005;44:700–708.

26. Weber DC, Rutz HP, Pedroni ES, et al. Results of spot-scanning proton radiation therapy for chordoma and chondrosarcoma of the skull base: the Paul Scherrer Institut experience. *Int J Radiat Oncol Biol Phys.* 2005;63:401–409.

27. Igaki H, Tokuuye K, Okumura T, et al. Clinical results of proton beam therapy for skull base chordoma. *Int J Radiat Oncol Biol Phys.* 2004;60:1120–1126.

28. Castro JR, Linstadt DE, Bahary JP, et al. Experience in charged particle irradiation of tumors of the skull base: 1977–1992. *Int J Radiat Oncol Biol Phys.* 19994;29:647–655.

29. Hug EB, Loredo LN, Slater JD, et al. Proton radiation therapy for chordomas and chondrosarcomas of the skull base. *J Neurosurg.* 1999;91:432–439.

30. Terahara A, Niemierko A, Goitein M, et al. Analysis of the relationspip between tumor dose inhomogeneity and local control in patients with skull base chordoma. *Int J Radiat Oncol Biol Phys.* 1999;45:351–358.

31. Debus J, Schulz-Ertner D, Schad L, et al. Stereotactic fractionated radiotherapy for chordomas and chondrosarcomas of the skull base. *Int J Radiat Oncol Biol Phys.* 2000;47:591–596.

32. Rosenberg AE, Nielsen GP, Keel SB, et al. Chondrosarcoma of the base of the skull: a clinicopathologic study of 200 cases with emphasis on its distinction from chordoma. *Am J Surg Pathol.* 1999;23:1370–1378.

33. Noel G, Habrand JL, Jauffret E, et al. Radiation therapy for chordoma and chondrosarcoma of the skull base and the cervical spine. *Strahlenther Onkol.* 2003;179:241–248.

34. Schulz-Ertner D, Nikoghosyan A, Hof H, et al. Carbon ion radiotherapy of skull base chondrosarcomas. *Int J Radiat Oncol Biol Phys.* 2007;67:171–177.

35. Weber DC, Chan AW, Bussiere MR, et al. Proton beam radiosurgery for vestibular schwannoma: tumor control and cranial nerve toxicity. *Neurosurgery.* 2003;53:577–586.

36. Bush DA, McAllister CJ, Loredo LN, et al. Fractionated proton beam radiotherapy for acoustic neuroma. *Neurosurgery.* 2002;50:270–273.

37. Ronson BB, Schulte RW, Han KP, et al. Fractionated proton beam irradiation of pituitary adenomas. *Int J Radiat Oncol Biol Phys.* 2006;64:425–434.

38. Noel G, Bollet MA, Calugaru V, et al. Functional outcome of patients with benign meningioma treated by 3D conformal irradiation with a combination of photons and protons. *Int J Radiat Oncol Biol Phys.* 2005;62:1412–1422.

39. Vernimmen FJ, Harris JK, Wilson JA, et al. Stereotactic proton beam therapy of skull base meningiomas. *Int J Radiat Oncol Biol Phys.* 2001;49:99–105.

40. Wenkel E, Thornton AF, Finkelstein D, et al. Benign meningioma: partially resected, biopsied, and recurrent intracranialtumors treated with combined proton and photon radiotherapy. *Int J Radiat Oncol Biol Phys.* 2000;48:1363–1370.

41. Weber DC, Lomax AJ, Rutz HP, et al. Spot-scanning proton radiation therapy for recurrent, residual or untreated intracranial meningiomas. *Radiother Oncol.* 2004;71:251–258.

42. Gudjonsson O, Blomquist E, Nyberg G, et al. Stereotactic irradiation of skull base meningiomas with high energy protons. *Acta Neurochir (Wien).* 1999;41:933–940.

43. Hug EB, DeVries A, Thornton AF, et al. Management of atypical and malignant meningiomas: role of high-dose, 3D-conformal radiation therapy. *J Neurooncol.* 2000;48:151–160.

44. Thornton AF, Fitzek MM, Vavares M, et al. Accelerated hyperfractionated proton/photon irradiation for advanced paranasal sinus cancer. Results of a prospective phase I-II study. *Int J Radiat Oncol Biol Phys.* 1998;42:222.

45. Mizoe J, Tsujii H, Kamada T, et al. Dose escalation study of carbon ion radiotherapy for locally advanced head and neck cancer. *Int J Radiat Oncol Biol Phys.* 2004;55:358–364.

46. Laramore GE, Krall JM, Griffin TW, et al. Neutron versus photon irradiation for unresectable salivary gland tumors: final report of an RTOG-MRC randomized clinical trial. *Int J Radiat Oncol Biuol Phys.* 1993;27:235–240.

47. Krüll A, Schwarz R, Brackrock S, et al. Neutron therapy in malignant salivary gland tumors: results at European centers. *Recent Results Cancer Res.* 1998;150:88–99.

48. Pommier P, Liebsch NJ, Deschler DG, et al. Proton beam radiation therapy for skull base adenoid cystic carcinoma. *Arch Otolaryngol Head Neck Surg.* 2006;132:1242–1249.

49. Schulz-Ertner D, Nikoghosyan A, Didinger B, et al. Therapy strategies for locally advanced adenoid cystic carcinomas using modern radiation therapy techniques. *Cancer.* 2005;104:338–344.

50. Slater JD, Yonemoto LT, Mantik DW, et al. Proton radiation for treatment of cancer of the oropharynx: early experience at Loma Linda University Medical Center using a concomitant boost technique. *Int J Radiat Oncol Biol Phys.* 2005;62:494–500.

51. Tokuuye K, Akine Y, Kagei K, et al. Proton therapy for head and neck malignancies at Tsukuba. *Strahlenther Onkol.* 2004;180:96–101.

52. Hof H, Muenter M, Oetzel D, et al. Stereotactic single-dose radiotherapy (radiosurgery) of early stage nonsmall-cell lung cancer (NSCLC). *Cancer.* 2007;110:148–155.

53. Wulf J, Haedinger U, Oppitz U, et al. Stereotactic radiotherapy for primary lung cancer and pulmonary metastases: a non-invasive treatment approach in medically inoperable patients. *Int J Radiat Oncol Biol Phys.* 2004;60:186–196.

54. Shioyama Y, Tokuuye K, Okumura T, et al. Clinical evaluation of proton radiotherapy for non-samll-cell lung cancer. *Int J Radiat Oncol Biol Phys.* 2003;56:7–13.

55. Miyamoto T, Baba M, Yamamoto N, et al. Curative treatment of stage I non-small-cell lung cancer with carbon ion beams using a hypofractionated regimen. *Int J Radiat Oncol Biol Phys.* 2007;67:750–758.

56. Miyamoto T, Baba M, Sugane T, et al. Carbon ion radiotherapy for stage I non-small cell lung cancer using a regimen of four fractions during 1 week. *J Thorac Oncol.* 2007;2:916–926.

57. Nihei K, Ogino T, Ishikura S, et al. High-dose proton beam therapy for stage I non-small-cell lung cancer. *Int J Radiat Oncol Biol Phys.* 2006;65:107–111.

58. Hashimoto T, Tokuuye K, Fukumitsu N, et al. Repeated proton beam therapy for hepatocellular carcinoma. *Int J Radiat Oncol Biol Phys.* 2006;65:196–202.

59. Bush DA, Hillebrand DJ, Slater JM, et al. High-dose proton beam radiotherapy of hepatocellular carcinoma: preliminary results of a phase II trial. *Gastroenterology.* 2004;127(Suppl 1):S189–S193.

60. Hata M, Tokuuye K, Sugahara S, et al. Proton beam therapy for hepatocellular carcinoma with limited treatment options. *Cancer.* 2006;107:591–598.

61. Kawashima M, Furuse J, Nishio T, et al. Phase II study of radiotherapy employing proton beam for hepatocellular carcinoma. *J Clin Oncol.* 2005;23:1839–1846.

62. Kato H, Tsujii H, Miyamoto T, et al. Results of the first prospective study of carbon ion radiotherapy for hepatocellular carcinoma with liver cirrhosis. *Int J Radiat Oncol Biol Phys.* 2004;59:1468–1476.

63. Rutz HP, Weber DC, Sugahara S, et al. Extracranial chordoma: outcome in patients treated with function-preserving surgery followed by spot-scanning proton beam irradiation. *Int J Radiat Oncol Biol Phys.* 2007;67:512–520.

64. Schoenthaler R, Castro JR, Petti PL, et al. Charged particle irradiation of sacral chordomas. *Int J Radiat Oncol Biol Phys.* 1993;26:291–298.

65. Hug EB, Fitzek MM, Liebsch NJ, et al. Locally challenging osteo- and chondrogenic tumors of the axial skeleton: results of combined proton and photon radiation therapy using three-dimensional treatment planning. *Int J Radiat Oncol Biol Phys.* 1995;31:467–476.

66. Imai R, Kamada T, Tsujii H, et al. Carbon ion radiontherapy for unresectable sacral chordomas. *Clin Cancer Res.* 2004;10:5741–5746.

67. Kamada T, Tsujii H, Yanagi T, et al. Efficacy and safety of carbon ion radiotherapy in bone and soft tissue sarcomas. *J Clin Oncol.* 2002;20:4466–4477.

68. Sugahara S, Tokuuye K, Okumura T, et al. Clinical results of proton beam therapy for cancer of the esophagus. *Int J Radiat Oncol Biol Phys.* 2005;61:103–111.

69. Nomiya T, Tsuji H, Hirasawa N, et al. Carbon ion radiation therapy for primary renal cell carcinoma: initial clinical experience. *Int J Radiat Oncol Biol Phys.* 2008;72:828–833.

70. Kato S, Ohno T, Tsujii H, et al. Dose escalation study of carbon ion radiotherapy for locally advanced carcinoma of the uterine cervix. *Int J Radiat Oncol Biol Phys.* 2006;65:388–397.

# Life, Liberty, and the Pursuit of Protons

## An Evidence-Based Review of the Role of Particle Therapy in the Treatment of Prostate Cancer

Jason A. Efstathiou • Alexei V. Trofimov • Anthony L. Zietman

The introduction of serum prostate-specific antigen (PSA) as a marker for prostate cancer and its use beginning in the late 1980s has led to a dramatic increase in prostate cancer detection. Since the advent of the PSA era, however, a stage migration has occurred toward diagnosis at a younger age at a lower serum PSA level and less aggressive disease more likely to be confined to the prostate.[1] This has led to an increase in aggressive local therapy, including radiation therapy, intended to cure these small volume and low-grade cancers.[2]

External beam radiation therapy (EBRT) is commonly used for the definitive treatment of localized-prostate cancer. Radiation oncologists have employed advances in technology, such as computer based treatment planning, 3-dimensional conformal radiation therapy, and intensity modulated radiation therapy (IMRT), to reduce the morbidity associated with conventional EBRT, such as cystitis and proctitis, while escalating the radiation dose to the prostate. Higher radiation doses delivered to the prostate gland have been associated with improved tumor eradication and biochemical disease-free survival (on the order of 10%–20% benefit after 5–10 years) in randomized controlled trials.[3–6]

Proton beam therapy (PBT), a form of EBRT, offers the potential of achieving dose escalation in the treatment of prostate cancer and decreasing toxicity by capitalizing on the unique dose deposition characteristics of the Bragg peak to avoid normal tissue. Although PBT for prostate cancer has been in use for many decades, it has recently increased in popularity spawning the opening of new proton facilities. There is little published data, however, aside from some comparative planning studies, to support its use or superiority over other forms of conformal radiation for prostate cancer.

Currently, the evidence does not support any definitive benefit to PBT. There are no published patient-reported outcomes for prostate cancer patients treated with IMRT versus PBT and no prospective studies have been initiated comparing these modalities. Yet, radiation oncologists are coming under increasing pressure to justify the use of more sophisticated treatments. Organizations conducting technology assessments are evaluating the use of PBT in the treatment of prostate cancer, with the expectation that comparative data on these technologies will be available.

This review critically addresses the current status and promise of PBT for localized prostate cancer compared with other forms of conformal radiation.

## PROTON PHYSICS AND THEORETICAL CONSIDERATIONS

Protons are positively charged subatomic particles. The use of protons as a source of therapeutic radiation is attractive and stems from physical, not biologic, advantages. Although their biologic effect is similar to that of conventional radiation, protons offer a substantial advantage in terms of their unique depth-dose distribution as compared with photons (ie, x-rays) (Fig. 1).

The physical characteristics of protons result in the majority of energy being deposited at the end of a linear track, a sharp maximum called the Bragg peak. Radiation dose then falls off rapidly beyond the Bragg peak at the end of the particles' range with essentially no exit dose, and a much reduced dose proximal to the target volume. The position of the Bragg peak for protons is determined by beam energy. An individual peak is too narrow to cover any tumor of realistic dimensions, so often beams of differing energies are combined and modulated to broaden or spread out the Bragg peak so as to uniformly cover the full extent of the target at depth.

Photons, on the other hand, lack mass and charge, and the x-ray beams deposit dose in a continuous fashion such that there is some dose received in the beam's path beyond the target (Fig. 1).

These considerable advantages to protons were realized by Wilson[7] and, since about 1960, protons have been explored in a few facilities, primarily in the environment of physics research laboratories. Beginning in the 1990s, a number of hospital-based purpose-built proton medical facilities came into operation, and there has been a recent explosion in the number of such facilities that are operational, under construction, or proposed worldwide.

The theoretical potential to precisely deliver high doses to a tumor and increase the probability of tumor control, while limiting collateral damage caused by scatter and exit dose to surrounding normal tissue and reduce morbidity, is the promise of protons. This promise of favorable dose distribution and the ability to spare critical structures has proven safe and successful in the management of rare malignancies, such as ocular,[8] base of skull,[9] central nervous system, and pediatric tumors.[10]

The benefit in prostate cancer, however, remains unclear. Protons' sharp distal falloff of dose is potentially a 2-edged sword. On one hand, it allows the delivery of dose to the tumor while sparing distal tissues. On the other hand, an overestimate or underestimate of the path length for any reason could cause undershooting or overshooting of the beam, respectively, with consequent complete miss of a distal portion of the tumor or high dose being delivered to adjacent normal tissue. In fact, there can be some uncertainty about the particle range in tissue and exact location of the steep fall off because of sensitivity to tissue heterogeniety (ie, bone and air). Such concerns are especially pertinent in the delivery of PBT to deep-seated, mobile targets such as the prostate, which is dependent on variations in bladder and rectal filling, as well as bony-hip anatomy[11] (Fig. 2). Proton beams also have a significant penumbra (ie, gradual dose fall off at the lateral edge of the beam) at depth, compromising their ability to spare adjacent tissues.

The uncertainties in proton-particle penetration in tissue dictate certain beam configurations (different to IMRT delivery). They

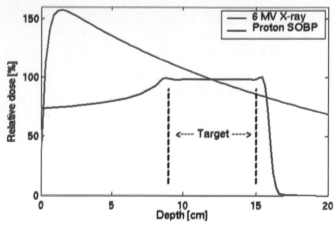

**FIGURE 1.** The relative physical advantage of protons is illustrated in this figure of depth-dose curves for typical therapeutic 6 megavolt (MV) photons (red) and spread-out Bragg peak (SOBP) protons (blue).

also require the use of liberal proximal and distal safety margins to ensure tumor coverage, at the expense of irradiating uninvolved normal tissue, such as portions of the bladder and rectum. Currently, given the range uncertainty in the anterior and posterior directions and to safely accommodate additional margins, opposed lateral proton beams are used so as not to increase the volume of rectum receiving high dose. This opposed lateral beam configuration travels through both femoral heads perpendicular to the rectum on an axial view. Such beam arrangement is associated with the largest radiologic depth of the target leading to higher scatter and wider-dose penumbra. Inevitably, this exposes the anterior rectal wall to some of the high-dose region and leads to not so insignificant hip dose. A range compensator, which is used to conform the dose to the distal surface of the target, needs to be modified ("smeared") to counter the possible effect of misalignment between bony anatomy and the prostate. In addition, the prostate has been observed to move significantly, not only from day-to-day treatment but also during a short treatment. This necessitates the employment of even more liberal safety planning margins to account for setup error as well as inter and intrafractional motion and ensure complete irradiation of the gland. Such insurance further dilutes any theoretical advantage of protons.

Thus, the potential benefit of protons as currently delivered is likely disease site specific and most readily realized when treating more superficial tumors surrounded by homogeneous tissue without any cavities, air pockets, or complex bones. Reproducible immobilization and daily localization using image guidance are key to exploiting the maximal precision of protons. Because protons remain a limited resource, it will be important to identify the sites in which PBT offers measurable and clinically significant advantages over other more readily available conformal treatments, such as IMRT or brachytherapy.

Although there are widespread reports of favorable clinical experiences with PBT, there has been a paucity of randomized studies and very few critical comparisons. This is largely because of the fact that, until quite recently, only a few centers have been engaged in PBT, and those that were had a number of constraints including limited capacity, limited energy, limited technology, and limited beam availability. Furthermore, in certain disease sites where the initial experience has been very favorable, subsequent randomized trials have not been considered feasible based on ethical grounds.

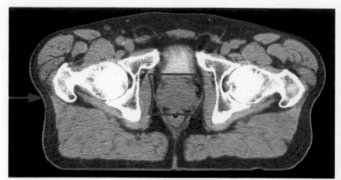

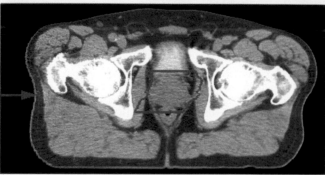

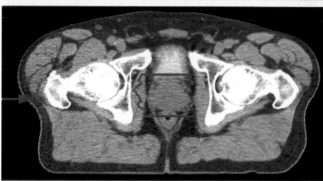

**FIGURE 2.** Sensitivity of the proton beam range to variations in the set up of soft tissue and bony anatomy. Arrows indicate the direction of the incoming proton beam. The red contour shows the approximate extent of the volume covered by the prescribed dose delivered with a single lateral beam for the planned patient set up (top). The proton range and the position of the prescription iso-dose curve are visibly affected when the hip is rotated by 10 degrees towards the anterior (middle) or posterior (bottom).

Although equipoise still exists, both by clinicians and patients, it would clearly be desirable to test protons against photons by means of an appropriately designed and powered prospective randomized clinical trial with validated quality of life endpoints for a commonly occurring tumor lying in close proximity to critical structures known to benefit from dose escalation, such as prostate cancer.

## COMPARATIVE PLANNING STUDIES

Although the unique dose distribution of protons suggests a potential dosimetric advantage, one must first ask against what is it being

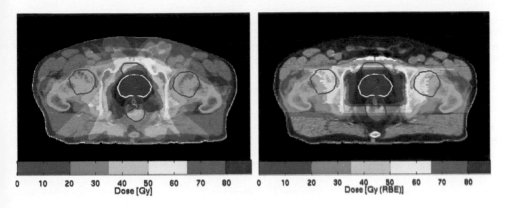

**FIGURE 3.** Dose distributions from photon IMRT (left) and proton therapy (right). Prostate (white contour) was irradiated to 79.2 Gy/CGE in both cases. Purple contours designate the critical organs: bladder, rectum, and femoral heads.

compared? IMRT has been in clinical use since the mid 1990s, and its dosimetric advantage over 3-dimensional conformal radiation therapy has been widely reported. IMRT has now become the most commonly used form of EBRT for prostate cancer in the United States, and thus should be the standard of reference for comparison with protons. IMRT employs advanced inverse treatment planning techniques and uses multiple photon beams of nonuniform intensity, which are combined to achieve a highly conformal dose distribution capable of sculpting around critical normal structures, such as the anterior rectum, in an elegant manner.

Trofimov et al[12] recently performed a treatment planning comparison of IMRT (seven equally spaced coplanar fields) with 3D conformal PBT (2 parallel-opposed lateral fields) to a dose of 79.2 Gy or cobalt Gray equivalent (CGE) taking into account range uncertainty (Fig. 3). IMRT plans yielded better dose conformity to the target (ie, ratio of the prescription isodose to the volume of target) and better sparing of the bladder in the high-dose range (>60 Gy/CGE). The bladder V70 (volume of bladder receiving 70 Gy/CGE) was 50% lower with IMRT than with PBT. Rectal sparing was similar between the 2 in the high-dose range, although other dose-volume comparison studies have suggested a significant benefit to rectal sparing with protons over IMRT.[13] Proton plans, on the other hand, achieved higher-dose homogeneity and better sparing of rectum and bladder in the low-dose range (<30 Gy/CGE). In addition, protons delivered a significantly lower total-body dose. IMRT, because of leakage radiation and more beams being used, exposes a substantially larger volume of normal tissue to low and medium dose. That is to say that IMRT creates a low-dose radiation bath that is significantly larger than that seen with PBT (Fig. 4).

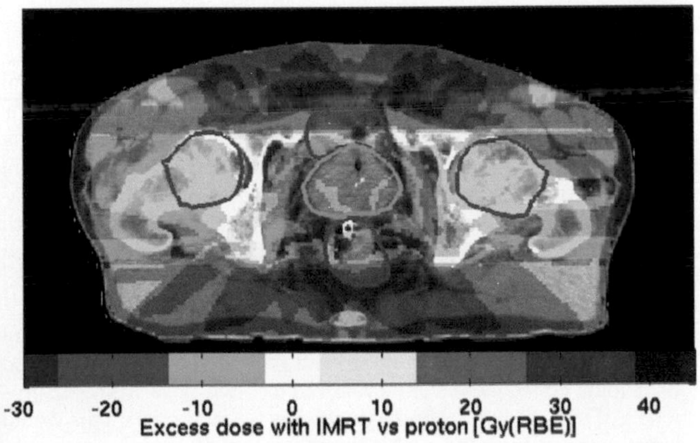

Whether the nuances that arise from such dosimetric comparisons between PBT and IMRT plans actually translate into tangible or measurable benefits for 1 modality over the other remains unknown. Does conventional PBT lead to more bladder bleeding and hip fractures? Does IMRT confer an increased risk of rectal bleeding? Does integral dose reduction with PBT mean fewer second malignancies?

A recent paper from the Hyogo Ion Beam Medical Center in Japan suggests that there is a low incidence of gastrointestinal toxicity and comparable genitourinary toxicity to photons.[14] Data from atomic bomb survivors estimate that patients receiving IMRT for prostate cancer may have a secondary malignancy risk of 1.75% at 10 years (compared with 1% with conventional photon EBRT).[15] Modeling studies from the Paul Scherrer Institut in Switzerland suggest that spot-scanned protons (which limit carcinogenic secondary neutron production) can halve the risk of secondary cancers with dose escalation.[16] Most centers in the United States, however, use passive scattering PBT which employs scattering foils, field-shaping apertures and range compensators, all sources of scatter, and neutron production.[15] The amount of such secondary neutron production and its significance in second tumor risk is a matter of debate.[15,17,18] Regardless, the risk of secondary malignancies from protons is unlikely to be higher than the risk from IMRT.[19] However, although a small absolute increase in the risk of second cancers with IMRT may be unacceptable for a pediatric patient with decades-long life expectancy,[20] the impact in older patients when balanced by excellent local tumor control and reduced acute toxicity has yet to be determined. Only a randomized comparison between protons and IMRT with careful acute and late toxicity profiling and patient-reported quality of life analyses can appropriately address all these important questions.

## CLINICAL EXPERIENCE WITH PBT FOR PROSTATE CANCER

Proton therapy was first delivered to prostate cancer patients in 1976 at the Harvard Cyclotron in Boston in conjunction with the Massachusetts General Hospital (MGH). The first publication of this experience in 1979 was based on 17 patients and demonstrated feasibility.[21] Clinical experience has since grown at centers in the United States, including the MGH and Loma Linda University Medical Center in California, and in Europe and Japan. Specifically, studies in prostate cancer have focused on escalating the dose with protons.

**FIGURE 4.** The dose distribution difference between the IMRT and proton plans shown in Figure 3, resulting in a low-dose bath with IMRT.

In 1995, the MGH reported on a phase III randomized trial of locally advanced prostate cancer treated to high dose of 75.6 CGE using a conformal proton boost compared with conventional dose irradiation to 67.2 Gy using photons alone.[22] In 2004, Loma Linda published their initial experience of 1277 patients with early disease treated with protons to 74 CGE. They found such treatment to be comparable in terms of disease outcome with other forms of local therapy with minimal morbidity.[23]

More recently, MGH and Loma Linda reported a randomized phase III dose-escalation trial (Proton Radiation Oncology Group/American College of Radiology 95-09) using mixed conformal photons with proton boost in 392 patients with early-stage prostate cancer. This study found that 79.2 CGE is superior to 70.2 CGE in terms of 5-year PSA failure-free survival without worse severe toxicity.[3] A long-term update will soon be reported and shows that the 10-year biochemical failure rates are 35.3% for the conventional dose arm and 16.3% for the high-dose arm ($P = 0.0001$) [ALZ by communication]. This advantage was achieved without any associated increase in grade $\geq 3$ late urinary or rectal morbidity. Parallel quality of life studies using the validated Prostate Cancer Symptom Index have shown similar levels of satisfaction with bowel and urinary function in both arms after a minimum follow-up of 8.3 years.[24] However, the contribution of the proton beam component is unclear, because the study did not compare the efficacy of protons versus photons and results are similar to those reported in a similar trial comparing 70 Gy versus 78 Gy using photon EBRT.[25]

The above studies show that PBT can be delivered to high doses without causing a significant difference in patient-reported quality of life. Whether PBT can be used to escalate radiation dose even further in the treatment of prostate cancer is unknown. Further dose escalation using protons alone to 82 CGE was the subject of a recently closed MGH/Loma Linda prospective pilot protocol,[26] and it seems that this may represent the ceiling on dose achievable using current PBT techniques. However, a key point remains in that there have been no randomized trials directly comparing the efficacy and tolerability of high-dose PBT with equally high-dose IMRT in the treatment of clinically localized-prostate cancer. Such a study with quality of life endpoints is currently under development by the MGH, University of Pennsylvania, and Midwest Proton Research Institute at Indiana University with support from the Radiation Therapy Oncology Group.

## COST EFFECTIVENESS

Enthusiasm for PBT must be tempered not only by clinical evidence but also by harsh economic reality. In this day and age of skyrocketing health-care expenditures, is PBT worth the cost? At a price tag of roughly $100 to 150 million ($20–30 million for significantly scaled-down units), a PBT facility represents a major financial investment for a hospital and health care system. The ability to repay the debt on a new proton center is heavily dependent on reimbursement. Although complex cases such as pediatric medulloblastoma benefit from PBT, these tumors are rare and require long-treatment times. Prostate cancer, on the other hand, is common and throughput can be rapid. Thus, a high volume of prostate cancer patients offers a tempting business model for the development of new proton centers.

Questions, however, have been raised as to the cost effectiveness of PBT relative to other options, such as IMRT. Konski et al[27] published a recent cost effectiveness analysis using Markov models of PBT compared with current state-of-the-art therapy in the treatment of patients with intermediate-risk prostate cancer. The model assumed a cost of $58,610 for protons and $25,846 for IMRT. Despite generous and unproven assumptions regarding achievable dose without any increase in toxicity (ie, that protons would permit a 10-Gy escalation of dose compared with IMRT [91.8 CGE vs. 81 Gy]) and efficacy (ie, 10% improvement in 5-year biochemical disease-free survival), PBT was not cost effective for most patients with prostate cancer when using the commonly accepted standard benchmark of $50,000 quality-adjusted life-years.

Currently, there are 5 gantry-based proton facilities open in the United States, and over a dozen under construction or in planning stages. While it is without a doubt that the United States needs PBT, ideally centers would be geographically well distributed, with a consortia based around academic centers placing a heavy emphasis on research and practicing evidence-based medicine divorced from commercial influence. Otherwise, PBT has the potential to distort patterns of health care, limit resources to other areas of medical need, and paradoxically lead to over treatment of patients. With the current debate over PSA screening having recently entered the public arena after the reporting of both American and European screening trials,[28,29] there is little doubt that prostate cancer is an over-diagnosed and over-treated disease.

Although PBT remains an excellent management option for prostate cancer, so do other viable options that come at a lower cost at this time. IMRT and brachytherapy are forms of conformal radiation that can deliver high doses to the prostate while effectively sparing normal tissue. Radical prostatectomy offers a surgical solution and active surveillance offers no treatment morbidity. Comprehensive evaluation of PBT is needed before opening too many new facilities that may be built around a potentially faulty business model and thus be at risk from their own exuberance.

## FUTURE DIRECTIONS

### Pencil Beam Scanning and Intensity-Modulated Proton Therapy

There are 2 ways of delivering proton therapy: passively scattered and intensity-modulated pencil beam. As pencil beam scanning replaces passive scattering for PBT and intensity-modulated proton therapy (IMPT) becomes possible, a significant dosimetric advantage for protons may yet manifest and a clinical advantage could possibly emerge.

Whereas passively scattered PBT is the analog of photon 3D conformal radiotherapy in that the incident beams have uniform profiles, IMPT is the analog of IMRT with photons except that there is an extra degree of control over the energy of each proton pencil beam. Similar to IMRT with photons, IMPT uses the inverse planning optimization technique (taking into account target and normal tissue constraints) and delivers individually inhomogeneous dose distributions from multiple different directions to yield a desired conformal composite distribution with the potential for sharp-dose gradients (Fig. 5). Such delivery can be achieved by magnetically scanning a narrow proton beam across the target volume. Beam intensity and speed are varied during the scan to achieve the desired-dose modulation, and the beam energy is adjusted for irradiation of varying depth within the target, thus conforming dose to proximal and distal edges of a target volume. IMPT may further sharpen the dose penumbra in tissue.[30]

Unlike 3D conformal PBT, IMPT dose not require a scattering foil, patient-specific compensators, and field-shaping apertures, and thus, avoids consequent scatter and reduces the dose from the production of undesirable secondary particles (ie, neutrons). This would address some of the concerns, including potential second tumor risk, that have been raised about the effect of whole-body dose neutron contamination produced in proton interactions with beam-shaping devices.

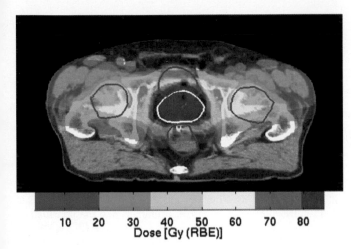

**FIGURE 5.** In intensity-modulated proton therapy (IMPT), several inhomogeneous dose distributions combine to achieve improved-dose conformality to the target.

IMPT is routinely used clinically at the Paul Scherrer Institut in Switzerland, namely for intracranial, nasopharyngeal, and paraspinal tumors. Treatment planning studies have shown exquisite-dose distributions achievable with IMPT for many treatment sites,[31–37] though given range uncertainty and other issues there is still a considerable amount of research and development required to improve IMPT and fully exploit its potential.[38]

The MGH recently delivered its first IMPT treatment to a sarcoma patient. IMPT treatment of prostate cancer has yet to be performed and optimized. Optimization of IMPT might allow for improved conformality, greater target dose homogeneity, reduced dose proximal to the target volume, sharpened beam boundaries, reduced margins, improved robustness of treatment plans to uncertainties, and increased efficiency.

## Higher-Dose Escalation

Currently, there is no suggestion that protons may afford further dose escalation more safely than IMRT given the exposure to dose-limiting structures, namely the bladder neck and anterior rectum. The hope would be that this may be possible with further technologic advances such as IMPT in concert with reproducible immobilization and daily localization. As discussed earlier, a prospective study (ACR 0312) of radiation dose escalation to 82 CGE in early prostate cancer has closed recently. Whether or not further dose escalation will materialize into improved cancer control and/or acceptable toxicity profiles remains unknown.

## Hypofractionation

The optimal radiation schedule for the curative treatment of prostate cancer remains unknown. Standard EBRT fractionation for prostate cancer entails roughly 40 treatments of 1.8 to 2.0 Gy/fraction delivered 5 days per week over 8 weeks or so. On the part of patients, this requires an obvious time commitment and sometimes even geographic relocation for treatment. On the part of health care economics, such protracted therapy represents a financial burden. There is a growing body of evidence suggesting that in slowly growing tumors, such as prostate cancer, the dose response of cancer cells and normal tissues to highly fractionated radiation (ie, the $\alpha/\beta$ ratio) is very low.[39,40] If

this is in fact true, then hypofractionated regimens (less frequent and larger fractions) may be more efficacious and less costly.

Randomized trials from Australia (55 Gy/20 fractions vs. 64 Gy/32 fractions)[41] and Canada (52.5 Gy/20 fractions vs. 66 Gy/33 fractions)[42] have demonstrated similar PSA outcome and acceptable toxicity with hypofractionated regimens. The Radiation Therapy Oncology Group (protocol 0415) is currently investigating 73.8 Gy at 1.8 Gy/fraction versus 70 Gy at 2.5 Gy/fraction. If noninferiority of the hypofractionated arm is demonstrated, this may have implications regarding health care savings and increased patient convenience. Extreme hypofractionation or stereotactic body radiotherapy using 5 to 7 fractions with doses in the range of 5.5 to 7 Gy/fraction has also been evaluated at some centers,[43] although this remains experimental without sufficient knowledge of late toxicity. The role for PBT in hypofractionated regimens for prostate cancer exists but remains largely unexplored.

## Focal Therapy and Partial Prostate Boosting

Prostate cancer is typically considered a multifocal disease; although, this is not always the case and not all foci are necessarily of the same volume.[44] Although current practice is to treat the entire prostate gland to the same uniform dose, dominant or bulky nodules may benefit from focal therapy or boosting to higher doses.

Focal therapy for prostate cancer in the form of cryosurgery, high-intensity focused ultrasound and photodynamic therapy have increased in use without much supporting evidence. As imaging of the tumor and target localization within the prostate is improving,[45,46] including dynamically enhanced MRI and 3-dimensional MR spectroscopy, it will be important to optimize conformal radiation therapy (ie, brachytherapy, IMRT, or PBT) and define its role in partial prostate boosting. Several centers have already studied the feasibility of such techniques with IMRT.[47–49] Improved conformal dose distribution and modulation, achievable with IMPT,[31] is potentially ideally suited for partial gland dose escalation while avoiding normal structures such as the urethra and nerves to the penis, with the goal of further improving disease control and reducing toxicity (Fig. 6). Reproducible immobilization, daily target localization with image guidance, and improved-range verification will become even more critical for such treatment delivery.

## In Vivo Treatment Verification With PET/CT

A potentially exploitable property of protons is their production of positron emitters along the beam path. These can be detected on a positron emission tomography (PET) or computed tomography scan taken shortly after a fraction is delivered. A recent study demonstrated the feasibility of postradiation PET or computed tomography for in vivo treatment verification and dosimetry.[50] Such advances could potentially provide real-time verification of dose delivered and targeting as well as quality assurance. One could further envision adaptive planning whereby adjustments are made to future fractions based on past dosimetry. Further technologic and methodologic refinements are needed for optimal clinical application in prostate cancer.

## Other Particle Therapies

Aside from protons, alternative particle irradiation has been explored, including neutron beam and carbon ion therapy. Carbon ions share a favorable physical dose distribution as defined by the Bragg peak similar to protons, with even less lateral scattering, although there is a small tail beyond the end of range. Carbon ions have another potential biologic advantage that may be exploited. This has to do with an increase in relative biologic effectiveness toward the end of the particle range, which theoretically would be located within the

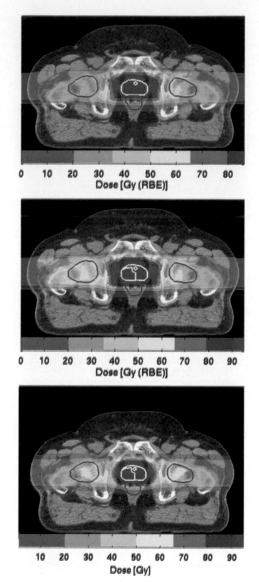

**FIGURE 6.**    Partial prostate dose escalation using 3D conformal proton therapy versus IMPT. The original 3D CPT plan (top) delivered 79.2 CGE and the dose to a hemisphere was then boosted to 91 CGE (middle). IMPT with beam scanning (bottom) allows for delivery of inhomogeneous dose and integration of the boost within a standard fractionated treatment while also improving the conformity of the dose to the target.

tumor volume and thus exaggerate effective dose with depth. The exact relative biologic effectiveness, however, remains unknown, so a certain degree of uncertainty persists. Another opportunity with carbon ions is their production of positron-emitting isotopes which can be detected by PET. As described earlier, this may allow for visualization of the high-dose treatment volume.

In 1994, the National Cancer Institute-sponsored Neutron Therapy Collaborative Working Group reported on their randomization of 178 men with locally advanced prostate cancer to photons (70–70.2 Gy) or fast neutron therapy alone (20.4 Gy).[51] Local-

regional control was superior for patients treated with neutrons (89% vs. 68%), as well biochemical control (83% vs. 55%), though survival was similar and severe late complications were worse (11% vs. 3%). It seems late morbidity was related to the degree of neutron beam shaping. Single institution studies using mixed neutrons and photons have shown a reduced rate of rectal complications and favorable tumor control.[52] Similarly, carbon ion radiation therapy has been evaluated in a phase II study from Japan that demonstrated local control with acceptable toxicity.[53] Neither neutrons nor carbon ions are widely used and additional data are needed to explore their role in the treatment of localized prostate cancer.

## CONCLUSIONS

There has been an explosion of interest in PBT for prostate cancer. Protons offer superior dose distributions and the potential for reduced morbidity. Experience to date has shown that PBT is safe and effective for a number of tumor sites including as a means for dose escalation in the treatment of prostate cancer. However, uncertainties remain surrounding their physical properties, perceived clinical gain, and economic viability. Future work will be aimed at optimizing this technology, including further development of IMPT. In prostate cancer, there exists the potential to further explore dose escalation, hypofractionation, partial prostate boosting, and verifying in real time the dose delivered to a reproducibly immobilized and localized target while maintaining maximal sparing of healthy organs. It is likely that the full clinical potential of PBT has not yet been realized. Currently, however, the evidence does not support any definitive benefit to PBT over other forms of high-dose conformal radiation in the treatment of localized prostate cancer. A prospective study comparing patient-reported outcomes for PBT and IMRT is needed to provide comparative data that may, or may not, justify the widespread use of such a sophisticated and costly resource.

## ACKNOWLEDGMENT

*We wish to thank Daphna Spiegel for assistance with manuscript preparation.*

## REFERENCES

1. Catalona WJ, Smith DS, Ratliff TL, et al. Detection of organ-confined prostate cancer is increased through prostate-specific antigen-based screening. *JAMA.* 1993;270:948–954.
2. Cooperberg MR, Broering JM, Kantoff PW, et al. Contemporary trends in low risk prostate cancer: risk assessment and treatment. *J Urol.* 2007;178(3 Pt 2): S14–S19.
3. Zietman AL, DeSilvio ML, Slater JD, et al. Comparison of conventional-dose vs high-dose conformal radiation therapy in clinically localized adenocarcinoma of the prostate: a randomized controlled trial. *JAMA.* 2005;294:1233–1239.
4. Kuban DA, Tucker SL, Dong L, et al. Long-term results of the M. D. Anderson randomized dose-escalation trial for prostate cancer. *Int J Radiat Oncol Biol Phys.* 2008;70:67–74.
5. Dearnaley DP, Sydes MR, Graham JD, et al. Escalated-dose versus standard-dose conformal radiotherapy in prostate cancer: first results from the MRC RT01 randomised controlled trial. *Lancet Oncol.* 2007;8:475–487.
6. Peeters ST, Heemsbergen WD, Koper PC, et al. Dose-response in radiotherapy for localized prostate cancer: results of the Dutch multicenter randomized phase III trial comparing 68 Gy of radiotherapy with 78 Gy. *J Clin Oncol.* 2006;24:1990–1996.
7. Wilson RR. Radiologic uses of fast protons. *Radiology.* 1946;47:487.
8. Gragoudas ES, Lane AM, Munzenrider J, et al. Long-term risk of local failure after proton therapy for choroidal/ciliary body melanoma. *Trans Am Ophthalmol Soc.* 2002;100:43–48, discussion 8–9.
9. Munzenrider JE, Liebsch NJ. Proton therapy for tumors of the skull base. *Strahlenther Onkol.* 1999;175(suppl 2):57–63.
10. MacDonald SM, Safai S, Trofimov A, et al. Proton radiotherapy for childhood ependymoma; initial clinical outcomes and dose comparisons. *Int J Radiat Oncol Biol Phys.* 2008;71:979–986.

11. Zhang X, Dong L, Lee AK, et al. Effect of anatomic motion on proton therapy dose distributions in prostate cancer treatment. *Int J Radiat Oncol Biol Phys.* 2007;67:620–629.

12. Trofimov A, Nguyen PL, Coen JJ, et al. Radiotherapy treatment of early-stage prostate cancer with IMRT and protons: a treatment planning comparison. *Int J Radiat Oncol Biol Phys.* 2007;69:444–453.

13. Vargas C, Fryer A, Mahajan C, et al. Dose-volume comparison of proton therapy and intensity-modulated radiotherapy for prostate cancer. *Int J Radiat Oncol Biol Phys.* 2008;70:744–751.

14. Mayahara H, Murakami M, Kagawa K, et al. Acute morbidity of proton therapy for prostate cancer: the Hyogo Ion Beam Medical Center experience. *Int J Radiat Oncol Biol Phys.* 2007;69:434–443.

15. Hall EJ. Intensity-modulated radiation therapy, protons, and the risk of second cancers. *Int J Radiat Oncol Biol Phys.* 2006;65:1–7.

16. Schneider U, Lomax A, Besserer J, et al. The impact of dose escalation on secondary cancer risk after radiotherapy of prostate cancer. *Int J Radiat Oncol Biol Phys.* 2007;68:892–897.

17. Wroe A, Rosenfeld A, Schulte R. Out-of-field dose equivalents delivered by proton therapy of prostate cancer. *Med Phys.* 2007;34:3449–3456.

18. Paganetti H, Bortfeld T, Delaney TF. Neutron dose in proton radiation therapy: in regard to Eric J. Hall (Int J Radiat Oncol Biol Phys 2006;65:1–7). *Int J Radiat Oncol Biol Phys.* 2006;66:1594–1595, author reply 5.

19. Zacharatou Jarlskog C, Lee C, Bolch WE, et al. Assessment of organ-specific neutron equivalent doses in proton therapy using computational whole-body age-dependent voxel phantoms. *Phys Med Biol.* 2008;53:693–717.

20. Miralbell R, Lomax A, Cella L, et al. Potential reduction of the incidence of radiation-induced second cancers by using proton beams in the treatment of pediatric tumors. *Int J Radiat Oncol Biol Phys.* 2002;54:824–829.

21. Shipley WU, Tepper JE, Prout GR Jr, et al. Proton radiation as boost therapy for localized prostatic carcinoma. *JAMA.* 1979;241:1912–1915.

22. Shipley WU, Verhey LJ, Munzenrider JE, et al. Advanced prostate cancer: the results of a randomized comparative trial of high dose irradiation boosting with conformal protons compared with conventional dose irradiation using photons alone. *Int J Radiat Oncol Biol Phys.* 1995;32:3–12.

23. Slater JD, Rossi CJ Jr, Yonemoto LT, et al. Proton therapy for prostate cancer: the initial Loma Linda University experience. *Int J Radiat Oncol Biol Phys.* 2004;59:348–352.

24. Talcott JA, Slater JD, Zietman AL, et al. Long-term quality of life after conventional-dose versus high-dose radiation for prostate cancer: results from a randomized trial (PROG-9509). *J Clin Oncol.* 2008;26(15S):264s.

25. Pollack A, Zagars GK, Starkschall G, et al. Prostate cancer radiation dose response: results of the M. D. Anderson phase III randomized trial. *Int J Radiat Oncol Biol Phys.* 2002;53:1097–1105.

26. Zietman AL, Bae K, Coen JJ, et al. A prospective phase I/II study using proton beam radiation to deliver 82 GyE to men with localized prostate cancer: preliminary results of ACR 0312. In: American Society of Therapeutic Radiology and Oncology. Boston: 2008:S77.

27. Konski A, Speier W, Hanlon A, et al. Is proton beam therapy cost effective in the treatment of adenocarcinoma of the prostate? *J Clin Oncol.* 2007;25:3603–3608.

28. Schroder FH, Hugosson J, Roobol MJ, et al. Screening and prostate-cancer mortality in a randomized European study. *N Engl J Med.* 2009;360:1320–1328.

29. Andriole GL, Grubb RL III, Buys SS, et al. Mortality results from a randomized prostate-cancer screening trial. *N Engl J Med.* 2009;360:1310–1319.

30. Safai S, Bortfeld T, Engelsman M. Comparison between the lateral penumbra of a collimated double-scattered beam and uncollimated scanning beam in proton radiotherapy. *Phys Med Biol.* 2008;53:1729–1750.

31. Lomax AJ, Pedroni E, Rutz H, et al. The clinical potential of intensity modulated proton therapy. *Z Med Phys.* 2004;14:147–152.

32. Weber DC, Lomax AJ, Rutz HP, et al. Spot-scanning proton radiation therapy for recurrent, residual or untreated intracranial meningiomas. *Radiother Oncol.* 2004;71:251–258.

33. Weber DC, Trofimov AV, Delaney TF, et al. A treatment planning comparison of intensity modulated photon and proton therapy for paraspinal sarcomas. *Int J Radiat Oncol Biol Phys.* 2004;58:1596–1606.

34. Weber DC, Rutz HP, Pedroni ES, et al. Results of spot-scanning proton radiation therapy for chordoma and chondrosarcoma of the skull base: the Paul Scherrer Institut experience. *Int J Radiat Oncol Biol Phys.* 2005;63:401–409.

35. Lomax AJ, Boehringer T, Coray A, et al. Intensity modulated proton therapy: a clinical example. *Med Phys.* 2001;28:317–324.

36. Timmermann B, Schuck A, Niggli F, et al. Spot-scanning proton therapy for malignant soft tissue tumors in childhood: first experiences at the Paul Scherrer Institute. *Int J Radiat Oncol Biol Phys.* 2007;67:497–504.

37. Rutz HP, Weber DC, Sugahara S, et al. Extracranial chordoma: outcome in patients treated with function-preserving surgery followed by spot-scanning proton beam irradiation. *Int J Radiat Oncol Biol Phys.* 2007;67:512–520.

38. Unkelbach J, Chan TC, Bortfeld T. Accounting for range uncertainties in the optimization of intensity modulated proton therapy. *Phys Med Biol.* 2007;52:2755–2773.

39. Brenner DJ, Hall EJ. Fractionation and protraction for radiotherapy of prostate carcinoma. *Int J Radiat Oncol Biol Phys.* 1999;43:1095–1101.

40. Fowler J, Chappell R, Ritter M. Is alpha/beta for prostate tumors really low? *Int J Radiat Oncol Biol Phys.* 2001;50:1021–1031.

41. Yeoh EE, Holloway RH, Fraser RJ, et al. Hypofractionated versus conventionally fractionated radiation therapy for prostate carcinoma: updated results of a phase III randomized trial. *Int J Radiat Oncol Biol Phys.* 2006;66:1072–1083.

42. Lukka H, Hayter C, Julian JA, et al. Randomized trial comparing two fractionation schedules for patients with localized prostate cancer. *J Clin Oncol.* 2005;23:6132–6138.

43. Madsen BL, Hsi RA, Pham HT, et al. Stereotactic hypofractionated accurate radiotherapy of the prostate (SHARP), 33.5 Gy in five fractions for localized disease: first clinical trial results. *Int J Radiat Oncol Biol Phys.* 2007;67:1099–1105.

44. Mouraviev V, Mayes JM, Sun L, et al. Prostate cancer laterality as a rationale of focal ablative therapy for the treatment of clinically localized prostate cancer. *Cancer.* 2007;110:906–910.

45. John SS, Zietman AL, Shipley WU, et al. Newer imaging modalities to assist with target localization in the radiation treatment of prostate cancer and possible lymph node metastases. *Int J Radiat Oncol Biol Phys.* 2008;71(1 suppl):S43–S47.

46. Rajesh A, Coakley FV, Kurhanewicz J. 3D MR spectroscopic imaging in the evaluation of prostate cancer. *Clin Radiol.* 2007;62:921–929.

47. Nederveen AJ, van der Heide UA, Hofman P, et al. Partial boosting of prostate tumours. *Radiother Oncol.* 2001;61:117–126.

48. Pickett B, Vigneault E, Kurhanewicz J, et al. Static field intensity modulation to treat a dominant intra-prostatic lesion to 90 Gy compared to seven field 3-dimensional radiotherapy. *Int J Radiat Oncol Biol Phys.* 1999;44:921–929.

49. Bos LJ, Damen EM, de Boer RW, et al. Reduction of rectal dose by integration of the boost in the large-field treatment plan for prostate irradiation. *Int J Radiat Oncol Biol Phys.* 2002;52:254–265.

50. Parodi K, Paganetti H, Shih HA, et al. Patient study of in vivo verification of beam delivery and range, using positron emission tomography and computed tomography imaging after proton therapy. *Int J Radiat Oncol Biol Phys.* 2007;68:920–934.

51. Russell KJ, Caplan RJ, Laramore GE, et al. Photon versus fast neutron external beam radiotherapy in the treatment of locally advanced prostate cancer: results of a randomized prospective trial. *Int J Radiat Oncol Biol Phys.* 1994;28:47–54.

52. Forman JD, Duclos M, Sharma R, et al. Conformal mixed neutron and photon irradiation in localized and locally advanced prostate cancer: preliminary estimates of the therapeutic ratio. *Int J Radiat Oncol Biol Phys.* 1996;35:259–266.

53. Ishikawa H, Tsuji H, Kamada T, et al. Carbon ion radiation therapy for prostate cancer: results of a prospective phase II study. *Radiother Oncol.* 2006;81:57–64.

# Current Clinical Evidence for Proton Therapy

Michael Brada • Madelon Pijls-Johannesma • Dirk De Ruysscher

Proton radiation therapy has gained popularity as a means of more localized delivery of ionizing radiation with increasing number of therapy units operational throughout the world. The initial driving force has been a desire to exploit improved dose distribution principally to achieve improved normal tissue avoidance. The magnitude of normal tissue sparing within individual tumor types and regions of the body is variable, and the potential clinical benefit of relevance to the individual patient is largely presumed. The potential improvement in normal tissue sparing can also be exploited by dose escalation to equitoxic levels to improve local tumor control and ideally survival and this aim is largely to be realized.

The proponents of proton beam therapy argue that the potential normal tissue sparing is of such importance to the future of radiation oncology that proof in the form of high-level clinical evidence is not required regardless of cost implications.[1,2] The frequently quoted example is a transition of radiation therapy from orthovoltage via cobalt to megavoltage therapy all of which proceeded without substantial clinical evidence of superiority.

The opposing argument requires robust clinical evidence in support of introduction of new expensive technology. Although high-level clinical evidence would be desirable, it is acknowledged that phase III trials testing different technologies would be difficult if not impossible to organize let alone complete. In the absence of prospectively designed randomized outcome studies, it is necessary to rely on available published clinical data to assess the potential benefit of protons. After all, many thousands of patients have already been treated, and it is not unreasonable to evaluate outcome data of proton therapy against best conventional standard of treatment using modern photon irradiation.

We present an update of our previous systematic review[3] of the published clinical outcome data on the efficacy and toxicity of proton beam therapy. This should provide as objective information as is currently possible to obtain on the efficacy and toxicity of this technique compared with best conventional external beam radiotherapy.

## METHODS

The methodology of systematic review was described in full previously.[4] It includes evaluation of all published articles dealing with protons in biologic abstracts, CINAHL, The Cochrane Library, Database of Abstracts of Reviews of Effects, EMBASE, Health Technology Assessment database, ISI Science and Technology Proceedings, MEDLINE, National Health Service Economic Evaluation Database, Office of Health Economics Health Economic Evaluations Database, and System for Information on Gray Literature in Europe, Medline, from 1980 to 2009 (previously from 1980 to September 2006). The articles included in the systematic analysis were only those of acceptable quality requiring at least 20 patients in the study with a follow-up period of at least 2 years. The initial review

identified 36 suitable publications. The updated review identified further 11 publications and the number of studies and the number of patients analyzed are shown in Table 1. In addition, a separate search on childhood tumors was performed, as proton therapy is believed by some to be the treatment of choice. As the number of patients in pediatric studies is often limited, no restriction on the number of patients was used. As previously, data on local tumor control [local progression free survival (PFS)], survival, and toxicity at specific time points was obtained from the publications. The outcome data was summarized using weighted means and these were compared with published outcome of the best available conventional treatment.

It should be acknowledged that patients offered novel treatment available at few selected sites worldwide are likely to be highly selected. Generally, they need to be sufficiently fit and well to travel long distances and having a tumor of appropriate size to be suitable for the novel technique. It is likely that in this case, the selection would have excluded worse prognosis patients not able to reach such specialist centers. Conversely, complex cases sometimes reaching the end of the treatment path may have also been referred for novel treatments, although personal experience suggests this is less frequently the case.

## Evidence for Efficacy of Protons for Different Types

### Chondrosarcomas and Chordomas of the Skull Base

Chondrosarcomas are rare skull base tumors perceived on the basis of histologic classification as aggressive malignant tumors. However, they are generally low-grade indolent tumors often presenting with long natural history, and the published series are usually small. The results after radical surgery with or without adjuvant external beam radiotherapy are reported as 90% to 100% 5-year local PFS.[5–8] The claims of superiority of proton therapy based on published studies[9–11] showing overall 5-year local PFS of 95% (Table 2) are, therefore, not substantiated as the results are no different to conventional management with surgery and photon radiotherapy.

Chordomas are more aggressive skull base tumors, which may also present in the axial skeleton particularly in the cervical region and the sacrum. Retrospective studies spanning over decades reported a 5-year PFS in the region of 20% to 30%.[12–14] The conclusion had been that conventional treatment with surgery and radiotherapy is considered poorly effective. However, after intensive management of patients with radical surgery, where only 20% received radiotherapy, the 5-year local PFS was 65%[8] and after fractionated stereotactic radiotherapy 50%.[6] In addition, predictors of outcome include the extent of surgery, brain stem involvement, and tumor size,[10] and patient selection is likely to be an important determinant of outcome.

The perception of the value of protons in the treatment of skull base chordoma comes principally from clinical experience of proton beam therapy in Boston. Reviews by proton practitioners reported 73% 5-year disease free survival apparently of 621 patients treated,[9]

**TABLE 1.** Clinical Studies of Proton Therapy With At Least 20 Patients and With a Follow-Up Period of At Least 2 yr

| Tumor Site | Number of Studies | Number of Patients |
|---|---|---|
| Head and neck tumors | 4 | 164 |
| Prostate cancer | 3 | 1642 |
| Ocular tumors | 15 | 10,328 |
| Gastrointestinal cancer | 5 | 375 |
| Lung cancer | 4 | 146 |
| CNS tumors | 15 | 880 |
| Sarcomas | 2 | 97 |
| Other sites | 4 | 104 |
| Total | 52 | 13,736 |

CNS indicates central nervous system.

**TABLE 3.** Actuarial Local Control in Adult Patients With Skull Base Chordoma Treated With Protons

| No. Patients | Median Follow-Up (yr) | 5-yr Local Progression Free Survival (%) | Publication |
|---|---|---|---|
| 100 | 2.3 | 50* | Noel et al 2005 |
| 33 | 2.8 | 59 | Hug et al 1999 |
| 169 | 3.4 | 64 | Munzenrider et al 1999 |
| 302 | 3.6 | 59 | Total (weighted mean) |

*Only 4 yr results of 54% local PFS given. Estimate for 5-yr PFS by extrapolation from graph.

which is undoubtedly impressive for such an uncommon tumor. However, a detailed analysis of the published chordoma data is disturbing. The only and last full peer-reviewed publication focusing on the treatment outcome of the full cohort of patients with chordoma (40 patients) is from 1989 where both chordoma and chondrosarcoma results are combined.[15] The data reporting 73% control rate comes from a review article of the Boston experience[11] where only 290 of 519 skull base tumor patients treated with protons had chordoma and of these only 169 were reported at a median follow-up 3.4 years. This means that 121 (42%) were excluded from the analysis presumably lost to follow up. In addition, although the text reports 73% local recurrence free survival, the value read from the published graph of actuarial local control is only 64%. Although even this figure is difficult to accept in the light of such incomplete follow up, the weighted mean 5-year control rate of 59% (Table 3), not taking into account the likely selection bias and the flawed reporting, is within the same range as the best published control rate after conventional treatment.

Since the previous systematic analysis, one further article has been published on the outcome of treatment of chordoma specifically in a pediatric population. The 5-year local control rate in 26 children with cervical spine and skull base chordoma was 77%[16] and this is in keeping with the suggestion that the outcome is better in children.[17]

Most publications reviewing the efficacy of protons come to a tacit conclusion that this is the treatment of choice for chordomas and chondrosarcomas. This is almost considered an unchallengeable fact; however, the available evidence in support of protons is tenuous and flawed. The present conclusion is that the widely held belief that proton beam therapy is superior to conventional treatment for skull base chordoma and chondrosarcoma is not supported by published literature.

**TABLE 2.** Actuarial Local Control in Adult Patients With Skull Base Chondrosarcoma Treated With Protons

| No. Patients | Median Follow-Up (yr) | 5-yr Local Progression Free Survival (%) | Publication |
|---|---|---|---|
| 25 | 2.8 | 75 | Hug et al 1999 |
| 165 | 3.4 | 98 | Munzenrider et al 1999 |
| 190 | 3.3 | 95 | Total (weighted mean) |

## Ocular Tumors

Proton beam therapy has been accepted as one of the treatment options for uveal melanoma with other radiation alternatives including stereotactic radiotherapy and brachytherapy. The review of published literature has been reported previously,[3] and outcome of 2 more peer-reviewed data has been identified.[19,20] The current conclusion, also noted by others, is that high-dose local proton beam therapy is effective with local control rate over 95%, 85% cause specific survival, and eye preservation rate of 90% although less than half of the patients retained reasonable vision. The results, at least in small tumors are not significantly different to other eye preserving radiation techniques, particularly stereotactic radiotherapy. In a randomized study of 151 patients with large uveal melanoma proton radiotherapy followed by transpupillary thermotherapy was associated with a reduction in the rate secondary enucleation.[21]

In conclusion, local irradiation with external beam techniques is effective in controlling growth of ocular melanoma with acceptable toxicity. Currently, there is no evidence that proton therapy is superior to high-precision photon irradiation.

## Prostate

Local radiotherapy is one of the principal options for localized prostate cancer, and proton beam therapy is a desirable candidate modality because of the perceived benefit in dose distribution. However, a detailed study of 3D dose distributions comparing protons with intensity-modulated radiation therapy (IMRT) failed to demonstrate better sparing of the bladder or the rectum, and the only apparent advantage in dose distribution terms was at doses not known to be associated with important adverse effects of radiation.[22] Although there is an apparent benefit in terms of volumes receiving low-dose radiation, the presumed risk is late radiation induced second tumor, which is of doubtful significance in the population of patients treated especially at the 10 year risk in adults in the region of 1.4%.[23]

In this context, it is therefore not surprising that there is currently no objective evidence of benefit in any of the important outcome measures for protons compared with photons. Although it is clear that modern photon external beam radiotherapy using best conformal techniques including IMRT achieve improved disease control with higher radiation doses, this can be accompanied by increased risk of toxicity.[24–28] It would certainly be attractive to employ protons with the aim of reducing the toxicity but the currently available trials do not show this and based on the radiation dose distribution such benefit is unlikely to be demonstrable.[22] More advanced proton techniques than those used in the published series may be worthwhile to investigate further. The largest published phase II study of prostate cancer stages I–III using combination of proton and photon therapy does not provide any information on comparative efficacy or toxicity of protons versus photons.[29] The 2 randomized studies of proton therapy specifically examine 2 dose levels of proton boost after photon irradiation and confirm the evidence from photon trials that high dose is associated with improved disease control albeit with increased late gastro-intestinal toxicity.[24,25] The studies were not designed to compare the efficacy of protons versus photons.

In summary, there is no evidence for benefit for proton beam therapy over photons in the treatment of localized prostate cancer. Currently, there is even lack of theoretical rationale, which would support its future use. However, prostate cancer remains one of the principal indications for treatment in a number of proton therapy centers.

## Other Tumors

We previously identified 2 studies of proton therapy in head and neck,[30,31] and further 2 studies reporting on the same patients have been published since.[32,33] The local tumor control rate ranged from 74% to 95% and 5 years survival from 39% to 90%. The treatment was not devoid of severe late toxicity with an incidence ranging from 10% to 18%. The mixture of tumor types and stages in such phase II trials makes the efficacy of protons largely not assessable, although the overall results are within the range seen following photon radiotherapy.

Four retrospective (360 patients) and 2 prospective studies (64 patients) of protons in patients with hepatocellular carcinoma[34–39] report results similar to those achieved with stereotactic photon radiotherapy.[40] One retrospective study reported outcome in 15 patients with osteogenic sarcoma and 12 patients with giant cell tumors, osteo- and chondroblastomas.[41] One prospective phase II study (50 patients)[42] investigated high-dose photon/proton therapy for spine sarcomas and reported satisfactory local tumor control although the benefit of exclusive proton therapy over conventional treatment is not clear.

To date, 2 prospective studies[43,44] of total of 58 patients with nonsmall cell lung cancer and 2 retrospective case studies[45,46] of 88 patients with nonsmall cell lung cancer were available for review. The overall outcome in terms of tumor control and survival is within the expected range in such selected patients when treated with modern high-dose conformal photon radiotherapy. As would be expected from such phase II studies, no conclusion about comparative efficacy can be made. There is certainly no clear evidence that proton beam therapy is superior to best available photon radiotherapy in this setting.

Brain tumors remain an attractive target for proton therapy because of the clear limitation of late radiation toxicity after doses beyond conventional tolerance (in the region of 60 Gy in 30 fractions at 2 Gy per fraction). Dose escalation studies in malignant gliomas (glioblastoma multiforme) have not demonstrated survival benefit and this is in keeping with dose escalation studies using modern photon techniques of conformal radiotherapy and IMRT.[47,48] Small cohorts of patients have been treated with acoustic neuroma, low grade astrocytoma, cavernous angiomas, and arteriovenous malformation, and the results in terms of comparative efficacy are not interpretable.[49–54] Although the perception remains that benign skull base meningiomas could be managed in a similar manner as skull base chordomas, the cohort of patients with benign meningioma treated with proton therapy did not demonstrate improved tumor control, whereas the late toxicity seemed higher than would be achieved with best conventional local photon irradiation.[55] A recent retrospective study of 24 patients with malignant meningiomas[56] suggested improved survival in patients receiving doses >60 Gy although the size of the study and potential selection of patients preclude definitive conclusion.

## Childhood Tumors

Radiotherapy is an integral component of management of childhood malignancies, such as central nervous system tumors and sarcomas of bone and soft tissues. Survival has improved with cure rates in the region of 60% to 70%, although this is accompanied by significant treatment related morbidity such as cognitive deficit, hearing impairment, endocrine, renal, and gonadal dysfunction, and second radiation induced malignancies.[57] Proton therapy is an attractive alternative to photon radiotherapy because it reduces both the irradiated volume particularly beyond the target and the dose to the normal tissue with better sparing of normal tissue and lower integral radiation dose compared with advanced photon techniques. Proton therapy should therefore lead to a reduction in the risk of second malignancy,[58–62] providing excess neutron exposure from some proton machines is taken care of.

Four studies of proton therapy in childhood skull base tumors (128 patients, mean age 11.5) reported a 5-year survival of 72% to 100% with limited acute and late treatment related toxicity.[16,17,63] Sixteen children (mean age 3.3) with soft tissue tumors (principally rhabdomysarcomas) were treated between 1999 and 2005 at the Paul Scherrer Institute with spot-scanning proton therapy. The local control and survival at a median follow-up of 18.6 months were 75% and 69%, respectively with grade 3 to 4 toxicity confined to bone marrow.[64]

Twenty-seven children with low-grade astrocytoma were treated in Loma Linda between 1991 and 1997 (mean age 8.7) and 5-year local control was 87% and overall survival were 93%,[65] which is within the range expected for these tumors treated with conventional therapy. Children with intracranial ependymoma treated in Boston between 2000 and 2006 had local control, PFS, and survival rates of 86%, 80%, and 89%, respectively at a median follow-up of 26 months.

The suggestion from early studies is that proton therapy is well tolerated and early local control rates are comparable with those achieved after conventional radiotherapy although direct comparison is difficult. The potential benefit in reducing late side effects will require in depth studies of large cohorts of children and longer follow-up.

## DISCUSSION

There is general agreement about the advantage of protons in terms of physical deposition of energy and potential sparing of tissues beyond the target. However, it is not always clear how this translates into specific advantage for an individual tumor type and site and what the magnitude of benefit is likely to be in any of the measurable and relevant clinical endpoints. In addition, most current proton treatment facilities do not routinely include the sophistication of modern photon therapy with limited regard for uncertainties such as target motion, tissue inhomogeneity, and temporal changes.

As demonstrated previously,[3] despite the potential technical advantage of proton beam therapy, no evidence even at a basic level shows improved outcome after protons compared with photons in any of the tumor types so far treated, and this is also confirmed by other authors.[4,66]

Most if not all modern technological advances in radiotherapy delivery aim to achieve normal tissue avoidance, and this in itself is laudable. However, the arguments put forward in favor of proton beam therapy frequently lack the detail to demonstrate tissue avoidance responsible for clinically relevant toxicity. Recent review publications discuss the consequences of reducing the overall dose to normal tissue, which may result in decreased incidence of second tumors.[2] This is of relevance to children and young adults with long-life expectancy and may not be applicable to the generality of patients with malignant disease affecting aging population. Similar arguments have been advanced in relation to the effect of low-dose irradiation on life expectancy demonstrated in primates.[2] Again, this is of potential relevance to young population with otherwise curable tumors and is not a sufficient justification for routine introduction of proton beam therapy into the treatment of common cancers in adults.

It is argued by proton therapy practitioners that the efficient use of proton facilities over extended hours and days (not generally achieved in radiotherapy facilities using photons, despite a compelling economic argument) the cost of treatment is roughly twice that of photon therapy.[67] At present, it is not clear whether the additional cost is worthwhile for the expected (and unproven) clinical gain.[68]

It is suggested that the apparently superior dose distribution that can be achieved with protons compared with photons is likely to result in a clinical benefit, and hence the real discussion about the introduction of proton beam therapy centers on treatment cost. If this is the case—and in many respects it is—the issue is not cost alone but cost benefit ratio (or cost effectiveness), and this should be assessable and measurable in real terms. The available clinical data based on treated cohorts of patients as presented here and reported by others[4,66] provides no evidence of superiority of protons in any of the parameters measured and hence whatever the additional cost, this is so far without real benefit and in health economic terms barely acceptable. A possibility remains that the confidence intervals for the relationship between dose-volume parameters and side effects are large, and the potential beneficial effect of protons may remain hidden. This would require improved trial design with better data on radiation-induced side effects and studies should focus on tumor sites where a large gain is expected.

However, at present it is not clear, which tumor sites they should be. A model-based approach using validated predictive normal tissue complication probability-models in combination with in silico dose planning comparative studies may provide useful information on which tumor types may benefit and to what extent. A proton treatment facility should therefore collect a prospective patient- and treatment-related data registry to expand the number of in silico analyses in addition to collecting solid clinical. Prospective data collection should start before the actual clinical introduction of proton therapy to determine baseline profile of side effects, quality of life, and other endpoints achieved with the present radiation techniques. Collaboration with other national and international proton treatment facilities is critical for exchange not only of expertise but also data and to identify patients who truly benefit from proton radiotherapy.

The potential merit of increasing radiation dose also requires appropriately powered studies as would be expected from any dose escalation studies using modern conformal and IMRT techniques.

Construction of new proton therapy facilities to improve the delivery of therapeutic radiation with potentially less toxic radiation therapy is to be welcomed as part of academic endeavor. With future advances in technology proton therapy may even become cost effective. However, in the absence of any convincing clinical data in favor of protons over photons the current focus on cost, which is based on belief alone, is not appropriate. Nevertheless, well-designed model-based economic evaluations can estimate the probability of cost effectiveness of protons over conventional radiotherapy for different tumor groups, which would aid medical decision making.

## CONCLUSIONS

Proton beam therapy is an innovative and technologically demanding method of delivery of therapeutic ionizing radiation. It has the potential for reducing normal tissue toxicity by better normal tissue avoidance, it may allow for equitoxic dose escalation to improve disease control or for a combination of both. The ultimate aim must be improved survival and/or quality of life. However, despite some tens of thousands of patients treated, the published peer-reviewed literature is devoid of any clinical data demonstrating benefit in terms of survival, tumor control, or toxicity in comparison with best conventional treatment.

The interest in proton therapy has led to an increasing number of treatment units becoming available. They are mostly set up as viable economic units requiring high throughput to achieve commercial success with scant regard for evidence-based medicine and consequent clinical need. Unfortunately, such facilities are poorly suited to noncommercial academically led clinical trials aiming to define the true benefit and the real need for proton beam therapy.

The current lack of evidence for benefit of protons is not a call to abandon the technique. It should provide a stimulus for a planned effort to identify suitable tumor targets with the greatest potential benefit in measurable and particularly clinically relevant endpoints. Well-designed in silico clinical trials using validated normal tissue complication probability-models are essential and can predict the magnitude of benefit. The perceived and largely theoretical benefit should be validated by clinical evidence from well-designed prospective studies, away from commercial influence, convincingly demonstrating improved outcome.

## REFERENCES

1. Goitein M, Cox JD. Should randomized clinical trials be required for proton radiotherapy? *J Clin Oncol.* 2008;26:175–176.
2. Suit H, Kooy H, Trofimov A, et al. Should positive phase III clinical trial data be required before proton beam therapy is more widely adopted? No. *Radiother Oncol.* 2008;86:148–153.
3. Brada M, Pijls-Johannesma M, De Ruysscher D. Proton therapy in clinical practice: current clinical evidence. *J Clin Oncol.* 2007;25:965–970.
4. Lodge M, Pijls-Johannesma M, Stirk L, et al. A systematic literature review of the clinical and cost-effectiveness of hadron therapy in cancer. *Radiother Oncol.* 2007;83:110–122.
5. Crockard A. Chordomas and chondrosarcomas of the cranial base: results and follow-up of 60 patients. *Neurosurgery.* 1996;38:420.
6. Debus J, Schulz-Ertner D, Schad L, et al. Stereotactic fractionated radiotherapy for chordomas and chondrosarcomas of the skull base. *Int J Radiat Oncol Biol Phys.* 2000;47:591–596.
7. Kondziolka D, Lunsford LD, Flickinger JC. The role of radiosurgery in the management of chordoma and chondrosarcoma of the cranial base. *Neurosurgery.* 1991;29:38–45; discussion 45–46.
8. Gay E, Sekhar LN, Rubinstein E, et al. Chordomas and chondrosarcomas of the cranial base: results and follow-up of 60 patients. *Neurosurgery.* 1995;36:887–896; discussion 896–897.
9. Noel G, Feuvret L, Calugaru V, et al. Chordomas of the base of the skull and upper cervical spine. One hundred patients irradiated by a 3D conformal technique combining photon and proton beams. *Acta Oncol.* 2005;44:700–708.
10. Hug EB, Loredo LN, Slater JD, et al. Proton radiation therapy for chordomas and chondrosarcomas of the skull base. *J Neurosurg.* 1999;91:432–439.
11. Munzenrider JE, Liebsch NJ. Proton therapy for tumors of the skull base. *Strahlenther Onkol.* 1999;(175 suppl 2):57–63.
12. Fuller DB, Bloom JG. Radiotherapy for chordoma. *Int J Radiat Oncol Biol Phys.* 1988;15:331–339.
13. Romero J, Cardenes H, la Torre A, et al. Chordoma: results of radiation therapy in eighteen patients. *Radiother Oncol.* 1993;29:27–32.
14. Zorlu F, Gurkaynak M, Yildiz F, et al. Conventional external radiotherapy in the management of clivus chordomas with overt residual disease. *Neurol Sci.* 2000;21:203–207.
15. Austin-Seymour M, Munzenrider J, Goitein M, et al. Fractionated proton radiation therapy of chordoma and low-grade chondrosarcoma of the base of the skull. *J Neurosurg.* 1989;70:13–17.
16. Habrand JL, Schneider R, Alapetite C, et al. Proton therapy in pediatric skull base and cervical canal low-grade bone malignancies. *Int J Radiat Oncol Biol Phys.* 2008;71:672–675.
17. Hoch BL, Nielsen GP, Liebsch NJ, et al. Base of skull chordomas in children and adolescents: a clinicopathologic study of 73 cases. *Am J Surg Pathol.* 2006;30:811–818.

19. Conway RM, Poothullil AM, Daftari IK, et al. Estimates of ocular and visual retention following treatment of extra-large uveal melanomas by proton beam radiotherapy. *Arch Ophthalmol.* 2006;124:838–843.
20. Lumbroso-Le Rouic L, Delacroix S, Dendale R, et al. Proton beam therapy for iris melanomas. *Eye.* 2006;20:1300–1305.
21. Desjardins L, Lumbroso-Le Rouic L, Levy-Gabriel C, et al. Combined proton beam radiotherapy and transpupillary thermotherapy for large uveal melanomas: a randomized study of 151 patients. *Ophthalmic Res.* 2006;38:255–260.
22. Trofimov A, Nguyen PL, Coen JJ, et al. Radiotherapy treatment of early-stage prostate cancer with IMRT and protons: a treatment planning comparison. *Int J Radiat Oncol Biol Phys.* 2007;69:444–453.
23. Hall EJ. Intensity-modulated radiation therapy, protons, and the risk of second cancers. *Int J Radiat Oncol Biol Phys.* 2006;65:1–7.
24. Shipley WU, Verhey LJ, Munzenrider JE, et al. Advanced prostate cancer: the results of a randomized comparative trial of high dose irradiation boosting with conformal protons compared with conventional dose irradiation using photons alone. *Int J Radiat Oncol Biol Phys.* 1995;32:3–12.
25. Zietman AL, DeSilvio ML, Slater JD, et al. Comparison of conventional-dose vs high-dose conformal radiation therapy in clinically localized adenocarcinoma of the prostate: a randomized controlled trial. *JAMA.* 2005;294:1233–1239.
26. Pollack A, Zagars GK, Starkschall G, et al. Prostate cancer radiation dose response: results of the M. D. Anderson phase III randomized trial. *Int J Radiat Oncol Biol Phys.* 2002;53:1097–1105.
27. Dearnaley DP, Hall E, Lawrence D, et al. Phase III pilot study of dose escalation using conformal radiotherapy in prostate cancer: PSA control and side effects. *Br J Cancer.* 2005;92:488–498.
28. Peeters ST, Heemsbergen WD, Koper PC, et al. Dose-response in radiotherapy for localized prostate cancer: results of the Dutch multicenter randomized phase III trial comparing 68 Gy of radiotherapy with 78 Gy. *J Clin Oncol.* 2006;24:1990–1996.
29. Slater JD, Rossi CJ Jr, Yonemoto LT, et al. Proton therapy for prostate cancer: the initial Loma Linda University experience. *Int J Radiat Oncol Biol Phys.* 2004;59:348–352.
30. Slater JD, Yonemoto LT, Mantik DW, et al. Proton radiation for treatment of cancer of the oropharynx: early experience at Loma Linda University Medical Center using a concomitant boost technique. *Int J Radiat Oncol Biol Phys.* 2005;62:494–500.
31. Igaki H, Tokuuye K, Okumura T, et al. Clinical results of proton beam therapy for skull base chordoma. *Int J Radiat Oncol Biol Phys.* 2004;60:1120–1126.
32. Pommier P, Liebsch NJ, Deschler DG, et al. Proton beam radiation therapy for skull base adenoid cystic carcinoma. *Arch Otolaryngol Head Neck Surg.* 2006;132:1242–1249.
33. Resto VA, Chan AW, Deschler DG, et al. Extent of surgery in the management of locally advanced sinonasal malignancies. *Head Neck.* 2008;30:222–229.
34. Fukumitsu N, Sugahara S, Nakayama H, et al. A prospective study of hypofractionated proton beam therapy for patients with hepatocellular carcinoma. *Int J Radiat Oncol Biol Phys.* 2009;74:831–836.
35. Hata M, Tokuuye K, Sugahara S, et al. Proton beam therapy for aged patients with hepatocellular carcinoma. *Int J Radiat Oncol Biol Phys.* 2007;69:805–812.
36. Mizumoto M, Tokuuye K, Sugahara S, et al. Proton beam therapy for hepatocellular carcinoma adjacent to the porta hepatis. *Int J Radiat Oncol Biol Phys.* 2008;71:462–467.
37. Nemoto H, Tokuue K, Onishi K, et al. Proton beam therapy for large hepatocellular carcinoma. *J JASTRO.* 2004;177:177–182.
38. Bush DA, Hillebrand DJ, Slater JM, et al. High-dose proton beam radiotherapy of hepatocellular carcinoma: preliminary results of a phase II trial. *Gastroenterology.* 2004;127:S189–S193.
39. Kawashima M, Furuse J, Nishio T, et al. Phase II study of radiotherapy employing proton beam for hepatocellular carcinoma. *J Clin Oncol.* 2005;23:1839–1846.
40. Choi BO, Jang HS, Kang KM, et al. Fractionated stereotactic radiotherapy in patients with primary hepatocellular carcinoma. *Jpn J Clin Oncol.* 2006;36:154–158.
41. Hug EB, Fitzek MM, Liebsch NJ, et al. Locally challenging osteo- and chondrogenic tumors of the axial skeleton: results of combined proton and photon radiation therapy using three-dimensional treatment planning. *Int J Radiat Oncol Biol Phys.* 1995;31:467–476.
42. Delaney TF, Liebsch NJ, Pedlow FX, et al. Phase II study of high-dose photon/proton radiotherapy in the management of spine sarcomas. *Int J Radiat Oncol Biol Phys.* 2009;74:732–739.
43. Bush DA, Slater JD, Bonnet R, et al. Proton-beam radiotherapy for early-stage lung cancer. *Chest.* 1999;116:1313–1319.
44. Hata M, Tokuuye K, Kagei K, et al. Hypofractionated high-dose proton beam therapy for stage I non-small-cell lung cancer: preliminary results of a phase I/II clinical study. *Int J Radiat Oncol Biol Phys.* 2007;68:786–793.
45. Nihei K, Ogino T, Ishikura S, et al. High-dose proton beam therapy for Stage I non-small-cell lung cancer. *Int J Radiat Oncol Biol Phys.* 2006;65:107–111.
46. Shioyama Y, Tokuuye K, Okumura T, et al. Clinical evaluation of proton radiotherapy for non-small-cell lung cancer. *Int J Radiat Oncol Biol Phys.* 2003;56:7–13.
47. Chan JL, Lee SW, Fraass BA, et al. Survival and failure patterns of high-grade gliomas after three-dimensional conformal radiotherapy. *J Clin Oncol.* 2002;20:1635–1642.
48. Floyd NS, Woo SY, Teh BS, et al. Hypofractionated intensity-modulated radiotherapy for primary glioblastoma multiforme. *Int J Radiat Oncol Biol Phys.* 2004;58:721–726.
49. Amin-Hanjani S, Ogilvy CS, Candia GJ, et al. Stereotactic radiosurgery for cavernous malformations: Kjellberg's experience with proton beam therapy in 98 cases at the Harvard Cyclotron. *Neurosurgery.* 1998;42:1229–1236; discussion 1236–1238.
50. Bush DA, McAllister CJ, Loredo LN, et al. Fractionated proton beam radiotherapy for acoustic neuroma. *Neurosurgery.* 2002;50:270–273; discussion 273–275.
51. Fitzek MM, Thornton AF, Harsh GT, et al. Dose-escalation with proton/photon irradiation for Daumas-Duport lower-grade glioma: results of an institutional phase I/II trial. *Int J Radiat Oncol Biol Phys.* 2001;51:131–137.
52. Fitzek MM, Thornton AF, Rabinov JD, et al. Accelerated fractionated proton/photon irradiation to 90 cobalt gray equivalent for glioblastoma multiforme: results of a phase II prospective trial. *J Neurosurg.* 1999;91:251–260.
53. Hug EB, Muenter MW, Archambeau JO, et al. Conformal proton radiation therapy for pediatric low-grade astrocytomas. *Strahlenther Onkol.* 2002;178:10–17.
54. Levy RP, Schulte RW, Slater JD, et al. Stereotactic radiosurgery—the role of charged particles. *Acta Oncol.* 1999;38:165–169.
55. Wenkel E, Thornton AF, Finkelstein D, et al. Benign meningioma: partially resected, biopsied, and recurrent intracranial tumors treated with combined proton and photon radiotherapy. *Int J Radiat Oncol Biol Phys.* 2000;48:1363–1370.
56. Boskos C, Feuvret L, Noel G, et al. Combined proton and photon conformal radiotherapy for intracranial atypical and malignant meningioma. *Int J Radiat Oncol Biol Phys.* 2009.
57. Geenen MM, Cardous-Ubbink MC, Kremer LC, et al. Medical assessment of adverse health outcomes in long-term survivors of childhood cancer. *JAMA.* 2007;297:2705–2715.
58. Chung CS, Keating N, Yock T, et al. Comparative analysis of second malignancy risk in patients treated with proton therapy versus conventional photon therapy. *Int J Radiat Oncol Biol Phys.* 2008;72:S8.
59. Hillbrand M, Georg D, Gadner H, et al. Abdominal cancer during early childhood: a dosimetric comparison of proton beams to standard and advanced photon radiotherapy. *Radiother Oncol.* 2008;89:141–149.
60. Kozak KR, Adams J, Krejcarek SJ, et al. A dosimetric comparison of proton and intensity-modulated photon radiotherapy for pediatric parameningeal rhabdomyosarcomas. *Int J Radiat Oncol Biol Phys.* 2009;74:179–186.
61. Lee CT, Bilton SD, Famiglietti RM, et al. Treatment planning with protons for pediatric retinoblastoma, medulloblastoma, and pelvic sarcoma: how do protons compare with other conformal techniques? *Int J Radiat Oncol Biol Phys.* 2005;63:362–372.
62. Merchant TE, Hua CH, Shukla H, et al. Proton versus photon radiotherapy for common pediatric brain tumors: comparison of models of dose characteristics and their relationship to cognitive function. *Pediatr Blood Cancer.* 2008;51:110–117.
63. Hug EB, Sweeney RA, Nurre PM, et al. Proton radiotherapy in management of pediatric base of skull tumors. *Int J Radiat Oncol Biol Phys.* 2002;52:1017–1024.
64. Timmermann B, Schuck A, Niggli F, et al. Spot-scanning proton therapy for malignant soft tissue tumors in childhood: First experiences at the Paul Scherrer Institute. *Int J Radiat Oncol Biol Phys.* 2007;67:497–504.
65. Hug EB, Slater JD. Proton radiation therapy for chordomas and chondrosarcomas of the skull base. *Neurosurg Clin N Am.* 2000;11:627–638.
66. Olsen DR, Bruland OS, Frykholm G, et al. Proton therapy—a systematic review of clinical effectiveness. *Radiother Oncol.* 2007;83:123–132.
67. Goitein M, Jermann M. The relative costs of proton and X-ray radiation therapy. *Clin Oncol (R Coll Radiol).* 2003;15:S37–S50.
68. Pijls-Johannesma M, Pommier P, Lievens Y. Cost-effectiveness of particle therapy: current evidence and future needs. *Radiother Oncol.* 2008;89:127–134.

# Comparison of Carbon Ions Versus Protons

Uli Weber • Gerhard Kraft

In 50 years of ion beam therapy, 50,000 patients have been treated worldwide mostly with protons and approximately 4000 using carbon ions. During this time, the beam application techniques were improved permanently in parallel to the conventional therapy.[1] The most recent development in particle therapy was the transition from passive to active beam forming systems where the target volume is divided in small volume elements (voxel), which are irradiated with a fine pencil beam, and where the intensity is modulated according to the dose needed for each voxel.[2] This intensity-modulated particle therapy produces extremely conformal target volumes tailored to the irregular shape of the tumors. But for intensity-modulated particle therapy, the physical and, more important, the biologic properties of the beam become more important determining the quality of the treatment.

## PHYSICAL PROPERTIES

### Depth Dose Distributions of Photons, Protons, and Carbon Ions

Particles like protons and ions show an inverted depth-dose profile compared with photons having a maximum (Bragg peak) at the end of the range[3] (Fig. 1). These Bragg curves are the result of a superposition of many individual depth-dose distributions of the individual particles. Because of energy straggling and consequently range straggling, these individual curves are shifted in respect to each other. This has 2 consequences: because the straggling for protons is larger than for carbon, the width of Bragg-maximum is larger for protons than for carbon. Secondly, for larger penetration depth for both ions, straggling increases and the Bragg maximum become broader and consequently smaller in amplitude. But the changes of the width of the Bragg curves and its absolute number are of minor importance when an extended target volume will be irradiated (Fig. 2).

For ions heavier than protons, like the carbon beams, the nuclear fragmentation as a second process beside the energy loss determines the depth-dose distribution.[4] In these nuclear reactions, lighter ions are created that continue their path with approximately the same velocity. However, because they are lighter, they have a larger penetration and create a dose tail at the distal side of the Bragg peak. This fragmentation process, however, produces also lighter carbon isotopes that are positron emitters. Their decay can be used to monitor the carbon ion range inside the patient, using positron emission tomography (PET) techniques.[5] For protons, there is no dose tail and also no projectile isotopes that can be used for a PET analysis.

The nuclear fragmentation increases with projectile mass, and consequently the amount of lighter particles in the beam increases, washing out the good biologic and physical properties. In addition, for these heavier ions and for larger penetration depth, this dose tail increases as well. For carbon ions, the contribution of fragments does not deteriorate the dose distribution in general, but allows monitoring the beam inside the patient applying PET observation. For ions much heavier than carbon, the fragmentation becomes a limiting factor, especially when passive beam shaping is used.

To irradiate an extended target volume, the natural width of the Bragg peak is too small, and the beams of different energies have to be superimposed. This can be done by using inhomogeneous absorbers (passive beam shaping)[1] or by requesting these different energies from the accelerator (active beam shaping).[2] In the optimal case, depth distribution so-called spread out Bragg peaks or extended maxima can be produced as shown in Figure 2.

These curves are calculated superimposing Bragg curves of different energies, which cover the appropriate range in depth. The calculations are performed for a homogenous water target not containing any inhomogeneity.

### Lateral Dose Profile (Beam Broadening by Multiple Scattering)

The pencil beam, which passes through the vacuum window, the monitors, air, and the patient, is continuously broadened by multiple scattering. In these materials, the ions undergo multiple interactions mostly with the target electrons. Because the mass of the projectiles is much greater than the electron mass, the net impact on the direction of the ions is small, but not negligible. The strength of this effect is roughly proportional to $Z_{proj}/(A_{proj} \times v_{proj}^2)$. In Figure 3, these effects are given for a typical beam scanning setup having exit windows, beam monitors, and a water phantom as tissue equivalent.[6] An initial beam width of 5 mm is assumed, and the broadening in these targets, but also in the air gap in-between, is calculated. The air contribution is large because of the divergence produced in the exit and monitors before. At a distance of 1.4 m from the exit window, the beam enters the patient and is scattered while slowing down. The broadening of a proton pencil beam is approximately 3.5 times larger than for a carbon beam compared for the same range. A factor of 2 is originating from the different charge-to-mass ratio and a factor of approximately 1.7 corresponding to the lower proton energies for the same range. Because of physical reasons, this cannot be influenced by any means, but the broadening in the air can be reduced slightly by reducing the air gap and bringing the patient closer to the exit window. To reduce the large scattering for low-energy protons, it is sometimes more efficient to use a greater energy from the accelerator and to put an absorber just in front of the patient.

For carbon ions, the beam-broadening is mostly in a tolerable limit and not of clinical concern, because even for the larger penetration depth it is smaller than 2 mm, but for protons it can interfere with the clinically wanted precision. For Helium ions, the beam widening is roughly half of that of proton. This is one of the arguments to use a helium beams instead of protons when other reasons ask for a low-linear energy transfer (LET) beam.

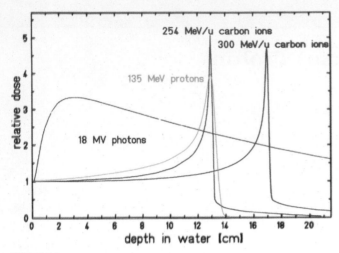

**FIGURE 1.**   Depth-dose profiles of radiotherapy beams like photons, protons, and carbon ions.

## ROLE OF INHOMOGENEOUS TARGETS

Therapy deals with inhomogeneous targets where bones, muscles, fat, and even vacuoles (antra) are close together. Especially, when exploiting the high precision of ion beams, the gradient and also internal accuracy of the dose plans become important. In treatment planning, the energy of a beam is calculated according to the penetration through the material of the central ray, ie, the range and the density of the tissue hit by the inner part of the beam. As the beam diameter is enlarged according to the lateral scattering, the outer fractions of the beam penetrate tissue of a different density than the central ray yielding a different range. Then the distal border shows spikes or holes in the dose distribution. This effect is widely independent from the type of beam application, active or passive, and becomes the larger the more the beam is spread out by multiple scattering. In this way, the lateral scattering of the beam is translated into range scattering, and the proton beams having a 3.5 times larger lateral straggling have a worse overall accuracy of the treatment conformity. This effect is mostly not shown on the treatment plans at the computer, but it is there in reality (Fig. 4). Even if the treatment planning software can handle the edge effects at density inhomogeneities, the optimization for carbon yields a much better conformation to the target volume.

## PET IMAGING

All possible drawbacks originating from the ion beam fragmentation causing a distal dose-tail are more than compensated by the possibility of the in situ beam monitoring using PET.[7] A frequent process of projectile fragmentation is the stripping of 1 or 2 neutrons producing lighter the lighter $^{10}C$ and $^{11}C$ isotopes, which are positron emitters with lifetimes of 19 seconds and 20 minutes, respectively. Detecting their positron decay with a PET camera, their range and consequently the range of the primary beam can be monitored. In addition, from the oxygen atoms of the target, the PET isotope $^{15}O$ is produced with very low recoil velocity having a broad distribution up to the maximum range. Figure 5 shows that the positron activity from the carbon isotopes as a single line at the position of the Bragg maximum, whereas the oxygen contribution is a broad continuum. This continuum is also produced by the protons beams and could be used to monitor proton ranges.[8] For ions heavier than carbon many different positron lines

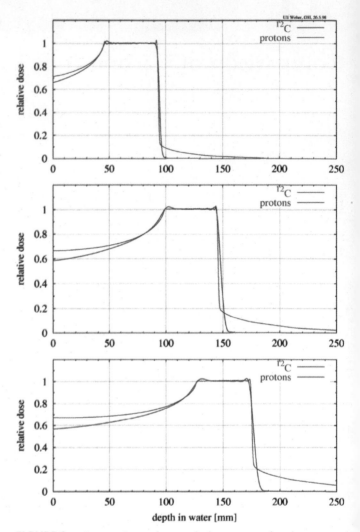

**FIGURE 2.**   Comparison of extended proton and carbon Bragg-curves of different penetration depth corresponding to tumors of a 5-cm extension located in various depths of 7.5, 12.5, and 15 cm.

contribute having different life times, which complicates the analysis of the measurements.

Up to now in the clinical practice, only the range of carbon beams has been determined routinely in the therapy for Gesellschaft für Schwerionenforschung. There, the positron decay was measured in and after each fraction and compared with an expected distribution that was calculated from the planned dose distribution (Fig. 6). With the present technique, a mispositioning and shifts in the dose distribution of approximately 2 mm could be detected, and the treatment plan could be corrected if necessary.

## THE BIOLOGIC ACTION OF ION BEAMS

The major reason for using carbon ions in tumor therapy is the elevated relative biologic effectiveness (RBE), enhancing the inactivation in the tumor volume while in the entrance channel RBE stays close to one.[9] This is different from neutrons used as high RBE radiation in

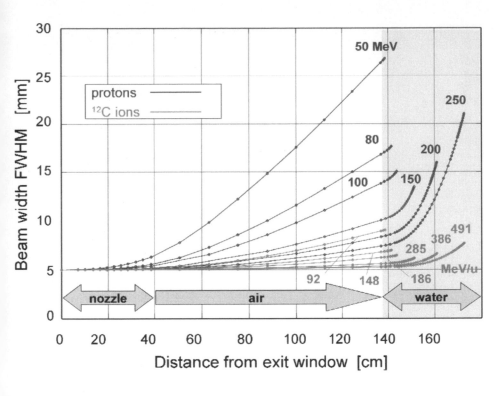

**FIGURE 3.** Lateral scattering in realistic scanning-therapy setups calculated for a nozzle based on GSI therapy facility. The beam penetrates through the exit windows and monitors and enters the patient body in a distance of 1.40 m from the exit.

the past. For neutrons, the elevated RBE is independent from penetration depth and combined with a photon like exponential depth-dose curve. Consequently, the neutron dose is amplified by the high RBE everywhere. This produced good tumor control values, but severe side effects in the normal tissue and neutron trials were finally terminated in most cases. In contrast, for the carbon beams, the RBE is selectively elevated in the target only, and the low dose in the entrance is associated with RBE values slightly greater than one. This combination

is perfect for therapy: low dose of low biologic effectiveness in the normal tissue combined with high dose of great biologic inactivation potential.

The reason for an RBE increase is a larger production of nonrepairable DNA damages (clustered lesions) in the region of high local ionization density at the end of the track of each individual ion. For photons (x-rays), an increase in ionization density can be reached only with an increase in the total dose. For particles, the local ionization

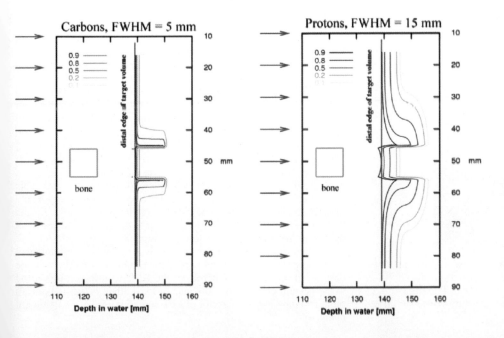

**FIGURE 4.** Edge effects in particle therapy. Realistic proton and carbon beams are passing the edges of a dense structure, such as bone. The 3-dimensional scanning pattern is optimized for best conformity of the 90% isodose to the distal edge of the target volume. The spikes behind the target are due to the increasing width of the pencil beam, which is shifted at the bone edge cannot be avoided. Accordingly, the integral dose of the spikes is much larger for protons than for carbons. Because the energy is adjusted for the central parts of the beam, the outer parts experience the wrong absorber, causing spikes in the dose profiles.

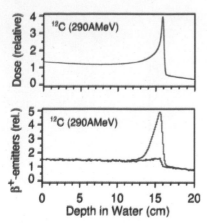

**FIGURE 5.**  The principles of in beam PET. The ß+ activity of a carbon beam has 2 components: the activated 15 oxygen from the tissue atoms (blue line in the lower panel) and the activated carbon isotopes (red line) that stop and decay nearly at the same depth as the primary carbon beam (upper panel).

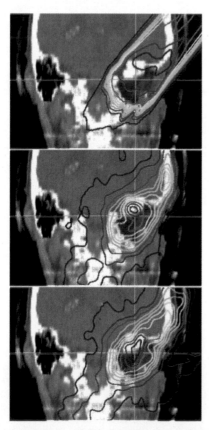

**FIGURE 6.**  Comparison of the planned physical dose distribution (top), measured PET activity (middle), and simulated PET activity from the treatment planning (bottom). The measurement shows good agreement with the simulation and no range differences.[18]

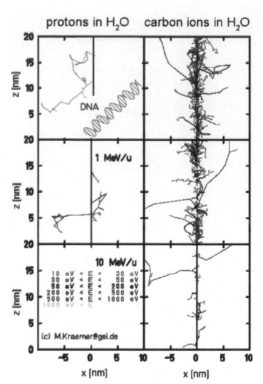

**FIGURE 7.**  Comparison of the microscopic track structure of protons and carbon ions at different energies corresponding to different positions in the depth–dose distribution. At higher energy before the Bragg maximum, the density of the emitted electrons is low, for energies of 1 MeV corresponding to the peak position the electron density is still low for protons but dense for carbon ions, causing multiple breaks. Finally, at very low energy, carbon ions produce more local damage than necessary to kill a cell (overkill) but for protons, the RBE starts to rise.[19]

density increases in each individual particle track with decreasing energy for 2 reasons: first the ionization increases according to the LET toward the end of the particle range up to the Bragg maximum, and, second, the diameter of the particle track shrinks with decreasing energies. Both effects together yield a higher local ionization density as shown in Figure 7. Correspondingly, the production of clustered lesions increases toward the end of range for all ions but at different energies and, consequently, at other positions in the depth dose curve.[10] For protons, the RBE maximum value occurs at 25 keV/$\mu$m, for Helium/$\alpha$ particles, at 100 keV/$\mu$m, and for carbon ions, at 200 keV/$\mu$m. When the ionization density increases further, RBE drops rapidly because more dose than necessary for killing is transferred to a cell in the track of a single ion (overkill effect). This general behavior is found for all ions from protons to the very heavy ones like Neon, but because of the different local LET values for the different ions, the increase of RBE occur at different distances from the end of the ions range as shown in Figure 8.

For protons, the RBE increases only in the last few micrometers of the range at the very distal part of the Bragg maximum where the dose rapidly decreases. Therefore, the RBE contributes very little to the general dose deposition, and its local effect is washed out. In proton therapy, a generic factor of RBE = 1.15 is used in the treatment planning.

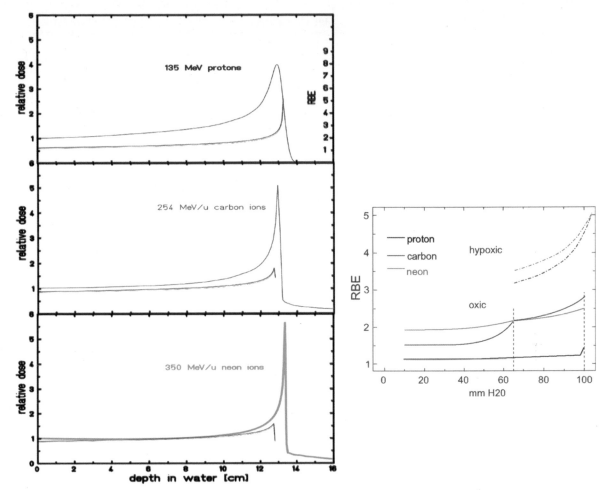

**FIGURE 8.**    In the left panel, the RBE (right scale) and the dose (left scale) are compared as function of depth: only for carbon ions dose- and the RBE-maximum coincide at the same depth, amplifying the high dose through the high effectiveness (data based on cell experiments of W.K. Weyrather). In the right panel, the RBE of different ions as function of depth are given. Solid lines represent RBE under oxic conditions, dashed line under hypoxic conditions.[20] Both graphs are based on experimental data, but they correspond to a specific cell sensitivity and should be viewed more as a schematic representation.

In contrast, for the very heavy Ne$^-$ ions, the RBE increases a few centimeters before the Bragg maximum, whereas the high-dose region of the Bragg maximum is already in the overkill regimen. This causes side effects in the normal tissue in the entrance channel and little or no benefit for the tumor treatment.

For carbon ions, the RBE and dose have their maximum almost at the same position, and the high dose of the Bragg maximum is amplified by an increased RBE. The therapeutic gain of this behavior becomes evident when the RBE for extended target volumes are compared (Fig. 8, right panel). In this graph, the RBE for hypoxic tissue is given: for protons, there is no significant difference, but for the heavy ions, the hypoxic RBE is much greater than under normoxic conditions.

As the action of the heavy ions interferes with the cellular repair system, all repair-related effects become of minor importance. This is true for the resistance induced by hypoxia, but it is also the case in a more general way: also other resistant populations for instance because of partial synchronization in the cell cycle become less influential for particle radiation. In a heterogeneous tumor, the radio-resistant compartments become more sensitive when irradiated with the high LET fraction of a heavy ion beam, ie, with the stopping ions. Therefore, the risk of surviving tumor cell decreases even in the radio-resistant part of the tumor, and recurrent tumor regrowth becomes less frequent.

The "inbuilt" adaptation according to the radiosensitivity of the tumor cells is a great advantage and cancels some important reasons for fractionated therapy. In conventional therapy, it is applied to reoxygenate hypoxic tissues and to redistribute partial cell-cycle synchronizations.[11] For high LET irradiation, these arguments are not valid, and the therapy fractionation can be accelerated. In fact, nonsmall cell lung cancer has been treated with hypofractionated regimen at National Institute for Radiological Science with great success, in which the curative dose was finally given in one fraction.[12] For carbon therapy, the repair of the normal tissue is the major argument to fractionate the treatment.

For a fair judgment, whether high- or low-LET radiation should be used, ie, whether proton or carbon beams would have a clinical benefit, both the normal tissue and the tumor sensitivity have to be taken

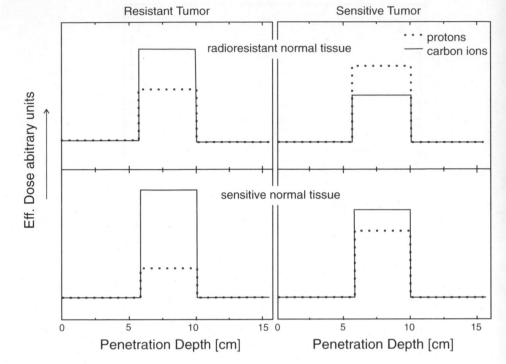

**FIGURE 9.** Schematic representation of the biologic effective dose for the irradiation of a tumor from 2 opposing sides. The biologic effective dose is given for the 4 possible combinations of sensitive or resistant normal tissue with the respective tumor sensitivities. The graphs are normalized for the same effect in the entrance channel.

into account. Because the RBE depends strongly on the repair capacity of the tissue, one has to differentiate not only between tumors of different sensitivity but also between the sensitivity of the surrounding normal tissue. In Figure 9, the biologic effective doses for the 4 possible combinations of resistant respective sensitive tumors and tissues are given in a very schematic way for a model tumor irradiated from 2 opposite entrance ports. The data are normalized to the same effective dose to the normal tissue in each case. For most combinations, the irradiation with carbon ions yields a biologic benefit when the tumor is of the same or greater resistance as the normal surrounding tissue. However, for the treatment of a sensitive tumor in a resistant normal tissue, the application of protons would bring a therapeutic gain. Because of the reduced targeting precision of protons, the use of helium ions instead is frequently discussed. In the first biologic experiments at the new HIT facility, the greater biological effectiveness of the carbon ions for the combination of resistant tumor and resistant normal tissue has been confirmed in cell experiments.[14]

## RBE AND TREATMENT PLANNING

In practice, the variation of RBE over the target volume has to be incorporated in the planning process to reach an isoeffective dose over the complete target volume. In the case of tumor-conforming treatment, the composition in energy and secondary particle will differ from each volume element (voxel) to the next. Consequently, the RBE has to be known with the same granularity.[14]

For these calculations of the local RBE values over the treatment volume corresponding to the mixture of the different energies in the treatment field (including the fraction of the secondary ions) and according to the radiobiological properties, the local effect model (LEM) has been developed.[15] LEM is based, on the physical side, on the dose distribution inside the particle tracks and, on the biologic side, on the cell-sensitivity measured against x-rays as parameterized in the $\alpha/\beta$ ratio of the survival curves. In dose effect curves for cell

survival, a shoulder is found for low doses of sparsely ionizing radiation. For repair proficient cells and tissues, this shoulder is larger; and for repair deficient cells and tissues, the shoulder decreases, and the irradiation becomes more efficient. Dose effect curves for cell inactivation (cell survival curves) are given as $S = S_0 \exp(-\alpha D - \beta^2)$, where S is the survival and D the dose. $\alpha$ and $\beta$ are individual parameters that describe the individual sensitivity. Because the coefficient $\alpha$ relates to the initial slope and $\beta$ to the slope at higher doses, the ratio $\alpha/\beta$ is a measure for the repair capacity. Cells having low $\alpha/\beta$ ratios have a large repair capacity and show a large shoulder in the dose effect curves, whereas large $\alpha/\beta$-ratios indicate a more exponential behavior.

From these parameters and the average size of the nucleus as the critical target inside the cell, the effect of the inhomogeneous dose distribution inside the particle tracks on the inactivation could be determined in a first approximation (LEM I). For example, for carbon treatment of chordomas and chondrosarcomas, the calculated RBE values range from 2 to 5 in the center of the target, but they are not constant over the irradiated target volume. In a second step, the diffusion of the radicals mostly out from the track center was incorporated. The interaction of single-strand breaks forming a double-strand break was then integrated as well (LEM II). Finally, in the latest version (LEM III) in which the energy dependence of the dose cut off in the very inner part of the tracks has been included. LEM I to LEM III brought smaller corrections for the calculation of the tumor RBE, but overestimates the expected damage in the low LET area in the entrance channel, as well as that for light ions. However, the LEM model is still under development. The main goal is to calculate the local RBE values for different particles like carbon and helium ions, as well as for protons, using the same set of parameters.

LEM has been tested extensively in radiobiological experiments, including animal studies, before therapy starts, and new additions are always checked in a series of experiments before applied in therapy. In addition, the LEM approach is in accordance with the

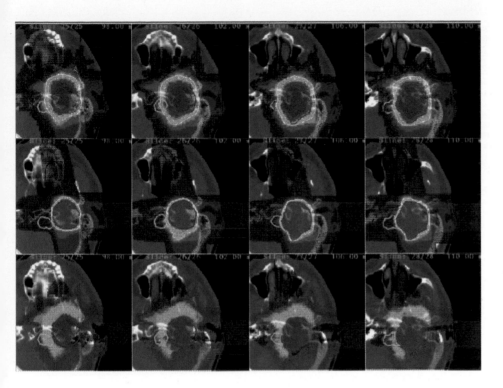

**FIGURE 10.** Comparison of dose distributions for proton therapy with passive dose conformation (upper row) and carbon ion therapy with beam scanning (middle row). The lower row shows the corresponding differences in dose (red: 0%–5%, orange: 5%–10%, and yellow: 10%–20%). Courtesy O. Jäkel and Ref. 17.

observation of the treatment response (toxicity, tumor control) of the patients at GSI. Up to now, no recurrent tumor has been observed in the target, and also no necrotic areas are found after treatment. This indicates the correctness of LEM.[16]

## COMPARISON OF TREATMENT PLANS FOR CARBON IONS AND PROTON

In Figure 10, the treatment plans for a clivus chordoma are compared for proton therapy with passive dose conformation with the planning for the same patient with a scanning carbon beam.[17] There are 2 effects influencing this comparison; first, the difference in beam delivery: the overall conformity between the target (red line) and the irradiated volume are better for the scanned beam than for passive system. Second, the dose gradients are less sharp for the protons, which are caused by the larger scattering of the proton beam inside the patient. The overall conformity of the high dose area is much better for carbon ions, which can be seen particularly in the area of the brainstem. Because of the lower scattering of ions, the dose fall-off at the border of the target volume is steeper.

## CONCLUSIONS

The comparison of protons with carbon ion beams for tumor therapy not only shows the great additional advantage of carbon beams but also confirms the positive properties of protons. Concerning the physical conformity, carbon has, at any depth, a dose gradient at least 3 times better than protons. Therefore, critical structures can be spared to a much better degree with carbon beams. Concerning the biologic selectivity, the situation is more complex: depending on the biologic sensitivity of the tumor, but also of the surrounding normal tissue, both ions can have some advantages. In this case, it is really important that the physician can choose either the one ion or the other. So, combined proton or carbon facilities seem to be the optimal choice, but require a greater initial investment. There is some agreement that a proton

alone therapy unit having the same number of treatment rooms, the cost reduction compared with a combined unit is 30% to 40%. However, for the overall treatment, the investment cost contributes only one third; the major costs are the personnel expenses and the consumables, like energy. In addition, in these estimations, the obvious possibility of shorter treatment times of carbon therapy because of hypofractionation is not included. In general, the combined facilities will have a greater future potential; however, at present, there is less experience with carbon ions than with protons. Therefore, more combined centers should be built to gain this knowledge.

## ACKNOWLEDGMENTS

*The authors thank all members of the GSI Biophysics Department for their discussions and constructive criticism. Especially, they thank W.K Weyrather, M. Scholz, Thilo Elsaesser, and Swetlana Ktitareva for their help in preparing the manuscript. They also thank the guest editors Drs. Theodore S. Lawrence and Benjamin Movsas for the invitation to contribute to this special issue on particle therapy.*

## REFERENCES

1. Chu WT, Ludewigt BA, Renner TR. Instrumentation for treatment of cancer using proton and light-ion beams. *Rev Sci Instr.* 1993;64:2055–2122.
2. Kraft G. Tumor therapy with charged particles. *Progr Part Nucl Phys.* 2000;45:473–544.
3. Tobias CA, Alpen EA, Blakely EA, et al. Radiobiological basis for heavy-ion therapy. In: Abe M, Sakamoto K, Phillips TJ, eds. *Treatment of Radioresistant Cancers.* New York: Elsevier; 1979:159–183.
4. Haettner E, Iwase H, Schardt D. Experimental fragmentation studies with 12C therapy beams. *Rad Prot Dosim.* 2006;122:485–487.
5. Tobias CA, Benton EV, Capp MP, et al. Particle radiotherapy and autoactivation. *Int J Radiat Oncology Biol Phys.* 1977;3:35–44.
6. Weber U. Volume conform irradiation in heavy ion tumor therapy, Ph.D. thesis. University of Kassel, 1996.
7. Enghardt W, Fromm WD, Geissel H, et al. The spatial distribution of positron-emitting nuclei generated by relativistic light ion beams in organic matter. *Phys Med Biol.* 1992;37:2127–2131.

8. Parodi K, Paganetti H, Shih HA, et al. Patient study of in vivo verification of beam delivery and range, using positron emission tomography and computed tomography imaging after proton therapy. *Int J Radiat Oncol.* 2007;68:920–934.

9. Blakely EA, Tobias CA, Ngo FQH, et al. Physical and cellular radiobiological properties of heavy ions in relation to cancer therapy application. In: Pirncello MD, Tobias CA, eds. *Biological and Medical Research With Accelerated Heavy Ions at the Bevalac.* CA: LBL-11220; 1980:73–88.

10. Price K. Use of radiation quality as a probe for DNA lesion quality. *Int J Radiat Biol.* 1994;65:43–48.

11. Scholz M, Matsufuji N, Kanai T. Test of the local effect model using clinical data: tumor control propability for lung tumors after treatment with carbon ion beams. *Rad Prot Dosim.* 2006;122:478–479.

12. Schulz-Ertner D, Tsujii H. Particle radiation therapy using protons and heavier ion beams. *J Clin Oncol.* 2007;25:953–964.

13. Weyrather WK, Debus J. Particle beams for cancer therapy. *Clin Oncol.* 2003;15:23–28.

14. Krämer M, Jäkel O, Haberer T, et al. Treatment planning for scanned ion beams. *Radiother Oncol.* 2004;73(Suppl 2):S80–S85.

15. Scholz M, Kraft G. A parameter-free track structure model for heavy ion action cross sections. In: Chadwick KH, Moschini G, Varma MN, eds. *Biophysical Modelling of Radiation Effects.* Bristol, UK: Adam Hilger; 1992:185–192.

16. Elsässer T, Krämer M, Scholz M. Accuracy of the local effect model for the prediction of biologic effects of carbon ion beams in-vitro and in-vivo. *Int J Radiat Oncol Biol Phys.* 2008;71:866–872.

17. Jäkel O. Treatment planning for heavy ion therapy, Habilitation thesis. University of Heidelberg, 2001.

18. Enghardt W, Debus J, Haberer T, et al. The application of PET to quality assurance of heavy-ion tumor therapy. *Strahlenther Onkol.* 1999;175(Suppl II):33–36.

19. Krämer M, Kraft G. Calculations of heavy ion track structure. *Radiat Environm Biophys.* 1994;33:91–109.

20. Scholz M. Basis of the biological treatment planning for heavy ion tumor therapy, Habilitation thesis. University of Heidelberg 2001.

# Proton Beam Therapy and the Convoluted Pathway to Incorporating Emerging Technology into Routine Medical Care in the United States

Michael L. Steinberg • Andre Konski

One of the most contentious and controversial issues for health policy decision makers, medical providers, and the healthcare technology industry in the United States is the pathway for incorporating new and emerging medical technologies into the healthcare delivery system. And one of the medical technologies that has proved most divisive and problematic on this pathway is proton beam therapy (PBT). Although not really new, PBT continues to be viewed as an "emerging" technology because of its high cost, which has been a barrier to entry and has led to a protracted ramp up. However, recently, interest in this technology and its implementation in the mainstream of cancer treatment has increased remarkably   driven as much by financial and market impetuses as by medical promise. In this regard, high startup of PBT and treatment-related costs and the conflicting evidence of its superior efficacy compared with less-expensive, conventional radiation treatments have put this technology's promise in question.

In consequence, the discourse among providers, payers, patients, and health policy experts about PBT and its place in medical care has become complicated and heated. There are allegations of unproved claims of medical superiority, assertions of meddling with personal choices of treatment, allegations of interference with physician judgment, pleas for evidence-based implementation, and expressions of anxious concern about the cost and other effects that widespread use of PBT will have on the healthcare delivery system. It is within this context that we explore, here, how the social, economic, and political milieu brought the issue of the incorporation of PBT into the healthcare delivery system to this point. We look at how new technologies are currently accepted into this system and discuss emerging trends—such as the use of evidence-based assessment of technology, coverage with evidence policies, and comparative effectiveness analysis—affecting PBT's effort to finds its place in the pantheon of available medical treatments for patients with cancer.

## THE CURRENT HEALTH POLICY CONTEXT

Serious challenges face the United States healthcare delivery system, including the fact that despite ever-increasing healthcare costs, the United States has not yet been able to achieve health outcomes as good as or as high value as those of other industrialized countries.[1] Moreover, this confounding situation continues while the number of medically uninsured in the United States grows. To date, most health policy experts agree that the United States has not coherently embraced policies and processes to simultaneously enhance value and address cost.[1]

The drivers of the rising cost of U.S. healthcare are often portrayed as fraud and abuse, bureaucratic inefficiencies, and inadequate free market influences in the business of healthcare delivery. However, the most significant contributor to the rising cost of healthcare (and, indirectly, to the increasing number of medically uninsured) is the rapid and uncontrolled demand for and introduction of new treatments, medical devices/technologies, and drugs, before their effectiveness, cost, and comparative value have been satisfactorily and acceptably evaluated.[2,3] Most cost-control efforts focus on payment issues, system abuse caused by patient and/or provider overuse, fraud (real and contrived), standardization-based discounting (eg, generic drugs and volume discounting of services by vendor selection), and control of demand via financing mechanisms, such as deductibles, patient self-funding, and provider gain sharing. However, these standard cost-control strategies and most new strategies (eg, disease management, health promotion, and "quality" purchasing) cannot change the behavior and mitigate the ever-rising costs of healthcare. In fact, the only strategy with a chance of doing so is that of changing the patient and provider attitudes toward the use of new healthcare interventions.[3] In other words, costs cannot be controlled in a milieu in which every promising but yet unproved "new" treatment, emerging technology, and "breakthrough" device is made available to patients through providers and a healthcare delivery system that inconsistently and only halfheartedly evaluate new advances in terms of absolute and marginal benefits and actual value.[3]

The United States has been slow to implement policies that directly and methodically address this critical aspect of healthcare spending and verification of value.[2] In the United Kingdom, however, the British National Institute for Health and Clinical Excellence (NICE) evaluates new and established drugs, devices, and diagnostic tests in an effort to compare treatment effectiveness in terms of cost and outcome.[4] Absent a hidden agenda asymmetrically slanted toward cost control, a U.S. approach akin to this one could bring needed information about relative effectiveness of medical treatments to a policy discussion on access of new technologies to routine healthcare use. At issue here in the minds of many policy makers, patients, and providers is whether such an approach can ever rise above the cost-control imperative.[5] Other stakeholders question whether the current situation, in which politics often overrides cogent policy, is economically sustainable.

## INSURANCE COVERAGE OF NEW MEDICAL TECHNOLOGY: POLITICS TRUMPS POLICY

Currently, politics is a stronger driver than policy when it comes to accepting and covering new medical treatments and devices. That is, policy and scientifically systematic pathways for transmitting new medical technology into routine use in the U.S. healthcare delivery system do not typify the process. Furthermore, the avenues that may lead to insurance coverage for such technology may even belie medical evidence and cogent policy.

The actors in this sociomedical drama are not only doctors and patients but also politicians, advocacy groups, hospitals, drug companies, device vendors, organized medicine, the media, and paid lobbyists. For example, consider the 1990s odyssey of bone marrow transplant (BMT) for patients with high-risk breast cancer, an odyssey that is instructive on the nuances of the current process by which new technology can make its way into routine use.

At the time, the circumstances were critical for the beleaguered patients, and the rationale for the treatment was sensible and medically possible. The argument was that the patients were at very high risk for disease recurrence and death after standard treatment and would benefit from very high-dose chemotherapy with BMT rescue. BMT would be expensive and toxic, but it would eradicate the cancer cells remaining in the patient's body after conventional treatment, thus rendering the patient cured. Initial studies had no control groups but were encouraging; and early on, many doctors said that the use of randomized clinical trials (RCTs) to address the efficacy of the treatment would be unethical and called for the procedure to be immediately added to the armamentarium for breast cancer treatment.[3]

The insurance industry initially insisted on high-level evidence as proof that this expensive treatment worked and, in the absence of such data, frequently denied coverage. Physicians and, more significantly, patient advocacy groups enlisted media and political support to gain insurance coverage for what they saw as a "life-saving" procedure. The media, in what has become a customary response, bashed the insurance companies for what was portrayed as unforgivable motives, framing them in terms of the corporate insurance industry trying to save money and boost profits by withholding payment for desperately needed care. The responses in some cases took the form of state-legislated mandates for insurance coverage for the procedure. In other cases, the legal system forced insurance companies to cover the treatment. In one famous legal decision, more than $74 million was awarded for a patient denied coverage for BMT. Coverage for the procedure soon followed, with insurance companies citing lawsuits—not medical evidence—as the primary motivation.[3]

During this time, academic centers and cooperative groups in the United States, Europe, and South Africa mounted RCTs to determine the efficacy of BMT in high-risk patients. However, given the reigning environment of compulsory coverage and groupthink on the part of patients and providers who were embracing the "obvious" benefits of BMT, numerous patients refused to participate in the RCTs. Accrual initially estimated to take 3 years for one U.S. trial ended up taking 8 years. European data started to become available in 1998, U.S. data in 2000. In the end, the "obvious" benefits proved illusive. Five RCTs showed that BMT for this clinical setting offered no advantage over standard therapy and that the treatment itself caused substantially greater toxicity and risk of death.[3]

This case is not an unusual example of the powerful social effect that a convergence of physician and patient advocacy groups, the media, the pharma/device industry, the legal system, and political/legislative groups can have on U.S. health policy as it relates to the uptake of emerging medical treatments. Basically, in the absence of a sensible systematic process, societal forces were for a time able to trump good medical science. And as it turned out, the expensive new treatment that was brought mainstream proved to be ineffective and toxic. Although this episode is often cited as an example of the system's inadequacies and the need for evidence-based coverage, its effect on policy has remained limited.

## MEDICARE POLICY AND NEW TECHNOLOGY

Medicare policy on the assimilation of new medical technology and treatments has determinative and formative effects on the coverage and payment policies of the entire U.S. healthcare delivery system. CMS (Centers for Medicare and Medicaid Services) has statutory authority to cover a wide range of physician- and hospital-based healthcare services that are reasonable or necessary for the diagnosis or treatment of illnesses or injury (Social Security Act, 1965. Section 1862(a)(1)(A)). The process through which Medicare determines coverage and payments for medical services and technology continues to evolve but remains somewhat arcane. Surprisingly, it has historically limited the direct consideration of cost and cost effectiveness for individual treatments and devices.[2]

The broad language of the Medicare Statute states that treatments must be "reasonable and necessary" and should be "safe and effective" (the Federal Drug Administration [FDA] criteria for devices); it also tacitly suggests that there may be adequate evidence to conclude that treatments improve patient health outcomes. Although the statute provides no specific authority to take costs into account when deciding whether to cover a particular treatment, patient outcomes such as quality of life, morbidity, and mortality have been increasingly emphasized in recent years. One emerging CMS approach includes the notions that a service or device should be as good as or better than current covered alternatives and that a service should have broad relevance to the entire Medicare population.[6] This second notion does not specifically address the absolute cost of a service, but CMS recently began looking more carefully at high-cost services with small comparative benefit. The economic stimulus package that Congress passed in February 2009 allocated funding to the Agency for Healthcare Research and Quality, National Institutes of Health, and Department of Health and Human Sciences to begin addressing the comparative effectiveness of medical treatments.

Any such evaluative process must deal with the complex problem of how to synthesize and value medical evidence. One mechanism that CMS uses is the Medicare Evidence Development & Coverage Advisory Committee (MEDCAC), which was established to provide CMS with independent external guidance and expert advice on new and emerging technologies and treatments. Implicit in the MEDCAC function are considerations of absolute and comparative effectiveness. To address the question of what evidence is necessary to deem a treatment or device ready for routine use in the Medicare population, MEDCAC has explored what it calls *evidentiary priorities* and the complexities of evidence development, trial design, and evidence thresholds for agency coverage of new medical treatments. MEDCAC considered practical arguments for flexibility of methodology, even noting the drawbacks of RCTs and the potential role and limitations of registries. MEDCAC has also identified a clear need to define standards for threshold of evidence but has not reached agreement on the use of generic standards, some members suggesting that evidence criteria must be applied on the basis of specific technologies and conditions.[7]

Unlike the commercial insurance industry, CMS has avoided definitive criteria for evidence in favor of flexibility in its technology assessments, the objective being to avoid a politically unpopular proliferation of noncoverage decisions.[8] The resulting de facto policy de-emphasizes the importance of analyzing effectiveness and its cost component. After all, if a healthcare financing system covers the cost of new technology and has few mechanisms for evaluating the effectiveness of innovations, vendors of new medical technologies have little to gain by self-submitting to evaluations of comparative effectiveness.[4] In addition, the current circumstances and payment system encourage hospitals and doctors to use more and more expensive treatments and encourage patients to continue to see health-care as a free good—all in the face of little evidence-based information about treatment effectiveness. Many people consider this to be inefficient and, in terms of its cost to society, poor policy.

## CPT, RUC, AND CMS ROLES IN THE VALUATION PROCESS

Both Medicare and the commercial insurance industry look to the American Medical Association's (AMA) current procedural terminology (CPT) coding and nomenclature process and the AMA/Specialty Society Relative Value Scale Update Committee's (RUC) valuation process to provide structure and input for the U.S. healthcare delivery payment system. By statute, CMS is required to define the healthcare services covered for Medicare beneficiaries and adjudicate appropriate payment for those services. CMS has looked to these AMA processes to inform its decisions in these matters.

The CPT nomenclature for coding medical services and procedures used in routine clinical care is designated as category I CPT codes. The criteria for these codes are that the service/procedure has received FDA approval, is a distinct service/procedure performed by many physicians/practitioners across the United States, and has had its clinical efficacy well established and documented in U.S. peer-reviewed literature.[9]

In recent years, the CPT editorial panel, which oversees the CPT process, has substantially raised the evidence standard for category I applications by closely scrutinizing the supporting peer-reviewed literature and ascertaining the veracity of claims that a new procedure has been widely accepted within the medical community. Many purveyors of new medical technology, especially small startup companies, find this raised standard daunting and at times insurmountable; and the venture capital community, which financially backs many medical technology developments in the United States, finds the raised standard at odds with its goal for time-based return on investment. The problem is further complicated by the fact that even though the evidence bar has been raised, the AMA and CMS still have not provided a specific, precisely defined standard of evidence.

In 2002, the CPT panel implemented category III CPT codes for emerging technology: "category III CPT codes are a temporary set of tracking codes for new and emerging technologies."[9] Intended initially for data collection purposes in the FDA approval process and to substantiate widespread use, this category does not require conformity with the category I evidence and usage criteria. Instead, it requires support from the specialties that would use the procedure, availability of U.S. peer-reviewed literature, and descriptions of current U.S. trials outlining the efficacy of the procedure or service.[9] Procedures designated as category III are not priced but have increasingly gained carrier-based and third-party insurance pricing and payment.

After a procedure or service gains category I CPT status, it is forwarded to the RUC for valuation. The RUC values physician work associated with the procedure and gathers, but does not validate, "direct" practice expense for the associated service. The work valuations are transmitted as recommendations to CMS, which accepts more than 90% of them without alteration. The practice expense data are included as inputs to CMS's valuation of the technical component of the reimbursement for the procedure. The actual process for valuing the technical fee is arcane and complex. Practitioners and the purveyors of new medical technology sometimes note surprise at final valuations that turn out lower or higher than expected.

In the less-stringent environment of the 1990s, CPT codes were granted for PBT. They were subsequently edited to adjust for changes in the technology and to enhance valuation, but there has never been an official CPT/RUC valuation of PBT's technical costs. In 2007, CMS requested inputs of practice expense information, but the evaluation did not occur. To date, PBT has not been priced in the national Medicare fee schedule. Instead, PBT pricing is done only by local Medicare carriers for nonhospital-based providers and by insurance companies.

Ambulatory payment classifications (APCs) are the mechanism for payment of the technical component of hospital-based outpatient procedures. This payment system parallels the Medicare fee schedule. Its reimbursement rates are developed by averaging and bundling procedures described by CPT, Healthcare Common Procedure Coding System Level II, and other revenue codes, and then grouping the codes based on clinical resource homogeneity and established payment rates. CMS gathers cost and charge information from individual hospital providers on particular procedures and then uses a complex "cost-to-charge ratio" methodology to set reimbursement values each year. Unlike the CPT/RUC process, this payment system gives vendors of new and otherwise unpriced medical technology the opportunity to be reimbursed through the "new technology APC" or the CMS-established G-code for the technical component of a hospital-based outpatient procedure—without providing more than a modicum of evidence of a technology's efficacy. The evidence criteria for granting APC/G-code standing in this circumstance is consistent with the more lenient CMS criteria noted earlier. Admittedly, this path to reimbursement may be fraught with technical nuances and bureaucratic barriers that can delay the realization of reimbursement. However, even though such codes are without the professional component of reimbursement, hospitals, often supported by their physicians, may be quick to take up newly reimbursed technology, for reasons that are both competitive and economic. So, even without the incentive of physician reimbursement, emerging medical technology endures as the driver of increased revenue for the hospital and increased cost to the healthcare delivery system—often, once again, without substantial evidence of a technology's effectiveness.

## THE CASE OF PROTON BEAM THERAPY

In 1946, 17 years after University of California Nobel Prize–winning physicist Ernest Lawrence invented the cyclotron, one of his protégés, Harvard professor Robert Wilson, proposed the use of protons for the treatment of cancer. Eight years later, the first patient was treated with protons at the Berkeley Radiation Laboratory; and in 1961, the Harvard Cyclotron Laboratory, initially established as a physics research facility, began treating patients with cancer. Thirty years later, in 1991, the first hospital-based proton facility was established at Loma Linda University Medical Center (LLUMC).

In the early 1990s, only 3 operational units consistently treated patients. Taking clinical advantage of the conformal superiority of PBT over the conventional photon-based radiation therapy of the day, these facilities developed notoriety for treating rare and unusual diseases—such as base of skull sarcomas, inoperable arteriovenous malformations in the brain, and intraocular melanoma—for which conventional radiation therapy was impossible or ineffective. The treatment results were anecdotally promising and at times even impressive. The series were observational and without control groups for comparison. Reimbursement was mostly based on individually negotiated agreements with the local Medicare carriers and insurance companies. Favorable payment-negotiation outcomes were facilitated by the exceptional nature of the patients' diagnoses when treated with the new modality and the associated low volume of services.

For this infrequently used treatment modality, payment was based on crosswalk methodology that would set PBT reimbursement by equating the total surgical costs for management of the same condition discounted to parity or was a multiple of conventional radiation therapy to cover estimated costs. This approach to setting payment for new technology was not unusual at the time, especially when the technology in question was being used for rare and unusual indications. However, 2 factors began to change payer attitudes toward PBT.

The first of these factors was the growing use of PBT as providers expanded the medical indications for this new, promising, and expensive technology. The cost of PBT began to be questioned, mostly by the nongovernmental health insurance industry. The second factor that affected payer attitudes was a change and an increased sophistication in the coding and valuation methodology related to new medical treatments. Realizing this, in 1997, the facility related to Harvard/Massachusetts General Hospital and the LLUMC applied for 6 new CPT codes for PBT to reflect the resources to provide PBT, which was described at the time as a new, proved, and necessary treatment modality supplied by only a few centers. A cost ratio for PBT was estimated to be 2 to 2.5 times that for conventional photon therapy. After that application was turned down, the facilities submitted a subsequent application, in 1999, requesting 3 new codes to capture the cost of the additional capital for equipment and manpower needed to operate the highly complex facilities. Of note is the fact that both applications were carried to the CPT editorial panel not, as was customary, by the representing specialty society but by the applicants themselves.

In retrospect, the 1997 and 1999 PBT CPT applications were early warnings of the significant costs associated with the modality's potential growth in the United States. Increasing use of PBT, driven by providers applying the modality to ever more diagnoses (notably in prostate cancer) and by patient demand, dramatically increased the number of insurance claims for PBT. Initial efforts by the insurance industry to limit coverage to the diagnoses associated with the apparent efficacy noted in the rare medical conditions in which PBT was pioneered stood in counterpoint to CMS's more lenient stance of accepting the new indications. Similar to what happened with BMT, PBT advocacy groups successfully sought legal remedies to secure coverage from the insurance industry. PBT advocates in the medical community presented the rational case for the enhanced efficacy and even potential superiority of PBT compared with other radiation modalities based on astute and rigorous modeling of physical characteristics of PBT.[10] Today, the LLUMC Website notes that the advantages of PBT include higher accuracy, which reduces healthy tissue damage, significantly fewer side effects, and lower risk of secondary cancer.[11]

The truth is that, despite PBT's potential physical advantage and the potential physical and biologic advantage of carbon ion therapy, there is virtually no evidence of superior effectiveness compared with existing radiation modalities, such as IMRT and brachytherapy.[12-16] Furthermore, the conflict over PBT deepened when people associated with PBT facilities began to question the need for empirical evidence to demonstrate effectiveness, as well as the ethics of randomization, when, in their view, PBT was better on a hypothetical basis.[10] In 2007 and 2008, articles and communications in the medical literature argued and rebutted the position that RCTs for PBT violated equipoise, the ethical notion that there must be genuine uncertainty in a clinical trial about any treatment arm being superior to another.[17-19]

In addition, Suit et al[20] have questioned the need for positive phase III data before PBT is more widely adopted, contending that if PBT were less expensive than photon therapy, there would be no interest in conducting RCTs. In the current economic context, that contention is neither valid nor realistic. From a historical CMS standpoint, cost is not a significant issue. However, a serious debate on comparative effectiveness in healthcare is beginning, and cost is important and even critical to those seeking rational healthcare policy.

The increasing demand for PBT can be attributed, in part, to marketing by PBT facilities and patient support groups advocating for PBT. In this regard, moral hazard—the prospect that an individual or groups of individuals may behave differently if insulated from a risk compared with how that individual or group would behave if fully exposed to that risk—contributes to the increased health expenditures associated with PBT. To understand how moral hazard relates to healthcare treatment, consider the treatment of early-stage prostate cancer, a prime driver in business pro formas for PBT facilities. Treatments for an otherwise healthy male with localized prostate cancer include interstitial seed implant, open or robot-assisted prostatectomy, external beam photon therapy with intensity-modulated conformal technique, or PBT, and reimbursement for the treatments run from lowest to highest, with PBT being the most expensive. Currently, there are no data to support the superiority of one of these treatments over another in terms of survival or significant morbidity,[14] so in terms of healthcare policy, cost is the sole difference among them. A man with health insurance can thus choose any one of these treatments and, if it is performed properly, will have a similarly acceptable health outcome. However, because this man does not bear the responsibility for payment, he can choose PBT, the most expensive of the equally effective therapies, at no cost to himself, but at increased cost to his insurance company and ultimately to society.

Moral hazard and the lack of systematic evaluation of treatment effectiveness are thought to contribute to the high costs of U.S. healthcare. As an example of an extreme consequence of these 2 factors, consider the patient choosing the PBT option who has a single focus of prostate cancer with a very low prostate-specific antigen. Such a patient likely would never have an unfavorable outcome from his prostate cancer, but because he has insurance that will pay for treatment, he is consuming healthcare resources that he would not consume in the absence of insurance. Those who argue the moral hazard imperative would say that this healthcare-consumer behavior would change if payers paid only for the least expensive among options with equal outcomes.

In an environment of impending significant growth in PBT's availability, rising patient demand stoked by claims of PBT's medical superiority that are not supported by high-level evidence, and ever-increasing costs to the system, payers are beginning to seriously question the existing basis of coverage. In late 2008, CMS announced its intent to consider PBT in prostate cancer for a so-called national coverage determination. If this action is taken, CMS could decide not to pay for PBT or to pay only under the auspices of a defined clinical trial, a circumstance called "coverage with evidence."

## THE BUSINESS OF PROTON BEAM THERAPY

Claims of PBT's medical superiority are well received by patients. And many physicians and forward-looking hospitals see PBT as a cutting-edge technology that offers an opportunity for clinical and research excellence in cancer care, as well as a concomitant business opportunity for potential market dominance and excellent return on investment. More than 20 proton-facility development companies currently exist, and more than 30 such facilities are in various phases of development in the United States.

From a medical perspective, a principal driver of PBT's development is its ability to conform radiation dose to the intended target while limiting radiation-induced morbidity—theoretically, a technological advantage over existing modalities. Powerful business-related imperatives also drive PBT's development. Being the first to offer the modality confirms the advantage of market differentiation, which has the collateral benefit of avoiding the risk of competitive displacement, the loss of market share. However, the primary impetus for many medical institutions and investors is the financial opportunity evidenced by the perceived economic success of the early adopters, the historically strong reimbursements, and the presence of financing models affording limited risk to the medical institution.

Yet, despite the anticipated favorable return on investment based on assumptions of stability of current reimbursement, the broadening of the technology's application to increasingly more medical conditions, and the possibility of shift in market share, there are enthusiasm-mitigating factors. For example, the barriers and costs of hiring and retaining the clinical and technical expertise needed to create the treatment throughput essential for achieving the modeled results of the pro forma are significant. New, "low-cost" PBT technologies may dramatically change the market landscape. Market shifts resulting from the technology's potential proliferation can occur during the long lead time needed to develop a large multivault PBT project. Changes in reimbursement and coverage for PBT can occur, adding to the financial risk.

The cost of PBT centers can range from around $20 million for a single-room facility to more than $125 million for a multiroom/gantry facility. The annual cost for electricity can vary from $50,000 to more than $200,000; maintenance may range from $1.7 million to $5 million. Carbon ion facilities, estimated to cost $250 million to $300 million, are a magnitude of expense greater than proton beam centers. These large multiroom/gantry facilities can require more than 100 full-time employees for staffing and maintenance.

Cuts in APC reimbursement of 30% and 16% year over year occurred from 2007 to 2009. This recent decline in compensation for the daily technical charge for PBT may force a reevaluation of centers ordered but not yet built. The 2009 APC rate for daily PBT resulted in a 16% decrease for both level I and level II proton therapy, with level I now being reimbursed at $703.38 per fraction and level II at $840.56 per fraction. These daily APC rates may actually increase as the newer centers, whose cost structure is higher than that of the facilities now in operation, come on line. It should be noted that when the first carbon ion projects come on line in the United States, they will have to obtain reimbursement de novo for carbon beam treatment, although the business models for these facilities include the concurrent use of protons in the projects' early stages to fund operations while awaiting reimbursement for the heavy ion.

## COST EFFECTIVENESS OF PROTON BEAM THERAPY

Because of the high costs associated with PBT, economic analyses should be performed alongside clinical trials of PBT. A well-done analysis of cost effectiveness compares the costs and outcomes of one treatment to the costs and outcomes of another (standard or otherwise). To date, all published cost-effectiveness analyses of PBT have compared PBT to photon beam therapy or brachytherapy.

Europe has provided the majority of the PBT economic analyses. Lundkvist et al[21,22] published an economic analysis of PBT compared with conventional therapy in the treatment of left-sided breast cancer, prostate cancer, head and neck cancer, and medulloblastoma. A Markov model was used to perform the analysis, and a societal perspective was used in estimating costs. Cost savings were realized for patients with medulloblastoma who were treated with PBT rather than with conventional radiation. Patients with a high risk of cardiac disease and left-sided breast cancer that were treated with PBT had an incremental cost-effectiveness ratio (ICER) of 34290 Euro/quality-adjusted life year (QALY) compared with those treated with conventional radiation. In addition, patients with prostate cancer had an ICER of 26776 Euro/QALY compared with those treated with conventional

radiation; patients with head and neck cancer had an ICER of 3811 Euro/QALY. The authors made a number of assumptions to inform the model, including a 20% reduction in cancer recurrence and in cancer mortality in patients with prostate cancer treated with PBT. At the current time, there are no data to support these 2 assumptions. In addition, a mortality risk reduction of 24% was assumed for patients with head and neck cancer treated with PBT. Sensitivity analysis found an ICER of 66608 Euro/QALY when an average breast cancer patient was treated, and an ICER of 105474 Euro/QALY when only a 50% reduction in cardiac events was used instead of the 76%. PBT was superior to conventional radiation in patients with medulloblastoma in all variables tested.

Konski et al[23] compared PBT with IMRT in the treatment of a man with intermediate-risk prostate cancer. Given the cost difference between the 2 modalities, it was assumed that to achieve a benefit of PBT, 91 Gy would need to be given to achieve a 10% improvement in freedom from biochemical failure. The ICER at 15 years for PBT compared with IMRT was $63,578/QALY, with only a 54% probability of cost effectiveness. It must be pointed out that no PBT cohort has successfully been treated to 91 Gy to date.

Comparative effectiveness, a concept that attempts to provide insight into the benefits of new treatments, can be defined as the evaluation of multiple treatments for a single disease or condition to identify the best option.[24] Comparative effectiveness has existed in one form or another for approximately 20 years and was originally intended as a way to provide information that patients and families needed to make informed decisions.[25]

## CLINICAL TRIALS PRIOR TO ADOPTION OF NEW TECHNOLOGY

Stevens and Glatstein,[26] in an editorial entitled "Beware of the Medical-Industrial Complex," were the first to elucidate the seduction of adopting new technology in hopes of improved local control or cure rates. As healthcare expenditures have become an increasing portion of gross domestic product, healthcare providers have been increasingly pressured to prove the value of new technology introduced into clinical care. Some have argued that RCTs are not necessary before introducing a new technology.[20,27] Proponents of PBT point to its superior dosimetric properties compared with photon radiation but have offered no high-level data to support a clinically meaningful difference between the 2 treatments.

Dahl[28] expressed concern about the adaption of a PBT facility in Sweden, given the current literature. Analyzed critically, PBT was estimated to be suitable for only 15% of the irradiated Swedish cancer population. In addition, Halperin and other radiation oncologists favor randomized prospective trials of innovative radiation therapy technology.[29] Halperin, for example, cautions about the objectivity of all parties involved in adoption of new technology—from machine manufacturers needing to improve shareholder value, to physicians concerned about their academic reputation in promoting new technology, to hospitals needing to recoup investments in the new technology. Emanuel et al[30] point out that "an intervention's value resides in its ability to reduce mortality, morbidity, or save money, not in its unique mechanism of action." Unfortunately, no data demonstrating any particle therapy's ability to reduce mortality or morbidity or to save money currently exist.

## CONCLUSION

The path that emerging technologies, such as PBT, take to incorporation in the U.S. healthcare delivery system is a product of the social, economic, and political milieu. For example, payment practices for emerging technologies have modulated health policy and have moderated market diffusion. However, given the current environment of dramatically rising healthcare costs and the growing numbers of persons lacking healthcare insurance, U.S. health policy makers have begun to embrace policies aimed at improving healthcare value while addressing cost, including cost-effectiveness and comparative effectiveness analysis. In this milieu, the effectiveness of PBT and other emerging, expensive medical technology can only be determined after substantial capital has been invested for facility development and significant ongoing operating revenue is made available for the clinical activity needed to evaluate treatment efficacy. Policies going forward will need to address the economic realities of healthcare delivery in the United States. To do this, these policies must embrace the use of evidence-based assessment of technology to ensure the solvency of the system and must find ways to pay for the development and clinical testing of new and emerging medical advancements.

## REFERENCES

1. Davis K. Slowing the growth of health care costs—learning from international experience. *N Engl J Med.* 2008;359:1751–1755.
2. Neumann PJ, Kamae MS, Palmer JA. Medicare's national coverage decisions for technology, 1999–2007. *Health Aff.* 2008;27:1620–1631.
3. Deyo RA, Patrick DL. *Hope of Hype.* New York: AMACOM Press; 2005.
4. Steinberg ML. Health policy and healthcare economics observed. *Semin Radiat Oncol.* 2008;18:149–151.
5. Steinbrook R. Saying No isn't NICE—travails of Britain's National Institute for Health and Clinical Excellence. *N Engl J Med.* 2008;359:1977–1981.
6. Tunis S. Medicare Coverage of New Technology. PowerPoint presentation. September 3, 2003.
7. Tunis S. Testimony to Medicare Evidence Development & Coverage Advisory Committee. April 30, 2008.
8. Staube B. Testimony to Medicare Evidence Development & Coverage Advisory Committee. April 30, 2008.
9. American Medical Association. CPT Process—How a Code Becomes a Code. Available at: http://www.ama-assn.org/ama/no-index/physician-resources/3882.shtml. Accessed March 31, 2009.
10. Glimelius B, Ask A, Bjelkengren G, et al. Number of patients potentially eligible for proton therapy. *Acta Oncol.* 2005;44:836–849.
11. Loma Linda University Medical Center. Welcome to Proton Therapy! Available at: http://www.protons.com/proton-therapy. Accessed March 31, 2009.
12. Nguyen PL, Trofimov A, Zietman AL. Proton-beam vs. intensity-modulated radiation therapy: which is best for treating prostate cancer? *Oncology (Williston Park).* 2008;22:748–754.
13. Olsen DR, Bruland OS, Fryholm G, et al. Proton therapy—a systematic review of clinical effectiveness. *Radiother Oncol.* 2007;83:123–132.
14. Institute for Clinical and Economic Review. *Brachytherapy & Proton Beam Therapy for Treatment of Clinically-Localized, Low-Risk Prostate Cancer.* Final appraisal document. December 22, 2008.
15. Brada M, Pijls-Johannesma M. Proton therapy in clinical practice. *J Clin Oncol.* 2007;25:965–970.
16. Pljls-Johannesma M. Cost-effectiveness of particle therapy: current evidence and future needs. *Radiother Oncol.* 2008;89:127–134.
17. Freedman, B. Equipoise and the ethics of clinical research. *N Engl J Med.* 1987;317:141–145.
18. Goitein M, Cox JD. Should randomized clinical trials be required in proton therapy? *J Clin Oncol.* 2008;26:175–176.
19. Tepper J. Protons and Parachutes. *J Clin Oncol.* 2008;26:2436–2437.
20. Suit H, Kooy H, Trofimov A, et al. Should positive phase III clinical trials be required before proton therapy is more widely adopted? *Radiother Oncol.* 2008;86:148–153.
21. Lundkvist J, Ekman M, Ericsson, SR, et al. Proton therapy of cancer: Potential clinical advantages and cost-effectiveness. *Acta Oncol.* 2005;44:850–861.
22. Lundkvist J, Ekman M, Ericsson SR, et al. Economic evaluation of proton radiation therapy in the treatment of breast cancer. *Radiother Oncol.* 2005;75:179–185.
23. Konski A, Speier W, Hanlon A, et al. Is proton therapy cost-effective in the treatment of adenocarcinoma of the prostate? *J Clin Oncol.* 2007;25:3603–3608.
24. Medicare's coverage with evidence development: a policy-making tool in evolution. *J Oncol Prac.* 2007;3:296–301.
25. Comparative effectiveness: Its origin, evolution, and influence on health care. *J Oncol Prac.* 2009;2:80–82.
26. Stevens CW, Glatstein E. Beware the medial-industrial complex. *Oncologist.* 1996;1:IV–V.
27. Bentzen SM. Randomized controlled trials in health technology assessment: overkill or overdue? *Radiother Oncol.* 2008;86:142–147.
28. Dahl O. Protons: a step forward or perhaps only more expensive radiation therapy? *Acta Oncol.* 2005;44:798–800.
29. Halperin EC. Randomized prospective trials of innovative radiotherapy technology are necessary. *J Am Coll Radiol.* 2009;6:33–37.
30. Emanuel EJ, Fuchs VR, Garber AM. Essential elements of a technology and outcomes assessment initiative. *JAMA.* 2007;298:1323–1325.

CHAPTER

# 46

# Monitoring of Therapeutic Response to Cancer Treatment

Tito Fojo

I still remember that December day 10 years ago when I asked my colleague Michael Bishop what had thrilled him most about the recent American Society of Hematology meeting. The imatinib presentation by Brian Druker in chronic myeloid leukemia, he replied. This was more than a home run, he added, it was a grand slam. Not long after that I found myself in Marbella in Southern Spain at the European Spring Oncology Conference-1 meeting organized by Bruce Chabner and Hernán Cortés-Funes where emerging therapies were the focus. The most exciting presentation was given by Jean Pierre Armand, as experienced a clinical researcher as there is. He had been as excited as Brian Druker had been when his first patient was treated with imatinib. Jean Pierre had been given the opportunity to work with a drug called sunitinib, the ugly duckling of the Sugen armamentarium, and he had observed dramatic responses in patients with renal cell carcinoma. His seminal observations with sunitinib in renal cell carcinoma would eventually be confirmed by an international consortium and lead to regulatory approval. Yes, there were a few problems with hypertension and even life-threatening hemorrhage, but he was confident this would be resolved, and he was confident that this was a very good drug for renal cell carcinoma.

I relate these 2 observations because as I read and thought about the excellent submissions that comprise this special issue of *The Cancer Journal*, I could not help but think that more than 30 years after a group of doctors treating lymphoma gathered to agree on a method for reporting responses, we are still arguing about the best way to make these assessments. Why is this? The simple answer may lie in the fact that cancer is complex, treatment has made it even more complex, and not all cancers behave in the same way. Other answers lie in the difficulty assessing end points such as progression-free survival (PFS) and response rate and of course those pesky statisticians who are continually more and more demanding. However, the real answer—a sad fact of cancer therapy—is that, our therapies have been and continue to be incremental and increasingly that increment is all too often smaller and smaller. After all why else would we want to count stable disease as a measure of anything when it lasts for 6 weeks?, or why would we argue that a PFS of 1 or 2 months, lost

in the overall survival (OS) analysis, should be considered a measure of drug efficacy? Were our therapies curative or paradigm changing as imatinib and sunitinib were, the majority of what we discuss here would be irrelevant. Brian Druker did not need to wait years to publish the long-term follow-up of imatinib-treated patients to know that imatinib was effective. He actually knew it after he had treated his first patient. In addition, Jean Pierre Armand knew that spring in 2000, long before the randomized trail that led to sunitinib's approval was designed that this was an active drug in renal cell carcinoma. So too did those treating lung cancer come to realize that a subset of patients receiving gefitinib or erlotinib were experiencing "significant benefit" even though they lacked a *P* value or hazard ratio to support their intuition.

So that while the challenge is to find more drugs that make us look as intuitive as Brian and Jean Pierre, the reality is that progress in the therapy for cancer remains incremental, and all the articles in this issue are thus extremely important. They are important to the clinical researcher who must identify active drugs early and invest their energies in the most promising. They are important to the pharmaceutical companies that now dominate drug development who must decide where to invest their often-limited resources and what endpoints to choose in the hopes of regulatory approval. They are important to the agencies that bless our efforts, which must agree that what we have measured as an effective end point is of value. Additionally, above all, they are important to our patients who should participate in trials that will hopefully lead to more effective and better-tolerated therapies.

The articles in this issue have been contributed by an excellent group of international investigators with diverse backgrounds who bring to these issues different perspectives. The pros and cons for response rate, stable disease, PFS and OS are both balanced and forceful. Admittedly, proponents are easier to find and hold stronger feelings. However, the opposing views teach us that an argument should not be judged by the decibels of its supporters. In the discussion of biomarkers and meta-analyses, the authors have presented very credible and balanced viewpoints in 1 article, and this should be valuable to both the novice and the seasoned investigator. "Other paradigms" present promising strategies to improve our research enterprise and are written by very knowledgeable and reasoned contributors who have thought about these problems with an eye to improving outcomes. The hope is that the newcomer will read these contributions and help move the field forward, whereas the experienced investigator will find useful information that challenges a long-held bias and stimulates thinking. In the end, we all hope for the day when OS, the gold standard, is replaced by an even higher standard—cures.

Thank you to all my colleagues for their hard work and spirited presentations.

# Tumor Shrinkage and Objective Response Rates

## Gold Standard for Oncology Efficacy Screening Trials, or an Outdated End Point?

Penelope Bradbury • Lesley Seymour

With greater understanding of the molecular aberrations underlying cancer, there has been a rapid expansion in the number of drugs entering clinical evaluation. In 2005, it was estimated that while almost 2000 drugs were in development,[1] only 8% of drugs ultimately receive regulatory approval. The phase III clinical trial is responsible for over two-thirds of the total cost of the clinical assessment of a new therapy,[2] however, only 40% to 50% of phase III trials are positive.[3] Failure at the phase III stage has enormous implications, for patients who may have received an ineffective treatment, and for financial and patient resources, which are consumed from an already constrained research environment. It is not surprising that decisions made regarding, which agents or combinations of agents to select for phase III trials (go, no-go decisions) have been criticized in many instances.[4]

Traditionally, for a new cytotoxic agent, a single arm phase II trial was used to ascertain whether the agent produced tumor shrinkage in a sufficiently high number of patients to result in survival benefit.[5] Further, randomized designs, when used (for example, to evaluate the addition of a new drug to standard therapies) usually had objective response rate (RR) as the primary end point.

Although this strategy was largely successful for cytotoxic agents, newer molecularly targeted agents were often noted to result in slowing of tumor growth rather than tumor shrinkage in preclinical studies and were hypothesized to be unlikely to result in tumor shrinkage in the clinic. In some instances, phase II studies of such agents were not planned.[6-8] In other instances, data from the phase II setting were used to justify phase III trials, which failed.[9-11] Criticism of the designs of recent development plans for new agents has focused on 3 main areas: phase II end points [response versus progression free survival (PFS)], assessment of response [response evaluation criteria in solid tumor (RECIST) versus functional imaging], and phase II design (single arm versus randomized design, adaptive designs). In this review, we focus on objective response as an end point, as well as the assessment of response.

## OBJECTIVE RESPONSE

### WHO and RECIST Criteria

Although "response" has long been a clinical end point for any cancer therapy, investigators soon realized that the utility of RRs is reliant on a standardized and robust mechanism of measuring and defining response. The first internationally accepted criteria for assessing response was established by the World Health Organization (WHO) in the 1980s, as part of an initiative to standardize reporting across cancer clinical trials.[12] Response was categorized into complete response (CR), partial response (PR), stable disease (SD), or progressive disease (PD). Boundaries to define PR and PD were arbitrarily set at a ≥50% decrease (PR) and a ≥25% increase (progression) in the sum of the product of the bidimensional measurements of all lesions, respectively (Table 1). The objective RR used as an end point in clinical trials is defined as the sum of the number of CRs and PRs. The definitions for a CR, PR, or PD were influenced by the margins that would minimize inaccurate response assessment through measurement error, rather than on biologic significance. These criteria, although significantly increasing the interpretability of clinical trial results from different groups and investigators, were associated with some difficulties, for eg, in the interpretation of small lesions (a 25% increase in disease, which has shrunk to near normal limits may not be clinically significant). A number of cooperative groups developed their own refinements of the WHO response criteria, leading again to difficulty in interpretation.[13,14] Other issues included the difficulty in reproducibly measuring lesion bidimensionally.

These and other issues led to the development of the RECIST guidelines.[15] The RECIST criteria were modeled from the WHO criteria, but required unidimensional measurements only, and the boundaries for PR and PD were adjusted to a ≥30% reduction and a ≥20% increase, respectively (Table 1). Volumetrically, this adjustment had a greater impact on the definition of PD, from a 40% increase in the disease volume using the WHO definition of PD, to a 73% increase using the RECIST definition of PD. For example, a lung metastasis that is 1 cm in diameter an assumed to be spherical, the WHO criteria defines progression as a 25% increase in the product of 2 perpendicular diameters. This equates to an increase in diameter from 1 cm to ≈1.12 cm ($1.12 \times 1.12 \approx 1.25$). The volume of this spherical tumor would have increased from 0.52 cm$^3$ to 0.74 cm$^3$ or ≈44%. By comparison using the RECIST criteria, an increase in the diameter of the spherical lesion to 1.2 cm would be classed as progressive disease, which equates to a volume of 0.90 cm$^3$ or a 73% increase in volume. Coming at the time of the introduction of targeted therapies, the change incorporated in RECIST (20% in one dimension versus the WHO guideline of 25% increase in the sum of 2 perpendicular diameters) has allowed for a much greater volumetric increase before disease is scored as progressive disease.

The guidelines have recently undergone a minor revision and further major revisions are planned.[16]

### Response Rate as an End Point

The primary purpose of a phase II clinical trial is to provide sufficient information on the efficacy of a new therapy to determine whether further evaluation is warranted. Traditionally, phase II trials have been considered as screening tests rather than definitive assessments of efficacy, although occasionally initial regulatory approval has been granted based on data from larger phase II studies (either single arm or randomized).[17-20] The most efficient design would require a small number of patients and yield results quickly, although providing robust data sufficient to support decision making.

**TABLE 1.** Comparison of WHO Response Evaluation Criteria in Solid Tumors (RECIST) 1.0 and RECIST 1.1

|  | WHO | RECIST 1.0 | RECIST 1.1 |
|---|---|---|---|
| Measurement criteria |  |  |  |
|   Measurement criteria | Sum of product of bidimensional measurements | Sum of unidimensional measurements | Sum of unidimensional measurements |
|   Number of lesions | All lesions | Maximum of 10 lesions, 5 per organ | Maximum of 5 lesions, 2 per organ |
| Response definitions |  |  |  |
|   Complete response | Complete resolution of all clinical and radiologic disease | Complete resolution of all radiologic, clinical and biochemical evidence of disease | Complete resolution of all radiologic, clinical and biochemical evidence of disease |
|   Partial response | ≥50% reduction of sum of products | ≥30% reduction of sum of unidimensional measurements | ≥30% reduction of sum of unidimensional measurements |
|   Stable disease | <50% reduction or <25% increase of sum of products | <30% reduction or <20% increase of unidimensional measurements | <30% reduction or <20% increase of unidimensional measurements |
|   Progressive disease | ≥25% increase of sum of product | ≥20% increase of sum of unidimensional measurements | ≥20% increase of sum of unidimensional measurements |

For cytotoxic agents, this has, albeit with some limitations, been achieved using RR as an end point. Trials have been powered to detect a RR in the order of 20%, adjusted for the disease type and setting (for example, a RR of 20% may be "of interest" for a new agent for breast cancer, whereas lower RRs may be of interest for tumor types with no effective therapies, such as melanoma). Certainly, in some tumor types, for cytotoxic agents, RR seems to be a validated surrogate of real clinical benefit,[21–23] although not in all malignancies.[24]

There are 3 limitations to RR as an end point. First, not all malignant lesions are easily measurable[25–27]; second, not all clinically efficacious therapies lead to significant tumor regression as measured by computed tomography (CT) or magnetic resonance imaging (MRI) scans[27,28]; and third, RR does not evaluate the duration, or "quality" of response.

## Measurability

Mesothelioma is a malignancy, which arises from the mesothelial cells of serosal membranes.[29] In the chest, mesothelioma progresses by forming a rind of tissue around the pleura with ill-defined margins, therefore, measurement of the longest dimension is virtually impossible. Although investigators have proposed modified criteria for mesothelioma in which the short axis of the lesion perpendicular to the chest or mediastinum is measured at 3 sites, initiatives such as this are unvalidated.[25] The assessment of response in mesothelioma continues to be a challenge. Similar difficulties have been described in the measurement of soft tissue sarcomas,[27] prostate cancer[26] and gliomas.[30]

Another consideration is inter and intra measurement variability, which can be substantial. In a study to evaluate the variability of measurements of non–small cell lung cancer (NSCLC) CT images read by thoracic radiologists, the interobserver measurement change ranged from 0% to 194%, corresponding to an average of 11.9 misclassifications/reader pair for unidimensional measurements.[31] The need to account for measurement error not only influenced the definitions of PR or PD in the WHO response guidelines but also is one reason that response guidelines have required that response is confirmed in nonrandomized studies with RR as a primary end point. This increases the cost and workload of a clinical trial, and imposes an additional burden on patients, and however, the necessity of this approach is unclear. Perez-Gracia et al[32] evaluated the correlation between a single assessment of response and the confirmed response assessment method and found the degree of correlation to be high

(Kappa coefficient 0.89). The authors suggested that a single determination may be sufficient. However, it is argued that if objective RR is the primary end point in a small phase II trial, even minor discrepancies may impact on the conclusions of that study, with implications regarding the future development of the drug.[33] The requirement for response to be confirmed in nonrandomized trials with RR as the primary end point has been retained in the current version of the RECIST guidelines.

## Residual or Unchanged Disease

The measurement of lymph nodes poses additional challenges. Normal physiologic lymph nodes can range in size from 6 mm to 12 mm across different nodal stations, and not all lymph nodes can be visualized on CT imaging.[34] Further, residual lymphadenopathy after treatment may not be reflective of active disease.[35] It is estimated between 30% and 60% of patients with non-Hodgkin or Hodgkin lymphoma may have residual disease after treatment, however, only a small proportion of these patients relapse.[36] In addition, CT imaging may underestimate the RR of other malignancies, for example, in the case of gastrointestinal stromal tumors (GIST) after therapy with imatinib, if lesions change in density rather than size during therapy.[27]

## Setting the Bar—Response Rates of "Interest"

Although it is hoped that data arising from a phase II trial will be predictive of a positive phase III trial, it is important that false negative results, which could inappropriately end the development of a potentially efficacious drug, be avoided (Table 2). This is highlighted with the experience of sorafenib for the treatment of renal cell carcinoma.[39] Sorafenib is a multitargeted receptor tyrosine kinase inhibitor (TKI) with antitumoral and antiangiogenic targets that include Raf and the vascular endothelial growth factor receptors 1–3. In a phase III, randomized, double blind placebo controlled study of sorafenib in patients with metastatic renal cell carcinoma, the RR in the sorafenib arm at the time of the first interim analysis was 2% [with a PR rate of 10% at time of the overall survival (OS) analysis]. However, this corresponded to an improvement in PFS from 2.8 months in the control arm to 5.5 months in the sorafenib arm.[39]

Interestingly, the phase II trial of sorafenib did not use RR as the primary end point,[40] because clinical benefit was hypothesized to arise from disease stabilization. Instead, the phase II clinical trial used a randomized discontinuation design in which all patients initially received sorafenib for a 12-week period, after which patients with

**TABLE 2.** Examples of the Response Rate and Overall Survival of Single Agent Targeted Therapies in Solid Tumors

| Reference | Drug | Disease | Response Rate (%CR + PR Combined) | Median Overall Survival (mo) |
|---|---|---|---|---|
| Escudier et al.[39] | Sorafenib vs. placebo | Renal cell carcinoma | 2%* | PFS, 5.5 mo vs. 2.8 mo (HR 0.44, 0.35–0.55, $P < 0.01$)* |
| Llovet et al.[62] | Sorafenib vs. placebo | Hepatocellular carcinoma | 2% | 10.7 mo vs. 7.9 mo (HR 0.69, 95% CI 0.55–0.87, $P < 0.001$) |
| Motzer et al.[63] | Sunitinib vs. interferon-$\alpha$ | Renal cell carcinoma | 31% vs .6% | PFS, 11 mo vs. 5 mo (HR 0.42, 95% CI 0.32–0.54, $P < 0.001$) |
| Shepherd et al.[37] | Erlotinib vs. placebo | Non–small cell lung cancer | 8.9% | 6.7 mo vs. 4.7 mo (HR 0.70, 95% CI 0.58–0.85, $P < 0.001$) |
| Jonker et al.[38] | Cetuzimab vs. placebo | Metastatic colon cancer | 8% | 6.1 mo vs. 4.6 mo (HR 0.77, −0.64–0.92, $P = 0.005$) |

*At first interim analysis.

at least SD were randomized to continue sorafenib or placebo. The PR rate for patients with renal cell carcinoma was 4%, a level which by traditional standards would not have reached the bar for further evaluation.[40]

El-Maraghi and Eisenhauer[5] evaluated the association between phase II trials of targeted agents and ultimate regulatory approval. Although they reported an increase in RR correlated with a greater chance of regulatory approval, they also demonstrated that agents with no evidence of response did not go on to receive regulatory approval.[5] Although this observation may help to inform on the future development of some agents, the challenge of interpreting the efficacy of agents with a low RR persists. Lowering the RR of "interest" would avoid false negative results, but would inevitably require an increase in sample size, increase the risk of false positive results and failure at phase III evaluation, or yield a small improvement in outcome at phase III evaluation, which is of uncertain clinical benefit and low cost effectiveness. In addition, some malignancies (including renal cell carcinoma and melanoma) are associated with a low incidence of spontaneous remissions, which may compound the interpretation of the efficacy of an agent with a low RR.[41,42]

Given these limitations of RR as an end point, what are the potential solutions?

## ALTERNATIVE WAYS TO MEASURE, ANALYZE, AND REPORT RESPONSE

One potential solution is to refine the assessment of response by adopting alternative methods of response measurement by using emerging functional imaging techniques, or technology to enumerate circulating tumor cells (CTC), which have the potential to yield more rapid and sensitive assessment of disease efficacy (Table 3). Alternatively, in addition to evaluating the proportion of patients that respond to a therapy, clinical trial design could incorporate an analysis of the proportion of patients that have early PD, as illustrated by the multinomial stopping rule.

## Multinomial Evaluation of Response

Although it is important that phase II clinical trials are designed to have a low false negative rate (ie, wrongly concluding that a drug does not have efficacy worthy of further evaluation), it is also desirable to limit the number of patients that are exposed to a drug if it truly is ineffective. To address the latter concern, phase II clinical trials commonly use a multistage design (for example, as described by Fleming[43] or Gehan[44]) in which a small number of patients are enrolled in the first stage, after which the RR is evaluated, and the trial only proceeds to

enroll further patients in a second stage if a preset level of responses have been seen. However, as discussed the multistage design does not address agents that are predominantly cytostatic resulting in a low RR but high SD rate. This is addressed by the multinomial stopping rule, which uses both the objective RR and early progression rate within a 2-stage phase II design.[45] The inclusion of the early progression rate (for example, the number of patients with PD at or before an 8 week disease assessment time point), may reduce the risk of concluding the agent has no activity, when in fact the proportion of patients that have SD on therapy is high, and correspondingly the proportion of patients that progress early is low, which may indicate the agent has clinical efficacy worthy of further evaluation. The benefit of using the multinomial stopping rule compared with the Fleming or Gehan rules was investigated in a retrospective study of 16 National Cancer Institute of Canada (NCIC) Clinical Trials Group and 23 European Organization for Research and Treatment of Cancer Early Clinical Studies Group, phase II trials.[46] In this study, the outcome of applying the multinomial stopping rule, compared with using the Fleming or Gehan rule, demonstratd that the multinomial stopping rule would have appropriately signaled the discontinuation of 8 of the 39 studies at the first stage, that the actual rule (Fleming or Gehan rule) failed to stop. This rule has subsequently been incorporated into a number of clinical trials.[47,48]

## Response as a Continuous Variable

Tumor size is a continuous variable that is categorized in the WHO and RECIST criteria to simplify data handling and reporting and minimize the impact of measurement error. However, converting a continuous variable into a categorical variable reduces statistical power and assumes the categories have biologic significance, which may not always be valid. For example, SD defined by the RECIST criteria is a default category encompassing a 29% reduction in the size of a lesion, to a 19% increase. These extremes are likely to have a fundamentally different biologic significance.

The concept of assessing radiologic response as a continuous variable (commonly referred to as a waterfall plot, Fig. 1) was described almost 30 years ago,[49] but there has been renewed interest in this concept as a tool for evaluating the efficacy of cytostatic therapies.[40,50] It has also been postulated that analyzing response as a continuous variable would maximize statistical efficiency and reduce the number of patients required in a phase II trial.[50]

The impact of assessing response as a continuous variable was assessed by Dhani et al[51] in a retrospective study of 2 randomized controlled clinical trials conducted by the NCIC Clinical Trials

**TABLE 3.** Summary of the Advantages and Disadvantages of Phase II Trial End Points and Response Evaluation Techniques

| Endpoint/Method of Response Assessment | Advantages | Disadvantages | Validation |
|---|---|---|---|
| **Endpoint** | | | |
| Objective response rate | Proven to be technically feasible for multicentre trials. Readily available imaging equipment. Enables small sample size and timely completion of trial | Targeted agents may have a low response rate. Does not include stable disease, address change in density (eg, cavitation) or assess duration of response. Some malignancies difficult to measure. Some patients do not have measurable disease. Response may not correlate with improved outcome | Association with overall survival validated in some malignancies |
| Progression free survival/time to progression | Addresses stable disease and duration of response. Not confounded by salvage therapy | Requires larger sample size compared with ORR. Takes longer time to achieve end point. May not correlate with improved outcome. Subject to bias | Association with overall survival validated in some malignancies |
| Multinomial Endpoint | Includes assessment of stable disease. May have greater efficiency than objective response rate alone. May be of utility in diseases for which response is difficult to assess | Subjective assessment of appropriate rate of progression and response required. Excludes patients without measurable disease | Progressive disease rate validated with overall survival in some malignancies |
| **Method of response assessment** | | | |
| PET | Assesses functional change. May enable more rapid assessment of response. May have benefit in some malignancies difficult to assess by CT imaging | Limited availability of imaging equipment. Lack of standardized protocols. Expensive. More time consuming per scan. Not all lesions PET positive | Some evidence may be superior to CT but further validation required |
| Response as a continuous variable | May improve statistical efficiency and reduce sample size. Includes stable disease | Sensitive to measurement error. Methodology to account for CR or a new lesion arbitrary | Not validated |
| Change in volume of disease | Includes data in "z" dimension may enable better assessment of disease difficult to measure bidimensionally (eg, mesothelioma) | Time consuming semiautomated, requires some manual measurement with risk of measurement variability/error | Not validated as an end point in phase II clinical trials |
| Enumeration of CTC | May provide an early assessment of response/biomarker status. Assess patients with nonmeasurable disease | Optimum platform unknown/limited sensitivity. Lack of availability of equipment. Expensive/time consuming. No standardized definition of CTC | Not validated as an end point in phase II clinical trials |

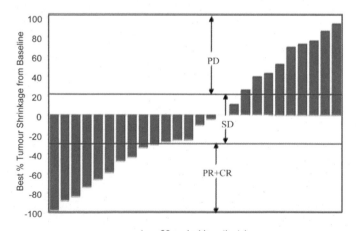

(n = 26 evaluable patients)

**FIGURE 1.** Simulated waterfall plot. In this simulated example, 10 patients have a tumor shrinkage of ≥30%; however, the waterfall plot depicts 5 patients who have at least disease stability. CR, complete response; PR, partial response; SD, stable disease; PD, progressive disease.

Group (CTG) and the North Central Clinical Treatment Group. The NCIC CTG Pancreas 1 (PA.1) trial randomized patients with advanced pancreatic cancer to a novel metalloproteinase inhibitor (BAY 12-9566) or single agent gemcitabine.[8,51] At the first interim analysis, the number of patients with PD (assessed using WHO criteria) was sufficiently low to allow the trial to continue, however, at the second interim analysis the study was terminated because of inferior outcome of patients randomized to the experimental BAY 12-9566 arm. In a retrospective analysis, the association between measurement of radiologic response on a continuous scale (using the methodology described by Karrison et al)[50] and clinical outcome was evaluated. In this methodology, the logarithm of the sum of the longest dimension of the lesions at baseline and at a specified time point eg, 8 weeks is collected, and the difference between these measurements is calculated for each patient. The mean of these measurements is taken for the patient cohort of interest and evaluated against that of a comparator group by means of simple statistical test.[50] Dhani et al demonstrated that there was a statistically significant difference in tumor size between the BAY-12-9566 arm (log difference between baseline and 8 weeks 0.087) and gemcitabine (log difference −0.066), $P < 0.0001$), in line with the final OS results. If used the trial would have stopped appropriately at the 1st decision point.[51]

## Assessment of Tumor Volumes

Neither the WHO nor the RECIST criteria include axial measurements, which may be important for the measurement of tumors that are not spherical. Thin section CT enables the reconstruction of the volume of disease, and this approach has become of interest in the evaluation of NSCLC or mesothelioma. In a study by Zhao et al,[52] unidimensional and bidimensional measurements were compared with a semiautomated technique of tumor volume assessment in 15 patients with NSCLC. They reported 1/15 patients had a ≥20% change in unidimensional measurements compared with 4/15 for bidimensional measurements and 11/15 when tumor volumes were assessed. Similar techniques are being evaluated in mesothelioma with CT or MRI imaging.[53] However, this technique is time consuming and requires validation to determine whether tumor volumes provide a better predictor of response than the less cumbersome conventional imaging techniques.

## Assessment of Tumor Density

Central cavitation of lesions is associated with antiangiogenic agents. This may arise from the inhibition of new vessel formation resulting in central necrosis. Although the clinical impression may be one of a reduction in the burden of viable cells, consistent with an effective therapy, response as assessed with RECIST criteria may be SD.

Crabb et al[54] reviewed an alternate method for assessing tumor response in the setting of central necrosis (Fig. 2). In short, the unidimensional measurement of the central necrosis is subtracted from the unidimensional measurement of entire length of the lesion. PD was defined as a refilling of the central area of necrosis. In a retrospective study of 33 patients treated with a combination chemotherapy and cediranib, a novel VEGR TKI,[54,55] cavitation was noted in 24% of cases but not in any control cases drawn from a clinical trial, which evaluated the same chemotherapy regimen but without cediranib (NCIC CTG BR.18).[56] Using this methodology, the best response changed from SD to a confirmed PR in one case and an unconfirmed PR in a second case. The duration of response assessed by RECIST versus the alternate method of assessment was also found to differ in some cases.[54]

A change in tumor density without an apparent change in tumor size has also been recognized in patients with GIST during therapy with imatinib, which has led to the under-reporting of response when assessed by computerized tomography (CT), for which positron emission tomography (PET) seems superior.[27] However, not all GISTs are PET positive, and not all patients have access to PET imaging. Choi et al evaluated an alternative CT based response criteria, classifying a response as ≥10% change in the longest dimension of the lesions or a ≥15% reduction in the density of the lesion by CT in Hounsfield Units, at 8 weeks compared with baseline. In a study of 40 patients with metastatic GIST who underwent both PET and CT imaging, 17 of the patients were classified as responders (best response at any time point) by RECIST. However, response by RECIST did not correlate to a statistcically significant difference in time to progression compared with the 23 patients that did not respond by RECIST ($P = 0.35$). However, when the response was defined by PET or the modified CT criteria (≥10% reduction in the size of the longest dimension of the target lesions or a ≥15% reduction in the density of the lesions by CT), the number of responders was higher using both methods [33 for fluorodcoxyglucose (FDG) PET and 32 for CT], and responders were associated with a statistically significant improvement in time to progression compared with the nonresponders ($P = 0.01$ for PET and $P = 0.04$ for modified CT). This modification of RECIST may increase the sensitivity of the assessment of the efficacy of a therapy; however, this approach is experimental and requites validation.

**RECIST**

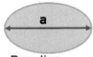

Baseline

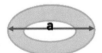

First response assessment
a=Stable disease

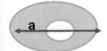

Second response assessment
a=Stable disease

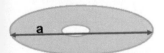

Third response assessment
a=Progressive disease

**Alternate response evaluation method**

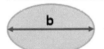

Baseline

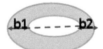

First response assessment
b1+b2 = Partial response

Second response assessment
b1+b2 = progressive  disease

Left panel RECIST measurement. Lesion forms a cavity suggestive of anti-tumour activity, but is classified as stable disease by RECIST.

Right panel alternative response evaluation.

Necrotic centre is not included in measurement resulting in classification of a partial response at first assessment. Subsequent "in filling" of  necrotic centre at second assessment is consequently classified as progressive disease

**FIGURE 2.** Diagram to illustrate an alternate to assess tumor response of lesions with central cavitation. Left Panel to illustrate the response assessment of a lesion that cavitates during therapy using the standard Response Evaluation Criteria in Solid Tumors (RECIST) and right panel to illustrate an alternative method as described by Crabb et al.[54]

## Functional and Molecular Imaging

Functional imaging (the measurement of physiologic events within a lesion) and molecular imaging (the measure of intratumoral molecular events) differ from CT or MRI because they yield information regarding the metabolic, and not anatomic, change within a tumor. This may provide a solution to the disadvantages of anatomic imaging already discussed and enable a more rapid assessment of response to therapy, as it is postulated that metabolic changes may precede morphologic change.

This field is rapidly advancing, with multiple imaging techniques and molecular imaging probes under evaluation (reviewed in Ref. 57). The most advanced platforms are PET with [18]F-FDG tracer, and dynamic contrast enhanced MRI. FDG PET exploits the high-glucose uptake that occurs within metabolically active tumors relative to normal tissue. A decline, in tracer uptake or standardized uptake value may reflect a decrease in viable tumor cells. FDG PET has an established role in the staging of several malignancies and an emerging role in the assessment of response to cytotoxic and targeted therapy.[57] FDG-PET has played an important role in the assessment of GIST to the TKI imatinib,[27] and there is emerging data that PET may also have a role in the assessment of other targeted agents including antiangiogenic agents and epidermal growth factor receptor pathway inhibitors.[57]

Although there are potential significant advantages to these imaging techniques compared with anatomic imaging, there is a need to standardize protocols and ensure reproducibility of results across centers before it can play a more prominent role in clinical trials. For example, change in standardized uptake value is sensitive to patient characteristics (glucose level, fasting state, and change in body weight), machines and technical aspects (dose of tracer, time from injection to scan, and scanner), and need for a standardized reporting guideline. The European Organization for Research and Treatment of Cancer and National Institute Health have strived to move forward with these challenges,[58] however, as noted in the updated RECIST guideline, research needs to progress in this area before functional or molecular imaging can be incorporated into the future RECIST criteria.[16]

## Circulating Tumor Cells and Nucleic Acids

Patients without measurable disease are currently excluded from clinical trials with RR as the primary end point. Technology now allows for the serial enumeration of CTC, which may enable the assessment of response to therapy in patients without radiologically evaluable diseases.[59–61] In a study of 46 patients with nonmeasurable metastatic breast cancer before starting a new therapy, the CTC count at first follow-up was found to correlate with OS and PFS.[62] In addition, in a cohort of patients with prostate cancer, the CTC count was found to predict OS better than decrement in prostate-specific antigen.[61] It is also possible to identify the expression of biomarkers within CTCs, which may predict for response to therapy, or emerging acquired resistance during treatment.[63] This may enable the prediction of resistance to therapy before anatomic evidence of relapse. However, the most robust platform for the enumeration of CTCs has yet to be determined, and there is no consensus definition for a CTC, so this remains an exploratory method of assessing treatment efficacy.

## CONCLUSIONS

RR, as assessed by standard criteria such as RECIST, remains the most commonly used end point in phase II clinical trials, despite concerns that some newer agents may result in a survival advantage in spite of a low RR. Although some of these concerns can be overcome to some extent by incorporating additional information, such as SD or functional imaging into the evaluation, these methods are as yet not fully validated. Larger phase II trials, randomizing patients between different therapies, doses or schedules, especially those incorporating other end point such as PFS, overcome many of these issues, but cannot always take the place of smaller single arm screening trials, especially for rare tumor types, or in selected patient populations such as pediatric patients.

Although response remains one of the standard validated end points of phase II trials, it seems appropriate to consider the further refinement of classic response criteria, such as RECIST, to include emerging technologies as they become validated.

## REFERENCES

1. Parmar MK, Barthel FM, Sydes M, et al. Speeding up the evaluation of new agents in cancer. *J Natl Cancer Inst.* 2008;100:1204–1214.
2. DiMasi JA, Hansen RW, Grabowski HG. The price of innovation: new estimates of drug development costs. *J Health Econ.* 2003;22:151–185.
3. Kola I, Landis J. Can the pharmaceutical industry reduce attrition rates? *Nat Rev Drug Discov.* 2004;3:711–715.
4. Ratain MJ. Phase II oncology trials: let's be positive. *Clin Cancer Res.* 2005;11:5661–5662.
5. El-Maraghi RH, Eisenhauer EA. Review of phase II trial designs used in studies of molecular targeted agents: outcomes and predictors of success in phase III. *J Clin Oncol.* 2008;26:1346–1354.
6. Giaccone G. The role of gefitinib in lung cancer treatment. *Clin Cancer Res.* 2004;10:4233s–4237s.
7. Herbst RS, Giaccone G, Schiller JH, et al. Gefitinib in combination with paclitaxel and carboplatin in advanced non-small-cell lung cancer: a phase III trial—INTACT 2. *J Clin Oncol.* 2004;22:785–794.
8. Moore MJ, Hamm J, Dancey J, et al. Comparison of gemcitabine versus the matrix metalloproteinase inhibitor BAY 12–9566 in patients with advanced or metastatic adenocarcinoma of the pancreas: a phase III trial of the National Cancer Institute of Canada Clinical Trials Group. *J Clin Oncol.* 2003;21:3296–3302.
9. Kindler HL, Niedzwiecki D, Hollis D, et al. A double-blind, placebo-controlled, randomized phase III trial of gemcitabine plus bevacizumab versus gemcitabine plus placebo in patients with advanced pancreatic cancer: a preliminary analysis of Cancer and Leukemia Group B (CALGB) 80303. Presented at ASCO Gastrointestinal Cancers Symposium, Orlando, FL. 2007: Abstract 108.
10. Philip PA, Benedetti J, Fenoglio-Preiser C, et al. Phase III study of gemcitabine [G] plus cetuximab [C] versus gemcitabine in patients [pts] with locally advanced or metastatic pancreatic adenocarcinoma [PC]: SWOG S0205 study. *J Clin Oncol.* 2007;25:Abstract LBA4509.
11. Hirsh V, Boyer M, Rosel R, et al. Randomized phase III trial of paclitaxel/carboplatin with or without PF-3512676 as first line treatment of advanced non-small cell lung cancer (NSCLC). *J Clin Oncol.* 2008;26s:Abstract 8016.
12. Miller AB, Hoogstraten B, Staquet M, et al. Reporting results of cancer treatment. *Cancer.* 1981;47:207–214.
13. Green S, Weiss GR. Southwest Oncology Group standard response criteria, endpoint definitions and toxicity criteria. *Invest New Drugs.* 1992;10:239–253.
14. Oken MM, Creech RH, Tormey DC, et al. Toxicity and response criteria of the Eastern Cooperative Oncology Group. *Am J Clin Oncol.* 1982;5:649–655.
15. Therasse P, Arbuck SG, Eisenhauer EA, et al. New guidelines to evaluate the response to treatment in solid tumors. European Organization for Research and Treatment of Cancer, National Cancer Institute of the United States, National Cancer Institute of Canada. *J Natl Cancer Inst.* 2000;92:205–216.
16. Eisenhauer EA, Therasse P, Bogaerts J, et al. New response evaluation criteria in solid tumours: revised RECIST guideline (version 1.1). *Eur J Cancer.* 2009;45:228–247.
17. Kris MG, Natale RB, Herbst RS, et al. Efficacy of gefitinib, an inhibitor of the epidermal growth factor receptor tyrosine kinase, in symptomatic patients with non-small cell lung cancer: a randomized trial. *JAMA.* 2003;290:2149–2158.
18. Fukuoka M, Yano S, Giaccone G, et al. Multi-institutional randomized phase II trial of gefitinib for previously treated patients with advanced non-small-cell lung cancer (The IDEAL 1 Trial) [corrected]. *J Clin Oncol.* 2003;21:2237–2246.
19. Cohen MH, Williams G, Johnson JR, et al. Approval summary for imatinib mesylate capsules in the treatment of chronic myelogenous leukemia. *Clin Cancer Res.* 2002;8:935–942.
20. Dagher R, Johnson J, Williams G, et al. Accelerated approval of oncology products: a decade of experience. *J Natl Cancer Inst.* 2004;96:1500–1509.

21. Paesmans M, Sculier JP, Libert P, et al. Response to chemotherapy has predictive value for further survival of patients with advanced non-small cell lung cancer: 10 years experience of the European Lung Cancer Working Party. *Eur J Cancer.* 1997;33:2326–2332.

22. Buyse M, Thirion P, Carlson RW, et al. Relation between tumour response to first-line chemotherapy and survival in advanced colorectal cancer: a meta-analysis. Meta-Analysis Group in Cancer. *Lancet.* 2000;356:373–378.

23. Goffin J, Baral S, Tu D, et al. Objective responses in patients with malignant melanoma or renal cell cancer in early clinical studies do not predict regulatory approval. *Clin Cancer Res.* 2005;11:5928–5934.

24. Grothey A, Hedrick EE, Mass RD, et al. Response-independent survival benefit in metastatic colorectal cancer: a comparative analysis of N9741 and AVF2107. *J Clin Oncol.* 2008;26:183–189.

25. Byrne MJ, Nowak AK. Modified RECIST criteria for assessment of response in malignant pleural mesothelioma. *Ann Oncol.* 2004;15:257–260.

26. Scher HI, Morris MJ, Kelly WK, et al. Prostate cancer clinical trial end points: "RECIST"ing a step backwards. *Clin Cancer Res.* 2005;11:5223–5232.

27. Choi H, Charnsangavej C, Faria SC, et al. Correlation of computed tomography and positron emission tomography in patients with metastatic gastrointestinal stromal tumor treated at a single institution with imatinib mesylate: proposal of new computed tomography response criteria. *J Clin Oncol.* 2007;25:1753–1759.

28. Vos MJ, Berkhof J, Postma TJ, et al. Thallium-201 SPECT: the optimal prediction of response in glioma therapy. *Eur J Nucl Med Mol Imaging.* 2006;33:222–227.

29. Jeong YJ, Kim S, Kwak SW, et al. Neoplastic and nonneoplastic conditions of serosal membrane origin: CT findings. *Radiographics.* 2008;28:801–817; discussion 817–808; quiz 912.

30. Vos MJ, Uitdehaag BM, Barkhof F, et al. Interobserver variability in the radiological assessment of response to chemotherapy in glioma. *Neurology.* 2003;60:826–830.

31. Erasmus JJ, Gladish GW, Broemeling L, et al. Interobserver and intraobserver variability in measurement of non-small-cell carcinoma lung lesions: implications for assessment of tumor response. *J Clin Oncol.* 2003;21:2574–2582.

32. Perez-Gracia JL, Munoz M, Williams G, et al. Assessment of the value of confirming responses in clinical trials in oncology. *Eur J Cancer.* 2005;41:1528–1532.

33. Therasse P, Eisenhauer E. Confirmation of response in cancer clinical trials: a meaningless exercise? *Eur J Cancer.* 2005;41:1501–1502.

34. Hampson FA, Shaw AS. Response assessment in lymphoma. *Clin Radiol.* 2008;63:125–135.

35. Cheson BD, Pfistner B, Juweid ME, et al. Revised response criteria for malignant lymphoma. *J Clin Oncol.* 2007;25:579–586.

36. Spaepen K, Stroobants S, Dupont P, et al. Prognostic value of positron emission tomography (PET) with fluorine-18 fluorodeoxyglucose ([18F]FDG) after first-line chemotherapy in non-Hodgkin's lymphoma: is [18F]FDG-PET a valid alternative to conventional diagnostic methods? *J Clin Oncol.* 2001;19:414–419.

37. Shepherd FA, Rodrigues Pereira J, Ciuleanu T, et al. Erlotinib in previously treated non-small-cell lung cancer. *N Engl J Med.* 2005;353:123–132.

38. Jonker DJ, O'Callaghan CJ, Karapetis CS, et al. Cetuximab for the treatment of colorectal cancer. *N Engl J Med.* 2007;357:2040–2048.

39. Escudier B, Eisen T, Stadler WM, et al. Sorafenib in advanced clear-cell renal-cell carcinoma. *N Engl J Med.* 2007;356:125–134.

40. Ratain MJ, Eisen T, Stadler WM, et al. Phase II placebo-controlled randomized discontinuation trial of sorafenib in patients with metastatic renal cell carcinoma. *J Clin Oncol.* 2006;24:2505–2512.

41. Kalialis LV, Drzewiecki KT, Mohammadi M, et al. Spontaneous regression of metastases from malignant melanoma: a case report. *Melanoma Res.* 2008;18:279–283.

42. Lekanidi K, Vlachou PA, Morgan B, et al. Spontaneous regression of metastatic renal cell carcinoma: case report. *J Med Case Reports.* 2007;1:89.

43. Fleming TR. One-sample multiple testing procedure for phase II clinical trials. *Biometrics.* 1982;38:143–151.

44. Gehan EA. The determinatio of the number of patients required in a preliminary and a follow-up trial of a new chemotherapeutic agent. *J Chronic Dis.* 1961;13:346–353.

45. Zee B, Melnychuk D, Dancey J, et al. Multinomial phase II cancer trials incorporating response and early progression. *J Biopharm Stat.* 1999;9:351–363.

46. Dent S, Zee B, Dancey J, et al. Application of a new multinomial phase II stopping rule using response and early progression. *J Clin Oncol.* 2001;19:785–791.

47. Chu QS, Forouzesh B, Syed S, et al. A phase II and pharmacological study of the matrix metalloproteinase inhibitor (MMPI) COL-3 in patients with advanced soft tissue sarcomas. *Invest New Drugs.* 2007;25:359–367.

48. Knox JJ, Gill S, Synold TW, et al. A phase II and pharmacokinetic study of SB-715992, in patients with metastatic hepatocellular carcinoma: a study of the National Cancer Institute of Canada Clinical Trials Group (NCIC CTG IND. 168). *Invest New Drugs.* 2008;26:265–272.

49. Lavin PT. An alternative model for the evaluation of antitumor activity. *Cancer Clin Trials.* 1981;4:451–457.

50. Karrison TG, Maitland ML, Stadler WM, et al. Design of phase II cancer trials using a continuous endpoint of change in tumor size: application to a study of sorafenib and erlotinib in non small-cell lung cancer. *J Natl Cancer Inst.* 2007;99:1455–1461.

51. Dhani N, Tu D, Sargent DJ, et al. Alternate endpoints for screening phase II studies. *Clin Cancer Res.* 2009;15:1873–1882.

52. Zhao B, Schwartz LH, Moskowitz CS, et al. Lung cancer: computerized quantification of tumor response—initial results. *Radiology.* 2006;241:892–898.

53. Plathow C, Klopp M, Thieke C, et al. Therapy response in malignant pleural mesothelioma-role of MRI using RECIST, modified RECIST and volumetric approaches in comparison with CT. *Eur Radiol.* 2008;18:1635–1643.

54. Crabb SJ, Patsios D, Sauerbrei E, et al. Tumor cavitation: impact on objective response evaluation in trials of angiogenesis inhibitors in non-small-cell lung cancer. *J Clin Oncol.* 2009;27:404–410.

55. Laurie SA, Gauthier I, Arnold A, et al. Phase I and pharmacokinetic study of daily oral AZD2171, an inhibitor of vascular endothelial growth factor tyrosine kinases, in combination with carboplatin and paclitaxel in patients with advanced non-small-cell lung cancer: the National Cancer Institute of Canada clinical trials group. *J Clin Oncol.* 2008;26:1871–1878.

56. Leighl NB, Paz-Ares L, Douillard JY, et al. Randomized phase III study of matrix metalloproteinase inhibitor BMS-275291 in combination with paclitaxel and carboplatin in advanced non-small-cell lung cancer: National Cancer Institute of Canada-Clinical Trials Group Study BR. 18. *J Clin Oncol.* 2005;23:2831–2839.

57. Desar IM, van Herpen CM, van Laarhoven HW, et al. Beyond RECIST: Molecular and functional imaging techniques for evaluation of response to targeted therapy. *Cancer Treat Rev.* 2009;35:309–321.

58. Shankar LK, Hoffman JM, Bacharach S, et al. Consensus recommendations for the use of 18F-FDG PET as an indicator of therapeutic response in patients in National Cancer Institute Trials. *J Nucl Med.* 2006;47:1059–1066.

59. Allard WJ, Matera J, Miller MC, et al. Tumor cells circulate in the peripheral blood of all major carcinomas but not in healthy subjects or patients with nonmalignant diseases. *Clin Cancer Res.* 2004;10:6897–6904.

60. Cristofanilli M, Budd GT, Ellis MJ, et al. Circulating tumor cells, disease progression, and survival in metastatic breast cancer. *N Engl J Med.* 2004;351:781–791.

61. de Bono JS, Scher HI, Montgomery RB, et al. Circulating tumor cells predict survival benefit from treatment in metastatic castration-resistant prostate cancer. *Clin Cancer Res.* 2008;14:6302–6309.

62. Budd GT, Cristofanilli M, Ellis MJ, et al. Monitoring circulating tumor cells (CTC) in nonmeasurable metastatic breast cancer (MBC). *J Clin Oncol.* 2005;23:16s.

63. Maheswaran S, Sequist LV, Nagrath S, et al. Detection of mutations in EGFR in circulating lung-cancer cells. *N Engl J Med.* 2008;359:366–377.

# Response Rates

## A Valuable Signal of Promising Activity?

Xavier Pivot • Antoine Thierry-Vuillemin • Cristian Villanueva • Fernando Bazan

The development of oncology drugs has become a highly dynamic field due in part to the increase in knowledge of both tumor and host biology. As a result, an increasing number of anticancer compounds have become available for the therapy for cancer with numerous agents currently under development. Criteria that allow investigators to assess a drug's potential are needed and these criteria must satisfy 3 objectives: (1) establish a hierarchy in terms of activity and efficacy among therapies; (2) lead to regulatory approval; and (3) become an established standard therapy. The ultimate goal of every anticancer therapy is to cure patients or to significantly prolong their survival. Commonly, the identification of the magnitude for such benefit is based on the results of phase III trials. Those phase III studies are designed to determine to what extent a treatment improves patient's survival and the quality of their lives.

Phase III trials represent the ultimate step of clinical research. It is critical to underscore the distinction between confirmatory trials such as phase III trials whose goal is to impact patient survival and exploratory trials including phase I and phase II studies designed to identify candidates for further drug development. A successful phase III drug development program depends on a careful and well-conducted exploratory program. The goals and criteria are very different. The main objective of phase I trials is to determine a safe dose either as a single agent or in a combination that will then be taken forward into phase II trials. Once a recommended dosage is established, it is taken into a phase II trial where the goal is to investigate the activity of a single agent or a combination in a variety of tumor types at various stages of disease evolution and/or after exposure to various treatment modalities. The objective of these phase II trials is on the one hand to assess antitumor activity in patients with a given tumor type to decide the wisdom of bringing the agent or more often the combination forward into confirmatory trials, and on the other hand to establish the optimal condition of use to achieve a benefit. However, in exceptional circumstances of unmet medical need, a phase II study demonstrating unequivocally an outstanding benefit with a new agent can serve as a basis for granting an authorization for use and for its eventual acceptance as a standard treatment.

Phase II trials generally generate and/or test hypotheses. They define a suitable target population for phase III studies and provide indispensable data needed for optimal clinical design in subsequent development. An important criterion that helps to identify activity in phase II studies is the response rate achieved in a well-defined subset of patients.

The response rate can be defined as a measure of tumor shrinkage. Taking into account that cytotoxic treatments are developed to kill cancer cells, a decrease in tumor size reflects cell killing and confirms the ability of the drug to achieve its goal. One might expect a drug able to induce reliable and reproducible tumor shrinkage will ultimately lead to true patient benefit. This response criterion is a predominant end point of phase II trials. Because of the importance of measuring tumor growth and shrinkage in clinical trials, metric methods have been developed to assess this response.

## Emergence of a Stringent Definition for Response

In 1976, Moertel and Hanley[1] tried to establish a level of tumor shrinkage that could be reliably and reproducibly detected by palpation. They placed rubber spheres under a piece of cloth and asked oncologists to decide, which spheres were different in size. They concluded that a minimum 50% decrease in the bidimensional measurement of a sphere was necessary for the difference to be discerned by those examining the spheres with <10% error. Thus, a 50% decrease (in 2-dimensions) became the threshold to identify tumor shrinkage as a response or to conclude there was no response. It is important to note this criterion was based on the precision of the measurements and not on any relationship between this measurement and patient outcome![2]

In 1977, Hayward et al,[3] advanced through the Programme on Clinical Oncology of the International Union Against Cancer a proposal to assess response to therapy in advanced breast cancer based on similar shrinkage criteria using skin metastases as the index lesions. Knowing therapeutic efficacy is often decided based on "progression" of the cancer, criteria for establishing progression were also proposed.[4] A 25% increase in bidimensional measurements or the appearance of any new lesion(s) were proposed as definitions of progressive disease (PD). Subsequently, these clinical criteria were extended to every cancer type, at every location, and to most radiologic assessment methods including computerized tomography scan, magnetic resonance imaging, and ultrasound imaging.

The World Health Organization (WHO) convened a consensusworking panel to provide definitions of tumor response. The following definitions, commonly known as the WHO criteria were proposed (Fig. 1).[5]

- Complete response (CR): disappearance of all clinical and radiologic evidence of target lesions and nontarget lesions with no new lesions confirmed.
- Partial response (PR): 50% or greater decrease in the overall sum of the products of diameters of all target lesions in reference to the baseline sum, persistence of 1 or more nontarget lesions with no new lesions confirmed.
- "Stable disease" (SD): failure to observe CR or PR as described earlier, in the absence of any evidence of PD or new lesions.
- PD: a 25% or greater increase in the overall sum of the products of diameters of all target lesions in reference to the smallest sum recorded at or following baseline or unequivocal progression of existing nontarget lesions overall or presence of new lesion.

The notion of objective response arose from the addition of the percent of patients whose tumor measurements met criteria for CR and

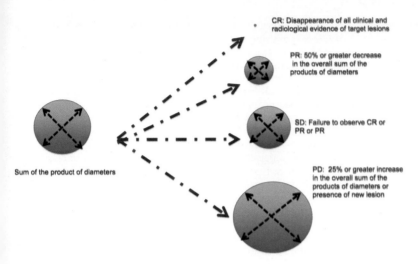

**FIGURE 1.** WHO criteria for response. CR, complete response; PR, partial response; SD, stable disease; PD, progressive disease.

PR. Subsequently, the need to "confirm" the response status at a defined interval emerged so as to increase the reliability of the results. The need for a similar (or better) evaluation on at least 2 consecutive observations at least 4 weeks apart became a requirement to score an objective reduction in tumor size as a response.[5] The WHO criteria influenced the development of oncology therapeutics from the time of their implementation to the beginning of the year 2000 and the introduction of Response Evaluation Criteria in Solid Tumors (RECIST) discussed later. Furthermore, these criteria influenced the clinical decision making process to interrupt, change, or prolong a therapy when assessable disease was available. So that often when administering a therapy, if there was no evidence of tumor progression, the therapy was continued.

Because tumors assessed by radiologic tests are not always spheres and their shrinkage might not occur uniformly in all dimensions, a 1-dimensional criterion that uses the longest tumor dimension was proposed. In 1999, the European Organization for the Research and Treatment of Cancer, the National Cancer Institute of the United States, and the National Cancer Institute of Canada proposed the RECIST as a revision of the WHO criteria to achieve a unified, objective set of criteria for assessing antitumor activity (Fig. 2).[6]

The RECIST guidelines recommend a 30% decrease in the sum of 1-dimensional measurements as the criterion for response. This cutoff was chosen simply because it represents the geometric equivalent of a sphere that shrinks by 50% in the sum of its orthogonal bidimensional measurements ($0.7 \times 0.7 = 0.49 \approx 50\%$).

The RECIST criteria are the following:

- CR: disappearance of all clinical and radiologic evidence of target lesions.
- PR: a 30% or greater decrease in the sum of LD of all lesions in reference to the baseline sum.
- SD: neither sufficient increase to qualify for PD nor sufficient shrinkage to qualify for PR.
- PD: a 20% or greater increase in the sum of LD of all target lesions, taking as reference the smallest sum recorded at or following baseline.

Subsequently, 1-dimensional RECIST has been widely accepted and their value confirmed in an attempt to simplify the standardized bidimensional WHO criteria.[7–9] A complete accord between these 2 measurement systems was established in a large comparative study that demonstrated the validity and performance of the RECIST criteria.[10]

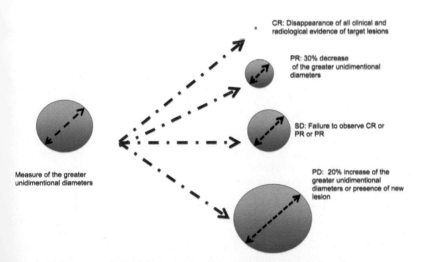

**FIGURE 2.** RECIST. CR, complete response; PR, partial response; SD, stable disease; PD, progressive disease.

Developments were made to define measurable and non-measurable lesions, target and non-target lesions, the maximal number of measurable lesions required with the aim of providing an accurate estimation of the response.[8] Nevertheless, several limitations of use and criticisms have emerged concerning the response criteria.

## Criticisms and Limits of Response Criterion

Several criticisms of response criteria have been advanced and these are discussed later. They can be summarized as follows: (1) the arbitrary assignment into "response" and "no response" categories; (2) its poor value as a surrogate for efficacy; (3) variability in response measurements; and (4) its lack of value for drugs that might inhibit growth without causing tumor shrinkage.

A first criticism of response rates as a measure of drug efficacy has been the arbitrary assignment into response and no response categories. For example, in RECIST, the arbitrary cutoff distinguishes patients whose tumors shrink by 29% from those whose tumors decrease by 31% without evidence of differences in the clinical behavior or tumor biology between these 2 patients. Similarly, there is no distinction between the patient whose tumors shrink by 31% and the patient whose tumors decrease by 99% although there might be differences of clinical import.[2] These categorizations are arbitrary and discard information available from a naturally continuous variable. A suggestion to use the tumor burden as a continuous variable has been proposed.[11] But the statistical exploitation requires large and unrealistic sample sizes. Subsequently, a proposal to use a log transformation of the sum of 1-dimensional measurements as the metric for tumor burden was made. The log transformation is a mathematic manipulation that turns the distribution of tumor measurements into a normal distribution, making the values more amenable to standard statistical testing.[12] The latter have not been widely adapted.

A second criticism has been its lack of validity as a surrogate of valuable clinical activity. However, we must remember that these response criteria were based on principles of measurement precision— the size of spheres oncologists could reliably score as different. They were not based on the identification of criteria for true activity or any relationship between this response measurement and patient outcome and indeed this remains a major criticism. This discordance emphasized by several authors has led some oncologist to question the value of the response rate as a measure of a drug's activity.[13–15] However, response criteria have generally been used to clarify in exploratory clinical trials the potential anticancer activity of drugs. With the exception of rare cases where tumor response may be a reasonable primary measure of patient benefit, (eg, breast preservation surgery or limb sparing surgery) response criteria have generally not been deemed sufficient to support a therapy as a new standard or to allow a marketing authorization for clinical use by the US Food and Drug Administration or the European Medicines Agency. The latter are usually achieved when a phase III trial determines the extent to which a new treatment improves a patient's survival. However, in many clinical settings, the latter could be affected due to a number of reasons, such as availability of effective poststudy treatment and the possibility of "crossover" to the investigational therapy among others. Faced with this clinical reality, one can consider as acceptable primary endpoints the progression free survival or disease free survival or time to treatment failure. These issues are discussed elsewhere in this monograph. Thus, the response rate remains a tool for estimating potential activity but is not a surrogate marker for either treatment benefit or survival. With rare exceptions, response rate is not valid as a measure for establishing a therapy as "standard" but only to help in the selection of interesting anticancer drugs.

A third criticism that might be expected is that, measurements of tumor size using the RECIST (or WHO) guidelines can be quite variable.[16] For example, large differences have been observed when the response rates for a drug reported in phase II studies are compared with the response rates in large randomized trials. In many cases, the response rates observed in phase II trials exceed those found in subsequent randomized trials by 30% to 80%. Because investigator bias may occur, attempts have been made to address the variability of those measurements. The need to confirm a response with a second assessment obtained within at least 4 weeks has been one of the improvements suggested. But despite the standardization of criteria for measurements, rigorous identification of experienced centers, stringent radiologic quality control, and other interventions, it remains difficult to avoid all possible biases. Because of this, in addition to investigator assessment, independent confirmation by a panel of experts has been advocated. However, the assessments performed by the investigators are essential for 2 principal reasons. First, because the investigator assessment is the basis for interruption of treatment, it is in effect the decision to crossover to the experimental arm or proceed to subsequent therapies. Second, the investigator assessment reflects most faithfully the ultimate use of the drug in routine clinical practice. Therefore, efforts need to be made to address the discrepancy between the investigator and the independent review committee so as to reduce their differences.

Interestingly, with the advent of sophisticated computerized tomography scans and associated tumor measurement software, it is possible to more accurately determine the tumor volume and to obtain a more accurate response rate.[17] But is the extra effort worth the possible enhancement in the accuracy of the analysis? Would more accurate assessments in the early phases reduce the discrepancies now observed? This is debatable because there is evidence that suggests the reliability of the response rate is not the only variable that explains the discordance between the observed response rates in phase II and phase III studies. Indeed the variability may be more related to the subset of patients selected for enrollment on a study and to the sample size. Given this, some have argued that to assess the role of an anticancer drug, one can perform a single arm phase II study and try to place the result in the context of historical control. However, interpreting results from single arm studies might be problematic given that numerous factors can affect the interpretation. An alternative approach discussed elsewhere in this monograph is to conduct a randomized phase II study with a control arm.[18]

Finally, a fourth criticism of response criteria is the argument that it ignores growth inhibition, a property that for some agents might be important than reduction in size.[19] For noncytotoxic compounds that are proposed to inhibit growth and not necessarily result in tumor shrinkage, some have advocated the use of a "clinical benefit" criterion that includes all responders with the addition of patients scored as having SD.[20] However, this suggestion may include among those scored as having SD a group with an increase of as much as 20% in their disease that obviously have not benefited from the treatment. Numerous biases could also occur in the identification of PD with a significant impact in the reliability of the assessment. Furthermore, in addition to the variability in measurement discussed earlier for response assessment, the presence of inflammatory or bleeding phenomena around the tumor could lead to a wrong status of progression. A variation of these criteria was suggested that considers the length of time until this arbitrary progression status occurs. This analysis could be of interest and some studies have reported that this length until progression might be a possible predictor of survival.[21] Some hormonal therapies and some targeted therapies might be suitable for this response criterion if their mechanism of action is one of growth inhibition and not cell killing with its attendant tumor shrinkage. Nevertheless, it is advisable to consider using time to event endpoints such as time to treatment failure, time to disease progression, or time to survival. These latter endpoints are more likely to allow the investigator to detect the antitumor activity of putative cytostatic agents.[22]

## Needs and Advantages of Response Criteria

Despite the potential shortcomings discussed earlier, advocates point to the attributes of response rate as a measure of activity and these are discussed in detail later. These attributes can be summarized as: (1) the ease with which it can be determined and the rapidity with which it can be gathered compared with other parameters of efficacy; (2) the ability to use the information to rank a given drug in hierarchy of activity.

A first and most important attribute is that the determination of a response rate is the easiest assessment that can be routinely performed using either clinical or imaging measures.[8] This evaluation can be done in every tumor type and in all tumor locations. Importantly, this response criterion allows an estimation of a drug's activity, sooner than all survival parameters. If response rates can be estimated by several investigators and methods, its reliability is wellestablished even if in need of further refinement.[14] Currently, no equivalent simple parameter linked to drug activity is available for most tumors. An exception might be surrogate biologic markers such as serum PSA or CA-125 in prostate and ovarian cancer.[23–25] These biologic surrogate markers represent an interesting, easy, and valuable alternative able to compete with metric response assessments.[25] Numerous investigators are actively searching for such biologic predictors of activity in most tumors. However, in most cases to date when such parameters have been identified, they have been rarely shown to be superior to response rates analyses.

A second attribute of response rates is that it allows for an easy estimation of activity that allows investigators to place the drug in the hierarchy of treatments. False positive results are unlikely because the response rate with observation or with an inactive agent is expected to be zero. Spontaneous regressions sufficient to qualify as a response using the RECIST guidelines are statistically unlikely. Thus, if an agent has an objective response rate >5%, it has at least some antitumor activity. This reasoning is the basis for the lower bound (null hypothesis) of 5% in most single-arm phase II trial designs. In contrast, a false result is possible if one relies on the lack of tumor growth or SD rate over any arbitrary time frame.

An exploratory trial is based on the premise that it is far worse to discard an agent with even modest activity than to accept an ultimately ineffective agent for further study.[2] The rejection of the null hypothesis in single-arm trials occurs only when no activity against a cancer is observed. Commonly, a large range of response rates are reported and stated as encouraging or promising by the authors. They are unlikely to be clinically significant when assessed by criteria of improvement in survival in subsequent phase III trials. Thus, numerous encouraging results observed in phase II studies never achieved confirmation in subsequent phase III studies. This point regularly provides a bad reputation for response rates as a valuable criterion for patient benefit. However, it must be stressed that a response rate should only be seen as a measure of activity to support the selection of active agents for further development. A response rate is rarely sufficient to support the advancement of a therapy as a new standard or to allow a marketing authorization for clinical use.

## CONCLUSION

To perform a successful randomized phase III trial, the first crucial step is to have solid data from exploratory studies that clearly identify the disease setting and the modalities of use for the experimental treatment under evaluation. With this information in hand, attention is then turned to the statistical considerations necessary to achieve valid and robust conclusions. Response rates remain one of the most useful tools to identify potential candidates for further randomized clinical trials. Even though its reliability is not perfect, even if the relationship with patients survival benefit is doubtful, even if all agents do not lead to tumor shrinkage. This response criterion seems to be the easiest assessment available to detect some level of activity.

A large number of anticancer compounds have been or are currently under development after achieving response rates that reflected at least a modest level of activity against cancer. However, only a minority has received or will receive a marketing authorization for clinical use. The majority of these new anticancer drugs fail to win marketing authorization because of insufficient evidence of efficacy or a detrimental safety profile. These failures are observed, despite preliminary encouraging activity reported in phase II studies based on response rates. We must not forget that exploratory trials in oncology are based on the premise that it is far worse to eliminate an agent with modest activity than to select an ultimately ineffective agent for further study. A well-balanced status is required between the need to reduce the current marketing authorization failure rate of new anticancer agents, although reducing the risk of discarding a future drug early in its development. A key component in the decision to assess a drug in a phase III trial remains the interpretation of the value of the response rates observed in exploratory phase II studies. The preclinical data, clinical data, statistical analysis, oncologist's intuition, science of medicine, and luck are required to decide if the response rates observed in the exploratory studies warrant future development. Thus, response rates reflecting a drug's activity remain promising parameters of efficacy.

Finally, we should remember that these response criteria evolved from criteria that were based on the ability to measurement precisely. They were not based on criteria of patient outcome or antitumor efficacy. We should use these parameters as measures of tumor reduction; we should not assign them other roles.

## REFERENCES

1. Moertel CG, Hanley JA. The effect of measuring error on the results of therapeutic trials in advanced cancer. *Cancer.* 1976;38:388–394.
2. Stadler W. *Tumor Burden Endpoint and Phase II Clinical Trial Design.* Chicago, IL: 44th American Society of Clinical Oncology; 2008:89–93.
3. Hayward JL, Carbone PP, Heusen JC, et al. Assessment of response to therapy in advanced breast cancer. *Br J Cancer.* 1977;35:292–298.
4. Hayward JL, Carbone PP, Heuson JC, et al. Assessment of response to therapy in advanced breast cancer: a project of the Programme on Clinical Oncology of the International Union Against Cancer, Geneva, Switzerland. *Cancer.* 1977;39:1289–1294.
5. World Health Organistaion. *WHO Handbook of Reporting Result of Cancer Treatment.* Geneva, Switzerland: World Health Organistaion; 1979.
6. Therasse P, Arbuck SG, Eisenhauer EA, et al. New guidelines to evaluate the response to treatment in solid tumors. European Organization for Research and Treatment of Cancer, National Cancer Institute of the United States, National Cancer Institute of Canada. *J Natl Cancer Inst.* 2000;92:205–216.
7. Bogaerts J, Ford R, Sargent D, et al. Individual patient data analysis to assess modifications to the RECIST criteria. *Eur J Cancer.* 2009;45:248–260.
8. Eisenhauer EA, Therasse P, Bogaerts J, et al. New response evaluation criteria in solid tumours: revised RECIST guideline (version 1.1). *Eur J Cancer.* 2009;45:228–247.
9. Therasse P, Eisenhauer EA, Verweij J. RECIST revisited: a review of validation studies on tumour assessment. *Eur J Cancer.* 2006;42:1031–1039.
10. Therasse P, Le Cesne A, Van Glabbeke M, et al. RECIST vs. WHO: prospective comparison of response criteria in an EORTC phase II clinical trial investigating ET-743 in advanced soft tissue sarcoma. *Eur J Cancer.* 2005;41:1426–1430.
11. Lavin PT. An alternative model for the evaluation of antitumor activity. *Cancer Clin Trials.* 1981;4:451–457.

12. Karrison TG, Maitland ML, Stadler WM, et al. Design of phase II cancer trials using a continuous endpoint of change in tumor size: application to a study of sorafenib and erlotinib in non small-cell lung cancer. *J Natl Cancer Inst.* 2007;99:1455–1461.

13. Michaelis LC, Ratain MJ. Measuring response in a post-RECIST world: from black and white to shades of grey. *Nat Rev Cancer.* 2006;6:409–414.

14. Jaffe CC. Measures of response: RECIST, WHO, and new alternatives. *J Clin Oncol.* 2006;24:3245–3251.

15. Eisenhauer EA. Response evaluation: beyond RECIST. *Ann Oncol.* 2007;18 (suppl 9):ix29–ix32.

16. Erasmus JJ, Gladish GW, Broemeling L, et al. Interobserver and intraobserver variability in measurement of non-small-cell carcinoma lung lesions: implications for assessment of tumor response. *J Clin Oncol.* 2003;21:2574–2582.

17. Zhao B, Schwartz LH, Moskowitz CS, et al. Lung cancer: computerized quantification of tumor response—initial results. *Radiology.* 2006;241:892–898.

18. Rosner GL, Stadler W, Ratain MJ. Randomized discontinuation design: application to cytostatic antineoplastic agents. *J Clin Oncol.* 2002;20:4478–4484.

19. Ratain MJ, Eckhardt SG. Phase II studies of modern drugs directed against new targets: if you are fazed, too, then resist RECIST. *J Clin Oncol.* 2004;22:4442–4445.

20. Johnston SPJ, Pivot X, Lichinitser M, et al. Lapatinib combined with letrozole vs letrozole and placebo as first-line therapy for postmenopausal hormone receptor-positive metastatic breast cancer. *J Clin Oncol.* In press.

21. Johnson KR, Ringland C, Stokes BJ, et al. Response rate or time to progression as predictors of survival in trials of metastatic colorectal cancer or non-small cell lung cancer: a meta-analysis. *Lancet Oncol.* 2006;7:741–746.

22. Ratain MJ, Eisen T, Stadler WM, et al. Phase II placebo-controlled randomized discontinuation trial of sorafenib in patients with metastatic renal cell carcinoma. *J Clin Oncol.* 2006;24:2505–2512.

23. Duffy MJ, Bonfrer JM, Kulpa J, et al. CA125 in ovarian cancer: European Group on Tumor Markers guidelines for clinical use. *Int J Gynecol Cancer.* 2005;15:679–691.

24. Tannock IF, de Wit R, Berry WR, et al. Docetaxel plus prednisone or mitoxantrone plus prednisone for advanced prostate cancer. *N Engl J Med.* 2004;351:1502–1512.

25. Scher HI, Morris MJ, Kelly WK, et al. Prostate cancer clinical trial end points: "RECIST"ing a step backwards. *Clin Cancer Res.* 2005;11:5223–5232.

# Stable Disease Is Not Preferentially Observed With Targeted Therapies and as Currently Defined Has Limited Value in Drug Development

Tatiana Vidaurre • Julia Wilkerson • Richard Simon • Susan E. Bates • Tito Fojo

As the number of "targeted therapies" (TAR) in preclinical development increased, the expectation that they would soon enter clinical trials led to several publications focusing on the design of clinical trials for TAR.[1-3] Noting that, "preclinical data suggests that some new anticancer agents directed at novel targets demonstrate tumor growth inhibition but not tumor shrinkage," numerous authors concluded that "such cytostatic agents may offer clinical benefits for patients in the absence of tumor shrinkage."[2] Early results seemed to support this concept. Sorafenib in renal cell cancer produced increases in progression-free survival despite a low-response rate; whereas in gastrointestinal stromal tumors, tumor size often did not initially change with therapy although metabolic studies demonstrated marked reduction in "activity." These studies led to a more general sense that classic response measures were inadequate. As other TAR began clinical trials, often with disappointing results, many asserted their efficacy could not be assessed by traditional response measures. This idea has become conventional wisdom, influencing clinical trial design and interpretation. Because stable disease (SD) as a "measure of activity" was being increasingly reported with traditional cytotoxic (CTX) agents, we set about to methodically compare the occurrence of SD in phase II trials of novel TAR and CTX agents.

As noted more than a decade ago, "an end point is that which can be measured to assist in reaching the stated trial goal; efficacy must reflect meaningful benefit at the level of the patient with the disease."[3] Here, we present data that raises questions about whether SD, as currently reported, has any value in assessing drug efficacy. We argue that if cytostasis is to be used as an end point, then either a randomized control group is necessary or SD definitions should be carefully developed appropriate to specific tumor types based on careful evaluation of the distribution of time to progression (TTP) in comparable historical control groups. Otherwise, proven indicators of clinical benefit should be used.

## MATERIALS AND METHODS

We catalogued response assessments in 143 phase II studies reported between October 2006 and March 2008 in 5 journals (*Cancer*, *British Journal of Cancer*, *Clinical Cancer Research*, *The Journal of Clinical Oncology*, and *Lancet Oncology*). Eighty-five used "cytotoxic therapies," and 58 used TAR. The journals were chosen to represent a spectrum of international clinical trials encompassing a range of malignancies recognizing other equally valuable journals were not selected. The time period was chosen to retrieve sufficiently diverse reports of TAR as single agents or in combination with other TAR, while also trying to avoid the expected evolution to studies combining TAR with "traditional cytotoxic compounds." All journals were examined "manually" and also using the individual journal's online search engine. All phase II studies in advanced, locally advanced, unresectable, or metastatic diseases were tabulated. Forty-seven reports that used combinations with either radiotherapy or radioactive therapies were excluded, as were half that many because they combined CTX and TAR. All data were entered on an Excel spreadsheet and checked for accuracy twice. The majority were not randomized comparisons. However, if a study had 2 or more treatment arms, each arm was entered as a separate entry. Finally, although most studies reported the analyses as "intention to treat," a few did not; however, similar results were obtained using the data as reported or after adjusting to reflect an intention to treat analysis and thus we used the reported data. Thirty-eight properties including complete response (CR), partial response (PR), SD, progression free survival (PFS), and overall survival (OS) were recorded for each study. The references can be found in Supplemental Material (http://links.lww.com/PPO/A2). The agents used were as follows:

CTX agents.
Amrubicin, capecitabine, carboplatin, cisplatin, cyclophosphamide, docetaxel, doxorubicin, epirubicin, estramustine, etoposide, 5FU, gemcitabine, ifosfamide, (indisulam), irinotecan, ixabepilone, pegylated liposomal doxorubicin, methotrexate, mitomycin-C, oxaliplatin, paclitaxel, topotecan, pemetrexed, S-1, SPI-77, temozolomide, treosulfan, trabectedin (ecteinascidin 743 or ET-743, Yondelis), ZT-1027 (Soblidotin), uracil-tegafur, vinblastine, vinflunine, and vinorelbine.

Targeted agents.
ABT-510, axitinib, bevacizumab, bexarotene, cetuximab, CI-1033 (PD 183805), erlotinib, gefitinib, (IFN-alfa-2b), imatinib, lapatinib, lenalidomide, midostaurin, sorafenib, sunitinib, thalidomide, temsirolimus, octreotide, panitumumab, perifosine, pertuzumab, and PF-3512676.

## RESULTS

Eighty-five of the studies used only CTX therapies and 58 used only TAR. As shown in Figure 1, the 2 groups were comparable in several ways. The median number of patients per study was 45.5 and 42.5 for studies administering CTX and TAR, respectively (mean 47.4 and 51.5). Both groups had a similar distribution of histologies, with the exception of breast or gastro-esophageal histologies, which were more prevalent in studies administering CTX therapies and renal cell carcinoma (RCC), which was over-represented in TAR. The previous therapies allowed were grouped into 1 of 4 categories (none, chemotherapy, radiation therapy, and other) and, as shown in Figure 1, the distribution was similar although more studies with CTX agents

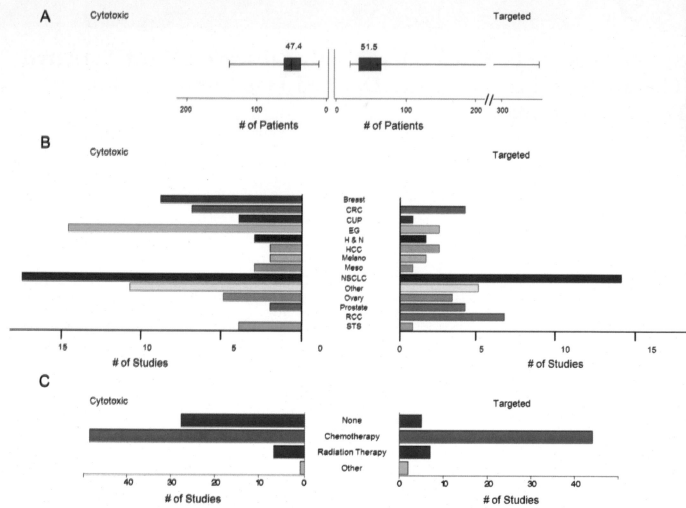

**FIGURE 1.** Comparisons between studies where patients received cytotoxic therapy (left) or targeted therapy (right) (A) box plot of the mean number of patients per study, (B) bar chart of the total number of studies by cancer type, (C) bar chart of the total number of studies by prior therapy category. All differences were found nonsignificant except for the following pairs within each panel: panel B, CTX/esophagogastric versus TAR/esophagogastric ($P = 0.0047$), and CTX/breast versus TAR/breast ($P = 0.0027$); panel C, CTX/none versus TAR/none ($P = 0.001$). CRC indicates colorectal cancer; CUP, carcinoma of unknown primary; EG, esophagogastric; H&N, head and neck; Melano, melanoma; Meso, mesothelioma; STS, soft tissue sarcoma.

had no previous therapy required, a difference that did not impact the subsequent analysis.

We next evaluated the PFS and OS for the 2 groups. The PFS (mean 5.6, median 4.8) and OS (mean 12.8, median 10.9) with CTX agents were similar to the PFS (mean 4.5, median 2.35) and OS (mean 12.6, median 9.15) with TAR. As shown in Figure 2, the OS of the various histologies overlapped and were not significantly different, suggesting patients with solid tumors who enroll in phase II clinical trials present a relatively homogenous group. Similarly, the percent SD, PFS, and OS were similar across the "prior therapy" groups whether they had enrolled on a clinical trial administering CTX or TAR. These similarities allowed us to explore response and prognostic correlations using patients with tumors comprising a broad histologic profile. Also note here the similar rates of SD across the different previous therapies categories.

Remarkably, although all studies scored SD, in fact the duration of SD was defined in only 28.6% (41/143) of studies. The definitions varied, requiring lack of progression for a median of 10 weeks (range 4 weeks to 6 months) with medians of 11 and 9 weeks for studies employing CTX and TAR, respectively. The rates of SD were nearly identical for the 2 groups—medians of 34.7% and 31.05% for CTX and TAR, respectively (mean 35% versus 32.34%). If patients in all studies were individually counted, the rates of SD were also similar, 34% (1356/3982) and 32.8% (982/2992) for CTX and TAR, respectively. Furthermore, as shown in Figure 3A, the distribution of percent SD was similar. Also similar was their distribution by histology (Fig. 3B). All of this suggests properties other than therapy determine SD. As shown in Figure 4, we found no real relationships between the percent SD observed with any therapy and PFS or OS. The apparent correlations seen between SD and PFS or OS with CTX therapies

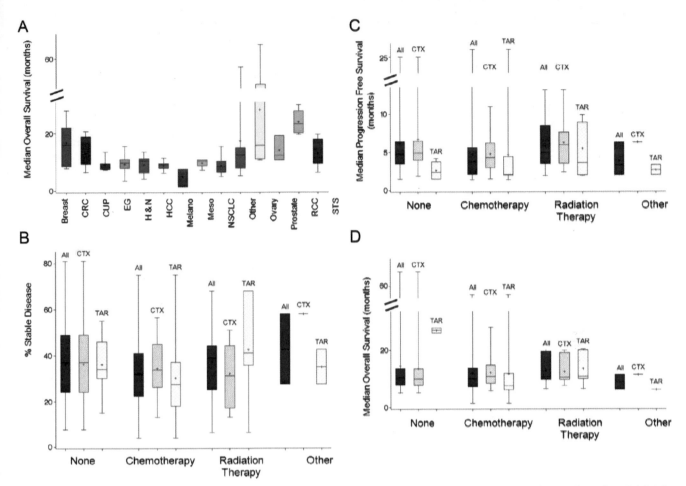

**FIGURE 2.** A, Box plots of median OS by 14 histologies. B-D, Box plots of percent SD (B), median PFS (C), and median OS (D) for 4 categories of prior treatment: none, other, radiation therapy, and chemotherapy. Within each category of prior treatment, groups are calculated; All refers to all patients from both the cytotoxic and targeted therapies groups, CTX refers to patients from the cytotoxic therapies group and TAR refers to patients from the targeted therapies group. All differences were found nonsignificant except for the following pairs within each panel: panel A, RCC versus all other cancers ($P < 0.05$); ovarian versus all other cancers ($P < 0.05$); breast cancer versus EG ($P = 0.0494$), breast cancer versus melanoma ($P = 0.0472$), and breast cancer versus NSCLC ($P = 0.0254$). Panel B, none/CTX versus chemotherapy/All ($P = 0.0351$). Panel C, radiation therapy/TAR versus chemotherapy/TAR ($P = 0.0476$); Panel D, none/TAR versus radiation therapy/All ($P = 0.0361$), none/TAR versus radiation therapy/CTX ($P = 0.0406$), and none/TAR versus radiation therapy/TAR ($P = 0.0359$). CRC indicates colorectal cancer; CUP, carcinoma of unknown primary; EG, esophagogastric; H&N, head and neck; Melano, melanoma; Meso, mesothelioma; STS, soft tissue sarcoma.

($P = 0.0132$ and $P = 0.0144$) are anomalous "negative correlations" that actually reflect the correlation of PFS and OS with CR + PR.

In contrast to the similarity in values for SD, the overall response rate (ORR) (CR + PR) was higher with CTX than with TAR (28% versus 13.1%) and as shown in Figure 5 demonstrated a strong correlation ($P < 0.0001$ for all variables) with PFS and OS for all therapies.

Although the similarities allowed us to compare results across a range of histologies, we were also able to examine a single histology, nonsmall cell lung cancer (NSCLC), in more detail because 35 NSCLC studies (18 CTX therapies/17 TAR) were part of the studies evaluated. In this subset, as in the group as a whole, there were no differences between the rate of SD reported for regimens using

CTX (median 34.9%; 269/882 = 30.4%) and those using TAR (median 22.2%; 224/883 = 25.3%). Similarly, as shown in Figure 6, in NSCLC there was no correlation between the rate of SD and PFS or OS, although as shown in the lower panels, there was a correlation between CR + PR with both PFS and OS for all the NSCLC data.

Finally, to examine an additional histology in depth we expanded the survey to cover the period of 1/04 to 12/08 for phase II studies in breast cancer. In this period of time, we identified in the same 5 journals a total of 46 breast cancer studies including 30 that used CTX and 16 that employed TAR. In breast cancer, as in the group as a whole and the NSCLC subset, there were no differences between the rates of SD reported for regimens using CTX (median 34.9%;

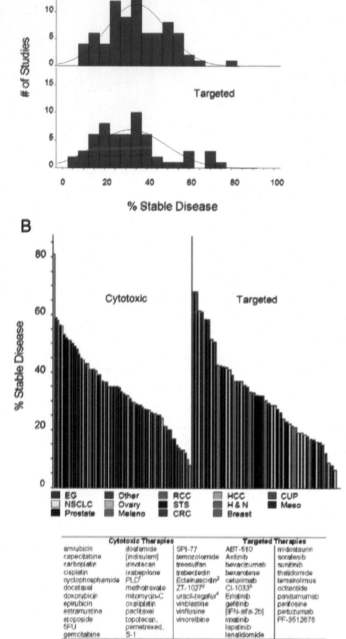

**FIGURE 3.** A, Histograms of percent SD within studies where patients received cytotoxic (top) and targeted therapies (bottom). Each bar represents a 5% increment. B, Plots of percent SD, color-coded by cancer type, reported for studies where patients received cytotoxic (left) and targeted therapies (right). For visual symmetry, each bar on the right is approximately 45% wider. CRC indicates colorectal cancer; CUP, carcinoma of unknown primary; EG, esophagogastric; H&N, head and neck; Melano, melanoma; Meso, mesothelioma; STS, soft tissue sarcoma.

570/1569 = 36.3%) or those using TAR (median 22.5%; 257/900 = 28.5%). Again, as in all the foregoing analyses, SD was not correlated with either PFS or OS, whereas CR + PR was strongly correlated (data not shown).

## DISCUSSION

The era of TAR has included both successes and disappointments.[4-8] Some have argued the disappointments are due in part to difficulties evaluating TAR in phase II clinical trials because SD and not OR were expected, a consequence of the "cytostatic" properties these agents have been said to possess. In its extreme, this has led to "cancer as a chronic disease" proposals. As noted in one publication, a "major challenge . . . is the lack of impressive response rates for many of the novel agents. Response rates may not be helpful at all in evaluating targeted agents that have growth inhibition as their primary effect (ie, cytostatic agents)."[9] Assertions that TAR are primarily growth inhibitory or "cytostatic" have usually not been referenced, however, because scientific support for the concept of targeted agents as "cytostatic" especially compared with "traditional" CTX therapies has been generally lacking.

SD as a valid endpoint was assigned to antiangiogenic agents since they would "starve tumors." Investigators wrote "it may be difficult to demonstrate a conventional antitumor response (ie, objective response) with antiangiogenic therapies in cohorts of patients with advanced disease."[10] Thus, they argued, "phase II trials designed to demonstrate the clinical activity (including durable stable disease) . . . would be ideal." Subsequently, SD as a measure of activity was advanced for numerous other targeted agents. For example, investigators reporting early results with erlotinib concluded "disease stabilization with a median duration of 16.1 weeks . . . in 38% of patients" demonstrated "the static effects of erlotinib against refractory HNSCC."[11] Although those who reported early experience with lapatinib noted "twelve patients . . . had SD and 8 of 14 patients with clinical activity remained on lapatinib therapy for >3 months," whereas "twenty-two patients with various tumors, most expressing either ErbB1 or ErbB2, experienced SD with a median duration of 4 months . . . . Together, these studies indicate the potential clinical activity of lapatinib in patients with a variety of solid tumors."[12] Numerous other examples can be cited.[13-15]

To be sure while some entertained, the possibility of SD as a measure of activity they did so with skepticism and advocated the need to test this concept using randomized control groups and novel trial designs.[16,17] Unfortunately, as the studies tabulated in this analysis demonstrate, despite the recognized need for randomized trial designs or novel paradigms for interpretation,[1] the design of choice has remained a "traditional" phase II design often with an emphasis on SD as a "signal of clinical activity."

Remarkably, although all studies reported the percent of patients scored as having SD, in fact the duration of what constitutes SD was defined in only 28.6% (41/143) of studies. We would note that in the initial description of response evaluation criteria in solid tumor (RECIST) the authors wrote, "The clinical relevance of the duration of stable disease varies for different tumor types and grades. Therefore, it is highly recommended that the protocol specify the minimal time interval required between 2 measurements for determination of stable disease. This time interval should take into account the expected clinical benefit that such a status may bring to the population under study."[18] Among the studies reporting a definition, the median was 10 weeks—a value that many oncologists and most patients would not consider meaningful, especially, without impact on PFS or OS. Indeed, periods as short as 4 to 6 weeks have been scored as SD in reporting phase III trials, a value many find unsatisfactory.

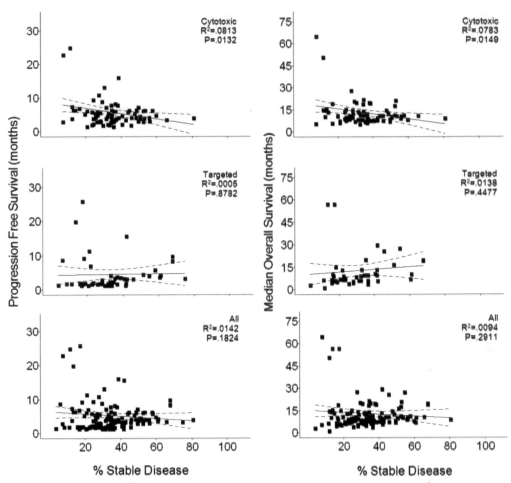

**FIGURE 4.** Plots of median PFS (left) and median OS (right) as a function of percent SD. Within each comparison, 3 groups are plotted. Cytotoxic refers to the group of studies where patients received cytotoxic therapy, Targeted therapies refers to the group of studies where patients received targeted, and All refers to patients from both the cytotoxic and targeted therapies groups combined. The only significant correlations found were anomalous "negative correlations" within the cytotoxic group for percent SD with median PFS ($P = 0.0132$) and with median OS ($P = 0.0144$) (see text for details).

(Sorafenib in advanced RCC, "Table 2: Stable disease was defined as disease that remained unchanged for 28 days"; and Sorafenib in RCC first line: "disease control rate (DCR); ie, stable disease [SD] for $\geq 6$ weeks ....")[19,20]

The lack of a definition in >2/3 of studies is especially disappointing because it is used in the context of precise RECIST-driven response measurements. As others have previously noted, "Standardized response criteria are essential for the conduct of clinical research. They facilitate interpretation of data, comparisons of the results among various clinical trials, and identification of new agents with promising activity, and provide a framework on which to evaluate new biologic and immunologic insights into the diseases being studied. The availability of uniform guidelines ensures a reliable analysis of comparable patient groups among studies and acquisition of similar data".[21] The lack of such definitions in most studies means the information provided—the rate of SD—is of no value because it has not been defined and those reading a report cannot assess its import. Although seasoned investigators, like Supreme Court Justice Potter Stewart, may argue, "they know SD when they see it" lacking a definition or better yet a randomized trial, such information is

merely anecdotal. (From the opinion of Potter Stewart (January 23, 1915 to December 7, 1985), Associate Justice of the United States Supreme Court, in the obscenity case of Jacobellis V. Ohio (1964). Stewart wrote in his short concurrence that "hard-core pornography" was hard to define, but that "I know it when I see it.") Similarly, an experienced clinician might argue that a patient with documented disease progression who enrolls on a study and has modest regression has had "clinical benefit." However, this type of data has seldom been gathered before study enrollment, and we do not know whether such an observation, if true, would translate to PFS or OS. In this regard, we would note again that the reported SD values had no correlation with PFS or OS. This is further evidence of the limitations of current SD designations. One would expect it would be correlated at a minimum with PFS because both measures are based on TTP. Although a positive correlation of SD with PFS or OS would not unequivocally establish that SD measured antitumor effect, the lack of correlation raises serious questions about the current definition and measurement of SD.

It is not certain that defining SD would add much value to that currently provided by PFS or TTP; these are values that are currently

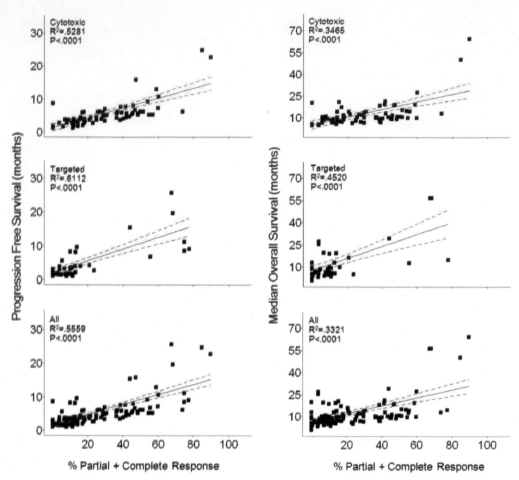

**FIGURE 5.**    Plots of median PFS (left) and median OS (right) as a function of percent PR + CR. Within each comparison, 3 groups are plotted. Cytotoxic refers to the group of studies where patients received cytotoxic therapy, targeted therapies refers to the group of studies where patients received targeted therapies and All refers to patients from both the cytotoxic and targeted therapies groups combined. In all plots, Percent PR + CR is significantly correlated ($P < 0.0001$) with both median PFS and median OS.

reported in a majority of studies, including 90.9% (130/143) of those surveyed for this analysis. It is rather clear that PFS results cannot be interpreted in terms of therapeutic effect without a control group. Reporting SD tends to obscure this fact. Furthermore, as has been previously noted, "we should not rush to falsely define drugs as active on the basis of stable disease, since stable disease is a composite outcome consisting of inherent tumor growth kinetics and potential drug effect."[22]

The nearly identical SD rates for the 2 therapy groups and their similar distribution and median durations suggests properties other than therapy are responsible for SD. Indeed, the near identity of the profiles with a median duration of PFS of 4.05 months suggests this duration of SD is likely to be similar across many refractory solid tumors.

In contrast to the values for SD, the ORR (CR + PR) was higher with CTX than with TAR (mean 28% versus 13.1%; median 25% versus 5.3%) and demonstrated a strong correlation ($P < 0.0001$) with PFS and OS for both CTX and TAR. Although one could argue this suggests these measures of drug activity are more meaningful and should be sought in all clinical trials, we can-

not be confident that trials with higher ORR and longer PFS and OS did not contain more prognostically favorable patients than the other trials.

Our results are consistent with and extend a recent review of phase II trial designs used in studies of TAR, which concluded that "even relatively low rates of objective response may signal that an agent has potential for achieving regulatory approval" and inferred "that agents affecting targets that are meaningful in one or more cancer types should reasonably be expected to cause tumor shrinkage in at least some patients."[23] The authors concluded, "Failing to see any evidence of response at all suggests that the drug is likely to fail in subsequent development." Similarly, in a recent review of CTX agents the authors reported a relationship between phase II response rate and eventual regulatory approval—with approval more likely the higher the response rate.[24] Although our data in general agree with these conclusions we would caution against redefining the level of shrinkage needed to qualify as a response to a value that is much less than current RECIST standards. Using a reduced level of shrinkage, as the response threshold can be problematic with regard to measurement error unless more accurate imaging is used.

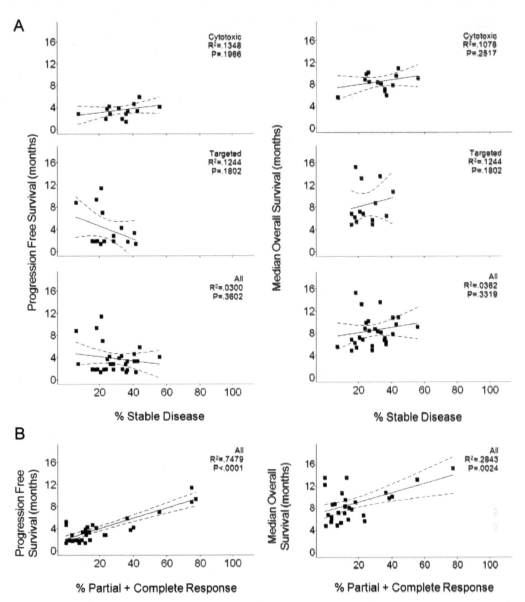

**FIGURE 6.** NSCLC analysis: (A) plots of median PFS (left) and median OS (right) as a function of percent SD. Within each comparison, 3 groups are plotted. Cytotoxic (top) refers to the group of studies where patients received cytotoxic therapy, targeted therapies (middle) refers to the group of studies where patients received targeted therapies, and All (bottom) refers to patients from both the cytotoxic and targeted therapies combined. B, Plot of median PFS (left) and median OS (right) as a function of Percent PR + CR. For each, 1 comparison is plotted, All, which refers to patients from both the cytotoxic and targeted groups. Percent PR + CR is significantly correlated with median PFS ($P = 0.0001$) and median OS ($P = 0.0024$).

Thus, we conclude that SD as currently defined and measured, occurs as frequently with CTX as with TAR and likely often reflects the natural course of the disease, not a therapeutic effect of the drug regimen. Responses are observed with TAR as with CTX, and this analysis suggests that even for TAR it is a measure of activity that should be sought. Assertions that targeted agents are generally cytostatic should be discouraged. Indeed given that there will likely never be a targeted agent more specific than any of our "cytotoxic" microtubule-targeting agents, and few agents more CTX than sunitinib in renal cell carcinoma or flavopiridol in CLL, 2 TAR, we would argue that this artificial divide should be ended.[6,25,26] Finally, whether a clinically meaningful definition of SD can be identified remains to be determined. Generally, if one wishes to reliably evaluate the potential cytostatic effect of a treatment, then a randomized phase II trial using PFS as an end point is recommended.

### REFERENCES

1. Gelmon KA, Eisenhauer EA, Harris AL, et al. Anticancer agents targeting signaling molecules and cancer cell environment: challenges for drug development? *J Natl Cancer Inst.* 1999;91:1281–1287.

2. Korn EL, Arbuck SG, Pluda JM, et al. Clinical trial designs for cytostatic agents: are new approaches needed? *J Clin Oncol.* 2001;19:265–272.
3. Eisenhauer EA. Phase I and II trials of novel anti-cancer agents: endpoints, efficacy and existentialism. *Ann Oncol.* 1998;10:1047–1052.
4. Druker BJ, Guilhot F, O'Brien SG, et al; IRIS Investigators. Five-year follow-up of patients receiving imatinib for chronic myeloid leukemia. *N Engl J Med.* 2006;355:2408–2417.
5. Blanke CD, Rankin C, Demetri GD, et al. Phase III randomized, intergroup trial assessing imatinib mesylate at two dose levels in patients with unresectable or metastatic gastrointestinal stromal tumors expressing the kit receptor tyrosine kinase: S0033. *J Clin Oncol.* 2008;26:626–632.
6. Motzer RJ, Hutson TE, Tomczak P, et al. Sunitinib versus interferon alfa in metastatic renal-cell carcinoma. *N Engl J Med.* 2007;356:115–124.
7. Tol J, Koopman M, Cats A, et al. Chemotherapy, bevacizumab, and cetuximab in metastatic colorectal cancer. *N Engl J Med.* 2009;360:563–572.
8. Hecht JR, Mitchell E, Chidiac T, et al. A randomized phase IIIB trial of chemotherapy, bevacizumab, and panitumumab compared with chemotherapy and bevacizumab alone for metastatic colorectal cancer. *J Clin Oncol.* 2009;27:672–680.
9. Roberts TG Jr, Lynch TJ Jr, Chabner BA. The phase III trial in the era of targeted therapy: unraveling the "go or no go" decision. *J Clin Oncol.* 2003;21:3683–3695.
10. Gasparini G, Longo R, Fanelli M, et al. Combination of antiangiogenic therapy with other anticancer therapies: results, challenges, and open questions. *J Clin Oncol.* 2005;23:1295–1311.
11. Soulieres D, Senzer NN, Vokes EE, et al. Multicenter phase II study of erlotinib, an oral epidermal growth factor receptor tyrosine kinase inhibitor, in patients with recurrent or metastatic squamous cell cancer of the head and neck. *J Clin Oncol.* 2004;22:77–85.
12. Burris HA III, Hurwitz HI, Dees EC, et al. Phase I safety, pharmacokinetics, and clinical activity study of lapatinib (GW572016), a reversible dual inhibitor of epidermal growth factor receptor tyrosine kinases, in heavily pretreated patients with metastatic carcinomas. *J Clin Oncol.* 2005;23:5305–5313.
13. Wolf M, Swaisland H, Averbuch S. Development of the novel biologically targeted anticancer agent gefitinib: determining the optimum dose for clinical efficacy. *Clin Cancer Res.* 2004;10:4607–4613.
14. Brachmann S, Fritsch C, Maira SM, et al. PI3K and mTOR inhibitors: a new generation of targeted anticancer agents. *Curr Opin Cell Biol.* 2009;21:194–198.
15. Strumberg D, Clark JW, Awada A, et al. Safety, pharmacokinetics, and preliminary antitumor activity of sorafenib: a review of four phase I trials in patients with advanced refractory solid tumors. *Oncologist.* 2007;12:426–437.
16. Stadler WM, Ratain MJ. Development of target-based antineoplastic agents. *Invest New Drugs.* 2000;18:7–16.
17. Ratain MJ, Stadler WM. Clinical trial designs for cytostatic agents. *J Clin Oncol.* 2001;19:3154–3155.
18. Therasse P, Arbuck SG, Eisenhauer EA, et al. New guidelines to evaluate the response to treatment in solid tumors. European Organization for Research and Treatment of Cancer, National Cancer Institute of the United States, National Cancer Institute of Canada. *J Natl Cancer Inst.* 2000;92:205–216.
19. Escudier B, Eisen T, Stadler WM, et al; TARGET Study Group. Sorafenib in advanced clear-cell renal-cell carcinoma. *N Engl J Med.* 2007;356:125–134.
20. Escudier B, Szczylik C, Hutson TE, et al. Randomized phase II trial of first-line treatment with sorafenib versus interferon Alfa-2a in patients with metastatic renal cell carcinoma. *J Clin Oncol.* 2009;27:1280–1289.
21. Cheson BD, Horning SJ, Coiffier B, et al. Report of an International Workshop to standardize response criteria for non-Hodgkin's lymphomas. *J Clin Oncol.* 1999;17:1244–1253.
22. Ratain MJ, Eckhardt SG. Phase II studies of modern drugs directed against new targets: if you are fazed, too, then resist RECIST. *J Clin Oncol.* 2004;22:4442–4425.
23. El-Maraghi RH, Eisenhauer EA. Review of phase II trial designs used in studies of molecular targeted therapies: outcomes and predictors of success in phase III. *J Clin Oncol.* 2008;26:1346–1354.
24. Goffin J, Baral S, Tu D, et al. Objective responses in patients with malignant melanoma or renal cell cancer in early clinical studies do not predict regulatory approval. *Clin Cancer Res.* 2005;11:5928–5934.
25. Byrd JC, Lin TS, Dalton JT, et al. Flavopiridol administered using a pharmacologically derived schedule is associated with marked clinical efficacy in refractory, genetically high-risk chronic lymphocytic leukemia. *Blood.* 2007;109:399–404.
26. Phelps MA, Lin TS, Johnson AJ, et al. Clinical response and pharmacokinetics from a phase I study of an active dosing schedule of flavopiridol in relapsed chronic lymphocytic leukemia. *Blood.* 2009;113:2637–2645.

# Stable Disease Is a Valid End Point in Clinical Trials

Anthony W. Tolcher

In reality, antitumor response is a continuous rather than categorical variable. Although by convention we have categorized response based on an arbitrary metric of the difference in tumor length, such as complete, or partial response, stable disease, or progression, there is little evidence in the age of targeted therapies that these arbitrarily derived measures accurately predict clinical benefit (complete response notwithstanding) or identify a drug worthy of further development.

## WHAT CONSTITUTES BENEFIT?

What is clinical benefit? This is far more than a rhetorical question. To the patient, clinical benefit may represent shrinkage of tumor, whereas to the treating physician, clinical benefit may be palliation of symptoms. In contrast, in new drug development, clinical benefit refers to a regulatory outcome that is used for the basis of all drug approvals. It is generally accepted that response rate alone, for most indications, does not qualify as a sufficient regulatory end point for clinical benefit, and therefore overall survival (OS) or progression-free survival (PFS) are the most appropriate end points used in clinical trial design to meet regulatory approval. In essence then, one achieves benefit following the application of a treatment, a treatment effect occurs which persists over the passage of time, and thereby changes the natural history of disease progression.

Intuitively, a decrement in tumor size should confer benefit and the converse, and absence of a decrement, little benefit. However, the change in tumor size as a function of treatment is a continuous variable, which arbitrarily has been converted into a categorical variable. Using response evaluation criteria in solid tumors (RECIST), responding patients are those who achieve at least a 30% reduction of the sum of the longest diameters and is an arbitrary cut off that significantly discounts a 29% reduction or gives greater value to a 60% reduction.[1] Stable disease, by contrast, includes the tumor measurement changes that encompass a 29% decrease all the way to a 20% increase. Therefore, stable disease can mean anything from a minor reduction all the way to frank progression. It is self-evident that the value placed on a 15% reduction is greater than 1 of a 10% increase despite both being classified by the term stable disease. The imprecision in the term "stable disease" results in most clinicians having little confidence in the interpretation of this as a clinical trial result. The perception, rightly or wrongly, is that the stable disease, even though tumor regression occurs, is a failure of treatment compared with that of a partial response.

To understand the somewhat meaningless value we place on achieving a partial response compared with a minor response in cancer, one merely needs to be reminded of a common high school example of exponential growth. To paraphrase the problem posed to students, if a lily pad in a pond doubles every 24 hours and covers the pond in 50 days, how long does it take to cover one-half the pond?

The correct answer (although frequently guessed wrong by students), 49 days, suggests that in an exponential growth system, the incremental time difference between one-half and complete coverage is small. So too, the analogy fits our misguided belief in benefit associated with a partial response compared with a lesser regression. We dismiss the value of a minor response compared with achieving a partial response. However, in the lily pad analogy, we are arguing over the difference of only a few hours!

It stands to reason then that if treatment does not change the exponential growth/regrowth rate, little is to be gained by a minor regression versus a partial regression. In contrast, if we can change the growth/regrowth rate, the problem described above becomes much more interesting. In oncology, although we find it gratifying to reduce the tumor by 30% or 50%, the impact on survival time may be small, and our incentives for trying, as well as the gratification achieved, is overly naive. Treatment that alters the exponential growth rate, even without shrinking the tumor, may have a greater impact on PFS or OS than response.

In the era of single-agent targeted therapies, the mechanism of action may be an antiproliferative, antiangiogenic, proapoptotic, or some combination thereof. The biologic effect observed may not fit the categorical criteria of a partial response, but nonetheless the result can be meaningful to the investigator, the clinician, and most importantly the patient. Those patients with the optimal molecular biology for a particular targeted therapy may respond, but this tends to be the minority. In contrast, a proportion of patients with less optimal tumor biology for that agent may have, at best, stable disease (SD). Other subjects, with absent target or redundant pathways will achieve no response at all to the therapeutic intervention. These distinct groups and the credibility of the argument for stable disease even in the absence of categorical responses can be supported by the results of recent clinical trials.

## THE ARGUMENT FOR STABLE DISEASE

It should be relatively easy to refute stable disease as a factor contributing to clinical benefit. In the analysis of a randomized study with both responders (a small number) and nonresponders (the majority of patients), intuitively the survival benefit should accrue strictly to the population of patients who had an objective response whereas the proportion of patients who failed to achieve a response contributing little to an improvement in survival benefit. The ability to detect a survival difference therefore would require the study to be powered accordingly (eg, large numbers to detect small differences). Such an example should have been the experience with erlotinib in nonsmall lung cancer. Several phase II studies demonstrated a reproducible but marginal response rate of 10% or less, with a nearly equal proportion of patients with stable disease.[2,3] In the randomized phase III study of erlotinib versus placebo, the response rate was equivalent to that observed in the phase II experience (9%), but the survival end point, based on a prospectively designed 33% increase in median survival, was achieved.[4] If the assumption that only the responding patient population contributed to the survival benefit was correct, the incremental survival gain for this responding patient population would have to been truly remarkable to reach statistical significance. Otherwise, the study would have been severely underpowered to detect an OS difference (would require several thousand patients). As we know from the results of the study, the magnitude of the survival gain to the responding population was not sufficiently large for the study size to detect the difference.[4] Based on this retrospective exercise, a population of "nonresponders" must have contributed to the survival benefit observed.

Furthermore, if the premise is correct that survival benefit can accrue to a overall treated patient population who have few, if any responses, but have a significant population that experiences stable disease, then this should be evident in a study comparing survival among 2 treatment populations when the response rate difference between the 2 arms is quite marginal. This is best illustrated by the development of the agents targeting mammalian target of rapamycin. In the development of sirolimus analogs, durable stable disease was observed in patients with renal cell carcinoma while objective responses were few.[5] A single-agent phase II study confirmed a substantial proportion of patients with stable disease and a marginal single agent response rate for both temsirolimus and everolimus. In the randomized phase III study of everolimus versus placebo, a PFS benefit was observed despite a marginal objective response rate (1%) for the everolimus arm.[6] The logical conclusion of this study was that response rate was not relevant to the difference in outcome between the populations and that a change in the natural history (tumor growth) of the disease process was induced in patients otherwise classified as stable disease.

Although the aforementioned single-arm phase II and III clinical trials illustrate indirectly the impact of stable disease on survival as an end point, they do not directly refute the argument that stable disease is not a result of drug effect. The most common confounding variable is due to the selection of naturally indolent disease patients, the observation of stable disease in single-arm studies is no more than over enthusiastic optimism. Randomized studies incorporating stable disease as an intermediate end point, with drug withdrawal used as the ultimate test of drug-effect eliciting stable disease is perhaps the only mechanism to irrefutably address this question.

## THE SORAFENIB RANDOMIZED DISCONTINUATION STUDY

The randomized discontinuation study with sorafenib in metastatic renal cell carcinoma patient population directly supports the validity of stable disease as a valid end point. In early clinical studies of sorafenib, persistent stable disease was observed in a diverse number of clinical indications. To further address this, a randomized discontinuation trial design was adopted. The specific results of this study have been published and discussed elsewhere, but the key design features were the following: patients with response or progression at 12 weeks were either continued or discontinued from treatment, respectively, whereas the patients with persistent stable disease were randomized in a double blind manner to continued treatment with either sorafenib or placebo.[7] Freedom from progression was the primary end point in this randomized subgroup. If stable disease was due solely to the indolent behavior of a particular patient's tumor, the 2 groups, treatment or drug withdrawal with placebo, would have similar in outcomes. However, if sorafenib altered the progression of disease and induced stable disease, an incremental improvement would accrue to the patients who were randomized to active drug compared with the withdrawal group. The results of this study confirmed the effect of sorafenib on the randomized patient population with an improvement in the rate of progression, and this later mirrored the effect seen in the randomized phase III study in patients with metastatic renal cell carcinoma.[8] This study design, more than any other in contemporary oncology, supported the argument that stable disease could be induced by drug treatment and was a valid end point in clinical drug development and is reviewed by Stadler elsewhere in this issue: Other Paradigms: Randomized Discontinuation Trial Design.

Although the widespread utility of this design for other agents currently in early development can be questioned for its practicality due to the large number of patients that must be initially entered (502 patients) and the small number of patients with SD eventually randomized (65 patients with renal cell carcinoma), the outcome supports the use of this design with certain agents and clearly demonstrates the impact of stable disease in sorafenib-treated patients.

Table 1 summarizes an ever expanding list of targeted therapies with low single-agent response rates in phase II studies that mirrored response rates in phase III studies had a significant proportion of patients classified as stable disease, yet had improvement in the end points of PFS or OS in pivotal studies, and were successful in regulatory approval.[3–16]

**TABLE 1.** Selected Targeted Therapies With Low Objective Response Rates in Phase II Studies That Later Had Success in Survival End Points

| Agent | Indication | Phase II Response Rate (%) | Phase II Stable Disease (%) | Phase III Response Rate (%) | Successful Phase III End Point | References |
|-------|-----------|---------------------------|----------------------------|----------------------------|-------------------------------|-----------|
| Erlotinib | NSCLC | 10 | 41 | 9 | OS | 2 and 3 |
| Bevacizumab | RCC | 10 | NS | 25* | PFS | 8 and 9 |
| Temsirolimus | RCC | 7 | 44 | 8.6 | OS | 4 and 10 |
| Everolimus | RCC | 14 | 57 | 1 | PFS | 5 and 11 |
| Sorafenib | RCC | 4 | 34 | 2 | PFS | 6 and 7 |
| Sorafenib | HCC | 2 | 39 | 2 | OS | 13 and 14 |
| Sunitinib | GIST | 11.7[†] | 46[†] | 7 | PFS | 15 and 16 |

*Combination with interferon $\alpha$.
[†]Based on initial group of 77 patients.
NS indicates not stated in publication; NSCLC, nonsmall cell lung cancer; RCC, renal cell carcinoma; HCC, hepatocellular carcinoma; GIST, gastrointestinal stromal tumor.

## YOU FIND WHAT YOU SEEK: WHY STABLE DISEASE IS THE LOGICAL OUTCOME USING CURRENT DRUG SCREENING METHODOLOGY

Candidate agents selected to enter clinical development are based largely on a convention of tumor growth inhibition (TGI) in preclinical in vivo models, with tumor regression the exception, rather than the rule. The benchmark of >63% TGI, indicative of an active compound is therefore a relatively low hurdle that can be achieved with a decrement in tumor growth rate. The clinical correlate therefore would be progression of tumor burden, but at a slower rate, rather than tumor response. The finding of TGI does not rule out the observation of antitumor activity because tumor regressions may be observed when patients with optimal biology presents itself, but, similar to conventional screening methodology, the majority of patients will achieve less. It remains a point of discussion whether the minimum benchmark for selection should be raised to require tumor regression in several tumor models, or at least an understanding of the molecular biology of those experimental tumors that do undergo regressions, before entry into the clinic, so that we can improve the number of agents that induce clinical responses.

If stable disease is the logical result from our preclinical screening end points, we must develop methods of analysis to improve our ability to discriminate clinically meaningful stable disease from nonmeaningful stable disease.

## IMPROVING THE CONFIDENCE AND PRECISION IN STABLE DISEASE AS A CLINICAL END POINT

The 3 clinical examples above demonstrate the validity of stable disease as an end point for new drug development. However, can the observations of stable disease be refined in earlier (phase II studies) to improve the precision around what constitutes "valuable" stable disease, provide confidence to initiate a phase III study, and reduce the risk of a failed phase III study?

If we assume stable disease has merit, the 2 aspects of clinical trial results that require close scrutiny and analysis (and will improve confidence in stable disease that predicts meaningful biologic effect) are (1) the proportion of treated patients who have some level of tumor regression including minor and partial responses and (2) the durability of stable disease, measured by sufficient passage of time in any study population, that implies drug effect on the natural history of the disease and the expectation of clinical benefit.

To address the first point, the adoption and increasing use of the waterfall plot analysis that displays the individual patient's maximal change in tumor size from baseline has permitted the rapid evaluation of the proportion of patients who have some level of tumor regression and correctly treats response as a continuous variable. Figures 1A, B portray the same hypothetical results in a phase II study with equal objective response rates, different stable disease proportions, and yet

indicate 2 very different outcomes. The interpretation of the data portrayed in Figure 1B indicates a substantial proportion of patients are classified as having stable disease and clinical benefit has occurred. On the basis of the appearance of the proportion of patients with a reduction of tumor size depicted as columns below the *x* axis, one would likely make a value judgment that the results for the drug depicted in Figure 1B has greater likelihood for success than the data for the drug depicted in Figure 1A.

Waterfall plot analysis is largely subjective but, nonetheless, is a useful tool to rapidly evaluate the continuous variable, tumor regression, and progression in a study population. Waterfall plots should therefore be considered in any phase II clinical trial publication that reports a low-response rate but proposes further development of the agent beyond phase II. The reviewer, and perhaps the oncology community, can rapidly determine whether the data justifies, or not, the authors recommendation by examining the illustration.

Despite the usefulness described for waterfall plot analysis, they still portray the data in unidimensional terms. Waterfall plots graphically reflect the antitumor activity, much like response criteria, in a binary manner, is the result above or below where the *x* axis intersects the *y* axis? The data presented does not include duration of response, or lack thereof, as a variable. However, it is the durability of both response and stable disease that will likely have the greatest relevance on, and engender confidence in, the data used to estimate clinical benefit measures in later studies such PFS and OS. To address the second question noted above and refine stable disease to a valid end point, the durability of stable disease should be incorporated into the waterfall plot analysis.

## THE DURATION OF SD AS A PREDICTOR OF CLINICAL BENEFIT

As mentioned before, response is defined as a categorical variable when in truth it is a continuous variable. Response definitions incorporate only rudimentary duration values as a covariable, and with the latest iteration of RECIST (1.1), this is now absent.[17] However, it is the duration of response that has implicit relevance to the outcomes of PFS and OS, because these 2 latter outcomes are time dependent. As stated earlier, altered tumor growth may be the critical end point in noncurative tumors, and the value of the durable stable disease and decreased tumor growth rate may equal or exceed the value of tumor regression in the right biologic circumstance. It is self-evident that biologic behavior trumps response if the growth of the tumors is different. The short lived response in a rapidly progressive tumor (eg, Burkitt's lymphoma) results in an inferior outcome compared with suboptimal response in an indolent tumor (follicular non-Hodgkin lymphoma). Perhaps in contemporary oncologic drug development, we should try to alter the biology to emulate indolent lymphomas and be able to discern when we have achieved this or not.

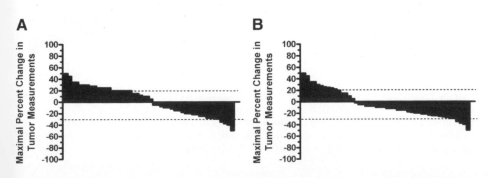

**FIGURE 1.** A, Hypothetical waterfall plot of the maximal percent change in tumor measurements for each individual entered onto a clinical trial. B, Identical results for objective response rate for same hypothetical clinical trial but different proportion of patients experiencing minor regressions classed as stable disease.

Nonetheless, despite the importance of time as end point in oncology, the duration of stable disease is often reported without a uniform means to decide the merit of the observation. In publications, statements are included that using landmarks such as 4, 6, or 8 courses of therapy or patients with SD combined with responding patients at 6 months as a measure of clinical benefit response. If by convention, in RECIST 1.0, a partial response must have a duration of 4 weeks, then it is logical to assign a duration to SD. Nevertheless, all these conventions remain arbitrary. Although it may be useful in the future to define a uniform benchmark for duration for stable disease duration to improve the confidence in SD, the data need to be portrayed and analyzed in a manner that recognizes both the continuous variable of response and therapy duration.

To facilitate more accurate assessment of a drug's impact in a phase II study, a modification of the waterfall plot is proposed.

## THE 2 DIMENSIONAL WATERFALL PLOT

The hypothetical waterfall plots illustrated in Figures 2A, B convey identical data with respect to the maximal change in tumor size. However, Figure 2B also conveys the duration the individual patient remained on study before discontinuing therapy due to progressive disease (as determined by the investigator). The narrowest column representing 1 course and the expansion of each column along the *x* axis reflecting proportionally the duration the individual was on study in courses. The value of durable stable disease can be weighed against short-lived responses and also short-lived stable disease (minor regressions) that likely will contribute little to PFS or OS and are of no consequence. Furthermore, the diverse groups of patients can be viewed as a collection of distinct categories: patients with a response, long or short duration; minor regressions of long or short durations; and rapid progressing patients versus those whose disease slowly progresses. Furthermore, minor regressions of short duration can now be discounted in contrast to the equal weight afforded them in the standard waterfall diagram. Similarly, examining the wide columns above the *x* axis representing patients who attained no tumor reduction but had prolonged time on study, one can quickly ascertain either the indolent nature of the disease in question or, alternatively, the biologic effect of the drug on growth rate that will provide useful information in the decision-making process.

The interpretation of the results from a clinical study depicted in Figures 2A versus 2B would be quite different, despite the fact that both had equal response rates and equal magnitudes of tumor regression or progression. Duration, depicted along the *x* axis, is now fully visualized.

Furthermore, this illustration permits the reader to rapidly assess the area under the curve (AUC) for both the progressing and the responding patients and through visual comparisons of the area under the curves, readily substantiate ones judgment of this drugs value in the particular indication. Perhaps more useful, a comparison of this data illustrated in this manner, by treatment arm, from a randomized phase II, may allow a more confident prediction of success in a later randomized phase III study. Two-dimensional waterfall plots are currently being explored in several phase II data sets to determine the utility of this analysis.

Improvements in waterfall plots notwithstanding, the dismal success rate of phase III studies in oncology remains a great concern among investigators, the pharmaceutical industry and society. Although it is self-evident that patient enrichment for the optimal molecular genetics for response is necessary to improve the success of late stage clinical studies, the identification of a distinct patient population that exhibits durable stable disease, and enriching this patient group, will no doubt contribute successful end points of PFS and OS. To recognize the importance of some patients with stable disease, categorize and determine those patients with meaningful SD in early studies, and characterize the biology of this distinct group of patients, the oncology community will no doubt improve the level of sophistication in clinical trial analysis and improve the success rate of new agents in oncology.

In conclusion, clinical trial results indicate that a proportion of patients with stable disease contribute to the survival benefit observed with targeted therapies, and stable disease can be considered a valid end point in early clinical studies. Ongoing studies are required to further refine strategies to identify distinct populations of patients with meaningful stable disease from those whose tumors fail to gain

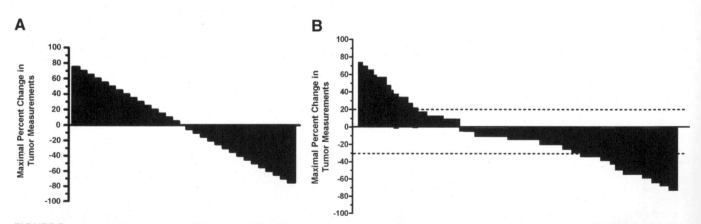

**FIGURE 2.** A, Hypothetical waterfall plot with symmetrical proportions of tumor growth and regression for a population entered into the clinical trial with no weighting for duration on trial. (B) Two-dimensional waterfall plot with identical proportions of patients with tumor growth and regressions from Figure 1A but illustrating the duration that each individual remained on study represented by width of column. Individuals have variable durations on study but the duration of patient population on study with regressions having 2-fold greater duration on study than nonregressing population for illustrative purposes.

therapeutic benefit and thereby improve the success rate in oncologic drug development.

## REFERENCES

1. Therasse P, Arbuck SG, Eisenhauer EA, et al. New guidelines to evaluate the response to treatment in solid tumors. European Organization for Research and Treatment of Cancer, National Cancer Institute of the United States, National Cancer Institute of Canada. *J Nat Cancer Inst.* 2000;92:205–216.
2. Giaccone G, Gallegos Ruiz M, Le Chevalier T, et al. Erlotinib for frontline treatment of advanced non-small cell lung cancer: a phase II study. *Clin Cancer Res.* 2006;12:6049–6055.
3. Jackman DM, Yeap BY, Lindeman NI, et al. Phase II clinical trial of chemotherapy-naive patients > or = 70 years of age treated with erlotinib for advanced non-small-cell lung cancer. *J Clin Oncol.* 2007;25:760–766.
4. Shepherd FA, Rodrigues Pereira J, Ciuleanu T, et al; National Cancer Institute of Canada Clinical Trials Group. Erlotinib in previously treated non-small-cell lung cancer. *N Engl J Med.* 2005;353:123–132.
5. Atkins MB, Hidalgo M, Stadler WM, et al. Randomized phase II study of multiple dose levels of CCI-779, a novel mammalian target of rapamycin kinase inhibitor, in patients with advanced refractory renal cell carcinoma. *J Clin Oncol.* 2004;22:909–918.
6. Motzer RJ, Escudier B, Oudard S, et al; RECORD-1 Study Group. Efficacy of everolimus in advanced renal cell carcinoma: a double-blind, randomised, placebo-controlled phase III trial. *Lancet.* 2008;372:449–456.
7. Ratain MJ, Eisen T, Stadler WM, et al. Phase II placebo-controlled randomized discontinuation trial of sorafenib in patients with metastatic renal cell carcinoma. *J Clin Oncol.* 2006;24:2505–2512.
8. Escudier B, Eisen T, Stadler WM, et al; TARGET Study Group. Sorafenib in advanced clear-cell renal-cell carcinoma. *N Engl J Med.* 2007;356:125–134.
9. Yang JC, Haworth L, Sherry RM, et al. A randomized trial of bevacizumab, an anti-vascular endothelial growth factor antibody, for metastatic renal cancer. *N Engl J Med.* 2003;349:427–434.
10. Rini BI, Halabi S, Rosenberg JE, et al. Bevacizumab plus interferon alfa compared with interferon alfa monotherapy in patients with metastatic renal cell carcinoma: CALGB 90206. *J Clin Oncol.* 2008;26:5422–5428.
11. Hudes G, Carducci M, Tomczak P, et al; Global ARCC Trial. Temsirolimus, interferon alfa, or both for advanced renal-cell carcinoma. *N Engl J Med.* 2007;356:2271–2281.
12. Amato RJ, Jac J, Giessinger S, et al. A phase 2 study with a daily regimen of the oral mTOR inhibitor RAD001 (everolimus) in patients with metastatic clear cell renal cell cancer. *Cancer.* 2009;115:2438–2446.
13. Abou-Alfa GK, Schwartz L, Ricci S, et al. Phase II study of sorafenib in patients with advanced hepatocellular carcinoma. *J Clin Oncol.* 2006;24:4293–4300.
14. Llovet JM, Ricci S, Mazzaferro V, et al; SHARP Investigators Study Group. Sorafenib in advanced hepatocellular carcinoma. *N Engl J Med.* 2008;359:378–390.
15. Heinrich MC, Maki RG, Corless CL, et al. Primary and secondary kinase genotypes correlate with the biological and clinical activity of sunitinib in imatinib-resistant gastrointestinal stromal tumor. *J Clin Oncol.* 2008;26:5352–5359.
16. Demetri GD, van Oosterom AT, Garrett CR, et al. Efficacy and safety of sunitinib in patients with advanced gastrointestinal stromal tumour after failure of imatinib: a randomised controlled trial. *Lancet.* 2006;368:1329–1338.
17. Eisenhauer EA, Therasse P, Bogaerts J, et al. New response evaluation criteria in solid tumours: revised RECIST guideline (version 1.1). *Eur J Cancer.* 2009;45:228–247. Available at: http://www.eortc.be/recist/.

# Progression-Free Survival Is Simply a Measure of a Drug's Effect While Administered and Is Not a Surrogate for Overall Survival

Julia Wilkerson • Tito Fojo

A clinical end point is a characteristic or variable that reflects how a patient feels, functions or survives, whereas a surrogate end point is a biomarker or other measure used as a substitute for a clinical end point.[1,2] A surrogate end point should be predictive of clinical benefit or harm. Potential surrogates may not necessarily be accurate predictors of an end point but may well correlate with an end point. A surrogate will be of most value if it fully captures the effect of the treatment on the clinical end point.[3] Progression-free survival (PFS) is a surrogate measure, defined as the time from randomization to objective tumor progression or death from any cause. On the other hand, overall survival (OS) is an objective, clinically significant end point defined as the time from randomization to the time of death from any cause. Although OS is held as a dependable, clinically meaningful end point, the use of PFS as an end point is widely debated, there being conflicting reports as to its efficacy.[4-7] For the Food and Drug Administration to accept an end point as a surrogate in the process of a cancer drug's approval, evidence must be presented of improvement of survival or quality of life in the patients. However, a recent option for end point approval, in refractory metastatic cancer patients with no known alternative treatment, is through a process called accelerated approval (AA).[8] A clear improvement in PFS, shown in a randomized trial for such refractory metastatic cancer patients, can be a foundation for AA. Marketing approval, by the AA route, is given when the drug demonstrates a clear, meaningful, and statistically significant benefit in the clinical setting through controlled, well-conducted trials[6] even without evidence for an improvement in OS.

Many reviewers have argued for and against the validity of PFS as a surrogate end point for OS through qualitative or quantitative analyses.[9-29] Two of the main arguments made for the use of PFS as an end point in a clinical trial are that such studies require a shorter period of time and fewer patients than a study that looks for an OS advantage.[20,29] There are problems with using OS itself as an end point. These include confounding post trial therapies or cross over designs, loss to follow-up, insufficient sample size to detect differences in therapies, and skewing because of the inclusion of death from any cause (even if it is not therapy related).[17,20,24]

However, there are many drawbacks to the use of a PFS end point. First is the lack of concordance between a statistically significant effect on PFS and either an important clinical benefit or a conclusion of "reasonably likely to provide a clinical benefit."[30] Second, the use of time to progression or disease-free survival, interchangeably with PFS, can lead to confounding interpretation of results because time to progression and disease free survival are themselves 2 different measures.[31] Third, the lack of standardization of PFS evaluation methodology is another confounding variable in the use of PFS as a surrogate end point.[13] Fourth, drug holidays, whereby an evaluation time point is skipped over (thereby falsely increasing PFS), further reduce the accuracy of PFS as a true measure of treatment effect.[9] Fifth, the proxy for true progression time is the date when the radiologic or other evaluation of first progression is detected. This interval-censored data can overestimate the median PFS because it could lead to statistically significant differences that are more a reflection of the evaluation interval than the treatment.[32] Given these caveats, some argue that OS is superior to PFS due to (1) a lack of investigator bias, with the end point being a known data point (date of death); (2) the fact that the initial population used for calculation is the "intention to treat" population (regardless of whether or not treatment was given); and (3) the fact that a statistically significant improvement in OS is the most meaningful clinically significant measure.

Some investigators have performed quantitative analyses and concluded there is association between PFS and OS[5,15,17,19,22,24-27,29,33-37]. Some of these reviewers and others have concluded that OS can be predicted by PFS,[5,14,16-19,22,24,26,27,36] whereas others have reported no such predictive capability.[10-13,17,25,28,29,35] Some that find a predictive capability of OS by PFS, warn that marginally significant differences in PFS may not translate to OS and are often context dependent.[12,16,27,28] However, the quantitative analysis methods used in the reviewed literature are highly variable across studies, regardless of the conclusion drawn. Correlation coefficients, Wald statistics, Kappa statistics, linear regression models, metaregression models, maximum likelihood estimation using accelerated failure time model, Monte Carlo simulations, and other statistical methods have been used in the assessment of PFS as a surrogate for OS making comparisons or a clear conclusion difficult. Reviews that have addressed this topic qualitatively have similarly produced conflicting conclusions with some reporting there is no association of PFS with clinical benefit[12,16,30,32] and others supporting the validity of PFS as a surrogate for OS.[10,30,38-40]

Our contribution to this debate is more straightforward. It arises out of our observation that the amount of time of improvement in PFS usually mirrors the amount of time of OS benefit. We confirm this observation and come to the obvious conclusion that in patients with metastatic cancer, the extent of improvement is OS depends on the improvement in PFS and that the latter is simply a measure of a drug's effect while it is administered and nothing more.

## METHODS

### For Data Entry

Criteria for inclusion were (1) a randomized trial conducted in patients with metastatic cancer, (2) a difference in either PFS or OS (or both) or the hazard ratio (HR) for PFS and OS between the control arm, and the experimental arm had achieved statistical significance. Canvassing the literature using numerous search entries identified potential studies for inclusion. Studies were also identified from references in reviews or in other randomized studies. Although extensive and unbiased in that all studies encountered during the search process were assessed, we do not consider the search exhaustive and recognize that some studies may have inadvertently been omitted. Older studies that antedated the era of modern imaging evaluations were not included. Each comparison of treatment arms was entered into the data table as 1 observation (Supplementary Digital Content, http://links.lww.com/PPO/A3). We extracted variables of interest, where available, for each entry [Author, year of publication, journal, disease, treatment comparison (arm 1 versus arm 2), total number patients, number of patients in each arm, % stable disease for each arm, % progressive disease for each arm, % complete response for each arm, % partial response for each arm, % response rate (RR)/(complete response + PR) for each arm, *P* value for difference in % RR, median PFS for each arm, HR for PFS, 95% confidence interval (CI) for PFS HR, *P* value for difference in PFS between arms, median OS for each arm, HR for OS, 95% CI > for OS HR, *P* value for difference in OS between arms, and citation]. Data was checked for errors twice after initial entry.

## For Data Analysis

### End Point Marker Analysis

The final data table with 82 entries was imported to SAS version 9.1 software[41] for analysis. Before conducting any analyses, we calculated 3 variables from our table: delta RR, delta OS, and delta PFS. We calculated the delta by subtracting the value for arm 2 from arm 1 (arm 1 − arm 2) for each of the 3 end point markers, respectively. To examine the correlation between endpoints, we ran linear regressions between delta OS and delta PFS, delta RR and delta PFS, delta RR and delta OS, HR OS and HR PFS, delta RR and HR PFS, and delta RR and HR OS. In addition to these 6 analyses performed on the whole dataset, we also examined delta OS and delta PFS as well as HR OS and HR PFS in the 3 subgroups of cancer with the largest numbers of studies (Colon, Ovarian, and Breast).

## Comparative Gene Analysis

To examine the association between genes associated with cell growth and those associated to cell death, we searched the Gene Ontology database AmiGo.[42] After examining the Gene Ontology tree of biologic processes/molecular functions/cellular component, we selected several Gene Ontology terms (specific biological processes/molecular functions/cellular components) that pertained to cell growth and cell death. These Gene Ontology terms were cell proliferation, cell cycle, cell growth, cell death, apoptosis, regulation of cell growth, regulation of cell death, and signal transduction. The parameters set for each Gene Ontology term search were *Homo sapiens* (species), all data sources, all ontology types, all gene product types, all evidences, and direct association to the term. We downloaded the set of genes annotated to each of the selected Gene Ontology terms for our comparative analysis. Using the Gene List Venn Diagram Web site,[43] we produced Venn diagrams to analyze a series comparisons between the GO terms listed above using respective gene lists [list comparisons, X versus X: (A) cell proliferation versus apoptosis, (B) cell growth versus apoptosis, (C) cell proliferation versus cell death, (D) cell growth versus cell death, (E) cell proliferation versus cell death versus apoptosis, (F) cell growth versus cell death versus apoptosis, (G) cell cycle versus cell death versus apoptosis, and (H) signal transduction versus cell death versus apoptosis].

## RESULTS

Sixty-six studies returned by the searches and related references met criteria for inclusion. Of these, 55 had 1 comparison and 11 had 2 or more comparisons (2 comparisons [N = 6], 3 comparisons [N = 5]). Therefore, the final data table consisted of 82 entries. Figure 1 presents a straightforward analysis of the difference in time of progression PFS versus the difference in time of OS for the 59 entries that had information on time for both PFS and OS (some studies provided only HRs for 1 or both endpoints). We would emphasize here as we did in Methods,

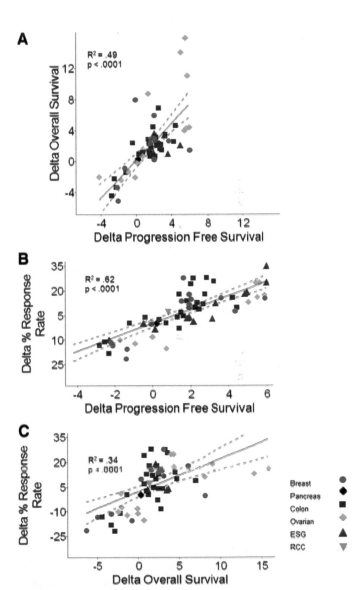

**FIGURE 1.** A, Plot of delta OS (change in overall survival, treatment group 1 − treatment group 2) versus delta PFS (change in Progression-Free Survival: treatment group 1 − treatment group 2). B, Plot of delta RR [change in response rate (%PR + %CR) treatment group 1 − treatment group 2] versus delta PFS. C, Plot of delta RR versus delta OS. RCC, renal cell carcinoma; ESG, esophagogastric cancer.

that for inclusion in this analysis, a study had to have had the difference in either PFS or OS achieve statistical significance, although in 54% of the comparisons, both had achieved significance. The histologies evaluated consisted of breast, pancreatic, colon/colorectal (colon), ovarian, renal (renal cell carcinoma), and esophagogastric. The control arm was usually designated as such, although in a few cases in which neither arm was clearly the control that designation was arbitrarily assigned to 1 of the 2 arms. As can be seen, there is concordance between the gain or loss of time in PFS and the gain or loss of time in OS. The slope of the line is 1.214 (95% CI; [+0.8902, +1.5376], a value near unity that underscores the concordance between the gains or losses in both PFS and OS. Note here that a greater gain in PFS, a value often thought to be "overestimated" does not seem to occur, but this is not surprising because both arms of a study would have had a similar "overestimation" of PFS and this would then not impact the difference. Panels B and C show the correlation between the delta in RR and the delta in PFS (B) and OS (C). Here again one can see concordance between these 2 measures of a drug's activity and not unexpectedly the correlation is higher with the delta in PFS. The latter would be more likely to be impacted by the RR, because barring rapid growth after the nadir was achieved, PFS would likely correlate well with RR.

Figure 2 shows a similar analysis performed this time by comparing the HR for PFS, OS, and RR. Again a strong correlation between the HR for PFS and that for OS is seen (panel A), in agreement with the findings in Figure 1. We would note here that this also agrees with similar observations by others in some cancers.[19,25,27,29] Also as in Figure 1, there is a correlation between the HR for RR and that for PFS (panel B) and OS (panel C), and again the values for RR correlate better with the values for PFS than for those with OS.

Figure 3 shows the results for the 3 histologies with the highest numbers of entries–colorectal, ovarian, and breast cancer. The results in these subsets are similar to that in the entire group of diseases.

## DISCUSSION

Although many have argued, and will continue to argue, that PFS is or should be a surrogate for OS, we would argue that the present analysis underscores what is perhaps the obvious: PFS is only a measure of a drug's effect while it is being administered. To the extent that PFS is prolonged, so too is OS prolonged. If this is the case, then some might argue that PFS can stand alone as a measure of drug efficacy, provided the extent to which it delays progression is both meaningful and of good quality. As we discuss later, we would disagree with this assessment.

Given what we know about the biology of cancer and the drugs used to treat it, the observation that the improvement in OS is similar to that in PFS is not unexpected. The reason is that a tumor's growth and its drug sensitivity are 2 distinct properties. Although we would like to have therapies that alter the intrinsic "biology" of tumors and promote the emergence of a cancer that is not "as bad as it was before therapy," our therapies are not designed to do that preclinical development strategies do not select for this property. Instead, current strategies aim to eradicate the tumor. Consequently, the biology of the malignant cells that "survive" both arms of a randomized clinical trial is the same. In short, any survival advantage that will accrue occurs only while such an experimental agent is administered. Current drugs do not have a significant effect on the biology of the tumor once the therapy is discontinued. In this argument consider that by the time a patient presents for therapy for their metastatic cancer, a selection process has been ongoing that has streamlined tumor growth such that most of the cells comprising a tumor mass have the capacity to grow

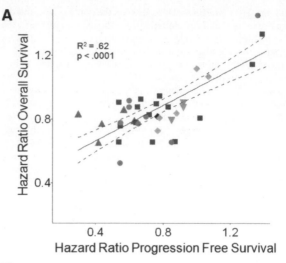

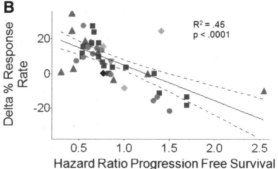

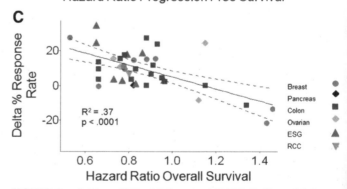

**FIGURE 2.** A, Plot of HR of OS versus HR PFS. B, Plot of delta RR versus HR PFS. C, Plot of delta RR versus HR OS.

at comparable rates, although for a given cell, its blood supply and other local factors can obviously affect this rate. Slow growing cells have been left behind, so that more rapidly growing cells comprise an increasing fraction of a tumor. Note that during the period when the tumor had been growing, and before a patient presents for therapy, a selection for drug sensitivity has not taken place. Unlike the strong selective pressure for growth that has been ongoing, the tumor cells have not been exposed to any therapeutic agents. The administration of a therapy then selects a drug-resistant fraction, because it eliminates drug-sensitive cells. That such a selection can occur is a result of the fact that the selection for growth abilities has not simultaneously

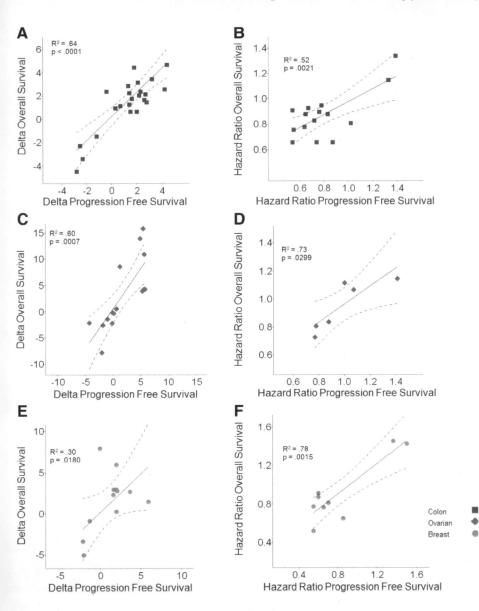

**FIGURE 3.** A, Plot of delta OS versus delta PFS in the subgroup of colon/colorectal cancer studies. B, Plot of HR OS versus HR PFS in the subgroup of colon/colorectal cancer studies. C, Plot of delta OS versus delta PFS in the subgroup of ovarian cancer studies. D, Plot of HR OS versus HR PFS in the subgroup of ovarian cancer studies. E, Plot of delta OS versus delta PFS in the subgroup of breast cancer studies. F, Plot of HR OS versus HR PFS in the subgroup of breast cancer studies. Note: Power (alpha = 0.05) for A = 0.999, B = 0.941, C = 0.984, D = 0.698, E = 0.498, and F = 0.989.

selected for genes that affect drug sensitivity and the genes that confer these properties need not be "homogenously expressed" in all the cells that comprise a tumor. Genes involved in "cell growth" and "cell proliferation" differ from those involved in "cell death" and "apoptosis," the latter comprising genes that might modulate "drug sensitivity." They comprise "different cassettes" of genes, a point illustrated by the data in Figure 4. In this figure, we can see a minimal overlap between the genes involved in apoptosis and those classified as involved either in cell proliferation (panel A) or in cell growth (panel B). Genes involved in apoptosis have been shown in numerous drug resistance studies to be the mediators of drug sensitivity.[44-47] Similarly, genes involved in cell proliferation (panel C) or in cell growth (panel D) overlap very little with genes involved in cell death. Panels E and F demonstrate that the cell growth and cell proliferation cassettes are not overlapping and that A/B and C/D are not overlapping analyses. These comparisons allow one to understand how a selection for cell growth, during the years that a tumor has been developing,

will not select for drug sensitivity. The tumor may demonstrate a PR to the drug, while leaving the surviving cells to grow at the same rate as the initial tumor, this rate being independent of the therapy received in the clinical trial. Further evidence for this standpoint can be found in the abundant literature that comprises the study of drug resistance, where for years countless investigators have identified hundreds of putative drug resistance genes, the majority of which have never been implicated in cellular growth. Included among these are genes that mediate apoptosis, drug transporters, drug metabolizing genes, genes involved in DNA repair, and the autocrine/paracrine pathways among others.[48-51] We would also note that studies examining the growth rate constants of tumors have reached similar conclusions, in that the growth rates of tumors that break through from therapy correlate with their growth rates before therapy,[52] Stein et al, TCJJPPO 2009. Finally, we would note the lack of overlap between genes involved in the cell cycle (panel G) and in signal transduction (panel H) and those involved in cell death and apoptosis, underscoring the fact that

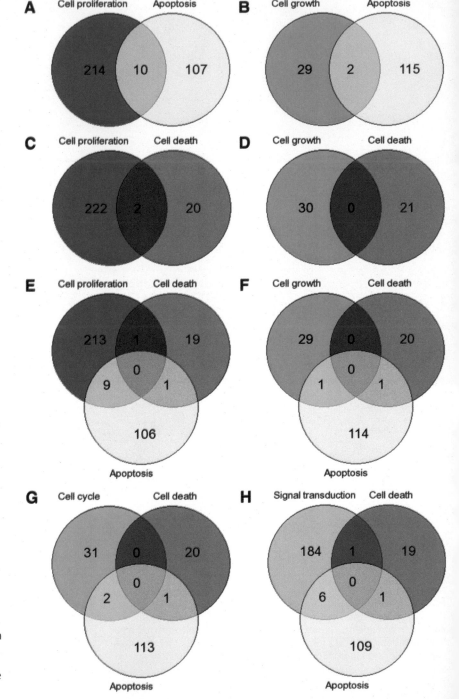

**FIGURE 4.**   Venn diagrams of genes annotated to Go terms (genes in common noted in parentheses): (A) cell proliferation and apoptosis (CDC2L1, CSE1L, E2F1, IL2RA, LY86, RAF1, SRA1, TNFSF9, TSPO) (B) cell growth and apoptosis (RRAGC), (C) cell proliferation and cell death (MLTK), (D) cell growth and cell death (none) (Ea) cell proliferation and cell death (MLTK) (Eb) cell proliferation and apoptosis (CDC2L1, CSE1L, E2F1, IL2RA, LY86, RAF1, SRA1, TNFSF9, TSPO) (Ec) cell death and apoptosis (IL17A) (Fa) cell growth and cell death (none) (Fb) cell growth and apoptosis (RRAGC) (Fc) cell death and apoptosis (IL17A) (Ga) cell cycle and cell death (none) (Gb) cell cycle and apoptosis (AHR, RPS27A) (Gc) cell death and apoptosis (IL17A) (Ha) signal transduction and cell death (NUP62) (Hb) signal transduction [combination of genes annotated to cell surface receptor signal transduction and intracellular signaling cascade] and apoptosis (CD14, IL2RA, MAG13, SEMA6A, SQSTM1, YWHAE) Hc. Cell death and apoptosis (IL17A). Note: In diagrams of 2 comparisons (A–D), the number of genes in common is the number shown in the overlap minus one (N-1). In diagrams of 3 comparisons (E–H), the number of genes in common is the number shown in the overlap (N).

our current "novel targeted therapies" are unlikely to be any better at modifying post-treatment growth.

The obvious question that arises then from these observations is whether longer administration of a therapy might offer greater benefit. If the extension in OS is driven by the extension in PFS, and this is a consequence of an "on-therapy" benefit, then might OS be further prolonged if therapy is continued longer, even beyond an arbitrarily

designated point of progression?[52] Stein et al, TCJJPPO 2009. The articles collected in the present monograph describe different methodologies for measuring success and disagreements as to their value. Nevertheless, there is (nearly) universal agreement that the values we currently use for determining therapeutic efficacy—whether "WHO" or Response Evaluation Criteria in Solid Tumors—are arbitrary. Using the Response Evaluation Criteria in Solid Tumors criterion, we score a therapy as ineffective when the size of the largest tumor dimension has increased 20%. This is difficult to support and, (nearly) everyone would agree, arbitrary. We note that for a patient with metastatic cancer, few options often exist, none of them curative. For such patients, the longer administration of an agent that can delay progression, beyond the currently defined arbitrary point of "progressive disease," might confer greater survival benefit. We would note in this regard that all chemotherapeutic agents, not just "targeted therapies", could slow tumors, a property we have called "cytolentic."[53] True "cytostatic" effects are rarely if ever observed, because mitosis and for that matter phases of the cell cycle other than $G_0$ are not places to "pause" and wait. We would argue that a cytolentic effect occurs because even therapies that cannot bring about cell death can inflict sufficient damage to slow the growth of tumors as they cope with the damage inflicted[52] Stein et al, TCJJPPO 2009. Such a prediction could be tested clinically and is supported by a recent study in non–small cell lung cancer where continued treatment with pemetrexed prolonged OS.[54,55] Additional similar studies are planned.[56]

Given the observation that the magnitude of gain in PFS is likely to be the gain in OS, why do we argue that PFS should not be considered a valid surrogate? Our reasons include the well-recognized fact that unlike OS that has a clear end point, assessment of PFS is subject to bias that may be important and the possibility that a subsequent therapy may alter the course of disease.

The allegations that because PFS is interval-censored data it is subject to bias has been addressed in the introduction and in other contributions found in this monograph and will not be discussed in detail further. We would only note here as we did in the Results section that in studies where investigator bias can be avoided, any overestimation of PFS could occur for both arms and should "cancel out."

As for the possibility that a therapy may alter the course of disease, we would disagree with investigators who advocate that PFS should replace OS in regulatory approval because the expanding number of therapeutic options can abolish a PFS advantage, because these are likely to be administered equally to patients enrolled in both arms of a clinical trial. It is thus unlikely they will prolong the life of patients enrolled on the control arm to a greater extent than that of patients enrolled on the experimental arm. As for the argument that cross over designs can eradicate the benefits, we believe this to be valid. However, if a gain in PFS "disappears" when OS is tabulated, and this is ascribed to the cross over design, the most straightforward conclusion is that administration of the experimental agent can be delayed without adversely impacting outcome or compromising the agent's ability to benefit a patient.

We would finally express a concern that some therapies might have detrimental long-term effects making PFS irrelevant and underscoring the need for assessing OS. Consider as an example the use of bevacizumab in breast cancer. In combination with paclitaxel, bevacizumab was reported to prolong PFS by a statistically significant 5.9 months compared with paclitaxel alone (median PFS, 11.8 versus 5.9 months; HR for progression, 0.60; $P < 0.001$).[57] However, the benefit in PFS did not translate into an increase in OS (median, 26.7 versus 25.2 months; HR, 0.88; $P = 0.16$). Although the disappearance of a large PFS benefit was difficult to explain, ascertainment bias has been proposed as 1 factor. But other factors raised by the authors include the possibility "that resistance to bevacizumab results in relative resistance to subsequent therapies, or that discontinuation of bevacizumab could result in more aggressive disease." A subsequent analysis demonstrated an association of vascular endothelial growth factor and vascular endothelial growth factor receptor-2 genetic polymorphisms with median OS and more troubling found single nucleotide polymorphisms combinations that seemed more likely to loose the gains in PFS.[58] These observations support our analysis of patients with metastatic renal cell carcinoma treated with single agent bevacizumab, where a significant advantage in PFS likewise disappeared when OS was assessed, suggested being a consequence of accelerated growth after the discontinuation of bevacizumab.[52] Together with basic science observations describing an impact on host-tumor interactions,[59–61] the bevacizumab results in breast cancer argue for at most using PFS to support a "conditional approval" pending documentation that OS has not been adversely impacted.

In summary, we would argue that PFS is not a surrogate for OS but rather a straightforward measure of how a therapy can delay growth while it is administered. Because the data that comprises this analysis includes a large number of traditional "cytotoxic agents," this underscores the fact that such "growth retardation" is not an exclusive property of "novel targeted agents." The extent of improvement in PFS becomes the extent of improvement in OS and whether this achieves statistical significance depends on the heterogeneity of clinical courses and whether over the longer period that comprise the OS the distribution around the mean OS is as tight as that around the mean PFS. Concerns that the post-therapy clinical course may be adversely impacted by some of our newer therapies argue against using PFS as an end point and ignoring OS. PFS is not a surrogate for the latter but a valuable measure of a drug's effect on a tumor while it is administered. Finally, barring the emergence of a curative alternative, we would argue that experimental therapies should be tried early and often or that continued treatment with a therapy that has had some benefit should be explored as an alternative, guided by a measure such as the growth rate constant (Stein et al, TCJJPPO) to ensure that growth remains on a trajectory consistent with a prolonged survival.

## REFERENCES

1. Biomarkers and surrogate endpoints: preferred definitions and conceptual framework. *Clin Pharmacol Ther.* 2001;69:89–95.
2. Buyse M, ed. Is PFS a "Valid" Surrogate for OS in Advanced Ovarian Cancer? A Meta-Analysis. *Presented In FDA/ASCO/AACR Public Workshop on Endpoints for Ovarian Cancer 2006*; North Bethesda, MD; 2006.
3. Cleophas TJ, Zwinderman AH, Chaib AH. Novel procedures for validating surrogate endpoints in clinical trials. *Curr Clin Pharmacol.* 2007;2:123–128.
4. Beckman M. More clinical cancer treatments judged by progression-free rather than overall survival. *J Natl Cancer Inst.* 2007;99:1068–1069.
5. Bast RC, Thigpen JT, Arbuck SG, et al. Clinical trial endpoints in ovarian cancer: report of an FDA/ASCO/AACR Public Workshop. *Gynecol Oncol.* 2007;107:173–176.
6. Chakravarty A, Sridhara R. Use of progression-free survival as a surrogate marker in oncology trials: some regulatory issues. *Stat Methods Med Res.* 2008; 17:515–518.
7. Lassere MN, Johnson KR, Boers M, et al. Definitions and validation criteria for biomarkers and surrogate endpoints: development and testing of a quantitative hierarchical levels of evidence schema. *J Rheumatol.* 2007;34:607–615.
8. Johnson JR, Williams G, Pazdur R. End points and United States Food and Drug Administration approval of oncology drugs. *J Clin Oncol.* 2003;21:1404–1411.
9. Allegra C, Blanke C, Buyse M, et al. End points in advanced colon cancer clinical trials: a review and proposal. *J Clin Oncol.* 2007;25:3572–3575.
10. Christensen E. Choosing the best endpoint. *J Hepatol.* 2008;49:672–673.
11. Dhani N, Tu D, Sargent DJ, et al. Alternate endpoints for screening phase II studies. *Clin Cancer Res.* 2009;15:1873–1882.
12. Grothey A. Surrogate endpoints for overall survival in early colorectal cancer from the clinician's perspective. *Stat Methods Med Res.* 2008;17:529–535.
13. Hughes MD. Practical issues arising in an exploratory analysis evaluating progression-free survival as a surrogate endpoint for overall survival in advanced colorectal cancer. *Stat Methods Med Res.* 2008;17:487–495.
14. Piedbois P, Buyse M. Endpoints and surrogate endpoints in colorectal cancer: a review of recent developments. *Curr Opin Oncol.* 2008;20:466–471.
15. Sargent DJ, Hayes DF. Assessing the measure of a new drug: is survival the only thing that matters? *J Clin Oncol.* 2008;26:1922–1923.
16. Shi Q, Sargent DJ. Meta-analysis for the evaluation of surrogate endpoints in cancer clinical trials. *Int J Clin Oncol.* 2009;14:102–111.

17. Buyse M, Burzykowski T, Carroll K, et al. Progression-free survival is a surrogate for survival in advanced colorectal cancer. *J Clin Oncol.* 2007;25:5218–5224.

18. Burzykowski T, Buyse M, Piccart-Gebhart MJ, et al. Evaluation of tumor response, disease control, progression-free survival, and time to progression as potential surrogate end points in metastatic breast cancer. *J Clin Oncol.* 2008;26:1987–1992.

19. Buyse M, Burzykowski T, Michiels S, et al. Individual- and trial-level surrogacy in colorectal cancer. *Stat Methods Med Res.* 2008;17:467–475.

20. Di Leo A, Buyse M, Bleiberg H. Is overall survival a realistic primary end point in advanced colorectal cancer studies? A critical assessment based on four clinical trials comparing fluorouracil plus leucovorin with the same treatment combined either with oxaliplatin or with CPT-11. *Ann Oncol.* 2004;15:545–549.

21. Golfinopoulos V, Salanti G, Pavlidis N, et al. Survival and disease-progression benefits with treatment regimens for advanced colorectal cancer: a meta-analysis. *Lancet Oncol.* 2007;8:898–911.

22. Hackshaw A, Knight A, Barrett-Lee P, et al. Surrogate markers and survival in women receiving first-line combination anthracycline chemotherapy for advanced breast cancer. *Br J Cancer.* 2005;93:1215–1221.

23. Korn EL, Liu PY, Lee SJ, et al. Meta-analysis of phase II cooperative group trials in metastatic stage IV melanoma to determine progression-free and overall survival benchmarks for future phase II trials. *J Clin Oncol.* 2008;26:527–534.

24. Michiels S, Le Maitre A, Buyse M, et al. Surrogate endpoints for overall survival in locally advanced head and neck cancer: meta-analyses of individual patient data. *Lancet Oncol.* 2009;10:341–350.

25. Miksad RA, Zietemann V, Gothe R, et al. Progression-free survival as a surrogate endpoint in advanced breast cancer. *Int J Technol Assess Health Care.* 2008;24:371–383.

26. Sargent DJ, Patiyil S, Yothers G, et al. End points for colon cancer adjuvant trials: observations and recommendations based on individual patient data from 20,898 patients enrolled onto 18 randomized trials from the ACCENT Group. *J Clin Oncol.* 2007;25:4569–4574.

27. Sargent DJ, Wieand HS, Haller DG, et al. Disease-free survival versus overall survival as a primary end point for adjuvant colon cancer studies: individual patient data from 20,898 patients on 18 randomized trials. *J Clin Oncol.* 2005;23:8664–8670.

28. Sertdemir Y, Burgut R. Does the decision in a validation process of a surrogate endpoint change with level of significance of treatment effect? A proposal on validation of surrogate endpoints. *Contemp Clin Trials.* 2009;30:8–12.

29. Tang PA, Bentzen SM, Chen EX, et al. Surrogate end points for median overall survival in metastatic colorectal cancer: literature-based analysis from 39 randomized controlled trials of first-line chemotherapy. *J Clin Oncol.* 2007;25:4562–4568.

30. Fleming TR, Rothmann MD, Lu HL. Issues in Using Progression-Free Survival When Evaluating Oncology Products. *J Clin Oncol.* 2009;27:2874–2880.

31. Saad ED, Katz A. Progression-free survival and time to progression as primary end points in advanced breast cancer: often used, sometimes loosely defined. *Ann Oncol.* 2009;20:460–464.

32. Panageas KS, Ben-Porat L, Dickler MN, et al. When you look matters: the effect of assessment schedule on progression-free survival. *J Natl Cancer Inst.* 2007;99:428–432.

33. Burzykowski T. Surrogate endpoints: wishful thinking or reality?. *Stat Methods Med Res.* 2008;17:463–466.

34. Ballman KV, Buckner JC, Brown PD, et al. The relationship between six-month progression-free survival and 12-month overall survival end points for phase II trials in patients with glioblastoma multiforme. *Neuro Oncol.* 2007;9:29–38.

35. Johnson KR, Ringland C, Stokes BJ, et al. Response rate or time to progression as predictors of survival in trials of metastatic colorectal cancer or non-small-cell lung cancer: a meta-analysis. *Lancet Oncol.* 2006;7:741–746.

36. Milella M, Bria E, Carlini P, et al. Surrogate endpoints for overall survival (OS) in advanced pancreatic cancer (APC): Analysis of randomized clinical trials (RCTs) exploring gemcitabine (G)-based combinations. *J Clin Oncol* [meeting abstracts]. 2007;25(18 suppl):4575.

37. Sargent D. General and statistical hierarchy of appropriate biologic endpoints. *Oncology (Williston Park).* 2006;20(6 suppl 5):5–9.

38. Dodd LE, Korn EL, Freidlin B, et al. Blinded independent central review of progression-free survival in phase III clinical trials: important design element or unnecessary expense? *J Clin Oncol.* 2008;26:3791–3796.

39. Pazdur R. Endpoints for assessing drug activity in clinical trials. *Oncologist.* 2008;13(suppl 2):19–21.

40. Yothers G. Toward progression-free survival as a primary end point in advanced colorectal cancer. *J Clin Oncol.* 2007;25:5153–5154.

41. SAS version 9.1 software. SAS Institute, Inc. Cary, NC. Copyright 2002–2003, SAS Institute Inc.

42. Ashburner M, Ball CA, Blake JA, et al. Gene Ontology: tool for the unification of biology. *Nat Genet.* 2000;25:25–29.

43. Nagarajan V. Gene List Venn Diagram. Available at: http://www.bioinformatics.org/gvenn/index.htm.

44. Stordal B, Davey R. A systematic review of genes involved in the inverse resistance relationship between cisplatin and paclitaxel chemotherapy: role of BRCA1. *Curr Cancer Drug Targets.* 2009;9:354–365.

45. Wilson TR, Johnston PG, Longley DB. Anti-apoptotic mechanisms of drug resistance in cancer. *Curr Cancer Drug Targets.* 2009;9:307–319.

46. Hector S, Prehn JH. Apoptosis signaling proteins as prognostic biomarkers in colorectal cancer: a review. *Biochim Biophys Acta.* 2009;1795:117–129.

47. Savage P, Stebbing J, Bower M, Crook T, et al. Why does cytotoxic chemotherapy cure only some cancers? *Nat Clin Pract Oncol.* 2009;6:43–52.

48. Broxterman HJ, Gotink KJ, Verheul HM. Understanding the causes of multidrug resistance in cancer: a comparison of doxorubicin and sunitinib. *Drug Resist Updat.* In press.

49. El Maalouf G, Le Tourneau C, Batty GN, et al. Markers involved in resistance to cytotoxics and targeted therapeutics in pancreatic cancer. *Cancer Treat Rev.* 2009;35:167–174.

50. Muggia F. Platinum compounds 30 years after the introduction of cisplatin: implications for the treatment of ovarian cancer. *Gynecol Oncol.* 2009;112:275–281.

51. Borst P, Rottenberg S, Jonkers J. How do real tumors become resistant to cisplatin? *Cell Cycle.* 2008;7:1353–1359.

52. Stein WD, Yang J, Bates SE, et al. Bevacizumab reduces the growth rate constants of renal carcinomas: a novel algorithm suggests early discontinuation of bevacizumab resulted in a lack of survival advantage. *Oncologist.* 2008;13:1055–1062.

53. Rixe O, Fojo T. Is cell death a critical end point for anticancer therapies or is cytostasis sufficient? *Clin Cancer Res.* 2007;13:7280–7287.

54. National Cancer Institute. FDA Approval for Pemetrexed Disodium. 2009. Available at: http://www.cancer.gov/cancertopics/druginfo/fda-pemetrexed-disodium. Accessed September 2, 2009.

55. Belani CP, Brodowicz T, Ciuleanu T, et al. Maintenance pemetrexed (Pem) plus best supportive care (BSC) versus placebo (Plac) plus BSC: A randomized phase III study in advanced non-small cell lung cancer (NSCLC) [meeting abstracts]. *J Clin Oncol.* 2009;27(18 suppl):CRA8000.

56. Patel JD, Bonomi P, Socinski MA, et al. Treatment rationale and study design for the pointbreak study: a randomized, open-label phase III study of pemetrexed/carboplatin/bevacizumab followed by maintenance pemetrexed/bevacizumab versus paclitaxel/carboplatin/bevacizumab followed by maintenance bevacizumab in patients with stage IIIB or IV nonsquamous non-small-cell lung cancer. *Clin Lung Cancer.* 2009;10:252–256.

57. Miller K, Wang M, Gralow J, et al. Paclitaxel plus bevacizumab versus paclitaxel alone for metastatic breast cancer. *N Engl J Med.* 2007;357:2666–2676.

58. Schneider BP, Wang M, Radovich M, et al. Association of vascular endothelial growth factor and vascular endothelial growth factor receptor-2 genetic polymorphisms with outcome in a trial of paclitaxel compared with paclitaxel plus bevacizumab in advanced breast cancer: ECOG 2100. *J Clin Oncol.* 2008;26:4672–4678.

59. Paez-Ribes M, Allen E, Hudock J, et al. Antiangiogenic therapy elicits malignant progression of tumors to increased local invasion and distant metastasis. *Cancer Cell.* 2009;15:220–231.

60. Ebos JM, Lee CR, Cruz-Munoz W, et al. Accelerated metastasis after short-term treatment with a potent inhibitor of tumor angiogenesis. *Cancer Cell.* 2009;15:232–239.

61. Loges S, Mazzone M, Hohensinner P, et al. Silencing or fueling metastasis with VEGF inhibitors: antiangiogenesis revisited. *Cancer Cell.* 2009;15:167–170.

# Progression-Free Survival

## Gaining on Overall Survival as a Gold Standard and Accelerating Drug Development

David Lebwohl • Andrea Kay • William Berg • Jean Francois Baladi • Ji Zheng

Overall survival (OS) is considered the gold standard for efficacy evaluation in randomized, controlled clinical trials of anticancer agents, because increased OS represents a direct measure of patient benefit and is assessed easily and objectively.[1–3] Regulatory agencies such as the United States Food and Drug Administration (US FDA) and the European Medicines Agency (EMEA) accept OS as an appropriate measure of clinical benefit.[3,4] However, with the advent of more effective therapies in a variety of cancer types, a benefit in OS is becoming more difficult to demonstrate in clinical trials, and its use could impede the rapid development of novel effective therapies. First, measurement of OS typically requires a long follow-up period, particularly as patients are living longer with improved therapies. Second, a large patient population is required to ensure that significant differences in OS between treatment arms will be detectable. Third, measurement of OS is vulnerable to the confounding effects of subsequent therapy; patients who show progressive disease after treatment with the drug of interest are typically discontinued from that agent and switched to another, the effects of which may contribute to OS.[1] In addition, for ethical reasons, many cancer clinical trials now incorporate a cross-over design, such that patients whose disease progresses in one arm of the trial may be crossed over to another arm to receive a more effective treatment; this practice confounds OS assessments for both arms.[3] As a result, reliance on OS as a primary end point for oncology drug approval may delay or even impede patient access to new effective treatments for a life-threatening illness.

Progression-free survival (PFS) is also an important end point for patients in whom it may reflect clinical benefit, directly or indirectly, in terms of the length of time to disease progression or death.[3] In some cancers for which PFS has been shown to be reasonably likely associated with clinical benefit, such as ovarian cancer, PFS may be used as a surrogate for OS in clinical trials.[5] Measurement of PFS requires a shorter period of time and a smaller population than measurement of OS, and PFS results are not confounded by the use of subsequent therapy.[3] For these reasons, PFS is a useful measure that has served as a primary end point for drug approval by both the US FDA and the EMEA.[1,3,4]

The aims of this study are to discuss the limitations of using OS as a primary efficacy end point in the setting of evolving cancer therapies and to put forth PFS as an alternative efficacy end point in cancer types to which it is best suited.

## METHODS

Published articles and other reference materials were identified through PubMed searches and a general Internet search. Search terms included PFS, primary end point, efficacy, OS, surrogate, cancer, approval, guidelines, and oncology.

## RESULTS

### Current Challenges to Using OS to Assess Cancer Treatments

#### OS: Definition and Attributes as an Endpoint for Clinical Trials in Oncology

OS is defined as the time from subject randomization to the time of death from any cause and is an objective, reliable clinical trial end point.[1,3] First, it is measured in the intent-to-treat population, which includes all subjects randomized to treatment, regardless of whether they receive the treatment. A second advantage of OS over other end points used in cancer clinical trials is that the subject's date of death is an exact, known data point that is not subject to investigator bias.[3] A third attribute is that statistically significant improvements in OS are considered clinically significant, provided the drug does not have unacceptable toxicity.[3] For these reasons, OS is accepted as the gold standard for efficacy evaluation in clinical trials of oncology agents.

#### Limitations of OS as an Endpoint in Clinical Trials

Although OS as an end point has clear and attractive attributes, it also suffers from limitations, some of which are increasingly problematic. These are discussed in this section, but can be summarized as (1) the problem of increased OS in cancer patients, (2) the need for large populations, (3) the confounding effect of posttrial therapies, and (4) the problem of cross-over designs. Despite its strengths, OS is not always the most appropriate primary end point to use in some cancer clinical trials.

First, in recent years, OS has improved in many types of cancer as a result of the development of more effective agents; thus, its measurement now requires increasingly longer follow-up periods. For example, results of a retrospective, population-based study conducted in Canada demonstrated that median OS in subjects with metastatic breast cancer increased from 14 months in subjects diagnosed in 1991–1992 to almost 22 months in subjects diagnosed in 1999–2001.[6] Improved OS has also been observed in colorectal cancer with the availability of irinotecan- and oxaliplatin-based combinations. Grothey et al conducted a review of seven phase III trials evaluating first-line therapy with various combinations of 5-fluorouracil/leucovorin, irinotecan, and oxaliplatin to determine the effects of active salvage therapies, and more specifically, the availability of all three treatments, on OS in patients with advanced colorectal cancer. Studies in which a high percentage of patients had access to all three treatments during the course of their treatment demonstrated a strong correlation with reported median OS (ie, patients with access to all three treatment had the longest OS; $P = 0.0008$). In addition, patients treated with first-line combinations had a predicted 3.5-month improvement in median OS versus monotherapy.[7] Consequently, if regulatory approval of a new agent in settings such as these is based on a demonstrated improvement in OS, patients will be required to wait a long time, and longer than in previous years, for access to a medication that is more effective than those currently available.

A second hurdle to the use of OS as a primary end point is that a large patient population is required to show statistically significant differences among treatments, and as comparator treatments continue to improve, statistical rules dictate that the sample size required to show significant differences among treatments will increase.[8] Some cancer types associated with limited clinical trial accruals would have considerable difficulty in obtaining study populations of a size necessary to show significant differences. Long survival durations often lead to subjects becoming lost to follow-up, which also impacts statistical analyses.

Third, the measurement of OS may be skewed by other events, posttrial treatment protocols, and ethically mandated clinical trial designs. By definition, the deaths measured are due to any cause; therefore, the time of death of a subject who dies from unrelated causes is included in the OS calculation, even though disease- or treatment-related death may not have occurred until much later. The influence of subsequent therapy that a subject receives after showing disease progression on the experimental agent may skew the OS, which will be attributed solely to the experimental agent. This may happen after the subject completes the trial or within the confines of the trial itself, because clinical trials with a cross-over design enable patients receiving less-effective therapy to switch to more effective therapy on disease progression.

Fourth, the confounding effects of subsequent therapy on OS remain a challenge, particularly as more trials adopt a cross-over design or allow cross-over at the time that the trial result for PFS is positive. Recently, in an attempt to circumvent the effect of cross-over on treatment-effect estimates for OS, investigators invoked a statistical method, the rank-preserving structural failure time (RPSFT) analysis, in a post hoc analysis of data from a phase III trial of the multikinase inhibitor sunitinib in imatinib-refractory patients with advanced gastrointestinal stromal tumors.[9] In the RPSFT model (and other failure time models), the subjects of the trial assume that they remain on the treatment to which they were randomized in its prediction of OS, making this analysis potentially valuable in trials with a cross-over design. However, this method is new to use in clinical oncology trials and has not yet been accepted by the FDA or the EMEA for use in drug labeling.

### OS and Regulatory Agencies

In 2003, the FDA reported that it had granted 71 new cancer drug approvals from 1990 to 2002 based on several end points and not just OS. OS was the basis for approval of 18 of 57 drugs that received regular approval; the remaining 39 received regular approval based on direct or indirect evidence of clinical benefit and 14 received accelerated approval, meaning that they showed evidence of benefit over available agents for a serious or life-threatening disease, but had not yet met the standard for regular approval (Table 1).[10] This is a testimony to the fact that OS is not the unique outcome required by the FDA to be the primary efficacy end point in every case. The current Guidance on Clinical Trial End points for the Approval of Cancer Drugs and Biologics recommends that applicants meet with the FDA before submitting protocols to support a new drug application or a biologics license application to discuss planned clinical trial end points.[3] Similarly, the EMEA does not require OS to be the primary efficacy end point in every case. In 2005, the EMEA reported that of 28 cancer drug approvals between 2000 and 2004, six were

based on OS, with 11 based on PFS and 11 on response rate.[11] The EMEA Guideline on the Evaluation of Anticancer Medicinal Products in Man recommends that OS should be used as the primary end point if major differences in toxicity are expected in favor of the control regimen, if no evidence-based, next-line therapies are available, and if the time from disease progression to death is expected to be short.[4] Both agencies recommend that if PFS is used as the primary end point, OS should be included as a secondary end point.[2,4,5]

In summary, OS is an appropriate and preferred efficacy end point in situations for which it is achievable (eg, clinical trial that does not contain a cross-over design, cancer type associated with short OS), but in situations where its measurement is not feasible, PFS may be a clinically meaningful and relevant alternative primary efficacy end point.

## The Validity and Use of PFS

### PFS: Definition and Attributes as an Endpoint for Clinical Trials in Oncology

PFS is defined as the time from subject randomization to objective tumor progression or death from any cause.[3] PFS is a time-dependent end point based on tumor measurements[3]; therefore, the precise way PFS is measured varies among clinical trials according to the definition of progression used and the time points for assessment established.[3,12]

First, PFS is a valid efficacy end point that has clinical relevance, because it reflects tumor growth. Second, its measurement requires a shorter time (ie, before death) and a smaller population than that of OS (ie, for a given sample size, the magnitude of effect on PFS can be greater than that of OS). Third, the measurement of PFS is subject to fewer uncontrolled variables affecting its outcome, and it is not affected by the effects of subsequent therapies because it is measured before their initiation.[3] Finally, PFS is accepted by both the FDA and the EMEA as a credible end point in clinical oncology trials.[2,4,10] The FDA recommends that PFS can be considered as a primary efficacy end point on a case-by-case basis,[2] and the EMEA considers PFS to be an acceptable primary end point in cases in which subsequent treatments are expected to affect OS in which demonstration of noninferiority is the goal of the trial and in which evidence-based next-line therapies are available.[4]

### Limitations of PFS as an Endpoint in Clinical Trials

Similar to OS, PFS as an end point has clear and attractive attributes but also suffers from limitations. These are discussed in this section, but can be summarized as (1) the need to assess the relationship with OS for every cancer, (2) the need for clear definitions, and (3) the problems of errors and bias therapies. Although there are many advantages of PFS, investigators must be aware of the caveats to the use of PFS when designing clinical trials.[2,3,12]

First, it is important to understand that the relationship between PFS and OS must be assessed thoroughly for each cancer type; not all cancers or all anticancer agents for which an improvement in PFS is observed will demonstrate an improvement in OS.[2,3] Second, a clear definition of disease progression is needed in each case. No standard regulatory criteria for defining progression exist[3]; definitions of progression typically rely on criteria such as the Response Evaluation Criteria in Solid Tumors[13] or the World Health Organization response criteria.[14]

Third, one must recognize that regardless of the definition chosen, the data obtained are subject to measurement error and bias.[12] It has been recommended that results could be analyzed by blinded independent central review as opposed to investigator review to minimize potential bias.[3] In fact, central review has been recommended

**TABLE 1.** Endpoints for Approval of Oncology Drug Marketing Applications January 1, 1990 to November 1, 2002

| Drug (yr, Application Type) | Indication | Approval Type | Endpoints Supporting Approval | Trial Design |
|---|---|---|---|---|
| Altretamine (1990, N) | Refractory ovarian cancer | Regular | RR | SAT |
| Altretinoin gel (1999, N) | Kaposi sarcoma, cutaneous lesions | Regular | RR, cosmesis | RCT |
| Amifostine | | | | |
|   1995, N | To decrease cisplatin-induced renal toxicity in refractory ovarian cancer | Regular | Creatinine clearance, CR and TTP to assess potential tumor protection | RCT |
|   1996, S | To decrease cisplatin-induced renal toxicity in lung cancer | AA | Creatine clearance, RR to assess tumor protection | SAT |
|   1999, S | To decrease xerostomia after radiation therapy for head and neck cancer | Regular | Salivary production and xerostomia scores | RCT |
| Anastrozole | | | | |
|   1995, N | Breast cancer, second-line treatment | Regular | RR, TTP | DB RCT |
|   2000, S | Breast cancer, first-line treatment | Regular | RR, TTP | DB RCT |
|   2002, S | Breast cancer, adjuvant therapy of postmenopausal patients with ER-positive tumors | AA | DFS | DB RCT |
| Arsenic trioxide (2000, N) | Acute promyelocytic leukemia, second-line treatment | Regular | CR and CR duration | SAT |
| Bexarotene capsules (1999, N) | Cutaneous T-cell lymphoma, skin lesions | Regular | RR, composite assessment of index lesion severity | SAT |
| Bexarotene gel (2000, N) | Cutaneous T-cell lymphoma, skin lesions | Regular | RR, composite assessment of index lesion severity | SAT |
| Bleomycin (1996, S) | Malignant pleural effusions | Regular | Recurrence of effusion | RCT |
| Busulfan injection (1999, S) | CML, conditioning regimen for stem-cell transplantation | Regular | DFS, time to engraftment | RCT |
| Capecitabine | | | | |
|   1998, N | Breast cancer, refractory | AA | RR | SAT |
|   2001, S | Colon cancer, first-line treatment | Regular | Survival | RCT |
|   2001, S | Breast cancer, with docetaxel after failed anthracycline treatment | Regular | Survival | RCT |
| Carboplatin (1991, S) | Ovarian cancer, first-line treatment | Regular | Pathologic CR, PFS, survival | RCT |
| Carmustine wafer (1996, N) | Recurrent glioblastoma multiforme | Regular | Survival | Placebo RCT |
| Cladribine (1993, N) | Hairy cell leukemia | Regular | CR and CR duration | SAT |
| Dexrazoxane (1995, N) | To decrease doxorubicin-induced cardiotoxicity | AA | Cardiotoxicity (clinical and MUGA scans), RR to assess potential tumor protection | Placebo RCT |
| Docetaxel | | | | |
|   1996, N | Breast cancer, second-line treatment | AA | RR | SAT |
|   1996, S | Breast cancer, second-line treatment | Regular | RR, TTP, survival | RCT |
|   1999, S | NSCLC, second-line treatment | Regular | TTP and survival | RCT |
| Epirubicin (1999, N) | Breast cancer, adjuvant treatment | Regular | DFS and survival | RCT |
| Exemestane (1999, N) | Breast cancer, second-line treatment | Regular | RR and TTP | DB RCT |
| Fludarabine (1991, N) | Refractory chronic lymphocytic leukemia | Regular | CR and PR, improvement in anemia and thrombocytopenia | SAT |
| Fulvestrant (2002, N) | Breast cancer, second-line treatment | Regular | RR and TTP | DB RCT |

*(continued)*

**TABLE 1.** *(Continued)*

| Drug (yr, Application Type) | Indication | Approval Type | Endpoints Supporting Approval | Trial Design |
|---|---|---|---|---|
| Gemcitabine | | | | |
| 1996, N | Pancreatic cancer | Regular | Survival, clinical benefit response (composite end point including pain, performance status, and weight gain) | RCT |
| 1998, S | NSCLC | Regular | RR, TTP, survival | RCT |
| Gemtuzumab ozogamicin (2000, N) | Acute myelogenous leukemia, second-line treatment in elderly patients | AA | CR and CRp (CR with decreased platelets) | SAT |
| Idarubicin (1990, N) | Acute myelogenous leukemia | Regular | CR and survival | RCT |
| Imatinib mesylate | | | | |
| 2001, N | CML, blast phase, accelerated phase, and failing interferon | AA | Hematologic response and cytogenetic response | SAT |
| 2002, S | Gastrointestinal stromal tumors (GISTs) | AA | RR | SAT |
| Irinotecan | | | | |
| 1996, N | Colon cancer, second-line treatment | AA | RR | SAT |
| 1998, S | Colon cancer, second-line treatment | Regular | Survival | RCT |
| 2000, S | Colon cancer, first-line treatment | Regular | Survival | RCT |
| Letrozole | | | | |
| 1997, N | Breast cancer, second-line treatment | Regular | RR, TTP | DB RCT |
| 2001, S | Breast cancer, first-line treatment | Regular | RR, TTP | DB RCT |
| Leucovorin (1991, S) | In combination with FU for metastatic colon cancer | Regular | Survival | RCT |
| Liposomal cytarabine (1999, N) | Lymphomatous meningitis | AA | Cytologic response | RCT |
| Liposomal daunorubicin (1996, N) | Kaposi sarcoma | Regular | RR, TTP, cosmesis | RCT |
| Liposomal doxorubicin | | | | |
| 1995, N | Kaposi sarcoma, second-line treatment | AA | RR | SAT |
| 1999, S | Ovarian cancer, refractory | AA | RR | SAT |
| Methoxsalen (1999, N) | Cutaneous T-cell lymphoma, skin lesions | Regular | RR based on overall skin scores, improvement in edema and scaling, and fissure resolution | SAT |
| Mitoxantrone (1996, S) | Patients with pain from hormone-refractory advanced prostate cancer | Regular | Decrease in pain | RCT |
| Oxaliplatin (2002, N) | Colon cancer progression after bolus 5-FU/LV and irinotecan | AA | RR and TTP | RCT |
| Paclitaxel | | | | |
| 1992, N | Refractory ovarian cancer | Regular | Durable PRs in bulky tumors | SAT |
| 1994, S | Breast cancer, second-line treatment | Regular | TTP | Dose-response RCT |
| 1997, S | Kaposi sarcoma | Regular | RR and clinical benefit (assessed by evaluating photographs) | SAT |
| 1998, S | Ovarian, first-line | Regular | Survival | RCT |
| 1998, S | NSCLC | Regular | TTP and survival | RCT |
| 1999, S | Breast cancer, adjuvant therapy | Regular | DFS and survival | RCT |
| Pamidronate | | | | |
| 1995, N | Skeletal morbidity of osteolytic bone metastases of myeloma | Regular | SRE | Placebo RCT |
| 1996, S | Skeletal morbidity of osteolytic bone metastases of breast cancer | Regular | SRE | Placebo RCT |

*(continued)*

**TABLE 1.** *(Continued)*

| Drug (yr, Application Type) | Indication | Approval Type | Endpoints Supporting Approval | Trial Design |
|---|---|---|---|---|
| Pentostatin | | | | |
| 1991, N | Hairy cell leukemia, second-line treatment | Regular | CR and CR duration, improvement in hemoglobin, WBC, platelets | SAT |
| 1993, S | Hairy cell leukemia, first-line treatment | Regular | CR and CR duration | RCT |
| Porfimer sodium | | | | |
| 1995, N | For PDT in completely obstructed esophageal cancer | Regular | Luminal response and palliative response | SAT |
| 1998, S | For PDT of CIS and microinvasive NSCLC | Regular | CR and CR duration | SAT |
| 1998, S | For PDT of completely or partially obstructing endobronchial NSCLC | Regular | Luminal response and pulmonary symptom severity scale | RCT |
| Talc (1997, N) | To prevent recurrence of malignant pleural effusion | Regular | Recurrence of effusion | RCT |
| Tamoxifen | | | | |
| 1990, S | Node-negative breast cancer, adjuvant therapy | Regular | DFS | Placebo RCT |
| 1998, S | To reduce the incidence of breast cancer in women at high risk | Regular | Occurrence of breast cancer | Placebo RCT |
| 2000, S | To reduce the incidence of breast cancer after treatment of DCIS | Regular | Occurrence of breast cancer | Placebo RCT |
| Temozolomide (1999, N) | Anaplastic astrocytoma, refractory | AA | RR | SAT |
| Teniposide (1992, N) | Refractory childhood acute lymphoplastic leukemia | Regular | CR and CR duration | SAT |
| Topotecan | | | | |
| 1996, N | Ovarian cancer, second-line treatment | Regular | RR, TTP, survival | RCT |
| 1998, S | Small-cell lung cancer, second-line treatment | Regular | RR and response duration, symptom improvement | RCT |
| Toremifene (1997, N) | Breast cancer, first-line treatment | Regular | RR, TTP | RCT |
| Tretinoin (1995, N) | Acute promyelocytic leukemia, second-line treatment | Regular | CR | SAT |
| Vinorelbine (1994, N) | NSCLC | Regular | Survival | RCT |
| Zoledronic acid (2002, N) | Multiple myeloma and bone metastases from solid tumors | Regular | SRE | |

N indicates new drug application; RR, response rate; SAT, single-arm trial; RCT, randomized controlled trial; S, supplement; CR, complete response; TTP, time to progression; AA, accelerated approval; DB, double blind; ER, estrogen receptor; DFS, disease-free survival; CML, chronic myelogenous leukemia; PFS, progression-free survival; MUGA, multiple-gated acquisition; FU, fluorouracil; LV, leucovorin; PDT, photodynamic therapy; CIS, carcinoma-in-situ; NSCLC, non-small-cell lung cancer; DCIA, ductal carcinoma-in-situ; SRE, skeletal-related event.

as the gold standard for pivotal studies in solid tumors in which objective response or PFS is the primary end point. The discrepancy rates between central and local review usually range from 24% to 40%.[15,16] The most common reasons for these discrepancies are the reviewer's selection of different lesions and/or differences in classification of lesions as measurable versus nonmeasurable but evaluable. In addition, obvious differences occur if films are available for local review but missing for the central review. However, blinded independent central review may not provide an unbiased estimate of treatment effectiveness. Within the independent central reviewers, interreader discordance rates of up to 38.6% have been reported.[16] Furthermore, in a review of phase III oncology trials that used blinded independent central review, differences between the local and central review did not result in different conclusions about treatment efficacy, despite the relatively high discrepancy rates.[17] Nevertheless, PFS by independent

central review remains the gold standard for industry-sponsored phase III studies submitted for health authority approval.

PFS is subject to evaluation-time bias (ie, differences in evaluation times according to treatment arms), and thus appropriate time points for measuring progression must be established. The Response Evaluation Criteria in Solid Tumors and World Health Organization criteria, as well as other sets of criteria, do not specify time intervals for tumor assessment. Unlike the situation for OS, the exact date of tumor progression is unknown, representing another source of measurement error.[12] The FDA recommends assigning the progression date to the earliest time progression documented without prior missing assessments and censoring at the date when the last radiologic assessment showed lack of progression.[3] Given that the actual time of progression occurs at some point between two scheduled assessments, the frequency with which progression is measured must be based on

**TABLE 2.** FDA-Identified Issues to Consider in PFS Analysis[3]

| Issue | Key Points |
|---|---|
| Definition of progression date | Suggested recorded progression dates include: |
| | That assigned to the first time at which progression can be declared (first observation of new lesion or date of predefined increase in the sum of the target lesion measurements) |
| | That of the protocol-scheduled clinic visit immediately after all radiologic assessments that collectively document progression have been carried out |
| Definition of censoring date | Last date on which progression status was adequately assessed in patients with no documented progression before data cutoff or dropout |
| Definition of an adequate PFS evaluation | Includes adequacy of target lesion assessments and radiologic tests to evaluate nontarget lesions and search for new lesions |
| Analysis of partially missing tumor data | Describe the method for calculating progression status when data are partially missing from adequate tumor assessment visits |
| Completely missing tumor data | Detail primary and secondary PFS analyses to evaluate the potential effect of missing data, incorporating reasons for dropouts |
| Progression of nonmeasurable disease | Specify criteria for each assessment modality |
| | Scans documenting progression based on nonmeasurable disease should be verified by blinded review |
| Suspicious lesions | Include an algorithm for evaluating and following indeterminate lesions for progression assessment |

the characteristics of the type of cancer being treated and must be balanced across treatment arms.[2,3,12] To enable informative results to be generated, the definition of progression and the time points identified for its measurement must be consistent across trials within a specific cancer type. Table 2 summarizes issues that the FDA recommends investigators to consider when planning a PFS analysis.[3]

PFS as a Surrogate and the View of Regulatory Agencies

PFS has been suggested as a surrogate to OS in oncology clinical trials. A validated surrogate end point is one that accurately predicts clinical efficacy; validation has been defined as the formal establishment that the effect of the intervention on the surrogate end point reliably predicts the effect of the intervention on the clinical end point.[18] The process of validating a surrogate end point is burdensome, time-consuming, and, from a statistical perspective, requires a pooled or meta-analysis of clinical trial data to demonstrate a consistency of effect.[18] However, in addition to its potential role as a surrogate OS in some types of cancer, PFS may itself represent a measure of clinical benefit of a treatment. The FDA guidance states that an improvement in PFS represents a direct clinical benefit or a surrogate of clinical benefit depends on the magnitude of the effect and the risk-benefit of

the treatment compared with existing treatments.[2,3] According to the EMEA guidelines, if PFS is the primary end point then OS must be reported as a secondary end point, with sufficient data collection to ensure that there are no relevant negative effects on OS.[4] Regardless of the end point chosen, a favorable risk-benefit should be established.[4] The potential clinical benefit of prolonged PFS could also include the patient perspective of the treatment effect. Prolonged PFS may be associated with improvements in quality of life (QOL) or disease symptoms. For example, if tumor progression is associated with disease symptoms and the patient's assessment of their QOL, and if delaying tumor progression delays the occurrence of symptoms, then prolonged PFS could be considered a clinical benefit, provided the toxicity of the treatment is acceptable.

## Examples of Cancer Types in Which PFS has Gained Value Versus OS

### Ovarian Cancer

A series of public workshops were undertaken by the FDA, in conjunction with the American Society of Clinical Oncology, the American Association for Cancer Research, the American Society of Hematology, and the National Cancer Institute to obtain feedback on clinical trial efficacy end points for anticancer agents in a variety of cancers.[1] Issues identified, including goals of therapy and trial end points that reflect those goals, were subsequently discussed in meetings of the Oncologic Drugs Advisory Committee, and the outcomes were used to draft guidances on clinical end points for oncology drug approvals in specific types of cancer.

As a result of this process, the FDA has accepted PFS as a surrogate for OS in advanced ovarian cancer in assessments of first-line therapies.[19] Data from seven US-based trials (Gynecologic Oncology Group Trials 97, 111, 152, 52, 158, 114, and 172) and six ex-US trials (ICON 2, ICON3, AGO/GINECO, AGO OVAR 3, OV 10, and EORTC Surg) demonstrated an association of PFS with OS, particularly when the PFS effect was large. Thus in this clinical setting, PFS predicts survival improvement. It was agreed that the availability of improved treatments for recurrent ovarian cancer will make significant increases in OS with first-line therapy more difficult to achieve. PFS was also recognized by the FDA as an independent measure of clinical benefit in first-line therapy for advanced ovarian cancer, because it enabled patients to have increased time of therapy without experiencing disease progression.[5,19]

### Colorectal Cancer

The improvements in OS achieved with current treatments for advanced colorectal cancer (CRC) complicate the use of OS as a primary efficacy end point for the evaluation of new drugs. To identify appropriate alternative end points for OS, a literature-based analysis of 39 randomized controlled trials of first-line therapy for advanced CRC in 18,668 patients was carried out. Results demonstrated an association of PFS with OS; each of the trials that found a significant difference in OS also found a significant difference in PFS or time to progression. A strong correlation between PFS and OS was reported ($r_s = 0.79$), which was significantly higher than that for time to progression and OS ($r_s = 0.24$, $P = 0.001$).[20] Shortly thereafter, PFS was validated as a surrogate end point for OS in advanced CRC using data from 10 historical trials and three validation trials. Each trial had a fluorouracil + leucovorin treatment group, and comparators were fluorouracil or raltitrexed in the historical trials and irinotecan or oxaliplatin in the validation trials.[21] The validity of PFS was assessed with a correlation approach. Correlations between treatment effects were estimated in the historical trials and used to predict effects on OS in the validation

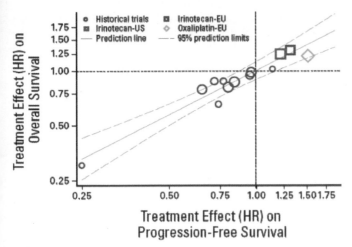

**FIGURE 1.** PFS is a validated surrogate for OS in advanced colorectal cancer: correlation of treatment effects on PFS with treatment effects on OS. Reprinted from Buyse et al,[21] with permission. Copyright American Society of Clinical Oncology, 2008. All rights reserved.

trials based on PFS effects in the validation trials. Results indicated a correlation coefficient of 0.82 between PFS and OS. Treatment effects on PFS and OS were also highly correlated, as shown in Figure 1, providing evidence of validation of PFS as a surrogate for OS in advanced CRC.[21] It has been argued that PFS is a credible primary end point in advanced CRC independent of its validation as a surrogate for OS, because PFS is a more sensitive indicator of treatment effect, because it counts progression events and is less sensitive to subsequent therapy compared with OS.[22] The findings in advanced ovarian cancer and advanced CRC set a precedent for the use of PFS as a primary end point in oncology trials, and the applicability of PFS in other types of cancers is currently under investigation.

**Breast Cancer**

Attempts to validate PFS as a surrogate for OS in advanced breast cancer have shown that although an association of PFS with OS was present, the ability of treatment effects on PFS to predict treatment effects on OS was not strong enough to confer surrogacy.[23,24] However, it was suggested that the effects of subsequent therapies, including those from cross-over trials, interfered with establishment of

surrogacy of PFS for OS in these analyses and that PFS may be an appropriate primary end point on its own merit in advanced breast cancer.[8] Supporting this, the antivascular endothelial growth factor monoclonal antibody bevacizumab, in combination with paclitaxel, was granted accelerated approval by the FDA for the first-line treatment of metastatic HER2-negative breast cancer on the basis of its prolongation of median PFS versus paclitaxel alone (11.3 vs. 5.8 months, respectively, hazard ratio [HR] = 0.48, $P < 0.0001$).[25]

**Renal Cell Carcinoma**

During the past decade, research into new treatments for advanced renal cell carcinoma (RCC) has expanded rapidly. Given the number of potentially effective therapies, it has become more difficult for a new therapy to show a benefit in OS during current treatments for advanced RCC. In a review of 24 RCC clinical trials conducted at Memorial Sloan-Kettering Cancer Center between 1975 and 1996 (n = 670), the median OS was 10 months.[26] The introduction of molecular targeted therapies for advanced RCC has nearly doubled the observed median OS[27] and, thus, has called attention to PFS as a valuable primary efficacy end point (Table 3).[27–32] In 2005, the multikinase inhibitor sorafenib received regular approval for the treatment of advanced RCC based on a significant improvement in median PFS (5.5 vs. 2.8 months with placebo, $P < 0.001$) with acceptable toxicity.[27,33] Measurement of OS was confounded as a result of the trial's cross-over design. Although no previous studies in metastatic RCC had indicated that the magnitude of PFS prolongation was a clinical benefit or a predictor of OS, the FDA reviewed the outcomes of six previous trials with interferon (IFN)-$\alpha$ and various comparators and noted that they provided evidence of a link between PFS and OS improvement.[33] In 2007, the multikinase inhibitor, sunitinib, received regular approval for the treatment of advanced RCC, based on its prolongation of median PFS in a planned second interim analysis of a phase III trial (11 vs. 5 months with IFN-$\alpha$, HR = 0.42, $P < 0.001$).[28] Again, the OS result was confounded by crossover after a positive interim result for PFS, as in the case for sorafenib. A statistically significant difference in OS between the two treatment arms was not achieved at the final analysis presented at American Society of Clinical Oncology 2008, despite the results being clinically relevant.[34]

In Europe, the combination of bevacizumab and IFN-$\alpha$ was approved for first-line treatment of metastatic RCC based on a significant improvement in PFS (10.2 vs. 5.4 months with placebo + IFN-$\alpha$, HR = 0.63, $P = 0.0001$) in a phase III trial.[29] OS was the primary end point of the trial, but PFS was considered for regulatory submission, because new therapies had become available during the study and could have confounded the OS data.

**TABLE 3.** Use of PFS in Phase III Trials of Targeted Therapies for Advanced RCC

| Comparison (n) | Study Population | Basis for Regulatory Approval | Median PFS (mo) | References |
|---|---|---|---|---|
| Sorafenib (n = 384) Placebo (n = 385) | Metastatic RCC that had progressed after 1 systemic treatment | PFS | 5.5 2.8 | Escudier et al[27] |
| Sunitinib (n = 375) IFN-$\alpha$ (n = 375) | Untreated metastatic RCC | PFS | 11 5 | Motzer et al[28] |
| Bevacizumab + IFN-$\alpha$ (n = 327) Placebo + IFN-$\alpha$ (n = 322) | Untreated metastatic RCC | PFS | 10.2 5.4 | Escudier et al[29] |
| Temsirolimus (n = 209) IFN-$\alpha$ (n = 207) | Untreated, poor-prognosis, metastatic RCC | OS | 5.5 3.1 | Hudes et al[30] |
| Everolimus (n = 272) Placebo (n = 138) | Metastatic RCC that had progressed on sunitinib, sorafenib, or both | PFS | 4.9 1.9 | Motzer et al[31]; Kay et al[32] |

The oral mammalian target of rapamycin inhibitor everolimus was recently approved by the FDA for the treatment of advanced RCC that has progressed after targeted therapy with sorafenib or sunitinib, based on demonstration of a significant improvement in PFS (4.9 vs. 1.9 months with placebo, HR = 0.33, $P < 0.0001$) with acceptable toxicity in a phase III trial.[32] Because the trial design allowed crossover to everolimus on disease progression on placebo, >80% of the patients randomized to placebo crossed over to everolimus and the OS data from this trial were confounded.

The totality of the data in metastatic RCC suggests an association of PFS with OS, and PFS has been proposed as a clinically meaningful and relevant end point in metastatic RCC.[35] Delea et al[36] conducted a systematic review of 21 controlled studies involving patients with metastatic RCC to evaluate the association between treatment effects on disease-progression end points and treatment effects on OS. The 21 studies reviewed included 6182 patients and 52 treatment groups; 35 comparisons were identified. The median difference between disease-progression end points and median OS averaged 2.8 months. The correlation between differences in median time to disease progression and differences in median OS was 0.69 ($P < 0.0001$). In a weighted ordinary least squares regression model, a 1-month difference in disease progression was associated with a 1.4-month difference in OS ($P < 0.001$). Thus, treatment effects on disease-progression end points seem to be predictive of treatment effects on OS in patients with metastatic RCC.

## Alternative Endpoints

The value of other alternative primary end points in oncology is also under investigation. For instance, disease-free survival (DFS), which is defined as the time from randomization until recurrence of the tumor or death from any cause,[3] has been shown to be associated with OS in adjuvant therapy for CRC. In this setting, which has a long timeline and typically involves many subsequent therapies, OS is time consuming to measure. A pooled analysis of data from 18 randomized phase III clinical trials of almost 21,000 patients validated 3-year DFS as a surrogate end point for 5-year OS. Results indicated that 80% of CRC recurrences occurred within the first 3 years of an 8-year follow-up period and that the correlation coefficient between DFS and OS at the patient level was high (0.87),[37] leading Oncologic Drugs Advisory Committee to accept 3-year DFS as a primary end point on which to base full-drug approval in CRC. This decision enabled patients with CRC to have access to new, more effective drugs a full 2 years earlier than before.[18]

## DISCUSSION

Although OS is a universally accepted efficacy end point that is a direct indication of clinical benefit, it has limitations as a primary end point in clinical trials of some cancers. If lack of a statistical difference in OS among treatment arms in such trials prevents an agent from becoming approved, the potential exists for patients to be denied access to a new effective treatment. PFS, although not a replacement for OS, is a credible end point that can be evaluated faster, with fewer patients, and with less susceptibility to confounding results than OS. The patient's perspective may identify clinical benefits of prolonged PFS in terms of improvements in QOL and disease symptoms, despite the presence of treatment toxicity. Data from clinical trials in advanced CRC, advanced breast cancer, advanced ovarian cancer, and metastatic RCC suggest that PFS represents a clinically meaningful end point. Relationships between PFS and OS in these cancers suggest that PFS may be analyzed to help understand the effect of an agent on OS in trials that incorporate cross-over in their designs. Recently, PFS has been accepted as a surrogate for OS in the first-line therapy for advanced

ovarian cancer and in advanced CRC. Even in cases when it does not meet the requirements for a validated surrogate end point, PFS may be an appropriate alternative end point to OS, specifically in cancers for which OS is prolonged, for which subsequent treatments are expected to have an effect on OS, for which crossover therapy is required, and for which evidence-based next-line therapies are available.

## ACKNOWLEDGMENT

*The authors thank Roseanne Degnan, Scientific Connections, for her editorial assistance with this manuscript.*

## REFERENCES

1. Pazdur R. Endpoints for assessing drug activity in clinical trials. *Oncologist.* 2008;13(suppl 2):19–21.
2. Beckman M. More clinical cancer treatments judged by progression-free rather than overall survival. *J Natl Cancer Inst.* 2007;99:1068–1069.
3. US Department of Health and Human Services, Food and Drug Administration, Center for Drug Evaluation and Research (CDER), Center for Biologics Evaluation and Research (CBER). Guidance for industry: clinical trial endpoints for the approval of cancer drugs and biologics. *Biotechnol Law Rep.* 2007;26:375–386.
4. European Medicines Agency. Committee for Medicinal Products for Human Use. Guideline on the evaluation of anticancer medicinal products in man. December 2005. Document CPMP/EWP/205/95/Rev.3/Corr. Available at: http://www.tga.gov.au/docs/pdf/euguide/ewp/020509enrev3.pdf. Accessed September 22, 2009.
5. Bast RC, Thigpen JT, Arbuck SG, et al. Clinical trial endpoints in ovarian cancer: report of an FDA/ASCO/AACR public workshop. *Gynecol Oncol.* 2007;107:173–176.
6. Chia SK, Speers CH, D'yachkova Y, et al. The impact of new chemotherapeutic and hormone agents on survival in a population-based cohort of women with metastatic breast cancer. *Cancer.* 2007;110:973–979.
7. Grothey A, Sargent D, Goldberg RM, et al. Survival of patients with advanced colorectal cancer improves with the availability of fluorouracil-leucovorin, irinotecan, and oxaliplatin in the course of treatment. *J Clin Oncol.* 2004;22:1209–1214.
8. Sargent DJ, Hayes DF. Assessing the measure of a new drug: is survival the only thing that matters? *J Clin Oncol.* 2008;26:1922–1923.
9. Demetri GD, Huan X, Garrett CR, et al. Novel statistical analysis of long-term survival to account for crossover in a phase III trial of sunitinib (SU) vs. placebo (PL) in advanced GIST after imatinib (IM) failure [abstract]. *J Clin Oncol.* 2008;26(15S):10524.
10. Johnson JR, Williams G, Pazdur R. End points and United States Food and Drug Administration approval of oncology drugs. *J Clin Oncol.* 2003;21:1404–1411.
11. Pignatti F. *EMEA Experience with Endpoints for Oncology Drug Approval.* EMEA/CHMP Biomarkers Workshop. December 16, 2005. Available at: http://www.emea.europa.eu/pdfs/human/biomarkers/04PIGNATTI.pdf. Accessed June 3, 2009.
12. Panageas KS, Ben-Porat L, Dickler NM, et al. When you look matters: the effect of assessment schedule on progression-free survival. *J Natl Cancer Inst.* 2007;99:428–432.
13. Therasse P, Arbuck SG, Eisenhauer EA, et al. New guidelines to evaluate the response to treatment in solid tumors. *J Natl Cancer Inst.* 2000;92:205–216.
14. *WHO Handbook for Reporting Results of Cancer Treatment.* Geneva, Switzerland: World Health Organization Offset Publication No. 48;1979.
15. Thiesse P, Ollivier L, Di Stefano-Louineau D, et al. Response rate accuracy in oncology trials: reasons for interobserver variability. *J Clin Oncol.* 1997;15:3507–3514.
16. Ford R, Schwartz L, Dancey J, et al. Lessons learned from independent central review. *Eur J Cancer.* 2009;45:268–274.
17. Dodd LE, Korn EL, Friedlin B, et al. Blinded independent central review of progression-free survival in phase III clinical trials: important design element or unnecessary expense? *J Clin Oncol.* 2008;26:3791–3796.
18. Sargent D. General and statistical hierarchy of appropriate biologic endpoints. *Oncology (Williston Park).* 2006;20:5–9.
19. US Food and Drug Administration, American Society of Clinical Oncology, American Association of Cancer Research. Meeting Summary. *Ovarian Cancer Endpoints Workshop.* 2006. Available at: http://www.fda.gov/CDER/drug/cancer_endpoints/ovarian_summary.pdf Accessed April 23, 2009.
20. Tang PA, Bentzen SM, Chen EX, et al. Surrogate end points for median overall survival in metastatic colorectal cancer: literature-based analysis from 39 randomized controlled trials of first-line chemotherapy. *J Clin Oncol.* 2007;25:4562–4568.

21. Buyse M, Burzykowski T, Carroll K, et al. Progression-free survival is a surrogate for survival in advanced colorectal cancer. *J Clin Oncol.* 2007;25:5218–5224.

22. Yothers G. Toward progression-free survival as a primary end point in advanced colorectal cancer. *J Clin Oncol.* 2007;25:5153–5154.

23. Miksad RA, Zietemann V, Gothe R, et al. Progression-free survival as a surrogate end point in advanced breast cancer. *Int J Technol Assess Health Care.* 2008;24:371–383.

24. Burzykowski T, Buyse M, Piccart-Gebhart MJ, et al. Evaluation of tumor response, disease control, progression-free survival, and time to progression as potential surrogate end points in metastatic breast cancer. *J Clin Oncol.* 2008;26:1987–1992.

25. *AVASTIN®(Bevacizumab) Prescribing Information.* South San Francisco, CA: Genentech, Inc.; 2008.

26. Motzer RJ, Mazumdar M, Bacik J, et al. Survival and prognostic factors of 670 patients with advanced renal cell carcinoma. *J Clin Oncol.* 1999;17:2530–2540.

27. Escudier B, Eisen T, Stadler WM, et al. Sorafenib in advanced clear-cell renal-cell carcinoma. *N Engl J Med.* 2007;356:125–134.

28. Motzer RJ, Hutson TE, Tomczak P, et al. Sunitinib versus interferon alfa in metastatic renal-cell carcinoma. *N Eng J Med.* 2007;356:115–124.

29. Escudier B, Pluzanska A, Koralewski P, et al. Bevacizumab plus interferon alfa-2a for treatment of metastatic renal cell carcinoma: a randomized, double-blind phase III trial. *Lancet.* 2007;370:2103–2111.

30. Hudes G, Carducci M, Tomczak P, et al. Temsirolimus, interferon-alfa, or both for advanced renal-cell carcinoma. *N Eng J Med.* 2007;356:2271–2281.

31. Motzer RJ, Escudier B, Oudard S, et al. Efficacy of everolimus in advanced renal cell carcinoma: a double-blind, randomised, placebo-controlled phase III trial. *Lancet.* 2008;372:449–456.

32. Kay A, Motzer R, Escudier B, et al. Updated data from a phase III randomized trial of everolimus (RAD001) versus PBO in metastatic renal cell carcinoma (mRCC). ASCO 2009 Genitourinary Cancers Symposium. Abstract 278.

33. Kane RC, Farrell AT, Saber H, et al. Sorafenib for the treatment of advanced renal cell carcinoma. *Clin Cancer Res.* 2006;12:7271–7278.

34. Figlin RA, Hutson TE, Tomczak P, et al. Overall survival with sunitinib versus interferon (IFN)-alfa as first-line treatment of metastatic renal cell carcinoma (mRCC). *J Clin Oncol.* 2008;26(May 20 suppl): Abstract 5024 and Oral Presentation. Available at: http://www.asco.org/ASCOv2/MultiMedia/Virtual+Meeting?&vmview=vm_session_presentations_view&confID=55&sessionID=363. Accessed June 3, 2009.

35. Knox JJ. Progression-free survival as endpoint in metastatic RCC? *Lancet.* 2008;372:427–429.

36. Delea TE, Khuu A, Kay A, et al. Association between treatment effects on disease progression (DP) endpoints and overall survival (OS) in patients with metastatic renal cell carcinoma (mRCC). *J Clin Oncol.* 2009;27(15s):Abstract 5105.

37. Sargent DJ, Wieand HS, Haller DG, et al. Disease-free survival versus overall survival as a primary end point for adjuvant colon cancer studies: individual patient data from 20,989 patients on 18 randomized trials. *J Clin Oncol.* 2005;23:8664–8670.

# Overall Survival: A Gold Standard in Search of a Surrogate

## The Value of Progression-Free Survival and Time to Progression as End Points of Drug Efficacy

Sen H. Zhuang • Liang Xiu • Yusri A. Elsayed

## OVERALL SURVIVAL: THE GOLD STANDARD

The difference between a surrogate and a true end point is like the difference between a check and cash. You can often get the check earlier, but then, of course, it may bounce.

—Stephen Senn, 2008[1]

The incisive analogy of Stephen Senn argues the value of true end points, while underscoring the uncertainties of surrogate end points. In the complex world of cancer drug development, surrogate end points are being increasingly advocated as indicators of efficacy and regulatory end points. However, surrogates attempt to replace the end point that is of greatest interest, and in oncology drug development, this remains overall survival (OS).

An improvement in OS remains the gold standard end point for a new oncology drug and the most appropriate measure of drug efficacy[2] (Table 1). The importance of a clinically meaningful survival improvement is unquestioned and universally accepted; in the extreme, it should translate into cures. OS, defined as time from randomization to time of death from any cause, remains the gold standard because it represents a true end point, a direct measure of drug benefit. Its value can be assessed easily and accurately, with 100% accuracy for the event and nearly 100% accuracy for the time of the event. Survival is essentially assessed on a daily basis, not at predetermined intervals, and can be easily documented through direct contact, and confirmed through registries. Additionally, because it is not measured in a subset but rather in the intent-to-treat population, it includes all randomized subjects in a clinical trial independent of their treatment outcome.

The Biomarkers Definitions Working Group defines a clinical end point as a "characteristic or variable that reflects how a patient feels, functions, or survives."[3] They note that clinical end points are "distinct measurements or analyses of disease characteristics observed in a study or a clinical trial that reflect the effect of a therapeutic intervention." Furthermore, "clinical end points are the most credible characteristics used in the assessment of the benefits and risks of a therapeutic intervention in randomized clinical trials." When one contrasts this with a surrogate end point that is "expected to predict clinical benefit (or harm or lack of benefit or harm)," it becomes easy to argue strongly for the use of OS as the end point of oncology drug development that while often "ignored" remains the principal goal in pharmaceutical drug development.

## IN SEARCH OF A SURROGATE

Despite the recognized eminence of OS as the gold standard, end points other than survival are increasingly being advocated and now comprise the approval basis for more than 3/4 of oncology drug marketing applications granted regular approval in the United States.[2]

The shrinking number of drug approvals based on OS recognizes several issues associated with the use of OS end points in cancer studies. First, OS may be affected by crossover therapy, sequential therapy, and the ever increasing number of available effective subsequent therapies that make isolating the contribution of 1 agent or treatment on survival difficult. Second, OS also includes noncancer deaths even if the cause of death is clearly not related to the cancer or the therapy received. This confounds the measurement of drug efficacy, particularly in certain cancer types with long natural history and in elderly patients.[4] Third, OS studies require large clinical trials with extended follow-up, leading to exponential increases in both the cost and time required before a new cancer drug is available to patients. The current estimate on the average time and cost for a new cancer therapy is more than 10 years and at least 1 billion dollars, respectively.[5]

In an effort to accelerate cancer drug development and to decrease the time before a new effective agent is available to patients, surrogate end points are of vital importance. The use of surrogate end points such as CD4 count and human immunodeficiency virus (HIV) viral load in AIDS drug evaluation in the last 2 decades has made available to patients several effective anti-HIV drugs that helped transform AIDS from a universally lethal disease to a controllable chronic condition.[6] It is important to remember that these surrogate end points (eg, CD4 count and HIV viral load) were neither perfect nor always predictive of clinical outcomes in all settings studied. For example, in the Concorde study (randomized, double-blinded controlled trial of immediate and deferred zidovudine in symptom-free HIV infection), there was a clear and persistent difference between the groups in CD4 count, but this did not translate into a difference in clinical outcomes.[7] Similarly, in the Delta study (a randomized, double-blinded controlled trial comparing the combination of zidovudine plus didanosine or zidovudine plus zalcitabine with zidovudine alone in HIV-infected individuals), short-term viral load changes were not adequate surrogates for clinical outcomes.[8]

Progression-free survival (PFS) and time to progression (TTP) are surrogate end points for cancer studies that are based on direct measurement of tumor growth. Compared with TTP, PFS is usually preferred because it includes deaths of all causes, takes into account potential drug toxicity-related deaths, and can better correlate with OS. Therefore, the remainder of this article will focus on PFS. Similar to other surrogate end points such as the case of CD4 and viral loads in HIV drug development, PFS is not a perfect surrogate for OS or improvement in clinical symptoms or physical functions. In some settings studied, it correlates with OS; in others, it does not. Although it is often difficult to identify the exact reasons why improvements in PFS do not result in OS benefits, several factors such as subsequent or crossover therapies and noncancer causes of death may contribute to the lack of correlation in some clinical settings. Patients and

**TABLE 1.** Attributes of Overall Survival

1. 100% accurate event
2. 100% accurate time
3. Assessed daily
4. Importance unquestioned
5. Assesses both safety and efficacy

**TABLE 2.** PFS as an Endpoint

| Advantages | Disadvantages |
|---|---|
| 1. Based on objective and quantitative assessments | 1. Not validated as surrogate for overall survival or improvement in symptoms in all tumor type |
| 2. Sample size can be smaller and follow-up shorter than in survival studies | 2. Uncertainty in some tumor type types whether improvement in PFS represents clinical benefit |
| 3. Ability to assess both cytostatic and cytotoxic drugs | 3. Assessment can be affected by the methodology (interval and symmetry of assessment schedules) |
| 4. Indifference to crossover or subsequent therapies after disease progression | 4. Requires randomized design, meticulous planning, and execution (particularly in open-label studies) |
| | 5. Difficulties estimating magnitude of the effect size accurately |

physicians view cancer as a deadly disease and they enter into treatment to reduce tumor size or prevent it from progressing with the hope that these intermediate effects will prolong patient life and reduce the suffering associated with continued tumor progression. It is logical to assume that prolonged control of tumor growth should lead to physical and psychologic benefits for the patient and the healthcare system. However, because of lack of validated and accepted methodology and logistical difficulties, most of the large oncology clinical trials with PFS as the primary end point have not been designed to document the improvement in cancer-related symptoms, quality of life measures, and medical resource utilization that should be expected with an improvement in PFS.

In the discussion, we will argue that an improvement in PFS of sufficient magnitude demonstrated by well designed and conducted studies can be considered direct evidence of clinical benefit independent of a benefit in OS. We will also discuss potential issues with PFS as the primary end point of cancer clinical trails and propose mitigation strategies that can strengthen this valuable clinical end point. Acceptance of PFS improvement as a direct benefit will accelerate cancer drug development and make effective therapy available sooner to patients with cancer. The availability of multiple effective drugs that could be administered sequentially, each delivering incremental tumor control, may collectively lead to transformation of cancer to controllable chronic disease.

## PFS: A COMPOSITE SAFETY AND EFFICACY ENDPOINT

PFS is defined as the time from randomization until objective tumor progression or death, whichever occurs first. PFS is a composite end point because it measures both the direct effect of treatment on the tumor growth and the impact of treatment effects on patient's survival by incorporating death in the end point analysis. Because PFS analysis includes death of all causes, it also takes into account the safety impact of treatment, eg, patients who die due to drug toxicity are included as an event.

The advantages of PFS as an end point include (Table 2): (1) it is based on objective and quantitative assessment, (2) the need for smaller sample size and shorter follow-up compared with survival studies, (3) the ability to assess both cytostatic and cytotoxic drugs because it also measures an experimental agent's impact on disease stabilization, and (4) its indifference to crossover or subsequent therapies after disease progression.

However, PFS also has several drawbacks including (Table 2): (1) the fact it is not yet validated as a surrogate for OS or improvement in symptoms in all tumor types, and there is uncertainty in some tumor type types as to whether an improvement in PFS represents clinical benefit for patients; (2) the problem that assessment of PFS can be affected by the methodology of assessment such as the interval and symmetry of assessment schedule. Therefore, PFS studies require a randomized design and meticulous planning and execution to avoid assessment bias, particularly in open-label studies; (3) difficulties in accurately estimating the magnitude of the effect size, especially when

different methodologies lead to discrepant results, eg, investigator assessment versus Independent Review Committee (IRC) assessment. These potential issues have been extensively studied. In the later part of this article, we will discuss key elements to minimize the impact of these issues by appropriate trial design, conduct, and analytical methodologies.

## PFS IMPROVEMENT AS DIRECT EVIDENCE OF CLINICAL BENEFIT

### The Lack of a Consensus on PFS as a Surrogate

For several decades, the US Food and Drug Administration (FDA) has maintained the position that cancer drug approval should be based on direct evidence of clinical benefit, such as improvement in survival, the quality of a patient's life, physical functioning, or the amelioration of tumor-related symptoms.[1] The question of whether a PFS improvement by itself can be considered a clinical benefit is one of the most important and debated questions in cancer drug development in recent time. This is primarily due to the fact that there is no consensus on whether an improvement in PFS can translate into an improvement in clinically meaningful outcomes such as OS, cancer-related symptoms, or physical functioning.

There is substantial literature examining whether PFS is a valid surrogate for OS. In certain tumors types and clinical settings, PFS has been shown to be a surrogate for OS; in other settings, a correlation has not been confirmed. Conceptually, if a therapy effectively slows tumor progression without a harmful effect on survival because of toxicity, it should translate into a survival benefit. Unfortunately, a benefit in OS has often been lacking. Several factors may have contributed to the observation that in some tumors, PFS improvements do not translate into OS benefits (Table 3). These mitigating factors include (1) a confounding of OS by effective subsequent or cross over therapy;

**TABLE 3.** Reasons Why PFS Improvements May Not Translate Into OS Benefits

1. Effective subsequent or cross over therapy
2. Deaths due to non-cancer causes in diseases with long survivals
3. Lack of power to detect significant OS differences
4. PFS improvement insufficient to translate into an OS benefit

(2) deaths due to noncancer causes in diseases where patients have long survivals; (3) a lack of power to detect significant OS differences in some studies; and (4) a magnitude of PFS improvement insufficient to translate into an OS benefit. Similarly, a prolongation in tumor growth control with no added toxicity should lead to improvement in cancer-related symptoms and quality of life. However, because of methodology, practical limitations, and poor trial design, there is very limited data adequately documenting an association between improved symptoms, quality of life improvements, and a prolonged PFS in patients with cancer.

Many patients and their caregivers clearly see the benefit of rapid, effective tumor control and the lack of progression in tumor burden, irrespective of the benefits in OS. This is particularly true when there is a need for immediate control of a rapidly progressing tumor or a tumor that threatens a vital organ. Prolongation of PFS can also translate into several tangible benefits such as the lessening of emotional stress that results from a constant awareness of disease progression and a delay in the need for additional therapy and its associated toxicities. However, it is important to emphasize that the value of PFS to patients, treating physicians, and regulators also depends largely on the magnitude of the delay in progression and the safety and tolerability of the treatment regimen.

One should note that a lack of data and philosophical and historical differences drive the debate on whether, by itself, an improvement in PFS should be considered direct evidence of clinical benefit. When a tumor progresses, it is usually associated, even if not immediately, with at least 1 of the following: a shortening of survival, a worsening of physical or emotional well being, and a worsening of physical performance. As demonstrated extensively in the literature, patients who have poor prognostic factors have tumor that progresses more rapidly and die sooner than those with good prognostic factors. The speed of tumor progression generally determines how much the patient suffers from cancer-related symptoms and how long the patient lives. Shortening of life expectancy of patients with cancer can ultimately be traced back to the progression of the tumor. PFS directly measures the effects of treatment on cancer growth using objective and quantitative methodology. It assesses both cytostatic (disease stabilization) and cytotoxic effects (tumor shrinkage). Therefore, in the context of a favorable risk benefit ratio, a clinically meaningful PFS improvement should be considered a clinical benefit on its own.

## Settings Where an Improvement in PFS Represents a Clinical Benefit

There are several clinical settings where an improvement in PFS should be considered a direct clinical benefit. First, tumor types where PFS has been demonstrated to be a surrogate end point for OS including advanced colorectal cancer,[9,10] glioblastoma multiforme,[11] locally advanced head and neck cancer,[12] advanced pancreatic cancer,[13] and metastatic nonsmall cell lung cancer.[14] In these tumor types, PFS improvement in the context of favorable risk benefit ratios should be considered clinical benefit. Second, tumors where patients have long survival (eg, follicular non-Hodgkin lymphoma and chronic lymphocytic leukemia) and an OS end point may not be feasible due to the indolent nature of the disease and its long natural history. In these tumors, an improvement in PFS should be an acceptable end point for clinical benefit. Third, tumors where although in individual clinical trials PFS has not been demonstrated to be a surrogate for OS (eg, metastatic breast cancer or ovarian cancer), the sequential use of drugs with improved PFS has resulted in a cumulative improvement in OS that has changed the natural history of the disease in recent decades. In these clinical settings, we would argue that a clinically meaningful improvement of PFS demonstrated by well designed and conducted studies and associated with an overall favorable risk benefit ratio should be considered direct evidence of clinical benefit, regardless of the impact of an individual drug on OS. This is particularly relevant in relapsed and refractory disease settings. During the American Society of Clinical Oncology 2008 annual meeting, the FDA presented an overview of the approvals in metastatic breast cancer and concluded that TTP and PFS alone can serve as the basis for regulatory approval in the second and third line settings of metastatic breast cancer.[15]

## POTENTIAL ISSUES IN PFS ASSESSMENT AND RECOMMENDATIONS FOR THEIR MITIGATION

As discussed earlier, methodological issues can impact the assessment of a PFS. Given the importance of controlling potential biases to maintain a robust clinical end point, we will focus on the major issues associated with assessment of PFS and propose solutions to address these issues.

### Evaluation and Measurement Bias

Bias in the evaluation and measurement of PFS could result in variability of PFS measurement and lead to difficulty in assessing the real magnitude of a PFS benefit. Multiple factors could result in systematic evaluation and measurement bias (Table 4). These are usually unintentional errors in the conduct of tumor assessments and include (1) the timing of tumor assessments; (2) asymmetry of evaluation periods; (3) subjective bias in open label studies; and (4) attrition bias.

First, time to disease progression is not a precise measurement, because the assessment cannot be performed on a daily basis. In oncology practice, various tumor assessment intervals (commonly 6–12 weeks) are used according to the tumor type and the aggressive nature of the disease. The timing of tumor assessments can have a significant impact on the degree of precision of the PFS measurement. A longer assessment interval such as 12 weeks can significantly overestimate the PFS length if the right side of the interval is chosen as the progression date. Although it is not clinically feasible to standardize the assessment interval across various tumor types or even different stages of the same tumor, it is possible to design clinical trials to limit the effect of the assessment interval on PFS results. It is even more important to understand the potential effect of the assessment interval on the treatment comparison in a controlled study. Several factors including the expected median PFS, the expected difference in median PFS in a comparative study, and the scheduling of assessments by calendar time or by treatment cycle should be considered at the study design stage in determining the assessment interval. A smaller treatment difference in median PFS tends to be more sensitive to the assessment interval. It is recommended that the tumor assessment interval should not exceed the expected improvement in median PFS in the experimental arm compared with the control arm. Other approaches could include reporting of progression as a binary (yes/no) outcome at a certain follow-up point (eg, 1-year and 2-year PFS rates).[16] Using this method, the evaluation of treatment

**TABLE 4.** Factors Responsible for Evaluation and Measurement Bias in PFS

1. Timing of tumor assessments
2. Asymmetry of evaluation periods
3. Subjective bias in open label studies
4. Attrition bias

effectiveness could be based on the proportion of patients whose cancer has progressed at 2 time points, rather than using an analysis based on a survival model. Two time points for imaging assessments would be determined prospectively, corresponding to the approximate median PFS and approximately twice the median PFS of the control arm on conventional therapies. Summary statistics would include the proportion alive and progression free at each time point. Progressions that have been documented before the designated imaging assessment time would be counted as an event for the rate of progression or death, and independent review of images would occur at the 2 time points. To properly analyze any effect of different assessment interval on the final PFS results, interval sensitivity analyses should also be conducted using established statistical methods.[17-19]

A second, potential issue in assessment of progression is asymmetry of the tumor evaluation intervals.[20] Asymmetric assessment of tumor between the 2 treatment arms will result in progression being systematically declared earlier in 1 arm than in the other, even when there is really no difference in efficacy. Although the importance of symmetrical assessment is well recognized now and is addressed in almost all well-designed comparative studies, asymmetry can still occur when the study is actually conducted. One example, mentioned above, may occur when the assessments are scheduled around the treatment cycle and 1 study arm experiences more cycle delays. Disparity in unscheduled visits between 2 treatment arms also can result in asymmetry. Studies should be designed and monitored closely to minimize the possibility of asymmetry. The actual tumor evaluations in a clinical trial should be analyzed and formally reported to assess any discrepancy in tumor assessment between the 2 treatment arms. It is important to analyze and report progression events declared at preplanned time points and those declared at unscheduled visits. Sensitivity analyses should also be performed to analyze the effect of asymmetric assessment on PFS measurement. Other approaches suggested in the literature to mitigate this bias is restricting PFS data analysis to 2 scheduled evaluation times at approximately the median PFS and twice the median PFS of the control arm.[20]

Although disease progression is often defined according to objective criteria, a third source of bias, a subjective bias, can be introduced in open-label studies when patients and treating physicians know the treatment assignment. If blinding is not possible, assessment methods and schedules should be well defined in the study protocol and closely followed by the study sites. Blinded IRC is often desired for studies intended for regulatory submissions. Issues with IRC review will be discussed in details in later part of this article.

A fourth source of bias, attrition bias, occurs when too many patients withdraw or are lost to follow-up from the study, especially if the attrition is larger in 1 arm than the other. Attrition bias is particularly common in clinical trials when there is a defined set of treatment cycles followed by a long follow-up period. It is usually impossible to document progression in patients who withdrew from the study or are lost to follow-up, and PFS data are censored at the time of the last available appropriate tumor evaluation. Adequate but short enough tumor assessment intervals and continuous patient and physician education regarding the goal of treatment have been shown to help minimize patient withdrawal and loss to follow-up. To assess the magnitude of any potential attrition bias, the proportion of censored patients should be reported for both treatment arms. The reason for censorship including withdrawal from study and lost to follow-up should also be summarized and discussed.

## Independent Review Committee

Blinded independent central review by an IRC to assess progression is commonly used in clinical trials and particularly open-label trials

seeking approval of a new regimen. The use of an IRC may be recommended by regulatory agencies.[4,21-23] Independent review is often performed for radiologic images but can also be conducted for efficacy measures other than radiologic images such as determination of response based on multiple laboratory tests as in multiple myeloma or pathologic confirmation of response in patients with minimal disease. Independent review by committee is a valuable approach to minimizing investigator bias in determining PFS in open-label clinical trials. However, an IRC introduces significant cost and operational complexity and can introduce new biases that could result in less reliable PFS measurements. These include (1) informative censoring and (2) discrepancies between local investigators and IRCs.

Informative censoring is the first major concern for the validity of PFS assessment in open label studies where the primary PFS data is generated by an IRC.[24] With the IRC process, the local investigator's assessment is used for "real time" local treatment decisions, whereas the IRC reassessment is routinely done later. If the IRC does not agree that a patient has progressed by the time the patient is off protocol, the patient is censored for the purpose of analysis. However, this patient is more likely to be assessed as having progressed sooner by the IRC than those remaining in the at-risk cohort if additional follow-up is obtained. However, when the investigator declares disease progression, the patient is discontinued from study, receives subsequent anticancer therapy, and no additional radiologic scans are obtained. This informative censoring violates the standard assumptions for censoring subjects, which assumes the progression course of censored individuals is the same as those remaining under observation, and leads to significant bias in the measurement of PFS.

Second, the use of IRCs can result in discrepancy in the assignment of and timing of progression between the IRC determination and the local investigator determination.[24] These discrepancies are approximately 50% in recently reported clinical trials that led to regulatory approval,[25-30] and there is no consensus on how these discrepancies should be reconciled or handled in determining the true occurrence of progression events. Furthermore, as a part of standard IRC review process, 2 radiologists independently review the same radiographic material. The discrepancy between the 2 primary IRC radiologists has been as high as 30% to 40% in recently published studies. These discrepancies result from variability in selection of target lesions and clinical judgments of radiologist based on the radiographic information available to them. Most of these discrepancies do not indicate systematic bias in the evaluation of the treatment effect and the final efficacy outcome conclusion,[24,30] but they raise concerns regarding the robustness of PFS as an end point.

## Approaches in Open-Label Trials to Minimize the Bias Associated With IRCs

Several approaches could be undertaken in open-label trials to minimize the bias associated with IRCs and strengthen the PFS data (Table 5). These include the following.

**TABLE 5.** Approaches in Open-Label Trials to Minimize the Bias Associated With Independent Review Committees (IRCs)

1. Real-time IRCs
2. Blinded local radiologist review
3. Intermediate step country/region IRC
4. Additional CT scans after local progression

### Real-Time IRCs

Real-time IRCs could eliminate bias associated with informative censoring and also minimize the number of patients censored due to subsequent therapy or lost to follow-up.[24,31] However, this approach is operationally not feasible in most large multicenter studies. Image retrieval, submission, standardization, and data reconciliation will need to be flawless to allow timely review of scans by IRC and reporting of results to investigators. Investigators and patients may not be willing to wait for the required length of time particularly if they believe that the patient's cancer is progressing. Additional issues that can rise from this approach are ethical and legal concerns about who is responsible for making treatment decisions about the patient? What will happen if the investigator does not agree with the IRC assessment?

### Blinded Local Radiologist Review

Blinding the local radiologist to treatment assignment could help eliminate investigator's bias and informative censoring. This approach would add some logistical complexity for the clinical site in preparing patients for local review and will require agreement from the investigator that the radiologist assessment of progression will be followed in making decisions regarding the patient.

### Intermediate Step Country/Region IRC

This intermediate step has been reported to be useful in multicountry clinical trials where ethical and legal concerns may prevent a centralized IRC from making treatment decision. In this scenario, the images are reviewed by a locally organized IRC (by country) that is blinded to treatment assignment, and the investigator agrees to follow this IRC assessment decision in patient care. This approach eliminates the legal and ethical concerns about the standards used to make treatment decisions for a specific patient, but it is not clear if it provides faster feedback to the clinical site.

### Additional Computed Tomography Scans After Local Progression

This approach is based on the assumption that patients removed from study by the investigator due to progression are very likely to be deemed to have progressed by the IRC if they are followed for an additional short period. In this scenario, the protocol requires the investigator to perform and submit at least 1 additional scan (at the protocol specific assessment interval) after local progression is determined even if the patient started subsequent therapy. For patients who receive subsequent treatment, PFS will be censored at the time of subsequent therapy. Submission of this additional computed tomography scan has been shown to minimize informative censoring.

## Scenarios Where No or Limited IRC May Provide Adequate Audit for PFS

Dodd et al[24] reviewed randomized cancer studies reported in the last few years and clearly showed that there was consistent agreement between investigator and IRC assessment of efficacy. It was concluded that the systematic use of an IRC may not be necessary, and several scenarios have been suggested where no or limited IRC may provide adequate audit for PFS while reducing the cost and complexity of clinical trials (Table 6). These include

1. Double-blinded clinical trials.
2. Open-label trials where the treatment effect size is expected to be large enough to mitigate any perceived bias in PFS assessment.
3. Two-point PFS evaluation. This approach requires IRC evaluation of PFS at only 2 time points (the approximate median and twice median PFS of the control arm). Treatment effectiveness

**TABLE 6.** Scenarios Where No or Limited IRC May Provide Adequate Audit for PFS While Reducing the Cost and Complexity of Clinical Trials

1. Double-blinded clinical trials
2. Open-label trials where the treatment effect size is expected to be large enough to mitigate any perceived bias in PFS assessment
3. Trials with two-point PFS evaluation (the approximate median and twice median PFS of the control arm)
4. IRC assessment of a sample of the study population (~10%)

is reported based on the proportion of patients whose cancer has progressed at the 2 time points, rather than using an analysis based on a survival model.[20]

4. IRC assessment of a sample of the study population. In this approach, only a prospectively determined sample (~10%) of the study patients will be selected randomly for IRC audit. If a meaningful difference in hazard ratios between the local review and IRC assessment is detected indicating a bias, then the IRC assessment will be expanded to the whole study population.

## PFS AS BASIS OF CANCER DRUG APPROVAL

All major regulatory agencies have recognized PFS as a valuable end point in cancer drug clinical trials and have provided guidelines for appropriate measurement of PFS.[4,21,22] In the last few years, the US FDA has shown increasing flexibility in accepting PFS end points for full approval. In May 2007, the FDA issued its most recent version of Guidance for Industry: Clinical Trial Endpoints for the Approval of Cancer Drugs and Biologics,[4] which offers recommendations on end points for cancer clinical trials submitted to the FDA. The guidance provided detailed discussion on PFS and suggestions to strengthen the PFS measurement. In addition to the role of PFS in accelerated approval, the document also indicates that PFS may serve as a basis for regular approval. Recently, cancer drug approvals have been granted solely on evidence of PFS. Examples include (1) the December 2005, FDA approval of sorafenib for the treatment of advanced kidney cancer based on an increase in PFS, despite the absence of a statistically significant benefit in OS; (2) the 2006 approval of gemcitabine in combination with carboplatin for the treatment of patients with advanced ovarian cancer that has relapsed at least 6 months after completion of platinum-based therapy; and (3) the 2007 FDA approval of ixabepilone for the treatment of patients with metastatic or locally advanced breast cancer.

When PFS is used as a primary end point, most regulatory agencies around the world[4,21,22] advocate blinded IRC review and prior consultation with the agency to agree on the methodological issues related to the definition and assessment of PFS.[21] In addition, adequacy of PFS improvement as basis of approval is highly dependent on other factors, such as effect size, effect duration, and benefits of other available therapy.

## CONCLUSION

OS remains the gold standard for cancer drug approval. However, given the growing number of available effective oncology drugs and the increasing OS of many cancers, reliance on OS as the only acceptable end point to measure efficacy is not logical and could result in many useful drugs delayed for many years before they are made available to patients. Clinical benefit could be documented in ways other than an increase in OS, and delaying progression may be clinically beneficial even if OS is not affected.

PFS is a valuable end point that can adequately measure the direct treatment effect and facilitate drug development. The theoretical and practical issues in PFS measurement are well studied, and there are many available design and statistical approaches to mitigate the impact of these issues and help generate robust and reliable PFS data. The availability of a series of effective therapies, each of which delivers incremental progress in tumor control, may collectively lead to transformation of cancer to a curable or controllable chronic disease.

## ACKNOWLEDGMENTS

*The authors thank Christopher Enny of Ortho Biotech Oncology Research and Development for editorial assistance in the development of this manuscript.*

## REFERENCES

1. Senn S. Statistical Issues in Drug Development, Second Edition. Statistics in Practice Series. 8.2.7: Using Surrogate Endpoints. NJ: Wiley; 2008:125.
2. Johnson JR, Williams G, Pazdur R. End points and United States food and drug administration approval of oncology drugs. *J Clin Oncol.* 2003;21:1404–1411.
3. Biomarkers Definitions Working Group. Biomarkers and surrogate endpoints: preferred definitions and conceptual framework. *Clin Pharmacol Ther.* 2001;69:89–95.
4. US Food and Drug Administration. *Guidance for Industry Clinical Trial Endpoints for the Approval of Cancer Drugs and Biologics.* Rockville, MD: Food and Drug Administration; 2007.
5. Adams CP, Brantner VV. Estimating the cost of new drug development: is it really 802 million dollars? *Health Aff (Millwood).* 2006;25:420–428.
6. Darbyshire J. Clinical trials of antiretroviral drugs: the role of the MRC AIDS Therapeutic Trials Committee (ATTC) and the MRC Clinical Trials Unit (CTU). *Br J Clin Pharmacol.* 2003;55:469–472.
7. Concorde: MRC/ANRS randomised double-blind controlled trial of immediate and deferred zidovudine in symptom-free HIV infection. Concorde Coordinating Committee. *Lancet.* 1994;343:871–881.
8. An evaluation of HIV RNA and CD4 cell count as surrogates for clinical outcome. Delta Coordinating Committee and Virology Group. *Aids.* 1999;13:565–573.
9. Buyse M, Burzykowski T, Carroll K, et al. Progression-free survival is a surrogate for survival in advanced colorectal cancer. *J Clin Oncol.* 2007;25:5218–5224.
10. Tang PA, Bentzen SM, Chen EX, et al. Surrogate end points for median overall survival in metastatic colorectal cancer: literature-based analysis from 39 randomized controlled trials of first-line chemotherapy. *J Clin Oncol.* 2007;25:4562–4568.
11. Ballman KV, Buckner JC, Brown PD, et al. The relationship between six-month progression-free survival and 12-month overall survival end points for phase II trials in patients with glioblastoma multiforme. *Neuro Oncol.* 2007;9:29–38.
12. Michiels S, Le Maitre A, Buyse M, et al; MARCH and MACH-NC Collaborative Groups. Surrogate endpoints for overall survival in locally advanced head and neck cancer: meta-analyses of individual patient data. *Lancet Oncol.* 2009;10:341–350.
13. Milella M, Bria E, Carlini P, et al. Surrogate endpoints for overall survival (OS) in advanced pancreatic cancer (APC): analysis of randomized clinical trials (RCTs) exploring gemcitabine (G)-based combinations. JCO *Proc Am Soc Clin Oncol.* 2007;25:4575.
14. Johnson KR, Ringland C, Stokes BJ, et al. Response rate or time to progression as predictors of survival in trials of metastatic colorectal cancer or non-small-cell lung cancer: a meta-analysis. *Lancet Oncol.* 2006;7:741–746.
15. Cortazar P, Johnson JR, Justice R, et al. Metastatic breast cancer (MBC): FDA approval overview. *Proc Am Soc Clin Oncol.* 2008;26:1013.
16. Beckman M. More clinical cancer treatments judged by progression-free rather than overall survival. *J Natl Cancer Inst.* 2007;99:1068–1069.
17. Lindsey JC, Ryan LM. Tutorial in biostatistics methods for interval-censored data. *Stat Med.* 1998;17:219–238.
18. Odell PM, Anderson KM, D'Agostino RB. Maximum likelihood estimation for interval-censored data using a Weibull-based accelerated failure time model. *Biometrics.* 1992;48:951–959.
19. Panageas KS, Ben-Porat L, Dickler MN, et al. When you look matters: the effect of assessment schedule on progression-free survival. *J Natl Cancer Inst.* 2007;99:428–432.
20. Freidlin B, Korn EL, Hunsberger S, et al. Proposal for the use of progression-free survival in unblinded randomized trials. *J Clin Oncol.* 2007;25:2122–2126.
21. European Medicines Agency. Methodological Considerations for Using Progression-Free Survival (PFS) as Primary Endpoint in Confirmatory Trials for Registration. London, UK: European Medicines Agency; 2008.
22. Health Canada. Issues Analysis Summary: The Use of Progression-Free Survival as the Efficacy Endpoint for Approval of Targeted and Chemotherapeutic Agents for Advanced Cancer. Ottawa, Canada: Health Canada; 2007.
23. Ford R, Schwartz L, Dancey J, et al. Lessons learned from independent central review. *Eur J Cancer.* 2009;45:268–274.
24. Dodd LE, Korn EL, Freidlin B, et al. Blinded independent central review of progression-free survival in phase III clinical trials: important design element or unnecessary expense?. *J Clin Oncol.* 2008;26:3791–3796.
25. Escudier B, Eisen T, Stadler WM, et al; TARGET Study Group. Sorafenib in advanced clear-cell renal-cell carcinoma. *N Engl J Med.* 2007;356:125–134.
26. Geyer CE, Forster J, Lindquist D, et al. Lapatinib plus capecitabine for HER2-positive advanced breast cancer. *N Engl J Med.* 2006;355:2733–2743.
27. Miller KD, Chap LI, Holmes FA, et al. Randomized phase III trial of capecitabine compared with bevacizumab plus capecitabine in patients with previously treated metastatic breast cancer. *J Clin Oncol.* 2005;23:792–799.
28. Motzer RJ, Hutson TE, Tomczak P, et al. Sunitinib versus interferon alfa in metastatic renal-cell carcinoma. *N Engl J Med.* 2007;356:115–124.
29. Thomas ES, Gomez HL, Li RK, et al. Ixabepilone plus capecitabine for metastatic breast cancer progressing after anthracycline and taxane treatment. *J Clin Oncol.* 2007;25:5210–5217.
30. Van Cutsem E, Peeters M, Siena S, et al. Open-label phase III trial of panitumumab plus best supportive care compared with best supportive care alone in patients with chemotherapy-refractory metastatic colorectal cancer. *J Clin Oncol.* 2007;25:1658–1664.
31. Fleming TR, Rothmann MD, Lu HL. Issues in using progression-free survival when evaluating oncology products. *J Clin Oncol.* 2009;27:2874–2880.

# Overall Survival: Still the Gold Standard

## Why Overall Survival Remains the Definitive End Point in Cancer Clinical Trials

James J. Driscoll • Oliver Rixe

The primary goal of clinical trials in the field of medical oncology is to give definitive evidence with regard to the benefit-to-risk ratio of an experimental intervention relative to a placebo or the existing standard-of-care to then provide optimal patient care and improve patient survival.[1] A challenging aspect of such trials is to provide convincing, pivotal evidence that a given therapy is superior (or noninferior) to the existing standard-of-care with acceptable risk, cost, and access and to permit regulatory approval. A crucial question is the choice of primary end point to assess clinical trial efficacy to then provide appropriate evaluation and approval. Although the efficacy of traditional cytotoxic chemotherapy-based clinical trials can be measured by standard radiologic measures response evaluation criteria in solid tumors (RECIST criteria), the advent of targeted, vaccine-, and cell-based therapies requires more disease- and drug-specific biomarkers to assess patient response and, thus, to evaluate such clinical trials. A second fundamental question is whether better outcome markers, eg, surrogates, can be established to replace overall survival (OS) and expedite accelerated drug approval.

Improvement in OS is considered by the US and European regulatory agencies to be the gold standard for drug approval, although alternative end points, eg, such as disease-free survival (DFS), progression-free survival (PFS), time-to-progression (TTP), objective response rate (ORR), may also be acceptable when the proposed indication is use in the adjuvant setting. It is noteworthy that from 1990 to 2002, 39 of 57 (68%) trials that led to drug approval for oncologic indications and 100% of the 14 trials that led to approval of small molecule compounds were approved through an accelerated process and such approval was based on end points other than OS. However, OS and the currently available validated surrogate markers remain the main primary end points presently used to evaluate and assess the temporal benefit of cancer treatment regimens. Alternative trial end points, with new clinical designs, have been evaluated to expedite the drug approval process required by US and European authorities. It is obvious that an accelerated approval mechanism for refractory cancers can reduce the time needed for marketing and regulatory approval. Accordingly, an analysis conducted in 2003 has demonstrated that the median time to marketing approval is 5.5 years shorter using the fast-track process. However, the quickest approval time observed with either the accelerated or standard processes were equal and suggest that a well-designed clinical development plan using conventional end points can similarly lead to a rapid approval process based on convincing, robust results.[2] The relevance of these biologic end points, the differences between conventional therapies, eg, cytotoxics, and molecular targeted therapies, and pertinent differences in end points used between oncology and nononcology clinical trials is discussed herein.

## DEFINITIONS AND HISTORICAL ASPECTS

OS is a term that denotes the chances of staying alive for a group of individuals that suffer from a specific cancer (or a subtype of that cancer). It denotes the percentage of individuals in a group likely to be alive after a fixed duration of time. At a basic level, OS is representative of cure rates. The first clinical trial of a novel therapy was conducted by the Renaissance surgeon Ambroise Paré in 1537 when he used a concoction of turpentine, rose oil, and egg yolk to treat battlefield wound infections and noted that the new treatment was more effective than the existing method. Paré's treatments may actually qualify historically as the earliest documented trial to use OS as an outcome.

A surrogate or intermediate outcome is intended to capture the treatment effect on an important clinical end point but does not directly measure the main clinical benefit of the intervention. For example, DFS, PFS, and TTP are currently surrogates for OS in a defined group of malignancies. However, survival is defined by clear-cut mutually exclusive outcomes, is an unambiguous end point, is not subject to investigator bias or subjective interpretation, and can be assessed without reliance on tumor measurements. Moreover, OS can be assessed with 100% accuracy for the event and with nearly 100% accuracy for the time of the event. Surrogate biomarker end points, eg, elevated tumor markers, may provide strong statistical association with tumor growth or OS for specific agents used to treat selected tumor types. When it is not feasible to achieve the necessary statistical power for a robust clinical end point such as OS, a valid surrogate may be used as the primary objective, with the main end point then becoming a secondary objective. However, in contrast to OS, the use of a surrogate end point in a trial does necessitate a clear statement of its method of evaluation, the degree of benefit expected from the intervention, or a precise definition of the patients for whom the benefit is sought and thus is inferior to OS.

Recent examples of targeted therapies approved based on improvement in end points that did and did not include OS are listed in Table 1. The first example, bevacizumab, was initially approved by the Food and Drug Administration (FDA) in 2004 as a first-line treatment for metastatic colorectal cancer based on improved OS of 5 months in patients treated with irinotecan/5-FU-leucovorin plus bevacizumab. Subsequently, in 2006, the FDA granted approval for bevacizumab in combination with 5 fluorouracil–based chemotherapy, for the second-line treatment of metastatic carcinoma of the colon or rectum, an approval that was based on improvement in OS in patients who received bevacizumab plus FOLFOX4. In 2006, the FDA granted approval for bevacizumab in combination with carboplatin and paclitaxel, for the initial treatment of unresectable, locally advanced, recurrent, or metastatic, nonsquamous, nonsmall cell lung cancer. However, in 2008, the FDA granted accelerated approval for bevacizumab used

**TABLE 1.** End Points Used for FDA-Approval of Molecularly Targeted Therapies

| Targeted Therapy | Indication | End Point | Benefit | Year |
|---|---|---|---|---|
| Bevacizumab | Metastatic colorectal cancer | Overall survival | 5 mo | 2004 |
| Bevacizumab | Metastatic colorectal cancer | Overall survival | 2.2 mo | 2006 |
| Bevacizumab | Unresectable, locally advanced and metastatic nonsmall cell lung cancer | Overall survival | 2 mo | 2006 |
| Bevacizumab | HER2 negative breast cancer | Progression-free survival | 5.5 mo | 2008 |
| Bevacizumab | Metastatic renal cell carcinoma | Progression-free survival | 5 mo | 2009 |
| Bevacizumab | Glioblastoma | Overall response rate WHO radiologic criteria | Improved | 2009 |
| Trastuzumab | Node-positive breast cancer | Disease-free survival | Prolonged | 2006 |
| Sunitinib | Advanced renal cell carcinoma | Progression-free survival | 6 mo | 2009 |

HER2, human epidermal growth factor receptor 2.

in combination with paclitaxel for the treatment of patients who have not received chemotherapy for metastatic human epidermal growth factor receptor 2-negative breast cancer with approval based on improvement in PFS and not OS. Similarly, approval of bevacizumab for metastatic renal cell carcinoma was based on improved PFS in patients treated with bevacizumab, again not based on OS improvement. The FDA granted accelerated approval to bevacizumab for patients with glioblastoma based on durable ORR observed in 2 single-arm trials, AVF3708g and NCI 06-C-0064E. A second targeted therapy to receive FDA approval was trastuzumab, approved as part of a regimen for the adjuvant treatment of women with node-positive, human epidermal growth factor receptor 2-overexpressing breast cancer based on DFS prolongation. A third targeted therapy, sunitinib, was recently granted regular FDA approval for the treatment of advanced renal cell carcinoma patients who failed prior cytokine-based therapy, upgrading it from the accelerated approval granted in January 2006.

Guidance promulgated in the 1980s by the FDA recommends that drug efficacy should be demonstrated by increasing patient survival, improving the quality of life, or increasing the level of an established surrogate end point for at least 1 of these outcomes.[3] From this initial statement, the FDA has added 3 amendments that have significantly modified the drug development process and have challenged OS as the single robust, most reliable end point. In 1992, an addition called Accelerated Approval Subpart H allowed more rapid regulatory approval of drugs for life-threatening diseases.[4] This was based on a given drug's effect on a surrogate end point likely to predict clinical benefit or demonstrated evidence of a clinical benefit other than survival. Oncology is included in this category of life-threatening diseases and, thus, tumor response rates and TTP have often been viewed as such surrogate end points. Durable complete responses have also been accepted as evidence of clinical benefit in hematologic malignancies. Second, in 1996, a document from the Office of the President of the United States described the accelerated regulations by the FDA to new anticancer drug approval.[5] The accelerated process is based on the determination of tumor size shrinkage in patients with refractory disease or in patients with no proven effective treatment. However, this process requires postapproval confirmatory studies to examine the effect of the experimental therapy on survival and/or to demonstrate that the surrogates correspond to clinical benefit. Finally, trial designs, the populations enrolled in these studies and the design of the confirmatory studies recommended for the accelerated approval were discussed and summarized in a FDA meeting in 2003. These administrative perspectives underline the limits of the alternative end points to OS and the need for improvements in drug development process.

## SURROGATE END POINTS: FACTS AND LIMITATIONS

Over the last decade, ORR has been the primary end point used for almost 50% of the approved anticancer agents from 4 different indications (Table 2). The first indication was the recognition of durable complete responses for refractory malignant hematologic disease, second was the validation of partial response rates for individual hormonal therapies in metastatic breast cancer, and third was partial response supported by tumor-specific symptomatic relief. More recently in a 4th indication, the tyrosine kinase inhibitor (sunitinib) was approved for patients with metastatic renal cell carcinoma based on the high-partial response rates obtained in 2 consecutive single-arm phase 2 studies, which enrolled a total of 136 patients.[6]

Based on the original work of Miller et al[7] in 1980, ORR became a widely accepted measure of efficacy for cytotoxic agents, based on tumor response assessed by bidimensional measurements. Twenty years later, these arbitrary criteria have been reevaluated on the basis of unidimensional parameters and are universally used in protocols to support drug evaluation and approval. Significant tumor shrinkage in the absence of treatment of metastatic solid tumors is a very rare phenomenon that supports the use of objective response as a valid surrogate marker of antitumor activity. Several examples have illustrated this hypothesis, such as accelerated approvals based on response rate that were then converted to regular approvals based on a randomized trial using a comparator arm to demonstrate a significant survival advantage. By contrast, marketing approval for gefitinib in the treatment of patients diagnosed with nonsmall cell lung cancer was based on 2 uncontrolled randomized studies and convincing ORRs of 11% and 19%, respectively.[8,9] However, the combination of gefitinib with chemotherapy in 2 randomized phase 3 studies failed to demonstrate a significant survival advantage (or any other positive parameter of clinical outcome) superior to standard chemotherapy and resulted in a withdrawal of FDA approval.[10,11] Such results emphasize the limitations of an approval process based on a single method of tumor response and evaluation.

**TABLE 2.** New Drug Approval in Oncology From 1990 to 2002: End Points for Anticancer Agents[15]

| Class of Agent | No. New Approvals | Type of Approval | Major End Point |
|---|---|---|---|
| Cytotoxics | 18 | Accelerated: 6 Regular: 12 | Response rate: 10, survival: 8 |
| Hormonal therapy | 5 | Regular: 5 | Response rate: 5 |

However, response rate is seldom a valid surrogate for clinical benefit. There is a lack of clear evidence to demonstrate that response rate captures the full effect of treatment benefit. In addition to RECIST criteria,[12] additional parameters need to be integrated to provide a more comprehensive picture of treatment efficacy. It could include not only the type of the response, eg, complete versus partial, site of response, and duration of response, but also the reproducibility of the tumor measurement. Standardized criteria should be used to ascertain response. However, in a provocative analysis, Hillman et al[13] have demonstrated that the measurement of 10 different lesions (as was initially requested by the RECIST criteria) does not improve the precision of the evaluation. Computer-based determination of the tumor volume currently has been implemented to eliminate human parameters and other biases that interfere with the real tumor volume modifications. In an innovative mathematical model, Fojo and coworkers[14] demonstrated that tumor regression after bevacizumab therapy in metastatic renal cell carcinoma did not correlate with survival in this specific setting. By contrast, the ability of the drug to modify the growth rate constant was highly correlated with patient survival. This approach noted the limits of drug evaluation using ORR and yielded a more robust surrogate marker that may correlate with clinical outcome. ORR could also underestimate treatment effects on clinical end points such as survival by failing to capture the magnitude and the duration of effects on tumor burden.[3] ORR can also overestimate the potential impact on survival if responses are brief or if this measure fails to capture unintended harmful mechanisms of action of treatment and mechanisms of acquired drug resistance. Bruzzi et al[15] have evaluated the ORR as a surrogate end point for survival in metastatic breast carcinoma. The authors performed a meta-analysis based on 10 randomized trials and 2126 patients treated with epirubicin-based regimens (high vs. standard dose). They reported that the experimental therapy (high-dose epirubicin regimens) provides a statistically nonsignificant benefit in duration of survival. They showed that tumor response is a highly significant predictor of survival but that the treatment effects on response poorly predict the treatment effects on survival. Interestingly, the authors do not recommend the use of response rate as the primary end point in clinical trials, based on limits previously noted—modest effect on survival, treatment-associated toxicity, cost, and lack of identification of the drug sensitive population. These findings were similar to the recent analysis performed by Burzykowski on 3953 patients treated with anthracycline alone or in combination with taxanes in metastatic breast cancer.[16] Tumor response was strongly associated with OS. However, response and disease control (log ORs) were poorly correlated with the log of hazard ratios for OS. The authors concluded that, even if tumor response is an acceptable surrogate for survival in this setting, "the clinical implications of this finding are rather limited." As the effectiveness of a new agent requires a demonstration of clinical benefit, objective response represents a partial and limited evaluation of the numerous ways to evaluate the entire benefit, including safety, quality of life, and superiority over the standard treatment.

## LIMITATIONS ON PROGRESSION-FREE SURVIVAL AS A SURROGATE MARKER

There are several challenges associated with the use of end point PFS in oncologic trials. PFS is defined as the time to detection of progressive disease or death and does not directly measure whether a patient survives but does provide insight on whether an intervention affects the tumor burden process, ie, the intended mechanism of the agent to provide benefit. PFS is a direct measure of the treatment on tumor burden, measures the effect of both cytostatic and cytotoxic interventions and includes the clinically relevant event of death. To determine whether an intervention has an effect on PFS, clinical trials are conducted whereby patients are followed to progression and death. The US FDA underlined the importance of DFS and response rates or TTP definitions and a complete randomized controlled trial report to approve new cancer drug applications. When OS is a trial's end point, the date of death of each patient is a fixed event that can be accurately measured, but when PFS is used, the outcome depends on when and how often patients are monitored for signs of disease. Five-year rates are reported for many cancers, because those who survive 5 years are quite likely to be cured of their disease. In some slow growing and low-grade malignancies such as follicular lymphoma where late relapses are common, the 10 year OS is more representative of cure rates. On the other hand, PFS may be a blurry yardstick for the efficacy of cancer drugs because (1) the definition of when progression begins is subjective; (2) it does not measure immunologic response to treatment; and (3) it measures disease only at the primary site or metastatic site but does not measure micrometastatic disease or circulating tumor cells. However, PFS is often an attractive measure because it is available earlier than OS and can hasten drug development. PFS assessment intervals should be standardized by the type of cancer studied and cancer stage. A determination that cancer has progressed is usually on the basis of radiographic findings from studies conducted at fixed intervals.

The intent of adjuvant therapy is to eradicate micrometastatic residual disease after curative resection with the goal of preventing or delaying recurrence. The time-honored standard for demonstrating efficacy of new adjuvant therapies is an improvement in OS not event-driven surrogates. This typically requires phase 3 trials of large sample size with lengthy follow-up. Salvage regimens for solid tumors remain under constant study, and longer follow-up is required to demonstrate that adjuvant treatments improve OS compared with other clinical end points.

## BIOMARKERS AND THE ACCELERATION OF DRUG DEVELOPMENT: LIMITATIONS

Because newer targeted, cell- or vaccine-based agents may not act directly at the tumor traditional methods of monitoring efficacy may be inadequate. Surrogate end points, as used in scientific and regulatory communities, are findings or measurements that may be used in clinical trials to evaluate the safety or effectiveness of a medical therapy for treating disease. Biomarkers are anatomic, physiologic, biochemical, or molecular parameters that ideally are associated with the presence and severity of specific disease states. Biomarkers analyzed in tissue or by imaging modalities may serve as nontraditional end points, though many if not most surrogate end points do not involve the imaging of biomarkers, and the concepts are not synonymous. Examples that correlate biomarker response and OS are scarce or do not exist. New surrogate markers that reflect efficacy are essential to accelerate the evaluation and approval of oncologic treatments.

To reduce the time and cost required for new drug development, biologic markers have been proposed as surrogate end points in oncology clinical trials. Such surrogates should reflect the mechanism of action of the investigational agent and validation should include the use of a specific and reproducible assay for target modulation with accessibility of the tumor tissue to perform the assay. Biomarkers must be incorporated in the early phases of drug development to determine toxicity and to select an enriched patient population whose tumors express the target of interest and are more likely to demonstrate benefit. Unfortunately this is still not done as frequent as it should be. The ultimate challenge to be met with biologic end points is to know

| **TABLE 3.** Biomarkers as a Surrogate End Point: Reasons for Putative Unreliability |
|---|
| **Limits** |
| Reproducibility of the assay |
| Access to tumor tissues |
| Absence of link between the evaluated pathway and the process of tumor growth |
| Multiplicity of pathways/mechanisms involved in tumor growth and/or drug resistance |
| Multiple mechanisms of drug action |

whether they are surrogate markers of not only drug efficacy but also clinical benefit. Unfortunately, demonstration of a beneficial effect on a biologic end point may not provide reliable evidence of an effect of the intervention on OS (Table 3). The unreliability of proposed biomarkers as surrogate end points has been described by Fleming et al[17] and can be summarized as follows. First, the absence of a link between expression of the biomarker and the pathway by which the tumor grows or metastasizes. In the absence of such a link, the active modulation of the biomarker and its expression will not influence the clinical end point and will not correlate with OS. For example, elevated tumor serum markers such as carcinoma embryonic antigen and prostate-specific antigen are correlated with advancing tumor burdens in colon and prostate cancer, respectively. However, these biomarkers do not reflect biologic mechanisms by which those 2 solid tumors progress or become refractory to treatment. Consequently, treatment-induced modifications of these markers cannot predict with certainty the impact of a therapy on clinical end points such as OS. Additionally, the absence of a relationship between the pathway targeted by the agent and the mechanism of tumor growth may not be valid. In this case, a valid method of evaluation of the biomarker modulation after drug exposure would not be correlated with OS. Many examples have been reported in the literature, in oncology or in cardiology, to illustrate this phenomenon. In this situation, the biomarker is a surrogate of drug activity but is not a surrogate of drug efficacy.

A second factor in the unreliability of biomarkers is the fact that anticancer agents, including cytotoxic compounds and biologics, could target cell components at different levels. This is probably true for tyrosine kinase inhibitors. A recent article from Karaman et al[18] described the multiplicity of tyrosine kinases hit by most of these small molecules. It suggests the paradoxical absence of selectivity on a unique pathway of these molecular targeted therapies. Consequently, beneficial effects due to the multiplicity of the mechanisms of action are not captured by determination of a drug's effect on a single biologic pathway. Furthermore, the drug could have mechanisms of action that are independent of its effect on the disease process.

Finally, we cannot be sure whether once a surrogate biomarker has been validated for a given targeted therapy for a specific tumor that same biomarker will be valid for other targeted therapies and other tumor types. Indeed, eventually the surrogates may be disease and drug class specific.

## ALTERNATIVE END POINTS USED IN NONONCOLOGIC CLINICAL TRIALS

Historically, there has been extensive interest in using surrogate end points in clinical trials to more rapidly evaluate new biologic agents, drugs, devices, or procedures in the treatment of all diseases that afflict humans.[19] To reduce the cost and duration of trials outside of oncology, surrogates that have been used include changes in cholesterol level, bone mineral density, blood pressure control, CD4 cell count, and decreased viral load. In theory, for a surrogate end point to be an effective substitute for the clinical outcome, effects of the intervention on the surrogate must reliably predict the overall effect on the clinical outcome, but in practice, this requirement frequently fails. As Fleming has stated, surrogate end points can be useful in phase 2 screening trials to identify whether a new drug or intervention is biologically active and to guide whether the intervention demonstrates sufficient promise to justify a large definitive trial. Moreover, in definitive phase 3 trials, except for rare circumstances in which the validity of the surrogate end point has already been rigorously established, the primary end point should remain the true clinical outcome such as OS.[20]

Clinical trials, particularly in cardiology, often use composite end points to reduce sample size requirements and to capture the overall impact of therapeutic interventions. Composite end points capture the number of patients who have 1 or more events of interest to increase the event rate and thus the statistical power of the study. However, they may mislead if component end points are of widely differing importance to patients, the number of events in the components of greater importance is small, and the magnitude of effect differs markedly across components. In 1986, the Gruppo Italiano per lo Studio della Streptochinasi nell'Infarto Miocardico group published a report of a large randomized clinical trial, demonstrating that intravenous streptokinase reduces the risk of death among patients with acute myocardial infarction.[21] The study investigated a single treatment, intravenous streptokinase, the control group received no streptokinase, there was no blinding, no placebo, and the end point was death from any cause. Failure to focus on all-cause mortality in the past has led to misleading impressions, as shown by the finding that amiodarone may be beneficial in survivors of myocardial infarction because it reduced the rate of arrhythmic death but had no impact on all-cause death. Furthermore, because of advances in treatment, placebo, or nontreatment controls are often no longer ethically permissible, meaning that the differences in outcomes between newer and older treatments will be relatively small, again mandating very large sample sizes. Nonetheless, more efficient trials with smaller sample sizes assembled to show a desired statistical effect do not necessarily compromise validity. Any end point that requires a measurement involving human judgment is inherently subject to bias and hence mandates a blinded end points committee, a core laboratory, or both. A composite end point that includes death and nonfatal events is subject to biases related to competing risks. Obviously, patients who die cannot later experience nonfatal myocardial infarction or be hospitalized. A treatment that leads to an increased risk of death may therefore seem to reduce the risk of nonfatal events. Although formal methods have been developed to analyze competing risks in an unbiased manner, the optimal approach to this problem is unclear. Quite often, the effects of a new drug, intervention, or procedure on a surrogate end point do not predict the true clinical effect, benefit, or intervention. Frequently, the reasons for a lack of consistency are unintended, unanticipated, and explained by the rationalization that the drug or intervention has mechanisms that are independent of the disease process.

## CONCLUSIONS

Cancer clinical trials constantly seek to define end points that are more rapidly available, more easily measured, and highly predictive of a definitive end point.[22] The rapidly expanding number of promising new anticancer agents in a current development for the treatment of solid tumors encourages clinicians, biologists, and statisticians to identify end points that are relevant and more rapidly observed than OS. However, with the steadily increasing number of novel molecules directed at "druggable" targets emerging, it is also imperative to design trials that appropriately evaluate such novel treatments in a valid and timely fashion. Moreover, the steady increase and refinement in diagnostic methods available allows for a more defined analysis of the effect of treatment modalities at the cellular and molecular level. The clinical implementation of any biologic marker has 2 major requirements: scientific validation and logistic feasibility. This approach should also improve the selection of patients who would benefit from adjuvant systemic treatment, reducing the rate of both overtreatment and undertreatment. Retrospective studies show that DNA microarray-based genomics represents a promising era of research in the field of prognosis and prediction of therapeutic response of ovarian cancer and other solid tumors.[23] Today, this approach remains in the research field, and there is no breakthrough that is close to become clinically applicable. The use of the reported predictors in clinical routine is premature, and no targeted therapy has yet emerged from the genomic results. However, there is no reason that the recent genomics-based advances obtained in breast cancer will not occur for other cancers. Other predictors will be identified in the coming years, and the challenge will be to demonstrate clinical benefits for patients. The scientific, medical, and pharmaceutical potential is enormous and could transform cancer management into a structured and logical science and a more successful medicine. This is all the promise of genomics medicine: to give the right treatment (and drug) to the right person at the right time. Until then, OS remains the gold standard.

## REFERENCES

1. Daugherty CK, Ratain MJ, Emanuel EJ, et al. Ethical, scientific, and regulatory perspectives regarding the use of placebos in cancer clinical trials. *J Clin Oncol.* 2008;26:1371–1378.
2. Hirschfeld S, Nagamura F, Keegan P. Food and Drug Administration with the accelerated approval program for oncology drugs. *Proc Am Soc Clin Oncol.* 2003;22:520, abstract no. 2094.
3. Johnson JR, Williams G, Pazdur R. End points and United States Food and Drug Administration approval of oncology drugs. *J Clin Oncol.* 2003;21:1404–1411.
4. Dagher R, Johnson J, Williams G, et al. Accelerated approval of oncology products: a decade of experience. *J Natl Cancer Inst.* 2004;96:1500–1509.
5. Clinton W, Gore A. Reinventing the Regulation of Cancer Drugs: National Performance Review. 1996. Available at: http://www.fda.gov/ohrms/dockets/ac/03/briefing/3936B1_01_C-Attachment%202.pdf.
6. Motzer RJ, Rini BI, Bukowski RM, et al. Sunitinib in patients with metastatic renal cell carcinoma. *JAMA.* 2006;295:2516–2524.
7. Miller AB, Hoogstraten B, Staquet M, et al. Reporting results of cancer treatment. *Cancer.* 1981;47:207–214.
8. Fukuoka M, Yano S, Giaccone G, et al. Multi-institutional randomized phase II trial of gefitinib for previously treated patients with advanced non-small-cell lung cancer (The IDEAL 1 Trial) [corrected.] *J Clin Oncol.* 2003;21:2237–2246.
9. Kris MG, Natale RB, Herbst R, et al. A phase II trial of ZD1839 in advanced non small cell lung cancer patients who had failed platinum and docetaxel-based regimens. *Proc Am Soc Clin Oncol.* 2002;21:292a, abstract no. 1116.
10. Herbst RS, Giaccone G, Schiller JH, et al. Gefitinib in combination with paclitaxel and carboplatin in advanced non-small-cell lung cancer: a phase III trial—INTACT 2. *J Clin Oncol.* 2004;22:785–794.
11. Giaccone G, Herbst RS, Manegold C, et al. Gefitinib in combination with gemcitabine and cisplatin in advanced non-small-cell lung cancer: a phase III trial—INTACT 1. *J Clin Oncol.* 2004;22:777–784.
12. Eisenhauer EA, Therasse P, Bogaerts J, et al. New response evaluation criteria in solid tumours: revised RECIST guideline (version 1.1). *Eur J Cancer.* 2009;45:228–247.
13. Hillman SL, An MW, O'Connell MJ, et al. Evaluation of the optimal number of lesions needed for tumor evaluation using the response evaluation criteria in solid tumors: a north central cancer treatment group investigation. *J Clin Oncol.* 2009;27:3205–3210.
14. Stein WD, Yang J, Bates SE, et al. Bevacizumab reduces the growth rate constants of renal carcinomas: a novel algorithm suggests early discontinuation of bevacizumab resulted in a lack of survival advantage. *Oncologist.* 2008;13:1055–1062.
15. Bruzzi P, Del Mastro L, Sormani MP, et al. Objective response to chemotherapy as a potential surrogate end point of survival in metastatic breast cancer patients. *J Clin Oncol.* 2005;23:5117–5125.
16. Burzykowski T, Buyse M, Piccart-Gebhart MJ, et al. Evaluation of tumor response, disease control, progression-free survival, and time to progression as potential surrogate end points in metastatic breast cancer. *J Clin Oncol.* 2008;26:1987–1992.
17. Fleming TR. Surrogate endpoints and FDA's accelerated approval process. *Health Aff (Millwood).* 2005;24:67–78.
18. Karaman MW, Herrgard S, Treiber DK, et al. A quantitative analysis of kinase inhibitor selectivity. *Nat Biotechnol.* 2008;26:127–132.
19. Lauer MS, Topol EJ. Clinical trials—multiple treatments, multiple end points, and multiple lessons. *JAMA.* 2003;289:2575–2577.
20. Ray ME, Bae K, Hussain MHA, et al. Potential surrogate endpoints for prostate cancer survival: analysis of a phase III randomized trial. *JNCI J Natl Cancer Inst.* 2009;101:228–236.
21. Effectiveness of intravenous thrombolytic treatment in acute myocardial infarction. Gruppo Italiano per lo Studio della Streptochinasi nell'Infarto Miocardico (GISSI). *Lancet.* 1986;1:397–402.
22. Schilsky RL. Hurry up and wait: is accelerated approval of new cancer drugs in the best interests of cancer patients? *J Clin Oncol.* 2003;21:3718–3720.
23. Minna JD, Girard L, Xie Y. Tumor mRNA expression profiles predict responses to chemotherapy. *J Clin Oncol.* 2007;25:4329–4336.

# Biomarker-Driven Early Clinical Trials in Oncology

## A Paradigm Shift in Drug Development

Daniel S. W. Tan • George V. Thomas • Michelle D. Garrett • Udai Banerji • Johann S. de Bono • Stan B. Kaye • Paul Workman

Following on from 3 decades of basic molecular oncology research, the complete sequencing of the human genome has led to a rapidly increasing understanding of the molecular pathogenesis of cancer.[1,2] Genetic and epigenetic control of signal transduction pathways involved in cell proliferation, apoptosis, invasion, senescence, and autophagy are deregulated in cancer and have emerged as key candidates for molecularly targeted therapy.[3] Identification of mission-critical drivers of the oncogenic process and improved understanding of the interactions and mediators of signaling pathways has opened up new vistas for developing rational individualized therapeutic strategies.[4–6] The expectation is that the new molecularly targeted agents will be more effective and less toxic than the previous generations of anticancer drugs.[7]

Important advances in drug discovery technologies have also been made over recent years. Modern approaches to small molecule drug discovery usually involve high-throughput screening using large or focused compound libraries and structure-based design strategies.[5,8,9] Technologies for the discovery of biologic agents, particularly engineered antibodies have also advanced.[10] The integrated use of new drug discovery technologies has shortened the time from selection of a new molecular target to the identification of a potent, selective, pharmacologically, pharmacokinetically, and pharmacodynamically optimized clinical candidate. Furthermore, molecular approaches, such as the development of transgenic animal models of cancer and more recently functional RNA interference screens, have greatly enhanced target validation, including the discovery of synthetically lethal combinations of drugs and genomic abnormalities that can be potentially exploited therapeutically.[11,12]

However, despite the high yield of potential new agents through integrative approaches in drug discovery, there remains a high rate of clinical failure, with only around 5% to 8% of first-in-human compounds reaching registration.[13,14] As a result, the investment needed for each successful new chemical entity has escalated to more than $800 million.[15] Of particular concern is the rising percentage of late-stage clinical failures, estimated at approximately 50% of oncology agents tested in phase III trials.[16] Such failures are especially expensive and deprive many patients of potentially more effective treatments.

## ONE DRUG DOES NOT FIT ALL

Emerging data suggest that targeted therapies are best used in the appropriate molecular context.[17] Despite this, the majority of randomized phase III trials—the defining hurdle for regulatory approval—continue to be designed for unselected patient populations. Furthermore, the traditional end points of overall survival or progression-free survival require protracted periods of follow-up for ascertaining benefit or indeed lack of benefit. Recent examples of negative trials include the IRESSA Survival Evaluation in Lung Cancer (ISEL) study, which examined the epidermal growth factor receptor (EGFR) inhibitor gefitinib versus placebo in advanced non–small cell lung cancer[18] and the Cetuximab Combined With Irinotecan in First-Line Therapy for Metastatic Colorectal Cancer (CRYSTAL) trial, where the combination of cetuximab, the EGFR-targeted antibody, with 5-fluorouracil and irinotecan failed to improve overall survival in metastatic colorectal cancer.[19] With both agents, retrospective analysis of available tissue led to the discovery that selected molecular subgroups attained greater benefit—presence of *EGFR* mutations with gefitinib[20] and *KRAS* wild type with cetuximab.[21] It follows that the inability to define an appropriate patient population for treatment in large phase III trials can lead to a substantial number of patients receiving ineffective treatment. Indeed, with the exception of a few targeted agents in molecularly well-defined diseases (eg, imatinib in gastrointestinal stromal tumors with activating *KIT* mutations), outcomes of clinical trials of targeted therapies have been at best modest, probably reflecting the hitherto lack of individualized, treatment approaches based on genetic alterations.[22]

However, recent key successes coupled with the large number of potential drug targets arising from genomic studies, and the wealth of interesting, innovative agents in development, suggests that the promise of personalized medicine is increasingly becoming a reality. Individual cancers are likely to have distinct biologic drivers, which can be exploited therapeutically by an appropriate targeted agent or a suitable combination of drugs. An excellent and well-known illustration is the incorporation of the cell membrane receptor human epidermal growth factor-2 targeting antibody trastuzumab in treatment regimens for breast cancer in the subgroup of patients who are human epidermal growth factor-2 positive.[23,24] In addition to patient selection markers, biomarkers that provide proof of target inhibition and facilitate the demonstration of downstream biologic effects are also extremely important in drug development.

The key challenge lies in increasing the odds for successful and efficient transition of a compound through the drug development pipeline. The incorporation of scientifically and analytically validated biomarkers into rationally designed hypothesis-testing clinical trials offers a promising way forward to achieving this objective.

## BIOMARKER-DRIVEN EARLY CLINICAL TRIALS

Phase I trials represent the first introduction of a drug or combination of drugs into the clinical setting and seek to define the optimal or recommended phase II dose for further testing. In phase I trials, dose escalation is usually carried out until excess clinical toxicities ensue, thus defining the maximal tolerated dose (MTD). However, the era of targeted therapies is challenging the utility of such simple dose-escalation paradigms. The relationship between toxicity and activity may be less linear than with conventional cytotoxics. In up to a third of phase I trials of molecularly targeted drugs, the MTD is not reached.[25]

Therapeutic activity may be seen at the low-dose levels used in the early stages of clinical trials with molecular therapeutics (as may also be observed with low doses of conventional cytotoxic drugs).[26] Moreover, although regressions have been observed because of induction of apoptosis by some molecularly targeted agents, in other cases, the predominant effect at the cellular level may be cytostasis, leading to disease stabilization that can be prolonged. Thus, in the setting of single agent phase I/II trials, drug activity does not always translate to typical response parameters according to the Response Evaluation Criteria in Solid Tumors (RECIST), underscoring the importance of incorporating measures of antitumor effect other than changes in tumor size into early clinical trials.[27]

Pharmacodynamic (PD) biomarkers, which assess the effect a drug has on the body, can provide a useful indicator of drug activity, including both proximal effects on the molecular target and also effects on more distal downstream events. Such PD biomarkers allow the demonstration of proof of concept for intended target modulation and achievement of the desired biologic effects. Especially when coupled with pharmacokinetic (PK) measurements of drug exposure, PD end points can help us to understand better the dose-response relationship and provide a rational basis for dose and schedule selection.[28,29] Increasingly, the incorporation of mechanism-based biomarker end points into phase I/II clinical trials is improving our ability to make early "go-no go" decisions.[30]

Efficiency of the drug development process can be enhanced by optimizing patient selection, demonstrating treatment effects earlier, eg, target modulation or cellular and tissue effects, and establishing science-based surrogate end points that correlate with response and survival.[30,31] With improved methods of tumor evaluation, including noninvasive functional imaging[32] and analysis of circulating tumor cells (CTCs),[33] biomarker-driven early phase trials not only promise to accelerate the drug development process but also importantly provide a unique opportunity to interrogate human disease biology in the patient and gain mechanistic insights into targeted molecular cancer therapeutics. The success of this new biomarker-driven approach demands close collaboration between academia, industry, and regulatory agencies.

## THE DRUG APPROVAL PROCESS AND FDA

Underpinning the conduct of clinical trials is the requirement for regulatory and marketing approval, a task undertaken by the Food and Drug Administration (FDA) in the United States, and equivalent bodies such as the European Medicines Agency in Europe. Such regulatory bodies have dual roles in protecting and promoting health—on one hand ensuring that new investigational agents are rigorously tested for safety, whereas on the other, facilitating expedient marketing approval if they are shown scientifically to be effective.[34] The accelerated drug approval program was adopted in 1992 to improve access to new drugs for life-threatening diseases based on surrogate end points such as response rates or symptom improvement.[35] Recognizing the need for the involvement of all stakeholders, the FDAs critical path initiative was launched in 2004. The primary objective of this initiative was to foster collaboration between clinicians, academic scientists, and the pharmaceutical industry as well as regulatory authorities, so as to integrate the preclinical scientific process with all stages of clinical trials.[36] Key areas identified for improvement include better development and utilization of biomarkers of safety and efficacy, modernization of clinical trial methodologies, and the aggressive use of bioinformatics, including disease modeling and trial simulation.[34] To ensure consistency in appraising the utility of biomarkers, it is important to accurately distinguish the various categories and the extent of validation.

## BIOMARKERS: SOME DEFINITIONS

One of the complications in the field of biomarker development has been the lack of uniformity in describing the various types of biomarkers. A biomarker can be broadly defined as "a characteristic that is objectively measured and evaluated as an indicator of normal biologic processes, pathogenic processes, or pharmacologic response to a therapeutic intervention."[37] They can be further subclassified into other major categories, such as (1) risk biomarkers, (2) biologic progression markers, or (3) PD biomarkers (Table 1).

1. Risk biomarkers can be prognostic or predictive. Prognostic biomarkers are often implicated in the mechanisms of disease causality or the oncogenic process. They describe risks of developing cancer or of cancer progression, and they encompass carcinogen exposure, genetic predisposition, pharmacogenomic parameters, previous disease or precursor lesions, and multifactorial risk models.[31] Their effect on outcome is usually independent of exposure to drug. A predictive biomarker is a pretreatment characteristic that can be assessed or measured, that predicts for response to a specific therapy, eg, estrogen receptor positivity and tamoxifen sensitivity. However, there are some biomarkers that are both prognostic and predictive, eg, HER-2 overexpression in breast cancer, which while portending a poor prognosis,[38,39] also predicts response to trastuzumab.[23]

2. Biologic progression markers measure tumor burden. Examples include the use of circulating cellular proteins such as

**TABLE 1.** Classification of Biomarkers

| Category | Application |
|---|---|
| **Risk** | |
| Prognostic | Pretreatment patient selection |
| Predictive | |
| **Pharmacodynamic** | |
| Proximal | Posttreatment |
|   Target modulation (eg, phosphorylation of downstream protein) | Disease monitoring |
| Distal* | Proof of treatment effect |
|   Genomic and proteomic expression profiles | |
|   Proliferation markers (eg, Ki-67, PCNA) | |
|   Apoptosis markers (eg, BCL-2 expression, TUNEL) | |
|   Histopathologic changes (eg, microvessel density) | |
|   Functional imaging (eg, $K_{trans}$, FDG) | |
| **Biological progression markers** | |
| Tumor markers (eg, PSA-doubling time) | Posttreatment |
| Anatomical imaging markers (eg, computer tomography scans) | Measure of tumor burden |
| Surrogate clinical end points Response rate, disease free survival | Correlates of overall survival |

*Consequence of drug action downstream from molecular target.
FDG indicates fluorodeoxyglucose; TUNEL, terminal deoxynucleotidyl transferase dUTP nick end labeling; and PCNA, proliferating cell nuclear antigen.

carcinoembryonic antigen (CEA), CA-125 and prostate-specific antigen (PSA), and more recently, CTC counts in certain cancer types, eg, breast and prostate.[40] Such biomarkers are often used to monitor the effect of a therapeutic intervention, where they are termed response biomarkers, and increasingly have been adopted as surrogate or intermediate end points. To meet the requirements of a surrogate end point, the biomarker must first be modulated by a therapy and then be shown to correlate with a clinically meaningful end point.[31] For example, PSA doubling time postlocal treatment has been shown to predict survival in locally advanced prostate cancer, as have CTC counts in metastatic disease.[31,41] It is anticipated that such biomarker end points will provide better estimates of clinical benefit in shorter timeframes, when compared with traditional end points such as progression-free survival and overall survival.

3. PD biomarkers are markers of drug effect that are usually on the pathway associated with the molecular target or alternatively represent downstream consequences of target and pathway modulation; they can include molecular, cellular, histopathologic, and imaging parameters.[30] It is important to emphasize that PD biomarkers, while characterizing the molecular and functional effects of a drug, may not necessarily have any correlation with biologic or clinical effects.[32] For example, even if the phosphorylation of the substrate of the target kinase is modulated, other factors may control the therapeutic response of the cancer cell, as observed with current mitogen-activated protein kinase kinase and phosphatidylinositide-3 (PI3) kinase inhibitors.[42,43]

It is noteworthy that the described biomarker categories are by no means mutually exclusive, and that any given biomarker can belong to different categories depending on the context in which they are used. For instance, in prostate cancer, high baseline CTC counts are associated with a poor prognosis, whereas a fall in cell counts may serve as a biologic progression marker for patients on treatment.[44] Moreover, molecular characterization of CTCs in prostate cancer can be also predictive of response to specific interventions, eg, prostate cancer patients with TMPRSS2-ERG translocations in their CTCs are more responsive than wild type to the promising 17α-hydroxylase/17,20 lyase inhibitor, abiraterone[45] (Fig. 1). In the context of phase I trials, PD end points form a crucial link between PK and response biomarkers and allows for the construction of what we have described as the pharmacologic audit trail.[29,30,46,47]

## THE PHARMACOLOGIC AUDIT TRAIL

With rapidly advancing methods for assessing PD effects, we are now in a position where we can construct a hierarchy of sequential connected questions that depict the target status; the effects of the body on the drug (PK and metabolism); the effects of the drug on the molecular target, biochemical pathway, and cellular and tissue function; and the subsequent therapeutic and toxicologic effects of the drug. First proposed in 2002, the pharmacologic audit trail provides a conceptual and practical framework to correlate clinical observations with scientifically measurable end points.[29,30,46,47] In this framework, each successive question, when answered appropriately, increases the likelihood of success with a particular drug. Importantly, the audit trail provides a means to assess and manage risk in a drug development program and thus increases the rationality of the decision-making process. The success of such an approach necessitates integration of preclinical and clinical phases of drug development, so that questions and hypotheses concerning biologic mechanisms of response and resistance may be examined seamlessly and simultaneously. An example of the use of a pharmacologic audit trail in this way is pro-

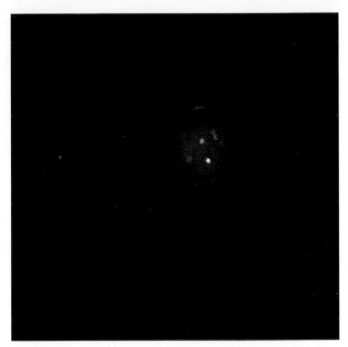

**FIGURE 1.** FISH detection of TMPRSS2 and *ERG* gene status on a circulating prostate tumor cell using Veridex Cell Search system. The status of the *ERG* gene was examined using the ERG "break-apart" assay revealing splitting of *TMPRSS2* (green) and *ERG* (red) gene in one of the alleles, representing translocation of 5′ ERG to another part of the nucleus. Emerging data suggest that such rearrangements are associated with a poor prognosis[154] but may also have a predictive role—with ERG rearrangements being associated with improved PSA responses to abiraterone, when compared with wild type.[45] (Courtesy of Dr Gerhardt Attard.)

vided by a phase I trial of 17-allyamino-17-demethoxygeldanamycin (17-AAG), a heat shock protein-90 inhibitor (HSP90, Fig. 2).[47–49]

A caveat to the PK-PD-effect audit trail model arises if the mechanisms of the drug in question are not fully elucidated or if there are unanticipated "off target" effects. For example, sorafenib was initially developed as a drug most likely acting as a B-RAF kinase inhibitor only to later achieve marketing approval as a vascular endothelial growth factor receptor tyrosine kinase inhibitor in renal cancer.[50,51] However, it is envisaged that with modern methods of drug discovery and sophisticated compound profiling, new agents emerging from the preclinical pipeline will have undergone thorough characterization of their activity spectrum, and their major pharmacologic targets will be defined in considerable detail in relevant experimental models. For example, in the case of kinase inhibitors, this will include profiling against large panels of kinases and other pharmacological targets, which often yields valuable information.

## BIOMARKER DISCOVERY AND VALIDATION

Advances in genomic and proteomic technologies and powerful bioinformatic tools have changed the face of both biomarker and target discovery.[52,53] Although early cancer biomarkers were based mainly on simple empirical observations, modern platforms offer the advantage of massively parallel analyses, resulting in the emergence of multiple markers with unique patterns rather than single markers.[54]

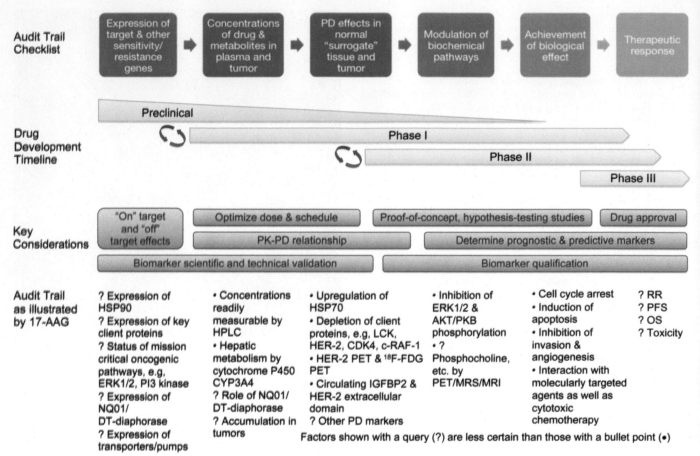

**FIGURE 2.**   The pharmacologic audit trail in the context of the drug development timeline and key considerations at each stage. The development of the molecular chaperone HSP90 inhibitor 17-AAG demonstrates the importance of using PK/PD relationships in adaptive phase I trial design. Before trial initiation, all biomarkers and assays were validated in preclinical models. A molecular signature of drug activity had been determined through gene expression profiling using microarrays, and this was corroborated with a set of Western blot assays developed for protein measurement in the clinical setting. During dose escalation, drug levels were measured by liquid chromatography mass spectrometry assay. Once plasma concentrations reached levels required for drug efficacy, PBMCs were obtained from blood samples, and the molecular signatures associated with target modulation were measured. Having demonstrated that 17-AAG was indeed inhibiting the target in PBMCs, pretreatment and posttreatment tumor biopsies were initiated, and these confirmed that the drug was working in the exact same way as preclinical models, resulting in a characteristic molecular signature assessed by Western immunoblotting and IHC. Additional assays are also being evaluated, as shown.

High-throughput functional genomics approaches, particularly small interfering RNA (siRNA) screens, have also facilitated comprehensive annotation of the consequences of deregulated genes through biologic assays. This enhances the identification of the mediators of drug response and resistance,[11] and potential predictive markers. Despite the large number of candidate biomarkers in the pipeline, the majority have yet to be adopted into routine clinical practice, with as few as 0 to 2 biomarkers per year achieving FDA approval across all diseases.[55] In a review in 2005, only 24 FDA-approved cancer biomarkers were described[54]—examples include HER-2 expression and copy number changes, circulating tumor markers, eg, CA-125 and CEA. One of the reasons for this is the high bar that is set for the clinical validation of biomarkers. This is usually achieved through a stepwise process of verification or qualification.[56,56a]

It is important to emphasize that the application of biomarkers should not be undertaken trivially and demands rigorous scientific and technical validation and very thorough assay standardization. Indeed, lack of appropriate technical validation pervades the field of biomarker research. Incorporation of poorly validated biomarkers will invariably yield misleading results, and can lead to subsequent disregard for a potentially useful marker or an inappropriate decision being made about the drug. It has been suggested that one of the reasons for the paucity of reliable assays and methods for validation studies is the failure to initiate their development sufficiently early to allow them to be validated and implemented in early clinical trials.[32]

## SYNERGISM IN BIOMARKER AND DRUG DEVELOPMENT

It is increasingly acknowledged that the drug and biomarker pipelines should be developed in tandem. Early discovery and clinical evaluation of biomarkers is a crucial step to their eventual qualification.

Indeed, biomarkers are increasingly used during the preclinical drug discovery phase and in clinical development.[5] Like drugs, biomarkers require several phases of development. After initial discovery and scientific validation of a given biomarker in exploratory preclinical or clinical studies, laboratory-based technical development of the particular biomarker assay should then ensue. During this phase, the assay is optimized, so that it is accurate, robust, and reproducible, especially for use in the clinical setting.[29,56] Further verification and qualification is then typically required through prospective evaluation, replication, and eventual regulatory approval.

The relatively small number of patients involved in early clinical trials makes it important to obtain corroborative biomarker information at this stage, so as to elucidate methodological limitations and obtain initial indications of utility. In addition, the availability of biomarker data from preclinical models serves as an avenue for cross-validation, as illustrated by our own work on HSP90 inhibitors,[48,49,57,58] PI3 kinase inhibitors,[45,59] and CDK inhibitors.[60-62] As in the HSP90 studies, it is very important that the emerging clinical biomarker data are compared with results from preclinical models in which the pharmacologic audit trail would ideally have been established. These preclinical models must be chosen carefully to parallel the clinical setting as accurately as possible, particularly in terms of relevant molecular pathology, and may involve human tumor xenografts or genetically engineered mouse models.[63,64]

The value of early introduction of biomarkers is further emphasized by the fact that determining assay variability is crucial with respect to appropriate statistical considerations when applied to the design of future clinical trials.[65] In this regard, there is increasing onus on pharmaceutical companies to develop companion diagnostics in tandem with new agents, so as to be able to better define the scope of clinical application if a drug is eventually approved.

We have argued that the degree of validation of a biomarker should not only be related to the stage of clinical development, ie, early versus late, but more importantly, should be proportionate to the intended role of the biomarker—for example whether or not it will be used in decision-making within the trial.[29] Hence, the requisite extent of validation should be "fit-for-purpose". In addition to established biomarkers, we propose that, in many instances, early stage but nevertheless fit-for-purpose biomarkers should be considered for use in early phase trials, where they can be designated as exploratory end points.[29,30] This allows for early hypothesis-testing or hypothesis-generating studies to be carried out using the biomarker in the clinic, without directly impacting on the key decision-making primary or secondary end points of a drug trial.

On the other hand, for scientifically validated biomarkers that are intended for decision making in the clinic, it is important to ensure an adequate degree of technical standardization. In the UK, the minimal standard is determined by Good Clinical Laboratory Practice,[65a] which embodies a set of principles that provides a framework within which laboratory studies are planned, performed, monitored, recorded, reported, and archived. This includes consistency in the collection, handling, and processing of clinical material, as well as ensuring uniformity of methodology and technology platforms. Such an approach minimizes technical confounders and permits a more accurate depiction of the pharmacologic audit trail.[30] There is an increasing trend toward companion diagnostic assays being performed in "accredited" laboratories. In the United States, such laboratories conform to the quality standards stipulated by Clinical Laboratory Improvement Amendments, ensuring accuracy, reliability, and timeliness to test. To gain consensus on international clinical laboratory operations, there are present efforts to harmonize the multitude of existing guidelines from goverment and accrediting and non-accrediting organizations, so as to increase implementation guidance.[56a]

## CHALLENGES OF INCORPORATING FIT-FOR-PURPOSE BIOMARKERS

We have previously discussed in detail the issues involved in the application of biomarkers that are fit for the intended purpose, including validation to GCLP requirements. This is especially crucial where the prescribed biomarker will be used to make decisions, eg, concerning dose and schedule, during the trial.[29] In addition to the technical hurdles, biomarkers have their inherent limitations. Ideally, biomarkers should be repeatable, reproducible, minimally invasive, and entail negligible or no risk when measured. They should at the same time yield sufficient material for analytical studies and be able to generate valuable data for the audit trail. The extent to which a biomarker depicts the biology of the entire tumor is also a key consideration, although the issue of tumor heterogeneity is a pervasive problem even with routine diagnostic biopsies.

The next section will elaborate on examples of commonly used sources of biomarkers in early phase trials and emerging technology platforms, including their limitations. Examples of commonly used biomarkers as applied to early phase trials are summarized in Table 2.

### Normal "Surrogate" Tissue

Normal "surrogate" tissues are commonly used for biomarker studies in phase I trials. They typically include superficial accessible tissue, such as plucked hair follicles,[76] skin biopsies,[66] and buccal mucosa scrapings[73]; or alternatively they may entail venepuncture to obtain peripheral blood mononuclear cells (PBMCs, see Table 2 for examples). Normal "surrogate" tissue is particularly suited for the pharmacogenomic analysis of germline DNA, eg, studies of single nucleotide polymorphisms. These are often stored and analyzed only after completion of trials, when toxicity and efficacy data emerge.

Increasingly, because of the ease of obtaining normal "surrogate" tissue, they are extensively used to examine the PD effects of drugs and to determine the changes that occur over time through repeated sampling. PBMCs are commonly used for the measurement of the expression levels or posttranslational modifications of particular proteins, and the methods may be qualitative (eg, Western immunoblotting), semiquantitative (eg, immunohistochemistry [IHC]), or quantitative (eg, ELISA-based). The most frequent assays performed with molecularly targeted agents examine target modulation with Western blots or IHC, where for example, PBMCs or skin biopsies are evaluated for phosphorylation of kinase substrates in response to kinase inhibitors[95,97] or the acetylation of histones with histone deacetylation inhibitors.[78]

It is also possible to correlate changes in gene expression profiles associated with target modulation to protein levels in PBMCs. In the development of the HSP90 inhibitor 17-AAG (tanespimycin), a molecular signature of drug activity was initially determined in vitro through gene expression profiling using cDNA microarrays.[57] Results were corroborated and extended in a set of Western blot assays that were subsequently developed for protein measurement in the clinical setting, in which depletion of the levels of chaperone client proteins, together with an increase in the stress response protein HSP72 in PBMCs provided a specific, scientifically validated molecular signature indicative of target modulation.[48,49] The PK-PD-efficacy relationship was validated in a preclinical model.[49] The initial dose level at which target modulation is seen might indicate that a pharmacologically active exposure has been reached, at which point further investigations may be introduced to examine the drug effect. In the 17-AAG phase I trial, pretreatment and posttreatment tumor biopsies were initiated within the dose escalation scheme only after target modulation had been demonstrated in PBMCs.[48] Interestingly,

**TABLE 2.** Examples of Biomarkers Used to Interrogate Specific Pathways and Biological Processes

| | Normal "Surrogate" Tissue | Blood/Plasma | Tumor Tissue | Imaging Techniques |
|---|---|---|---|---|
| **Pathways** | | | | |
| EGFR | Paired skin biopsies: p-EGFR, p-ERK1/2 (MAPK activation), Ki-67, p27[KIP1], keratin 1, p-STAT3[66] | CTCs: EGFR L858R, T790M mutations, exon 19 deletions[67] | Paired tumor biopsies: EGFR (IHC and FISH), p-EGFR, p-MAPK, p-AKT, p27, Ki-67, K-RAS[68] | *EGFR kinase PET* [69,70] |
| | Buccal mucosa epithelial cells: p-AKT, p-EGFR and p-MAPK[73] | Plasma DNA: EGFR-activating or T790M mutations[71] | Biopsy: EGFR T790M mutation (secondary resistance)[72] | |
| IGF-1 | PBMC: IGF-IR expression[74] | Plasma: IGF-1 levels[74,75] CTCs: IGF-IR expression[33] | Paired tumor biopsies: p-AKT, p-MAPK and p-S6[75] | [18]FDG-PET/CT[75] |
| PI3K | PBMC: p-AKT, PRAS40[76] | Platelet-rich plasma: p-AKT[77] | Paired tumor biopsies: p-AKT and p-S6[77] | [18]FDG-PET/CT[77] |
| | Hair follicles: p-AKT, PRAS40, p-4EBP1, p-S6[76] | | Paired tumor biopsies: p-AKT, p-4EBP1, p-ERK, Ki-67, TUNEL[76] | |
| Histone deacetylation inhibitors (epigenetic regulation) | PBMC: histone H3 and H4 acetylation[78] *Serial fat pad FNA sampling: histone H3 acetylation[81]* | Nil | NY-ESO-1, MAGE-3, p16, histone H4 acetylation, p21, Ki-67, p-ERK, cleaved caspase-3 protein levels[79] | *P-magnetic resonance spectroscopy[80]* |
| **Biological processes** | | | | |
| Angiogenesis | Skin biopsy: microvessel density, blood vessel maturity[82] | Serum: decreases in VEGFR2, and increases in VEGF and PlGF[83] Blood: circulating endothelial cells[86,87] | Biopsy: microvessel density, IHC for angiogenic factors eg, VEGF, HIF1α, proteomics, gene expression profiling[84] | DCE-MRI[85] DCE-CT[88] |
| Apoptosis | PBMC: XIAP mRNA levels[89] | Blood: M30 ELISA (caspase-cleaved neo-epitope on CK18) and M65 ELISA (both intact and cleaved soluble CK18)[90] | Biopsy: overexpression of Bcl-2 family members (BCL-2, BCL-X_L, BCL-w, MCL-1); Inhibitors of apoptosis proteins (survivin or XIAP); Pro-apoptotic proteins, such as Bax, caspase 8, death receptors, p53/p73/p21[waf-1]; TUNEL[91] | DWI-MRI *(necrosis)*[92,122] |
| Proliferation | Buccal mucosa swabs and punch skin biopsies: polyploidy and histone H3 phosphorylation (mitotic arrest)[93] | CTCs: histone H3 phosphorylation (mitotic arrest)[94] | Biopsy: p-MAPK, p27, Ki-67[68,95] | [18]FLT-PET[96] |

Italicized modalities remain in preclinical development.
FDG inditaces fluorodeoxyglucose; CT, computer tomography; TUNEL, terminal deoxynucleotidyl transferase dUTP nick-end labeling; VEGF, vascular endothelial growth factor; IGF-1R, insulin-like growth factor1 receptor; DWI, diffusion weighted imaging; FLT, fluoro-L-thymidine; FNA, fine needle aspiration.

in this same PK-PD guided study, reproducible PD changes in patient PBMC samples that led to incorporation of biopsies were triggered by the achievement of plasma levels shown to be active in preclinical studies.[48,49]

In contrast to their application in guiding decision making with respect to selection of the optimal dose and schedule, the effect of drug on surrogate tissue biomarkers may be carried out for hypothesis-testing or hypothesis-generating reasons. The hypothesis-generation biomarker approach is exemplified in our recent phase I study of the marine natural product ES-285, where exploratory cDNA expression profiling studies in blood and skin revealed dose-responsive changes in the expression of genes of potential mechanistic relevance.[98] The effect of drug on a surrogate biomarker may also be analyzed in a hypothesis-testing setting, such as the recent ARQ-197 c-Met inhibitor trial, where observed falls in circulating endothelial cells suggested an antiangiogenic effect and led to the incorporation of dynamic contrast-enhanced magnetic resonance imaging (DCE-MRI).[86,99] Adaptive designs of this last type ensure that more invasive or costly investigations, such as tumor biopsies or MRI scans, are incorporated in a rational manner.

Defining the dose range at which target modulation occurs using biomarkers in surrogate tissue is increasingly common in phase I trials of molecularly targeted therapies.[100] It remains controversial whether the recommended phase II dose should be established from MTD or an optimal biologic dose determined by PD effects.[101] Knowledge of drug targets should allow the discovery, validation, and application of biomarkers, which depict molecular and biochemical evidence of target engagement and their anticipated biologic effects. This should facilitate more informed choices about optimal dose levels and schedules for future studies, including combination trials. For example, in an ongoing phase Ib trial of a poly ADP-ribose polymerase (PARP) inhibitor combined with paclitaxel and carboplatin, the starting dose level of the PARP inhibitor was derived from the PD data from the phase I trial, using the lower limit of the dose range at which significant inhibition of PARP activity on PBMCs was demonstrated.[102]

With appropriate PK/PD modeling, the relationship between target modulation in PBMCs and tumors in animal models has been extrapolated to human subjects, without necessarily incorporating tumor biopsies in the clinical study. This was recently illustrated with the mammalian target of rapamycin (mTOR) inhibitor everolimus, where the relationship between plasma concentrations, S6K1 inhibition in PBMCs, and antitumor effect was first elucidated in treated CA20948 pancreatic tumor-bearing rats. Subsequently, a PK/PD model was developed that allowed selection of optimal dose and schedule based on the PBMC S6K1 inhibition time profiles in patients.

Importantly, however, the major drawback of the use of normal "surrogate" tissue is the lack of oncogenic molecular pathology that might be targeted by a drug, thereby potentially limiting the extent of demonstrable link to tumor tissue responses. In addition, it is possible that the qualitative or quantitative responses in normal tissue may be different from those seen in the tumor (Table 3). For example, inhibition of a pathway might result in a differential response, such as more cell death in tumor versus normal tissue, due to oncogene addiction or dependence or a synthetic lethal effect. The way forward on this is probably best based on experience with correlative studies in preclinical models. More comparative work is needed in this area.

## Tumor Biopsies

Pretreatment and posttreatment tumor biopsies afford direct assessments of drug effect on cancer cells. More importantly, they contain a

**TABLE 3.** Challenges of Incorporating Fit-for-Purpose Biomarkers: Normal "Surrogate" Tissue

| Attributes | Drawbacks |
| --- | --- |
| Generally safe; repeated sampling often possible allowing temporal evaluation of PD changes | Lack of oncogenic molecular pathology that may be found only in tumor tissue |
| Defines the dose range at which target modulation occurs using biomarkers | Limitations in the extent of demonstrable link to tumor tissue responses (although clinical relevance can be potentially elucidated by parallel correlative biopsies of tumor tissue) |
| Can be used for preliminary hypothesis-testing or hypothesisgenerating purposes | |
| Particularly suited for the pharmacogenomic analysis of germline DNA | Qualitative or quantitative responses in the normal surrogate tissue may be different from those seen in the tumor |

**TABLE 4.** Challenges of Incorporating Fit-for-Purpose Biomarkers: Tumor Biopsies

| Attributes | Drawbacks |
| --- | --- |
| Analysis of cancer tissue is likely to be molecularly and therapeutically more relevant compared to normal tissue | Procedural risks |
| Allows massively parallel high-throughput analysis of genetic and epigenetic events | Limited ability to perform multiple procedures to assess time points |
| IHC studies allow morphologic and spatial examination in the assessment of biologic effects | Tissue heterogeneity |
| Pretreatment and posttreatment biopsies can give insights into drug effects on cancer cells mediators of response (PD effect) or resistance to a targeted agent | Sampling bias |
| Allows for quantification of drug effects in tumor | |

wealth of molecular and genetic information that can be retrieved using conventional or high-throughput analysis platforms. In addition, in the case of IHC studies, they can also allow morphologic examination in the assessment of biologic effects, offering a unique insight to the cell-specific consequences of drug exposure or target modulation in the complex milieu of a solid tumor (Table 4). An example of this is illustrated in Figure 3A, B, where the consequences of target modulation by an mTOR inhibitor are demonstrated in the preclinical and clinical setting.

Despite the vast potential for translational research with tumor biopsies, some commentaries have been sceptical regarding their routine use and have, for example, questioned whether such additional procedures are justified ethically.[104] However, it has been reported that tumor biopsies are generally safe,[105] and that a significant proportion of patients on trials perceive the 5% to 10% risk of complications to be acceptable.[106] Furthermore, if the additional biopsies permit determination of key translational end points that can accelerate drug development and aid discovery and validation of biomarkers, one might argue that it is unethical to miss the opportunity to derive maximal information on the drug and its target.

Indeed, biopsy studies from trials involving tyrosine kinase inhibitors have generated useful preliminary data on both predictive and PD biomarkers. Candidate predictive biomarkers were identified in translational studies from early phase trials of EGFR inhibitors, even as the phase III trials were still ongoing. In a phase II study of erlotinib in advanced nonsmall cell lung cancer, EGFR fluorescent in situ hybridization (FISH)-positive status was found to be associated with improved outcome, and there was a further suggestion that median progression-free survival was longer in those with EGFR mutations.[68] Baseline expression of EGFR, p-EGFR, p-mitogen activated protein kinase (MAPK), p-AKT, p27, and Ki-67 was not related to clinical outcomes. Whether the high profile failure of the phase III trials of EGFR inhibitors in unselected patient populations could have been averted if these findings were incorporated, remains an open question.

As mentioned, analysis of posttreatment biopsies can also be informative with respect to PD markers that demonstrate target inhibition and their downstream consequences. For example, early studies with the EGFR tyrosine kinase inhibitors used a range of proximal and distal markers that showed evidence of inhibition of the target

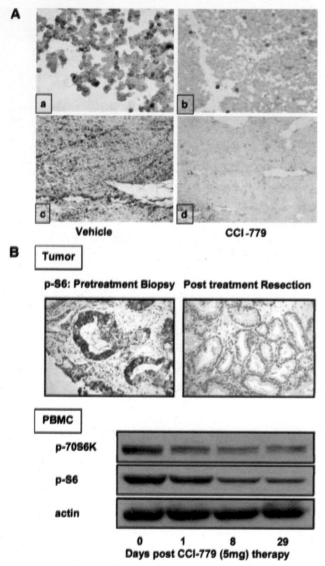

**FIGURE 3.** A, Inhibition of mTOR activity can be monitored by loss of phospho-S6 immunoreactivity. a and b, Human renal cell carcinoma cell lines treated with 10 nM CCI-779, an mTOR inhibitor, and subsequently trypsinized and cell pellets fixed in formalin. The pellets were paraffin embedded and tissue sections cut. c and d, Human renal cell carcinoma xenograft tumors from vehicle and CCI-779 treated mice were probed with anti–p-S6 antibody. B, p-S6 in the tumor (IHC) and PBMC (immunoblotting) as biochemical readouts for mTOR inhibition. Upper panels: loss of p-S6 staining after 29 days of CCI-779 therapy (5 mg/d) is documented in the pretreatment prostate biopsy and posttreatment prostatectomy tumor sections from a patient with prostate cancer. Lower panels: PBMCs were extracted from the peripheral blood samples of the same patient at specific days post-CCI-779 therapy initiation (per protocol); lysates prepared and stored in −80°F. At the end of the trial, the lysates were probed with both antip-70S6K (S6K1) and antip-S6 antibodies. Loss of both phospho-specific antibodies are documented and correlate with the loss of signal seen in the tumor tissue. Actin serves as loading control.

and blockade of proliferation, initially in skin biopsies, and then in tumor samples.[66,68] In some cases, proof of mechanism for target, pathway, and biologic effect modulation will translate into proof of concept for therapeutic activity. Alternatively, when successful target modulation in tumor does not translate into a therapeutic response and outcome, this may suggest that the degree of inhibition is not sufficient or that the molecular target is not valid in human subjects in that setting.[107] In a PD study of erlotinib in breast cancer, the expected downstream changes posttreatment were seen in skin biopsies (inhibition of p-MAPK, increased cell cycle inhibitor p27, and reduced proliferation marker Ki-67), whereas tumor biopsies revealed only inhibition of MAPK phosphorylation, with no effect on p27 and Ki-67, implying a lack of EGFR dependence in the tested population.[95]

Although early clinical trials involve small patient numbers, PD data from pretreatment and posttreatment biopsies can generate useful insights into mediators of response or resistance to a molecularly targeted agent. For example, in a phase I trial of the mTOR inhibitor RAD001, analysis of pretreatment and posttreatment tumor biopsies demonstrated the unexpected finding that mTOR inhibition resulted in activation of AKT.[108] This led to subsequent experiments that showed that AKT activation occurred through the induction of insulin receptor substrate-1, which in turn could be abrogated by insulin-like growth factor-1 receptor inhibition, representing a potential means of sensitizing tumor cells to mTOR inhibitors.

Such early exploratory studies are not limited to kinase inhibitors. In the phase I trial of 17-AAG, in addition to providing PD data, biopsies of melanoma lesions in a small cohort of patients who responded to therapy suggested an association with [V600E]*BRAF* or [G13D]*NRAS* mutations.[109]

Pretreatment and posttreatment biopsies provide us with an early opportunity not only to appraise the potential therapeutic value of an agent in the clinic through predicted on-target effects but also, in addition, to generate hypotheses with regard to feedback loops, off-target effects, or alternative mechanisms of resistance to target inhibition. Such data indicate the need for more wide-ranging profiling of the effects of a drug on multiple pathways in the clinic. The future use in the clinic of emerging technologies, such as phosphoprotein arrays, can facilitate the delineation of drug effects on a wide range of targets and on independent or interacting signaling pathways, thus guiding the development of rational therapeutic approaches, including synergistic combinations.[110] Indeed, it is likely that preclinical network systems biology studies will soon be extrapolated into corresponding clinical studies to better predict therapeutic success.[111]

Furthermore, it is conceivable that such tumor biopsies might facilitate better molecular classification of solid tumors and eventually help select patients best suited to a trial of a specific targeted drug.[112] Recently, Kim et al[113] reported a biomarker-directed randomized phase II trial in metastatic non–small cell lung cancer. In this study, 11 biomarkers were analyzed—*EGFR*, *KRAS*, and *BRAF* gene mutation (polymerase chain reaction-based sequencing), EGFR and Cyclin D1 copy number analyses (FISH), and the expression of 6 proteins by IHC (VEGF, VEGFR, retinoid X receptor-$\alpha$, $\beta$, $\gamma$, and Cyclin D1). Based on real time biomarker analysis, patients tumors were delineated into predominant molecular pathways that best predicted for response to 1 of 4 treatments—erlotinib, sorafenib, vandetanib, and erlotinib in combination with bexarotene—and subsequently subject to outcome-based adaptive randomization. Despite the need for 2 fresh core needle biopsy specimens, enrolment into this trial has been brisk, suggesting that the incorporation of biopsies to identify molecular characteristics for rational allocation to a trial treatment arm is feasible. Such an approach may be extended to phase I trials, particularly with the advent of modern DNA sequencing technology, eg, Sequenom Massarray, where detection of mutations in key cancer genes can potentially help identify subgroups of patients who may be more likely to benefit from novel therapies. An example could be the determination of *PI3KCA* activating mutations or *PTEN* loss for allocation to a PI3 kinase inhibitor trial, although this has yet to be confirmed. It is now readily achievable to determine the status of at least 200 common gene mutations in 17 cancer genes in patient tissue. As sequencing costs fall, the next stage would be whole genome resequencing in individual cancer patients.

A final and important consideration is the quantification of drug effects. The use of biomarkers to determine optimal drug dose can be further strengthened if markers used are quantitative, and where there is preclinical information concerning how inhibition of normal and tumor tissue are equated. Of particular significance is information on how much target modulation is needed and for how long to deliver a given biologic or therapeutic effect. For example, in the case of our recent studies with PI3 kinase inhibitors, including the clinical candidate GDC-0941, preclinical results (using MesoScale Discovery quantitative electrochemoluminescent immunoassay technology) indicated that more than 90% inhibition of protein kinase B substrate phosphorylation is needed for several hours to produce a 50% inhibitory antiproliferative effect in cancer cells in vitro and corresponding growth arrest of human tumor xenografts in athymic mice in vivo.[43,59]

The drawbacks of tumor biopsies include the procedural risks and limited ability to assess multiple time points, and the problem of tissue heterogeneity and sampling bias. In addition, tissue samples for analysis are frequently available only from the primary tumor, which might have different molecular features and drug response compared with metastatic lesions or vice versa.[114–117] This has been a perennial criticism of many studies that describe the prognostic or predictive value of molecular markers. It is important to be cognizant of this in the context of phase I trials, because false negative results can curtail progression of a drug to further phase trials. Unbiased, whole tumor assessments are thus desirable—a need that can potentially be met by advanced imaging methods.

## Minimally Invasive Functional and Molecular Imaging

Progress in new technologies for imaging the effects of cancer drugs has been prolific in the past decade. The ability to complement detailed morphologic data with information on function and metabolism provides a powerful tool for assessing novel mechanism-based therapeutics in both preclinical and clinical settings.[118] DCE-MRI and DCE computed tomography are now frequently applied to study the modulation of tumor vasculature in response to antiangiogenic agents, using changes in parameters, eg, $K_{trans}$ as PD end points.[119] Moreover, with the advent of high-resolution scanners, better processing software, and advanced mathematical modeling, it is now possible to delineate various dynamic components of tumor vasculature such as blood flow and permeability.[120] Furthermore, there is an expanding repertoire of MRI sequences that are capable of imaging key biologic phenomenon—such as hypoxia with blood oxygen level-dependent MRI[121] and tissue cellularity with diffusion-weighted MRI.[122] These sequences have broader relevance to nonangiogenic targeted therapies and may serve as predictive markers (eg, with chemoradiotherapy in rectal cancer) or biologic progression markers to monitor response to different therapies.[121]

Positron emission tomography (PET) allows dynamic, noninvasive measures of the 3-dimensional distribution of a positron-labeled compound within a living body. PET scanning can be used with a range of radiolabeled tracers that are able to appraise various biologic processes. For example, [$^{18}$F] fluorodeoxyglucose-PET is increasingly used as a means to assess early response and predict outcome to signal transduction inhibitors for patients with gastrointestinal stromal tumors treated with imatinib.[123] It can also be used as a PD marker of biochemical modulation by PI3 kinase/AKT/mTOR inhibitors, where activation of the pathway is associated with increased hexokinase activity and glycolysis, with inhibition of the pathway resulting in decreased fluorodeoxyglucose uptake.[124] Other positron-labeled markers that have been used examine particular biologic processes, such as monitoring changes in cellular proliferation ($^{11}$C-thymidine), tissue perfusion ($^{15}$O-H2O), blood volume ($^{15}$O-CO), and DNA synthesis and cellular proliferation ($^{18}$F-Fluoro-L-Thymidine).[32]

The role of PET has also been applied to evaluating intratumoral and normal tissue drug PK in patients. This is achieved by labeling drugs of interest with positron-emitting isotopes, such as $^{11}$C, $^{18}$F, or $^{13}$N. Examples of drugs for which PET has been used include: $^{18}$F 5-Fluorouracil,[125] $^{11}$C temozolomide,[126] $^{13}$N cisplatin,[127] and $^{18}$F tamoxifen.[128] More recently, PET has been explored as a method for imaging molecular characteristics of tumors, eg, HER-2 expression.[129]

The main disadvantages of using imaging biomarkers are radiation exposure (with the exception of MRI), and financial cost, operator dependency, and labor intensiveness. Furthermore, the lack of uniformity in scanners and varying expertise in different institutions limits intercenter comparisons, making validation and widespread adoption extremely challenging (Table 5). An in-depth discussion of each imaging modality is beyond the scope of this review, but the reader is directed to the following articles for a comprehensive overview of imaging biomarkers relevant to drug development.[32,129]

Finally, increasingly sophisticated imaging methods are becoming available to determine the molecular and biologic effects of anticancer agents, providing the advantages of spatial information, quantification of a drug's modulatory effect and repeatability of sampling to examine multiple time points.[118,130] Furthermore, it may be feasible to evaluate tumor heterogeneity using such approaches, potentially enhancing its accuracy as a predictive and PD marker.

**TABLE 5.** Challenges of Incorporating Fit-for-Purpose Biomarkers: Minimally Invasive Functional and Molecular Imaging

| Attributes | Drawbacks |
|---|---|
| Allow for dynamic, real-time, noninvasive measures of structure and function | Radiation exposure (with the exception of MRI) |
| Ability to complement detailed morphologic data with information on function and metabolism | Financial cost |
| Allows delineation of various dynamic components of tumor vasculature, such as blood flow and permeability | Operator dependency and labor intensiveness |
| Expanding repertoire of MRI and PET methods are capable of imaging key biologic phenomenon | Lack of uniformity in scanning methodology and varying expertise in different institutions limits intercentre comparisons |

## EMERGING TECHNOLOGY PLATFORMS: CIRCULATING BIOMARKERS

One of the most exciting avenues of biomarker research is the identification of circulating biomarkers that reflect the contemporaneous biology of the tumor. In the context of drug development, the ability to obtain circulating nucleic acids and enumerate CTCs has tremendous scope as a minimally invasive biomarker tool. Coupled with the "omics" revolution, this has the potential to demonstrate the evolution of cancer cells during a course of treatment.

### Circulating Nucleic Acids

Free nucleic acids have been detected in serum and proposed as a biologic progression marker in cancer.[131] Indeed, measurement of circulating nucleic acids has been found to be extremely useful in the context of chronic viral infections such as HIV.[132] In solid tumors, such as those from the colon or breast, it has been shown that, on average, approximately 80 genes harbor mutations that are present in virtually every cancer cell, but are not present in normal cells.[133] Such somatic mutations have the potential to serve as highly specific biomarkers, and indeed tumor-derived DNA from mutant cancer genes has previously been detected in the cell-free fraction of blood using standard real-time polymerase chain reaction techniques in individuals with malignancies.[134] Recently, in patients with colon cancer, Diehl et al[135] developed a highly sensitive approach, termed "BEAMing," to quantify circulating mutant DNA by proportional representation of mutant fragments over the total number of fragments. The authors went on to demonstrate that levels of tumor-derived mutant DNA declined with treatment intervention. In addition, compared with CEA, the tumor-derived mutant DNA was found to be more reliable and sensitive as a biologic progression biomarker. Furthermore, when measured postoperatively, detectable tumor-derived mutant DNA levels were a much better predictor of relapse than CEA. A drawback of this technique is that not all tumors bear the same aberrant gene, thereby precluding the applicability of this biomarker to unselected populations. There is also less scope for additional genetic studies other than sequencing, thereby limiting the ability to probe the basis of therapeutic effects. It is also unclear if changes in DNA levels are derived from stromal cell populations or cancer cells. At present, measurement of tumor DNA remains exploratory and technology for detection of circulating DNA has to yet to be commercially available. Larger scale clinical validation and qualification on patient samples are needed.

### Circulating Tumor Cells

Perhaps no biomarker of late has captured more attention than CTCs.[136] Advances in technology, such as automated and high-throughput separation of cells, eg, with CellSearch system (Veridex, LLC), have made visualization and semiautomated quantitation of epithelial cancer cells from blood feasible.[137] Recent studies in breast, colon, and prostate cancers underscore the clinical significance of CTCs, where cell counts at baseline and/or subsequent falls after treatment are highly predictive of outcome.[41,138,139]

At present, several methods for CTC detection exist. The 2 platforms that have generated the most interest of late are the CellSearch system (Veridex, LLC) utilizing an enrichment immunomagnetic bead assay and immunofluorescence staining[41,43,140] and a microfluidic platform (called the CTC chip).[67,141] Other platforms include the use of an automated scanning fluorescence microscope (Ikoniscope)[142] and filtration methods (with or without antibody enumeration).[143]

However, it is noteworthy that the criteria to define CTC events has not been uniform across platforms (eg, presence of 4,6-diaminidine-2-phenylindole staining, size and morphology, antibody panel used for identification) leading to substantial variations in the reported number of cells. This has complicated the interpretation of the significance of CTC events as detected by different groups in relation to clinical outcomes. Direct comparisons between these methods with uniform definitions of CTC events are urgently required. Until such cross validation studies are conducted, at the time of writing, only CTC counts as determined by the Veridex CellSearch system is FDA approved, specifically in the context of determining prognosis in breast, colorectal, and most recently castration resistant prostate cancer.[41,42,144]

There is now considerable interest in enabling rapid and accurate molecular characterization of CTCs. The feasibility of detecting *EGFR* mutation status on CTCs was recently reported using the microfluidic CTC chip platform.[118] Using the Veridex CellSearch system, it is now possible to perform fluorescence in situ hybridization on enumerated prostate cancer CTC to determine copy number changes of key genes like *MYC*, *AR*, and *PTEN*, as well as detect gene rearrangements, eg, *TMPRSS2/ERG*, using a break-apart assay.[43,140]

Present attempts to further enhance CTC platforms include the application of more precise technology to facilitate objective quantification of molecular changes on cancer cells and to improve sensitivity and specificity for the detection of genetic alterations, possibly through expanding on current methods for RNA and DNA analysis (eg, high-throughput gene expression arrays and genome sequencing).

### Circulating Proteomic and Metabolomic Biomarkers

High-throughput proteomic techniques have enhanced protein biomarker discovery, the most notable platform being the matrix-assisted laser desorption/ionization (MALDI), a soft ionization technique that uses a time-of-flight (TOF) mass spectrometer.[145] MALDI-TOF mass spectrometry can be used to analyze biomolecules to serve as classifiers—to delineate disease states, and responders or nonresponders. Taguchi et al[146] derived a prognostic and predictive algorithm based on MALDI-TOF mass spectrometry analysis of pretreatment serum of patients with non–small lung cancer, highlighting the potential for such platforms to facilitate patient selection. However, technical limitations are very significant, and variations in sample collection and preparation as well as instrument settings can potentially lead to nonreproducible data. Other obstacles include a lack of common reagents and public data sets, ineffective transfer of technologies to clinical applications, and limitations in the ability to manage the massive volume of data produced by proteomic techniques.

Simpler proteomic approaches based on individual circulating proteins have also been developed. Recently, measurement of the levels of a molecular target, eg, extracellular domain of HER-2 protein by ELISA, was reported, although no clear relationship was found between serum levels and response.[147] Nevertheless, there has been some success with the development of specific circulating protein biomarkers. Tumor markers, such as CEA, are a prime example. Further biomarkers of key biologic processes, eg, apoptosis, are also emerging (Table 2). Apoptotic biomarkers include cytokeratins CK 18 and 19, and M30 (an antibody to a caspase-cleaved neo-epitope on CK18) and M65 (which detects both intact and cleaved soluble CK18).[91] Measuring these proteins in the circulation using ELISA facilitates the estimation of apoptotic cell death after drug treatment and provides a useful method to assess and understand the mediators of response to cancer therapies. Other methods include commercial kits of multiplex biologic assays that are being developed for measurement of growth factors, cytokines, and phosphoproteins, eg, based on MesoScale Discovery technology.

Compared with gene and protein expression profiling, there have been relatively scanty data on the role of circulating metabolites, or metabolomic profiles, on malignant disease progression. Recently, using high throughput liquid and gas chromatography-based mass spectrometry, distinct metabolomic profiles were identified that distinguished benign, locally advanced and metastatic prostate cancer.[148] Differences in the metabolite profiles at each stage of progression, and subsequent RNA interference validation studies then identified sarcosine as a potential metabolic mediator of cancer cell invasion and aggressiveness. Sarcosine was also detected in urine, raising the possibility of its use as a noninvasive biomarker. Although this work requires independent corroboration, this example illustrates the utility of using novel platforms for discovery of new treatment targets and clinically relevant biomarkers.

## BEYOND TRADITIONAL ENDPOINTS: HYPOTHESIS-TESTING CLINICAL TRIALS

The revolution in molecular biology and genomics has resulted in numerous tools to interrogate the consequences of therapeutic intervention with novel biologics and targeted small molecule agents. Hence, we are now in a position to move beyond traditional end points of safety and toxicity, and to determine pharmacologically active dose ranges, improve our understanding of target biology in human subjects, and better characterize on-target and off-target effects, eg, using high-throughput analysis of posttreatment biopsies.

Close collaboration between scientists and clinicians facilitates rational design of trials that allow investigators to interrogate human tumor biology in the clinic, using targeted drugs as molecular probes, and to test biologic hypotheses such as mechanisms of resistance and synthetically lethal combinations. For example, underpinning the recently completed phase I trial of the PARP inhibitor olaparib (AZD2281) were the preclinical studies that found BRCA mutations and PARP inhibition to be synthetically lethal.[149] These findings led to the implementation of cohort enrichment for BRCA-mutated patients in a phase I trial, which in turn demonstrated antitumor responses in a substantial proportion of BRCA mutated patients.[150] In this study, evidence of PARP inhibition was demonstrated in PBMCs (with PARP activity measured through an ex vivo PARP activation assay), plucked hair follicles (induction of $\gamma$H2AX), and tumor biopsies (loss of PAR signal from tumor whole cell extracts). Importantly, such parallel correlative biomarker studies provide direct evidence for the relevance of normal "surrogate" tissue. Current efforts are aimed at measuring homologous recombination repair capacity in surrogate tissue as a predictive biomarker, so that patients with deficient BRCA1/2 function through nonhereditary mechanisms, eg, hypermethylation, might be identified for treatment with a PARP inhibitor.[151] Development of such an assay not only improves patient selection but also potentially further extends the application of PARP inhibitors to those with other functionally equivalent defects in homologous recombination repair.

Other examples of rational design in the setting of phase I trials were recently reported. In a trial involving a small molecule inhibitor of c-Met/HGFR and anaplastic lymphoma kinase receptor tyrosine kinase, promising clinical activity was seen in an enriched cohort of tumors harboring anaplastic lymphoma kinase rearrangements.[152] A similar enrichment strategy was used with the novel therapeutic target, oncogenic [V600E]*BRAF* kinase that is found mutated in up to 60% of melanomas. In the first-in-class phase I study with a mutant BRAF-specific kinase inhibitor, approximately 90% of the cohort comprised melanomas, and regression was reported in up to 83% of [V600E]*BRAF* mutant tumors.[153]

## SUMMARY AND CONCLUSIONS

The increasing use of new molecularly targeted agents demands new paradigms in early phase trials. High-tech, ideally minimally invasive, biomarkers have the potential ability to comprehensively characterize on-target and off-target drug effects, define enriched patient subsets, monitor treatment progress, and provide insights into tumor biology. There is an urgent need to design hypothesis-testing, biomarker-driven, early phase oncology trials, addressing key questions that provide mechanistic insights into target modulation, drug sensitivity, and resistance, as well as guiding decision making such as dose and schedule optimization, in addition to traditional dose finding objectives. Our burgeoning knowledge of the genetic landscape of cancer is revealing both the mysteries and complexities of malignant diseases and is providing the basis for a new generation of diagnostic and predictive tests.[2] These encompass the analysis of normal or tumor tissues, and body fluid samples ex vivo and molecular imaging methods that will enable improved disease characterization and treatment. The financial implications of incorporating biomarkers into clinical trials of molecularly targeted drugs are relatively modest compared with the overall cost of developing a drug, which is now in the region of one billion dollars. Indeed, the costs of biomarker studies can be more than compensated by the benefits obtained.

An extensive range of methods is now available to determine the effect of drugs on their intended molecular target and to evaluate the downstream effects on the corresponding biochemical pathway and resultant biologic process. Subject to appropriate scientific and technical validation, these PD end points should be incorporated in early clinical trials to show proof of concept for target modulation and help define the optimal dose and schedule. Equally important is the development of predictive markers of response to facilitate selection of the "right patients for the right drug." Incorporation of suitably qualified fit-for-purpose PD and predictive end points into early and later stage clinical trials can have profound implications on the drug approval process, reducing time, cost, and effort of attrition from phase III clinical trials.[13]

The challenge now lies in the discovery, validation, and clinical qualification of biomarkers that elucidate the molecular and biologic events linking a drug target to the clinical activity and benefit.[32] The PK/PD relationship remains the central tenet for early phase clinical trials, and early implementation of suitable biomarkers so as to allow time for scientific, technical, and clinical validation and qualification is crucial. The concept of the pharmacologic audit trail provides a framework for rational decision making and risk management in clinical drug development. In addition to PK-PD biomarkers, predictive assays for patient selection or at least the enrichment of trials with potentially responsive patients are now having a major impact. Looking to the future, there are exciting prospects for whole genome sequencing and systems network analysis, both during clinical trial evaluation and also in the subsequent use of approved drugs. There is tremendous scope for biomarkers to contribute to the drug development process, with the aim of increasing the success rate, accelerating the timeline of new molecularly targeted therapies to regulatory approval and patient benefit, and ultimately facilitating the implementation of personalized cancer medicine.

## ACKNOWLEDGMENTS

*The Drug Development Unit of the Royal Marsden NHS Foundation Trust and The Institute of Cancer Research is supported in part by a programme grant from Cancer Research UK. Support is also provided by the Experimental Cancer Medicine Center (programme grant) (to ICR) and the National Institute for Health Research Biomedical Research Center (jointly to the RMH NHS Foundation Trust and the ICR).*

## REFERENCES

1. Hanahan D, Weinberg RA. Hallmarks of Cancer. *Cell.* 2000;100:57–70.
2. Stratton MR, Campbell PJ, Futreal PA. The cancer genome. *Nature.* 2009; 458:719–724.

3. Gibbs JB. Mechanism-based target identification and drug discovery in cancer research. *Science.* 2000;287:1969–1973.

4. Vogelstein B, Kinzler KW. Cancer genes and the pathways they control. *Nat Med.* 2004;10:789–799.

5. Collins I, Workman P. New approaches to molecular cancer therapeutics. *Nat Chem Biol.* 2006;2:689–700.

6. Greenman C, Stephens P, Smith R, et al. Patterns of somatic mutation in human cancer genomes. *Nature.* 2007;446:153–158.

7. Workman P. Genomics and the second golden era of cancer drug development. *Mol Biosyst.* 2005;1:17–26.

8. Gershell LJ, Atkins JH. A brief history of novel drug discovery technologies. *Nat Rev Drug Discov.* 2003;2:321–327.

9. van Montfort R, Workman P. Structure-based design of molecular cancer therapeutics. *Trends Biotechnol.* 2009;27:315–328.

10. Reichert JM, Valge-Archer VE. Developmental trends for monoclonal antibody cancer therapeutics. *Nat Rev Drug Discov.* 2007;6:349–356.

11. Iorns E, Lord CJ, Turner N, et al. Utilizing RNA interference to enhance cancer drug discovery. *Nat Rev Drug Discov.* 2007;6:556–568.

12. Luo J, Emanuele M, Li D, et al. A genome-wide rnai screen identifies multiple synthetic lethal interactions with the ras oncogene. *Cell.* 2009;137:835–848.

13. Kola I, Landis J. Can the pharmaceutical industry reduce attrition rates? *Nat Rev Drug Discov.* 2004;3:711–715.

14. Reichert JM, Wenger JB. Development trends for new cancer therapeutics and vaccines. *Drug Discov Today.* 2008;13:30–37.

15. DiMasi JA, Hansen RW, Grabowski HG. The price of innovation: new estimates of drug development costs. *J Health Econ.* 2003;22:151–185.

16. DiMasi JA, Grabowski HG. Economics of new oncology drug development. *J Clin Oncol.* 2007;25:209–216.

17. Simon R. The use of genomics in clinical trial design. *Clin Cancer Res.* 2008;14:5984–5993.

18. Thatcher N, Chang A, Parikh P, et al. Gefitinib plus best supportive care in previously treated patients with refractory advanced non-small-cell lung cancer: results from a randomised, placebo-controlled, multicentre study (Iressa Survival Evaluation in Lung Cancer). *Lancet.* 2005;366:1527–1537.

19. Van Cutsem E, Nowacki M, Lang I, et al. Randomized phase III study of irinotecan and 5-FU/FA with or without cetuximab in the first-line treatment of patients with metastatic colorectal cancer (mCRC): the CRYSTAL trial. *J Clin Oncol.* 2007;25:4000.

20. Takano T, Fukui T, Ohe Y, et al. EGFR mutations predict survival benefit from gefitinib in patients with advanced lung adenocarcinoma: a historical comparison of patients treated before and after gefitinib approval in Japan. *J Clin Oncol.* 2008;26:5589–5595.

21. Van Cutsem E, Köhne CH, Hitre E, et al. Cetuximab and chemotherapy as initial treatment for metastatic colorectal cancer. *N Engl J Med.* 2009;360:1408–1417.

22. Stuart D, Sellers WR. Linking somatic genetic alterations in cancer to therapeutics. *Curr Opin Cell Biol.* 2009;21:304–310.

23. Slamon DJ, Leyland-Jones B, Shak S, et al. Use of chemotherapy plus a monoclonal antibody against HER2 for metastatic breast cancer that overexpresses HER2. *N Engl J Med.* 2001;344:783–792.

24. Piccart-Gebhart MJ, Procter M, Leyland-Jones B, et al. Trastuzumab after adjuvant chemotherapy in HER2-positive breast cancer. *N Engl J Med.* 2005;353:1659–1672.

25. Dowlati A, Manda S, Gibbons J, et al. Multi-institutional phase I trials of anticancer agents. *J Clin Oncol.* 2008;26:1926–1931.

26. Postel-Vinay S, Arkenau HT, Olmos D, et al. Clinical benefit in phase-I trials of novel molecularly targeted agents: does dose matter? *Br J Cancer.* 2009;100:1373–1378.

27. Kummar S, Gutierrez M, Doroshow JH, et al. Drug development in oncology: classical cytotoxics and molecularly targeted agents. *Br J Clin Pharmacol.* 2006;62:15–26.

28. Workman P. How much there is and what does it do?: the need for better pharmacokinetic and pharmacodynamic endpoints in contemporary drug discovery and development. *Curr Pharm Des.* 2003;9:891–902.

29. Sarker D, Pacey S, Workman P. Use of pharmacokinetic/pharmacodynamic biomarkers to support rational cancer drug development. *Biomark Med.* 2007;1:399–417.

30. Sarker D, Workman P. Pharmacodynamic biomarkers for molecular cancer therapeutics. *Adv Cancer Res.* 2007;96:213–268.

31. Kelloff GJ, Sigman CC. New science-based endpoints to accelerate oncology drug development. *Eur J Cancer.* 2005;41:491–501.

32. Workman P, Aboagye EO, Chung YL, et al. Minimally invasive pharmacokinetic and pharmacodynamic technologies in hypothesis-testing clinical trials of innovative therapies. *J Natl Cancer Inst.* 2006;98:580–598.

33. de Bono JS, Attard G, Adjei A, et al. Potential applications for circulating tumor cells expressing the insulin-like growth factor-I receptor. *Clin Cancer Res.* 2007;13:3611–3616.

34. Woodcock J, Woosley R. The FDA critical path initiative and its influence on new drug development. *Annu Rev Med.* 2008;59:1–12.

35. Belknap SM, Lyons EA, McKoy JM, et al. Report card for accelerated FDA approval oncology drugs (1995–2003): is it time for a make-up test? *J Clin Oncol.* 2004;22(14S):abstr 6002.

36. Amur S, Frueh F, Lesko L, et al. Integration and use of biomarkers in drug development, regulation and clinical practice: a US regulatory perspective. *Biomark Med.* 2008;2:305–311.

37. Biomarkers Definitions Working Group. Biomarkers and surrogate endpoints: preferred definitions and conceptual framework. *Clin Pharmacol Ther.* 2001;69:89–95.

38. Slamon DJ, Clark GM, Wong SG, et al. Human breast cancer: correlation of relapse and survival with amplification of the HER-2/neu oncogene. *Science.* 1987;235:177–182.

39. Press MF, Bernstein L, Thomas PA, et al. HER-2/neu gene amplification characterized by fluorescence in situ hybridization: poor prognosis in node-negative breast carcinomas. *J Clin Oncol.* 1997;15:2894–2904.

40. Park JW, Kerbel RS, Kelloff GJ, et al. Rationale for biomarkers and surrogate end points in mechanism-driven oncology drug development. *Clin Cancer Res.* 2004;10:3885–3896.

41. de Bono JS, Scher HI, Montgomery RB, et al. Circulating tumor cells predict survival benefit from treatment in metastatic castration-resistant prostate cancer. *Clin Cancer Res.* 2008;14:6302–6309.

42. Solit DB, Garraway LA, Pratilas CA, et al. BRAF mutation predicts sensitivity to MEK inhibition. *Nature.* 2006;439:358–362.

43. Raynaud FI, Eccles S, Patel S, et al. Biological properties of potent inhibitors of class I phosphatidylinositide 3-kinases: from PI-103 through PI-540, PI-620 to the oral agent GDC-0941. *Mol Cancer Ther.* 2009;8:1725–1738.

44. Olmos D, Arkenau HT, Ang JE, et al. Circulating tumour cell (CTC) counts as intermediate end points in castration-resistant prostate cancer (CRPC): a single-centre experience. *Ann Oncol.* 2009;20:27–33.

45. Attard G, Swennenhuis JF, Olmos D, et al. Characterization of ERG, AR and PTEN gene status in circulating tumor cells from patients with castration-resistant prostate cancer. *Cancer Res.* 2009;69:2912–2918.

46. Workman P. Challenges of PK/PD measurements in modern drug development. *Eur J Cancer.* 2002;38:2189–2193.

47. Workman P. Auditing the pharmacological accounts for Hsp90 molecular chaperone inhibitors: unfolding the relationship between pharmacokinetics and pharmacodynamics. *Mol Cancer Ther.* 2003;2:131–138.

48. Banerji U, O'Donnell A, Scurr M, et al. Phase I pharmacokinetic and pharmacodynamic study of 17-allylamino, 17-demethoxygeldanamycin in patients with advanced malignancies. *J Clin Oncol.* 2005;23:4152–4161.

49. Banerji U, Walton M, Raynaud F, et al. Pharmacokinetic-pharmacodynamic relationships for the heat shock protein 90 molecular chaperone inhibitor 17-allylamino, 17-demethoxygeldanamycin in human ovarian cancer xenograft models. *Clin Cancer Res.* 2005;11(19 pt 1):7023–7032.

50. Wilhelm SM, Carter C, Tang L, et al. BAY 43–9006 exhibits broad spectrum oral antitumor activity and targets the RAF/MEK/ERK pathway and receptor tyrosine kinases involved in tumor progression and angiogenesis. *Cancer Res.* 2004;64:7099–7109.

51. Wilhelm SM, Adnane L, Newell P, et al. Preclinical overview of sorafenib, a multikinase inhibitor that targets both Raf and VEGF and PDGF receptor tyrosine kinase signaling. *Mol Cancer Ther.* 2008;7:3129–3140.

52. Sauter G, Simon R, Hillan K. Tissue microarrays in drug discovery. *Nat Rev Drug Discov.* 2003;2:962–972.

53. Frank R, Hargreaves R. Clinical biomarkers in drug discovery and development. *Nat Rev Drug Discov.* 2003;2:566–580.

54. Ludwig JA, Weinstein JN. Biomarkers in cancer staging, prognosis and treatment selection. *Nat Rev Cancer.* 2005;5:845–856.

55. Paulovich A, Whiteaker J, Hoofnagle A, et al. The interface between biomarker discovery and clinical validation: the tar pit of the protein biomarker pipeline. *Proteomics Clin Appl.* 2008;2:1386–1402.

56. Gutman S, Kessler LG. The US Food and Drug Administration perspective on cancer biomarker development. *Nat Rev Cancer.* 2006;6:565–571.

56a. Goodsaid F, Frueh F. Biomarker qualification pilot process at the US Food and Drug Administration. *AAPS J.* 2007;9:E105–E108.

57. Clarke PA, Hostein I, Banerji U, et al. Gene expression profiling of human colon cancer cells following inhibition of signal transduction by 17-allylamino-17-demethoxygeldanamycin, an inhibitor of the hsp90 molecular chaperone. *Oncogene.* 2000;19:4125–4133.

58. Hostein I, Robertson D, DiStefano F, et al. Inhibition of signal transduction by the Hsp90 inhibitor 17-allylamino-17-demethoxygeldanamycin results in cytostasis and apoptosis. *Cancer Res.* 2001;61:4003–4009.

59. Guillard S, Clarke P, te Poele R, et al. Molecular pharmacology of phosphatidylinositol 3-kinase inhibition in human glioma. *Cell Cycle.* 2009;8:443–453.

60. Raynaud FI, Whittaker SR, Fischer PM, et al. In vitro and in vivo pharmacokinetic-pharmacodynamic relationships for the trisubstituted aminopurine cyclin-dependent kinase inhibitors olomoucine, bohemine and CYC202. *Clin Cancer Res.* 2005;11:4875–4887.

61. Whittaker SR, Walton MI, Garrett MD, et al. The Cyclin-dependent kinase inhibitor CYC202 (R-roscovitine) inhibits retinoblastoma protein phosphorylation, causes loss of Cyclin D1, and activates the mitogen-activated protein kinase pathway. *Cancer Res.* 2004;64:262–272.

62. Whittaker SR, Te Poele RH, Chan F, et al. The cyclin-dependent kinase inhibitor seliciclib (R-roscovitine; CYC202) decreases the expression of mitotic control genes and prevents entry into mitosis. *Cell Cycle.* 2007;6:3114–3131.

63. Sharpless NE, Depinho RA. The mighty mouse: genetically engineered mouse models in cancer drug development. *Nat Rev Drug Discov.* 2006;5:705.

64. Frese KK, Tuveson DA. Maximizing mouse cancer models. *Nat Rev Cancer.* 2007;7:645–658.

65. Pintilie M, Iakovlev V, Fyles A. Heterogeneity and power in clinical biomarker studies. *J Clin Oncol.* 2009;27:1517–1521.

65a. Sarzotti-Kelsoe M, Cox J, Cleland N. Evaluation and recommendations on good clinical laboratory practice guidelines for phase I–III clinical trials. *PLoS Med.* 2009;6:e1000067.

66. Albanell J, Rojo F, Averbuch S, et al. Pharmacodynamic studies of the epidermal growth factor receptor inhibitor ZD1839 in skin from cancer patients: histopathologic and molecular consequences of receptor inhibition. *J Clin Oncol.* 2002;20:110–124.

67. Maheswaran S, Sequist LV, Nagrath S, et al. Detection of mutations in EGFR in circulating lung-cancer cells. *N Engl J Med.* 2008;359:366–377.

68. Felip E, Rojo F, Reck M, et al. A phase II pharmacodynamic study of erlotinib in patients with advanced non-small cell lung cancer previously treated with platinum-based chemotherapy. *Clin Cancer Res.* 2008;14:3867–3874.

69. Pal A, Glekas A, Doubrovin M, et al. Molecular imaging of EGFR kinase activity in tumors with 124I-labeled small molecular tracer and positron emission tomography. *Mol Imaging Biol.* 2006;8:262–277.

70. Gelovani JG. Molecular imaging of epidermal growth factor receptor expression-activity at the kinase level in tumors with positron emission tomography. *Cancer Metastasis Rev.* 2008;27:645–653.

71. Kuang Y, Rogers A, Yeap BY, et al. Noninvasive detection of EGFR T790M in gefitinib or erlotinib resistant non-small cell lung cancer. *Clin Cancer Res.* 2009;15:2630–2636.

72. Pao W, Miller VA, Politi KA, et al. Acquired resistance of lung adenocarcinomas to gefitinib or erlotinib is associated with a second mutation in the EGFR kinase domain. *PLoS Med.* 2005;2:e73.

73. Loprevite M, Tiseo M, Chiaramondia M, et al. Buccal mucosa cells as in vivo model to evaluate gefitinib activity in patients with advanced non-small cell lung cancer. *Clin Cancer Res.* 2007;13:6518–6526.

74. Lacy MQ, Alsina M, Fonseca R, et al. Phase I, pharmacokinetic and pharmacodynamic study of the anti-insulinlike growth factor type 1 receptor monoclonal antibody CP-751,871 in patients with multiple myeloma. *J Clin Oncol.* 2008;26:3196–3203.

75. Atzori F, Tabernero J, Cervantes A, et al. A phase I, pharmacokinetic (PK) and pharmacodynamic (PD) study of weekly (qW) MK-0646, an insulin-like growth factor-1 receptor (IGF1R) monoclonal antibody (MAb) in patients (pts) with advanced solid tumors. *J Clin Oncol.* 2008;26(15S):abstr 3519.

76. LoRusso P, Markman B, Tabernero J, et al. A phase I dose-escalation study of the safety, pharmacokinetics (PK), and pharmacodynamics of XL765, a PI3K/TORC1/TORC2 inhibitor administered orally to patients (pts) with advanced solid tumors. *J Clin Oncol.* 2009;27(15S):abstr 3502.

77. Sarker D, Kristeleit R, Mazina KE, et al. A phase I study evaluating the pharmacokinetics (PK) and pharmacodynamics (PD) of the oral pan-phosphoinositide-3 kinase (PI3K) inhibitor GDC-0941. *J Clin Oncol.* 2009;27:abstr 3538.

78. de Bono JS, Kristeleit R, Tolcher A, et al. Phase I pharmacokinetic and pharmacodynamic study of LAQ824, a hydroxamate histone deacetylase inhibitor with a heat shock protein-90 inhibitory profile, in patients with advanced solid tumors. *Clin Cancer Res.* 2008;14:6663–6673.

79. Schrump DS, Fischette MR, Nguyen DM, et al. Clinical and molecular responses in lung cancer patients receiving Romidepsin. *Clin Cancer Res.* 2008; 14:188–198.

80. Chung YL, Troy H, Kristeleit R, et al. Noninvasive magnetic resonance spectroscopic pharmacodynamic markers of a novel histone deacetylase inhibitor, LAQ824, in human colon carcinoma cells and xenografts. *Neoplasia.* 2008;10:303–313.

81. Altiok S, Brazelle W, Gemmer J, et al. Subcutaneous adipose tissue as a surrogate for pharmacodynamic assessment of HDAC inhibitors. ASCO-NCI-EORTC Molecular Markers Meeting. 2008; abstract 123.

82. Mundhenke C, Thomas JP, Wilding G, et al. Tissue examination to monitor antiangiogenic therapy: a phase I clinical trial with endostatin. *Clin Cancer Res.* 2001;7:3366–3374.

83. Drevs J, Siegert P, Medinger M, et al. Phase I clinical study of AZD2171, an oral vascular endothelial growth factor signaling inhibitor, in patients with advanced solid tumors. *J Clin Oncol.* 2007;25:3045–3054.

84. Brown AP, Citrin DE, Camphausen KA. Clinical biomarkers of angiogenesis inhibition. *Cancer Metastasis Rev.* 2008;27:415–434.

85. Liu G, Rugo HS, Wilding G, et al. Dynamic contrast-enhanced magnetic resonance imaging as a pharmacodynamic measure of response after acute dosing of AG-013736, an oral angiogenesis inhibitor, in patients with advanced solid tumors: results from a phase I study. *J Clin Oncol.* 2005;23:5464–5473.

86. Yap TA, Harris D, Barriuso J, et al. Phase I trial to determine the dose range for the c-Met inhibitor ARQ 197 that inhibits c-Met and FAK phosphorylation, when administered by an oral twice-a-day schedule. *J Clin Oncol.* 2008;26: abstr 3584.

87. Willett CG, Duda DG, di Tomaso E, et al. Efficacy, safety, and biomarkers of neoadjuvant bevacizumab, radiation therapy, and fluorouracil in rectal cancer: a multidisciplinary phase II study. *J Clin Oncol.* 2009;27:3020–3026.

88. Ng QS, Goh V, Milner J, et al. Effect of nitric-oxide synthesis on tumour blood volume and vascular activity: a phase I study. *Lancet Oncol.* 2007;8: 111–118.

89. Dean E, Jodrell D, Connolly K, et al. Phase I trial of AEG35156 administered as a 7-day and 3-day continuous intravenous infusion in patients with advanced refractory cancer. *J Clin Oncol.* 2009;27:1660–1666.

90. Cummings J, Ranson M, Lacasse E, et al. Method validation and preliminary qualification of pharmacodynamic biomarkers employed to evaluate the clinical efficacy of an antisense compound (AEG35156) targeted to the X-linked inhibitor of apoptosis protein XIAP. *Br J Cancer.* 2006;95:42–48.

91. Ward TH, Cummings J, Dean E, et al. Biomarkers of apoptosis. *Br J Cancer.* 2008;99:841–846.

92. Thoeny HC, De Keyzer F, Chen F, et al. Diffusion-weighted magnetic resonance imaging allows noninvasive in vivo monitoring of the effects of combretastatin a-4 phosphate after repeated administration. *Neoplasia.* 2005;7:779–787.

93. Robert F, Hurwitz H, Verschraegen CF, et al. Phase 1 trial of SNS-314, a novel selective inhibitor of aurora kinases A, B, and C, in advanced solid tumor patients. *J Clin Oncol.* 2008;26:abstr 14642.

94. Olmos D, Allred A, Sharma R, et al. Phase I first-in-human study of the polo-like kinase-1 selective inhibitor, GSK461364, in patients with advanced solid tumors. *J Clin Oncol.* 2009;27:abstr 3536.

95. Baselga J, Albanell J, Ruiz A, et al. Phase II and tumor pharmacodynamic study of gefitinib in patients with advanced breast cancer. *J Clin Oncol.* 2005;23:5323–5333.

96. Liu G, Jeraj R, Perlman S, et al. Pharmacodynamic study of FLT-PET imaging in patients treated with sunitinib. *J Clin Oncol.* 2008;26:abstr 3515.

97. O'Donnell A, Faivre S, Burris HA III, et al. Phase I pharmacokinetic and pharmacodynamic study of the oral mammalian target of rapamycin inhibitor everolimus in patients with advanced solid tumors. *J Clin Oncol.* 2008;26:1588–1595.

98. Baird RD, Kitzen J, Clarke PA, et al. Phase I safety, pharmacokinetic, and pharmacogenomic trial of ES-285, a novel marine cytotoxic agent, administered to adult patients with advanced solid tumors. *Mol Cancer Ther.* 2009;8:1430–1437.

99. Yap TA, Frentzas S, Tunariu N, et al. Final results of a pharmacokinetic (PK) and pharmacodynamic (PD) phase I trial of ARQ 197 incorporating dynamic contrast-enhanced (DCE) magnetic resonance imaging (MRI) studies investigating the antiangiogenic activity of selective c-Met inhibition. *J Clin Oncol.* 2009;27:abstr 3523.

100. Booth CM, Calvert AH, Giaccone G, et al. Endpoints and other considerations in phase I studies of targeted anticancer therapy: recommendations from the task force on methodology for the development of innovative cancer therapies (MDICT). *Eur J Cancer.* 2008;44:19–24.

101. Parulekar WR, Eisenhauer EA. Phase I trial design for solid tumor studies of targeted, non-cytotoxic agents: theory and practice. *J Natl Cancer Inst.* 2004; 96:990–997.

102. Yap TA, Boss DS, Fong PC, et al. First in human phase I pharmacokinetic (PK) and pharmacodynamic (PD) study of KU-0059436 (Ku), a small molecule inhibitor of poly ADP-ribose polymerase (PARP) in cancer patients(p), including BRCA1/2 mutation carriers. *J Clin Oncol.* 2007;25:abstr 3529.

103. Tanaka C, O'Reilly T, Kovarik JM, et al. Identifying optimal biologic doses of everolimus (RAD001) in patients with cancer based on the modeling of preclinical and clinical pharmacokinetic and pharmacodynamic data. *J Clin Oncol.* 2008;26:1596–1602.

104. Helft P, Daugherty C. Are we taking without giving in return? The ethics of research-related biopsies and the benefits of clinical trial participation. *J Clin Oncol.* 2006;24:4793–4795.

105. Dowlati A, Haaga J, Remick SC, et al. Sequential tumor biopsies in early phase clinical trials of anticancer agents for pharmacodynamic evaluation. *Clin Cancer Res.* 2001;7:2971–2976.

106. Agulnik M, Oza A, Pond G, et al. Impact and perceptions of mandatory tumor biopsies for correlative studies in clinical trials of novel anticancer agents. *J Clin Oncol.* 2006;24:4801–4807.

107. Workman P. Using biomarkers in drug development. *Clin Adv Hematol Oncol.* 2006;4:736–739.

108. O'Reilly KE, Rojo F, She QB, et al. mTOR inhibition induces upstream receptor tyrosine kinase signaling and activates Akt. *Cancer Res.* 2006;66:1500–1508.

109. Banerji U, Affolter A, Judson I, et al. BRAF and NRAS mutations in melanoma: potential relationships to clinical response to HSP90 inhibitors. *Mol Cancer Ther.* 2008;7:737–739.

110. Vasudevan KM, Barbie DA, Davies MA, et al. AKT-independent signaling downstream of oncogenic PIK3CA mutations in human cancer. *Cancer Cell.* 2009;16:21–32.

111. Taylor IW, Linding R, Warde-Farley D, et al. Dynamic modularity in protein interaction networks predicts breast cancer outcome. *Nat Biotechnol.* 2009;27:199–204.

112. Swanton C, Caldas C. Molecular classification of solid tumours: towards pathway-driven therapeutics. *Br J Cancer.* 2009;100:1517–1522.

113. Kim ES, Herbst RS, LeeJJ, et al. Phase II randomized study of biomarker-directed treatment for non-small cell lung cancer (NSCLC): the BATTLE (Biomarker-Integrated Approaches of Targeted Therapy for Lung Cancer Elimination) clinical trial program. *J Clin Oncol.* 2009;27:abstr 8024.

114. Guarneri V, Giovannelli S, Ficarra G, et al. Comparison of HER-2 and hormone receptor expression in primary breast cancers and asynchronous paired metastases: impact on patient management. *Oncologist.* 2008;13:838–844.

115. Kalikaki A, Koutsopoulos A, Trypaki M. Comparison of EGFR and K-RAS gene status between primary tumours and corresponding metastases in NSCLC. *Br J Cancer.* 2008;99:923–929.

116. Lower EE, Glass E, Blau R, et al. HER-2/neu expression in primary and metastatic breast cancer. *Breast Cancer Res Treat.* 2009;113:301–306.

117. Klein CA. Parallel progression of primary tumours and metastases. *Nat Rev Cancer.* 2009;9:302–312.

118. Weissleder R, Pittet MJ. Imaging in the era of molecular oncology. *Nature.* 2008;452:580–589.

119. Leach MO, Brindle KM, Evelhoch JL, et al. Assessment of antiangiogenic and antivascular therapeutics using MRI: recommendations for appropriate methodology for clinical trials. *Br J Radiol.* 2003;76:S87–S91.

120. Jackson A, O'Connor JP, Parker GJ, et al. Imaging tumor vascular heterogeneity and angiogenesis using dynamic contrast-enhanced magnetic resonance imaging. *Clin Cancer Res.* 2007;13:3449–3459.

121. Padhani AR, Liu G, Mu-Koh D, et al. Diffusion-weighted magnetic resonance imaging as a cancer biomarker: consensus and recommendations. *Neoplasia.* 2009;11:102–125.

122. Patterson DM, Padhani AR, Collins DJ. Technology insight: water diffusion MRI–a potential new biomarker of response to cancer therapy. *Nat Clin Pract Oncol.* 2008;5:220–233.

123. Gayed I, Vu T, Iyer R, et al. The role of 18F-FDG PET in staging and early prediction of response to therapy of recurrent gastrointestinal stromal tumors. *J Nucl Med.* 2004;45:17–21.

124. Majewski N, Nogueira V, Robey B, et al. Akt inhibits apoptosis downstream of BID cleavage via a glucose-dependent mechanism involving hexokinases. *Mol Cell Biol.* 2004;24:730–740.

125. Saleem A, Yap J, Osman S, et al. Modulation of fluorouracil tissue pharmacokinetics by eniluracil: in-vivo imaging of drug action. *Lancet.* 2000;355:2125–2131.

126. Saleem A, Brown GD, Brady F, et al. Metabolic activation of temozolomide measured in vivo using positron emission tomography. *Cancer Res.* 2003;63:2409–2415.

127. Ginos JZ, Cooper AJ, Dhawan V, et al. [13N]Cisplatin PET to assess pharmacokinetics of intra-arterial versus intravenous chemotherapy for malignant brain tumours. *J Nucl Med.* 1987;28:1844–1852.

128. Inoue T, Kim EE, Wallace S, et al. Preliminary study of cardiac accumulation of F-18 fluorotamoxifen in patients with breast cancer. *Clin Imaging.* 1997;21:332–336.

129. Weber WA, Czernin J, Phelps ME, et al. Technology insight: novel imaging of molecular targets is an emerging area crucial to the development of targeted drugs. *Nat Clin Pract Oncol.* 2008;5:44–54.

130. Kelloff GJ, Krohn KA, Larson SM, et al. The progress and promise of molecular imaging probes in oncologic drug development. *Clin Cancer Res.* 2005;11:7967–7985.

131. Leon SA, Shapiro B, Sklaroff D, et al. Free DNA in the serum of cancer patients and the effect of therapy. *Cancer Res.* 1977;37:646–650.

132. Schooley RT. Correlation between viral load measurements and outcome in clinical trials of antiviral drugs. *AIDS.* 1995;9(suppl 2):S15–S19.

133. Wood LD, Parsons DW, Jones S, et al. The genomic landscapes of human breast and colorectal cancers. *Science.* 2007;318:1108–1113.

134. Sidransky D. Emerging molecular markers of cancer. *Nat Rev Cancer.* 2002;2:210–219.

135. Diehl F, Schdmt K, Choti M, et al. Circulating mutant DNA to assess tumor dynamics. *Nat Med.* 2008;14:985–990.

136. Mocellin S, Keilholz U, Rossi CR, et al. Circulating tumor cells: the 'leukemic phase' of solid cancers. *Trends Mol Med.* 2006;12:130–139.

137. Allard WJ, Matera J, Miller MC, et al. Tumour cells circulate in the peripheral blood of all major carcinomas but not in healthy subjects or patients with non malignant diseases. *Clin Cancer Res.* 2004;10:6897–6904.

138. Cristofanilli M, Budd GT, Ellis MJ, et al. Circulating tumour cells, disease progression, and survival in metastatic breast cancer. *N Engl J Med.* 2004;351:781–791.

139. Cohen SJ, Punt C, Iannotti N, et al. Relationship of circulating tumor cells to tumor response, progression-free survival, and overall survival in patients with metastatic colorectal cancer. *J Clin Oncol.* 2008;26:3213–3221.

140. Leversha MA, Han JL, Asgari Z, et al. Fluorescence in situ hybridization analysis of circulating tumor cells in metastatic prostate cancer. *Clin Cancer Res.* 2009;15:2091–2097.

141. Nagrath S, Sequist LV, Maheswaran S, et al. Isolation of rare circulating tumour cells in cancer patients by microchip technology. *Nature.* 2007;450:1235–1239.

142. Ntouroupi TG, Ashraf SQ, Mcgregor SB, et al. Detection of circulating tumour cells in peripheral blood with an automated scanning fluorescence microscope. *Br J Cancer.* 2008;99:789–795.

143. Tan SJ, Yobas L, Lee GY, et al. Microdevice for the isolation and enumeration of cancer cells from blood. *Biomed Microdevices.* 2009;11:883–892.

144. Scher HI, Jia X, de Bono JS, et al. Circulating tumour cells as prognostic markers in progressive, castration-resistant prostate cancer: a reanalysis of IMMC38 trial data. *Lancet Oncol.* 2009;10:233–239.

145. Zwierzina H. Biomarkers in drug development. *Ann Oncol.* 2008;19(supp 5):33–37.

146. Taguchi F, Solomon B, Gregorc V, et al. Mass spectrometry to classify non-small cell lung cancer patients for clinical outcome after treatment with epidermal growth factor receptor tyrosine kinase inhibitors: a multicohort cross-institutional study. *J Natl Cancer Inst.* 2007;99:838–846.

147. Lennon S, Barton C, Banken L, et al. Utility of serum HER2 extracellular domain assessment in clinical decision making: pooled analysis of four trials of trastuzumab in metastatic breast cancer. *J Clin Oncol.* 2009;27:1685–1693.

148. Sreekumar A, Poisson L, Rajendiran T, et al. Metabolomic profiles delineate potential role for sarcosine in prostate cancer progression. *Nature.* 2009;457:910–914.

149. Farmer H, McCabe N, Lord CJ, et al. Targeting the DNA repair defect in BRCA mutant cells as a therapeutic strategy. *Nature.* 2005;434:917–921.

150. Fong PC, Boss DS, Yap TA, et al. Inhibition of poly(ADP-ribose) polymerase in tumors from BRCA mutation carriers. *N Engl J Med.* 2009;361:123–134.

151. Weberpals JI, Clark-Knowles KV, Vanderhyden BC, et al. Sporadic epithelial ovarian cancer: clinical relevance of BRCA1 inhibition in the DNA damage and repair pathway. *J Clin Oncol.* 2008;26:3259–3267.

152. Kwak EL, Camidge Dr, Clark J, et al. Clinical activity observed in a phase I dose escalation trial of an oral c-met and ALK inhibitor, PF-02341066. *J Clin Oncol.* 2009;27:abstr 3509.

153. Flaherty K, Puzanov I, Sosman J, et al. Phase I study of PLX4032: proof of concept for V600E BRAF mutation as a therapeutic target in human cancer. *J Clin Oncol.* 2009;27:abstr 9000.

154. Attard G, Clark J, Ambroisine L, et al. Heterogeneity and clinical significance of ETV1 translocations in human prostate cancer. *Br J Cancer.* 2008;99:314–320.

# Use of Meta-Analysis for the Validation of Surrogate Endpoints and Biomarkers in Cancer Trials

Marc Buyse

The issue of which endpoints to choose when designing trials of new therapeutic anticancer agents is driven by the desire to speed up clinical development while at the same time ensuring that new drugs provide true clinical benefits to patients, not merely short-lived palliation or biomarker changes. Table 1 contrasts advantages of using survival or earlier endpoints as the primary endpoint of randomized trials.

Although survival remains the endpoint of choice for advanced disease with poor prognosis and few therapeutic options, and even though regulatory agencies still consider survival a gold standard because of its relevance and objectivity, it is fair to assume that survival will not remain a realistic primary endpoint to use for most tumor types in the near future.[1–5] The underlying reasons for such a claim are not only that survival takes too long to be observed but also that randomized trials of new agents increasingly allow patients who fail on the standard therapy to "cross-over" to the new agent, thus making it difficult for the trial to show any difference in survival even if large differences were seen in time to progressive disease (or some other intermediate endpoint). Paradoxically, a highly effective new drug is less likely, in such cross-over trials, to show any benefit on overall survival (OS), than one with only marginal activity (since a highly effective therapy would be able to prolong survival even if it was given after failure of some other, less-effective therapy). If survival progressively loses its unquestioned status of primary endpoint in most cancer clinical trials then the main question will be to choose among other possible endpoints those that either directly reflect clinical benefit or are good surrogates for survival (or some other clinically relevant endpoint). The issue of clinical relevance is discussed in great detail in other articles of this issue of *The Cancer Journal*. The issue of surrogacy is taken up in the present article.

## BIOMARKERS

We set the framework of this discussion by first defining the terminology used throughout. A biomarker can be formally defined as "a characteristic that is objectively measured and evaluated as an indicator of normal biologic processes, pathogenic processes, or pharmacologic responses to a therapeutic intervention."[6] Biomarkers can include biochemical markers, cellular markers, cytokines, genetic markers, gene expression profiles, imaging markers, physiological markers, or any other patient or tumor measurements. Because the focus of this article will be on biomarkers that can potentially be used as surrogates to assess the effect of new treatments on clinical endpoints, our interest will focus on biomarkers that can be measured repeatedly before, during, or after treatment. We will use prostate-specific antigen (PSA) in patients with hormone refractory prostate cancer as an illustrative example.

## ENDPOINTS

In contrast to biomarkers, clinical endpoints directly measure "how a patient feels, functions, or survives."[7] In metastatic cancer, commonly used endpoints, besides OS, are objective tumor response (assessed according to the Response Evaluation Criteria in Solid Tumours criteria[8]), clinical benefit (also known as duration of disease control) defined as the achievement of a tumor response or a stable disease for some predefined period of time (for instance 3 months), time to disease progression or progression-free survival (PFS),[9] and time to treatment failure. In the remainder of this article, we will focus on objective tumor response and PFS as potential surrogates for OS.

Note that the distinction between a biomarker and an endpoint is not always clear: for instance, tumor response may be viewed as a biomarker indicating that treatment has cytotoxic activity that causes the tumor to shrink, but it may also be viewed as an endpoint if the achievement of a response is accompanied by clinical benefit, such as symptom improvement or the possibility to undertake a surgical tumor resection of residual metastases. The term "endpoint" is itself somewhat ambiguous, because it may be understood as implying some terminal event; the term "outcome" could be used instead to avoid this ambiguity, but we will stick here to the conventional terminology.

## SURROGATE BIOMARKERS AND ENDPOINTS

The meaning of the term "surrogate" is highly context dependent. It is generally used in a rather informal way to indicate that a biomarker or intermediate endpoint can be used instead of a final endpoint of interest.[10–12] Our goal here is to discuss statistical methods that have been proposed to validate potential surrogates, and this requires the term surrogate to be given a precise meaning, so that the conditions required to establish its validity be defined as rigorously as possible. We shall call surrogate a biomarker or endpoint that is able to replace a clinical endpoint for the purposes of evaluating the effect of a specific treatment for a specific disease. Note that this definition implies that surrogacy is disease dependent as well as treatment dependent. We shall return to this important issue when we discuss actual examples.

The requirements for a surrogate to be considered "valid" have been a theme of debate in the statistical literature during the past years. In early discussions about surrogate endpoints, a common misconception was that it was sufficient for this endpoint to be prognostic for the clinical endpoint to establish surrogacy. For example, if it could be shown that treatment response was an independent prognostic factor for OS then tumor response could be considered a surrogate. As it turns out, tumor response does predict longer survival independent of other prognostic factors, yet it has been shown in several common solid tumors not to be a good surrogate for OS,[13–15] because the effect of a treatment on response poorly predicted the effect of the same treatment on survival.

**TABLE 1.** Reasons to Use Early Endpoints Instead of Survival as the Primary Endpoint of Randomized Clinical Trials

| Reasons to Use Early Endpoints | Reasons to Use Survival |
|---|---|
| Treatment effects can be confirmed sooner on the surrogate than on survival | Survival is the most relevant endpoint ultimately targeted by all treatments |
| Experimental treatments may show a larger benefit on the surrogate | Survival is measured objectively |
| The effects of experimental treatments on the surrogate are unconfounded by competing risks | Survival captures net treatment effects, including any untoward effects due to late toxicities (eg, second malignancies) |
| The effects of experimental treatments on the surrogate are unconfounded by other treatments | |

A formal definition of surrogacy was proposed long ago by Prentice,[16] and criteria for the validation of surrogates was defined by Schatzkin et al and Freedman et al.[17,18] More recently, Buyse and Molenberghs[19] proposed a validation approach based on randomized trials or, when possible, on meta-analyses of randomized trials.[20] Although there is still controversy as to what level of evidence is needed to consider a surrogate as valid,[21–23] the latter approach has produced informative results in the adjuvant setting,[24,25] in locally advanced tumors[26] as well as in metastatic disease.[13–15,27–30]

Essentially, this approach consist of estimating associations at two levels: the association between the surrogate and the clinical endpoint, called the individual-level association, and the association between the effects of treatment on the surrogate and the clinical endpoint, called the trial-level association.[31–33] A strong individual-level association implies that the clinical endpoint can be reliably estimated from the biomarker in individual patients, whereas a strong trial-level association implies that the effect of treatment on the clinical endpoint can be reliably estimated from the effect of treatment on the biomarker (Fig. 1). A good surrogate is one that has biologic plausibility and is shown, statistically, to have strong individual-level and trial-level associations with the final endpoint. The appropriate

statistics to quantify the strength of these associations are also a matter of debate. Standard correlation coefficients (or their squares, which are interpreted as proportions of variance explained) are currently most popular, but other measures derived from information theory have been proposed recently.[34,35]

It is important to emphasize that the strength of the association between a surrogate and a clinical endpoint in general does not provide information about the relationship between the effects of treatment on the biomarker and the clinical endpoint, ie, between treatment-induced changes in the biomarker and corresponding changes in the risk of the clinical endpoint. In many situations of clinical interest, one would expect effective treatments to "shift" patients from a high biomarker-risk group to a low biomarker-risk group, and the difference in prognosis between the two biomarker-risk groups would be expected to reasonably predict the impact of treatment on the clinical endpoint of interest. For example, there is some empirical evidence that treatment-induced cholesterol reductions lead to reductions in major cardiovascular events that parallel predictions made from population-based epidemiologic studies. It remains to be seen whether such biomarker-based predictions can successfully be identified in oncology.

## META-ANALYSIS

Meta-analysis is the statistical process of combining information from several trials addressing the same question.[36] A clear distinction must be made between different types of meta-analysis,[37] as summarized in Table 2.

- The first type of meta-analysis, which is unfortunately by far the most common, uses data extracted from the published reports of the trials, such as survival estimates read off the published curves at some time point, and hazard ratios (HR). Such meta-analyses are often severely flawed because of publication bias and/or exclusion bias; moreover, the data available in the publications may be inadequate to perform meaningful calculations.[38–41]
- The second type of meta-analysis uses summary data, such as the number of events of interest and the number of patients treated in each treatment group, obtained from the principal investigators of all trials, whether published or unpublished. In this way, both publication bias and exclusion bias can be avoided. Moreover, simple but unbiased summary statistics can be obtained even

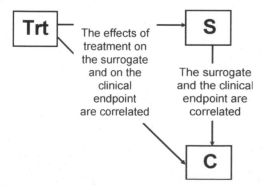

**FIGURE 1.** A surrogate (S) is acceptable if the surrogate and the clinical endpoint (C) are correlated (individual-level surrogacy) and if the effects of treatment (Trt) on the surrogate and the clinical endpoints are correlated (trial-level surrogacy).

**TABLE 2.** Comparison Between the 3 Main Types of Meta-Analysis

| Data Source | Literature | Summary Statistics* | Individual Patient Data* |
|---|---|---|---|
| Publication biases | Yes | No | No |
| Reporting biases | Yes | No | No |
| Data checks possible | No | No | Yes |
| Data up to date | No | Yes | Yes |
| Investigation of heterogeneity | No | Limited | Yes |
| Other analyses† | No | No | Yes |
| Difficulty of data collection | Low | Reasonable | High |
| Cost | Trivial | Low | High |

*Obtained from the principal investigator of the trials.
†Other analyses include subset analyses, validation of surrogate endpoints, and exploration of time patterns.

for outcomes that are time-related (eg, the absolute number of deaths per treatment group or the HR calculated from a life-table analysis).

- If the principal investigators of all trials can be contacted then a meta-analysis based on individual patient data (IPD) is undoubtedly the best approach. Such IPD meta-analyses have contributed to therapeutic progress in many ways, and they have recently been used to investigate whether early endpoints can be used as surrogates for later endpoints.[37]

## USING META-ANALYSES TO ASSESS POTENTIAL SURROGATES

As discussed earlier, a good surrogate is one for which there is a strong association between the surrogate and the clinical endpoint of interest, and there is a strong association between the effects of treatment on the surrogate and the clinical endpoint. The former condition can be verified easily using prospective or retrospective patient series. The latter condition, in contrast, requires data from prospective trials in which patients are randomized between two or more treatment groups. The comparison of these groups provides estimates of the effect of treatment both on the surrogate and the clinical endpoint. Ideally, several trials must be available, so that the effects of treatment can be repeatedly estimated; hence, a quantitative assessment of surrogacy is best performed in the context of a meta-analysis of several trials. It is the association between the treatment effects estimated in the various trials that will provide an assessment of the trial-level surrogacy.

For binary endpoints such as tumor response or clinical benefit, an appropriate measure of treatment effect is the odds ratio (OR). For time-related endpoints such as survival or PFS, an appropriate measure of treatment effect is the HR. Let us illustrate how to calculate these measures of treatment benefit in the simple situation where two treatment groups are being compared in terms of the incidence of an untoward event such as death, failure to achieve a tumor response, and some treatment toxicity. Table 3 presents the calculations required to calculate the relative risk (ie, the risk of the event in the treatment group divided by the risk of the event in the control group) and the OR (ie, the odds of the event in the treatment group divided by the odds of the event in the control group). Note that if the event of interest is death and about 10% of patients or more have died, then using the time to death into account may substantially increase the statistical power to detect a difference between the treatment groups. In this case, the relative risk is calculated as the ratio of the instantaneous risks (or "hazards") of death over time and is called the HR.

Now if we are interested, for instance, in validating tumor response as a surrogate for survival, we will estimate the association between the response ORs in a set of trials and the survival HRs in the same set of trials. If there is a strong association, we will claim that response is potentially a good surrogate for survival; we cannot make such a claim if the association is weak. We can in fact go one step

**TABLE 3.** Calculation of the Relative Risk and Odds Ratio for an Untoward Event in 2 Randomized Treatment Arms

|  | Treatment | Control |
|---|---|---|
| Risk of the event | 0.1 | 0.2 |
| Relative risk | 0.5 = 0.1/0.2 | |
| Odds ratio | 0.44 = (0.1/0.9)/(0.2/0.8) | |

No. events (No. patients) in the treatment and control groups are 10 (100) and 20 (100), respectively.

further and estimate the "surrogate threshold effect" (STE), which is the minimum treatment effect on the surrogate required to predict a nonzero treatment effect on the clinical endpoint in a future trial.[42] If the STE is small (ie, realistically achievable by future treatments) then the surrogate may be of potential interest. If, in contrast, the STE is large then the surrogate is unlikely to be of practical value. Finally, if the STE cannot be estimated at all then we have no statistical basis to make claims of surrogacy.

## RESPONSE AS A SURROGATE FOR SURVIVAL

Several meta-analyses have been conducted to investigate the usefulness of response as a surrogate for survival in patients with advanced colorectal,[13,14] breast,[15] and prostate cancer.[29,30] In colorectal and breast cancer, response was defined on the basis of repeated tumor measurements according to World Health Organization criteria. In prostate cancer, response was defined on the basis of repeated measurements of PSA levels. In all tumor types, the achievement of a response was associated with a better survival (suggesting good individual-level surrogacy), but there was a poor correlation between the treatment effects on tumor response and OS (suggesting poor trial-level surrogacy). Hence, although response may be useful for patient management, it does not qualify as a surrogate for survival in any of the solid tumors studied.

## PFS AS A SURROGATE FOR SURVIVAL

PFS has also been proposed as a potential surrogate for OS in patients with advanced colorectal,[28] breast,[15] prostate,[29,30] and ovarian cancer[27] (Table 4).

In colorectal, breast, and ovarian cancer, time to progression was defined on the basis of repeated tumor measurements according to World Health Organization criteria. In prostate cancer, time to progression was defined on the basis of repeated measurements of PSA levels. The correlation between PFS and OS was acceptably high (suggesting good individual-level surrogacy) in ovarian and colorectal cancer, as indicated by squared correlation coefficients of 0.70 and 0.82, respectively (Table 5). The squared correlation coefficient represents the proportion of variance in the clinical endpoint explained

**TABLE 4.** Data Used to Validate PFS as a Surrogate for OS in 4 Advanced Solid Tumors

| Tumor Type (Reference) | Treatment Comparison | No. Trials | No. Units of Analysis | No. Patients |
|---|---|---|---|---|
| Advanced colorectal cancer (28) | 5-Fluorouracil, leucovorin vs. 5-fluorouracil or ralitrexed | 10 | 10 Trials | 3089 |
| Advanced breast cancer (15) | Taxane vs. anthracycline regimens | 11 | 11 Trials | 3953 |
| Advanced prostate cancer (29) | Liarozole vs. cyproterone acetate or flutamide | 2 | 19 Countries | 596 |
| Advanced ovarian cancer (27) | Cyclophosphamide, adriamycin, platinum vs. cyclophosphamide, platinum | 4 | 50 Centers | 1189 |

**TABLE 5.** Squared Correlation Coefficients for Individual-Level and Trial-Level Surrogacy, and Surrogate Threshold Effects for PFS as a Surrogate for OS in 4 Advanced Solid Tumors

| Tumor Type (Reference) | $R^2$ Between PFS and OS (95% CI) | $R^2$ Between Treatment Effects on PFS and OS (95% CI) | Surrogate Threshold Effect |
| --- | --- | --- | --- |
| Advanced colorectal cancer (28) | 0.67 (0.67–0.69) | 0.98 (0.88–1.08) | 0.86 |
| Advanced breast cancer (15) | 0.47 (0.47–0.48) | 0.23 (0.12–1.69) | — |
| Advanced prostate cancer (29) | — | 0.22 (−0.14–0.58) | — |
| Advanced ovarian cancer (27) | 0.70 (0.69–0.72) | 0.95 (0.82–1.07) | 0.55 |

CI, confidence interval.

by the surrogate. In contrast, the correlation between PFS and OS was unacceptably low (suggesting poor individual-level surrogacy) in breast cancer, as indicated by a squared correlation coefficient of 0.47 (Table 5).

The trial-level surrogacy could be studied using individual trials as the units of analysis in the meta-analyses of breast and colorectal cancer trials, but not in the meta-analyses of ovarian and prostate cancer trials (because these included only four and two trials, respectively). Therefore, smaller units of analysis were chosen in these tumor types: centers for the ovarian cancer trials and countries for the prostate cancer trials (Table 4). The squared correlation coefficients for the treatment effects on PFS and OS were high for colorectal cancer (0.98) and ovarian cancer (0.95), again suggesting that PFS was a good surrogate for OS in these tumor types (Table 5). In contrast, the squared correlation coefficients for the treatment effects on PFS and OS were low for breast cancer (0.23) and prostate cancer (0.22), suggesting that PFS was not an acceptable surrogate for OS in these tumor types (Table 5).

In advanced colorectal cancer, the STE was an HR for PFS of 0.86, which implies that if a new treatment could reduce the risk of progression or death by at least 14% (= 1–0.86), it would be expected to have a statistical significant impact on OS.[28] In advanced ovarian cancer, the STE was an HR for PFS of 0.55, which suggested that more extreme treatment effects on PFS would be required in this tumor type to predict a statistical significant impact on OS. In other words, if a new treatment cut the risk of progression or death by about one half, one might be reasonably confident that this treatment would also lead to a survival benefit; if the new treatment had a smaller effect on PFS then no such claim could be made about its potential effect on survival.

## LONGITUDINAL BIOMARKER DATA AS A SURROGATE FOR SURVIVAL

Analyses of response and time to progression do not do full justice to the data collected in clinical trials, for these endpoints represent a summary of repeated measures (of the tumor surface area or PSA levels), and as such, they lose potentially valuable information. It is reasonable to wonder whether the full longitudinal data might represent a better surrogate endpoint for survival than response or time to progression. In advanced prostate cancer, repeated measures of PSA over time have been shown not to be a satisfactory surrogate for survival in two independent meta-analyses based on IPD.[29,30] Analyses conducted in single trials came to different conclusions.[43,44] However, these studies used potentially misleading statistical criteria to assess surrogacy,[23] and a meta-analysis based on IPD from several trials would provide a higher level of evidence to claim that PSA is or is not an acceptable surrogate for use in future trials in patients with advanced prostate cancer.[45]

## CONCLUSION

Clinical research in cancer is facing an unprecedented challenge. Advances in molecular biology send a fast rising number of potentially useful molecules to the clinic, yet the pace of new drug approval has remained almost unchanged during the past decade and shows no sign of picking up any time soon. One of the main reasons for the inefficiency of the clinical trials process is the lack of properly validated biomarkers that can replace or complement clinical endpoints such as survival to assess the benefits of new therapies. In this article, we have outlined some conditions that a valid surrogate should fulfill and shown that the ideal setting to verify these conditions is a meta-analysis of several trials with IPD on both the surrogate and the clinical endpoints.

## REFERENCES

1. DiLeo A, Bleiberg H, Buyse M. Overall survival is not a realistic endpoint for clinical trials in advanced solid tumors: a critical assessment based on recently reported phase III trials in colorectal and breast cancer. *J Clin Oncol.* 2003;21:2045–2047.
2. DiLeo A, Bleiberg H, Buyse M. Is overall survival a realistic primary endpoint in advanced colorectal cancer? A critical assessment based on four clinical trials comparing fluorouracil plus leucovorin with the same treatment combined either with oxaliplatin or with irinotecan. *Ann Oncol.* 2004;15:545–549.
3. Sargent DJ, Hayes DF. Assessing the measure of a new drug: is survival the only thing that matters? *J Clin Oncol.* 2008;26:1922–1923.
4. Schilsky RL. Endpoints in cancer clinical trials and the drug approval process. *Clin Cancer Res.* 2002;8:935–938.
5. Stewart DJ, Kurzrock R. Cancer: the road to Amiens. *J Clin Oncol.* 2009;27:328–333.
6. Biomarker Definition Working Group. (2001). Biomarkers and surrogate endpoints: preferred definitions and conceptual framework. *Clin Pharmacol Ther.* 2001;69:89–95.
7. Temple RJ. A regulatory authority's opinion about surrogate endpoints. In: Nimmo WS, Tucker GT, eds. *Clinical Measurement in Drug Evaluation.* New York: Wiley; 1995:3–22.
8. Eisenhauer EA, Therasse P, Bogaerts J, et al. New response evaluation criteria in solid tumors: revised RECIST guideline (version1.1). *Eur J Cancer.* 2009;45:228–247.
9. Dancey JE, Dodd LE, Ford R, et al. Recommendations for the assessment of progression in randomized cancer treatment trials. *Eur J Cancer.* 2009;45:281–289.
10. Lesko LJS, Atkinson AJ. Use of biomarkers and surrogate end-points in drug development and regulatory decision making: criteria, validation, strategies. *Ann Rev Pharmacol Toxicol.* 2001;41:347–366.
11. Sridhara R, Eisenberger MA, Sinibaldi VJ, et al. Evaluation of prostate-specific antigen as a surrogate marker for response of hormone-refractory prostate cancer to suramin therapy. *J Clin Oncol.* 1995;13:2944–2953.
12. Smith DC, Dunn RL, Stawderman MS, et al. Change in serum prostate-specific antigen as a marker of response to cytotoxic therapy for hormone-refractory prostate cancer. *J Clin Oncol.* 1998;16:1835–1843.
13. Buyse M, Thirion P, Carlson RW, et al, for the Meta-Analysis Group In Cancer. Relation between tumour response to first-line chemotherapy and survival in advanced colorectal cancer: a meta-analysis. *Lancet.* 2000;356:373–378.
14. Burzykowski T, Molenberghs G, Buyse M, et al. The validation of surrogate endpoints using data from randomized clinical trials: a case-study in advanced colorectal cancer. *J Roy Stat Soc A.* 2004;167:103–124.

15. Burzykowski T, Buyse M, Piccart-Gebhart MJ, et al. Evaluation of tumor response, disease control, progression-free survival, and time to progression as potential surrogate endpoints in metastatic breast cancer. *J Clin Oncol.* 2008;26:1987–1992.

16. Prentice RL. Surrogate endpoints in clinical trials: definitions and operational criteria. *Stat Med.* 1989;8:431–440.

17. Schatzkin A, Freedman LS, Schiffman MH, et al. Validation of intermediate end points in cancer research. *J Natl Cancer Inst.* 1990;82:1746–1752.

18. Freedman LS, Graubard BI, Schatzkin A. Statistical validation of intermediate endpoints for chronic diseases. *Stat Med.* 1992;11:167–178.

19. Buyse M, Molenberghs G. Criteria for the validation of surrogate end-points in randomized experiments. *Biometrics.* 1998;54:1014–1029.

20. Buyse M, Molenberghs G, Burzykowski T, et al. The validation of surrogate endpoints in meta-analyses of randomized experiments. *Biostatistics.* 2000;1:49–68.

21. Lassere M, Johnson K, Boers M, et al. Definitions and validation criteria for biomarkers and surrogate endpoints: development and testing of a quantitative hierarchical levels of evidence schema. *J Rheumatol.* 2007;34:607–615.

22. Weir CJ, Walley RJ. Statistical evaluation of biomarkers as surrogate endpoints: a literature review. *Stat Med.* 2006;25:183–203.

23. Molenberghs G, Buyse M, Geys H, et al. Statistical challenges in the evaluation of surrogate endpoints in randomized trials. *Control Clin Trials.* 2002;23:607–625.

24. Sargent D, Wieand S, Haller DG, et al. Disease-free survival (DFS) vs. overall survival (OS) as a primary endpoint for adjuvant colon cancer studies: individual patient data from 20,898 patients on 18 randomized trials. *J Clin Oncol.* 2005;23:8664–8670.

25. Burzykowski T, Buyse M, Sargent D, et al. Exploring and validating surrogate endpoints in colorectal cancer. *Lifetime Data Anal.* 2008;14:54–64.

26. Michiels S, Le Maître A, Buyse M, et al. Surrogate endpoints for overall survival in locally advanced head and neck cancer: meta-analyses of individual patient data. *Lancet Oncol.* 2009;10:341–350.

27. Burzykowski T, Molenberghs G, Buyse M, et al. Validation of surrogate endpoints in multiple randomized clinical trials with failure-time endpoints. *J Roy Stat Soc C Appl Stat.* 2001;50:405–422.

28. Buyse M, Burzykowski T, Carroll K, et al. Progression-free survival is a surrogate for survival in advanced colorectal cancer. *J Clin Oncol.* 2007;25:5218–5224.

29. Buyse M, Vangeneugden T, Bijnens L, et al. Validation of biomarkers as surrogates for clinical endpoints. In: Bloom JC, Dean RA, eds. *Biomarkers in Clinical Drug Development.* New York: Marcel Dekker; 2003:149–168.

30. Collette L, Burzykowski T, Carroll KJ, et al. Is prostate-specific antigen a valid surrogate end point for survival in hormonally treated patients with metastatic prostate cancer? *J Clin Oncol.* 2005;23:6139–6148.

31. Molenberghs G, Burzykowski T, Alonso A, et al. The meta-analytic framework for the evaluation of surrogate endpoints in clinical trials. *J Stat Plan Infer.* 2008;138:432–449.

32. Burzykowski T, Molenberghs G, Buyse M, eds. *The Evaluation of Surrogate Endpoints.* New York: Springer; 2005.

33. Buyse M, Burzykowski T, Michiels S, et al. Individual- and trial-level surrogacy in colorectal cancer. *Stat Methods Med Res.* 2008;17:5.

34. Alonso A, Molenberghs G, Geys H, et al. A unifying approach for surrogate marker validation based on Prentice's criteria. *Stat Med.* 2006;25:205–221.

35. Alonso A, Molenberghs G. Surrogate marker evaluation from an information theory perspective. *Biometrics.* 2006;63;180–186.

36. Buyse M, Piedbois P, Piedbois Y, et al. Meta-analysis: methods, strengths and weaknesses. *Oncology.* 2000;14:437–443.

37. Buyse M. Contributions of meta-analyses based on individual patient data to therapeutic progress in colorectal cancer. *Int J Clin Oncol.* 2009;14:95–101.

38. Buyse M, Piedbois P. Meta-analyses, use and misuse. *J Clin Oncol.* 1993;11:382.

39. Piedbois P, Buyse M. Meta-analyses need time, collaboration and funding. *J Clin Oncol.* 1994;12:878–879.

40. Buyse M, Carlson RW, Piedbois P. Meta-analyses of published results are unreliable. *J Clin Oncol.* 1999;16:1646–1647.

41. Piedbois P, Buyse M. Meta-analyses based on abstracted data: a step in the right direction, but only a first step. *J Clin Oncol.* 2004;22:3839–3841.

42. Burzykowski T, Buyse M. Surrogate threshold effect: An alternative measure for meta-analytic surrogate endpoint validation. *Pharm Stat.* 2006;5:173–186.

43. Petrylak DP, Ankerst DP, Jiang CS, et al. Evaluation of prostate-specific antigen declines for surrogacy in patients treated on SWOG 99–16. *J Natl Cancer Inst.* 2006;98:516–521.

44. Armstrong AJ, Garrett-Mayer E, Ou Yang YC, et al. Prostate-specific antigen and pain surrogacy analysis in metastatic hormone-refractory prostate cancer. *J Clin Oncol.* 2007;25:3965–3970.

45. Collette L, Buyse M, Burzykowski T. Are prostate-specific antigen changes valid surrogates for survival in hormone-refractory prostate cancer? A meta-analysis is needed! *J Clin Oncol.* 2007;25:5673–5674.

# Other Paradigms: Better Treatments Are Identified by Better Trials

## The Value of Randomized Phase II Studies

Manish R. Sharma • Michael L. Maitland • Mark J. Ratain

Before 1990, there were only 47 cytotoxic anticancer drugs approved by the Food and Drug Administration (FDA) to treat diverse tumor types. In 2 decades, that number has almost tripled to 138 approved drugs,[1] and many more are currently in clinical trials. Many of the newer drugs are molecularly targeted (ie, developed based on activity against a specific target) and can be used alone or in combination with traditional cytotoxic drugs to treat tumors more effectively. In select diseases (eg, chronic myelogenous leukemia), drugs are administered orally indefinitely, much like the management of chronic diseases outside of oncology. The changing landscape requires that we rethink the way that we conduct phase II trials in oncology, and perhaps learn from our peers in other fields.

When many diseases and stages had no clear standard of care, most phase II trials of new anticancer drugs used a single-arm design with a primary end point of tumor response, defined as a reduction in bidimensional size $\geq 50\%$ or a reduction of unidimensional size $\geq 30\%$ according to the Response Evaluation Criteria in Solid Tumors guidelines.[2,3] A 2-stage design was often used to distinguish whether a drug had an unpromising response rate (often $<5\%$) or a promising response rate (often $>20\%$), the latter being the criteria for further investigation in phase III trials.[4] In the era of molecularly targeted drugs, however, the assessment of response rate on a single-arm trial will leave out a number of promising drugs, whereas advancing others that may not improve outcomes in the phase III setting. In other fields of medicine, phase II trials have commonly been randomized studies, and this approach has helped identify promising therapies for a variety of chronic and progressive diseases.[3] At this time, we contend that randomization between an experimental arm and a control arm should be no less feasible or necessary in phase II oncology trials. Randomized studies will better enable us to identify those agents (or combinations) that are the most promising for a selected indication.

### THE PURPOSE OF PHASE II TRIALS

After establishing the safety and dose-limiting toxicities of new drugs in phase I trials, phase II trials must yield enough information about efficacy to determine whether a particular drug (or combination) justifies the investment of significant resources for designing and conducting a definitive phase III trial. Much like the selection of elite athletes, setting the bar too high will lead to many worthy candidates being left out, whereas setting the bar too low leads to a more dilute pool of candidates, a few of which will prove successful but most of which will fall short. Adjei et al[5] have detailed many recent negative phase III trials that followed promising phase II trials with targeted anticancer drugs, suggesting that the bar is currently too low. In modern oncology, there are 800 to 900 new drugs available for investigation, and resources will be quickly exhausted if we advance too many drugs to phase III trials. Both our patients' welfare and cost limitations in

our health care system require that we minimize the risk of failure in phase III trials.

With rapid advances in cancer science, phase II trials should not simply screen for which novel drug candidates continue to further investigation. These trials must also provide valuable information about the drug so that the design of a subsequent phase III trial is optimized. Only through randomized designs can we establish the relationship of dose to both efficacy and toxicity. In a typical cost/benefit analysis, we hope to find a dose at which the drug has both efficacy (potentially based on a biomarker end point) and acceptable toxicities. Randomization in phase II trials enables investigators to determine the optimal dose, to find the most sensitive end point, to analyze drug toxicity relative to a control arm, and to predict the effect size that might be expected in a phase III study. A single-arm design cannot yield any of this information with accuracy, because it fundamentally relies on comparisons with historical controls that are never completely comparable with respect to efficacy, toxicity, or choice of end point.

### COMPARISONS WITH OTHER DISEASES

Although cancer's unique heterogeneity depends on various tumor-specific (genetic, molecular, and histologic) and host-specific (genetic, environmental, and comorbid) factors, it shares common features with other chronic and progressive diseases. One natural comparison is with human immunodeficiency virus (HIV) infection, an incurable, progressively debilitating illness with diverse trajectories based on virus-specific and host-specific factors. The rapid progress of antiretroviral therapy during the last 2 decades surpasses the advances with molecularly targeted anticancer drugs, and much can be learned about clinical trial design from reviewing the HIV therapeutics literature. Inflammatory diseases, such as rheumatoid arthritis (RA), have traditionally been treated with some of the same cytotoxic drugs used to treat cancer. Recently, targeted therapies have altered treatment paradigms for RA and other inflammatory diseases, with many more drugs on the horizon. For devastating neurologic diseases, such as Alzheimer disease and multiple sclerosis, the focus of research has been on early detection and early treatment. Not unlike our most refractory cancers, there are few effective agents and many candidate therapies that require further testing. In each of these fields, randomized phase II studies have played a crucial role in improving patient care by advancing novel drugs to successful phase III trials and FDA approval.

### OPTIONS FOR RANDOMIZED PHASE II TRIAL DESIGNS

The most basic design for a randomized phase II trial is a study with a single experimental arm and a single control arm, where the control arm is a placebo and the experimental arm is a novel drug. Of course, this type of design can only be used in a study population in which there is no current standard of care. In an excellent example, patients with relapsing-remitting multiple sclerosis received a single course of rituximab or placebo in a double-blind study. Compared with placebo, rituximab reduced gadolinium-enhancing brain lesions and clinical relapses for 48 weeks.[6] A slight variation is a trial in which there are multiple experimental arms, involving different doses of the same drug. This was the strategy used in the recent phase II trial of tarenflurbil, a selective amyloid-beta peptide (42)-lowering agent, for mild to moderate Alzheimer disease.[7] In that study, patients with mild Alzheimer disease randomized to receive 800 mg of the drug twice daily had a slower rate of decline during a 12-month period, according to previously validated scales to assess activities of daily living and global cognitive function. Importantly, the study found that a lower dose (400 mg twice daily) did not have the same effect, nor did either dose have an effect on patients with moderate Alzheimer disease. After this phase II study, a phase III study can be optimally designed to assess the higher dose versus placebo in patients with mild Alzheimer disease.

A more complex design is a randomized discontinuation (or randomized withdrawal) study in which all participants initially receive the experimental drug, with disease assessment at a prespecified time point. Patients with stable disease are then randomized to continue the active drug or receive placebo in a blinded fashion, with the option to crossover from placebo to active drug at the time of progression. This design is most useful for drugs that are anticipated to have a low response rate but a significant disease-stabilizing effect, as the initial period allows the population to be enriched for patients most likely to benefit from the drug. This was the strategy used in a study of donepezil for the treatment of mild to moderate Alzheimer disease. All patients received donepezil 5 mg daily for 6 weeks followed by 10 mg daily for another 6 weeks, at which point they were assessed and randomized to 10 mg daily versus placebo. Patients who continued donepezil after randomization had significant improvements in neuropsychiatric symptoms (using a previously validated measure) compared with those in the placebo group.[8] A notable example of the randomized discontinuation design in oncology was the phase II trial of sorafenib, which demonstrated a marked effect on progression-free survival (PFS) in patients with metastatic renal cell carcinoma.[9] The results led rapidly to the design of a phase III trial that won FDA approval of sorafenib for advanced renal cell carcinoma.[10]

More complicated randomized phase II trials involve an experimental arm that adds a new drug to the current standard of care, where the control arm is the standard of care plus placebo. Such trials are very useful in modern oncology, because most cancers have treatments that are already the standard of care; however, there is still significant room for improvement of outcomes in some or all patients. Raltegravir, an HIV-1 integrase inhibitor, was initially studied in this fashion in patients on optimized standard antiretroviral regimens who had evidence of resistance to at least 1 drug from each class. In a randomized phase II study, patients receiving raltegravir versus placebo (in addition to background therapy) had better viral suppression at all 3 doses studied, with no significant toxicities at any dose.[11] Not surprisingly, a follow-up phase III trial showed that complete viral suppression could be achieved in significantly more patients receiving raltegravir than placebo (in addition to background therapy), and the drug was approved by the FDA even before the phase III results were published.[12]

In RA, for which methotrexate is a standard therapy, 2 recent studies have evaluated the combination of methotrexate and various doses of a targeted drug in patients with active RA despite methotrexate monotherapy. First, a combined phase I/II study showed that ocre-

lizumab (a humanized anti-CD20 monoclonal antibody) was well tolerated when combined with methotrexate, and randomization during phase II showed that higher doses of the drug plus methotrexate had more clinical activity (based on reduction in C-reactive protein) and better clinical responses than placebo plus methotrexate, without increased toxicity.[13] A phase III trial of the same combination is now underway.[14] Another randomized phase II study evaluated 2 doses of abatacept (CTLA-4Ig, a selective costimulation modulator) in combination with methotrexate for 1 year versus methotrexate plus placebo.[15] Both doses were safe and well tolerated, but the higher dose led to significant reductions in disease activity and improvements in physical function compared with placebo. A subsequent phase III study showed similar results,[16] whereas the initial phase II study has now been followed up for 5 years with consistent efficacy and safety.[17] These studies in RA had many of the same challenges faced in oncology trials, where multiple doses of a drug must be compared with each other and to a standard of care over an extended period of time.

## RANDOMIZED PHASE II TRIALS IN ONCOLOGY: THE EXAMPLE OF LUNG CANCER

In advanced nonsmall cell lung cancer (NSCLC), the longstanding challenge has been to improve on outcomes with conventional doublet chemotherapy, such as carboplatin and paclitaxel. Recent trials with targeted drugs in combination with chemotherapy have included examples of both randomized and nonrandomized phase II trial designs. The single example of a drug that has achieved FDA approval for use with first-line chemotherapy is bevacizumab, a vascular endothelial growth factor inhibitor. A randomized phase II trial was conducted with 2 different doses (7.5 mg/kg and 15 mg/kg) of bevacizumab in combination with carboplatin and paclitaxel, compared with carboplatin and paclitaxel alone. The bevacizumab 15 mg/kg arm resulted in a higher response rate and longer median time to progression, although identifying hemoptysis as a significant risk.[18] The subsequent phase III study used only the 15 mg/kg dose and excluded patients who were observed to have a higher bleeding risk in the phase II study. The results were similar to the phase II study and also showed an improvement in the primary end point of overall survival, leading to FDA approval for this indication.[19]

In contrast, the epidermal growth factor receptor (EGFR) inhibitor gefitinib was first studied in a pilot phase I trial in combination with carboplatin and paclitaxel and was found to be safely tolerated.[20] There were multiple phase II studies of gefitinib monotherapy in patients previously treated with chemotherapy with substantial response rates, but no randomized phase II study was conducted using the combination of gefitinib and chemotherapy. A phase III trial of gefitinib at 2 different dose levels versus placebo, in combination with carboplatin and paclitaxel, showed no difference in overall survival, time to progression or response rate, compared with standard chemotherapy alone.[21] Another EGFR inhibitor, erlotinib, is already approved as monotherapy for advanced NSCLC in the second-line setting. Like gefitinib, erlotinib did not improve outcomes when combined with carboplatin and paclitaxel chemotherapy in a phase III trial (the TRIBUTE trial).[22] The same group that ran negative trials for gefitinib and erlotinib later conducted a randomized phase II trial of vandetanib, a VEGFR and EGFR inhibitor, in combination with docetaxel in the second-line setting. The results showed that vandetanib (100 mg daily or 300 mg daily) plus docetaxel significantly improved PFS compared with placebo plus docetaxel.[23] The follow-up phase III trial was very recently reported and confirmed the improvement in PFS with vandetanib 100 mg daily plus docetaxel, making this the first doublet therapy demonstrated to improve outcomes in the second-line setting.[24] It is

**TABLE 1.** Examples of Successful Randomized Phase II Trials in Oncology

| Disease | Regimens Tested | Comments | Reference |
|---|---|---|---|
| NSCLC, (1st line) | Carboplatin plus paclitaxel ± bevacizumab | Two different doses of bevacizumab tested and higher dose found to be effective, based on time to progression. Risk of bleeding also identified. | 18 |
| NSCLC, (2nd line) | Docetaxel plus vandetanib or placebo | Addition of vandetanib, at either of 2 doses, significantly improved PFS. | 23 |
| RCC | Sorafenib vs. placebo | In a randomized discontinuation design, PFS was significantly improved in the sorafenib arm. | 9 |

RCC, renal cell carcinoma.

very likely that the drug will earn FDA approval in the near future on the basis of these findings.

The experience in advanced NSCLC illustrates the point that randomized phase II trials can maximize the probability of success in phase III. The results of a single arm phase II trial are difficult to interpret because the drug is not compared directly to an accepted standard of care, as was the case for gefitinib and erlotinib in the first-line setting. Moreover, randomized phase II trials present an opportunity to determine the optimal dose, dosing schedule, and target population that should be used in phase III, as was the case for bevacizumab and vandetanib. Moving forward, other targeted drugs will need to be studied in randomized phase II trials to avoid negative phase III trials. The same is true in cancers for which targeted therapies, rather than chemotherapy, are now the standard of care. A recent editorial addressed this issue in the field of hepatocellular carcinoma, where sorafenib has become the standard of care and, the authors argue, randomized phase II trials will be necessary to assess other targeted therapies.[25] Table 1 briefly summarizes examples of successful randomized phase II trials in oncology that have been discussed earlier.

## STATISTICAL CONSIDERATIONS

The major argument against randomized phase II trials is that they require much larger sample sizes than single arm trials, resulting in greater expense and longer accrual periods, with a potential delay in promising drugs making it to phase III trials and FDA approval. Although this is true, there is a direct relationship between expense and the amount of information obtained from a phase II trial. Smaller and less expensive studies yield less information, whereas larger and more expensive studies yield more information. The challenge in phase II design is to find the right balance, so that sufficient resources are spent to get valuable information without compromising efficiency. Fortunately, randomized phase II trials can be designed in ways that limit the sample size while maintaining the primary objective of evaluating drugs (or combinations) for advancement to phase III.

The issue of calculating sample sizes for the design of randomized phase II trials in oncology was addressed by Rubinstein et al,[26] who proposed a method using either the logrank test or binomial proportion test.[27] Given that the only goal is to evaluate the superiority of the experimental arm(s) to the control arm, a 1-sided testing framework is sufficient. Moreover, a type I error rate ($\alpha$) of 0.05 is not necessary, given that such a standard would later be used in a phase III trial. An $\alpha$ of 0.20 would theoretically result in a phase III success rate of 80%, which would be a dramatic improvement over the status quo. A type II error rate ($\beta$) of 0.20, which equates to a "power" (1-$\beta$) of 80% is also a reasonable assumption, as this means that we would only overlook a truly efficacious drug (or combination) for a specific indication 20% of the time. Assuming $\alpha = 0.20$ and $\beta = 0.20$, trials with a PFS end point and a hazard ratio of 1.5 (eg, increase in PFS from 4 months to 6 months) would only require 69 patients. Trials with a PFS rate end point, where PFS is measured at

a prespecified time point, and an increase in PFS rate from 20% to 40%, would only require 78 patients. Trials with a response rate end point and an increase in response rate from 20% to 40% would also only require 78 patients. Thus, randomized phase II trials can readily detect clinically relevant differences with fewer than 100 patients. In contrast, increasing the sample size of a single-arm phase II trial does not solve the problem of misleading results. A recently presented simulation-based analysis showed that the larger the single-arm phase II trial, the greater the false positive error rate, implying that the direct relationship between sample size and knowledge is only true for randomized trials.[28]

As we have discussed earlier, phase II trials of novel therapeutics in other chronic and progressive diseases routinely use randomization. As Figure 1 illustrates, the incidence of these diseases (HIV, RA, and multiple sclerosis) in the United States is substantially lower

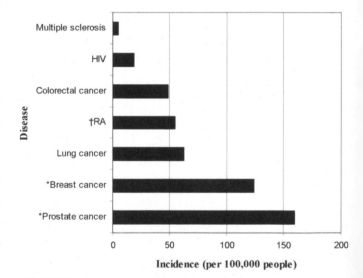

**FIGURE 1.** Incidence of the most common cancers in the United States, compared with those of HIV, RA, and multiple sclerosis. *Breast cancer incidence is per 100,000 women; prostate cancer incidence is per 100,000 men. †Incidence of RA ranges from 42 to 68.3, depending on the source. For purposes of the chart, the middle point of this range was used. Sources: (1) http://seer.cancer.gov/statfacts/ (data as of January 1, 2006), (2) http://www.cdc.gov/arthritis/arthritis/rheumatoid.htm, (3) http://www.cdc.gov/hiv/topics/surveillance/united_states.htm (data from 2006), (4) Alonso A, Hernán MA. Temporal trends in the incidence of multiple sclerosis: a systematic review. *Neurology.* 2008;71: 129–135.

than those of the most common cancers, suggesting that it should be even more difficult and expensive for investigators in these fields to recruit a similar number of patients. As oncologists, we certainly have no reason to hold ourselves to a lower standard than our peers in other therapeutic areas in the design of phase II trials. Although the drug-to-patient ratio might be higher in oncology than in other diseases, leading to competition between trials for accrual, this only strengthens the argument for raising the bar at the phase II level, so that there is less competition for patient and financial resources at the more important phase III level.

## BARRIERS TO CHANGE

Given what we have presented earlier, one may wonder why it has taken so long for oncologists to be convinced that randomized phase II trials should be the norm rather than the exception. The biggest reason is that single-arm phase II trials played a very important role in the era of cytotoxic chemotherapy drugs. In this era, response rate was a universally accepted end point and standards of care did not change very frequently, allowing for more reliable use of historical controls. Many experienced investigators continue to believe in the utility of single-arm phase II trials with response rate as the typical end point in the era of targeted drugs. El-Maraghi and Eisenhauer[29] reviewed 89 trials of 19 targeted drugs, and concluded that objective response predicted for eventual success, defined as FDA approval. Of the 89 trials, only 3 used randomization between a control (placebo or standard therapy) arm and an experimental arm. Four of the drugs that were eventually approved had response rates of <10%, whereas 2 of them (cetuximab and sorafenib) had response rates of <5% when used as monotherapy. As editorialists point out, one interpretation of the data is to propose that "the target response rate for the alternate hypothesis that prompts phase III testing may need to be lowered."[30] Ironically, this strategy would actually increase the sample size of single-arm trials, as more patients are needed to establish smaller differences in response rates with statistical significance. Moreover, the result of studying all such drugs in phase III trials would be an increase in the rate of negative phase III trials. Rather than lower the standards for advancement, we believe that drugs with relatively low anticipated response rates should be studied for efficacy using PFS (or related endpoints such as change in tumor volume[31]) as an end point, which can only be done in the setting of a randomized trial. This is especially true in an era where most new drugs are being studied in combination with standard therapies that already may have significant response rates, rather than as single agents. Acknowledging that there is still a role for single-arm phase II trials in rare cases, Table 2

contrasts drug development settings in which single arm designs may suffice versus those in which randomized designs are necessary.

## CONCLUSIONS

In the era of numerous targeted drugs available for clinical trials, patient care and financial considerations require that oncologists minimize the number of negative phase III trials. Doing so requires that we not only raise the bar for advancement of a drug from phase II to phase III, but also try to learn the optimal dose and dosing schedule for a drug in the phase II trial. This is best done by randomization between an experimental arm and a control arm, a strategy that has been successfully used in phase II trials for other chronic and progressive diseases in medicine. Randomized phase II trials are feasible, because they do not require an unrealistically large sample size when reasonable statistical standards are applied. Leaders in the field, including editors of high impact journals, are openly recognizing the need to prioritize randomized phase II trials over other designs.[32] Academic oncologists should emphasize quality over quantity in phase II trials and invest the resources necessary to conduct randomized trials that yield valuable information and eventually improve outcomes for our patients.

## REFERENCES

1. http://www.fda.gov/CDER/cancer/druglistframe.htm. Accessed May 12, 2009.
2. Eisenhauer EA, Therasse P, Bogaerts J, et al. New response evaluation criteria in solid tumours: revised RECIST guideline (version 1.1). *Eur J Cancer.* 2009;45: 228–247.
3. Michaelis LC, Ratain MJ. Phase II trials published in 2002: a cross-specialty comparison showing significant design differences between oncology trials and other medical specialties. *Clin Cancer Res.* 2007;13:2400–2405.
4. Simon R. Optimal two-stage designs for phase II clinical trials. *Control Clin Trials.* 1989;10:1–10.
5. Adjei AA, Christian M, Ivy P. Novel designs and end points for phase II clinical trials. *Clin Cancer Res.* 2009;15:1866–1872.
6. Hauser SL, Waubant E, Arnold DL, et al; HERMES Trial Group. B-cell depletion with rituximab in relapsing-remitting multiple sclerosis. *N Engl J Med.* 2008;358:676–688.
7. Wilcock GK, Black SE, Hendrix SB, et al; Tarenflurbil Phase II Study investigators. Efficacy and safety of tarenflurbil in mild to moderate Alzheimer's disease: a randomised phase II trial. *Lancet Neurol.* 2008;7:483–493.
8. Holmes C, Wilkinson D, Dean C, et al. The efficacy of donepezil in the treatment of neuropsychiatric symptoms in Alzheimer disease. *Neurology.* 2004;63: 214–219.
9. Ratain MJ, Eisen T, Stadler WM, et al. Phase II placebo-controlled randomized discontinuation trial of sorafenib in patients with metastatic renal cell carcinoma. *J Clin Oncol.* 2006;24:2505–2512.
10. Escudier B, Eisen T, Stadler WM, et al; TARGET Study Group. Sorafenib in advanced clear-cell renal-cell carcinoma. *N Engl J Med.* 2007;356:125–134.
11. Grinsztejn B, Nguyen BY, Katlama C, et al; Protocol 005 Team. Safety and efficacy of the HIV-1 integrase inhibitor raltegravir (MK-0518) in treatment-experienced patients with multidrug-resistant virus: a phase II randomised controlled trial. *Lancet.* 2007;369:1261–1269.
12. Steigbigel RT, Cooper DA, Kumar PN, et al; BENCHMRK Study Teams. Raltegravir with optimized background therapy for resistant HIV-1 infection. *N Engl J Med.* 2008;359:339–354.
13. Genovese MC, Kaine JL, Lowenstein MB, et al; ACTION Study Group. Ocrelizumab, a humanized anti-CD20 monoclonal antibody, in the treatment of patients with rheumatoid arthritis: a phase I/II randomized, blinded, placebo-controlled, dose-ranging study. *Arthritis Rheum.* 2008;58:2652–2661.
14. http://www.clinicaltrials.gov/ct2/show/NCT00406419?term=ocrelizumab&rank=3.
15. Kremer JM, Dougados M, Emery P, et al. Treatment of rheumatoid arthritis with the selective costimulation modulator abatacept: twelve-month results of a phase IIb, double-blind, randomized, placebo-controlled trial. *Arthritis Rheum.* 2005;52:2263–2271.
16. Kremer JM, Genant HK, Moreland LW, et al. Effects of abatacept in patients with methotrexate-resistant active rheumatoid arthritis: a randomized trial. *Ann Intern Med.* 2006;144:865–876.
17. Westhovens R, Kremer JM, Moreland LW, et al. Safety and efficacy of the selective costimulation modulator abatacept in patients with rheumatoid

**TABLE 2.** Drug Development Settings that Favor Randomized Versus Single-Arm Phase II Trials

| Randomized Phase II Trials | Single-Arm Phase II Trials |
| --- | --- |
| Combination study, in which toxicity needs to be assessed relative to a control arm | Single agent only, with preclinical or phase I data suggesting a potentially high response rate |
| Need to predict effect size for subsequent phase III study | Rare disease, making accrual difficult |
| Need to optimize dose for subsequent phase III study | No standard treatment options, limited value for comparator arm |
| Low response rate by tumor size, making alternative endpoints necessary (PFS, OS, time to progression, and other) | No standard treatment options, making high failure rate at phase III level tolerable |

arthritis receiving background methotrexate: a 5-year extended phase IIB study. *J Rheumatol.* 2009;36:736–742.

18. Johnson DH, Fehrenbacher L, Novotny WF, et al. Randomized phase II trial comparing bevacizumab plus carboplatin and paclitaxel with carboplatin and paclitaxel alone in previously untreated locally advanced or metastatic non-small-cell lung cancer. *J Clin Oncol.* 2004;22:2184–2191.

19. Sandler A, Gray R, Perry MC, et al. Paclitaxel-carboplatin alone or with bevacizumab for non-small-cell lung cancer. *N Engl J Med.* 2006;355:2542–2550.

20. Miller VA, Johnson DH, Krug LM, et al. Pilot trial of the epidermal growth factor receptor tyrosine kinase inhibitor gefitinib plus carboplatin and paclitaxel in patients with stage IIIB or IV non-small-cell lung cancer. *J Clin Oncol.* 2003;21:2094–2100.

21. Herbst RS, Giaccone G, Schiller JH, et al. Gefitinib in combination with paclitaxel and carboplatin in advanced non-small-cell lung cancer: a phase III trial—INTACT 2. *J Clin Oncol.* 2004;22:785–794.

22. Herbst RS, Prager D, Hermann R, et al; TRIBUTE Investigator Group. TRIBUTE: a phase III trial of erlotinib hydrochloride (OSI-774) combined with carboplatin and paclitaxel chemotherapy in advanced non-small-cell lung cancer. *J Clin Oncol.* 2005;23:5892–5899.

23. Heymach JV, Johnson BE, Prager D, et al. Randomized, placebo-controlled phase II study of vandetanib plus docetaxel in previously treated non small-cell lung cancer. *J Clin Oncol.* 2007;25:4270–4277.

24. Herbst RS, Sun Y, Korfee S, et al. Vandetanib plus docetaxel versus docetaxel as second-line treatment for patients with advanced non-small cell ung cancer (NSCLC): a randomized, double blind phase III trial (ZODIAC). *ASCO.* 2009: Abstract #CRA8003.

25. Llovet JM, Bruix J. Testing molecular therapies in hepatocellular carcinoma: the need for randomized phase II trials. *J Clin Oncol.* 2009;27:833–835.

26. Rubinstein LV, Korn EL, Freidlin B, et al. Design issues of randomized phase II trials and a proposal for phase II screening trials. *J Clin Oncol.* 2005;23:7199–7206.

27. Rubinstein L, Crowley J, Ivy P, et al. Randomized phase II designs. *Clin Cancer Res.* 2009;15:1883–1890.

28. Tang H, Foster NR, Grothey A, et al. Excessive false-positive errors in single-arm phase II trials: a simulation-based analysis. *ASCO.* 2009:Abstract #6512.

29. El-Maraghi RH, Eisenhauer EA. Review of phase II trial designs used in studies of molecular targeted agents: outcomes and predictors of success in phase III. *J Clin Oncol.* 2008;26:1346–1354.

30. Dowlati A, Fu P. Is response rate relevant to the phase II trial design of targeted agents? *J Clin Oncol.* 2008;26:1204–1205.

31. Karrison TG, Maitland ML, Stadler WM, et al. Design of phase II cancer trials using a continuous endpoint of change in tumor size: application to a study of sorafenib and erlotinib in non small-cell lung cancer. *J Natl Cancer Inst.* 2007;99:1455–1461.

32. Cannistra SA. Phase II trials in journal of clinical oncology. *J Clin Oncol.* 2009;27:3073–3076.

# Other Paradigms

## Randomized Discontinuation Trial Design

Walter Stadler

Phase II trials of novel antitumor agents have generally depended on the agent's ability to cause tumor shrinkage. The underlying assumption has always been that a certain degree of tumor shrinkage is necessary in order for patients to have any benefit from the drug and thus lack of such an effect should preclude further definitive phase III testing of the agent. Under this assumption, one must assure that the tumor size measurement is reliable, reproducible, and a direct result of the intervention. In an era before modern imaging technology when oncologists depended on palpation for assessing "response," a small reliability experiment demonstrated that oncologists could only consistently detect tumor shrinkage if the sum of the orthogonal dimensions of a sphere decreased by at least 50%.[1] This, thus, became the accepted criteria for response, which was then translated to the now familiar mathematically equivalent 30% decrease in unidimensional measurements,[2] despite the fact that modern imaging modalities are capable of measuring much more subtle changes in tumor size and are expected to be more accurate than clinical palpation.

Given these considerations, the extensive use of tumor measurements in oncology clinical trials, and the focus on standardization of measurements, it is surprising that there is rather limited data on variability of tumor size measurement using modern cross-sectional imaging. Furthermore, such measurements may be much more variable than generally supposed.[3] More important is the fact that measurement of changes in tumor size is a continuous variable and dichotomizing it at an arbitrary cut point into response versus "nonresponse" (or similarly into "progression" versus "not progression") discards important information.[4] In addition, without careful validation studies, any arbitrary cut point may or may not correlate with actual patient benefit, and such correlations are likely to be both disease and agent specific. Finally, agents with potent growth inhibitory properties may not cause dramatic tumor shrinkages but could still have significant patient benefit.

These considerations are not simply theoretical. A large number of agents in preclinical studies have been identified as being active based on their growth inhibitory properties. Antiangiogenic agents specifically have not led to dramatic tumor shrinkages in either the laboratory or patients and yet have demonstrated clinically important benefits. Perhaps the most relevant example is the vascular endothelial growth factor receptor inhibitor Sorafenib, which leads to response evaluation criteria in solid tumors (RECIST)-based response rates of <10% in both hepatocellular and renal carcinoma but has been demonstrated to benefit both of these patient populations in randomized phase III trials.[5,6] Thus, the lack of tumor shrinkage sufficient to meet "standard" criteria in a single-arm phase II trial is insufficient to determine that the agent is truly inactive.

On the other hand, variability considerations noted earlier make it difficult to choose any arbitrary decrease (or lack of increase) in tumor size much less than the standard RECIST criteria in a phase II trial as a signal sufficient to determine that an agent is active. For example, a variability study of baseline computed topography scans of patients enrolled in a lung cancer study suggested that 15% of patients in whom the tumor measurements were performed by 2 separate expert readers would be classified as "responders" by RECIST criteria simply based on interobserver variability in the measurements.[3] For progression endpoints in clinical trials, interpatient variability in tumor growth rates, in addition to observer and measurement variability, must also be considered. For example, the median time to progression of metastatic renal cancer treated with interferon, which is a modestly active agent at best, is 4.7 months but 14% of patients are progression free at 2 years.[7] The criteria for determining disease progression by standard RECIST criteria in renal cancer is furthermore highly dependent on including or excluding the primary tumor measurement in the calculation.[8] Finally, progression is typically determined only when a computed topography scan is performed and thus the time to progression is highly dependent on the scanning interval. Close attention to measurement metrics and use of clinical prognostic models can decrease but not eliminate these sources of variability. As a result, it is difficult to determine whether any tumor measurement endpoint that uses a progression metric or a metric of tumor size change that is less than standard criteria is different than would be expected with observation alone. Thus, historical controls for any such metric are insufficient and if used in a phase II trial will generally require a randomized study to determine whether the studied agent has the hypothesized effect.

The typical randomized study conducted for evaluation of a novel agent in the laboratory would be a study of agent versus placebo or control, and this could certainly be done in patients as well. However, in contrast to relatively homogeneous laboratory models, and as is the case with most approved antitumor agents, there is an underlying variability in the agent's ability to impact a specific patient's cancer. In fact, in the highly heterogeneous human disease, it is typical that only a subset of patients will benefit and a priori identification of patients likely to benefit is difficult to impossible. If the agent to be tested furthermore inhibits tumor growth (or tends to cause tumor shrinkages less than standard RECIST-based response), it becomes even more difficult to determine whether a lack of growth in an individual or even a population represents activity of the agent, selection of a patient or population with indolent disease, or some combination of both. Once again, this is not necessarily an unusual clinical scenario. The epidermal growth factor receptor (EGFR) pathway inhibitors have only modest antitumor effects in colorectal cancer with the predominate effect being growth inhibitory; however, it was only recently recognized that only those tumors with wild type RAS pathway are responsive to these agents.[9] This explains the lack of benefit with these agents in certain large phase III trials with broad entry criteria or with putative predictive biomarkers such as EGFR expression levels that were later shown to be invalid.

Given the expense of large phase III trials, and the increasing number of agents and targets being evaluated, it thus seems prudent to explore clinical trial designs that can provide more robust data in the phase II setting regarding antitumor activity of a putative agent that may be growth inhibitory or lead to only modest tumor shrinkages, especially, if this effect is observed in only a subset of patients. A design that meets these metrics is the randomized discontinuation trial design (RDT).[10,11]

## THE RANDOMIZED DISCONTINUATION TRIAL DESIGN

The general design is depicted in Figure 1. All patients receive the drug of interest upfront for a specified period of time. Those who experience a clear tumor shrinkage and apparent benefit, typically based on RECIST guidelines, would continue therapy, and those who have obvious tumor growth or are intolerant to the agent would discontinue. Patients who experience stable disease (which can include modest growth and/or shrinkage) are then randomized to continuing or discontinuing the therapy for an additional period of time with the primary endpoint being the fraction of patients in the randomized group who do not progress over that time period. In this manner, the agent selects a population that may be experiencing growth inhibitory effect from the drug, and the randomization then tests whether this population is truly a population in whom the agent induces stable disease or whether an indolent population with no or limited benefit from the agent was selected.

This design has several major advantages addressing the noted issues of variability in natural history, tumor size assessment, and antitumor effect of any specific agent. First, the agent and not incomplete scientific knowledge of the investigator selects the population most likely to benefit. For example, and as noted, many of the initial trials of EGFR-directed agents in colorectal cancer were limited to those whose tumors expressed EGFR, typically based on immunohistochemistry and an arbitrary cutoff. However, quantitative assessment of EGFR expression by immunohistochemistry has been extremely difficult to standardize. More importantly, further work demonstrated that RAS mutation was a much more important predictive marker for benefit from these agents.[9] The RDT design allows the agent to "select" the population with minimal a priori investigator input, and this enrichment markedly improves the power of the randomization phase.[10,12,13] In fact, previous and ongoing trials using the RDT design allow multiple tumor types to enroll in what may be considered

the most broad application of the investigator being agnostic to the population most likely to benefit.[14]

A second major advantage of the RDT is that a randomized concurrent control group is used. As noted earlier, heterogeneity in tumor natural history and measurement variability limits the utilization of historical controls for all but the most dramatic changes in tumor size. The placebo control in the randomized portion of the RDT allows unbiased assessment of essentially any chosen tumor-sized endpoint. Finally, and in contrast to upfront randomization, a much smaller number of patients are exposed to placebo, which has been a major issue for patients in phase II trials, who are typically participating because of the potential for therapeutic benefit. In fact, the ability for all participants to receive the investigational agent upfront has, in this investigator's anecdotal experience, made the RDT design more acceptable to potential subjects than upfront randomization. Some authors have emphasized the overall smaller size of RDT as opposed to upfront randomization trials, but this occurs only under a limited set of circumstances.[13]

The RDT design has been successfully used in cancer drug development to identify both active and confirmed inactive agents.[15,16] Nevertheless, in order for this design to be used most effectively, certain issues must be considered. First, the selection basis of the trial introduces several biases that require the results to be verified in an upfront randomized trial, hopefully in a more narrow population as "selected" by the agent in the RDT. This could be a standard new drug versus placebo trial or a standard therapy ± new drug trial if other data exists that the combination is safe. Presumably, such a trial would have a definitive endpoint demonstrating patient benefit, such as survival, rather than a tumor size endpoint, which in and of itself does not define a patient benefit. The aforementioned ability of the RDT to select the population most likely to benefit and the differences in timeline, regulatory oversight, and endpoints in the RDT phase II and the definitive phase III trial suggest that performing these sequential trials does provide important value in the drug development process. The RDT design does, however, require a large number of patients and resources and thus should not be undertaken until significant data on safety, pharmacology, and appropriate scheduling is available. On the other hand, because the RDT is a phase II design, it may be more efficient to move directly to a definitive phase III trial if there is already good evidence that the agent has antitumor activity, but patient benefit has not yet been confirmed, in a specific population.

The second major issue to consider is the duration of the prerandomization phase and the related issue of how broad the initial patient population should be. If the prerandomization phase is too long, or similarly the population is too large, the total trial size will be impractically large to randomize the necessary number of patients to meet the primary endpoint. On the other hand, if the prerandomization phase is too short or similarly the population is too highly preselected to benefit from the agent of interest then the RDT becomes no different than an upfront randomization scheme. Simulation studies suggest that a randomization rate of 20% to 50%, representing a sensitive population on the order of 10% to 30%, especially if more stringent criteria for lack of progression is used, provides the greatest overall trial power.[12] Some attention should be paid to the duration of the postrandomization phase as well. As originally conceived, the primary endpoint of the RDT was the fraction of patients progression free at an arbitrary time point.[10] There, thus, has to be sufficient time allowed for the control group to progress, but not so long that it exceeds an active agent's likely total duration of activity taking into account the prerandomization treatment duration as well. An estimated 20% to 30% free of progression in the control group is an appropriate goal. A continuous time-to-progression endpoint from the randomization

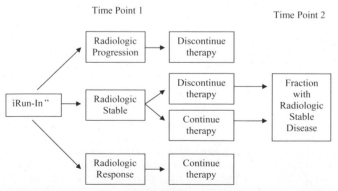

Time Point 1                                          Time Point 2

**FIGURE 1.**    General randomized discontinuation trial schema.

**TABLE 1.** Considerations in the Use of the RDT

| RDT Favored | Design Other Than RDT Favored |
| --- | --- |
| Larger number of patients available | Limited number of patients available |
| Good data on drug safety, pharmacology, and schedule available | Limited data on drug safety, pharmacology, and schedule |
| Drug with minimal to no antitumor activity after discontinuation | Drug with "carry-over effect" after discontinuation (eg, LHRH agonist) |
| Sensitive population predicted to be 10% to 30% | Sensitive population very low or very high |
| More heterogeneous population | Highly homogeneous population with highly stereotypical outcome |
| Agent expected to have "cytostatic properties" as its major mechanism of activity | "Cytotoxic agent" likely to effect RECIST measurable responses |
| Prolonged therapy with minimal to moderate toxicity | Significant cumulative toxicity |

RECIST, response evaluation criteria in solid tumors.

point could minimize some of these challenges but may inordinately increase the total trial duration. A related problem with the RDT is the potential for a drug to have a carry-over effect after treatment thus limiting the informativeness of discontinuing treatment. Depot luteinizing hormone-releasing hormone agonists, whose effect on sex hormones may be quite prolonged after administration, would for example not be appropriately studied in a RDT. A summary of patient and drug characteristics that favor utilization of the RDT as opposed to some other design is provided in Table 1.

Finally, the original description of the RDT as applied to oncology clinical trials did not use any early stopping rules, but such rules for both efficacy and futility seem to be necessary. For example if RECIST-based response rates similar to what would be considered sufficient for further agent development under classic cytotoxic agent development paradigms is observed, there is probably little reason to continue. Likewise, it is prudent to stop the trial early if the rate of randomization is lower than expected to manage the maximum size of the trial. Should that occur, and assuming the pre- and postrandomization time frames are chosen appropriately for the disease of interest, it would not be possible to determine whether the low randomization rate is due to a lower than expected population fraction sensitive to the agent or simply a agent not capable of inducing stable disease; however, it is clear that the drug development strategy needs to be markedly rethought and in this era of multiple agents likely abandoned.

## CONCLUSION

Oncology drugs have had one of the lowest success rates in phase III trials of any therapeutic area and one of the lowest rates of correlation between phase II and III results.[17] In order for phase II trials to be more informative there must be a greater focus on randomization and identification of the most sensitive subset of patients. This, by definition, requires larger trials and a greater emphasis on identification of useful agents rather than simply elimination of completely ineffective agents. In an era with limited options for oncologic therapy and even fewer agents to test, the most critical error to be made in drug development was to eliminate from further testing an agent that might have

even modest activity. This, and the fact that the available agents were all cytotoxic, led to the traditional paradigm of eliminating agents in phase II only if the objective tumor shrinkage rate was extremely low.

In the current era, there are multiple putative agents against multiple putative targets, many of which are predicted to be growth inhibitory. Paradigms for drug development must thus adapt. It will remain critical to identify single agent activity, hopefully identify the most sensitive population, and then subsequently confirm that this activity translates into true patient benefit. Given the high expense that these latter definitive phase III trials entail, and the multiple alternative agents to be tested, the expense of larger randomized phase II trials and a greater risk of excluding an agent from further development due to a false negative phase II trial seem to be low and acceptable. The randomized discontinuation trial design meets many of these criteria. It enriches the population for those most likely to benefit, rigorously identifies the growth inhibitory properties of an agent, and as an added benefit minimizes the number of patients exposed to placebo. With careful attention to pre- and postrandomization intervals, early stopping rules, and potential carry-over effects of the agent, this design should be a critical tool in the clinical trialist's armamentarium.

## REFERENCES

1. Moertel CG, Hanley JA. The effect of measuring error on the results of therapeutic trials in advanced cancer. *Cancer.* 1976;38:388–394.
2. Eisenhauer EA, Therasse P, Bogaerts J, et al. New response evaluation criteria in solid tumours: revised RECIST guideline (version 1.1). *Eur J Cancer.* 2009;45:228–247.
3. Erasmus JJ, Gladish GW, Broemeling L, et al. Interobserver and intraobserver variability in measurement of non-small-cell carcinoma lung lesions: implications for assessment of tumor response. *J Clin Oncol.* 2003;21:2574–2582.
4. Karrison TG, Maitland ML, Stadler WM, et al. Design of phase II cancer trials using a continuous endpoint of change in tumor size: application to a study of sorafenib and erlotinib in non small-cell lung cancer. *J Natl Cancer Inst.* 2007;99:1455–1461.
5. Escudier B, Eisen T, Stadler WM, et al. Sorafenib in advanced clear-cell renal-cell carcinoma. *N Engl J Med.* 2007;356:125–134.
6. Llovet JM, Ricci S, Mazzaferro V, et al. Sorafenib in advanced hepatocellular carcinoma. *N Engl J Med.* 2008;359:378–390.
7. Motzer RJ, Bacik J, Murphy BA, et al. Interferon-alfa as a comparative treatment for clinical trials of new therapies against advanced renal cell carcinoma. *J Clin Oncol.* 2002;20:289–296.
8. Schwartz LH, Mazumdar M, Wang L, et al. Response assessment classification in patients with advanced renal cell carcinoma treated on clinical trials. *Cancer.* 2003;98:1611–1619.
9. Allegra CJ, Jessup JM, Somerfield MR, et al. American Society of Clinical Oncology provisional clinical opinion: testing for KRAS gene mutations in patients with metastatic colorectal carcinoma to predict response to antiepidermal growth factor receptor monoclonal antibody therapy. *J Clin Oncol.* 2009;27:2091–2096.
10. Rosner GL, Stadler W, Ratain MJ. Randomized discontinuation design: application to cytostatic antineoplastic agents. *J Clin Oncol.* 2002;20:4478–4484.
11. Stadler WM. The randomized discontinuation trial: a phase II design to assess growth-inhibitory agents. *Mol Cancer Ther.* 2007;6:1180–1185.
12. Freidlin B, Simon R. Evaluation of randomized discontinuation design. *J Clin Oncol.* 2005;23:5094–5098.
13. Kopec JA, Abrahamowicz M, Esdaile JM. Randomized discontinuation trials: utility and efficiency. *J Clin Epidemiol.* 1993;46:959–971.
14. Galsky MD, Zaks T, Hassani H, et al. Target-specific randomized discontinuation trial design: a novel approach in molecular therapeutics. *Invest New Drugs.* In press.
15. Ratain MJ, Eisen T, Stadler WM, et al. Phase II Placebo-controlled randomized discontinuation trial of sorafenib in patients with metastatic renal cell carcinoma. *J Clin Oncol.* 2006;24:2505–2512.
16. Stadler WM, Rosner G, Small E, et al. Successful implementation of the randomized discontinuation trial design: an application to the study of the putative antiangiogenic agent carboxyaminoimidazole in renal cell carcinoma—CALGB 69901. *J Clin Oncol.* 2005;23:3726–3732.
17. Booth B, Glassman R, Ma P. Oncology's trials. *Nat Rev Drug Discov.* 2003;2:609–610.

# Other Paradigms: Health-Related Quality of Life as a Measure in Cancer Treatment

## Its Importance and Relevance

Peter C. Trask • Ming-Ann Hsu • Richard McQuellon

Health-related quality of life (HRQOL) is traditionally defined as the impact of an illness or treatment on an individual's physical, psychologic, social, and somatic functioning and general well being.[1] According to Ferrans,[2] the core element of several HRQOL definitions is an assessment by the patient of the impact that a medical condition or treatment has on some aspect of their functioning. These definitions are consistent with a conceptual model of HRQOL developed by Wilson and Cleary[3] to help explain the objective measurement of a subjective experience. Their model, which includes health outcomes such as psychologic factors, symptom status, functional health, general health perceptions, and overall QOL, has been applied to different patient populations including those with cancer.

During the past 15 years, there have been many articles that have defined HRQOL, how it can be measured, how it changes with different cancers and their treatments, and how to determine whether the change is significant.[1,4] General measures of HRQOL in cancer medicine, such as the European Organization for the Research and Treatment of Cancer (EORTC) Quality of Life Questionnaire-Core 30 (QLQ-C30) and the Functional Assessment of Cancer Therapy (FACT), have been developed that contain items that assess many of the symptoms that are experienced by individuals, regardless of the specific cancer with which they are affected. There are also tumor specific (eg, breast, colon, and lung), treatment specific (eg, bone marrow transplant, biologic response modifiers, and neurotoxicity), and symptom specific (eg, fatigue and lymphedema) subscales that can be added to these general measures.[5–7] These and other efforts have led clinicians and health care providers to conclude that consideration of the HRQOL of a patient with cancer is important when deciding whether a patient is doing well or is responding to a given treatment. Among researchers, there is a general consensus that HRQOL is also an important clinical trial end point. To illustrate, the US Food and Drug Administration (FDA) has named patient-reported outcomes (PROs) and HRQOL as an important end point for approval of new anticancer drugs.[8–10] A survey of 12 clinical trials' groups from the US, Canada, and Europe revealed that all had a major commitment to patient rated outcomes and included some type of quality of life (QOL) committee in their structure.[11] The American Society of Clinical Oncology has introduced recommended guidelines for HRQOL assessment,[12] and there is growing interest in HRQOL assessment in surgical oncology.[13,14] In addition, many of the large cooperative groups are beginning to adopt administrative structures that include HRQOL nested within their broader context. For example, the QOL subcommittee is part of the broader Cancer Control and Health Outcome committee in the Cancer and Leukemia Group B. Finally, most major cooperative groups in the US, Canada, and Europe have integrated HRQOL research into hundreds of treatment protocols.

The pharmaceutical industry has also started to include HRQOL end points, either general or specific to disease- or treatment-related symptoms into phase II to phase IV trials. To illustrate, Gondek et al reported that a search of the "clinicaltrials.gov" website using the selected terms of interest—cancer, symptom, QOL, PRO, and industry sponsored trials, produced 322 studies. In 2006, this comprised ~12% of all industry sponsored clinical trials in cancer care including phase I, I/II, II, II/III, III, IV, and pediatric studies.[15] It should be noted that the percentage of phase II/III and III studies with HRQOL end points was slightly higher (12.8% and 16.2%, respectively), and that this varied by cancer type, with roughly 1 of 5 brain, breast, and prostate studies including HRQOL end points. The authors note that HRQOL outcome measures may be underreported based on the search criteria they used. Nevertheless, HRQOL end points are not included in every cancer clinical trial, raising the question of when might HRQOL be important to the pharmaceutical industry. Some answers to this will be discussed later in the article.

Despite the recognition of the importance of measuring HRQOL in clinical trials and in conjunction with cancer treatments, there is no consistent use of HRQOL data by health care practitioners. Why? Presumably this is because providers are unsure how to use HRQOL information. The result of this discrepancy brings one back to the question of "Is HRQOL information important?" This and several related issues, including (1) the reasons to include HRQOL measurement in oncology treatments, (2) the importance of HRQOL in the absence of a clinical therapeutic benefit [ie, improved overall survival (OS), progression free survival, or overall response rate], (3) what is a meaningful difference in a HRQOL assessment, and (4) when it may not be important to measure HRQOL, are addressed in this article.

## Inclusion of HRQOL Assessment

The diagnosis of cancer, depending on the type and stage, may or may not result in immediate changes to an individual's HRQOL. It is more likely, however, that subsequent treatment for the cancer, be it surgery, radiation, chemotherapy, or biologic therapy will have an effect. Treatment that extends life while impairing QOL may be worth little to the patient. As such, one reason to assess HRQOL is to understand how an existing or novel treatment impacts an individual's functioning in the context of any improvement to survival. Similarly, if a new treatment is being compared with an existing standard of care (SOC), inclusion of a measure of HRQOL would allow for a comparison with the SOC, especially if there is existing knowledge of the impact the SOC has on HRQOL. Table 1 provides a concise summary of when HRQOL may be assessed.

Inclusion of HRQOL measures in early clinical trials (eg, phase 2) can also help in deciding whether the drug or intervention in question is worth progressing to a confirmatory full phase 3 trial. In a recent phase 2 trial in pancreatic cancer patients, results from the HRQOL assessment failed to demonstrate greater improvements in aspects of

| **TABLE 1.** Reasons to Include HRQOL Assessment | | |
|---|:---:|:---:|
| **Reason to Include HRQOL** | **In the Clinic** | **In Clinical Trials** |
| Understand how existing treatments (standard of care) impacts functioning | X | X |
| Understand how novel treatment impacts patient functioning | | X |
| Identify treatment-related symptoms that need management | X | X |
| Provide early indications of a treatments' effectiveness | X | X |
| Assist in determining whether a drug should progress from phase II to phase III | | X |
| Understand relation between HRQOL and OS/PFS | | X |
| Patient reports of symptoms frequently occur before AEs are observed | X | X |
| Patient reports and provider reports of patient symptoms are not highly correlated | X | |
| Differentiate 2 treatments with similar efficacy | X | X |
| Further complement and augment a products' efficacy and safety data | | X |

PFS, progression free survival; AE, adverse event.

HRQOL in the experimental arm than the control arm[16]; a lack of difference that was subsequently reflected in the clinical end points based on the futility analysis of the phase 3 study, thus resulting in its early termination. Inclusion of measures in a phase 2 study can also provide needed information to inform whether a HRQOL end point is important and/or to refine the measurement strategy for a phase 3 study. By having preliminary results, especially if the design of the subsequent study is the same, researchers will have a better idea of the degree of change they can expect to see with their intervention. Finally, the inclusion of HRQOL measures early in the development of a drug or intervention can help to identify what treatment-related symptoms are having a negative impact on patients, thus resulting in the creation of side effect management strategies. The optimal result is greater adherence to a medication with potentially beneficial effects on health and improvement in HRQOL. Indeed, in several studies, changes were observed on HRQOL measures before the corresponding changes were noted as adverse events.[17,18] Thus, observing a patient-reported change in a symptom such as diarrhea before a physician-reported adverse event could provide an early sign that there is a need for symptom management. Alternatively, if a symptom is a sign that a treatment is active, for example the presence of rash, patient report may provide an early indicator of effectiveness.

Another reason to include assessment of HRQOL in cancer treatments is that baseline HRQOL scores have predicted treatment outcomes including treatment benefit and OS in patients with metastatic and localized disease.[19] To illustrate, a recent article by Cella et al[20] revealed that baseline HRQOL scores predicted OS, with those having better HRQOL at baseline having a longer response to treatment. Thus, stratification by baseline HRQOL may be another approach to identifying who would respond well to a treatment and who would not.

Finally, inclusion of HRQOL measures, allows for the identification of short- and long-term sequelae of treatments, which can influence not only future communication and decision-making, but also treatment and assessment guidelines. This is particularly important as

the progress in treating many cancers has resulted in the development of chronic diseases. In pediatric oncology, successful treatments have unfortunately led to the development of neuropsychological late effects. The recognition of this has resulted in required discussion with patients about these potential effects, along with neuropsychological testing before treatment. In adult oncology, the assessment of HRQOL in women who have received mastectomies has resulted in additional information that can be provided to women when deciding upon their course of treatment, especially if that treatment is prophylactic.[21]

## Determining the Meaning of Results From HRQOL Assessment

If the decision is made to include HRQOL assessment, how does one go about interpreting the responses obtained by the patients? How does one determine whether the changes observed are meaningful to the patient? Guyatt[22] illustrates this problem with the following scenario. He analyzed a study by Mangione et al[23] on the HRQOL of lung cancer patients in which patients had been given the Medical Outcome Short Form Health Survey (SF-36), a general HRQOL measure, after 3 different surgical procedures. He noted that although the authors predicted deterioration in emotional functioning or health perceptions 1 month post operatively, this did not happen. As a result, he posited; "have the investigators discovered something we didn't know about how lung cancer patients feel after surgery, or have they discovered limitation in the SF-36's ability to measure emotional functioning?" (Ref. 24 p 720). This question exemplifies one of the problems with the SF-36, and why, when combined with its' reported psychometric instability in some cancer populations, the EORTC and FACT measures were developed specifically for assessing HRQOL in cancer populations.

Although one approach to interpreting the responses of patients would be to simply look at the mean of treatment A versus treatment B at any given point, or the change in means of one treatment at 2 timepoints, Joly et al[24] and others have argued that this strategy should be avoided, at least as it applies to palliative chemotherapy regimens, as it does not provide valuable information on the proportion of people who benefited from the treatment. A report of the statistical significance of the results from a HRQOL measure is unfortunately the approach that is usually provided. The result is a presentation of 2 means that although statistically different from each other, may not be either clinically significant or overly important from a HRQOL standpoint.

A preferred approach used by Joly et al[24] and earlier by Osoba et al,[25] would be to prespecify an improvement of a specific number of points (eg, $\geq 10$ or 15; usually one standard error of measurement or 10% of the scale) that would equate to a clinically important difference between groups or 2 time points for 1 group. Brundage et al suggested that a cut point of 10 points in improvement or deterioration could be used on a 100 point HRQOL instrument to avoid false positive responses. Given data from several sources, including patients reporting subjective differences in their status and the work of others on nonanchor-based assessment methods, this seems reasonable. Specific clinical contexts and different instruments may call for a modified cut point.[26] This suggestion, and that proposed by Joly et al[24] is consistent with what Osoba et al[25] and others[27-30] have identified as a minimally important difference (MID) that degree of change in a symptom or aspect of functioning that is recognizable and important to a patient, for other scales. Indeed, a review of the common HRQOL and symptom measures used in clinical trials with cancer patients shows that the most frequently used measures, the EORTC QLQ-C30 and the FACIT FACT, have specified MIDs.

**TABLE 2.**    HRQOL and Symptom Measures With Identified MIDs

| Measure | MID |
|---|---|
| EORTC QLQ-C30[25,56] | 5–10 points for a little change; 10–20 points for moderate change |
| FACT | |
|    G[57] | 8–10 for worsening in total score; 5–6 for improvement in total score |
|    L[27] | 2–3 points for LCS; 5–7 points for TOI |
|    B[29] | 2–3 points for BCS; 5–6 points for TOI; 7–8 points for total score |
|    BRM[58] | 2 points for SWB; 2–3 points for EWB; 5–8 points for TOI; |
|    C[30] | 2–3 points for the CCS; 4–6 points for the TOI; 5–8 points for total score |
|    P[28] | 2–3 for PCS; 1–2 for the 4 PCS pain-related questions; 2–3 for FAPSI; 5–9 for TOI; 6–10 for total score |
| Profile of mood states[59] | 5.6; 1.1 per item |
| Schwartz cancer fatigue scale[59] | 5.0; 0.8 per item |
| General fatigue scale[59] | 9.7; 1.0 per item |
| EQ-5D utility and EQ-VAS[60] | 0.05 to 0.12; 7 to 12 |

LCS, lung cancer subscale; TOI, trial outcome index; BCS, breast cancer subscale; SWB, social well-being; EWB, emotional well being; CCS, colorectal cancer subscale; FAPSI, FACT Advanced Prostate Symptom Index; PCS, Prostate Cancer Subscale.

(See Table 2 for a description of some representative measures and their MIDs.) Both of these measures have used a variety of techniques to obtain the MIDs, but in general, 10% of the scale seems to be the point at which patients are able to identify a significant change in aspects of their HRQOL. This is frequently the point when a patient moves from a different descriptive category on a Likert-type scale (eg, "a little" to "somewhat").

The determination of MIDs is increasingly being discussed as a part of measurement development. Among the guidelines put forth by the FDA in their draft guidance to industry[31] was the importance of ensuring that any patient-reported measure used could define an MID as a way of interpreting clinical trial results. They summarized 4 ways to derive an MID: (1) mapping to objective measures of interest (eg, number of morphine equivalent pain medications or pulse-oximeter score), (2) mapping to other patient-obtained scores (eg, a patient global impression of change question (ie, a question that asks how they think they are doing compared with a prior time point), (3) distribution based analysis (ie, an analysis which computes effect sizes from the distribution of scores on a measure), and (4) use of an empirical rule (eg, a specified percentage of the range of possible scores); along with the subsequent issues with the approaches, and concluded that the most useful approach would be to use several methods to obtain concordance. Additional research in this area is needed, and a final guidance from the FDA would clarify, which is the preferred method of analysis for a regulatory purpose.

Despite the fact that MIDs have been identified for the common HRQOL measures, most clinical trials that include HRQOL do not report findings in terms of MIDs; whether that is the proportion of patients who obtained an MID change, if the difference between groups exceeds an MID, or the time to a change in a symptom that exceeds an MID. Exceptions to this statement include: (1) results from a randomized phase 3 study of sorafenib versus placebo in metastatic renal cell carcinoma in which change was defined a priori according to the MID of the measure (the FACT—Kidney Symptom Index), and time to deterioration was in part how long it took patients to exceed that change[32]; and (2) results from the phase 3 study of erlotinib versus placebo in nonsmall cell lung cancer in which patients were classified as improved or worsened if they exhibited a difference from baseline score greater than or equal to 10 points on the QLQ-C30 and QLQ-LC13.[33] Both of these studies were able to show that the respective treatment was different than placebo in a manner that was clinically meaningful to the patient.

## Problems With Measuring and Interpreting Meaningful Change

Despite the benefit of using an MID to establish relevance of a HRQOL change, there remain several problems with measuring and interpreting meaningful change over time that could serve as a deterrent for inclusion of HRQOL in treatment studies. These issues were identified at a ground breaking symposium convened in 2000 devoted to assessing clinical significance in measuring oncology patient QOL.[4] The 6 articles that comprise this effort provide deep insight into the many problems in measuring and understanding meaningful HRQOL change over time. Specifically, the topics include (1) Methods to explain the clinical significance of health status measures.[34] (2) Group versus individual clinical significance differences.[35] (3) Single item versus summated scores.[36] (4) Patient, clinician, and population perspectives on clinical significance of HRQOL data.[37] (5) Assessing change over time.[38] (6) Interpreting the clinical significance of HRQOL results from 2 perspectives: clinical trial and clinical practice.[39]

These articles contain rich, detailed information, and a summary of them is beyond the scope of this article. However, there are several important points that relate to meaningful change in HRQOL scores and its relationship to therapeutic response to cancer treatment. First, almost all longitudinal HRQOL research with cancer patients is plagued with nonrandom missing data. Specifically, mortality in some cancer populations is as high as 50% at 6 months after the initiation of chemotherapy.[40] When as many as 50% of patients who started a protocol are missing because of death, what conclusions can be drawn? Even with advanced analytic techniques proposed by biostatisticians trained and experienced in cancer medicine, there are severe limitations to interpreting HRQOL data over the long term.[41,42] How should group HRQOL data be interpreted when so many patients do not complete the protocol? Fortunately, the problem of missing data is not the same for all HRQOL projects. Specifically, cross-sectional surveys of patients following different treatment approaches such as mastectomy versus lumpectomy plus radiation can yield robust findings given the near completeness of data sets in this context.[43]

Second, even when data is nearly complete for a specific group of patients, the unique clinically meaningful changes that can occur within individuals could be masked by only using overall scores on a particular instrument. For example, a patient's physical well-being subscale score may deteriorate by 5 points over the initial courses of chemotherapy, whereas their emotional well being could improve by 5 points. Deterioration in 1 domain, (physical well being) relative to improvement in a second domain, (emotional well being) would cancel each other out. Thus, a patient who scored a total of 80 on the FACT at baseline and 80 at 3 months would seem to have made no changes without close examination of their individual subscale scores. The interpretation of no change would be erroneous. However, if a researcher had set overall QOL score as their primary outcome, this difference would be obscured.

Third, patient "response shift" can alter how patients rate their HRQOL over the course of disease trajectory.[44] This phenomenon refers to the fact that internal standards for rating HRQOL can change over a long course of treatment.[45] For example, a patient may say "I really did not know what fatigue was until I came to the 4th course of my chemotherapy." Although this concept has yet to be researched in depth, it makes intuitive sense to think that cancer treatments over a period of months to years will shape the patient's perspective on how they understand, experience, and rate HRQOL. The complexity of this phenomenon is seen where individual patients with obvious and significant loss of functioning may nevertheless report relatively "normal" overall QOL relative to a comparison cohort.

## Additional Challenges to Using HRQOL as a Therapeutic Response to Cancer Treatment

Despite the general agreement on the importance of measuring HRQOL when examining cancer treatments and the relevance of understanding change through the use of MIDs, there remain several challenges regarding HRQOL as a therapeutic response. These include the lack of a common instrument, interpretability, patient burden, and financial/resource and logistical barriers.

### Lack of a Common Instrument

There is not one measure of HRQOL that is accepted as the "gold standard" when assessing the effect of cancer treatments. Nevertheless, as previously noted, there are both cancer specific and generic measures that have become widely accepted over the past 20 years of HRQOL measurement (ie, EORTC-QLC-C30, FACT, and the SF-36 although the latter is being used with less frequency in advanced cancer trials).[11] The EORTC and FACT instruments, in particular, have proven validity and utility in hundreds of clinical trials.

One single instrument for measuring HRQOL would make interpretation and application simpler. Keeping track of many instruments complicates matters for clinicians who do not use these tools regularly and must contend with different scoring methods and many subscales. This can be confusing. A single instrument would likely facilitate the application of HRQOL data by nurses, physicians, and allied health care workers in the clinical setting. However, it is unlikely that there will be a single instrument developed for measuring HRQOL that is as simple as the sphygmomanometer, used for measuring blood pressure. One common measure may also eliminate the creative development of the field, and actually limit the ability to effectively assess the most important aspects of HRQOL for a specific cancer or its treatment. Given that the reliability and validity questions that were central in the early development of HRQOL measures have been managed reasonably well as evidenced by the sound psychometric properties of the aforementioned measures in a variety of treatment settings, the issue of identifying "the" gold standard is less important.

### Belief That HRQOL Data Is "Soft" and Subjective

There are still individuals who believe that HRQOL assessment is "soft" and not as rigorous as other clinical end points. Nevertheless, there has been a growing appreciation for the validity of instruments that collect HRQOL data when compared with other medical testing.[46] This appreciation stems in part from a growing familiarity with the commonly used HRQOL instruments and research comparing the various instruments to normative scores.[47] Specifically, HRQOL end points meet all general requirements for incorporation into clinical research or practice when compared with similar laboratory studies used in clinical practice. These include a uniform description of the end point, a way to calibrate and standardize the instrument, guidelines

for interpretation, and clinical pathways or practices for actions that can be taken based on the end point.

### Patient Burden

Depending on where the patient is on their trajectory of diagnosis, treatment, and survivorship, they may have more or less interest and energy to complete HRQOL questionnaires. Consistent with the premise of "first, do no harm," it is important to consider these issues when determining whether administering a HRQOL measure would constitute an undue burden to the patient. HRQOL questionnaires can vary significantly in their number of items (10–139) and page length.[48] Lengthy questionnaires may tax the abilities of patients particularly in the palliative setting. Generally, long surveys should be used for long-term survivorship patients who may have near normal functioning. For a healthy survivor, length of questionnaires may make little difference in compliance level, but for those people initiating treatment, currently in active treatment or in acute palliative care completing long surveys may be quite difficult. Our clinical experience in consenting patients to studies that have 10 page follow-up questionnaires at baseline, discharge, 3, 6, 12, and 24 months in intensive treatment settings (ie, stem cell transplantation and cytoreductive surgery and intraperitoneal hyperthermic chemotherapy) has revealed a significant number of drop outs that may be related to burden.[49,50] With questionnaires of such length, it is common for patients to begin with great interest in providing their HRQOL data to researchers only to tire of the repetition and fail to see the use of such efforts over the course of multiple administrations. Furthermore, patients may be less willing to complete HRQOL questionnaires when they believe that this data will have no impact on their own care. Further contributing to patient burden is the notion that patients may fear that their data will not be kept confidential. A solution to the issue of burden would be to limit the length or number of questionnaires or to target questions based on issues of greatest salience to the patient in either that or a previous assessment. The National Institutes of Health Patient-Reported Outcomes Measurement Information System roadmap may hold great potential to such an approach.[50-52]

### Financial/Resource and Logistical Barriers

The cost to supply materials, human resources, and data analysis for HRQOL data is significant. The integration of HRQOL assessments in a large clinical trial could involve dozens of people at multiple clinical sites, work time of the HRQOL/outcomes committee members, biostatistical and coordinating center units, and cost. Initiation and completion of such ambitious efforts involve many players in the cooperative groups and may require a shift in group culture.[11]

There are 3 significant categories of barriers to assessing HRQOL in clinical practice.[53] First, provider inexperience. Applying HRQOL assessments requires familiarity with the instruments, something that is not generally a part of fellowship training in Hematology and Oncology. Second, methodologic barriers such as limited ability of instruments to detect meaningful clinical change for individuals or presentation of the data that is unfamiliar to practitioners. Third, feasibility and logistic barriers such as time constraints in a busy office. Who has time to score and interpret HRQOL instruments? Unless these can be overcome, the assessment of patients' HRQOL will likely not occur.

## CONCLUSION

The purpose of this article was to discuss the use of HRQOL as a therapeutic outcome in cancer and to provide some rationale for measuring HRQOL when assessing cancer treatments. In addition to that, we have addressed how to interpret HRQOL information, and what barriers might need to be managed to make the best use of HRQOL data. However, even with that, the question of "So What?" may still be asked. This question is related to meaning or interpretability and is the practical challenge for HRQOL researchers. Even if reliable and valid HRQOL data can be obtained in a timely manner, what good is it if it cannot be directly pegged to therapeutic response as defined by tumor shrinkage or stabilization? Moreover, how helpful is it to assess HRQOL if there are no services to help deal with issues that are identified through the assessment? To behavioral scientists and those mindful of a biopsychosocial model of patient care, the answer to the "so what" question seems obvious.[54] This is the question of a clinician attempting to integrate the best of empirical science with the art of medicine at the bedside. There is only one model that has been proposed to link clinical variables with HRQOL data.[55] If HRQOL instruments are so complex as to be cumbersome for the clinician, they will not be incorporated into practice. This raises the question of what might clinicians define as cumbersome. If the interest is in understanding many areas which may be affected by treatment (eg, physical and emotional functioning), a 30-item questionnaire may be required, whereas, if the desire is to gain an appreciation of change in a specific symptom, (eg, pain and distress) a single item NRS or thermometer may be all that is necessary. Psychometrically sound measures exist that satisfy both wishes.

The question of "so what" has to do with improving patient outcomes from the patient's perspective as recorded with HRQOL instruments which can then be translated into clinical practice during and after treatment. Reliable and valid HRQOL data can aid patients and clinicians with decision making prior to and during intensive chemotherapy regimens with information on what may be expected during and after treatment. This can be in the form of symptom management and tracking of patient-rated progress back to normal. If patients exceed established MIDs, this can further serve as an important "trigger" for receiving clinical interventions. Finally, as patients move from active treatment to surveillance, the assessment of HRQOL can help identify issues these survivors should address proactively, before they become bigger issues. Thus, even if HRQOL is not highly correlated with clinical variables, the wealth of information it can provide from the patient as to their condition makes its inclusion essential to modern medical care.

## REFERENCES

1. Revicki D, Osoba D, Fairclough D, et al. Recommendations on health-related quality of life research to support labeling and promotional claims in the United States. *Qual Life Res.* 2000;9:887–900.
2. Ferrans CE. Definitions and conceptual models of quality of life. In: Lipscomb J, Gotay CC, Snyder C, eds. *Outcomes Assessment in Cancer.* New York: Cambridge University Press; 2005:14–30.
3. Wilson IB, Cleary PD. Linking clinical variables with health-related quality of life: a conceptual model of patient outcomes. *JAMA.* 1995;273:59–65.
4. Sloan JA, Cella D, Frost M, et al. Assessing clinical significance in measuring oncology patient quality of life: introduction to the symposium, content overview, and definition of terms. *Mayo Clin Proc.* 2002;77:367–370.
5. Aaronson NK, et al., The European Organization for Research and Treatment of Cancer (EORTC) modular approach to quality of life assessment in oncology: an update. S. B., Editor. In: *Quality of Life and Pharmacoeconomics in Clinical Trials.* 2nd Ed. New York: Raven Press; 1996:179–189.
6. Aaronson NK, Ahmedzai S, Bergman B, et al. The European Organization for Research and Treatment of Cancer QLQ-C30: a quality-of-life instrument for use in international clinical trials in oncology. *J Natl Cancer Inst.* 1993;85:365–376.
7. Cella D. *F.A.C.I.T. Manual. Manual of the functional assessment of chronic illness therapy (FACIT) scales (version 4).* Evanston, IL: Center on Outcomes, Research and Education (CORE), Evanston Northwestern Healthcare and Northwestern University; 1997.
8. Johnson JR, Temple R. Food and Drug Administration requirements for approval of new anticancer drugs. *Cancer Treat Rep.* 1985;69:1155–1159.
9. Johnson JR, Williams G, Pazdur R. End points and United States Food and Drug Administration approval of oncology drugs. *J Clin Oncol.* 2003;21:1404–1411.
10. *Guidance for Industry Clinical Trial Endpoints for the Approval of Cancer Drugs and Biologics April 2005.* Rockville, MD: USDHHS, FDA; 2005.
11. Watkins Bruner D, Bryan CJ, Aaronson N, et al. Issues and challenges with integrating patient-reported outcomes in clinical trials supported by the National Cancer Institute sponsored clinical trials networks. *J Clin Oncol.* 2007;25: 5051–5057.
12. Outcomes of cancer treatment for technology assessment and cancer treatment guidelines. American Society of Clinical Oncology. *J Clin Oncol.* 1996;14: 671–679.
13. Blazeby JM, Avery K, Sprangers M, et al. Health-related quality of life measurement in randomized clinical trials in surgical oncology. *J Clin Oncol.* 2006;24: 3178–3186.
14. McQuellon R, Gavazzi C, Piso P, et al. Quality of life and nutritional assessment in peritoneal surface malignancy (PSM): recommendations for care. *J Surg Oncol.* 2008;98:300–305.
15. Gondek K, Sagnier PP, Gilchrist K, et al. Current status of patient-reported outcomes in industry-sponsored oncology clinical trials and product labels. *J Clin Oncol.* 2007;25:5087–5093.
16. Spano JP, Chodkiewicz C, Maurel J, et al. Efficacy of gemcitabine plus axitinib compared with gemcitabine alone in patients with advanced pancreatic cancer: an open-label randomised phase II study. *Lancet.* 2008;371:2101–2108.
17. Huschka MM, Mandrekar SJ, Schaefer PL, et al. A pooled analysis of quality of life measures and adverse events data in North Central Cancer Treatment Group lung cancer clinical trials. *Cancer.* 2007;109:787–795.
18. Morton RF, Sloan JA, Grothey A, et al. A comparison of simple single-item measures and the common toxicity criteria in detecting the onset of oxaliplatin-induced peripheral neuropathy in patients with colorectal cancer [abstract]. *J Clin Oncol.* 2005;23:8087.
19. Osoba D. The clinical value and meaning of health-related quality of life outcomes in oncology. In: Lipscomb J, Gotay CC, Snyder C, eds. *Outcomes Assessment in Cancer.* New York: Cambridge University Press; 2005:386–405.
20. Cella D, Cappelleri JC, Bushmakin A, et al. Quality of life predicts progression-free survival in patients with metastatic renal cell carcinoma treated with sunitinib versus interferon alfa. *J Oncol Pract.* 2009;5:66–70.
21. Montazeri A. Health-related quality of life in breast cancer patients: a bibliographic review of the literature from 1974 to 2007. *J Exp Clin Cancer Res.* 2008; 29:1–32.
22. Guyatt G. Insights and limitations from health-related quality-of-life research. *J Gen Intern Med.* 1997;12:720–721.
23. Mangione CM, Goldman L, Orav EJ, et al. Health-related quality of life after elective surgery: measurement of longitudinal changes. *J Gen Intern Med.* 1997;12:686–697.
24. Joly F, Vardy J, Pintilie M, et al. Quality of life and/or symptom control in randomized clinical trials for patients with advanced cancer. *Ann Oncol.* 2007;18: 1935–1942.
25. Osoba D, Rodrigues G, Myles J, et al. Interpreting the significance of changes in health-related quality of life scores. *J Clin Oncol.* 1998;16:139–144.
26. Brundage M, Osoba D, Bezjak A, et al. Lessons learned in the assessment of health-related quality of life: selected examples from the National Cancer Institute of Canada Clinical trials group. *J Clin Oncol.* 2007;25:5078–5081.
27. Cella D, Eton DT, Fairclough DL, et al. What is a clinically meaningful change on the Functional Assessment of Cancer Therapy-Lung (FACT-L) Questionnaire? Results from Eastern Cooperative Oncology Group (ECOG) Study 5592. *J Clin Epidemiol.* 2002;55:285–295.
28. Cella D, Nichol MB, Eton D, et al. Estimating clinically meaningful changes for the functional assessment of cancer therapy-prostate: results from a clinical trial of patients with metastatic hormone-refractory prostate cancer. *Value Health.* In press.
29. Eton DT, Cella D, Yost KJ, et al. A combination of distribution- and anchor-based approaches determined minimally important differences (MIDs) for four endpoints in a breast cancer scale. *J Clin Epidemiol.* 2004;57:898–910.
30. Yost KJ, Cella D, Chawla A, et al. Minimally important differences were estimated for the Functional Assessment of Cancer Therapy-Colorectal (FACT-C) instrument using a combination of distribution- and anchor-based approaches. *J Clin Epidemiol.* 2005;58:1241–1251.
31. Guidance for Industry. Patient-reported outcome measures: Use in medical product development to support labeling claims. Draft Guidance. 2006. USDHHS, FDA, Rockville, MD.
32. Bukowski R, Cella D, Gondek K, et al. Effects of sorafenib on symptoms and quality of life: results from a large randomized placebo-controlled study in renal cancer. *Am J Clin Oncol.* 2007;30:220–227.
33. Bezjak A, Tu D, Seymour L, et al. Symptom improvement in lung cancer patients treated with erlotinib: quality of life analysis of the National Cancer Institute of Canada clinical trials group study BR. 21. *J Clin Oncol.* 2006;24:3831–3837.

34. Guyatt GH, Osoba D, Wu AW, et al; the Clinical Significance Meeting Group. Methods to explain the clinical significance of health status measures. *Mayo Clin Proc.* 2002;77:371–383.

35. Cella D, Bullinger M, Scott C, et al; the Clinical Significance Consensus Meeting Group. Group vs individual approaches to understanding the clinical significance of differences or changes in quality of life. *Mayo Clin Proc.* 2002;77:384–392.

36. Sloan JA, Aaronson N, Cappelleri JC, et al; the Clinical Significance Consensus Meeting Group. Assessing the clinical significance of single items relative to summated scores. *Mayo Clin Proc.* 2002;77:479–487.

37. Frost MH, Bonomi AE, Ferrans CE, et al; the Clinical Significance Consensus Meeting Group. Patient, clinician, and population perspectives on determining the clinical significance of quality-of-life scores. *Mayo Clin Proc.* 2002;77:488–494.

38. Sprangers MAG, Moinpour CM, Moynihan TJ, et al; the Clinical Significance Consensus Meeting Group. Assessing meaningful change in quality of life over time: a users' guide for Clinicians. *Mayo Clin Proc.* 2002;77:561–571.

39. Symonds T, Berzon R, Marquis P, et al; the Clinical Significance Consensus Meeting Group. The clinical significance of quality-of-life results: practical considerations for specific audiences. *Mayo Clin Proc.* 2002;77:572–583.

40. Moore DH, Blessing JA, McQuellon RP, et al. Phase III study of cisplatin with or without paclitaxel in stage IVB, recurrent, or persistent squamous cell carcinoma of the cervix: a gynecologic oncology group study. *J Clin Oncol.* 2004;22:3113–3119.

41. Fairclough DL, Peterson HF, Cella D, et al. Comparison of several model-based methods for analysing incomplete quality of life data in cancer clinical trials. *Stat Med.* 1998;17:781–796.

42. Fairclough DL, Peterson HF, Chang V. Why are missing quality of life data a problem in clinical trials of cancer therapy? *Stat Med.* 1998;17:667–677.

43. Ganz PA, Schag AC, Lee JJ, et al. Breast conservation versus mastectomy. Is there a difference in psychological adjustment or quality of life in the year after surgery? *Cancer.* 1992;69:1729–1738.

44. Bar-On D, Lazar A, Amir M. Quantitative assessment of response shift in QOL research. *Soc Indic Res.* 2000;49:37–49.

45. Visser MR, Oort FJ, Sprangers MA. Methods to detect response shift in quality of life data: a convergent validity study. *Qual Life Res.* 2005;14:629–639.

46. Halyard MY, Frost MH, Dueck A, et al. Is the use of QOL data really any different than other medical testing? *Curr Probl Cancer.* 2006;30:261–271.

47. Brucker PS, Yost K, Cashy J, et al. General population and cancer patient norms for the Functional Assessment of Cancer Therapy-General (FACT-G). *Eval Health Prof.* 2005;28:192–211.

48. Ganz PA, Goodwin PJ. Quality of life in breast cancer-what have we learned and where do we go from here? In: Lipscomb J, Gotay CC, Snyder C, eds. *Outcomes Assessment in Cancer.* New York: Cambridge University Press; 2005:93–125.

49. McQuellon RP, Russell GB, Jesse MT, et al. Factors associated with long-term survival following stem cell transplantation (SCT) for non-Hodgkins lymphoma. *J Clin Oncol.* 2007;25:702s.

50. McQuellon RP, Russell GB, Shen P, et al. Survival and health outcomes after cytoreductive surgery with intraperitoneal hyperthermic chemotherapy for disseminated peritoneal cancer of appendiceal origin. *Ann Surg Oncol.* 2008;15:125–133.

51. Cella D, Yount S, Rothrock N, et al. The Patient-Reported Outcomes Measurement Information System (PROMIS): progress of an NIH Roadmap cooperative group during its first two years. *Med Care.* 2007;45:S3–S11.

52. Fries JF, Bruce B, Cella D. The promise of PROMIS: using item response theory to improve assessment of patient-reported outcomes. *Clin Exp Rheumatol.* 2005;23:S53–S57.

53. Davis K, Cella D. Assessing quality of life in oncology clinical practice: a review of barriers and critical success factors. *J Clin Outcomes Manage.* 2002;9:327–332.

54. Engel GL. The need for a new medical model: a challenge for biomedicine. *Science.* 1977;196:129–136.

55. Wilson IB, Cleary PD. Linking clinical variables with health-related quality of life. A conceptual model of patient outcomes. *JAMA.* 1995;273:59–65.

56. King MT. The interpretation of scores from the EORTC Quality of Life Questionnaire QLQ-C30. *Qual Life Res.* 1996;5:555–567.

57. Cella D, Hahn EA, Dineen K. Meaningful change in cancer-specific quality of life scores: differences between improvement and worsening. *Qual Life Res.* 2002;11:207–221.

58. Yost KJ, Sorensen MV, Hahn EA, et al. Using multiple anchor- and distribution-based estimates to evaluate clinically meaningful change on the Functional Assessment of Cancer Therapy-Biological Response Modifiers (FACT-BRM) instrument. *Value Health.* 2005;8:117–127.

59. Schwartz AL, Meek PM, Nail LM, et al. Measurement of fatigue. Determining minimally important clinical differences. *J Clin Epidemiol.* 2002;55:239–244.

60. Pickard AS, Neary MP, Cella D. Estimation of minimally important differences in EQ-5D utility and VAS scores in cancer. *Health Qual Life Outcomes.* 2007;5:70.

# Other Paradigms

## Growth Rate Constants and Tumor Burden Determined Using Computed Tomography Data Correlate Strongly With the Overall Survival of Patients With Renal Cell Carcinoma

Wilfred D. Stein • Hui Huang • Michael Menefee • Maureen Edgerly • Herb Kotz • Andrew Dwyer • James Yang • Susan E. Bates

In the United States, approximately 562,340 deaths due to cancer are projected for 2009, and the majority of these will succumb to chemotherapy-refractory solid tumors.[1] The advent and proliferation of targeted therapies has brought the hope that cancer survival data will improve in larger increments than observed in the past. Along with this advance, there has come the added problem of determining which therapies provide true patient benefit. The 2009 annual report by the Pharmaceutical Research and Manufacturers of America identifies 861 different agents currently in clinical development for cancer.[2] This is more than double the number of agents reported by Pharmaceutical Research and Manufacturers of America in 2001, when 402 drugs were identified.[3] With only a fraction of drugs tested in phase I ultimately achieving regulatory approval, there is an urgent need to identify better methods of selecting active agents. Herein, we present a novel paradigm for assessing the efficacy of anticancer therapy—measurement of tumor growth rate while a patient is receiving therapy. We have used data from a phase II trial of ixabepilone in renal cell cancer, a disease in which the activity of sunitinib and, in particular, sorafenib illuminated the problem of relying on traditional response measures.[4,5]

Metastatic renal cell carcinoma (mRCC) is a tumor that exemplifies our continued inability to cure solid tumors that have metastasized. Although the incidence of RCC has increased over time, no single "cytotoxic" agent or combination consistently produces responses justifying their routine use in patients with mRCC.[6–10] For the 2 decades before the approval of "targeted" therapies, interleukin-2 and interferon-alpha were the main treatments for mRCC despite their low response rates (5%–20%) and modest effects on median OS.[10–16] A shift in outcomes began with the demonstration of an effect of sorafenib (Nexavar) on mRCC, followed by reports of the effectiveness of sunitinib (Sutent) and then temsirolimus (Torisel).[17–19]

One interesting outcome of the sorafenib trial was the observation that a response rate that would traditionally be considered insignificant could be accompanied by an improvement in progression-free survival.[17] Visually, this was demonstrated in a "waterfall plot," which demonstrated the magnitude of tumor shrinkage in each patient, and included those with shrinkage that, while insufficient to qualify for a partial response, could confer clinical benefit.[5,20] This led us to ask whether an impact on tumor growth rate could be measured as an alternate efficacy end point. We used a mathematical analysis of tumor growth using kinetic parameters and in RCCs observed that radiologic tumor measurements could be fitted to an equation that incorporates both exponential growth and decay.[21,22] The equation provides both a regression (decay) rate constant that defines tumor regression and a growth rate constant that describes tumor progression. Data obtained from the National Cancer Institute's (NCI's) bevacizumab (Avastin) versus placebo randomized trial in mRCC not only confirmed an important impact of bevacizumab in reducing growth rate but also suggested that the growth rate returned at least to placebo levels after the drug was discontinued.[22] Subsequently, we noted that in prostate cancers, prostate-specific antigen (PSA) values could be fitted to the same equation.[21] These data could be mined for different biologic insights, some of which concurred with our fundamental understanding of cancer. For example, the growth rate constant correlated with survival, whereas the decay constant did not, implying that the biologic properties of tumor growth were more important for determining when a patient would die of cancer than the rate of response to therapy. Furthermore, in prostate cancer, the depth of PSA decline was mostly determined by the growth rate constant, implying that, to achieve a very low nadir, the drug must result in a profound reduction in cancer cell growth.

In this study, growth rate constants were derived from radiologic data obtained in a single-arm phase II trial of ixabepilone in renal cell cancer. Ixabepilone, a semisynthetic epothilone B analog and nontaxane microtubule stabilizing agent, exerts antiproliferative effects by binding tubulin and stabilizing microtubules, effecting mitotic arrest and impairing microtubule trafficking.[23–26] Epothilones are poor substrates for P-glycoprotein and exhibit activity in paclitaxel-resistant cell lines and paclitaxel-resistant tumor models.[23–27] Because of encouraging results and tolerable toxicity profiles in phase I studies, a phase II trial was initiated to determine the efficacy and safety of ixabepilone in patients with mRCC.[28,29] Response evaluation criteria in solid tumors (RECIST) guidelines were used as per protocol, and an overall response rate of 12.6% was observed. The growth rate constants calculated using these data again show a striking correlation with survival and suggest a new end point for clinical trial assessment.

## PATIENTS AND METHODS

### Clinical Trial and Study Design

The data for this analysis came principally from the phase II clinical trial of ixabepilone in RCC.[28,29] Limited comparisons were made with data obtained from the NCI randomized trial of bevacizumab versus placebo.[30,31] Both trials were conducted at Warren G. Magnusen Clinical Center and were approved by the Institutional Review Board, Center for Cancer Research, NCI. All patients provided written informed consent. The Cancer Therapy Evaluation Program, NCI, through Cooperative Research and Development Agreements with Bristol-Myers Squibb (Wallingford, CT) and Genentech (South San Francisco, CA) provided ixabepilone and bevacizumab, respectively. All patients had mRCC and most were treated before the approval of sorafenib (Nexavar), sunitinib (Sutent), or temsirolimus (Torisel) for the therapy for mRCC. Overall survival (OS) was calculated from the on-study date until date of death. Ixabepilone was administered at a dose of 6 mg/m$^2$ intravenously during a 1-hour infusion daily for 5 consecutive days every 3 weeks. Other details have been previously provided.[28,29]

## Response Assessment

Measurable disease in the ixabepilone trial was assessed by computed tomography using RECIST guidelines,[32] with baseline imaging within 4 weeks of enrollment and restaging after every 2 cycles. Responses were scored according to RECIST guidelines with the longest diameter of up to 5 lesions recorded and summated.

## Mathematical, Data, and Statistical Analyses

The use of first-order kinetics to derive a tumor growth rate constant, $g$, and a decay (tumor regression) constant, $d$, has been previously described[21,22] and is briefly summarized here, with more detail having been provided in the cited Refs. 21 and 22. Those sources provided an Excel spreadsheet into which radiologic measurements can be inserted; the Excel program immediately computing and reporting the appropriate growth rate constants.

### Mathematical Analysis

The regression-growth equation: We developed an equation based on the model that tumor quantity decreases exponentially (ie, as a first-order process) but that there is also independent exponential regrowth of the tumor reflected in larger tumor quantities. This equation is as follows:

$$f = \exp(-d \times t) + \exp(g \times t)^{-1} \quad (1)$$

where exp is the base of the natural logarithm, $e = 2.7182\ldots$, and $f$ is the tumor measurement at time $t$ in days, normalized to the value at day 0, the time at which treatment is commenced. The rate constant $d$ (decay/day) accounts for the exponential decrease in the sum of tumor measurements and can be considered a regression rate constant. The rate constant $g$ (growth/day) represents the exponential regrowth of the tumor during treatment. Figure 1 depicts a set of tumor measurement data through which lines were fitted on the basis of this model.

When the data showed a continuous decrease from the time of treatment, such that the parameter $g$ could not be extracted with probability $P$ of <0.05, Eq. (1) was replaced by the reduced form eliminating the growth rate constant:

$$f = \exp(-d \times t) \quad (2)$$

When tumor measurements showed a continuous increase, so that $d$ could not be extracted with a $P < 0.05$, Eq. (1) was replaced eliminating the decay constant:

$$f = \exp(g \times t) \quad (3)$$

Additional variations on Eq. (1) have been previously described.[21,22]

### Data Analysis

We attempted to fit Eq. (1) to the 75 data sets for which more than 1 data point was available. Curve fitting was performed using Sigmaplot (Systat Software). We extracted the parameters $g$ and $d$ and their associated Student's $t$ values and $P$ values. We declared significance at $P < 0.05$. When either $g$ or $d$ was not significant at this level, we used the respective reduced form of Eq. (1), namely, Eqs. (2) or (3). Data from 9 patients could not be fit to any equation at $P < 0.05$ and were not included in subsequent analyses. The ixabepilone

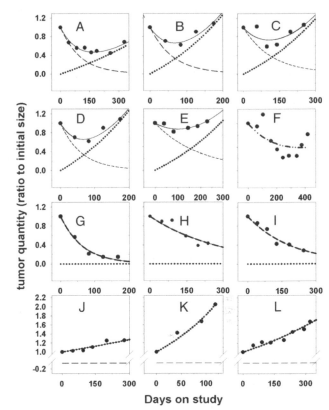

**FIGURE 1.** Plots for the regression/growth model using clinical data obtained from 12 patients treated with ixabepilone. Tumor measurements (solid circles) are fitted using Eq. (1), (2), or (3) as described in the Patients and Methods section. Measurements for patients (A) to (E) fit Eq. (1), such that rate constants for both regression and disease progression could be determined. This is displayed as concomitant regression (dashed curve) and growth (dotted curve) kinetically added together (solid line). Data obtained in patient (F) could not be fit by any equation. Measurements for patients (G) to (I) fit only the regression curve [dashed curve, Eq. (2)], whereas measurements (J) to (L) fit only the growth curve [dotted curve, Eq. (3)] without any evidence of disease regression.

data were also compared with measurements obtained from the earlier NCI trial designed to determine whether bevacizumab (Avastin) was superior to placebo in renal cell cancer.[30] In the latter trial, bidimensional measurements were obtained, and the data were recorded as the sum of the product of the perpendicular diameters. To compare the data obtained in the ixabepilone trial (longest diameter) with that of patients who received placebo in the bevacizumab trial (product of perpendicular diameters), we used the square of the largest diameter measured for the RECIST assessment in the ixabepilone trial. As noted in the Results section, this method of analyzing the data would likely overestimate the growth rate constant of tumors in the patients receiving ixabepilone.

### Statistical Analyses

Data were analyzed in Excel (Microsoft) and in Sigmaplot 9.0. Linear regressions to evaluate the relationship between the growth rate constant or other parameters and survival were implemented using the polynomial linear routine of Sigmaplot 9.0. Sample comparisons, were performed by Student's *t* test using SigmaStat 3.5 (Systat Software), with *P* set at 0.05 for significance. We wished to combine an analysis of the effect of the growth rate constant (*g*) and the initial tumor burden (ITB) on OS. To this end, we developed an autoscale, by first normalizing both sets of data by subtracting a set's median value from each data point in the set. Then, to scale the data, we divided each normalized data point by the standard deviation of the normalized data points for that set. To assess the regression of OS on the combination of *g* and ITB, we simply added, for each patient, the autoscaled normalized data value for *g* and for ITB and then regressed OS against this sum.

## RESULTS

Between February 2002 and April 2007, 81 patients with mRCC were enrolled on the ixabepilone trial. Clinical trial results are to be published separately.[29] Among the 81 patients enrolled on study, the overall response rate was 12.6%. One patient had a complete response, 9 patients experienced partial responses, and a best response of stable disease for at least 4 cycles (at least 12 weeks) per RECIST criteria was confirmed in 33 patients (37.9%).

Patients enrolled on the ixabepilone trial had extensive tumor burden at baseline. Taking the sum of the longest diameter of all measurable tumors (defined as those >1.0 cm), a median value of 21.7 cm of tumor was recorded. Taking the sum of the longest diameters of up to 5 tumors followed as part of the RECIST evaluations, a median value of 10.5 cm of tumor was recorded. The mean number of metastatic sites was 3, with lung, lymph nodes, liver, bones, and soft tissue the most common sites (a site of metastatic disease, such as "lung parenchyma," counted as 1 site, regardless of the number of nodules).

The equations described in the Patients and Methods section constitute a kinetic analysis that allows one to discern the growth rate constant when both regression and growth are occurring simultaneously. As noted under Patients and Methods section, we used the sum of the tumor diameters measured for the RECIST evaluation while patients were enrolled on study to determine the effect of ixabepilone on the kinetics of tumor growth, with an emphasis on the effect therapy had on the regression (*d*) and growth rate constants (*g*). Figure 1 depicts measurement of tumor behavior for 12 patients with mRCC treated with ixabepilone. The appropriate regression (*d*, dashed curve) and growth (*g*, dotted curve) curves, derived for each tumor, together model the measurements obtained in the clinical setting (solid line). The solid line here represents the sum of the fraction of tumor that is regressing and the fraction that is growing. Panels A to E depict data from ixabepilone-treated patients whose clinical course was characterized by tumor regression followed by subsequent regrowth and fit Eq. (1). Panel F depicts a case where neither *g* nor *d* could be extracted from the scattered data. Panels G to I depict the results obtained in patients who achieved a complete response and during the period on study had no evidence of regrowth and thus fit Eq. (2). Panels J to L depict the results obtained in patients who had no evidence of benefit from ixabepilone and whose disease progression fit Eq. (3). Two or more sets of response measurements were available in 75 patients and are individually plotted in Figure S1. The remaining 6 patients included 5 who did not have a follow-up tumor measurement and 1 patient who was still being treated at the time of study analysis.

As Figure 1 and the derivations described in the Patients and Methods section demonstrate, *g* represents the growth of the tumor that remains after the regression or disappearance of any drug sensitive cells. In both mRCC and in prostate cancer, we have previously

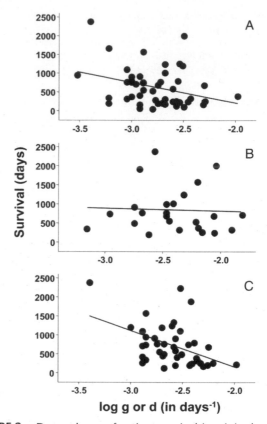

**FIGURE 2.** Dependence of patient survival (*y* axis in days) on the log of the growth and regression rate constants. All *x* axes are logarithmic scales. Growth rate constants (*g*, per day) were derived using Eq. (1) or (3), and regression rate constants (*d*, per day) were derived using Eq. (1) or Eq. (2). Panel A: log *g* calculated from the sum of linear tumor measurements (sum of RECIST measurements for all lesions assessed) is plotted against survival. The regression has *r* = 0.32; *P* = 0.023. Panel B: log *d* against survival. The regression has *r* = 0.042; *P* = 0.84. Panel C: log *g* calculated from linear tumor measurements of the fastest growing tumor (lesions) versus survival. The regression has *r* = 0.46; *P* = 0.0024.

demonstrated that *g* correlates with OS, whereas *d* does not,[21,22] and in this study, we found similar results. Figures 2A, B depict graphs plotting patient survival versus the logarithms of the rate constants *g* and *d*, respectively, for the patients treated with ixabepilone. As can be seen, survival was correlated with the logarithm of the growth rate constant (Fig. 2A, *r* = 0.32; *P* = 0.023) but not with the logarithm of the regression rate constant (Fig. 2B, *r* = 0.042; *P* = 0.84). These results confirm and extend our previous observations and lend support to our conclusion that the critical determinant in survival is the effect of therapy on the tumor growth rate constant not its effect on the regression rate constant. Figure 2C shows the correlation between the log *g* of the fastest growing lesion (among those measured for RECIST evaluation) and survival. Just as the log *g* of all measured lesions correlated with survival, so too did the log *g* of the fastest growing lesion correlate with survival (Fig. 2C, *r* = 0.46; *P* = 0.0024).

Gompertz suggested that biologic growth processes should slow with time to a plateau value, a suggestion sometimes thought

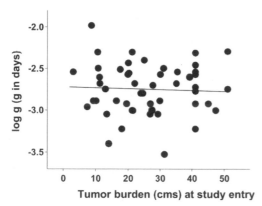

**FIGURE 3.** Lack of dependence of tumor growth rate constant (*g*) on initial tumor burden. *y* axis: log *g* as in Figure 2A; *x* axis: tumor burden as the RECIST sum of the lengths of visible tumors at time of admission (cm). The regression has $r = 0.03$; $P = 0.84$.

to be applicable also to tumor growth in vivo [A Gompertz curve or Gompertz function, named after Benjamin Gompertz, is a sigmoid function. It is a type of mathematical model for a time series, where growth is slowest at the start and end of a time period. $Y(t) = ae^{be(ct)}$, where *a* is the upper asymptote, *c* is the growth rate, *b*, *c* are negative numbers and *e* is Euler's Number ($e = 2.71828$).[33] We wondered whether this concept would, indeed, characterize the tumors in this study. Would the growth rate constant correlate inversely with the tumor burden? Would we find negative correlations between the growth rate constant and either the sum of all measurable lesions (total tumor burden) or the baseline RECIST measurement (the sum of up to 5 lesions)? In actuality, there was total independence between the growth rate constant and the quantity of tumor measured whether it was the amount followed as part of the RECIST assessment of response ($r = 0.03$; $P = 0.84$) or, as shown in Figure 3, the total tumor burden at study entry ($r = 0.047$; $P = 0.74$).

However, not surprisingly, Figure 4 shows that a strong correlation was observed between tumor burden and OS (Fig. 4A, $r = 0.49$; $P < 0.0001$). When both the tumor burden and the growth rate constant were combined mathematically, an even stronger correlation with survival was obtained (Fig. 4B, $r = 0.61$; $P < 0.0001$), indicating that, together, the amount of tumor at presentation and its growth rate constant, both values obtained from radiographic measurements, are excellent predictors of survival. We confirmed this result using multivariate analysis. Figure 4B highlights with different colored symbols the results in 14 patients who received other therapies or underwent surgical resection of residual disease after discontinuing ixabepilone. Interestingly, they represent a disproportionate fraction of the data points above the arc of 99% confidence representing patients who survived longer than predicted by the growth rate constant measured while receiving ixabepilone.

Although the ixabepilone study was a single-arm phase II trial, we had in hand data from a randomized study conducted a few years earlier at the NCI where patients enrolled on 1 arm received a placebo.[30] We decided to compare the growth rate constants of renal cell cancers on ixabepilone with that of the growth rate constants observed in renal cancers of patients randomized to bevacizumab or placebo. As noted in the Patients and Methods section, to compare the data obtained in the ixabepilone trial (the longest diameter for each tumor by RECIST) with that obtained in patients randomized

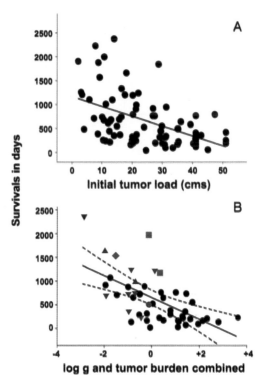

**FIGURE 4.** Dependence of survival on tumor load (panel A) and on the combination of the growth rate constant and tumor load (panel B). The *y* axis is the survival in days. In panel A, the *x* axis is the sum of the linear measurements of all visible tumors in each patient. In panel B, the *x* axis is the sum of the normalized, autoscaled tumor length and the normalized, autoscaled log *g* (see Statistical Analysis section). In both the figures, the regression has a $P < 0.0001$. In (A), the Pearson *r* is 0.49; in (B), the Pearson *r* is 0.61. Symbols relating to subsequent therapy: downward pointing red triangle (n = 7) = sorafenib (Nexavar); upward pointing blue triangle (n = 2): sunitinib (Sutent); green square (n = 2): gemcitabine (Gemzar); reddish-pink circle (n = 1): anti-CTL4; pink diamond (n = 1): surgical resection of disease; and downward pointing reddish brown triangle (n = 1): multiple therapies.

to bevacizumab or placebo in the NCI trial (product of perpendicular diameters), we used the squares of the longest diameter measured for the RECIST assessment in the ixabepilone trial. Note that the sum of the products of 2 measured diameters, as in the bevacuzimab trial, would be smaller than or, at most, equivalent to the sum of the squares of the longest diameter, as used in the ixabepilone calculation. Thus, this would likely overestimate the growth rate constant of tumors in the patients receiving ixabepilone. Figure 5 shows the individual growth (*g*) and regression rate (*d*) constants of the 66 patients treated with ixabepilone for whom *g* and/or *d* was extracted with a $P < 0.05$, depicted in dot plots. These results can be compared with the similar values obtained in the high-dose bevacizumab and placebo arms of the previous study. For patients treated with a placebo, the mean *g* value was $10^{-2.23}$/day compared with a mean value of $10^{-2.56}$ for bevacizumab and $10^{-2.53}$/day for patients treated with ixabepilone.[22] The difference in growth rate constants between the placebo and the ixabepilone treatment ($10^{-0.3}$ or approximately a 2-fold difference)

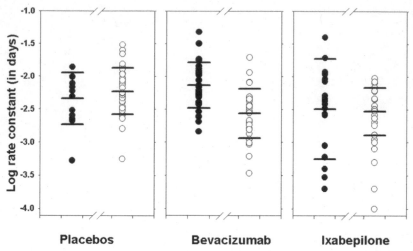

**FIGURE 5.**    Dot plots of the distribution of the best-fit regression rate constants ($d$, left side of each panel, filled circles) or growth rate constants ($g$, right side of each panel, open circles) for patients with mRCC who received placebo or bevacizumab in the randomized trial[17,25] (panels A and B, respectively) and patients on the ixabepilone study (panel C), where $g$ was calculated from the sum of the squares of the RECIST linear tumor dimensions. The horizontal lines in each set represent the mean values and standard deviations. The $y$ axis is the logarithm of the derived rate constant. Regression rate constants could be measured in a larger number of patients treated with ixabepilone compared with patients who received a placebo. The values for both $d$ and $g$ varied over at least a 50-fold range. For the patients who received placebo, the mean $g$ value was $10^{-2.23}$/day (SD $= 10^{-0.35}$) compared with mean values of $10^{-2.56}$/day for bevacizumab (SD $= 10^{-0.38}$) and $10^{-2.53}$/day (SD $= 10^{-0.37}$) for patients treated with ixabepilone. For the patients who received placebo, the mean $d$ value was $10^{-2.34}$/day (SD $= 10^{-0.39}$) compared with mean values of $10^{-2.14}$/day (SD $= 10^{-0.35}$) for patients treated with bevacizumab and $10^{-2.49}$/day (SD $= 10^{0.77}$) for patients treated with ixabepilone.

was statistically significant ($P < 0.001$). Turning to the regression ($d$, decay) rate constants for the patients on placebo, the mean $d$ value was $10^{-2.34}$/day, for patients treated with bevacizumab $10^{-2.14}$/day, compared with a mean value of $10^{-2.49}$/day for patients on ixabepilone. The regression rate constants for patients receiving therapy were not statistically significantly different from that for the placebo.

## DISCUSSION

This study using computed tomography measurements of tumors extends our previous conclusion that the growth of treatment-refractory cancer cells is responsible for the death of a patient with cancer, whereas regression of tumor ultimately has no effect on OS.[21,22] Although the former is intuitive, the latter underscores the discouraging fact that in a patient with a metastatic solid tumor, such as mRCC, where complete eradication of disease is usually not possible, the rate of tumor reduction is made irrelevant by the rate at which residual tumor regrows. Furthermore, these results again demonstrate that using data gathered while a patient is receiving therapy—and this applies here to data obtained by computed tomography—a growth rate constant can be calculated that can serve as an end point in clinical trials and as a surrogate to predict OS in patients with metastatic cancer.

The observation that the growth rate constants correlate strongly with OS concurs with our previous results where we found similar correlations.[21,22] Further supporting this conclusion was the observation that the growth rate constant derived from the fastest growing tumor from each data set was correlated with OS. Although the growth rate constant as a tool for clinical trial assessments needs independent validation, we have found a correlation with survival in every data set thus far examined, with the exception of a trial em-

ploying vaccine therapy, where the growth rate constant was obtained while the patient was actively receiving vaccine rather than later after an immune response had been established (manuscript in preparation). We have also found that the kinetic analysis is precise enough to see differences between therapies, notably, across a decade of prostate cancer studies (manuscript in preparation), such that we can also envision the growth rate constant being used as a tool for individual patients to confirm whether a new therapy has reduced the growth rate or not.

The biologic inferences that can be made from calculation of the growth rate constant are also worthy of note. The tumor that grows during therapy is the tumor that determines survival—a simple heuristic evident to clinicians but not always quantified in the RECIST-measured response rate. Furthermore, in this study, we found a strong negative correlation between the ITB and the OS (Fig. 4A). Because the growth rate constants are fully independent of the ITB (Fig. 3), we considered the possibility that there would be an additive effect of growth rate and tumor burden in predicting OS. This was, indeed, found (Fig. 4B) where the regression coefficient of 0.61 appeared as the largest of any in this study. Whether these observations would be true for all cancers or for only a subset that includes RCC, we do not know. Data sets in other diseases need to be analyzed.

The finding that tumor growth rate is of critical importance in determining outcome is consistent with other studies that have examined tumor doubling times, albeit in the absence of therapy.[34–37] It is important to note that there is a fixed ratio between any determined growth rate constant and the doubling time, a fact well known to enzyme kineticists. This value, $dt = 0.693/g$, means that the doubling time can be extrapolated from the growth rate constant. For PSA, for example, the doubling time has been very well accepted as indicative of survival and is often used in the clinical trial setting.[34-37] The value of Eq. (1) is that the growth rate constant can be determined even in the face of ongoing therapy as long as the nadir value has passed.

Our analysis also suggested that ixabepilone had a significant effect on the growth rate constant when compared with placebo. Even though the placebo group was not a concurrent cohort, we consider it valid for our comparisons for several reasons. First, neither the biology of mRCC nor its surgical management changed in the 5 years between studies (note that the majority of patients had undergone nephrectomy in both studies). Second, entry criteria in the 2 trials were similar. Further supporting the validity of this placebo group, their survival was nearly identical to that of the placebo group in the randomized sorafenib registration trial: 453 days (or 15.1 months) versus 15.9 months, respectively.[17,22] Limiting our comparison to the growth rate constants in the 2 settings, we believe that the data show ixabepilone to have a clear impact on slowing tumor growth.

Although we remarked above that a correlation between growth of treatment refractory cancer and survival is intuitive, it is not entirely clear how such a correlation would be preserved in the setting of a clinically effective agent. We would argue that the correlation of the on-study growth rate constants with survival could be explained either by the fact that a substantial portion of the remaining lifespan of these patients was spent receiving ixabepilone (median time on study 117 days) and hence what happened on study impacted OS or by the possibility that the on-study and off-study growth rate constants were related.

During the conduct of the ixabepilone trial, both sorafenib (Nexavar), and sunitinib (Sutent) became available first through clinical trials and, subsequently, by Food and Drug Administration approval. The data in Figure 4B show what happened to patients who went on to receive other therapies. In 7 of the 14 cases, the therapy did not impact their predicted survival, based on their inclusion within or below the 99% confidence intervals around the regression line. However, it is interesting that a few patients did "deviate," albeit only slightly, from the projected survival and survived longer than would have been predicted. We believe this can be attributed to the therapy administered after ixabepilone.

The analysis here again underscores the obvious to provide true clinical benefit, a therapy must either eradicate tumor in its entirety or significantly alter the growth rate of a tumor. It also demonstrates that the growth rate constant can be calculated from radiologic measurements gathered while a patient is undergoing therapy. We would emphasize here that the measurements used in these analyses were determined as the patients were being treated and were obtained by numerous radiologists—"the radiologist of the day." They were not re-measured after the study was concluded, which indicates similar valuable information could be generated in practice provided the lesion(s) that are measured are clearly identified so that sequential radiologists can measure the same lesion and transmit the values to the treating physician, who can calculate the growth rate constant. Importantly, the data suggest that tumor growth rate constants may be a valuable measure for determining the benefit of a new agent in the context of a clinical trial and may be added to the list of innovative strategies for assessment in drug development.

## REFERENCES

1. Jemal A, Siegel R, Ward E, et al. Cancer statistics, 2009. *CA Cancer J Clin.* 2009;59:225–249.
2. 2009 Report. *Medicines in Development for Cancer. Pharmaceutical Research and Manufacturers of America.* Washington, DC. Available at: http://www.phrma.org. Accessed September 15, 2009.
3. Update. *Health Affairs.* 2001;20(5):290.
4. Samlowski WE, Wong B, Vogelzang NJ. Management of renal cancer in the tyrosine kinase inhibitor era: a view from 3 years on. *BJU Int.* 2008;102:162–165.
5. Kane RC, Farrell AT, Saber H, et al. Sorafenib for the treatment of advanced renal cell carcinoma. *Clin Cancer Res.* 2006;12:7271–7278.
6. Chow WH, Devesa SS, Warren JL, et al. Rising incidence of renal cell cancer in the United States. *JAMA.* 1999;281:1628–1631.
7. Pantuck AJ, Zisman A, Belldegrun AS. The changing natural history of renal cell carcinoma. *J Urol.* 2001;166:1611–1623.
8. Nguyen MM, Gill IS, Ellison LM. The evolving presentation of renal carcinoma in the United States: trends from the surveillance, epidemiology, and end results program. *J Urol.* 2006;176:2397–2400; discussion 2400.
9. Yagoda AD, Petrylak D, Thompson S. Cytotoxic chemotherapy for advanced renal cell cancer. *Urol Clin North Am.* 1993;20:303–321.
10. Motzer RJ, Russo P. Systemic therapy for renal cell carcinoma. *J Urol.* 2000;163:408–417.
11. Rosenberg SA, Lotze MT, Muul LM, et al. A progress report on the treatment of 157 patients with advanced cancer using lymphokine-activated killer cells and interleukin-2 or high-dose interleukin-2 alone. *N Engl J Med.* 1987;316:889–897.
12. Yang JC, Topalian SL, Parkinson D, et al. Randomized comparison of high-dose and low-dose intravenous interleukin-2 for the therapy of metastatic renal cell carcinoma: an interim report. *J Clin Oncol.* 1994;12:1572–1576.
13. Fyfe G, Fisher RI, Rosenberg SA, et al. Results of treatment of 255 patients with metastatic renal cell carcinoma who received high-dose recombinant interleukin-2 therapy. *J Clin Oncol.* 1995;13:688–696.
14. Negrier S, Escudier B, Lasset C, et al. Recombinant human interleukin-2, recombinant human interferon alpha-2a, or both in metastatic renal-cell carcinoma. Groupe Français d'Immunothérapie. *N Engl J Med.* 1998;338:1272–1278.
15. Motzer RJ, Murphy BA, Bacik J, et al. Phase III trial of interferon alpha-2a with or without 13-cis-retinoic acid for patients with advanced renal cell carcinoma. *J Clin Oncol.* 2000;18:2972–2980.
16. McDermott DF, Regan MM, Clark JI, et al. Randomized phase III trial of high-dose interleukin-2 versus subcutaneous interleukin-2 and interferon in patients with metastatic renal cell carcinoma. *J Clin Oncol.* 2005;23:133–141.
17. Escudier B, Eisen T, Stadler WM, et al.; TARGET Study Group. Sorafenib in advanced clear-cell renal-cell carcinoma. *N Engl J Med.* 2007;356:125–134.
18. Motzer RJ, Hutson TE, Tomczak P, et al. Sunitinib versus interferon alfa in metastatic renal-cell carcinoma. *N Engl J Med.* 2007;356:115–124.
19. Hudes G, Carducci M, Tomczak P, et al.; Global ARCC Trial. Temsirolimus, interferon alfa, or both for advanced renal-cell carcinoma. *N Engl J Med.* 2007;356:2271–2281.
20. Ratain MJ, Eisen T, Stadler WM, et al. Phase II placebo-controlled randomized discontinuation trial of sorafenib in patients with metastatic renal cell carcinoma. *J Clin Oncol.* 2006;2505–2512.
21. Stein WD, Figg WD, Dahut W, et al. Tumor growth rates derived from data for patients in a clinical trial correlate strongly with patient survival: a novel strategy for evaluation of clinical trial data. *Oncologist.* 2008;10:1046–1054.
22. Stein WD, Yang J, Bates SE, et al. Bevacizumab reduces the growth rate constants of renal carcinomas: a novel algorithm suggests early discontinuation of bevacizumab resulted in a lack of survival advantage. *Oncologist.* 2008;10:1055–1062.
23. Kowalski RJ, Giannakakou P, Hamel E. Activities of the microtubule-stabilizing agents epothilones A and B with purified tubulin and in cells resistant to paclitaxel (Taxol(R)). *J Biol Chem.* 1997;272:2534–2541.
24. Lee FY, Borzilleri R, Fairchild CR, et al. BMS-247550: a novel epothilone analog with a mode of action similar to paclitaxel but possessing superior antitumor efficacy. *Clin Cancer Res.* 2001;7:1429–1437.
25. Goodin S, Kane MP, Rubin EH. Epothilones: mechanism of action and biologic activity. *J Clin Oncol.* 2004;22:2015–2025.
26. Bollag DM, McQueney PA, Zhu J, et al. Epothilones, a new class of microtubule-stabilizing agents with a taxol-like mechanism of action. *Cancer Res.* 1995;55:2325–2333.
27. Chou TC, Zhang XG, Harris CR, et al. Desoxyepothilone B is curative against human tumor xenografts that are refractory to paclitaxel. *Proc Natl Acad Sci USA.* 1998;95:15798–15802.
28. Abraham J, Agrawal M, Bakke S, et al. Phase I trial and pharmacokinetic study of BMS-247550, an epothilone B analog, administered intravenously on a daily schedule for five days. *J Clin Oncol.* 2003;21:1866–1873.
29. Huang H, Menefee M, Edgerly M, et al. A phase II clinical trial of ixabepilone (Ixempra®, BMS-247550, NSC 710428), an epothilone B Analog, in patients with metastatic renal cell carcinoma. *J Clin Oncol.* 2008;26(suppl 15):5053.
30. Yang JC, Haworth L, Sherry RM, et al. A randomized trial of bevacizumab, an anti-vascular endothelial growth factor antibody, for metastatic renal cancer. *N Engl J Med.* 2003;349:427–434.

31. Yang JC. Bevacizumab for patients with metastatic renal cancer: an update. *Clin Cancer Res.* 2004;10:6367S–6370S.

32. Therasse P, Arbuck SG, Eisenhauer EA, et al. New guidelines to evaluate the response to treatment in solid tumors. European Organization for Research and Treatment of Cancer, National Cancer Institute of the United States, National Cancer Institute of Canada. *J Natl Cancer Inst.* 2000;92:205–216.

33. Laird AK. Dynamics of tumor growth. *Br J Cancer.* 1964;13:490–502.

34. Egawa S, Arai Y, Tobisu K, et al. Use of pretreatment prostate-specific antigen doubling time to predict outcome after radical prostatectomy. *Prostate Cancer Prostatic Dis.* 2000;3:269–274.

35. Stephenson AJ, Aprikian AG, Souhami L, et al. Utility of PSA doubling time in follow-up of untreated patients with localized prostate cancer. *Urology.* 2002;59:652–656.

36. Ward JF, Blute ML, Slezak J, et al. The long-term clinical impact of biochemical recurrence of prostate cancer 5 or more years after radical prostatectomy. *J Urol.* 2003;170:1872–1876.

37. D'Amico AV, Moul J, Carroll PR, et al. Prostate specific antigen doubling time as a surrogate end point for prostate cancer specific mortality following radical prostatectomy or radiation therapy. *J Urol.* 2004;172:S42–S46; discussion S46–S47.

# The Evolving Treatment Paradigm in Multiple Myeloma

Kenneth C. Anderson

Thalidomide, lenalidomide, bortezomib, and doxil represent 4 novel drugs that provide the framework for 6 FDA/EMEA new drug registrations for treatment of multiple myeloma (MM) in the past 5 years. As a direct consequence, survival of patients with MM has doubled from 3 to 4 years to 7 to 8 years, and several promising novel agents, alone and in combination, offer even greater promise. The rapid evolution of bench to bedside translational research in MM highlights the need for this up to date description of cutting-edge advances in diagnosis, prognosis, and treatment of MM. Drs. San Miguel, Mateos, and Gutierrez first discuss conventional and cutting-edge genetically based stratification of standard- versus high-risk groups. Excitingly, novel therapies can overcome features associated with adverse prognosis to conventional therapies, highlighting the need to prospectively define risk groups in the era of novel treatments using technologies including genomics and multiparameter fluorescent analysis. Drs. Nooka, Kaufman, and Lonial next describe the accepted definition of complete response (CR), which is critical for comparison of outcome of novel versus conventional treatments. This definition of CR has become more stringent with time, because use of high-dose therapies and integration of novel therapies can for the first time achieve sustained CRs in a significant fraction of patients. Novel therapies targeting the MM cell in its bone marrow microenvironment first showed efficacy for treatment of relapsed refractory MM and have now achieved unprecedented frequency and extent of response in newly diagnosed patients. Drs. Kristinsson, Landgren, and Rajkumar describe how novel therapies have transformed initial treatment options for the elderly nontransplant candidates with newly diagnosed MM. Dr. Jean-Luc Harousseau describes that how novel therapies have impacted transplantation therapy for the newly diagnosed transplant candidate with MM. For example, the fraction of patients achieving very good partial response or better after high-dose therapy and a single stem cell transplant has increased with incorporation of novel therapies, thereby decreasing the need for a second transplant. Indeed, clinical trials are now evaluating the role of high-dose therapy and stem cell transplantation in the era of novel therapies. Despite the use of novel therapies as initial treatment, patients inevitably relapse. Drs. Thomas, Richards, and Weber next describe the very promising results using next-generation novel single agents, as well as using scientifically informed combinations of novel therapies, to overcome resistance and improve patient outcome. The track record for $\alpha$ interferon and corticosteroids has not established a standard maintenance therapy in MM; however, thalidomide has already shown its efficacy after high-dose therapy, and Drs. Magarotto and Palumbo here report the promise of other novel agents to sustain response and prolong both progression-free and overall survival. Although the promise of immunotherapy of cancer has never been realized, Dr. Yi describes very exciting preclinical and early clinical results of vaccination and adoptive immunotherapy to restore host anti-MM immunity. Finally, the progress to date has been very rapid, but the future is even brighter. Drs. Cristea and Raje report how MM now represents a paradigm for the development of next generation novel therapies targeting the tumor cell in its microenvironment, which has major implications for other hematologic malignancies and solid tumors as well.

# Risk Stratification in the Era of Novel Therapies

Jesus San-Miguel • M. Victoria Mateos • Norma C. Gutierrez

Novel insights into the biology of myeloma cells have led to the identification of relevant prognosis factors and the suggestion that multiple myeloma (MM) should no longer be considered as a single entity.[1-3] Accordingly, rather as occurs in other hematological malignancies, such as acute lymphoblastic and myeloblastic leukemias, and non-Hodgkin lymphomas, treatment should be adapted with respect to the different MM subtypes.[2,3] This concept, together with the recent discovery of new drugs with novel mechanisms of action,[4] seems likely to lead to the design of individualized treatment based on each patients' particular characteristics.[3]

In the first part of this article, we review the most relevant prognostic factors that may contribute to the definition of risk categories; in the second, we discuss whether novel drugs can overcome the adverse prognosis of high-risk patients.

## Prognostic Factors for Risk Stratification

Although most novel prognostic factors, which are discussed here, reflect the intrinsic characteristics of the malignant clone, it is important to mention that there are also relevant host-related factors that have a marked influence on disease outcome. These latter factors are mainly linked to age, performance status, and disease complications such as renal insufficiency. In fact, age is a parameter that already discriminates between transplant and nontransplant candidates ($\leq$ or >65–70 years, respectively). Moreover, although recent reports suggest that novel agents may overcome the adverse prognosis of advanced age, this would apply mainly to patients aged between 65 and 75 years,[5-8] whereas above this age survival continues to be short. A poor performance score is usually due to comorbidities or disease complications, which hamper the use of full treatment doses, and this finally translates into a reduced response rate and short survival. The most significant disease complication influencing survival is probably renal insufficiency, whereas the impacts of anemia, thrombocytopenia, and bone disease are less clear.[9,10]

Other prognostic factors are associated with tumor burden and disease activity. The Durie and Salmon classification was the first attempt to measure tumor burden while also considering renal function, and it remained the most widely accepted staging system for >30 years. Prognostic discrimination between stages I and III was clear, but the presence or absence of renal impairment had more prognostic weight in intermediate- and high-risk patients. This classification has been replaced by the international staging system (ISS), which is derived from a multivariate analysis of >11,000 patients and identifies B2 microglobulin and albumin as the most relevant independent prognostic factors.[11] An important advantage of the ISS system is that it is based on 2 easily reproducible parameters. B2 microglobulin increases as a result of both rising tumor burden and renal function deterioration, whereas low levels of albumin may reflect effects on the liver by the production of interleukin-6 by the

microenvironment of myeloma cells.[11] The ISS is able to discriminate 3 risk categories: low (B2 microglobulin <3.5 mg/dL and albumin $\geq$3.5 mg/dL), intermediate (B2 microglobulin 3.5–5.5 mg/dL or albumin <3.5 mg/dL), and high risk (B2 microglobulin $\geq$5.5 mg/dL) with median survivals of 62, 44, and 29 months, respectively.[11] The prognostic value of the ISS has been reproduced across trials and with different treatment approaches. Nevertheless, it should be noted that other important prognostic factors, such as cytogenetic abnormalities, were not included in the system because they were only available for a minority of patients.

## Genetic Prognostic Factors

Cytogenetics has become one of the most important prognostic factors of MM, as is the case with other hematological malignancies. Cytogenetic evaluation is now mandatory in all patients with newly diagnosed MM and should include interphase fluorescence in situ hybridization (FISH) in purified plasma cells (PCs) or in combination with immunofluorescent detection of light-chain–restricted PCs (cIg-FISH). In fact, molecular cytogenetic investigations of myeloma cells have demonstrated that almost all cases of MM are cytogenetically abnormal. Nowadays, immunoglobulin heavy-chain (IGH) translocations, which are detectable in 40% to 60% of patients, are considered an early event in PC disorders with significant prognostic implications. Thus, several groups have demonstrated that t(4;14)(p16;q32) and t(14;16)(q32;q23) are associated with poor survival[12] in patients receiving induction therapy with conventional chemotherapy (vincristine, adriamycin, and dexamethasone [VAD] or vincristine, BCNU, melphalan, cyclophosphamide, and prednisone/vincristine, BCNU, adriamycin, and dexamethasone) followed by autologous stem cell transplant (ASCT). Thus, in the experience of the French group, the median survival for patients with these abnormalities is 41 months versus not achieved for patients without t(4;14)[13]; a similar finding was reported by the Spanish group.[14] In contrast, the presence of t(11;14)(q13;q32) has either a favorable or a negligible influence on the prognosis.[13,14] Monosomy 13/13q deletions (present in ~50% of cases) are associated with short survival in almost all large series of patients treated with either conventional- or high-dose therapy.[15] However, the independent prognostic influence of monosomy 13 is currently under question because its adverse prognosis can be at least partially influenced by the association with other cytogenetic aberrancies such as 14q32 translocations or p53 deletions. Thus, the French and Spanish groups have both shown that the adverse prognostic value of 13q deletion disappears in the absence of t(4;14)[13,14] (Table 1).

Other relevant adverse cytogenetic features are 17p13 deletion (p53) and gains on 1q. In all series tested, 17p13 deletions confer a very negative effect on survival and the median survival in the French and Spanish trials was only 22 and 29 months, respectively.[13,14] Regarding chromosome 1, gains and amplifications on 1q have recently been

**TABLE 1.** Cytogenetic Tests With Prognostic Value in Patients With Myeloma

| Established Tests | Investigational Tests |
|---|---|
| FISH analysis | FISH analysis |
|   t(4;14) (p16;q32) |   1q amplifications |
|   t(14;16) (q32;q23) |   1p deletions |
|   17p13 |   Loss of 12q |
| |   Gains of Chr5 |
| |   Hyperdiploidy |
| Cytogenetic analysis | Gene expression profiling |
|   13q | |
|   Hypodiploidy | |
|   Complex karyotype | |

Another relevant test: proliferative activity of PC (PCLI on S-phase >3%).

proposed as major prognostic factors for MM.[16] However, some groups have failed to confirm this observation.[13,15] In addition, the presence of complex as well as hypodiploid karyotypes is also associated with short survival.[10,12,15] In fact, MM is divided into 2 main categories according to ploidy status: hyperdiploid MM (with a low prevalence of IGH translocations) and nonhyperdiploid MM encompassing hypodiploid, pseudodiploid and near-tetraploid MM (highly enriched in IGH translocations)[14] (Table 1). Recently, the French group has shown that the favorable prognostic impact of hyperdiploid MM is largely related to the gain of chromosome 5.[17]

Transformation of a normal into a malignant PC involves a multistep process in which genetic changes are sequentially accumulated.[15] Oncogenic events associated with disease progression include several genetic changes such as translocations, mutations, deletions, and epigenetic abnormalities. Some of these genetic abnormalities have an impact on the aggressiveness and prognosis of the disease. *P53* mutations and deletions are associated with progressive disease and relapse, and similarly, patients who display *K-RAS* mutations have significantly shorter survival compared with those who do not. The issue is less clear for *p16* methylation. Although some

original studies had suggested a negative association with prognosis, recent findings from large datasets suggest that *p16* methylation is prognostically neutral.[18]

## Gene Expression Profiling

Gene expression profiling (GEP) analysis of MM has confirmed the huge genetic diversity of this tumor. A genetic classification based on 7 groups has been proposed from a consideration of all this information. Each group displays a specific genetic signature, some of which are associated with a particular *IGH* translocation or ploidy status and with a characteristic clinical behavior. Table 2 summarizes this classification, which links genetic abnormalities, cell transcriptome, and clinical features of patients.[19] More recently, 2 gene expression models of high-risk myeloma (the Arkansas signature, based on 17 genes, and the French signature, which includes 15 genes) have been developed using 2 different array platforms.[20,21]

Furthermore, GEP has enabled the identification of some other genes that are potentially involved in the pathogenesis and clinical behavior of MM, such as *ZHX2* and *RCBTB2* (*CHC1L*) and *RAN*. In a recent article, we were able to confirm that *ZHX2* is weakly expressed in high-risk/proliferative forms of MM and correlates with poor response and short survival after high-dose therapy. In contrast, *RCBTB2* and *RAN* expression seems not to be as important in the prognosis of MM.[22]

## MicroRNAs

The prognostic importance of microRNA expression profiling has been demonstrated for several hematological malignancies. Recent studies have shown that microRNAs are also involved in myeloma pathogenesis[23,24] and that their expression profile in MM is associated with genetic abnormalities.[25] Their prognostic influence in MM remains to be shown.

## Dysregulation of Cyclin D Genes as a Potential Unifying Event in the Pathogenesis of MM

There seems to be no common genetic mechanism to explain MM pathogenesis. However, we may speculate that although *IGH* Tx induce up-regulation of different oncogenes, it is possible that all *IGH*

**TABLE 2.** Molecular Classification of Multiple Myeloma[19]

| Group | Specific Translocation | Percentage Prevalence | Cyclin D Expression | Genetic Signature | Prognosis | Other Characteristics |
|---|---|---|---|---|---|---|
| PR | — | 12 | CCND2 | ↑ *CCNB1, CCNB2, MCM2, BUB1*<br>↑ *MAGEA6, MAGEA3, GAGE1* | Unfavorable | Normal karyotypes |
| LB | — | 11 | CCND2 | ↑ *EDN1, IL6R*<br>↓ *DKK1, FRZB* | Favorable | Fewer bone lesions |
| MS | t(4;14): *FGFR3/MMSET* | 18 | CCND2 | ↑ *FGFR3, MMSET, PBX1 PAX5* | Unfavorable | |
| HY | — | 26 | CCND1 | ↑ *TRAIL, DKK1, FRZB*<br>↓ *CKS1B* | Favorable | Hyperdiploid karyoty<br>Bone lesions |
| CD-1 | t(11;14): *CCND1* or<br>t(6;14): *CCND3* | 8 | CCND1<br>CCND3 | ↑ *CEBPB, NID2, SET7* | Favorable | |
| CD-2 | t(11;14): *CCND1* or<br>t(6;14): *CCND3* | 17 | CCND1<br>CCND3 | ↑ *CD20, PAX5, CD27,*<br>*CXCR4* | Favorable | |
| MF | t(14;16): *c-MAF*<br>or t(14;20): *MAFB* | 8 | CCND2 | ↑ *c-MAF, MAFB, CXCR1,*<br>*ITGB7*<br>↓ *DKK1* | Unfavorable | Fewer bone lesions |

Modified from *Blood*. 2006;108:2020–2028.
PR indicates proliferation; LB, low bone disease; MS, MMSET; HY, hyperdiploid; CD-1, *CCND1/CCND3*; CD-2, *CCND1/CCND3*; MF, *MAF/MAFB*.

Tx involved in MM converge on a common pathway, resulting in the blocking of differentiation and an increase of cell survival and proliferation. Thus, GEP analysis has demonstrated that expression of *CCND1*, *CCND2*, and *CCND3* is increased in almost all patients with MM, giving rise to the recent hypothesis that there is a potential unifying event in MM pathogenesis.[26] Approximately 25% of cases with MM display overexpression of one of these cyclins that may be triggered by the direct effect of individual *IGH* Tx, such as t(11;14) and t(6;14) that directly dysregulate *CCND1* and *CCND3*, respectively, or by an indirect effect of individual *IGH* Tx involving *MAF* genes (*MAF*, 16q23 and *MAFB*, 20q23), which encodes a transcription factor that targets cyclin D2. Nearly 40% of MMs express higher levels of cyclin D1 through the biallelic dysregulation of *CCND1* and have no apparent t(11;14); most other MMs, including those with a t(4;14), have a lower level of expression of cyclin D2. The expression level of cyclin D has also been incorporated in the aforementioned molecular classification (Table 2).[26]

## Other Biologic Prognostic Factors

### DNA Ploidy Studies and Proliferative Activity of PCs

As mentioned earlier, hyperdiploidy is usually associated with a more favorable outcome, whereas hypodiploidy is associated with a poor response to treatment and short survival,[27–29] which is consistent with the high incidence of hypodiploid cases reported in PC leukemia.[28,30] In our experience, DNA hyperdiploidy is readily detected by flow cytometry and these patients with MM show a significantly better outcome than nonhyperdiploid cases.[31,32] The chromosome count of MMs with hypodiploidy is not very different from diploid cases, and therefore detection of hypodiploidy using flow cytometry is difficult.[33] Interestingly, using both standard karyotype analysis and comparative genomic hybridization, we have shown that several monosomies have important negative prognostic implications, and thus consistent with the clinical observation of the poor outcome of hypodiploid MM.[27,34]

The myeloma cell mass is the result of an imbalance between tumor cell proliferation and apoptosis. In most hematological malignancies, a high cell proliferation rate was associated with short survival. This led to the early introduction of proliferation assays as prognostic tools for MM. The growth rate can be measured using the PC labeling index (PCLI), a slide-based assay based on bromodeoxyuridine staining, capable of estimating the number of cells undergoing DNA replication.[35] The alternative is the use of propidium iodide staining for PC, and its subsequent analysis by flow cytometry, which enables discrimination of the PC distribution throughout all cell cycle phases and the enumeration of S-phase PC.[32,36] Both methods show a strong correlation between a high proliferation rate (>3%) and short survival.[32,37]

Recently, the availability of GEP has enabled the use of a new concept for PCLI because the proliferative activity of PC can be estimated using the normalized value of 11 genes associated with proliferation (*TOP2A*, *BIRC5*, *CCNB2*, *NEK2*, *ANAPC7*, *STK6*, *BUB1*, *CDC2*, *C10orf3*, *ASPM* and *CDCA1*).[19,26] This system has been validated by comparing PC from healthy donors, patients with MM, and MM cells lines, but no survival analysis has so far been undertaken.

### Antigen Expression

Discrepant results have been reported regarding the prognostic implications of the antigenic profile of PC.[38–40] These may be due to inappropriate study designs, based on small series of not uniformly treated patients, or to technical pitfalls, such as the use of single versus multiparametric labeling, differences in the clones of monoclonal antibodies and fluorochromes, criteria used to define positivity, and analytical strategy adopted.

In our experience, the most relevant antigens associated with disease outcome are CD19, CD28, and CD117. The expression of the first 2 is associated with adverse prognosis, whereas acquisition of CD117 is associated with a favorable outcome.[41] However, none of these antigens retained independent prognostic influence in multivariate analysis when cytogenetic characteristics were included in the model, because of the association of these surface proteins with t(4;14) deletion 17p and nonhyperdiploidy.[41]

### Response to Initial Therapy as a Prognostic Factor

In most hematological malignancies, response to front-line therapy is an important, if not the most important, prognostic factor. This is not so clearly the case for MM, probably because, until the introduction of high-dose chemotherapy, complete remission was extremely rare and the only available comparison was between responding (patients achieving partial or minor responses) and nonresponding patients, wherein the former category had the better outcome.

There is now a large body of evidence showing an association between optimal response to ASCT therapy and prolonged progression-free survival and overall survival (OS) in patients with MM.[42,43] This association is not as well established for elderly patients mainly because, in the era of melphalan–prednisone (MP), few patients achieved complete response (CR). Nevertheless, recent data from studies of novel agents such as bortezomib and lenalidomide also show that elderly patients achieving CR enjoy longer survival.[44,45] Despite this, the current definition of CR in MM is far from optimal because it is solely based on the disappearance of the monoclonal component by immunofixation and the presence of <5% PCs in bone marrow (BM); the incorporation of new criteria such as the normal free light chain ratio and the absence of clonal PCs, as revealed by immunohistochemistry (stringent CR), although representing a step forward, has not greatly improved on its low sensitivity.[46] To improve the assessment of treatment efficacy at the BM level, more sensitive tools are currently been investigated. These include multiparametric flow cytometry and real-time quantitative polymerase chain reaction, which may help define immunophenotypic and molecular remission, respectively.[47,48] In addition, imaging techniques, such as magnetic resonance imaging and positron emission tomography-computed tomography are worth investigating to detect residual disease outside the BM and to define CR in MM more accurately.

Despite these observations about the value of CR and how its assessment might be improved, it should be noted that within an apparently uniform diagnosis of myeloma, together with a large group of patients who may represent two thirds of all MMs, and whose quality of response is clearly associated with survival, 3 other small subgroups can be distinguished on the basis of their response pattern: (1) rapidly responding but early relapsing. This pattern is also observed in other hematological malignancies such as non-Hodgkin lymphoma, and patients exhibiting this pattern probably harbor distinct genotypic features that would require a different treatment approach; (2) nonresponding, nonprogressive patients; and (3) those that revert to a monoclonal gammopathy of undetermined significance profile after treatment. The final goal would be the design of "risk-adapted" treatment strategies for these singular patient subgroups.[3] Thus, although rapidly responding but early relapsing patients may benefit from intensive-sequential therapy, those developing a monoclonal gammopathy of undetermined significance profile and nonresponding, nonprogressing patients should probably not be overtreated. An additional treatment endpoint is to pay more attention to the individual response obtained with each line of therapy to avoid using consolidation or maintenance approaches with drugs that had low efficacy in that particular patient during previous treatment phases.

**TABLE 3.** Mayo Stratification of Myeloma and Risk-Adapted Therapy (mSMART)[56]

| High Risk: 25% | Standard Risk*: 75% |
|---|---|
| FISH | All others, including |
|   del 17p- |   Hyperdiploidy |
|   t(4;14) |   t(11;14) |
|   t(14;16) |   t(6;14) |
| Cytogenetic del 13 | |
| Hypodiploidy | |

*Standard risk also requires B2-microglobulin <5.5 and a normal upper limit for LDH.
LDH indicates lactate dehydrogenase.

### The Definition of High-Risk Myeloma Patients

Based on the above information, the term "high-risk MM" should include those patients with at least one of the following features: deletion of 17p or t(4;14) or t(14;16), detected by FISH analysis; deletion of 13q detected by conventional cytogenetics, or hypodiploidy or complex karyotype.[13,14,34,49] In addition, patients with high proliferative activity of PC ($\geq$3%) measured by the PCLI or S-phase by flow cytometry are also high risk. Overall, these make up around a one quarter of the myeloma population, whereas the remaining will be classified as standard risk (Table 3).

Patients with primary refractory disease (less than partial response after an optimized treatment, such as induction with novel agents followed by ASCT) or early relapses (<1 year after ASCT), together with those with renal insufficiency also form a poor prognostic category and accordingly should be considered as high-risk MM.

It is important to mention that the genetic high-risk categorization is based on patients treated with conventional chemotherapy and ASCT and therefore it is of great interest to determine whether the dismal outcome so far observed in these patients can be overcome by the novel drugs.

### Can Novel Drugs Overcome the Adverse Prognosis of Genetic Features?

Tables 4–7 summarize the results obtained with novel drugs in the setting of patients with MM with cytogenetic abnormalities.

As far as thalidomide is concerned, the pivotal initial study conducted by the Arkansas group on relapse and/or refractory patients showed that those with deletion 13q have short survival.[50] In the upfront setting, an abstract of an Italian study indicates that patients with coexisting deletion 13q and t(4;14) have a lower probability of response to thalidomide plus dexamethasone than do patients without these abnormalities, although the 3-year survival was similar.[51] The Hovon investigators, using thalidomide, adriamycin, and dexamethasone as an induction therapy before ASCT, reported that patients with deletion 13q detected by FISH or conventional karyotyping had no different outcomes.[52] In patients receiving thalidomide as maintenance therapy, the IFM group[53] reported benefit for the overall population but not for patients with 13q deletion. The Multiple Myeloma Research Consortium has found more resistant relapses after thalidomide maintenance and very short survival for patients with 17p deletion.[54] Finally, using the total therapy II program, which includes thalidomide throughout all treatment phases, the Arkansas group has shown that this treatment approach mainly favors patients with abnormal cytogenetics[55] (Table 4).

The efficacy of lenalidomide in high-risk patients has been mainly explored in the relapse setting (Table 5). Thus, Reece et al,[56] studying a series of 130 relapsed/refractory patients treated with lenalidomide plus dexamethasone, reported that those with deletion (13q) or t(4,14) had a similar overall response rate (ORR), time to progression (TTP), and OS as patients without these abnormalities, whereas the presence of deletion (17p13) was associated with significantly lower ORR, TTP, and OS. In contrast to these findings, Avet-Loiseau et al[57] found that both deletions 13 and t(4;14) had a significant adverse effect on ORR, TTP, and OS in 207 relapse/refractory patients treated with the same scheme. Kapoor et al[58] evaluated the outcome after initial therapy with lenalidomide/dexamethasone in 100 newly diagnosed patients who were risk stratified not only by cytogenetic abnormalities but also by PCLI. Response rates were similar in high- and standard-risk patients but the TTP was significantly shorter in the high-risk subgroup (18.5 vs. 36.5 months), although this has not so far resulted in a significant different 3-year OS (77 vs. 86%) (Table 5).

Bortezomib single-agent induced similar response rates in relapse/refractory patients with or without deletion 13, but survival information was not available[59,60] (Table 6). In newly diagnosed patients with either deletion 13q (204 cases) or t(4;14) with or without deletion 17p (69 cases), the efficacy of bortezomib plus dexamethasone versus VAD, as induction regimens before ASCT, were compared; in both scenarios, the response rates were significantly higher with the bortezomib plus dexamethasone scheme ($\geq$very good partial response: 47/40% vs. 15/17%). No data are so far available for TTP.[61] The Italian group[62] compared bortezomib plus thalidomide and dexamethasone (VTD) versus thalidomide and dexamethasone as induction

**TABLE 4.** Efficacy of Thalidomide-Based Combinations in Patients With Cytogenetic Abnormalities

| Regimen (and Cytogenetic Change) | Overall Response Rate (%) Cytogenetic Abnormalities | | PFS/TTP/OS Cytogenetic Abnormalities | | Reference |
|---|---|---|---|---|---|
| | Yes | No | Yes | No | |
| Thal-Dex (front line) del[13], t(4;14) | $\geq$VGPR: 12% | 41% | Nonsignificant impact on 3-yr OS | | 51 |
| Thal monotherapy (maintenance) del[17p] | Worse PFS and OS for patients with del[17p] (HR: 4.55, $P = 0.02$) | | | | 54 |
| Thal monotherapy (maintenance) Cytogenetic abnormalities | NA | | 5-yr OS: 46% | 34% | 55 |

Shorter OS for rel/ref patients with del[13] receiving Thal monotherapy.[50]
No prognostic effect in ORR and OS for newly diagnosed patients with del[13] receiving Thal-Adriamycine-Dex.[52]
Shorter OS for newly diagnosed patients with del[13] receiving Thal as maintenance therapy.[53]
PFS indicates progression-free survival; NA, not available; and VGPR, very good partial response.

**TABLE 5.** Efficacy of Lenalidomide-Based Combinations in Patients With Cytogenetic Abnormalities

| Regimen (and Cytogenetic Change) | Overall Response Rate (%) Cytogenetic Abnormalities | | PFS/TTP/OS Cytogenetic Abnormalities | | Reference |
|---|---|---|---|---|---|
| | Yes | No | Yes | No | |
| Len + Dex (rel/ref) | | | | | 56 |
| del[13] | 76 | | | | |
| t(4;14) | 78 | ORR for all patients: 83 | TTP and OS significantly worse with del[17] | | |
| del[17] | 58 | | | | |
| Len + Dex (rel/ref) | | | | | 57 |
| Del[13] | 43 | 71 | PFS/OS: 5 mo/10 mo | 12 mo/17 mo | |
| t(4;14) | 39 | 62 | PFS/OS: 5 mo/9 mo | 11 mo/15 mo | |
| Len + Dex (front line) | 81 | 89 | TTP: 18.5 mo | 36.5 mo | 59 |
| High risk* | | | 3 yr-OS: 77% | 86% | |

PFS indicates progression-free survival.
*High-risk hypodiploidy, del [13] by metaphase crytogenetics, del [17], IGH translocations [t(4;14) or t(14;16)] or PCLJ ≥ 3%.

**TABLE 6.** Efficacy of Bortezomib-Based Combinations in Patients With Cytogenetic Abnormalities

| Regimen (and Cytogenetic Change) | Overall Response Rate (%) Cytogenetic Abnormalities | | PFS/TTP/OS Cytogenetic Abnormalities | | Reference |
|---|---|---|---|---|---|
| | Yes | No | Yes | No | |
| Bz monotherapy (rel/ref) | | | | | |
| (del[13] by FISH) | 45 | 55 | DOR: 12.3 mo | 9.2 mo | 60 |
| Alternate Bz and Dex (front line) | | | | | |
| (del[13], t(4;14), t(14;16), by FISH) | 93 | 75 | NA | | 63 |
| Bz + Dex (front line) | | | | | |
| (del[13] by FISH) t(4;14), del[17p] | 54.5 | 41 | NA | | 61 |
| VMP front line (VISTA trial) | | | TTP: 19 mo | 23 mo | |
| t(4;14), t(14;16), del[17p] by FISH | 81 | 82 | OS: NR | NR | 8 |

NA indicates not available; DOR, duration of response.

**TABLE 7.** Efficacy of Bortezomib-IMiD-Based Combinations in Patients With Cytogenetic Abnormalities

| Regimen (and Cytogenetic Change) | Overall Response Rate (%) Cytogenetic Abnormalities | | PFS/TTP/OS Cytogenetic Abnormalities | | Reference |
|---|---|---|---|---|---|
| | Yes | No | Yes | No | |
| Bz + Thal + Dex (front line) | | | | | 62 |
| del[3q] by FISH | 71 (≥VGPR) | 48 | NA | | |
| t(4;14) | 79 (≥VGPR) | 55 | | | |
| del[17p]* | 27 (CR/nCR) | — | | | |
| Bz + Thal + Dex (front line) | | | | | 63 |
| t(4;14), t(14;16), del[17p] by FISH* | 79 | 80 | NA | | |
| Bz + Len + Dex (rel/ref) | | | | | 64 |
| Abnormal cytogenetic† | 73 | 63 | NA | | |
| Bz + Len + Dex (front line) | | | | | 65 |
| del[13] | 86 | 100 | NA | | |
| T(4;14)* | 100 | 98 | | | |

*High risk: hypodiploidy, del[13] by metaphase cytogenetics, del[17], IGH translocations [t(4;14) or t(14;16)] or PCLI ≥ 3%.
† Abnormal cytogenetics not specified by metaphase analysis.
NA indicates not available; PFS, progression-free survival; and VGPR, very good partial response.

regimens; VTD was associated with significantly higher CR + nCR rates than with TD, in patients with deletion 13q (39 vs. 12%), t(4;14) (40 vs. 8.5%) and 17p (27 vs. 0%) (Table 7). Again, no data are currently available for TTP, and it should also be noted that the CR in patients with 17p is slightly lower than that observed in other patients (Tables 6 and 7). The Spanish myeloma group compared VTD, TD, and conventional chemotherapy (vincristine, BCNU, melphalan, cyclophosphamide, and prednisone/vincristine, BCNU, adriamycin, and dexamethasone) followed by bortezomib; in the subgroup of patients with t(4;14), t(14;16) or deletion of 17p, VTD resulted in higher response rates than with TD and chemotherapy (79 vs. 45 vs. 45%); data on TTP and OS are not yet available[63] (Table 7). In newly diagnosed elderly patients, the use of bortezomib plus MP seems to overcome the adverse prognosis of high-risk cytogenetics because comparison of high- and standard-risk cases showed a similar CR rate, TTP, and OS (Table 4), although the number of high-risk patients (26 cases) was too small to conclude statistical significance for the magnitude of difference observed.[8] The combination of bortezomib plus lenalidomide and dexamethasone (BRD) is currently being explored. Preliminary data suggest that it is highly effective and responses are independent of cytogenetics (deletion 13q and t(4;14)) and ISS stage.[64,65]

Finally, in the total therapy III program (TT3), conducted by the Arkansas group, bortezomib was added in the induction, consolidation, and maintenance (VTD instead of TD). TT3 showed a major advantage over TT2 in low-risk myelomas but only a minor improvement was achieved in high-risk patients defined by GEP. Interestingly, TT3 was associated with a unique benefit for FGFR3 myelomas.[66]

## Should We Recommend Patient Stratification According to Risk Factors?

Overall, the aforementioned current data suggest that novel agents can overcome the initial adverse prognosis of high-risk cytogenetics for deletion 13q and t(4;14) but probably not for 17p deletion, at least when using immunomodulatory drugs. Nevertheless, the number of patients analyzed is rather limited and, more important, TTP is only available in a small number of studies.

On the basis of these data, it is probably premature to mandate specific therapies on the basis of cytogenetic abnormalities. Moreover, it is possible that the more intensive therapies selected for high-risk patients may be of even greater benefit to standard-risk cases. Accordingly, at present, we discourage treatment of high-risk patients with conventional schedules, such as VAD plus ASCT or MP because it is already well known that their outcome with these treatments is very poor. In contrast, we would not discriminate between high- and standard-risk patients if it were possible to include them in a large cooperative trial in which randomized treatments, based on novel agents, are compared; in fact in this setting, we currently recommend enrolling all patients (high and standard risk) and performing a comprehensive genetic analysis up-front, so that the patients benefiting most from each treatment can subsequently be identified. If there is no such possibility, treatment approaches including 1 or 2 novel agents (particularly bortezomib) plus corticosteroids and/or 1 alkylating agent, such as BRD or BRD plus cyclophosphamide, are attractive.

Although the use of ASCT after conventional chemotherapy has proved to be of little value to high-risk patients, its efficacy should be reexamined in combination with novel agents. Regarding allogeneic transplant, the IFM group has reported no benefit to high-risk patients (13q deletion and high levels of B2 microglobulin), although the numbers were very small. Because this therapeutic approach may offer the hope of long-term disease control, it should not be excluded as an option for high-risk patients in the design of well-controlled trials.

An attractive alternative experimental possibility for patients with specific genetic lesions is to include them in pilot studies in which a targeted therapy (such as FGFR kinase inhibitors in t(4;14) or cyclin-dependent kinase inhibitors) is added to an efficient scheme such as BRD. Another option for these patients would be to add experimental drugs with a complementary mechanism of action (eg, Hsp90 or histone deacetylase inhibitors) to proteasome inhibitors and/or IMiD combinations. If CR or very good partial response is achieved, these patients could be exposed to high-dose therapy (ASCT) or to the experimental possibility of a tandem ASCT plus Allo-trx with a reduced-intensity conditioning regimen. However, we must emphasize that whichever option is chosen, the patient should be treated in the context of a well-controlled clinical trial to reach a conclusion about the efficacy of a particular therapeutic approach.

## REFERENCES

1. Hideshima T, Bergsagel PL, Kuehl WM, et al. Advances in biology of multiple myeloma: clinical applications. *Blood.* 2004;104:607–618.
2. Stewart AK, Bergsagel PL, Greipp PR, et al. A practical guide to defining high-risk myeloma for clinical trials, patient counseling and choice of therapy. *Leukemia.* 2007;21:529–534.
3. San-Miguel J, Harousseau JL, Joshua D, et al. Individualizing treatment of patients with myeloma in the era of novel agents. *J Clin Oncol.* 2008;26:2761–2766.
4. San-Miguel JF, Mateos MV, Pandiella A. Novel drugs for multiple myeloma. *Hematol J.* 2006;2:205–211.
5. Richardson PG, Sonneveld P, Schuster MW, et al; Assessment of Proteasome Inhibition for Extending Remissions (APEX) Investigators. Bortezomib or high-dose dexamethasone for relapsed multiple myeloma. *N Engl J Med.* 2005;352:2487–2498.
6. Dimopoulos M, Spencer A, Attal M, et al; Multiple Myeloma (010) Study Investigators. Lenalidomide plus dexamethasone for relapsed or refractory multiple myeloma. *N Engl J Med.* 2007;357:2123–2132.
7. Weber D, Knight R, Chen C, et al. Prolonged overall survival with lenalidomide plus dexamethasone compared with dexamethasone alone in patients with relapsed or refractory multiple myeloma (ASH Annual Meeting Abstracts). *Blood.* 2007;110:128a.
8. San Miguel JF, Schlag R, Khuageva NK, et al. Bortezomib plus melphalan and prednisone for initial treatment of multiple myeloma. *N Engl J Med.* 2008;359:906–917.
9. San Miguel JF, Garcia-Sanz R. Prognostic features of multiple myeloma. *Best Pract Res Clin Haematol.* 2005;18:569–583.
10. Fonseca R, San MJ. Prognostic factors and staging in multiple myeloma. *Hematol Oncol Clin North Am.* 2007;21:1115–1140.
11. Greipp PR, San MJ, Durie BG, et al. International staging system for multiple myeloma. *J Clin Oncol.* 2005;23:3412–3420.
12. Fonseca R, Blood E, Rue M, et al. Clinical and biologic implications of recurrent genomic aberrations in myeloma. *Blood.* 2003;101:4569–4575.
13. Avet-Loiseau H, Attal M, Moreau P, et al. Genetic abnormalities and survival in multiple myeloma: the experience of the Intergroupe Francophone du Myelome. *Blood.* 2007;109:3489–3495.
14. Gutierrez NC, Castellanos MV, Martin ML, et al. Prognostic and biological implications of genetic abnormalities in multiple myeloma undergoing autologous stem cell transplantation: t(4;14) is the most relevant adverse prognostic factor, whereas RB deletion as a unique abnormality is not associated with adverse prognosis. *Leukemia.* 2007;21:143–150.
15. Fonseca R, Barlogie B, Bataille R, et al. Genetics and cytogenetics of multiple myeloma: a workshop report. *Cancer Res.* 2004;64:1546–1558.
16. Hanamura I, Stewart JP, Huang Y, et al. Frequent gain of chromosome band 1q21 in plasma-cell dyscrasias detected by fluorescence in situ hybridization: incidence increases from MGUS to relapsed myeloma and is related to prognosis and disease progression following tandem stem-cell transplantation. *Blood.* 2006;108:1724–1732.
17. Avet-Loiseau H, Li C, Magrangeas F, et al. Prognostic significance of copy-number alterations in multiple myeloma. *J Clin Oncol.* 2009;27:4585–4590.
18. Gonzalez-Paz N, Chng WJ, McClure RF, et al. Tumor suppressor p16 methylation in multiple myeloma: biological and clinical implications. *Blood.* 2007;109:1228–1232.
19. Zhan F, Huang Y, Colla S, et al. The molecular classification of multiple myeloma. *Blood.* 2006;108:2020–2028.
20. Shaughnessy JD Jr, Zhan F, Burington BE, et al. A validated gene expression model of high-risk multiple myeloma is defined by deregulated expression of genes mapping to chromosome 1. *Blood.* 2007;109:2276–2284.

21. Decaux O, Lode L, Magrangeas F, et al. Prediction of survival in multiple myeloma based on gene expression profiles reveals cell cycle and chromosomal instability signatures in high-risk patients and hyperdiploid signatures in low-risk patients: a study of the Intergroupe Francophone du Myelome. *J Clin Oncol.* 2008;26:4798–4805.
22. Armellini A, Sarasquete ME, Garcia-Sanz R, et al. Low expression of ZHX2, but not RCBTB2 or RAN, is associated with poor outcome in multiple myeloma. *Br J Haematol.* 2008;141:212–215.
23. Pichiorri F, Suh SS, Ladetto M, et al. MicroRNAs regulate critical genes associated with multiple myeloma pathogenesis. *Proc Natl Acad Sci USA.* 2008; 105:12885–12890.
24. Roccaro AM, Sacco A, Thompson B, et al. MicroRNAs 15a and 16 regulate tumor proliferation in multiple myeloma. *Blood.* 2009;113:6669–6680.
25. Gutierrez NC, Sarasquete ME, Delgado M. MicroRNA expression profiling in multiple myeloma: correlation with genetic abnormalities. *Blood.* 2008; 112:629a.
26. Bergsagel PL, Kuehl WM, Zhan F, et al. Cyclin D dysregulation: an early and unifying pathogenic event in multiple myeloma. *Blood.* 2005;106:296–303.
27. Debes-Marun CS, Dewald GW, Bryant S. Chromosome abnormalities clustering and its implications for pathogenesis and prognosis in myeloma. *Leukemia.* 2003;17:427–436.
28. Garcia-Sanz R, Orfao A, Gonzalez M, et al. Primary plasma cell leukemia: clinical, immunophenotypic, DNA ploidy, and cytogenetic characteristics. *Blood.* 1999;93:1032–1037.
29. Morgan RJ Jr, Gonchoroff NJ, Katzmann JA, et al. Detection of hypodiploidy using multi-parameter flow cytometric analysis: a prognostic indicator in multiple myeloma. *Am J Hematol.* 1989;30:195–200.
30. Shimazaki C, Gotoh H, Ashihara E, et al. Immunophenotype and DNA content of myeloma cells in primary plasma cell leukemia. *Am J Hematol.* 1992;39: 159–162.
31. Garcia-Sanz R, Orfao A, Gonzalez M, et al. Prognostic implications of DNA aneuploidy in 156 untreated multiple myeloma patients. Castelano-Leones (Spain) Cooperative Group for the Study of Monoclonal Gammopathies. *Br J Haematol.* 1995;90:106–112.
32. San Miguel JF, Garcia-Sanz R, Gonzalez M, et al. A new staging system for multiple myeloma based on the number of S-phase plasma cells. *Blood.* 1995; 85:448–455.
33. Greipp PR, Trendle MC, Leong T, et al. Is flow cytometric DNA content hypodiploidy prognostic in multiple myeloma? *Leuk Lymphoma.* 1999;35:83–89.
34. Gutierrez NC, Garcia JL, Hernandez JM, et al. Prognostic and biologic significance of chromosomal imbalances assessed by comparative genomic hybridization in multiple myeloma. *Blood.* 2004;104:2661–2666.
35. Greipp PR, Lust JA, O'Fallon WM, et al. Plasma cell labeling index and beta 2-microglobulin predict survival independent of thymidine kinase and C-reactive protein in multiple myeloma. *Blood.* 1993;81:3382–3387.
36. San Miguel JF, Garcia-Sanz R, Gonzalez M, et al. Immunophenotype and DNA cell content in multiple myeloma. *Baillieres Clin Haematol.* 1995;8:735–759.
37. Garcia-Sanz R, Gonzalez-Fraile MI, Mateo G, et al. Proliferative activity of plasma cells is the most relevant prognostic factor in elderly multiple myeloma patients. *Int J Cancer.* 2004;112:884–889.
38. San Miguel JF, Gonzalez M, Gascon A, et al. Immunophenotypic heterogeneity of multiple myeloma: influence on the biology and clinical course of the disease. Castellano-Leones (Spain) Cooperative Group for the Study of Monoclonal Gammopathies. *Br J Haematol.* 1991;77:185–190.
39. Pellat-Deceunynck C, Barille S, Puthier D, et al. Adhesion molecules on human myeloma cells: significant changes in expression related to malignancy, tumor spreading, and immortalization. *Cancer Res.* 1995;55:3647–3653.
40. Robillard N, Jego G, Pellat-Deceunynck C, et al. CD28, a marker associated with tumoral expansion in multiple myeloma. *Clin Cancer Res.* 1998;4:1521–1526.
41. Mateo G, Montalban MA, Vidriales MB, et al. Prognostic value of immunophenotyping in multiple myeloma: a study by the PETHEMA/GEM cooperative study groups on patients uniformly treated with high-dose therapy. *J Clin Oncol.* 2008;26:2737–2744.
42. Van de Velde H, Liu X, Chen G, et al. Complete response correlates with long-term survival and progression-free survival in high-dose therapy in multiple myeloma. *Haematologica.* 2007;92:1399–1406.
43. Lahuerta JJ, Mateos MV, Martinez-Lopez J, et al. Influence of pre- and post-transplantation responses on outcome of patients with multiple myeloma: sequential improvement of response and achievement of complete response are associated with longer survival. *J Clin Oncol.* 2008;26:5775–5782.
44. Harousseau JL, Weber D, Dimopoulos M, et al. Relapsed/refractory multiple myeloma patients treated with lenalidomide/dexamethasone who achieve a complete or near complete response have longer overall survival and time to progression compared with patients achieving a partial response (ASH Annual Meeting Abstracts). *Blood.* 2007;110:1052a.
45. Harousseau JL, Palumbo A, Richardson P. Superior outcomes associated with complete response: analysis of the phase III VISTA study of bortezomib plus melphalan-prednisone versus melphalan-prednisone. *Blood.* 2008;112:2778a.
46. Durie BG, Harousseau JL, Miguel JS, et al. International uniform response criteria for multiple myeloma. *Leukemia.* 2006;20:1467–1473.
47. Paiva B, Vidriales MB, Cervero J, et al. Multiparameter flow cytometric remission is the most relevant prognostic factor for multiple myeloma patients who undergo autologous stem cell transplantation. *Blood.* 2008;112:4017–4023.
48. Sarasquete ME, Garcia-Sanz R, Gonzalez D, et al. Minimal residual disease monitoring in multiple myeloma: a comparison between allelic-specific oligonucleotide real-time quantitative polymerase chain reaction and flow cytometry. *Haematologica.* 2005;90:1365–1372.
49. Dispenzieri A, Rajkumar SV, Gertz MA, et al. Treatment of newly diagnosed multiple myeloma based on mayo stratification of myeloma and risk-adapted therapy (mSMART): consensus statement. *Mayo Clin Proc.* 2007;82:323–341.
50. Singhal S, Mehta J, Desikan R, et al. Antitumor activity of thalidomide in refractory multiple myeloma. *N Engl J Med.* 1999;341:1565–1571.
51. Cavo M, Testoni N, Terragna C, et al. Up-front thalidomide-dexamethasone (THAL) and double autologous transplantation (Double TX) for multiple myeloma: comparison with double TX without added thalidomide and prognostic implications of chromosome 13 deletion and translocation t(4;14). *Blood.* 2006;108:3081a.
52. Lokhorst H, van der Holt B, Zweegman S. Final analysis of HOVON-50 randomized phase III study on the effect of thalidomide combined with adriamycine, dexamethasone (AD) and high dose melphalan (HDM) in patients with multiple myeloma (MM). *Blood.* 2008;112:157a.
53. Attal M, Harousseau JL, Leyvraz S, et al. Maintenance therapy with thalidomide improves survival in patients with multiple myeloma. *Blood.* 2006;108: 3289–3294.
54. Morgan G, Jackson GH, Davies FE. Maintenance thalidomide may improve progression free but not overall survival; results from the myeloma IX maintenance randomisation. *Blood.* 2008;112:656a.
55. Barlogie B, Pineda-Roman M, van RF, et al. Thalidomide arm of total therapy 2 improves complete remission duration and survival in myeloma patients with metaphase cytogenetic abnormalities. *Blood.* 2008;112:3115–3121.
56. Reece D, Song KW, Fu T, et al. Influence of cytogenetics in patients with relapsed or refractory multiple myeloma treated with lenalidomide plus dexamethasone: adverse effect of deletion 17p13. *Blood.* 2009;114:522–525.
57. Avet-Loiseau H, Soulier J, Fermand J. Impact of chromosomal abnormalities del(13), T(4;14), and del(17p) and prior treatment on outcomes in patients with relapsed or refractory multiple myeloma treated with lenalidomide. *Blood.* 2008;112:3685a.
58. Kapoor P, Kumar S, Fonseca R, et al. Impact of risk stratification on outcome among patients with multiple myeloma receiving initial therapy with lenalidomide and dexamethasone. *Blood.* 2009;114:518–521.
59. Jagannath S, Richardson PG, Sonneveld P, et al. Bortezomib appears to overcome the poor prognosis conferred by chromosome 13 deletion in phase 2 and 3 trials. *Leukemia.* 2007;21:151–157.
60. Sagaster V, Ludwig H, Kaufmann H, et al. Bortezomib in relapsed multiple myeloma: response rates and duration of response are independent of a chromosome 13q-deletion. *Leukemia.* 2007;21:164–168.
61. Harousseau J, Mathiot C, Attal M. Bortezomib/dexamethasone versus VAD as induction prior to autologous stem cell transplantation (ASCT) in previously untreated multiple myeloma (MM): updated data from IFM 2005/01 trial. *J Clin Oncol.* 2008;26:8505a.
62. Cavo M, Testoni N, Terragna C. Superior rate of complete response with up-front velcade-thalidomide-dexamethasone versus thalidomide-dexamethasone in newly diagnosed multiple myeloma is not affected by adverse prognostic factors, including high-risk cytogenetic abnormalities. *Blood.* 2008;112:1662a.
63. Rosinol L, Cibeira MT, Martinez J. Thalidomide/dexamethasone (TD) vs. bortezomib (velcade®)/thalidomide/dexamethasone (VTD)) vs. VBMCP/VBAD/velcade® as induction regimens prior autologous stem cell transplantation (ASCT) in younger patients with multiple myeloma (MM): first results of a prospective phase III PETHEMA/Gem trial. *Blood.* 2008;112:654a.
64. Richardson P, Jagannath S, Jakubowiak A. Lenalidomide, bortezomib, and dexamethasone in patients with relapsed or relapsed/refractory multiple myeloma (MM): encouraging response rates and tolerability with correlation of outcome and adverse cytogenetics in a phase II study. *Blood.* 2008;112:1742a.
65. Richardson P, Lonial S, Jakubowiak A. Lenalidomide, bortezomib, and dexamethasone in patients with newly diagnosed multiple myeloma: encouraging efficacy in high risk groups with updated results of a phase I/II Study. *Blood.* 2008;112:92a.
66. Barlogie B, Anaissie E, Shaughnessy J. Ninety percent sustained complete response (CR) rate projected 4 years after onset of CR in gene expression profiling (GEP)-defined low-risk multiple myeloma (MM) treated with total therapy 3 (TT3): basis for GEP-risk-adapted TT4 and TT5. *Blood.* 2008;112:162a.

# The Importance of Complete Response in Outcomes in Myeloma

Ajay Nooka • Jonathan Kaufman • Sagar Lonial

It is clear that perhaps not all patients who achieve complete response (CR) are the same, just as not all patients with myeloma are the same with regard to disease biology and host factors that may influence the clinical benefit of any given therapy. It is also clear that CR, as currently defined, does not represent eradication of all malignant plasma cells, and thus for most patients does not represent cure. Finally, in this era of "cure versus control" where does achievement of CR fall as a therapeutic goal and can it be a uniform approach that is suitable for all patients, or only applied to selected subsets of patients? To better address the issues surrounding this controversial endpoint, it is important that we first review how CR has been measured, in which contexts it has been shown to be relevant, and where future approaches in therapy may lead with regards to targeting the optimal endpoints for patients.

## DEFINITION OF CR

The Chronic Leukemia and Myeloma Task Force first defined objective response as at least a 50% reduction in the serum paraprotein.[1] Southwest Oncology Group (SWOG) subsequently redefined objective response as either a 75% reduction of the serum paraprotein and to a value $\leq$2.5 g/100 mL or 90% reduction of Bence-Jones protein excretion and to a value $\leq$200 mg/d or both.[2] Neither the Chronic Leukemia and Myeloma Task Force nor the SWOG response criteria included a definition of CR as few therapies achieved this endpoint. The next response criteria came from the European Group for Blood and Marrow Transplantation (EBMT) where CR was defined as absence of M-protein by immunofixation (IFX) and <5% plasma cells in bone marrow.[3] The definition of CR including IFX negativity is more sensitive than routine electrophoresis but also has its reliability issues. Patients in CR by electrophoresis as well as IFX had an overall 5-year survival rate of 72%, which was significantly different from 48% for the patients who achieved IFX-positive CR.[4] Subsequently, a new endpoint was defined for patients with no detectable protein by electrophoresis, but IFX positive was defined as a "near CR" (nCR).[3] However, because of the variability in IFX as a qualitative test, its reproducibility has often been limited.[5] Subsequently, the IFM identified the category of very good partial response (VGPR) that represents a 90% or greater reduction in the serum M-protein level along with urine paraprotein of <100 mg/24 h. The VGPR criterion does not depend on the vagaries of IFX interpretation, and data from the Francophone Myeloma Intergroup (IFM) suggest that achieving a VGPR results in similar progression-free survival (PFS) and overall survival (OS) to CR.

Most recently, the uniform response criteria was described by the International Myeloma Working Group (IMWG), resulting in proposal of the new response category "stringent CR" (sCR), which requires normalization of the free light-chain ratio and the absence of clonality by immunohistochemistry or IFX.[6,7] nCR and VGPR are considered as a single entity in the revised IMWG uniform criteria.

In all likelihood, the present definition of CR represents a threshold to the limits of current detection. Use of techniques such as quantitative polymerase chain reaction (qPCR) and multiplanar flow cytometry (MFC) to detect minimal residual disease (MRD) below the limits of current detection is necessary if we seek to eradicate evidence of all disease. Molecular CR can be attained in higher proportion of patients who have achieved CR after undergoing allogeneic transplant ($\approx$50%)[8,9] compared with a smaller fraction of patients after autologous transplant (<10%). However, allogeneic transplants are associated with high risk of early mortality and morbidity; and patients continue to relapse at 4, 5, and 6 years after transplant. The use of bortezomib, thalidomide, and dexamethasone (VTD) consolidation after autologous transplant has been shown to induce molecular remission in a higher proportion of patients with myeloma.[10] Among a group of 40 patients who received autologous transplantation, 94% were noted to have a PCR-positive bone marrow posttransplant. After treatment with 4 cycles of VTD, 36% of patients converted from VGPR to CR and 12% from nCR to CR. Overall, 22% of the patients transformed from PCR positivity to PCR negativity, suggesting that combinations of newer agents may be able to induce molecular responses, whereas conventional agents failed to achieve similar responses. Seven relapses occurred on the updated analysis, all in PCR-positive patients. Another prospective analysis demonstrating the benefit of achieving lower levels of MRD detection by MFC at day 100 after autologous transplant was reported by Paiva et al.[11] Persistent plasma cells were detected by MFC in 170 of 295 (58%) patients after autologous transplant. Median PFS (71 vs. 37 months; $P < 0.001$) and OS (median not reached vs. 89 months; $P < 0.002$) were significantly longer in patients who were MRD negative versus MRD positive, using MFC as a measure of CR. With the development of standardized flow cytometric approaches and a defined specificity and sensitivity, MFC could be a potential method for monitoring and establishing even lower levels of MRD and thus better predictive value of long-term remission.[12]

## CR AND OUTCOMES AMONG NONTRANSPLANT CANDIDATES

Although much has been made of the improvement in OS among younger patients with myeloma, there has been little tangible evidence that these improvements in OS have translated to older patients.[13] In the Eastern Cooperative Oncology Group (ECOG) trial E9486, 653 patients were randomized to 1 of the 3 treatment arms—vincristine, carmustine, melphalan, cyclophosphamide, and prednisone (VBMCP); VBMCP and recombinant interferon alfa-2 (INF$\alpha$-2); or VBMCP and high-dose cyclophosphamide. Objective response was achieved in 420 of the 628 (67%) eligible patients, and

85 of the 628 (14%) achieved a CR. Among them, the patients who achieved a CR had a 61 months median OS when compared with patients with less than CR with 44 months median survival ($P < 0.0001$). This study is an important landmark, because it helps to establish that CR is critical even when transplant is not the primary therapeutic modality.[14] Five randomized studies have assessed the combination of melphalan and prednisone (MP) plus thalidomide in patients with newly diagnosed multiple myeloma. The CR + VGPR rate was significantly higher in all the studies with addition of thalidomide yet only two of the studies demonstrated an improvement in OS.[15] The reason for this discrepancy may be methodology related (different more toxic doses of thalidomide in some studies), but may also relate to the fact that the CR difference with the addition of thalidomide is not high enough to consistently demonstrate a survival benefit.

In the absence of alkylation-based therapies, few studies have compared MP-based combinations with non-MP-based treatments among older nontransplant patients. A comparison of thalidomide and dexamethasone (TD) versus dexamethasone demonstrated a significant improvement in overall response rate (ORR) using TD, which did translate into improved time to progression (TTP) and PFS[16]; but when TD was compared with MP in elderly patients,[17] while the ORR favored TD, PFS was the same and OS favored the use of MP (41.5 vs. 49.4 months). In the E4A03 trial comparing lenalidomide with low-dose dexamethasone (Rd) versus lenalidomide with high-dose dexamethasone (RD) in newly diagnosed patients, 2-year OS rates clearly favored the Rd arm, a difference most marked among older patients. The 1- and 2-year OS rates for the Rd arm does compare favorably with other trials for nontransplant eligible patients and thus should be considered a reasonable treatment option for these patients. Notably, the VGPR and CR rates for the Rd arm improved with longer duration of therapy but were still inferior to the RD arm.[18]

In the VISTA trial comparing bortezomib, melphalan, and prednisone (VMP) versus MP,[19] CR rates were 30% versus 4% by EBMT criteria, and 33% versus 4% CR and 8% versus 4% VGPR, by IMWG criteria. CR by EBMT criteria was associated with significantly longer TTP, time to next therapy, treatment-free interval, and OS versus PR further supporting the benefit of CR in a nontransplant setting. The median duration of response among patients with CR was 24 versus 12.8 months without CR suggesting that patients who achieve CR stay in remission longer, despite the CR penalty that was present in the older response criteria.[5]

In the nontransplant population, achieving a CR in elderly patients is associated with improved outcomes and this benefit is more evident with the introduction of newer agents. However, in the older patient population, additional attention must be paid to toxicities. The ECOG trial suggests that not just rapid responses, but longer duration of therapy may be equally important in the older population and should be balanced with the drive to CR. Additional studies are clearly needed, but it is clear that we should not abandon aggressive therapy in suitable patients, because clearly, there can be improvements in OS associated with achieving CR even in the older patient population.

## CR AND OUTCOMES AMONG TRANSPLANT CANDIDATES

Three prospective randomized trials comparing conventional chemotherapy and high-dose therapy (HDT) provided evidence that achieving CR correlates with improved EFS and OS (Table 1). The IFM-90 study demonstrated CR rate of 22% versus 5% and OS benefit of 12 months with HDT.[20] When the results of a second study Medical Research Council VII[21] were combined with the others, the estimated treatment effect was consistent with a significant survival

**TABLE 1.** Survival and Response Rates With HDT vs. CT

| Study (N) | Median Follow-Up (mo) | CT Regimen | CT CR (%) | CT VGPR (%) | CT PR (%) | CT mEFS (mo) | CT mOS (mo) | HDT CT + Regimen | HDT CR (%) | HDT VGPR (%) | HDT PR (%) | HDT mEFS (mo) | HDT mOS (mo) |
|---|---|---|---|---|---|---|---|---|---|---|---|---|---|
| Attal et al[20] IFM-90 1996 (200) | 84 | Alt VMCP and BVAP | 5 | 9 | 43 | 18 | 44 | MEL140, TBI, IFN-α | 22 | 16 | 43 | 27 | 56 |
| Child et al[21] MRC VII 2003 (407) | 42 | BCAM | 8 | | 81 | 19.6 | 42.3 | MEL140 | 44 | 42 | | 31.6 | 54.1 |
| Fermand et al[44] GMA 2005 (190) | 10 | VMCP | 4.1 | 15.6 | 38.5 | 18.7 | 47.6 | MEL140 vs. MEL200 vs. MEL140 + Bu16 | 8.4 | 39.4 | 26 | 25.3 | 47.8 |
| Barolgie et al[22] S9321 2006 (516) | 76 | VBMCP | 15 | NR | NR | 14 | 38 | MEL140 + TBI | 17 | NR | NR | 17 | 38 |
| Blade et al[45] PETHEMA(164) | 44 | VBMCP and VBAD | 11 | NR | NR | 33 | 61 | MEL200 vs. MEL140 + TBI | 30 | NR | NR | 42 | 66 |
| Palumbo et al[46] (142) | 39 | MP | 5 | 44 | 44 | 17.7 | 48 | MEL100 | 47 | 41 | 41 | 34 | 56+ |
| Lenhoff et al[47] (548) | 32 | VAD | NR | NR | NR | NR | 44 | MEL200 | 41 | 48 | NR | 32 | NRe |
| Barolgie et al[48] (232) | 31 | VMCP/VBAP | NR | 52 | 52 | 22 | 48 | VAD, Cy EDAP, MEL200 | 25 | 85 | NR | 49 | 62+ |

VMCP indicates vincristine, melphalan, cyclophosphamide and prednisone; BVAP, BCNU, vincristine, doxorubicin, and prednisone; CT, conventional chemotherapy; VBMCP, vincristine, BCNU, melphalan, cyclophosphamide, and prednisone; VBAD, vincristine, BCNU, doxorubicin, dexamethasone; BCAM, BCNU, cyclophosphamide, doxorubicin and melphalan; EDAP, etoposide, dexamethasone, cytarabine, cisplatin; HDT, high-dose chemotherapy; TBI, total body irradiation; mEFS, median event-free survival; mOS, median overall survival; MEL100, melphalan 100 mg/m²; MEL140, melphalan 140 mg/m²; MEL200, Melphalan 200 mg/m²; MEL140 + Bu16, Melphalan 140 mg/m2 + Busulfan 16 mg/m²; Cy, high-dose cyclophosphamide; IFN-α interferon-α; NRe, not reached; and NR, not reported.

benefit with HDT compared with conventional therapy (OR 0.70; 95% CI 0.53–0.93; $P = 0.01$). In addition, it conferred an increase in median survival of approximately 1 year among patients in the HDT group. Although the US Intergroup Trial S9321[22] did not demonstrate a survival benefit for HDT, the conditioning was found to be toxic and the length of the time to enroll this trial was so prolonged that its results cannot be easily generalized.

Several meta-analysis reviewed the association between CR, PFS, and OS after HDT/autologous stem-cell transplantation (ASCT) in newly diagnosed[23] as well as relapsed patients.[24] A majority of studies reviewing the single (Table 2) or double ASCT (Table 3) demonstrated that achieving CR or at least VGPR was associated with a longer PFS and usually a longer OS.

In a large analysis from the IFM, Attal et al[20] evaluated the probability of extended event-free survival (EFS) and OS after HDT. In this analysis, the 5-year probability of survival after diagnosis was 72% among patients who achieved CR/VGPR, 39% among patients who achieved PR, and 0% among patients who achieved less PR after HDT. In the studies evaluating[25] double ASCT versus single ASCT, EFS was significantly higher for double-transplant group while lacked

significance for improvement in OS. The absence of a survival benefit for patients in the double-ASCT arm, despite their significantly higher CR or nCR rate and superior EFS, may be due to the long OS of patients assigned to the single-transplantation arm attributed to second salvage ASCT and usage of novel agents as salvage therapies.

Studies from University of Arkansas evaluating tandem transplants have demonstrated the importance of obtaining a CR or nCR. Among the patients treated with Total Therapy I,[26] patients with CR after the first transplant had longer EFS and OS when compared with patients with only a PR. The trend continued in Total Therapy II,[27] EFS and OS were significantly longer for those who had a CR than for those who had a PR or no response. The duration of CR was significantly longer in patients with early onset of CR.[28] Early onset CR before transplant[29,30] as well as sustained CR[31] are the other critical prognostic factors for improved OS; and in particular, CR duration is important among patients with high-risk disease.

Early intensification of therapy in patients already in CR was of no further benefit.[32,33] In the IFM study, patients who did not have at least a VGPR after the first transplant had a significant benefit from the second transplantation. The rates of survival at 7 years were

**TABLE 2.** Survival Outcomes With High Dose Chemotherapy (HDT) and Autologous Stem Cell Transplant (ASCT), by Response

| Study (N) | RR (Postinduction) | | | RR1 (Post-ASCT1) | | | Survival | | | |
|---|---|---|---|---|---|---|---|---|---|---|
| | CR (%) | VGPR (%) | PR (%) | CR1 (%) | VGPR1 (%) | PR1 (%) | Median EFS (mo) | Median OS (mo) | 5 yr EFS (%) | 5 yr OS (%) |
| Bjorkstrand et al[49] (130) | 12 | | 56 | 47 | | 47 | | | | |
| Attal et al[20] (100) | 22 | 16 | 43 | 30 | 22 | 43 | | | | CR1/VGPR1 72 PR1 39 <PR1 0 |
| Majolino et al[50] (290) | 19.7 | | 66.2 | 40 | | 50 | | | | |
| Lahuerta et al[4] (344) | | | | 24 + 19 nCR1 | 16 | 33 | | | CR1 35 nCR1 21 VGPR1 27 PR1 15 | CR1 72 nCR1 48 VGPR1 42 PR1 41 |
| Davies et al[51] (96) | 18 | | 70 | 53 | | 47 | CR1 49.4 PR1 41.4 | | | CR1 58 PR1 64 |
| Alexanian et al[52] (68) | 6 | | 37 | | | | PR → CR1 49.2 PR → PR1 27.6 | PR → CR1 99.6 PR → PR1 60 | | |
| Terpos et al[53] (127) | 6 | | 73 | 15 | | 81 | CR1 31 PR1 16.3 | CR/PR 50.2 <PR1 58.9 | | *CR1 77 PR1 69 |
| Child et al[21] (201) | | | | 44 | | 42 | | CR1 88.6 PR1 39.8 <PR1 25.6 | | |
| Alvares et al[54] (383) | 15 | | | 50 | | 10 | CR1 45.6 <PR1 22.4 | CR1 71 <PR1 64 | | |
| Fermand et al[44] (94) | | | | 36 | 26 | | CR1/VGPR1 59 < CR1/VGPR1 40 | | | |
| O'Shea et al[55] (211) | 5.2 | | 71.2 | 16 | | 68 | CR1 59 <PR1 22 | CR1 NR PR1 47 | | |
| Lenhoff et al[56] (247) | 13 | | 60 | 43 | | 47 | CR1 40 <CR1 27 | CR1 71 <CR1 64 | | |
| Lahuerta et al[30] (632) | 16 | 15 | 55 | 44 | 20 | 28 | CR1 61 nCR1 40 PR 34 | | | CR1 74 nCR1 63 PR 50 |

*3 yr overall survival.
HDT indicates high-dose chemotherapy; ASCT, autologous stem cell transplant; CR, complete response; nCR, near CR; PR, partial response; OS, overall survival; and VGPR, very good partial response.

**TABLE 3.** Survival Outcomes With High Dose Chemotherapy (HDT) and Double Autologous Stem Cell Transplant (ASCT2), by Response

| Study Yr (N)* | Regimen | RR (Post-HDT/Pre-ASCT) CR% | VGPR% | PR% | RR1 (Post-ASCT1/Pre-ASCT2) Transplant Regimen 1 | CR1% | VGPR1% | PR1% | RR2 (Post-ASCT2) Transplant Regimen 2 | CR2% | VGPR2% | PR2% | Survival EFS | OS |
|---|---|---|---|---|---|---|---|---|---|---|---|---|---|---|
| Barlogie et al[26] TT (231) | VAD Cy EDAP | 15 | | 50 | MEL200 | 26 | | 49 | MEL200 vs. MEL200 + TBI/Cy | 41 | | 42 | CR1 78 + m PR1 52 m | CR1 80 + m PR1 68 m |
| Attal et al[32] (399) | VAD | | 12 | | MEL140/TBI | | 42 | 42 | MEL140/TBI | 50 (NS) | | 38 | 30 m | 58 m |
| Galli et al[57] (110) | VAD | 15 | 11 | 57 | MEL200 | 39 | 28 | 20 | MEL200 v MEL140/TBI | 46 | 15 | 10 | [†]CR 65% PR 24% CR1 32% PR1 30% | [‡]CR 63% PR 47% CR1 50% PR1 58% |
| Cavo et al[25] (321) | VAD Cy | | | | MEL200 | 33 | | | MEL120 + Bu12 | 47 | | | 35 m | 71 m (NS) |
| Barlogie et al[27] TT2 (668) | VAD EDAP | 16 | 19 | 19 | MEL200 vs. MEL200 + EAP | 30 | 28 | 20 | MEL200 | 56 | 24 | 12 | [§]PR → nCR/ CR1 70% PR → PR1 26% | [¶]CR → CR1 70% PR/nCR → CR 62% |
| Harousseau et al[28] (849) | VAD | 4 | 12 | 49 | MEL140/200vs. MEL140/200 + Thalidomid | | | | Allogeneic SCT vs. MEL220 | 32 | 22.5 | 37 | CR 42 m VGPR 38 m | 5y CR 77% 5y VGPR 63% |
| Sonneveld et al[58] (155) | VAD | 2 | | | MEL140 Cy | 19 | | | Cy/TBI | 32 | | | 22 m | 50 m |

*All the studies are prospective except by Galli et al, which is a retrospective study.
[†]5-yr event-free survival.
[‡]5-yr overall survival.
[§]4-yr event-free survival.
[¶]4-yr overall survival.
VAD indicates vincristine, doxorubicin, and dexamethasone; Cy, high-dose Cyclophosphamide; EAP, etoposide, cytarabine, and cisplatin; VBMCP, vincristine, BCNU, melphalan, cyclophosphamide, and prednisone; VBAD, vincristine, BCNU, doxorubicin, dexamethasone EDAP, etoposide, dexamethasone, cytarabine, and cisplatin; TBI, total body irradiation; MEL140 Melphalan 140 mg/m² ; MEL200, Melphalan 200 mg/m² ; and MEL140 + Bu16, Melphalan 140 mg/m² + Busulfan 16 mg/m².

**TABLE 4.**  RR, PFS, OS From Various Studies With Novel Agents

| Study (N) | Median Age (yr) | Regimen | Median Follow-Up (mo) | RR CR % | RR VGPR% | RR PR % | Median PFS (mo) | Median OS (mo) | Comments |
|---|---|---|---|---|---|---|---|---|---|
| Palumbo et al[59] GIMEMA (331) | 72 | MPT vs. MP | 38.4 | 16 vs. 4 | 29 vs. 11 | 24 vs. 33 | 21.8 vs. 14.5 | 45 vs. 47.6 | ↑ $\beta2$-m treated with MPT HR = 0.70 95% CI, 0.45–1.08) $P = 0.05$ |
| Facon et al[60] IFM 99–06 (447) | <70 | MPT vs. MP | 51.5 | 13 vs. 2 | 47 vs. 7 | 16 vs. 27 | 27.5 vs. 17.8 | 51.6 vs. 33.2 | Third arm is MEL100; OS MEL100 vs. MP; $P = 0 \times 32$ (NS) |
| Hulin et al[61] IFM 01/01 (232) | >75 | MPT vs. MPPLACEBO | 47.5 | 7 vs. 1 | 21 vs 7 | 33 vs. 23 | 24.1 vs. 18.5 | 45.3 vs. 27.7 | |
| Waage et al[62] (362) | 75 | MPT vs. MPPLACEBO | NR | 13 vs. 4 | 44 vs 36 | | 14.5 vs. 14.5 | 30 vs. 30 | Interim analysis-better RR and TTP in MPT group ($P = 0.03$). No improvement in PFS/OS. |
| Wijermans et al[15] HOVON 49 (344) | >65 | MPT vs. MP | NR | 2 vs. 2 | 28 vs. 8 | 36 vs. 37 | 14 vs. 10 | 37 vs. 30 | PFS after 2 yr, 33% vs. 19% |
| Richardson et al[15] APEX (669) | 61 | Vel vs. Dex | 15.8 | 9 vs. <1 | 7 vs. 1 | 34 vs. 17 | 6.22 vs. 3.49 | 25.4 vs. NR | 1-yr survival rate is 80% vs. 66% ($P = 0.003$)-updated |
| Kyle et al[14] E9486 (653) | 63 | BCNU vs. VBMCP vs. VBMCP-IFN-α vs. VBMCP-CY | 157 | 14% | 53% | | NR | CR 61 vs. PR 40 | VBMCP-IFNα had higher CR (18%) than VBMCP alone (10%) CR rate VBMCP-CY-12% |
| San Miguel et al[19] VISTA (682) | 71 | VMP vs. MP | 16.3 | 30 vs. 4 | 41 vs. 31 | | 18.3 vs. 14 | NRe | 13% vs. 22% deaths |
| Palumbo et al[63] (511) | 71 | VMPT vs. VMP | 36 | 35 vs. 21 | 16 vs. 21 | | NRe | NRe | |
| Rajkumar et al[16] (470) | 64 | TD vs. D | >17 | 7.7 vs. 2.6 | 55.3 vs. 43.4 | | 15 vs. 6.5 | NR | 24.3% vs. 28.9% deaths |
| Ludwig et al[17] (289) | 72 | TD vs. MP | 28.1 | 2 vs. 2 | 24 vs. 11 | 42 vs. 37 | 16.7 vs. 20.7 | 41.5 vs. 49.4 | |
| Wang et al[64] (704) n = 430 | 64 | RD vs. D (No prior Thal exposure) | 74 | 19 vs. 2.5 | 19.5 vs. 4.4 | 26.1 vs. 20.6 | 13.2 vs. 4.7 | 36.1 vs. 32 | 39% of patients previously exposed to thalidomide; OS statistically NS |
| n = 274 | 63 | RD vs. D (prior Thal exposure) | | 7.9 vs. 1.4 | 13.4 vs. 0.7 | 32.3 vs. 12.2 | 8.4 vs. 4.6 | 33.3 vs. 28.7 | |
| Rajkumar et al[18] E4A03 (445) | 65 | RD vs. Rd | 24 | 52 vs. 42 | | 30 vs. 26 | NRe | NRe | 2 yr OS rates 87% (Rd) vs. 75% (RD). |
| Anderson et al[39] (64) | NR | RVD | NR | 21 | 47 | | 30 | NRe | |

NR indicates not reported; NRe, not reached.

11% versus 43% for single versus double transplantation ($P < 0.001$). Patients who had at least a VGPR did not benefit significantly from the second transplantation ($P = 0.70$). Similar results were noted in the retrospective evaluation of response and survival of 758 patients by Wang et al[34] and Dingli et al.[33]

## CR AND OUTCOMES WITH NOVEL AGENTS AS INDUCTION REGIMENS

Encouraging results are being seen with novel agents as induction regimens (Table 4). CR rates in the range of $>30\%$ and VGPR $>70\%$ with induction therapy alone before even receiving HDT/ASCT raise the hope that curability is in reach. In the IFM phase 3 randomized trial, CR + nCR/$\geq$VGPR response of 78% were seen with the randomized trial of bortezomib and dexamethasone (VD) compared with the vincristine, doxorubicin, and dexamethasone (VAD) arm.[35] After autologous transplant, VD arm continued to show superior results as given in Table 5. We reviewed results with VTD induction at our institution.[36] Of the 44 patients who were treated with VTD, we had ORR of 91% (increased to 94% in treatment naive patients). CR/VGPR rate of 57% was reported postinduction. After ASCT in 34 patients, the ORR is 100% and VGPR $\geq$76% (sCR/CR 53%). Median PFS was 27.4 months, and 2-year OS rate is 82%. Similar results were seen with Gruppo Italiano Malattie Ematologiche dell'Adulto (GIMEMA) trial that compared VTD with TD in 480 patients: ORR was 92%, of which 61% had CR + nCR/$\geq$VGPR postinduction, and 76% achieved VGPR or better after HDT.[37] Results with three drug regimens have demonstrated superior results that were deemed impossible a decade earlier. The combination of bortezomib with lenalidomide has been treated in the relapsed and upfront setting with impressive results. Lenalidomide, bortezomib, and dexamethasone (RVD) as induction therapy resulted in $\geq$PR in 100% patients, $\geq$VGPR in 74% patients, and CR/nCR in 44% patients.[38] RVD in refractory setting, at the time of presentation at ASCO 2009, achieved a response rate of 94% and PFS was reached at 30 months.[39] It seems that the combination of proteosome inhibition and immunomodulatory drugs would form the frontline therapy in the upcoming years. Although RVD is being tested in two ongoing phase III trials (ECOG evaluating RVD vs. VD and SWOG evaluating RVD vs. RD), the clinical benefit of the CR achieved with RVD is still to be validated.

## CORRELATION BETWEEN CR AND OUTCOMES IN MAINTENANCE THERAPY

By offering maintenance therapy, the primary goal is to prolong CR by decreasing the burden of residual tumor cells. Two randomized trials have been published demonstrating that post-ASCT treatment with thalidomide increases the rate of CR + VGPR, PFS, and OS.[40,41] From the Australian study that compared thalidomide and prednisone versus prednisone,[41] after a median follow-up of 3 years, the postrandomization 3-year PFS rates for thalidomide and control group were 42% and 23% (HR 0.5; 95% CI 0.35–0.71; $P < 0.001$) and the OS rates were 86% and 75% (HR, 0.41; 95% CI, 0.22–0.76; $P = 0.004$), respectively. The findings differed with IFM study comparing thalidomide versus placebo, where benefit was only evident in the patients not achieving CR or VGPR after HDT, and patients who did not have deletion of chromosome 13 [del (13)] by cytogenetics.

## CR AND OUTCOMES AMONG HIGH-RISK PATIENTS

In the era of novel agents, studies suggest that innovative combinations may overcome the unfavorable prognosis conferred by the high-risk features by improving RR and prolong the PFS and OS. In the IFM 2005 trial, where VAD was compared with VD, achievement of CR

**TABLE 5.** Novel Agents as Induction Regimens

| Study (N) | Median Age (yr) | Regimen | Median f/u (m) | CR % | RR VGPR% | RR PR % | Median PFS (mo) | Median OS (mo) | Comments |
|---|---|---|---|---|---|---|---|---|---|
| Lokhorst et al[65] HOVON-50 2007 (402) | 56 | TAD vs. VAD | NR | 4 vs. 2 | 29 vs. 13 | 39 vs. 39 | NR | NR | Post-HDT-76% vs. 79% ORR (NS) |
| Sonneveld et al[66] HOVON-65 | NR | PAD vs. VAD | NR | 5 vs. 1 (CR + nCR) | 37 vs. 14 | 41 vs. 44 | NR | NR | Post-ASCT responses of CR + nCR/$\geq$VGPR/$\geq$PR are 23%/80%/93% vs. 9%/50%/80% for PAD vs. VAD |
| Cavo et al[37] GIMEMA (480) | <65 | VTD vs. TD | 15 | 33 vs. 12 (CR + nCR) | 28 vs. 18 | 31 vs. 48.5 | 20 mo estimate 93% vs. 86%, $P = 0.04$ | 20 mo estimate 93% both arms | ITT basis-VTD vs. TD-CR (41% vs. 20%, $P < 0.001$), CR + nCR (54% vs. 29%, $P < 0.001$) and $\geq$VGPR (75% vs. 53%, $P < 0.001$) |
| Harousseau et al[35] IFM (482) | <65 | VD vs. VAD | NR | 21.3 vs. 8.3 (CR + nCR) | 46.7 vs. 18.6 | NR | NRe | NRe | CR + nCR/$\geq$VGPR Vd-post-ASCT, in pts → ASCT (40.8%/71.8% vs. 28.8%/51%, $P = 0.0089/<0.0001$) and in the ITT population (35%/61.7% vs. 23.6%/41.7%, $P = 0.0056/<0.0001$ |
| Kaufman et al[36] (44) | 58 | VTD | NR | 20 | 37 | 34 | 27.4 | 2-yr OS rate 82% | ORR post-ASCT in 34 patients-100%; 76% $\geq$VGPR (53% sCR/CR) |

VAD indicates vincristine, doxorubicin, dexamethasone; TAD, thalidomide, doxorubicin, dexamethasone; PAD, bortezomib, doxorubicin, dexamethasone; VTD, bortezomib, thalidomide, dexamethasone; NRe, not reached; and NR, not reported.

was independent of elevated $\beta_2$-microglobulin (International Staging System stage III).[35] In the GIMEMA trial of VTD versus TD, CR + nCR rates of 43% versus 4% were seen for patients with del (13) and 47% versus 8% for t(4;14).[37] Data from Richardson et al[38] evaluating RVD as induction therapy also showed efficacy independent of baseline cytogenetics or stage. Although these 3 trials show encouraging ORRs and high CR rates, durability of this response remains unknown.[42] From the VISTA trial, any high-risk chromosomal abnormality did not impact the efficacy of VMP ($\geq$PR of 81% vs. 82% for high risk vs. standard risk) or in terms of TTP or OS.[19] From UAMS data, CR correlates with OS in high-risk patients, suggesting that novel agents improve ORR and CR rate and overcome the unfavorable prognosis conferred by the high-risk features.[43] Because OS in high-risk patients is associated with CR, and higher CR rates were associated with VD, VTD than VAD or TD, newer combination RVD, whose efficacy is independent of baseline cytogenetics, may have better outcome with regards to OS. Overall, combination therapies resulted in improved OS for high-risk patients.

## CONCLUSION

The past 10 years have represented a time of unprecedented growth and improvements in therapeutic outcomes for patients with myeloma. As we have improved treatments, the measures of our success are changing as well. The definition of CR has been revised to include sCR; however, the current definition represents a threshold to the limits of current detection. To evaluate the disease below the limits of current detection to eradicate evidence of all disease, new techniques for assessing MRD with quantitative PCR or multiparameter flow cytometry to detect molecular remissions need to be validated and used. Specially, in the context of novel agents achieving molecular CRs, and the evidence that molecular CR represents translation to improved PFS and OS is essential if we are to eventually cure myeloma.

CR has been demonstrated as a relevant and meaningful endpoint among nontransplant eligible older patients; however, it must be balanced with safety and toxicity in this group of patients. Among younger transplant eligible patients, the data are much clearer. Achievement of CR or at least VGPR is generally associated with prolonged PFS and OS. Achieving CR or at least VGPR before transplant and sustained CR remained important prognostic factors for PFS and OS.

The future for our patients with current therapeutic tools and new technology to risk stratify has never looked better. As we further refine our treatment regimens and strive toward individualized therapy, it has never been more important to push measurable disease to lower limits. CR as currently defined is one of those limits that help us to improve outcomes and survival for patients.

## REFERENCES

1. Alexanian R, Haut A, Khan AU, et al. Treatment for multiple myeloma. Combination chemotherapy with different melphalan dose regimens. *JAMA.* 1969;208:1680–1685.
2. Alexanian R, Bonnet J, Gehan E, et al. Combination chemotherapy for multiple myeloma. *Cancer.* 1972;30:382–389.
3. Blade J, Samson D, Reece D, et al. Criteria for evaluating disease response and progression in patients with multiple myeloma treated by high-dose therapy and haemopoietic stem cell transplantation. Myeloma Subcommittee of the EBMT. European Group for Blood and Marrow Transplant. *Br J Haematol.* 1998;102:1115–1123.
4. Lahuerta JJ, Martinez-Lopez J, Serna JD, et al. Remission status defined by immunofixation vs. electrophoresis after autologous transplantation has a major impact on the outcome of multiple myeloma patients. *Br J Haematol.* 2000;109:438–446.
5. Lonial S, Gertz MA. Eliminating the complete response penalty from myeloma response assessment. *Blood.* 2008;111:3297–3298.
6. Dispenzieri A, Kyle R, Merlini G, et al. International Myeloma Working Group guidelines for serum-free light chain analysis in multiple myeloma and related disorders. *Leukemia.* 2009;23:215–224.
7. Durie BG, Harousseau JL, Miguel JS, et al. International uniform response criteria for multiple myeloma. *Leukemia.* 2006;20:1467–1473.
8. Corradini P, Voena C, Tarella C, et al. Molecular and clinical remissions in multiple myeloma: role of autologous and allogeneic transplantation of hematopoietic cells. *J Clin Oncol.* 1999;17:208–215.
9. Martinelli G, Terragna C, Zamagni E, et al. Polymerase chain reaction-based detection of minimal residual disease in multiple myeloma patients receiving allogeneic stem cell transplantation. *Haematologica.* 2000;85:930–934.
10. Palumbo FC, Pagliano G, Ferrero S, et al. Early consolidation with bortezomib, thalidomide and dexamethasone in mm patients in CR or VGPR following autologous transplantation induces molecular remissions. *Haematologica.* 2008;93(s1):76.
11. Paiva B, Vidriales MB, Cervero J, et al. Multiparameter flow cytometric remission is the most relevant prognostic factor for multiple myeloma patients who undergo autologous stem cell transplantation. *Blood.* 2008;112:4017–4023.
12. Rawstron AC, Orfao A, Beksac M, et al. Report of the European Myeloma Network on multiparametric flow cytometry in multiple myeloma and related disorders. *Haematologica.* 2008;93:431–438.
13. Kumar S, Rajkumar SV, Dispenzieri A, et al. Improving survival in multiple myeloma: impact of novel therapies (ASH Annual Meeting Abstracts). *Blood.* 2007;110:3594.
14. Kyle RA, Leong T, Li S, et al. Complete response in multiple myeloma: clinical trial E9486, an Eastern Cooperative Oncology Group study not involving stem cell transplantation. *Cancer.* 2006;106:1958–1966.
15. Wijermans P, Schaafsma M, van Norden Y, et al. Melphalan + prednisone versus melphalan + prednisone + thalidomide in induction therapy for multiple myeloma in elderly patients: final analysis of the Dutch Cooperative Group HOVON 49 Study (ASH Annual Meeting Abstracts). *Blood.* 2008;112:649.
16. Rajkumar SV, Rosinol L, Hussein M, et al. Multicenter, randomized, double-blind, placebo-controlled study of thalidomide plus dexamethasone compared with dexamethasone as initial therapy for newly diagnosed multiple myeloma. *J Clin Oncol.* 2008;26:2171–2177.
17. Ludwig H, Hajek R, Tothova E, et al. Thalidomide-dexamethasone compared with melphalan-prednisolone in elderly patients with multiple myeloma. *Blood.* 2009;113:3435–3442.
18. Rajkumar SV, Jacobus S, Callander N, et al. Randomized trial of lenalidomide plus high-dose dexamethasone versus lenalidomide plus low-dose dexamethasone in newly diagnosed myeloma (E4A03), a trial coordinated by the Eastern Cooperative Oncology Group: Analysis of response, survival, and outcome wi (Meeting Abstracts). *J Clin Oncol.* 2008;26:8504.
19. San Miguel JF, Schlag R, Khuageva NK, et al. Bortezomib plus melphalan and prednisone for initial treatment of multiple myeloma. *N Engl J Med.* 2008;359:906–917.
20. Attal M, Harousseau JL, Stoppa AM, et al. A prospective, randomized trial of autologous bone marrow transplantation and chemotherapy in multiple myeloma. Intergroupe Francais du Myelome. *N Engl J Med.* 1996;335:91–97.
21. Child JA, Morgan GJ, Davies FE, et al. High-dose chemotherapy with hematopoietic stem-cell rescue for multiple myeloma. *N Engl J Med.* 2003;348:1875–1883.
22. Barlogie B, Kyle RA, Anderson KC, et al. Standard chemotherapy compared with high-dose chemoradiotherapy for multiple myeloma: final results of phase III US Intergroup Trial S9321. *J Clin Oncol.* 2006;24:929–936.
23. van de Velde HJ, Liu X, Chen G, et al. Complete response correlates with long-term survival and progression-free survival in high-dose therapy in multiple myeloma. *Haematologica.* 2007;92:1399–1406.
24. Desikan R, Barlogie B, Sawyer J, et al. Results of high-dose therapy for 1000 patients with multiple myeloma: durable complete remissions and superior survival in the absence of chromosome 13 abnormalities. *Blood.* 2000;95:4008–4010.
25. Cavo M, Tosi P, Zamagni E, et al. Prospective, randomized study of single compared with double autologous stem-cell transplantation for multiple myeloma: Bologna 96 clinical study. *J Clin Oncol.* 2007;25:2434–2441.
26. Barlogie B, Jagannath S, Desikan KR, et al. Total therapy with tandem transplants for newly diagnosed multiple myeloma. *Blood.* 1999;93:55–65.
27. Barlogie B, Tricot G, Anaissie E, et al. Thalidomide and hematopoietic-cell transplantation for multiple myeloma. *N Engl J Med.* 2006;354:1021–1030.
28. Harousseau J-L, Attal M, Moreau P, et al. The prognostic impact of complete remission (CR) plus very good partial remission (VGPR) in a double-transplantation program for newly diagnosed multiple myeloma (MM). Combined results of the IFM 99 trials (ASH Annual Meeting Abstracts). *Blood.* 2006;108:3077.
29. Kim JS, Kim K, Cheong JW, et al. Complete remission status before autologous stem cell transplantation is an important prognostic factor in patients with

multiple myeloma undergoing upfront single autologous transplantation. *Biol Blood Marrow Transplant.* 2009;15:463–470.

30. Lahuerta JJ, Mateos MV, Martinez-Lopez J, et al. Influence of pre- and post-transplantation responses on outcome of patients with multiple myeloma: sequential improvement of response and achievement of complete response are associated with longer survival. *J Clin Oncol.* 2008;26:5775–5782.

31. Barlogie B, Anaissie E, Haessler J, et al. Complete remission sustained 3 years from treatment initiation is a powerful surrogate for extended survival in multiple myeloma. *Cancer.* 2008;113:355–359.

32. Attal M, Harousseau JL, Facon T, et al. Single versus double autologous stem-cell transplantation for multiple myeloma. *N Engl J Med.* 2003;349:2495–2502.

33. Dingli D, Pacheco JM, Nowakowski GS, et al. Relationship between depth of response and outcome in multiple myeloma. *J Clin Oncol.* 2007;25:4933–4937.

34. Wang M, Delasalle K, Feng L, et al. CR represents an early index of potential long survival in multiple myeloma. *Bone Marrow Transplant.* In press.

35. Harousseau JL, Mathiot C, Attal M, et al. Bortezomib/dexamethasone versus VAD as induction prior to autologous stem cell transplantation (ASCT) in previously untreated multiple myeloma (MM): updated data from IFM 2005/01 trial (Meeting Abstracts). *J Clin Oncol.* 2008;26:8505.

36. Kaufman J, Nooka A, Vrana M, et al. Bortezomib, thalidomide, and dexamethasone as induction therapy for patients with symptomatic multiple myeloma: a retrospective study. *Cancer.* In press.

37. Cavo M, Tacchetti P, Patriarca F, et al. Superior complete response rate and progression-free survival after autologous transplantation with up-front velcade-thalidomide-dexamethasone compared with thalidomide-dexamethasone in newly diagnosed multiple myeloma (ASH Annual Meeting Abstracts). *Blood.* 2008;112:158.

38. Richardson P, Lonial S, Jakubowiak A, et al. Lenalidomide, bortezomib, and dexamethasone in patients with newly diagnosed multiple myeloma: encouraging efficacy in high risk groups with updated results of a phase I/II study (ASH Annual Meeting Abstracts). *Blood.* 2008;112:92.

39. Anderson KC, Jagannath S, Jakubowiak A, et al. Lenalidomide, bortezomib, and dexamethasone in relapsed/refractory multiple myeloma (MM): Encouraging outcomes and tolerability in a phase II study (Meeting Abstracts). *J Clin Oncol.* 2009;27:8536.

40. Attal M, Harousseau JL, Leyvraz S, et al. Maintenance therapy with thalidomide improves survival in patients with multiple myeloma. *Blood.* 2006;108:3289–3294.

41. Spencer A, Prince HM, Roberts AW, et al. Consolidation therapy with low-dose thalidomide and prednisolone prolongs the survival of multiple myeloma patients undergoing a single autologous stem-cell transplantation procedure. *J Clin Oncol.* 2009;27:1788–1793.

42. Lonial S. Risky business in myeloma. *Blood.* 2009;114:496–497.

43. Haessler J, Shaughnessy JD Jr, Zhan F, et al. Benefit of complete response in multiple myeloma limited to high-risk subgroup identified by gene expression profiling. *Clin Cancer Res.* 2007;13:7073–7079.

44. Fermand JP, Katsahian S, Divine M, et al. High-dose therapy and autologous blood stem-cell transplantation compared with conventional treatment in myeloma patients aged 55 to 65 years: long-term results of a randomized control trial from the Group Myelome-Autogreffe. *J Clin Oncol.* 2005;23: 9227–9233.

45. Blade J, Rosinol L, Sureda A, et al. High-dose therapy intensification compared with continued standard chemotherapy in multiple myeloma patients responding to the initial chemotherapy: long-term results from a prospective randomized trial from the Spanish cooperative group PETHEMA. *Blood.* 2005;106: 3755–3759.

46. Palumbo A, Triolo S, Argentino C, et al. Dose-intensive melphalan with stem cell support (MEL100) is superior to standard treatment in elderly myeloma patients. *Blood.* 1999;94:1248–1253.

47. Lenhoff S, Hjorth M, Holmberg E, et al. Impact on survival of high-dose therapy with autologous stem cell support in patients younger than 60 years with newly diagnosed multiple myeloma: a population-based study. Nordic Myeloma Study Group. *Blood.* 2000;95:7–11.

48. Barlogie B, Jagannath S, Vesole DH, et al. Superiority of tandem autologous transplantation over standard therapy for previously untreated multiple myeloma. *Blood.* 1997;89:789–793.

49. Bjorkstrand B, Goldstone AH, Ljungman P, et al. Prognostic factors in autologous stem cell transplantation for multiple myeloma: an EBMT Registry Study. European Group for Bone Marrow Transplantation. *Leuk Lymphoma.* 1994;15:265–272.

50. Majolino I, Vignetti M, Meloni G, et al. Autologous transplantation in multiple myeloma: a GITMO retrospective analysis on 290 patients. Gruppo Italiano Trapianti di Midollo Osseo. *Haematologica.* 1999;84:844–852.

51. Davies FE, Forsyth PD, Rawstron AC, et al. The impact of attaining a minimal disease state after high-dose melphalan and autologous transplantation for multiple myeloma. *Br J Haematol.* 2001;112:814–819.

52. Alexanian R, Weber D, Giralt S, et al. Impact of complete remission with intensive therapy in patients with responsive multiple myeloma. *Bone Marrow Transplant.* 2001;27:1037–1043.

53. Terpos E, Apperley JF, Samson D, et al. Autologous stem cell transplantation in multiple myeloma: improved survival in nonsecretory multiple myeloma but lack of influence of age, status at transplant, previous treatment and conditioning regimen. A single-centre experience in 127 patients. *Bone Marrow Transplant.* 2003;31:163–170.

54. Alvares CL, Davies FE, Horton C, et al. Long-term outcomes of previously untreated myeloma patients: responses to induction chemotherapy and high-dose melphalan incorporated within a risk stratification model can help to direct the use of novel treatments. *Br J Haematol.* 2005;129:607–614.

55. O'Shea D, Giles C, Terpos E, et al. Predictive factors for survival in myeloma patients who undergo autologous stem cell transplantation: a single-centre experience in 211 patients. *Bone Marrow Transplant.* 2006;37:731–737.

56. Lenhoff S, Hjorth M, Turesson I, et al. Intensive therapy for multiple myeloma in patients younger than 60 years. Long-term results focusing on the effect of the degree of response on survival and relapse pattern after transplantation. *Haematologica.* 2006;91:1228–1233.

57. Galli M, Nicolucci A, Valentini M, et al. Feasibility and outcome of tandem stem cell autotransplants in multiple myeloma. *Haematologica.* 2005;90:1643–1649.

58. Sonneveld P, van der Holt B, Segeren CM, et al. Intermediate-dose melphalan compared with myeloablative treatment in multiple myeloma: long-term follow-up of the Dutch Cooperative Group HOVON 24 trial. *Haematologica.* 2007;92:928–935.

59. Palumbo A, Bringhen S, Caravita T, et al. Oral melphalan and prednisone chemotherapy plus thalidomide compared with melphalan and prednisone alone in elderly patients with multiple myeloma: randomised controlled trial. *Lancet.* 2006;367:825–831.

60. Facon T, Mary JY, Hulin C, et al. Melphalan and prednisone plus thalidomide versus melphalan and prednisone alone or reduced-intensity autologous stem cell transplantation in elderly patients with multiple myeloma (IFM 99–06): a randomised trial. *Lancet.* 2007;370:1209–1218.

61. Hulin C, Facon T, Rodon P, et al. Efficacy of melphalan and prednisone plus thalidomide in patients older than 75 years with newly diagnosed multiple myeloma: IFM 01/01 trial. *J Clin Oncol.* 2009;27:3664–3670.

62. Waage A, Gimsing P, Juliusson G, et al. Melphalan-prednisone-thalidomide to newly diagnosed patients with multiple myeloma: a placebo controlled randomised phase 3 trial (ASH Annual Meeting Abstracts). *Blood.* 2007;110:78.

63. Palumbo AP, Bringhen S, Rossi D, et al. A phase III study of VMPT versus VMP in newly diagnosed elderly myeloma patients (ASCO Meeting Abstracts). *J Clin Oncol.* 2009;27:8515.

64. Wang M, Dimopoulos MA, Chen C, et al. Lenalidomide plus dexamethasone is more effective than dexamethasone alone in patients with relapsed or refractory multiple myeloma regardless of prior thalidomide exposure. *Blood.* 2008;112:4445–4451.

65. Lokhorst HM, Schmidt-Wolf I, Sonneveld P, et al. Thalidomide in induction treatment increases the very good partial response rate before and after high-dose therapy in previously untreated multiple myeloma. *Haematologica.* 2008;93:124–127.

66. Sonneveld P, van der Holt B, Schmidt-Wolf IGH, et al. First analysis of HOVON-65/GMMG-HD4 randomized phase III trial comparing bortezomib, adriamycine, dexamethasone (PAD) vs VAD as induction treatment prior to high dose melphalan (HDM) in patients with newly diagnosed multiple myeloma (MM) (ASH Annual Meeting Abstracts). *Blood.* 2008;112:653.

# Novel Therapies in Multiple Myeloma for Newly Diagnosed Nontransplant Candidates

Sigurdur Yngvi Kristinsson • Ola Landgren • Vincent S. Rajkumar

Multiple myeloma is a malignant B-cell disorder characterized by a monoclonal proliferation of plasma cells in the bone marrow.[1,2] In a recent prospective cancer screening study including 77,469 healthy subjects, among whom 71 developed multiple myeloma during the course of the study, multiple myeloma was consistently preceded by the precursor condition monoclonal gammopathy of undetermined significance (MGUS).[3] Multiple myeloma accounts for about 10% of hematological malignancies.[4,5] The median age at diagnosis is about 65 to 70 years and is only occasionally diagnosed in patients aged below 40 years.[4–6] Men are affected more commonly than women[7]; compared with Caucasians, Blacks have higher rates of both MGUS and multiple myeloma.[8] MGUS and multiple myeloma are 2-fold to 3-fold more common among blood relatives of MGUS/multiple myeloma patients.[9–11] In the Western world, the annual age-adjusted incidence for multiple myeloma is 4.8 to 8 per 100,000.[5]

In multiple myeloma, the proliferation of B-cells commonly results in overproduction of monoclonal immunoglobulins, termed M-proteins. Approximately 8% of all patients are asymptomatic at diagnosis.[12] Clinical signs and symptoms may be caused by direct tumor growth or the monoclonal products. The malignant proliferation of plasma cells produces skeletal destruction that leads to bone pain and pathologic fractures. The M-protein may lead to renal failure, hyperviscosity syndrome, or result in recurrent infections through suppression of uninvolved immunoglobulins. Anemia and hypercalcemia are common complications.[13]

## Prognostic Factors

A number of prognostic factors have been identified in various multiple myeloma patient populations and in patients following different therapies. Today, the International Staging System (ISS) is the most widely used prognostic scoring system and provides a simple and reproducible three-stage classification: stage I is characterized by $\beta_2$-microglobulin less than 3.5 mg/L and serum albumin higher than 3.5 g per 100 mL and had a median survival of 62 months; stage II is represented by neither stage I nor III and showed a median survival of 44 months; and stage III is defined by $\beta_2$-microglobulin above 5.5 mg/L, with a median survival of 29 months (Table 1).[14]

Patients with symptomatic multiple myeloma may be classified into high-risk or standard-risk disease (Table 2).[15,16] Acquired chromosomal abnormalities significantly impact survival in myeloma patients. In current clinical practice, poor prognosis is associated with the presence of immunoglobulin heavy chain translocations t(4;14), t(14;16), t(14;20), deletion of 17p13, or deletion of 13. By contrast, a favorable prognosis has been observed in the presence of t(11;14), t(6;14), or hyperdiploidy.[17–20] In research settings, gene expression profiling has become an increasingly powerful tool with the

aim to characterize prognostic profiles[21] and define distinct multiple myeloma subtypes.[22,23]

It must be noted that the ISS and the adverse impact of cytogenetic abnormalities, as well as gene expression profiling, are established in the context of conventional therapies but not with novel treatments. Also, other factors, such as age at diagnosis, performance status, and response to therapy, are of importance in the prognosis of multiple myeloma patients.[24,25]

## Indications for Therapy

At this time, there are no data to support that asymptomatic multiple myeloma patients benefit from early treatment.[26] Therefore, therapy shall not be given to asymptomatic multiple myeloma patients in clinical practice. However, clinical trials are currently ongoing to determine if new agents can delay progression from asymptomatic to symptomatic myeloma and, thereby, prolong survival.

Patients with the diagnosis of multiple myeloma and with symptomatic disease are in need of therapy. Based on our overall aim to improve and develop new therapeutic strategies and novel drugs, we are in strong support of clinical trials in multiple myeloma. For patients who are not eligible for clinical trials, or if clinical trials are not available, in a standard clinical setting, one may separate multiple myeloma patients into those who are eligible versus those who are ineligible for high-dose melphalan therapy, followed by an autologous stem cell transplant.[16] In most institutions, patients considered ineligible for autologous stem cell transplantation are those aged more than 65 to 70 years, with a serum creatinine >2.5 mg/dL, Eastern Cooperative Oncology Group (ECOG) performance status 3 or 4, or New York Heart Association functional status class III or IV, or a combination. Patients with renal failure may be transplanted, but the morbidity and mortality is higher.[27] Given the high median age at diagnosis and concurrent morbidity, the majority of all multiple myeloma patients are not eligible for autologous stem cell transplantation.

## Development of Novel Treatments in Multiple Myeloma

Since the 1960s, oral melphalan and prednisone (MP) has been the standard of therapy for patients not eligible for autologous stem cell transplantation.[28,29] Until recently, MP was considered standard of care for symptomatic patients older than 65 to 70 years. Based on several clinical trials, the response rate with MP is only 50% to 60% and complete remissions (CR) are rare. This is reflected in a median overall survival of 24 to 48 months.[28,29] Consequently, through the years, many clinical trials have been conducted to develop treatment regimens with higher response rates and improved overall survival compared with those of MP. In a large meta-analysis of 4930 symptomatic myeloma patients in 20 prospective trials, the response rate was 60% for combination chemotherapy compared with 53% for MP

| TABLE 1. | International Staging System |
|----------|------------------------------|
| **Stage** | **Criteria** |
| I | Serum $\beta_2$-microglobulin <2.5 mg/L and serum albumin >35 g/L |
| II | Not stage I or III |
| III | Serum $\beta_2$-microglobulin >5.5 mg/L |

| TABLE 2. | High-Risk Cytogenetic Features |
|----------|-------------------------------|
| By fluorescent in-situ hybridization | |
|    Translocation t(4;14) | |
|    Translocation t(14;16) | |
|    Deletion 17p⁻ | |
| By conventional karyotyping | |
|    Hypodiploidy | |
|    Deletion chromosome 13 | |

($P < 0.001$). However, there was no difference in survival. Also, the meta-analysis failed to identify a subset of patients who benefited from additional combinations of chemotherapy.[28]

The discovery of novel therapies, including thalidomide, bortezomib, and lenalidomide, targeting both myeloma cells and the bone marrow microenvironment, has changed the paradigm of myeloma therapy, especially for the elderly population. Thalidomide and lenalidomide have been found to have antiangiogenesis properties, stimulate T-cells and natural killer cells, and interfere with cytokines. They suppress growth factors, such as interleukin-6, tumor necrosis factor-$\alpha$, and inhibit myeloma cell adhesion and blood vessel growth cytokines such as vascular endothelial growth factor.[30,31]

Bortezomib, a proteasome inhibitor, specifically interferes with the 26S proteasome, which is responsible for degrading protein that control transcription, the cell-proliferation cycle, and metabolism.[32] Interestingly, although the initial rationale for its use in multiple myeloma was inhibition of nuclear factor-$\kappa$B activity by blocking proteasomal degradation of I-$\kappa$B-$\alpha$, recent work indicates that bortezomib-induced cytotoxicity cannot be fully attributed to inhibition of canonical nuclear factor-$\kappa$B activity in multiple myeloma.[33]

Combinations of novel agents with steroids, alkylating agents, or anthracyclines have significantly improved response rates, progression-free survival (PFS), and overall survival in multiple myeloma.[34-40] There is also evidence that novel agents may overcome the poor prognosis induced by chromosomal abnormalities and ISS score. Below, we review and discuss results and toxicities from major studies based on novel multiple myeloma drugs.

## Thalidomide-Based Regimens

### Thalidomide Combined With Melphalan-Prednisone

Recently, MP has been combined with thalidomide (MPT) in five different randomized studies (Table 3). Palumbo et al[41] reported a

randomized trial (GIMEMA trial) comparing MPT with MP in 255 patients with newly diagnosed myeloma, aged 65 to 85 years, and who were considered ineligible for an autologous stem cell transplant. The patients were randomized to six 4-week cycles of melphalan (4 mg/m² on days 1–7) and prednisone (40 mg/m² on days 1–7) or MP plus thalidomide 100 mg daily (MPT) during the 6 cycles and then as maintenance until sign of relapse or progressive disease. The response rate was 76% and CR 16% in the MPT regimen compared with 48% and 2%, respectively, for MP. The 2-year event-free survival was 54% versus 27%, while the 3-year survival was 80% versus 64%, favoring the MPT regimen, although not significantly.[41] In a recent update of that trial, after a median follow-up of 38 months, there was still a significantly superior PFS in the MPT arm. However, the median overall survival was similar: 45 months in the MPT group and 47.6 months in the MP group.[42]

Grades 3 to 4 adverse events occurred in 48% with the MPT regimen, compared with 25% for MP. The risk of thromboembolic phenomena (12% vs. 2%) was significantly increased in the MPT group. Because of that, the protocol was amended and enoxaparin 40 mg per day was given during the first 4 cycles as anticoagulation prophylaxis, with a reduction in the number of events. In addition, infections (10% vs. 2%), peripheral neuropathy (8% vs. 0%), and constipation (6% vs. 0%) were greater in MPT compared with MP.

In the second study, the IFM 99-06, the French Myeloma Group reported on 447 previously untreated patients with myeloma, aged 65 to 70 years, and who were ineligible for autologous stem cell transplantation.[43] They were randomized to 12 cycles of 6-weeks melphalan (0.25 mg/kg) and prednisone (2 mg/kg; days 1–4) and

| TABLE 3. | Recent Randomized Trials in Nontransplant Candidates With Newly Diagnosed Myeloma | | | | | |
|----------|--------|--------|--------|--------|--------|--------|
| | **GIMEMA** | **IFM 99-06** | **IFM 01-01** | **NMSG** | **HOVON** | **VISTA** |
| No. patients | 331 | 447 | 232 | 363 | 344 | 682 |
| Median age (range) (yr) | 72 (60–85) | 69 (65–75) | 78.5 (75–89) | 75 (49–92) | 72 | 71 (48–91) |
| MP regimen | Six 4-wk cycles | 12 6-wk cycles | 12 6-wk cycles | 6-wk cycles until plateau | Eight 4-wk cycles | Nine 6-wk cycles |
| Melphalan dose | 4 mg/m2; d 1–7 | 0.25 mg/kg; d 1–4 | 0.2 mg/kg; d 1–4 | 0.25 mg/kg; d 1–4 | 0.25 mg/kg; d 1–5 | 9 mg/m²; d 1–4 |
| Prednisone dose | 40 mg/m²; d 1–7 | 2 mg/kg; d 1–4 | 2 mg/kg; d 1–4 | 100 mg; d 1–4 | 1 mg/kg; d 1–5 | 60 mg/m²; d 1–4 |
| Thalidomide dose (mg) | 100 | Up to 400 | 100 | Up to 400 | 200 | Bortezomib* |
| Maintenance | Yes | No | No | Yes | Yes | No |
| PR (%) | 60.4 vs. 45.2 | 76 vs. 35 | 62 vs. 31 | 27 vs. 22 | 36 vs. 37 | 33 vs. 31 |
| CR (%) | 15.5 vs. 2.4 | 13 vs. 2 | 21 vs. 7 | 15 vs. 6 | 2 vs. 2 | 30 vs. 4 |
| PFS (mo) (median) | 21.8 vs. 15.5 | 27.5 vs. 17.8 | 24.1 vs. 18.5 | 16 vs. 14 | 13 vs. 10 | 24 vs. 16† |
| Overall survival (mo) (median) | 45.0 vs. 47.6 | 51.6 vs. 33.2 | 44.0 vs. 29.1 | 29 vs. 33 | 37 vs. 30 | Not reached‡ |

*Bortezomib 1.3 mg/m² on days 1, 4, 8, 11, 22, 25, 29, and 32 in cycles 1–4 and on days 1, 8, 22, and 29 during cycles 5–9.
†Time to progression.
‡Hazard ratio 0.61 ($P = 0.008$) in favor of MPV.

thalidomide (given in an increasing dosage to a maximum of 400 mg daily if tolerated during the cycles and then stopped); or MP in the same dosage and schedule; or vincristine, doxorubicin, and dexamethasone followed by melphalan 100 mg/m$^2$ × 2 and then followed by stem cell rescue. A higher partial response (PR) rate was seen in the MPT and in the melphalan 100 mg/m$^2$ groups, compared with MP (76% vs. 65% vs. 35%, respectively). Similarly, the CR rates were significantly higher with MPT (13%) and intermediate-dose melphalan (18%) compared with MP (2%). Median PFS was 27.5 months in the MPT patients and 17.8 months in the MP group ($P < 0.0001$), and median overall survival was significantly better in the MPT group compared with the MP group (51.6 and 33.2 months, respectively ($P < 0.001$) and the melphalan 100 mg/m$^2$ group ($P = 0.027$).[43]

Compared with the MP group, MPT was associated with higher rates of grade 3 or 4 neutropenia (48%), constipation (10%), and somnolence, fatigue, or dizziness (8%). Patients did not receive anticoagulation, and 12% of the patients in the MPT arm developed venous thromboembolism.

In another French study (IFM 01-01), 229 patients with previously untreated multiple myeloma, who were aged older than 75 years, were randomized to melphalan (0.2 mg/kg) plus prednisone (2 mg/kg) on days 1 to 4 for every 6 weeks for 12 cycles or MP in the same dosage plus thalidomide 100 mg daily (MPT) without maintenance.[44] The PR rate was 62% in the MPT group and 31% in the MP group, and CR was observed in 7% and 1%, respectively. Median PFS was 24.1 months for MPT and 19.0 months for MP ($P = 0.001$), and median overall survival was 45.3 months for MPT and 27.7 months for MP ($P = 0.03$).[44]

Toxicity in this elderly population was similar to that observed in earlier trials. Peripheral neuropathy was seen in 39% in the MPT group compared with 21% in the MP group. Grades 3 to 4 neutropenia was greater in the MPT arm. No anticoagulation was prospectively planned, and no significant difference was observed in thrombosis complication between the arms, possibly related to more frequent use of antithrombotic treatments for other comorbidity in this age group.[44]

In a study by the Nordic Myeloma Study Group, 362 patients with a mean age of 75 years (range, 49–92) were randomized to receive melphalan (0.25 mg/kg) and prednisone (100 mg) for 4 days every 6 weeks until plateau phase.[45] The MPT arm received additionally thalidomide at a starting dose of 200 mg, escalating to 400 mg if possible, and then given as maintenance as 200 mg in plateau phase. Results of an interim analysis showed better PR (27% vs. 22%) and CR/nCR (6% vs. 3%) in the MPT group compared with MP. No difference was observed in PFS or overall survival (29 vs. 33 months) in this study. Furthermore, in patients above 75 years, there was a tendency to higher early mortality in the MPT group.

No thrombosis prophylaxis was given, and there was no difference in the incidence of thromboembolic complications, however, approximately 30% of the patients had antithrombotic treatment for other reasons.[45]

In the HOVON study, 344 patients aged 65 years and older were randomized to receive eight 4-week cycles of melphalan (0.25 mg/kg; days 1–5) and prednisone (1 mg/kg; days 1–5), with or without 200 mg of thalidomide, until plateau.[46] The MPT arm additionally received thalidomide as maintenance, 50 mg per day. The overall response rates were higher in MPT group (66% vs. 47%) and CR was 2% in both arms. The PFS was significantly improved in the MPT group ($P < 0.001$). Median overall survival was 37 months in the MPT group compared with 30 months in MP (not significant).

Grades 2 to 4 toxicity was seen in 60% of the patients in the MP arm and in 88% of the MPT patients, and was mainly because

of peripheral neuropathy. No differences between the two arms were seen for other toxicities.[46]

Taken together, results from these five randomized studies have been consistent with regard to response rate being superior in the MPT arms compared with MP, however, all but one have shown an improvement in PFS. Only the two French studies have shown a survival benefit. Comparisons between different studies are difficult to make because of differences in patient populations, duration of treatment, and use of maintenance regimens. Despite these differences, data strongly support the MPT regimen as the new standard of care for elderly myeloma patients. In all studies, the MPT patients showed a higher incidence of extrahematological toxicities compared with the MP regimen, especially neurologic adverse events, infections, and thromboembolism. Antithrombotic prophylaxis is recommended when using MPT, and aspirin seems to be a safe option.[24] The higher toxicity rate significantly reduced the efficacy of the MPT combination. Randomized studies that used more strict inclusion criteria showed better outcome. In the French studies, a higher incidence of grades 3 to 4 hematological toxicity (neutropenia and thrombocytopenia) was also observed, probably because of a higher number of MP cycles administered (12 cycles) and a higher dose of thalidomide (median dose 200 mg). The duration of MP treatment may also be reduced from 12 cycles to 6 cycles, because prolonged melphalan exposure induces thrombocytopenia that hampers the delivery of subsequent effective salvage regimens.

## Other Thalidomide Combinations

In younger patients, thalidomide/dexamethasone (Thal/Dex) significantly improves PFS in comparison with high-dose dexamethasone alone.[34] In 289 elderly patients, Thal/Dex was compared with MP in a randomized study. Patients in the Thal/Dex arm had a significantly higher response rate but failed to show any advantage in PFS. In fact, overall survival was inferior with Thal/Dex compared with MP ($P = 0.024$).[47] Patients on Thal/Dex experienced more grades 2 to 3 neuropathy (25%) and skin toxicity (12%) compared with those on MP (8% vs. 3%, respectively), particularly in patients older than 75 years with poor performance status. Thromboembolic complications were seen in 8% of patients receiving Thal/Dex and in 3% of patients receiving MP. The higher toxicity rate of Thal/Dex regimen can explain the lower efficacy of Thal/Dex in the elderly population.

In the Medical Research Council Myeloma IX trial, cyclophosphamide, thalidomide, and dexamethasone (CTD) was been compared with MP in 900 patients. In the CTD group, the PR rate (82% vs. 49%) and the CR rates (23% vs. 6%) were significantly superior.[48] Data on remission durations are not available, and mature survival data are needed on this trial before making recommendations for clinical practice.

## Bortezomib-Based Regimens

### Bortezomib Combined With Melphalan-Prednisone

The Spanish Cooperative Group conducted a large phase I/II trial of melphalan, prednisone, and bortezomib (MPV), with encouraging results.[49] This study formed the basis for the VISTA trial, where 682 patients, median age 71 years (range 48–91), were randomized to receive nine 6-week cycles of bortezomib (1.3 mg/m$^2$) intravenously on days 1, 4, 8, 11, 22, 25, 29, and 32 during cycles 1 to 4 and bortezomib (1.3 mg/m$^2$) on days 1, 8, 22, and 29 during cycles 5 to 9 plus melphalan (9 mg/m$^2$) and prednisone (60 mg/m$^2$) on days 1 to 4 of each cycle (MPV) or to MP in the same dosage and schedule.[50] The response rates were better in the MPV arm, both PR (71% vs. 4%) and, importantly, a very high CR were observed in the MPV arm (30% vs. 4%). Median survival was not reached in either group, but at

16 months, the survival was significantly improved in the MPV arm ($P = 0.008$). Furthermore, the efficacy seemed not to be influenced by poor prognostic factors, including ISS stage, renal failure, and high-risk cytogenetic profiles.[50]

As expected, neutropenia, thrombocytopenia, anemia, and gastrointestinal symptoms were more common with the MPV regimen. Peripheral neuropathy occurred in 44% of the MPV group and in 5% with MP. This included 13% risk of grade 3 neuropathy in the MPV arm. The peripheral neuropathy resolved or improved in 74% of patients within a median of 2 months.[50] Preexisting neuropathy or previous neurotoxic therapy increases the risk of peripheral neuropathy, which can be reduced or resolved by prompt dose reduction of the drug. The incidence of neuropathy can also be reduced greatly by once-weekly administration of bortezomib instead of the twice-weekly schedule. There is an increased risk of herpes zoster infection with MPV, and prophylactic antiviral medications are recommended. There was no difference in the incidence of venous thromboembolism between the groups.

## Lenalidomide-Based Regimens

### Lenalidomide Combined With Melphalan-Prednisone

The Italian group evaluated in a phase I/II trial, dosing, safety, and efficacy of melphalan plus prednisone and lenalidomide (MPR) in newly diagnosed elderly myeloma patients.[51] The maximum tolerated dose was considered to be melphalan at 0.18 mg/kg on days 1 to 4, prednisone at a 2-mg/kg dose on days 1 to 4, and lenalidomide at 10 mg on days 1 to 21, every 28 days for 9 cycles. Aspirin was given as a prophylaxis for thrombosis. Eighty-five percent of patients achieved at least a PR, and 23.8% achieved immunofixation-negative CR. The 1-year event-free and overall survival was 92% and 100%, respectively. Preliminary results showed that the event-free survival of patients with deletion of chromosome 13 or chromosomal translocation[4,14] was not significantly different from those who did not have such abnormalities.[51] The results of an international phase III study comparing MP versus MPR are awaited. An ECOG study comparing MPT versus MPR is ongoing.

Grades 3 to 4 adverse events in the Italian study were mainly related to hematologic toxicities (neutropenia 66%). Severe nonhematologic side effects were less frequent and included febrile neutropenia (8%), cutaneous rash (10%), and thromboembolism. Neutropenia and deep vein thrombosis are the major complications with lenalidomide, although the addition of aspirin markedly reduced the risk of thromboembolic events in newly diagnosed patients treated with lenalidomide in association with dexamethasone or chemotherapy.[51] Recommendations for thromboprophylaxis in patients treated with thalidomide or lenalidomide have been published, and aspirin seems to be the preferred choice in the absence of additional risks of thromboembolism.[24] The addition of granulocyte colony-stimulating factor is recommended in case of neutropenia, and melphalan dose reduction (from 0.18 to 0.13 mg/kg) should be applied in the presence of severe neutropenia despite granulocyte colony-stimulating factor.

### Lenalidomide With High-Dose Versus Low-Dose Dexamethasone

A randomized trial from the ECOG group studied 445 previously untreated symptomatic multiple myeloma. Patients were assigned to lenalidomide (25 mg daily on days 1–21) plus high-dose dexamethasone (40 mg daily on days 1–4, 9–12, and 17–20) or to lenalidomide in the same dose and schedule plus dexamethasone (40 mg) given weekly for each 28-day cycle.[52] The median age was 66 years and included 233 patients older than 65 years. Among all patients, preliminary results show that the 1-year survival was 96% for lenalidomide/low-dose

dexamethasone compared with 88% for lenalidomide plus high-dose dexamethasone. Early deaths were more common in the high-dose arm. The 2-year survival probability was 87% and 75%, respectively.[52] Among elderly patients, the 2-year survival was also superior in the low-dose group.

There was significantly more grades 3 to 4 toxicity among patients in the low-dose dexamethasone group (35% vs. 52%), including infections, fatigue, and venous thrombosis. The risk of deep venous thrombosis was less in the low dexamethasone regimen (12% vs. 26%), as was the incidence of infections (9% vs. 16%).[52] Based on these results, a randomized trial comparing lenalidomide plus low-dose dexamethasone and MPT has been initiated, and accrual is ongoing.

## Maintenance Therapy

There are a few studies on thalidomide maintenance after autologous stem cell transplantation, suggesting that it may improve outcome in a subset of patients with high-risk myeloma or a poor response after autologous stem cell transplantation.[36,53–56] However, there are no studies supporting maintenance therapy after MPT or MPV. Currently, patients are treated for a fixed duration of 18 months with MPT with no maintenance based on the French studies.[43,44] Similarly, with MPV, the treatment duration is for 12 months, followed by no maintenance. Lenalidomide is better suited to maintenance, but little data are available. At Mayo Clinic, if patients are treated with lenalidomide plus low-dose dexamethasone, patients are offered the option of continuing lenalidomide until progression after 12 to 18 months of treatment.

## Summary and Future Directions

Similar to historical drugs, the efficacy of novel multiple myeloma regimens have to be balanced against their higher toxicities. At present, in elderly patients, MPT, MPV, MPR, and lenalidomide plus low-dose dexamethasone have all shown to possess significant clinical activity. Treatment with MPT and MPV are supported by phase III trials showing superiority in overall survival compared with MP. Lenalidomide and low-dose dexamethasone had the advantage of low toxicity. Randomized trials have not compared these regimens, and in the absence of such trials, the choice of regimen should take into account several factors. Although the numbers are small, it appears that MPV overcomes the adverse effect of chromosomal abnormalities.[50] Thus, in the presence of high-risk cytogenetic features (Table 2), as well as in patients at high risk for thromboembolism, and in patients with renal insufficiency, MPV is the preferred option, whereas MPT is preferred for patients with standard-risk disease. Lenalidomide plus low-dose dexamethasone is a reasonable alternative to MPT. MPR is also an emerging alternative. There is no evidence that continued chemotherapy with MP is of benefit after achieving a plateau state, and hence, treatment with MPT and MPV is given for a fixed duration of time. There is a risk of myelodysplasia from continued treatment with alkylating agents.

Management of complications in patients with multiple myeloma is also important, especially in the elderly with more comorbidity. Recommendations on the management of complications such as skeletal disease, hypercalcemia, anemia, renal insufficiency, infections, and thrombosis have been published.[13,24,57]

Results from three population-based studies (one registry-based Swedish study, one registry-based U.S. SEER study, and one hospital-based study from the Mayo Clinic, MN), indicate that survival in multiple myeloma has improved in recent years after the introduction of the novel agents.[58–60] However, in all, the improvement was predominantly observed in the younger patients. A limitation of these investigations is the fact that none of the three studies had detailed information on individual patients' clinical characteristics or therapy. Underlying causes of the absence of improvement in long-term survival among elderly patients remain unclear and are probably multifactorial, including increased comorbidity among older patients. Early mortality has been reported to be higher among elderly patients.[61] In addition to the fact that patients do not tolerate aggressive treatment such as high-dose therapy, it has also been proposed that elderly patients present with a more advanced disease at diagnosis.[62,63] Results from randomized studies indicate that survival has improved in elderly patients with multiple myeloma with the introduction of novel agents. Innovative agents and procedures suitable for the older patient (>70 years) coupled with better prognostic markers used to guide individualized treatment in multiple myeloma are greatly needed.

In the shorter perspective, a key clinical challenge will be to better define the optimal sequence, combination(s), and use of available novel multiple myeloma drugs. In the future, molecular diagnostics/prognostics together with more targeted designed drugs and integrated molecular monitoring will likely become increasingly important to explain clinical heterogeneity, to provide more personalized treatment strategies, and, thereby, to improve survival for multiple myeloma patients.[21]

# REFERENCES

1. Kyle RA, Rajkumar SV. Monoclonal gammopathy of undetermined significance. *Br J Haematol.* 2006;134:573–589.
2. Swerdlov SH, Campo E, Harris NL, et al, eds. *WHO Classification of Tumours of Haematopoietic and Lymphoid Tissues.* Lyon: IARC; 2008.
3. Landgren O, Kyle RA, Pfeiffer RM, et al. Monoclonal gammopathy of undetermined significance (MGUS) consistently precedes multiple myeloma: a prospective study. *Blood.* 2009;113:5412–5417.
4. Ries LAG, Eisner MP, Kosary CL, eds. *SEER Cancer Statistics Review, 1975–2001.* Bethesda, MD: National Cancer Institute; 2004.
5. Socialstyrelsen. *Cancer Incidence in Sweden 2006.* Stockholm, Sweden: Socialstyrelsen; 2007.
6. Kyle RA, Gertz MA, Witzig TE, et al. Review of 1027 patients with newly diagnosed multiple myeloma. *Mayo Clin Proc.* 2003;78:21–33.
7. Landgren O, Kyle RA. Multiple myeloma, chronic lymphocytic leukaemia and associated precursor diseases. *Br J Haematol.* 2007;139:717–723.
8. Landgren O, Weiss BM. Patterns of monoclonal gammopathy of undetermined significance and multiple myeloma in various ethnic/racial groups: support for genetic factors in pathogenesis. *Leukemia.* 2009;23:1691–1697.
9. Kristinsson SY, Bjorkholm M, Goldin LR, et al. Patterns of hematologic malignancies and solid tumors among 37,838 first-degree relatives of 13,896 patients with multiple myeloma in Sweden. *Int J Cancer.* 2009;125:2147–2150.
10. Landgren O, Kristinsson SY, Goldin LR, et al. Risk of plasma cell and lymphoproliferative disorders among 14621 first-degree relatives of 4458 patients with monoclonal gammopathy of undetermined significance in Sweden. *Blood.* 2009;114:791–795.
11. Vachon CM, Kyle RA, Therneau TM, et al. Increased risk of monoclonal gammopathy in first-degree relatives of patients with multiple myeloma or monoclonal gammopathy of undetermined significance. *Blood.* 2009;114:785–790.
12. Kyle RA, Remstein ED, Therneau TM, et al. Clinical course and prognosis of smoldering (asymptomatic) multiple myeloma. *N Engl J Med.* 2007;356:2582–2590.
13. Kyle RA, Rajkumar SV. Multiple myeloma. *N Engl J Med.* 2004;351:1860–1873.
14. Greipp PR, San Miguel J, Durie BG, et al. International staging system for multiple myeloma. *J Clin Oncol.* 2005;23:3412–3420.
15. Dispenzieri A, Rajkumar SV, Gertz MA, et al. Treatment of newly diagnosed multiple myeloma based on mayo stratification of myeloma and risk-adapted therapy (mSMART): consensus statement. *Mayo Clin Proc.* 2007;82:323–341.
16. Stewart AK, Bergsagel PL, Greipp PR, et al. A practical guide to defining high-risk myeloma for clinical trials, patient counseling and choice of therapy. *Leukemia.* 2007;21:529–534.
17. Smadja NV, Bastard C, Brigaudeau C, et al. Hypodiploidy is a major prognostic factor in multiple myeloma. *Blood.* 2001;98:2229–2238.
18. Fonseca R, Blood E, Rue M, et al. Clinical and biologic implications of recurrent genomic aberrations in myeloma. *Blood.* 2003;101:4569–4575.
19. Gertz MA, Lacy MQ, Dispenzieri A, et al. Clinical implications of t(11;14) (q13;q32), t(4;14)(p16.3;q32), and – 17p13 in myeloma patients treated with high-dose therapy. *Blood.* 2005;106:2837–2840.
20. Avet-Loiseau H, Attal M, Moreau P, et al. Genetic abnormalities and survival in multiple myeloma: the experience of the Intergroupe Francophone du Myelome. *Blood.* 2007;109:3489–3495.
21. Anguiano A, Tuchman SA, Acharya C, et al. Gene expression profiles of tumor biology provide a novel approach to prognosis and may guide the selection of therapeutic targets in multiple myeloma. *J Clin Oncol.* 2009;27:4197–4203.
22. Zhan F, Tian E, Bumm K, et al. Gene expression profiling of human plasma cell differentiation and classification of multiple myeloma based on similarities to distinct stages of late-stage B-cell development. *Blood.* 2003;101:1128–1140.
23. Carrasco DR, Tonon G, Huang Y, et al. High-resolution genomic profiles define distinct clinico-pathogenetic subgroups of multiple myeloma patients. *Cancer Cell.* 2006;9:313–325.
24. Palumbo A, Rajkumar SV, Dimopoulos MA, et al. Prevention of thalidomide- and lenalidomide-associated thrombosis in myeloma. *Leukemia.* 2008;22:414–423.
25. Attal M, Harousseau JL, Stoppa AM, et al. A prospective, randomized trial of autologous bone marrow transplantation and chemotherapy in multiple myeloma. Intergroupe Francais du Myelome. *N Engl J Med.* 1996;335:91–97.
26. Hjorth M, Hellquist L, Holmberg E, et al. Initial versus deferred melphalan-prednisone therapy for asymptomatic multiple myeloma stage I—a randomized study. Myeloma Group of Western Sweden. *Eur J Haematol.* 1993;50:95–102.
27. Badros A, Barlogie B, Siegel E, et al. Results of autologous stem cell transplant in multiple myeloma patients with renal failure. *Br J Haematol.* 2001;114:822–829.
28. Combination chemotherapy versus melphalan plus prednisone as treatment for multiple myeloma: an overview of 6,633 patients from 27 randomized trials. Myeloma Trialists' Collaborative Group. *J Clin Oncol.* 1998;16:3832–3842.
29. Alexanian R, Haut A, Khan AU, et al. Treatment for multiple myeloma. Combination chemotherapy with different melphalan dose regimens. *JAMA.* 1969;208:1680–1685.
30. Corral LG, Haslett PA, Muller GW, et al. Differential cytokine modulation and T cell activation by two distinct classes of thalidomide analogues that are potent inhibitors of TNF-alpha. *J Immunol.* 1999;163:380–386.
31. Dredge K, Marriott JB, Macdonald CD, et al. Novel thalidomide analogues display anti-angiogenic activity independently of immunomodulatory effects. *Br J Cancer.* 2002;87:1166–1172.
32. Mitra-Kaushik S, Harding JC, Hess JL, et al. Effects of the proteasome inhibitor PS-341 on tumor growth in HTLV-1 Tax transgenic mice and Tax tumor transplants. *Blood.* 2004;104:802–809.
33. Hideshima T, Ikeda H, Chauhan D, et al. Bortezomib induces canonical nuclear factor-kappaB activation in multiple myeloma cells. *Blood.* 2009;114:1046–1052.
34. Rajkumar SV, Blood E, Vesole D, et al. Phase III clinical trial of thalidomide plus dexamethasone compared with dexamethasone alone in newly diagnosed multiple myeloma: a clinical trial coordinated by the Eastern Cooperative Oncology Group. *J Clin Oncol.* 2006;24:431–436.
35. Cavo M, Zamagni E, Tosi P, et al. Superiority of thalidomide and dexamethasone over vincristine-doxorubicindexamethasone (VAD) as primary therapy in preparation for autologous transplantation for multiple myeloma. *Blood.* 2005;106:35–39.
36. Barlogie B, Pineda-Roman M, van Rhee F, et al. Thalidomide arm of total therapy 2 improves complete remission duration and survival in myeloma patients with metaphase cytogenetic abnormalities. *Blood.* 2008;112:3115–3121.
37. Jagannath S, Durie BG, Wolf J, et al. Bortezomib therapy alone and in combination with dexamethasone for previously untreated symptomatic multiple myeloma. *Br J Haematol.* 2005;129:776–783.
38. Richardson PG, Sonneveld P, Schuster MW, et al. Bortezomib or high-dose dexamethasone for relapsed multiple myeloma. *N Engl J Med.* 2005;352:2487–2498.
39. Dimopoulos M, Spencer A, Attal M, et al. Lenalidomide plus dexamethasone for relapsed or refractory multiple myeloma. *N Engl J Med.* 2007;357:2123–2132.
40. Weber DM, Chen C, Niesvizky R, et al. Lenalidomide plus dexamethasone for relapsed multiple myeloma in North America. *N Engl J Med.* 2007;357:2133–2142.
41. Palumbo A, Bringhen S, Caravita T, et al. Oral melphalan and prednisone chemotherapy plus thalidomide compared with melphalan and prednisone alone in elderly patients with multiple myeloma: randomised controlled trial. *Lancet.* 2006;367:825–831.
42. Palumbo A, Bringhen S, Liberati AM, et al. Oral melphalan, prednisone, and thalidomide in elderly patients with multiple myeloma: updated results of a randomized controlled trial. *Blood.* 2008;112:3107–3114.
43. Facon T, Mary JY, Hulin C, et al. Melphalan and prednisone plus thalidomide versus melphalan and prednisone alone or reduced-intensity autologous stem

cell transplantation in elderly patients with multiple myeloma (IFM 99-06): a randomised trial. *Lancet.* 2007;370:1209–1218.

44. Hulin C, Facon T, Rodon P, et al. Efficacy of melphalan and prednisone plus thalidomide in patients older than 75 years with newly diagnosed multiple myeloma: IFM 01/01 trial. *J Clin Oncol.* 2009;27:3664–3670.

45. Waage A, Gimsing P, Juliusson G, et al. Melphalan-prednisone-thalidomide to newly diagnosed patients with multiple myeloma: a placebo controlled randomized phase 3 trial. *Blood.* 2007;110:Abstract 78a.

46. Wijermans P, Schaafsma M, van Norden Y, et al. Melphalan + prednisone versus melphalan + prednisone + thalidomide in induction therapy for multiple myeloma in elderly patients: final analysis of the Dutch C ooperative Group HOVON 49 study. *Blood.* 2008;112:Abstract 649.

47. Ludwig H, Hajek R, Tothova E, et al. Thalidomide-dexamethasone compared with melphalan-prednisolone in elderly patients with multiple myeloma. *Blood.* 2009;113:3435–3442.

48. Morgan G, Davies FE, Owen RG, et al. Thalidomide combinations improve response rates: results from the MRC IX study. *Blood.* 2007;110:Abstract 3593.

49. Mateos MV, Hernandez JM, Hernandez MT, et al. Bortezomib plus melphalan and prednisone in elderly untreated patients with multiple myeloma: results of a multicenter phase $^{1}/_{2}$ study. *Blood.* 2006;108:2165–2172.

50. San Miguel JF, Schlag R, Khuageva NK, et al. Bortezomib plus melphalan and prednisone for initial treatment of multiple myeloma. *N Engl J Med.* 2008;359:906–917.

51. Palumbo A, Falco P, Corradini P, et al. Melphalan, prednisone, and lenalidomide treatment for newly diagnosed myeloma: a report from the GIMEMA—Italian Multiple Myeloma Network. *J Clin Oncol.* 2007;25:4459–4465.

52. Rajkumar SV, Jacobus S, Callander N, et al. Lenalidomide plus high-dose dexamethasone versus lenalidomide plus low-dose dexamethasone as initial therapy for newly diagnosed multiple myeloma: an open-label randomised controlled trial. *Lancet Oncol.* October 22, 2009. doi: 10.1016/S1470-2045(09)70284-0.

53. Barlogie B, Tricot G, Anaissie E, et al. Thalidomide and hematopoietic-cell transplantation for multiple myeloma. *N Engl J Med.* 2006;354:1021–1030.

54. Attal M, Harousseau JL, Leyvraz S, et al. Maintenance therapy with thalidomide improves survival in patients with multiple myeloma. *Blood.* 2006;108:3289–3294.

55. Abdelkefi A, Ladeb S, Torjman L, et al. Single autologous stem-cell transplantation followed by maintenance therapy with thalidomide is superior to double autologous transplantation in multiple myeloma: results of a multicenter randomized clinical trial. *Blood.* 2008;111:1805–1810.

56. Spencer A, Prince HM, Roberts AW, et al. Consolidation therapy with low-dose thalidomide and prednisolone prolongs the survival of multiple myeloma patients undergoing a single autologous stem-cell transplantation procedure. *J Clin Oncol.* 2009;27:1788–1793.

57. Kyle RA, Yee GC, Somerfield MR, et al. American Society of Clinical Oncology 2007 clinical practice guideline update on the role of bisphosphonates in multiple myeloma. *J Clin Oncol.* 2007;25:2464–2472.

58. Kristinsson SY, Landgren O, Dickman PW, et al. Patterns of survival in multiple myeloma: a population-based study of patients diagnosed in Sweden from 1973 to 2003. *J Clin Oncol.* 2007;25:1993–1999.

59. Brenner H, Gondos A, Pulte D. Recent major improvement in long-term survival of younger patients with multiple myeloma. *Blood.* 2008;111:2521–2526.

60. Kumar SK, Rajkumar SV, Dispenzieri A, et al. Improved survival in multiple myeloma and the impact of novel therapies. *Blood.* 2008;111:2516–2520.

61. Augustson BM, Begum G, Dunn JA, et al. Early mortality after diagnosis of multiple myeloma: analysis of patients entered onto the United Kingdom Medical Research Council trials between 1980 and 2002—Medical Research Council Adult Leukaemia Working Party. *J Clin Oncol.* 2005;23:9219–9226.

62. Anagnostopoulos A, Gika D, Symeonidis A, et al. Multiple myeloma in elderly patients: prognostic factors and outcome. *Eur J Haematol.* 2005;75:370–375.

63. Lenhoff S, Hjorth M, Westin J, et al. Impact of age on survival after intensive therapy for multiple myeloma: a population-based study by the Nordic Myeloma Study Group. *Br J Haematol.* 2006;133:389–396.

# CHAPTER

# 65

# Integrating Novel Therapies in the Transplant Paradigm

Jean-Luc Harousseau

## AUTOLOGOUS STEM CELL TRANSPLANTATION

Until now high-dose therapy (HDT) supported by autologous stem cell transplantation (ASCT) has been considered the standard of care for frontline therapy for multiple myeloma (MM) in younger patients with normal renal function and without severe comorbidities.[1]

However, the introduction of novel agents thalidomide, bortezomib, and lenalidomide is changing the scenario in 2 ways. First, these agents can be added to HDT before and/or after ASCT with the objectives of increasing the complete remission (CR) rate and of prolonging first remission duration.

Second, the use of novel agents as frontline therapy in combination with either dexamethasone or alkylating agents yield CR rates and progression-free survival (PFS) rates that are comparable with those achieved with HDT. Therefore, the role of ASCT is again a matter of debate: should it be used upfront or only as salvage treatment at progression in patients initially treated with novel agents?

### ASCT Before the Era of Novel Therapies

Two randomized studies showed the superiority of HDT with ASCT compared with conventional chemotherapy in patients younger than 65 years of age.[2,3] In these trials, HDT significantly improved the response rate, event-free survival (EFS), and overall survival (OS). However, other randomized studies were published in the past 10 years and not all were that positive. A meta-analysis of all randomized trials indicated that HDT significantly improved the EFS but not the OS.[4] This was partly explained by the impact of ASCT after relapse in patients initially treated with conventional chemotherapy.[1] Overall, the use of ASCT either initially or at relapse was a major factor in the survival improvement described in the nineties for patients aged younger than 60 years.[5]

An important finding from these studies was the strong relationship between quality of response and OS.[2,3] Patients achieving CR or at least very good partial remission (VGPR) had longer OS than patients who had only partial remission. The relationship between the magnitude of response and the outcome was confirmed in most clinical trials on HDT.[6] The consequences of this finding are

- Response criteria have been redefined to introduce the concepts of CR (negative immunofixation) and VGPR ($\geq$90% reduction of the M-component).[7,8]
- Achievement of at least VGPR is a simple and robust prognostic factor in the context of HDT and is now considered an objective of any treatment.[9]

With HDT, median EFS was 24 to 30 months but there was no plateau of the EFS curves and almost all patients did ultimately relapse.[1] Therefore, the concept of double ASCT was developed by the Arkansas group in the late eighties with the objective of improving ASCT results by further increasing the CR rate.[10]

The IFM conducted a randomized trial comparing single and double ASCT in 599 patients up to 60 years of age.[11] On an intent-to-treat basis, the 7-year EFS and OS were significantly improved in the double ASCT arm. The benefit in EFS but not in OS was confirmed by 2 other randomized studies.[12,13] However, many investigators considered the benefit of this approach to be marginal, and were concerned by cost and morbidity. Therefore, defining which patients benefit more from this aggressive management seemed important. In 2 studies, patients achieving CR or VGPR after the first transplant did not benefit from the second.[11,12] Even more importantly, although results of double ASCT were very satisfactory for patients with good-risk MM, patients with poor-risk characteristics still did poorly, despite this more intensive regimen. As an example in the IFM 99 trial, patients with both a high beta-2 microglobulin level and cytogenetic abnormalities associated with poor outcome, either t(4;14) or del 17p, had a median OS inferior to 2 years.[14] For those patients, other solutions were clearly needed.

### ASCT in the Era of Novel Agents: Novel Agents in Combination With ASCT

The introduction of novel agents (thalidomide, bortezomib and more recently Lenalidomide) has provided a new opportunity to improve ASCT results. They have been evaluated both after and before ASCT.

### Novel Agents After ASCT

Because even with double ASCT almost all patients ultimately relapse, maintenance therapy was a logical approach to prolong remission duration and thalidomide was the first to be evaluated in this indication. Six randomized trials have evaluated the impact of thalidomide maintenance after ASCT in MM.[15–20] These trials differed by their design and by the dose and duration of thalidomide maintenance (Table 1). Despite these disparities, all 6 studies showed a benefit in favor of thalidomide in terms of response rate (CR or $\geq$VGPR) and PFS (Table 2).

Results are not that clear cut as regards OS. While in the initial publication of the French and Tunisian studies,[16,17] OS was significantly longer in the thalidomide arm, with longer follow-up this survival advantage disappeared and the Tunisian authors did retract recently.[21] On the contrary, the first publication from the Arkansas group showed no significant difference in OS between the 2 arms, due to a shorter OS after relapse in patients initially treated with thalidomide.[15] However, in the updated analysis, the OS curves segregated after 5 years, and there was actually a trend in favor of thalidomide and a significant benefit in the subgroup of patients with karyotypic abnormalities.[22]

In the Dutch and in the British studies, the PFS benefit did not translate into a significant OS benefit, again due to a shorter OS after relapse in the thalidomide arm.[18,19]

**TABLE 1.**   Post-ASCT Maintenance With Thalidomide. Randomized Studies

| Author | Induction | ASCT | Thalidomide Administration | Design |
|---|---|---|---|---|
| Attal et al[16] | No Thal | Double | Starting dose 400 mg/D until relapse | After ASCT (if no progression) No treatment vs. Thal + pamidronate |
| Barlogie et al[15] | 50% Thal | Double | Starting dose 400 mg/D until relapse | Initial randomization Thal vs. no Thal |
| Abdelkefi et al[17] | Thal | Single + Thal vs. double | 100 mg/D 6 mo | After ASCT |
| Spencer et al[18] | No Thal | Single | 200 mg/D 1 yr | After ASCT (if no progression) |
| Morgan et al[19] | 50% Thal | Single | 100 mg/D until relapse | After ASCT |
| Lokhorst et al[20] | 50% Thal | Double | 200 mg/D until relapse | Initial randomization TAD → Thal VAD → IFN |

Thal indicates thalidomide; TAD, thalidomide adriamycin dexametasone; and IFN, interferon.

## How Can We Analyze These Differences?

The first message is that OS data should not be analyzed and published too early. In the past, the only possibility at relapse was conventional chemotherapy. Currently, we have more possibilities (ASCT, thalidomide and lenalidomide, bortezomib) and survival after relapse may be longer than duration of first response.

Second, OS obviously depends on salvage treatments. If thalidomide is prescribed until relapse or severe toxicity, one can imagine that thalidomide should not be used at relapse. Therefore, more patients received thalidomide at relapse in the no-thalidomide arms and the design of these studies was rather early (upfront) thalidomide versus late (at relapse) thalidomide. Moreover, the risk of thalidomide-induced peripheral neuropathy is clearly related to the cumulative dose and prolonged exposure carries the risk of severe neuropathy precluding or limiting the use of bortezomib at relapse. Prolonged exposure to thalidomide might also select clones resistant to thalidomide but also to others agents. We already know that lenalidomide is less effective in patients resistant to thalidomide than in thalidomide-naive patients.[23]

Finally salvage treatment depends on the availability of novel agents. When the British trial was performed, in UK there was a limited access to bortezomib and lenalidomide was not available out of a clinical trial. Therefore, there were less therapeutic possibilities at relapse in the thalidomide arm (including thalidomide).

These considerations clearly raise the issue of the optimal duration of maintenance therapy. Should it be fixed as in the Tunisian or Australian studies[17,18] or unlimited as in the other 4 studies.[15,16,19,20] The theoretical interest of prolonged maintenance is to further improve the level of tumor burden reduction, hence prolonging PFS, but on the other hand, this benefit might be hampered by reduced salvage possibilities, hence a shorter OS after relapse. A randomized study addressing this question might be extremely useful.

## Additional Questions

### What Is the Optimal Dose?

In the first 2 studies, the initial daily dosage was high (400 mg) and the duration of treatment was unlimited, which explains the high incidence of severe neuropathy (grade $\geq 3$) and the high number of patients who discontinued treatment because of toxicity.[15,16] Although no randomized study has compared different schedules of administration, doses of 100 mg or 200 mg/d during 6 to 12 months seem to be effective and better tolerated.[17,18]

**TABLE 2.**   Results of Randomized Studies on Post-ASCT Maintenance With Thalidomide

| Author | No. Patients | Median Follow-Up | Response Rate | PFS or EFS | OS Initial Publications | OS Updated Results (Reference) |
|---|---|---|---|---|---|---|
| Barlogie et al[15] | 668 | 42 m | 62% vs. 43%, $P < 0.001$ | 5 yr EFS, 56% vs. 44%, $P = 0.01$ | 5 yr OS, 65% vs. 65% | $P = 0.09$[21] |
| Attal et al[16] | 597 | 40 m | *67% vs. 55% or 57%, $P = 0.03$ | 3 yr EFS, 52% vs. 37%, $P = 0.002$ | 4-yr, 87% vs. 75%, $P = 0.04$ | NS |
| Abdelkefi et al[17] | 195 | 33 m | *68% vs. 54%, $P = 0.04$ | 3-yr PFS, 85% vs. 57%, $P = 0.02$ | 3 yr, 85% vs. 65%, $P = 0.04$ | NS[22] |
| Spencer et al[18] | 269 | 3 yr | 65% vs. 44%*, $P < 0.001$ | 3 yr PFS, 42% vs. 23%, $P < 0.001$ | 3 yr, 86% vs. 75%, $P = 0.004$ | ND |
| Morgan et al[19] | 820[†] | 32 mo | NA | Better in patients with <VGPR, $P < 0.007$ | Median OS, NS | ND |
| Lokhorst et al[20] | 556 | 52 mo | *66% vs. 54%, $P = 0.005$ | Median EFS, 34 m vs. 22 m, $P < 0.001$ | 73 m vs. 60 m, $P = 0.77$ | ND |

*Complete response + very good partial response (VGPR).
[†]Including patients receiving nonintensive induction.
NA indicates not available; ND, not done; and NS, not significant.

## Is Thalidomide Maintenance Useful for All Patients and Are We Able to Predict Patients Who Will Benefit From Maintenance Therapy?

Unfortunately, there is no clear response to this question. In the French study, patients with del(13) apparently did not benefit from thalidomide maintenance, but at the time of this trial, other abnormalities that are frequently associated with del(13), such as t(4;14) or 17p del were not routinely studied.[16] We now know that the negative prognostic impact of del(13) is mostly due to these 2 additional abnormalities.[14] We have no data on the impact of thalidomide in the subgroup of patients with these poor-risk abnormalities, although in a preliminary report of the British study, thalidomide seemed to do poorly in patients with del (17p).[19]

In the updated analysis of the Arkansas study, thalidomide significantly improved OS of patients with cytogenetic abnormalities as defined by conventional karyotyping.[22] This heterogeneous subgroup of patients is generally considered as poor risk, because the possibility of studying mitoses is associated with a more proliferative disease.

Finally, in the French and British studies, only patients who did not achieve at least a VGPR after transplant did benefit from thalidomide maintenance,[16,19] but this was not confirmed in the Australian study.[18]

### Other Novel Agents as Maintenance Therapy After ASCT

Lenalidomide, which is better tolerated than thalidomide and can be prescribed safely for long periods of time appears to be an ideal candidate. However, this agent is more myelotoxic than thalidomide, and the optimal dose of lenalidomide after high-dose therapy is not known. Two large randomized trials from the IFM and the CALGB groups have tested lenalidomide as maintenance after ASCT, but results of these studies are not available.

Bortezomib has also been evaluated in this setting by the Dutch and the Spanish groups. Because bortezomib is associated with a high incidence of peripheral neuropathy when used on a bi-weekly schedule at a dose of 1.3 mg/m$^2$, the interval between bortezomib injections is increased in this indication.

### Consolidation or Maintenance?

In all studies, PFS prolongation was associated with a CR or CR/VGPR increase. Therefore, thalidomide might act more by increasing the post-ASCT CR rate than by controlling the residual clone. In other words, post-ASCT thalidomide might be considered as a consolidation therapy and might be administered with the objective of further decreasing the tumor burden. If that is true, we still have to determine the optimal level of response. Is CR with negative immunofixation the requested level or should we try to obtain higher

levels of response (stringent response, immunophenotypic response, or even molecular response)? Again this important question should be addressed in future trials. The Spanish group has already shown that immunophenotypic CR as assessed by multiparameter flow cytometry is associated with a better outcome than CR as defined only by immunofixation.[24]

If consolidation is needed, a combination might be more active than thalidomide alone and could be given for a limited period of time. The Italian group has shown that post-ASCT consolidation with a combination of bortezomib, thalidomide, and dexamethasone (VTD) may improve the level of remission and yield molecular remissions in some patients with already were at least in VGPR after ASCT.[25] This might translate into longer PFS. The role of short-term consolidation with novel agents is currently evaluated in clinical trials.

## Novel Agents as Induction Treatment Before ASCT

The standard induction therapy in patients who are candidates for ASCT was dexamethasone-based, either dexamethasone alone or VAD-like therapy. The primary objective of novel agents given in this context is to increase the CR rate not only before but also after ASCT. The increased CR rate might be converted into longer EFS and OS. Another interest would be to reduce the proportion of patients needing a second ASCT because of a less than VGPR after the first.

## Double Combinations

### Thalidomide-Dexamethasone (TD)

Thalidomide was the first novel agent to be used in this setting, in combination with dexamethasone (TD) (Table 3). This combination has been compared with Dexamethasone or VAD[26–28] in a historical control and in 2 randomized studies.

In all 3 studies, TD was superior to dexamethasone alone or VAD in terms of response rate or VGPR rate. However, the thalidomide-based regimens did not increase the CR rate before ASCT, which remained very low ≤10%). In the French trial, post-ASCT VGPR rates with TD and VAD were similar.[28] Moreover, these combinations with thalidomide induced a high incidence of deep-vein thrombosis. Therefore, the benefit of TD compared with VAD seems to remain modest.

### Bortezomib-Dexamethasone (VD)

The IFM has performed a randomized trial (IFM 2005–01) comparing 4 courses of induction treatment before ASCT with either VAD or VD in 482 patients with newly diagnosed MM.[29] Compared with VAD, VD regimen increased not only the overall response rate but also CR plus n-CR rate and the CR plus VGPR rate. More importantly, this higher pre-ASCT efficacy translated into a higher post-ASCT CR

**TABLE 3.** Novel Agents for Induction Therapy Before ASCT. Comparative Studies on 2-Drug Combinations

|  | TD vs. VAD | TD vs. D | VD vs. VAD | VD vs. VAD | RD vs. Rd |
|---|---|---|---|---|---|
| Author | Cavo et al[27] (historical control) | Rajkumar et al[26] (randomized) | Macro et al[28] (randomized) | Harousseau et al[29] (randomized) | Rajkumar et al[30] (randomized) |
| No. patients | 200 | 201 | 204 | 424 | 421 |
| Response rate after induction | ORR 76% vs. 52% CR = NS | ORR 69% vs. 59% CR = NS | ≥VGPR 35% vs. 17% | ORR 82% vs. 65% ≥ VGPR 39% vs. 16% | ORR 79% vs. 69% ≥ VGPR 42% vs. 24% |
| Response rate after ASCT | — | — | ≥VGPR 44% vs. 42% | CR + n-CR 37% vs. 19% ≥ VGPR 57 % vs. 38% | NA |
|  | NA | NA |  |  |  |

ORR indicates overall response rate; RD, lenalidomide plus high-dose dexamethasone; n-CR, near-complete response; Rd, lenalidomide plus low-dose dexamethasone; VGPR, very good partial response; NS, not significant; NA, not available; and D, dexamethasone.

plus n-CR or CR plus VGPR rates. This better efficacy was observed across all prognostic subgroups, including poor-risk cytogenetics such as t(4;14) and del (17p). The VD regimen was well tolerated with no more adverse events than with the standard VAD except peripheral neuropathy (27% grade $\geq$2). Stem cell collection after priming with G-CSF alone was sufficient to allow one ASCT in 97% of patients.

Therefore, VD is superior to VAD and seems to be more effective than TD at least in terms of post-ASCT VGPR. VD is a new standard induction treatment before ASCT to which other more complex regimens should be compared.

### Lenalidomide-Dexamethasone (RD)

In the absence of randomized comparisons with other induction regimens, the role of lenalidomide-dexamethasone is unclear. In clinical trials that have evaluated this combination as initial therapy, only part of the patients were actually candidates for ASCT. However, high response rates (including CR + VGPR rate) after 4 cycles have been reported.[30] Concerns regarding the hematopoietic quality of stem cell collection in relation with the myelotoxicity of lenalidomide[31,32] have been solved by the use of cyclophosphamide as part of the mobilization regimen.[33]

## Triple Combinations

The addition of a 3rd agent (cyclophosphamide or doxorubicine) to either thalidomide or bortezomib looks very attractive (Table 4). The TAD (thalidomide, doxorubicine, and dexamethasone), TCD (thalidomide, cyclophosphamide, and dexamethasone), and PAD (bortezomib, doxorubicine, and dexamethasone) regimens have been compared with VAD in large randomized trials.[34-36] All 3 new combination were significantly superior to VAD in terms of CR plus VGCR rates both before and after ASCT, but in the absence of a randomized study, it is not currently possible to, which is the best and whether they are superior to VD.

Finally, the combinations of 2 novel agents might be even more effective. The Italian group recently showed results of a randomized trial comparing VTD and TD.[37] The CR plus VGPR rates were significantly superior to those achieved with TD both before (60% vs. 27%) and after ASCT (77% vs. 42%). Preliminary results of the Spanish group also show impressive CR rates.[38]

To summarize, induction regimens including novel agents look very promising because they increase the response rate compared with classic regimens like VAD. Preliminary results with VD and VTD indicate that this higher-tumor burden reduction might translate into prolonged PFS.[29,37] However, longer follow-up is needed before drawing definite conclusions.

## Novel Agents Before and After ASCT

A number of groups are currently evaluating novel therapies both before and after ASCT but the only mature results come from the Arkansas group investigators. They have integrated thalidomide and bortezomib in their complex approach including tandem ASCT called total therapy programs.

In the total therapy 2 trial, patients were randomly assigned to receive thalidomide throughout their treatment (induction, consolidation, and maintenance).[22]

More recently, in the total therapy 3 program, the same group has added bortezomib. Preliminary results show impressive CR rates and 2-year PFS.[39] Again longer follow-up is needed but an important message is that the addition of bortezomib might overcome the poor prognosis associated with t(4;14).[40]

## ASCT in the Era of Novel Agents: Novel Agents in Place of ASCT

Frontline therapy with novel agents is markedly improving the outcome in patients who are not candidates for ASCT, especially elderly patients. Several European groups have evaluated the combination melphalan-prednisone with,[41,42] bortezomib,[43] or lenalidomide.[44] Combinations of lenalidomide plus dexamethasone have been evaluated by US investigators.[30,45,46]

Although most of these studies have been performed in elderly patients (older than 65 years), the CR plus VGPR rates ranges from 40% to >70%. In one of these studies, the CR rate was 30%, which is even better that what was achieved in younger patients with single ASCT before the introduction of novel agents.[42] In the most mature studies, median PFS are around 2 years,[41-43] and preliminary results with lenalidomide plus dexamethasone show promising PFS and OS data.[30,45] Therefore, some investigators already state that ASCT should no longer be used in frontline therapy, but that stem cells could be collected during the first month of therapy with novel agents and used only as a rescue at time of relapse or progression. However, although these results are impressive, they do not necessarily indicate the end of ASCT as primary therapy in MM for a number of reasons.

- Follow-up is still short in several studies with novel agents.
- In studies with upfront lenalidomide, older patients and patients who are not willing to undergo ASCT are mixed with patients who receive HDT plus ASCT.
- ASCT results have recently improved with double ASCT and with the addition of novel agents.

Therefore, randomized studies comparing novel agents with or without early transplantation are needed.

**TABLE 4.**    Novel Agents for Induction Therapy Before ASCT: Randomized Studies on 3-Drug Combinations

|  | TAD vs. VAD | RD vs. c-VAD | PAD vs. VAD | VTD vs. TD |
|---|---|---|---|---|
| Author | Lokhorst et al[34] | Morgan et al[35] | Sonneveld et al[36] | Cavo et al[37] |
| No. patients | 402 | 251 | 300 | 460 |
| Response after induction | ORR 72% vs. 54% $\geq$ VGPR 32% vs. 15% | CR 19% vs. 9% $\geq$ VGPR 39% vs. 27% | ORR 83% vs. 59% $\geq$ VGPR 42% vs. 15% | ORR 94% vs. 79% $\geq$ 62% vs. 29% |
| Response after ASCT | CR 16% vs. 11% $\geq$ VGPR 49% vs. 32% | CR 51% vs. 40% $\geq$ VGPR 67% vs. 43% | CR + n-CR 23% vs. 9% $\geq$ VGPR 59% vs. 50% | CR 43% vs. 23% $\geq$ VGPR 76% vs. 58% |

ORR indicates overall response rate; CR, complete response; n-CR, near-complete response; TD, thalidomide-dexamethasone; c-VAD, cyclophosphamide plus VAD; TAD, thalidomide adriamycine dexamethasone; PAD, bortezomib adriamycin dexamethasone; and VTD, bortezomib thalidomide dexamethasone.

## ALLOGENEIC STEM CELL TRANSPLANTATION

Allogeneic SCT following myeloablative preparative regimen can induce molecular remissions and seems to be the only available therapy with a potential for cure or long-term disease control in at least some patients. However, toxicity is excessively high with transplant-related mortality (TRM) of up to 50% in some studies. Therefore, allogeneic BMT after myeloablative conditioning is abandoned by a large majority of investigators.[47]

Much of the clinical impact of allogeneic SCT has been attributed to the immunologic effect of donor lymphoid cells which is called graft-versus-myeloma (GVM). This antitumor effect of donor immunocompetent cells, which is unfortunately linked to graft-versus host disease (GVHD), is the basis of reduced intensity conditioning (RIC) allogeneic SCT. The principle of RIC allogeneic transplantation is to reduce transplant-related toxicity, while harnessing GVM effect.

Preliminary experience showed that RIC allogeneic SCT is possible in MM, with reduced TRM even in older patients (older than 60 years of age) and with matched-unrelated donors.[48] However, it seemed rapidly that relapses were frequent when RIC allotransplants were used in relapsed/refractory patients.[49] These results suggested that the allogeneic GVM effect is not sufficient and that it remains important to reduce tumor burden. Therefore, RIC allotransplantation is now mostly used after HDT followed by ASCT.

The Seattle group recently updated results obtained with tandem ASCT-RIC allogeneic SCT.[50] Although the CR rate was 59% and the TRM 11% at 1 year, grades 2 to 4 acute GVHD was 42% and extensive chronic GVHD was 74%. The 5-year PFS and OS were, respectively, 36% and 64%. Large prospective trials comparing double ASCT and tandem ASCT-RIC allotransplantation have been performed in the United States and in Europe but all results are not yet fully available. Three of these studies have been published but selection of patients, preparative regimen and GVHD prophylaxis were different.[51–53] The Italian study was the only one to show a significant benefit in favor of RIC allo.

Even though TRM is reduced with RIC allogeneic SCT compared with standard myeloablative regimens, it remains in the order of 10% to 15% at 1-year for newly diagnosed patients and the incidence of chronic GVHD is still very high.

Moreover, relapses still remain too frequent, especially in the absence of chronic GVHD.[48] Novel agents have been used to treat relapses after allogeneic SCT.[54–56] The next step is to use them as posttransplant immunotherapy before relapse with the objective of upgrading the level of response. In a preliminary experience, Kroger et al[57] have proposed novel agents (thalidomide, bortezomib, or lenalidomide) to patients who were not in CR after allo-SCT and donor lymphocyte infusions. They could convert partial remission to CR in 59% of patients and to molecular remissions in 50% of patients.

There are still too many areas of uncertainty and the risk of GVHD-associated severe toxicity remains too high with tandem ASCT-RIC allotransplantation; therefore, this strategy should not be proposed in the upfront setting out of a clinical trial, especially for patients without adverse prognostic factors, considering the very good results achieved in this subgroup of patients with single or tandem ASCT plus novel agents or even with novel agents without ASCT.

## REFERENCES

1. Harousseau J-L, Moreau P. Autologous stem-cell transplantation in multiple myeloma. *N Engl J Med.* 2009;360:2645–2654.
2. Attal M, Harousseau JL, Stoppa AM, et al. A prospective randomized trial of autologous bone marrow transplantation and chemotherapy in multiple myeloma. *N Engl J Med.* 1996;335:91–97.
3. Child JA, Morgan GJ, Davies FE, et al. High-dose chemotherapy with hematopoietic stem-cell rescue for multiple myeloma. *N Engl J Med.* 2003;348: 1875–1883.
4. Koreth J, Cutler CS, Djulbegovic B, et al. High-dose therapy with single autologous transplantation versus chemotherapy for newly diagnosed multpiple myeloma. A systematic review and meta-analysis of randomized controlled trials. *Biol Blood Marrow Transplant.* 2007;13:183–196.
5. Kumar S, Rajkumar SV, Dispenzieri A, et al. Improved survival in multiple myeloma. *Blood.* 2008;111:2516–2520.
6. Harousseau J-L, Attal M, Avet-Loiseau H. The role of complete response in multiple myeloma. *Blood.* 2009;114:3139–3146.
7. Blade J, Samson D, Reece D, et al. Criteria for evaluating disease response and progression in patients treated with high-dose therapy and haematopoietic stem cell transplantation. *Br J Haematol.* 1998;102:1115–1123.
8. Durie BG, Harousseau JL, San Miguel JS, et al. International uniform response criteria for multiple myeloma. *Leukemia.* 2006;20:1467–1473.
9. Harousseau JL, Avet-Loiseau H, Attal M, et al. Achieving at least very good partial remission is a simple and robust prognostic factor in patients with multiple myeloma treated with high-dose therapy: long-term results if the IFM 99–02 and 99–04 trials. *J Clin Oncol.* In press.
10. Barlogie B, Jagannath S, Desikan KR, et al. Total therapy with tandem autotransplants for newly diagnosed multiple myeloma. *Blood.* 1999;93:55–65.
11. Attal M, Harousseau JL, Facon T, et al. Intergroupe Francophone du Myeloma:single versus double autologous stem cell transplantation for multiple myeloma. *N Engl J Med.* 2003;349:2495–2425.
12. Cavo M, Tosi P, Zamagni E, et al. Prospective randomized study of single compared with double autologous stem cell transplantation for multiple myeloma: Bologna 96 clinical study. *J Clin Oncol.* 2007;25:2434–2441.
13. Sonneveld P, van der Holt B, Segeren CM, et al. Intermediate-dose melphalan compared with myeloablative treatment in multiple myeloma: long-term results of the Dutch Cooperative group HOVON 24 trial. *Haematologica.* 2007;92:928–935.
14. Avet-Loiseau H, Attal M, Moreau P, et al. Genetic abnormalities and survival in multiple myeloma: the experience of the Intergroupe Francophone du Myélome. *Blood.* 2007;109:3489–3495.
15. Barlogie B, Tricot G, Anaissie E, et al. Thalidomide and hematopoietic stem cell transplantation for multiple myeloma. *N Engl J Med.* 2006;354:1021–1030.
16. Attal M, Harousseau JL, Leyvraz S, et al. Maintenance therapy with thalidomide improves survival in multiple myeloma patients. *Blood.* 2006;15:3289–3295.
17. Abdelkefi A, Ladeb S, Torjman L, et al. Single autologous stem cell transplantation followed by maintenance therapy with thalidomide is superior to double autologous transplantation in multiple myeloma: results of a multicenter randomized clinical trial. *Blood.* 2008;111:1805–1810.
18. Spencer A, Prince HM, Roberts A, et al. Consolidation therapy with thalidomide and prednisolone prolongs the survival of multiple myeloma patients undergoing a single ASCT procedure. *J Clin Oncol.* 2009;27:1788–1793.
19. Morgan GJ, Jackson GH, Davies FE, et al. Maintenance thalidomide may improve progression free but not overall survival: results from the myeloma IX maintenance randomisation. *Blood.* 2008;112:656.
20. Lokhorst HM, van der Holt B, Zweegman S, et al. Hovon-50. Final analysis of thalidomide combined with adriamycin,dexamethasone and high-dose melphalan. *Clin Lymphoma Myeloma.* In press.
21. Abdelkefi A, Ladeb S, Torjman L. Retraction of reference 17. *Blood.* 2009;113:6265.
22. Barlogie B, Pineda-Roman M, van Rhee F, et al. Thalidomide arm of Total therapy 2 improves complete remission and survival in myeloma patients with metaphase cytogenetic abnormalities. *Blood.* 2008;112:3115–3121.
23. Wang M, Dimopoulos MA, Chen C, et al. Lenalidomide plus dexamethasone is more effective than dexamethasone alone in patients with relapsed or refractory multiple myeloma regardless of prior thalidomide exposure. *Blood.* 2008;112:4445–4451.
24. Paiva B, Vidriales MB, Cervero J, et al. Multiparameter flow cytometry is the most relevant prognostic factor relevant prognostic factor for multiple myeloma patients who undergo autologous stem cell transplantation. *Blood.* 2008;112:4017–4023.
25. Ladetto M, Pagliano G, Ferrero S, et al. Major shrinking of residual tumor cell burden and achievement of molecular remissions in myeloma patients undergoing post-transplant consolidation with bortezomib, thalidomide and dexamethasone: a qualitative and quantitative PCR study (abstract). *Blood.* 2008;112:3683.
26. Rajkumar SV, Blood E, Vesole D, et al. Phase III clinical trial of Thalidomide plus Dexamethasone compared with Dexamethasone alone in newly diagnosed multiple myeloma: a clinical trial coordinated by the Eastern Cooperative Oncology Group. *J Clin Oncol.* 2006;24:431–436.
27. Cavo M, Zamagni E, Tosi P, et al. Superiority of thalidomide and dexamethasone over vincristine-doxorubicine-dexamethasone (VAD) as primary therapy

in preparation for autologous transplantation for multiple myeloma. *Blood.* 2005;106:35–39.

28. Macro M, Divine M, Uzunban Y, et al. Dexamethasone + thalidomide compared to VAD as pre-transplant treatment in newly diagnosed multiple myeloma: a randomized trial (abstract). *Blood.* 2006;108:22a.

29. Harousseau J-L, Mathiot C, Attal M, et al. Velcade/dexamethasone versus VAD as induction treatment prior to autologous stem cell transplantation in newly diagnosed multiple myeloma: updated results of the IFM 2005–01 trial. *Presented at ASH/ASCO Symposium During ASH 2008.* Atlanta, GA: ASH; 2008.

30. Rajkumar SV, Jacobus S, Callander N, et al. A randomized trial of lenalidomide plus high-dose dexamethasone versus lenalidomide plus low-dose dexamethasone in newly diagnosed multiple myeloma (E4A03): a trial coordinated by the Eastern Cooperative Oncology Group (abstract). *Blood.* 2007;110:74.

31. Mazumder A, Kaufman J, Niesvizky R, et al. Effect of lenalidomide therapy on mobilization of peripheral blood stem cells in previously untreated multiple myeloma patients. *Leukemia.* 2008;22;1280–1281.

32. Paripati H, Stewart AK, Cabou S, et al. Compromised stem cell mobilization following induction therapy with lenalidomide in myeloma. *Leukemia.* 2008;22;1282–1284.

33. Mark T, Stern J, Furst JR, et al. Stem cell mobilization with cyclophosphamide overcomes the suppressive effect of lenalidomide therapy on stem cell collection in multiple myeloma. *Biol Blood Marrow Transplant.* 2008;14:795–798.

34. Lokhorst HM, Schidt-Wolf I, Sonneveld P, et al. Thalidomide in induction treatment increases the very good partial remission rate before and after high-dose therapy in previously untreated multiple myeloma. *Haematologica.* 2008;93:124–127.

35. Morgan GJ, Davies FE, Owen RG, et al. Thalidomide combinations improve response rates: results from the MRC IX study (abstract). *Blood.* 2007;110: 1051a.

36. Sonneveld P, van der Holt B, Schmidt-Wolf IGH, et al. First analysis of HOVON-65/GMMG-HD4 randomized phase II trial comparing bortezomib, adriamycine, dexamethasone (PAD) vs VAD as induction treatment prior to high-dose melphalan in patients with newly diagnosed multiple myeloma (abstract). *Haematologica.* 2009;94:473.

37. Cavo M, Tachetti P, Patriarca F, et al. Superior complete response rate and progression-free survival after autologous transplantation with up-front velcade-thalidomide dexamethasone (VTD) compared with thalidomide-dexamethasone in newly diagnosed multiple myeloma (abstract). *Blood.* 2008; 112:158.

38. Rosinol L, Cibeira MT, Martinez J, et al. Thalidomide/dexamethasone vs bortezomib/thalidomide/dexamethasone vs VBMCP/VBAP/velcade as induction regimens prior to autologous stem cell transplantation in younger patients with multiple myeloma: first results of a prospective phase III PETHEMA/GEM trial (abstract). *Blood.* 2008;112:654.

39. Barlogie B, Anaissie E, Van Rhee F, et al. Incorporating Bortezomib into upfront treatment for multiple myeloma: early results of total therapy 3. *Br J Haematol.* 2007;138:176–185.

40. Pineda-Roman M, Zangari M, Haessler J, et al. Sustained complete remission in multiple myeloma linked to bortezomib in total therapy 3: comparison with total therapy 2. *Br J Haematol.* 2008;140:625–634.

41. Facon T, Mary JY, Hulin C, et al. Intergroupe Francophone du Myélome. Melphalan and prednisone plus thalidomide versus melphalan and prednisone alone or reduced-intensity autologous stem cell transplantation in elderly patients with multiple myeloma (IFM 99–06): a randomised trial. *Lancet.* 2007;307:1209–1218.

42. Palumbo A, Bringhen S, Liberati A, et al. Oral melphalan, prednisone, and thalidomide in elderly patients with multiple myeloma: updated results of a randomized, controlled trial. *Blood.* 2008;112:3107–3114.

43. San Miguel JF, Schlag R, Khuageva NK, et al. Bortezomib plus melphalan and prednisone for initial treatment of multiple myeloma. *N Engl J Med.* 2008;35: 906–917.

44. Palumbo A, Falco P, Corradini P, et al. Melphalan, prednisone, lenalidomide treatment for newly diagnosed myeloma: a report from the GIMEMA-Italian Multiple Myeloma Network. *J Clin Oncol.* 2007;25:4459–4465.

45. Niesvizky R, Jayabalan DS, Christos PJ, et al. BiRD (Biaxin/Revlimid/Dexamethasone) combination therapy results in high complete and ovaerall response rates in treatment-naïve symptomatic multiple myeloma. *Blood.* 2008; 111:1101–1109.

46. Richardson PG, Lonial S, Jakubowiak S, et al. Safety and efficacy of lenalidomide, bortezomib and dexamethasone in patients with newly diagnosed multiple myeloma. *J Clin Oncol.* 2008;26:459s.

47. Harousseau J-L. The allogeneic dilemma. *Bone Marrow Transplant.* 2207;40: 1123–1128.

48. Crawley C, Lalancette M, Szydlo R, et al. Outcomes of reduced-intensity allogeneic transplantation for multiple myeloma: an analysis of prognostic factors from the Chronic Leukemia Working Party of the EBMT. *Blood.* 2005;105: 4532–4539.

49. Crawley C, Iacobelli S, Björkstrand B, et al. Reduced-intensity conditioning for myeloma: lower nonrelapse mortality but higher relapse rates compared with myeloablative conditioning. *Blood.* 2007;109:3588–3594.

50. Rotta M, Storer BE, Sahebi F, et al. Long-term outcome of patients with multiple myeloma after autologous hematopoietic cell transplantation and nonmyeloablative allografting. *Blood.* 2009;113:3383–3391.

51. Bruno B, Rotta M, Patriarca F, et al. A comparison of allografting with autografting for newly diagnosed myeloma. *N Engl J Med.* 2007;356:1110–1120.

52. Moreau P, Garban F, Attal M, et al. Long-term follow-up results of IFM 99–03 and IFM 99–04 trials comparing nonmyeloablative allotransplantation with autologous transplantation in high-risk de novo multiple myeloma. *Blood.* 2008;112:3914–3915.

53. Rosinol L, Perez-Simon JA, Sureda A, et al. A prospective Pethema study of tandem autologous transplantation versus autograft followed by reduced-intensity conditioning allogeneic transplantation in multiple myeloma. *Blood.* 2008;112:3591–3592.

54. Bruno B, Patriarca F, Sorasio R, et al. Bortezomib with or without dexamethasone in relapsed multiple myeloma following allogeneic hematopoietic cell transplantation. *Haematologica.* 2006;91:837–839.

55. Tosi P, Zamagni E, Cangini B, et al. Complete remission upon bortezomib-dexamethasone therapy in three heavily pretreated multiple myeloma patients relapsing after allogeneic stem cell transplantation. *Ann Hematol.* 2006;85: 549–558.

56. Van de Donk NW, Kroger N, Hegenbart U, et al. Remarkable activity of novel agents bortezomib and thalidomide in patients not responding to donor lymphocyte infusions following nonmyeloablative allogeneic stem cell transplantation in multiple myeloma. *Blood.* 2006;107:3415–3416.

57. Kroger N, Badbaran A, Lioznov M, et al. Post-transplant immunotherapy with donor-lymphocute infusions and novel agents to upgrade partial into complete and molecular remission in allografted patients with multiple myeloma. *Exp Hematol.* 2009;37:791–798.

# Novel Agents for Relapsed and/or Refractory Multiple Myeloma

Sheeba K. Thomas • Tiffany A. Richards • Donna M. Weber

Almost a decade ago, Singhal et al[1] conducted a landmark phase II trial of single-agent thalidomide in 84 patients with relapsed, refractory multiple myeloma, resulting in an overall response rate (ORR) of 25%. This promising result led to many subsequent studies of thalidomide both alone and in combination with other agents.[2-6] In patients with relapsed and/or refractory disease, response rates with single-agent thalidomide have been 15% to 36%, with a median overall survival (OS) of 14 to 58 months.[7]

When combined with dexamethasone, between 25% and 50% of patients have achieved partial response (PR) or better; notably, even among patients whose disease has become refractory to thalidomide or dexamethasone monotherapy, up to one third of patients have responded to the doublet.[2,8] This additive, and possibly synergistic, activity between thalidomide and dexamethasone, has led to numerous trials combining these agents with other novel drugs and conventional chemotherapeutics (Tables 1 and 2).

When combined with alkylating agents and steroids, ORRs (ie, complete response (CR) + PR rates) have ranged from 32% to 86%, with CR rates up to 20%.[3-6,9-11] Similarly, high rates of response have been seen when thalidomide has been combined with anthracyclines and steroids (ORR 56%–76%, CR 0%–22%).[12,13]

Unlike most available treatment options for multiple myeloma, myelosuppression is not a prominent feature of thalidomide's adverse event profile. In addition, its use does not require dose adjustment in the setting of renal or hepatic impairment. However, thalidomide is not without associated adverse events. In addition to its well-known teratogenic potential, thalidomide is associated with a significant rate of peripheral neuropathy (actuarial incidence at 12 months, 81%), and at least one third of patients also experience constipation, fatigue, and somnolence.[1,14] Thromboembolic events are also a concern when thalidomide is combined with corticosteroids or anthracyclines, and in this setting, prophylaxis with an anticoagulant is essential.[15]

## MECHANISM OF IMMUNOMODULATORY DRUGS

Both thalidomide and its analog, lenalidomide, act on the bone marrow microenvironment, disrupting cell adhesion-mediated drug resistance through down-regulation of adhesion molecules, such as intercellular adhesion molecule-1. These agents also inhibit the activity of interleukin (IL)-6, insulin-like growth factor-1, and vascular endothelial growth factor induced by adhesion of multiple myeloma cells to the bone marrow stroma, making the bone marrow microenvironment less hospitable to myeloma cell growth and proliferation.[16]

Lenalidomide was developed in an effort to improve the rate of response seen with thalidomide and increase the potency of its tumor necrosis factor-$\alpha$ inhibition, while also providing a different side effect profile. It is a structural analogue of thalidomide, created by adding an amino group to the fourth carbon of the phthaloyl ring of thalidomide. In addition to the mechanisms it shares with thalidomide, lenalido-

mide effects apoptosis by down-regulating nuclear factor (NF)-$\kappa$B signaling, and activating the intrinsic apoptotic pathway. By moderating the NF-$\kappa$B activity, it also reduces expression of the antiapoptotic proteins, cellular inhibitor of apoptosis protein 2, and Fas-associated protein with death domain–like IL-1 $\beta$–converting enzyme inhibitory protein.[16]

## LENALIDOMIDE

### Lenalidomide Monotherapy

In phase I clinical trials of patients with relapsed and/or refractory multiple myeloma, single-agent lenalidomide yielded response rates of 20% to 29%.[17,18] These early studies established the maximum tolerated dose (MTD) of lenalidomide at 25 mg once daily and provided the basis for a phase II study of 102 patients. In this study, lenalidomide monotherapy produced an ORR of 17%; however, with the addition of dexamethasone to patients with either stable or progressive disease after 2 cycles, the response rate rose to 22%.[19]

### Lenalidomide Combination Therapy

Based on the activity of lenalidomide-dexamethasone in these phase I and II studies, randomized, double-blind, placebo-controlled phase III clinical trials of this couplet were conducted in North America and internationally (Australia, Europe, and Israel) (Table 3).[20,21] Patients were randomized to receive dexamethasone 40 mg orally on days 1 to 4, 9 to 12, and 17 to 20 together with either lenalidomide 25 mg orally on days 1 to 21 or a placebo. These trials both demonstrated a benefit in overall response, progression-free survival, and OS for patients who received lenalidomide-dexamethasone compared with counterparts who received placebo-dexamethasone.[20,21] An updated pooled analysis of the 704 patients treated on these studies demonstrated superior ORR (60.6% vs. 21.9%), median time to disease progression (TTP; 11.2 vs. 4.7 months, $P < 0.001$), and median OS (35 vs. 31 months, $P = 0.02$) for patients treated with lenalidomide-dexamethasone compared with those who received placebo-dexamethasone.[22] It is noteworthy that 14.7% and 11.4% of patients on these studies developed venous thromboembolic events (VTEs) during the course of the studies, emphasizing the need for prophylaxis against VTE with aspirin, warfarin, or low molecular weight heparin, as recommended in the International Myeloma Working Group guidelines.[15,20,21]

Subset analysis of these studies examined outcomes of the 126 patients with previous thalidomide exposure and showed reduced response rates among those whose disease was resistant to thalidomide (43%) when compared with those whose disease was still sensitive (63%, $P < 0.05$).[23] The fact that responses were still achieved among thalidomide-resistant patients suggests that despite the overlapping mechanism of action of these drugs, there is not complete cross resistance between lenalidomide and thalidomide.

**TABLE 1.** Thalidomide/Alkylating Agent Combinations

| Author | Regimen | Sample Size | ORR (%) | CR (%) | TTP/PFS/EFS (mo) | Median OS (mo) | Zoster (%) | VTE (%) |
|---|---|---|---|---|---|---|---|---|
| Garcia-Sanz et al[3] | T 200–800 mg/d PO, d 1–28<br>Cy 50 mg/d PO, d 1–28<br>D 20 mg/m²/d PO, d 1–4 and 15–18 | 71 | 57 | 2 | 57% PFS at 2 yr | 66% at 2 yr | NR | 7 |
| Roussou et al[6] | T 400 mg/d PO, d 1–5, 14–18<br>D 20 mg/m²/d PO, d 1–5, 14–18<br>Cy 150 mg/m²/BID PO, d 1–5 | 43 | 67 | 0 | 10 | NA | 7.5 | 4 |
| Kyriakou et al[4] | T 50–300 mg/d PO, d 1–28<br>D 40 mg/d PO, d 1–4<br>Cy 300 mg/m²/d PO d 1, 8, 15, 22 | 52 | 78 | 17 | 34% EFS at 2 yr | 73% at 2 yr | NR | 11.5 |
| Suvannasankha et al[11] | T 200 mg/d, d 1–28<br>Cy 50 mg PO BID d 1–21<br>P 50 mg PO QOD, d 1–28 | 35 | 63 | 20 | 13.2 | NA | NR | 8.6 |
| Palumbo et al[5] | T 50–100 mg/d PO, d 1–28<br>M 20 mg/m²/d IV, d 1 every 4th month<br>P 50 mg/d PO, QOD | 24 | 42 | 0 | 9 PFS | NA | 0 | 4.2 |
| Ponisch et al[10] | T 50–200 mg/d PO, d 1–28<br>B 60 mg/m² /d IV, d 1, 8, 15<br>P 100 mg/d PO, d 1, 8, 15, 22 | 28 | 86 | 14 | 11 PFS | 19 | 0 | 0 |
| Lee et al[9] | D 40 mg/d PO, d 1–4<br>T 400 mg/d PO, d 1–28<br>Cis 10 mg/m²/d IVCI d 1–4<br>Do 10 mg/m²/d IVCI d 1–4<br>Cy 400 mg/m²/d IVCI d 1–4<br>E 40 mg/m²/d IVCI d 1–4 | 229 | 32 | 7 | NR | NR | NR | 15 |

T indicates thalidomide; Cy; cyclophosphamide; D, dexamethasone; P, prednisone; M, melphalan; B, bendamustine; Cis, cisplatin; Do, doxorubicin; E, etoposide; PFS, progression-free survival; VTE, venous thromboembolism; NR, not reached; PO, orally; BID, twice daily; IV, intravenous; IVCI, intravenous continuous infusion; and EFS, event-free survival.

The utility of lenalidomide-dexamethasone in patients with high-risk features has recently been explored in retrospective studies of patients receiving salvage therapy on the Lenalidomide Expanded Access Program (EAP) by Reece et al, and in previously untreated patients, by Kapoor et al.[24,25] In the study by Reece et al, fluorescence in situ hybridization (FISH) was used to probe for deletion of chromosome 13q, t(4;14), and del 17p13 among 130 patients enrolled on the Lenalidomide EAP. Median TTP and OS were comparable for patients with and without del(13q) or t(4;14), but outcomes for patients with del 17p13 were significantly worse (TTP 2.22 vs. 8.17 months, hazard ratio, 2.82; $P < 0.001$; OS 4.67 vs. 23.7 months, hazard ratio, 3.23; $P < 0.001$). Because studies by Barlogie et al[26] and the Intergroupe Francophone du Myélome showing the poor prognostic risk of del 13q and t(4;14) were performed using metaphase cytogenetics, it is unclear if these chromosomal abnormalities bear the same significance when identified by FISH. Prospective studies are needed to understand whether lenalidomide-dexamethasone truly overcomes the poor prognosis associated with del 13q and t(4;14), or

**TABLE 2.** Thalidomide + Pegylated Liposomal Doxorubicin Combinations

| Author | Regimen | No. Evaluable Patients | ORR (%) | CR (%) | TTP/PFS/EFS (mo) | Median OS (mo) | Zoster (%) | VTE (%) |
|---|---|---|---|---|---|---|---|---|
| Offidani et al[13] | T 100 mg/d PO, d 1–28<br>D 40 mg/d PO, d 1–4, 9–12<br>PLD 40 mg/m²/d IV, d 1 | 47 | 75.5 | 0 | 21 PFS | 35.5 | NR | 12.8 |
| Hussein et al[12] | PLD 40 mg/m²/d IV, d 1<br>V 2 mg IV, d 1<br>D 40 mg/d PO, d 1–4<br>T 50–400 mg/d PO, d 1–28 | 49 | 75 | 20 | 15.5 PFS | 39.9 | NR | 25* |

*Combined rate for newly diagnosed and relapsed-refractory patients.
T indicates thalidomide; D, dexamethasone; PLD, pegylated liposomal doxorubicin; V, vincristine; PFS, progression-free survival; VTE, venous thromboembolism; NR, not reached; PO, orally; IV, intravenous; and EFS, event-free survival.

**TABLE 3.**  Pivotal Studies

| Author | Regimen | No. Patients | ORR (%) | CR (%) | TTP/PFS/EFS (mo) | Median OS (mo) | Zoster (%) | VTE |
|---|---|---|---|---|---|---|---|---|
| Dimopoulos et al[20] | L 25 mg/d PO, d 1–21 | 351 | 60 | 15.9 | TTP 13 | NR | NR | 11.4 |
| | D 40 mg/d PO, cycles 1–4: d 1–4, 9–12, 17–20; cycles = 5–9: d 1–4 only | | | | | | | |
| Weber et al[21] | Same as above | 354 | 61 | 14 | TTP 11 | NR | 1.7 | 14.7 |
| Richardson[45] (APEX) | Bz 1.3 mg/m$^2$/d IV d 1, 4, 8, 11 | 333 | 43 | 9 | TTP 6.2 | 29.8 | 13 | 0 |
| | D 40 mg/d PO, d 1–4, 9–12, 17–20 for four cycles, then d 1–4 | 336 | 18 | 1 | TTP 3.5 | 23.7 | 5 | 1 |
| Orlowski et al[50] | Bz 1.3 mg/m$^2$/d IV, d 1, 4, 8, 11 | 322 | 44 | 4 | TTP 9.3 | 76% at 15 mo | NR | 1 |
| | PLD 30 mg/m$^2$/d IV, d 2 | | | | | | | |
| | Bz 1.3 mg/m$^2$ /d IV, d 1, 4, 8, 11 | 324 | 41 | 2 | TTP 6.5 | 65% at 15 mo | | 1 |

L indicates lenalidomide; Bz, bortezomib; D, dexamethasone; PFS, progression-free survival; VTE, venous thromboembolism; NR, not reached; PO, orally; IV, intravenous; and EFS, event-free survival.

whether these abnormalities are not associated with poor prognosis by FISH.

As discussed in an editorial by Lonial, data from patients having the highest risk are not included in analyses of salvage therapy, because they do not survive long enough to participate in such studies.[27] Accordingly, information about this subset of patients must be gleaned from trials of induction therapy. Among 100 previously untreated patients reviewed by Kapoor et al, 16% had high-risk multiple myeloma (as defined by the presence of hypodiploidy, del (13q) by metaphase cytogenetics, del (17p), immunoglobulin heavy chain translocations t(4;14) or t(14;16) by cytogenetics or FISH, or plasma cell labeling index ≥3%). Median progression-free survival (PFS) was shorter in

the high-risk group (18.5 vs. 36.5 months, $P < 0.001$), but OS was comparable.[24] This suggests that lenalidomide-dexamethasone may not overcome the risk associated with these features, but that subsequent salvage with other agents may account for the benefit in OS. Further confirmation with prospective studies is necessary to make definitive conclusions.

Because of the significant clinical activity of lenalidomide-dexamethasone and its in vitro synergy with anthracyclines and alkylating agents, investigators have combined these 2 drugs with agents from the aforementioned "conventional" drug classes (Table 4).[28] In a phase II study of lenalidomide, doxorubicin, and dexamethasone, Knop et al[29] reported an ORR of 73% among 66 patients evaluable

**TABLE 4.**  Lenalidomide + Alkylating Agent/Anthracycline Combinations

| Author | Regimen | Sample Size | ORR (%) | CR (%) | TTP/PFS/EFS (mo) | Median OS (mo) | Zoster (%) | VTE (%) |
|---|---|---|---|---|---|---|---|---|
| Schey et al[30] | L 10 mg/d PO, d 1–21 | 31 | 81 | 36 (CR/VGPR) | NA | NA | NR | NR |
| | Cy 300–700 mg/d PO, d 1, 8 (MTD 600 mg/d) | | | | | | | |
| | D 20 mg/d PO, 1–4, 8–11 | | | | | | | |
| Reece et al[72] | Cy 150–300 mg/d PO, d 1, 8, 15 | 15 | 76 | 6 (nCR) | NA | NA | 6.7 | 6.7 |
| | P 100 mg/d PO, QOD | | | | | | | |
| | L 15–25 mg/d PO, d 1–21 | | | | | | | |
| Palumbo et al[33] | L 10 mg/d PO, d 1–21 | 44 | 75.8 | 30 VGPR | 48.6% 1 yr PFS | 90% 1 yr survival | NR | 0 |
| | M 0.18/kg/d PO, d 1–4 | | | | | | | |
| | P 2 mg/kg/d PO, d 1–4 | | | | | | | |
| | T 50–100 mg/d PO, d 1–28 | | | | | | | |
| | ASA 100 mg/d PO d 1–28 | | | | | | | |
| Knop et al[29] | L 25 mg/d PO, d 1–21 | 66 | 73 | 15 | TTP 45 wk | 88% 1 yr survival probability | NR | 1.4 |
| | Do 9 mg/m$^2$/d IVCI, d 1–4 | | | | | | | |
| | D 40 mg/d PO, d 1–4 and 17–20 | | | | | | | |
| Baz et al[73] | PLD 40 mg/m$^2$/d IV, d 1 | 52 | 75 | 29 (CR/nCR) | 12 PFS | NR | NR | 9 |
| | V 2 mg/d IV, d 1 | | | | | | | |
| | D 40 mg/d PO, d 1–4 | | | | | | | |
| | L 5–25 mg/d PO, d 1–21 | | | | | | | |

L indicates lenalidomide; Cy, cyclophosphamide; D, dexamethasone; P, prednisone; M, melphalan; ASA, aspirin; Do, doxorubicin; PLD, pegylated liposomal doxorubicin; V, vincristine; IVCI, intravenous continuous infusion; PFS, progression-free survival; VTE, venous thromboembolism; NR, not reached; nCR, near complete remission; PO, orally; IV, intravenous; and EFS, event-free survival.

for response; CR was achieved in 15% of patients. Median time to progression was 45 weeks, and probability of survival at 1 year was 88%. Similar to the findings of Reece et al from review of data from the EAP, multivariate analysis of this study showed no significant difference in the outcomes of patients with deletion of 13q or t(4;14) by FISH; however, those with deletion of 17 p had a lower rate of response (20% vs. 87%, $P = 0.001$).[25,29] The most prominent toxicities were hematologic, with 48% of patients experiencing $\geq$grade 3 neutropenia, 38% $\geq$grade 3 thrombocytopenia, and 16% $\geq$grade 3 anemia. Despite prophylaxis with aspirin or enoxaparin, 4.5% of patients developed thromboembolic events.[29]

When lenalidomide (25 mg orally on days 1–21) and dexamethasone (20 mg orally on days 1–4 and 8–11) were combined with cyclophosphamide in a dose escalation study by Schey et al,[30] the MTD of cyclophosphamide was 600 mg orally on days 1 and 8 of a 28-day cycle. Among 31 enrolled patients, PR or better was noted in 81% of patients, and 36% achieved either CR or very good partial remission (VGPR). Neutropenia (grade $\geq$3) was the most common reason for dose delays and reductions. Other grade $\geq$3 adverse events seen were pneumonia, syncope and pancytopenia. A similar study, combining cyclophosphamide, lenalidomide, and prednisone, by Reece et al found an MTD of cyclophosphamide 300 mg/m$^2$ on days 1, 8, and 15, lenalidomide 25 mg on days 1 to 21, and prednisone 100 mg every other day. Neutropenia was the most common hematologic toxicity. One patient experienced varicella zoster, and another developed a deep vein thrombosis despite aspirin prophylaxis.

In previously untreated patients with myeloma, the addition of either thalidomide or lenalidomide to melphalan and prednisone has yielded significant improvement in patient outcomes.[31–33] Building on these regimens, Palumbo et al[34] combined lenalidomide, melphalan, prednisone, and thalidomide in patients with relapsed and/or refractory disease. On days 1 to 4 of each 28 day cycle, patients received oral melphalan 0.18 mg/kg and prednisone 2 mg/kg, together with lenalidomide 10 mg on days 1 to 21 and were then randomized to receive either 50 or 100 mg of thalidomide on days 1 to 28. All patients received thromboembolic prophylaxis with aspirin. Among patients who received 100 mg of thalidomide per day, 93.3% achieved at least PR (including VGPR 46.7%), compared with 64.7% of those who received 50 mg per day of thalidomide. The 1-year progression-free survival was 48.6%, and the 1-year OS was 90%. Grade 3 to 4 neutropenia was seen in 66.6% of patients, thrombocytopenia in 36.3% of patients, and anemia in 30.2% of patients. Grade 3 to 4 infections occurred in 21.2% of patients, whereas neurologic toxicity and fatigue were seen in 6% and 9%. No thromboembolic events were observed.

## BORTEZOMIB

Bortezomib is a first-in-class proteasome inhibitor, designed to inhibit the function of the 26S proteasome complex. It is believed to exert its effect in part by down-regulating NF-$\kappa$B signaling. This in turn reduces the expression of cytokines, such as tumor necrosis factor-$\alpha$, IL-1, and IL-6, as well as stress response enzymes, cell adhesion molecules, and antiapoptotic proteins.[35–39]

Because malignant cells have a higher rate of proliferation than normal cells, rates of protein translation and degradation in these cells are accordingly increased. The proteasome, a multicatalytic protease present in all eukaryotic cells, is the primary mechanism of protein degradation in cells. Each human cell contains approximately 30,000 proteasomes that regulate such cell functions as transcription, stress response, cell cycle progression, cellular differentiation, antigen processing, and DNA repair.[35–41] Proteasome inhibition was explored

as a therapeutic strategy because of its potential for interfering with these processes, thereby inducing apoptosis in malignant cells.

## Bortezomib Monotherapy

Promising preclinical data led to a phase I trial of bortezomib in 27 patients with hematologic malignancies, of whom 9 had relapsed and/or refractory plasma cell dyscrasias.[42] Among those with plasma cell dyscrasias, 1 achieved a CR, and the remaining 8 had reductions of their paraprotein levels and/or marrow plasmacytosis. These findings led to the subsequent phase II, Clinical Response and Efficacy Study of Bortezomib in the Treatment of Relapsing Multiple Myeloma (CREST) and Study of Multiple Myeloma Managed With Proteasome Inhibition Therapy (SUMMIT) trials, which showed ORRs of 27% to 38% in patients who had previously received 1 (CREST) and 2 or more (SUMMIT) prior lines of therapy, respectively.[43,44] In CREST, patients received either 1.0 or 1.3 mg/m$^2$ intravenously (IV) on days 1, 4, 8, and 11 of a 21-day cycle; 20 mg of dexamethasone was added on the day of and day after each bortezomib dose for those with stable or progressive disease after 2 cycles of therapy. ORRs were 30% and 38% at the 1.0 and 1.3 mg/m$^2$ doses, respectively, with no statistically significant difference in OS between arms (26.8 vs. 60 months, $P = 0.13$), suggesting that even lower doses of bortezomib might be beneficial in patients who cannot tolerate the standard 1.3 mg/m$^2$.[43]

Based on the success of these phase I and II studies, the phase III Assessment of Proteasome Inhibition for Extending Remissions (APEX) pivotal trial of 669 patients comparing bortezomib with dexamethasone was reported and demonstrated superior response (43% vs. 18%), TTP (6.2 vs. 3.5 months), and median OS (29.8 vs. 23.7 months, $P = 0.027$) with bortezomib compared with dexamethasone (Table 3).[42–45] The improvement in OS is particularly noteworthy, because 62% of the patients initially randomized to receive dexamethasone, subsequently crossed over and received bortezomib.[45] Impaired renal function (creatinine clearance [CrCl] >50 mL/min vs. $\leq$50 mL/min) was associated with significantly poorer OS among those treated with dexamethasone but did not affect outcome (ORR, TTP, OS) among those who received bortezomib.[46]

In a retrospective-matched pairs analysis, the impact of del (13q) identified by metaphase cytogenetics based on the outcomes of patients treated on the phase II and III bortezomib studies was also evaluated. The presence of this cytogenetic abnormality did not affect the OS of those treated with bortezomib, but it was associated with reduced survival among those treated with dexamethasone, suggesting that bortezomib may reduce the impact of del (13q) on survival.[47]

The most common grade 3 to 4 adverse events observed in these studies of bortezomib were thrombocytopenia, lymphopenia, neutropenia, fatigue, and neuropathy.[45] Subset analysis of the APEX study also showed an increased incidence of varicella zoster among those who received bortezomib, highlighting the need for antiviral prophylaxis among patients treated with this drug.[48]

## Bortezomib Combination Therapy

The development of myeloma cell resistance to conventional chemotherapy is due in part to up-regulation of NF-$\kappa$B expression. By moderating the NF-$\kappa$B activity, bortezomib may reduce this mechanism of chemoresistance. Bortezomib also reduces expression of P-glycoprotein, which is encoded in the *multidrug resistance gene 1* and may overcome cell adhesion-mediated drug resistance. In addition, it seems to sensitize myeloma cells to DNA damage, by down-regulating the transcription of DNA repair enzymes.[49]

Resistance to bortezomib may in turn be overcome by combining it with conventional chemotherapy. One of several mechanisms of proteasome inhibitor-induced apoptosis is through activation of Jun

*N*-terminal kinase. However, bortezomib induces mitogen-activated protein kinase phosphatase-1, which can dephosphorylate and inactivate Jun *N*-terminal kinase. Anthracyclines and alkylators have been shown to inhibit mitogen-activated protein kinase phosphatase-1 activity, potentially contributing to the synergy of these agents with bortezomib. These preclinical observations have led the investigators to develop clinical trials, evaluating the combination of bortezomib with these chemotherapeutic classes.[49]

A phase III trial, by Orlowksi et al,[50] comparing bortezomib monotherapy with bortezomib-pegylated liposomal doxorubicin (PLD) showed comparable ORR between arms (41% vs. 44%), but higher rates of CR + VGPR (19% vs. 27%) (*P* = 0.0157), longer TTP (9.3 vs. 6.5 months) and improved 15 month OS (76% vs. 65%) with the combination (Table 3). This improvement in median TTP and OS, despite similar overall response, suggests that the degree of response may be important even among patients with relapsed and refractory disease. Gastrointestinal toxicities (nausea, vomiting, and diarrhea), neutropenia, thrombocytopenia, peripheral neuropathy, and palmar-plantar erythrodysesthesia were the most common grade 3 to 4 adverse events seen with bortezomib-PLD.[50] When dexamethasone (40 mg on days 1–4) was added to bortezomib and either doxorubicin or PLD in a more recent study of 64 patients, 67% achieved at least PR, 1 year event-free survival was 34%, and 1 year OS was 66%.[51]

Several investigators have combined bortezomib with alkylating agents, with or without steroids (Table 5).[52–56] In 1 study by Reece et al,[56] bortezomib (1.5 mg/m$^2$/d IV on days 1, 8, and 15 or 1.3 mg/m$^2$ days 1, 4, 8, and 11) was given together with cyclophosphamide (300 mg/m$^2$ IV on days 1, 8, 15, and 22) and prednisone (100 mg orally every other day). Among 37 patients, the ORR was 68%, and 32% achieved CR/near complete remission. Median OS was 24.3 months. Patients treated with the weekly schedule of bortezomib experienced lower rates of peripheral neuropathy and myelosuppression. However, the rate of infections was notable across this study and included 6 episodes of pneumonia and 11 episodes of varicella zoster reactivation.

Another bortezomib-alkylating agent study was performed by Berenson et al,[52,53] who evaluated the steroid sparing combination of bortezomib and melphalan. The MTD of this study was defined as 1.0 mg/m$^2$ of bortezomib on days 1, 4, 8, and 11 with 0.10 mg/kg of melphalan on days 1 to 4. Of 46 evaluable patients, 50% achieved PR or better, including 15% who achieved either CR or nCR. Median OS was 32 months. The most common grade 3 toxicities were neutropenia (31%), thrombocytopenia (25%), and anemia (13%). Given the activity of this regimen, Popat et al[55] examined a similar regimen of bortezomib 1.3 mg/m$^2$ on days 1, 4, 8, and 11 with escalating doses of IV melphalan (2.5–10.0 mg/m$^2$) on day 2 of a 28-day cycle, for a maximum of 8 cycles. Dexamethasone 20 mg was added for progressive or stable disease. Among 53 patients who had received a median of 3 prior lines of chemotherapy, the MTD was defined at melphalan 7.5 mg/m$^2$ and bortezomib 1.3 mg/m$^2$. The ORR was 68%, including 23% CR or near-CRs. Among those treated at the MTD, the ORR was higher, at 76%, and 27% achieved CR. Median PFS of patients treated at the MTD was 12 months, and median OS for this cohort had not been reached. Patients who obtained a CR/nCR had a superior PFS to

**TABLE 5.** Bortezomib + Alkylating Agent/Anthracycline Combinations

| Author | Regimen | No. Evaluable Patients | ORR (%) | CR (%) | TTP/PFS/EFS (mos.) | Median OS (mos) | Zoster (%) | VTE (%) |
|---|---|---|---|---|---|---|---|---|
| Davies et al[54] | Bz 1.3 mg/m$^2$/d IV, d 1, 4, 8, 11 | 11 | 27 | 0 | | | 9* | |
| | Above B+ | | | | | | | |
| | D 40 mg PO d 1, 2, 4, 5, 8, 9, 11, 12 | 20 | 47 | 5 | | | 35* | |
| | Above B/D+ | 16 | 75 | 31 | NR | NR | 6* | NR |
| | Cy 500 mg POD 1, 8, 15 | | | | | | | |
| Reece et al[56] | Bz 1.5 mg/m$^2$/d IV, d 1, 8, 15, or 1.3 mg/m$^2$/d IV, d 1, 4, 8, 11 | 37 | 68 | 32 CR/nCR | 1 yr PFS 83% | 24.3 | 29.7 | NR |
| | Cy 300 mg/m$^2$ d 1, 8, 15, 22 | | | | | | | |
| | P 100 mg/d once q2d | | | | | | | |
| Berenson et al[53] | Bz 0.7–1.3 mg/m$^2$/d IV, d 1, 4, 8, 11 | 46 | 50 | 4 | 9 PFS | 32 | NR | NR |
| | M 0.025–0.25 mg/kg PO d 1–4 | | | | | | | |
| Popat et al[55] | Bz 1.3 mg/m$^2$/d IV, d 1, 4, 8, 11 | 53 | 68 | 19 | 10 PFS | NR | NR | NR |
| | M 7.5 mg/m$^2$/d IV, d 2 | | | | | | | |
| | D 20 mg/d PO d 1, 2, 4, 5, 8, 9, 11, 12 for progressive disease | | | | | | | |
| Palumbo et al[51] | Bz 1.3 mg/m$^2$/d IV, d 1, 4, 8, 11 | 64 | 67 | 0 | 34% 1 yr EFS | 66% 1 yr OS | 5 | 3 |
| | Do 20 mg/m$^2$ IV, d 1, 4 or PLD 30 mg/m$^2$/d IV, d 1 | | | | | | | |
| | D 40 mg/d PO, d 1–4 | | | | | | | |
| Di Raimondo et al[74] | Bz 1.3 mg/m$^2$/d IV, d 1, 4, 8, 11 | 15 | 40 | 0 | NA | NA | 0 | 0 |
| | PLD 20 mg/m$^2$/d IV, d 1, 15 | | | | | | | |
| | Cy 100 mg/d PO, d 1–15 | | | | | | | |
| | D 40 mg/d IV, d 1, 4, 8, 11 | | | | | | | |

*Includes incidence of chicken pox and herpes simplex infections.
Bz indicates bortezomib; Cy, cyclophosphamide; D, dexamethasone; M, melphalan; Do, doxorubicin; PLD, pegylated liposomal doxorubicin; PFS, progression-free survival; VTE, venous thromboembolism; NR, not reached; nCR, near complete remission; PO, orally; IV, intravenous; and EFS, event-free survival.

those who had less optimal responses (14 vs. 10 months, $P = 0.0485$). More mature data are needed to determine whether this difference in PFS will translate into a statistically significant difference in OS.

## Combinations of Novel Agents

Proteasome inhibitors and IMiDs have also been combined in an effort to improve the patient outcomes (Table 6). One of the earliest of these studies evaluated 85 patients treated on a phase I/II trial of bortezomib, thalidomide, and dexamethasone.[57] The MTD was defined as 1.3 mg/m$^2$ of bortezomib (given on days 1, 4, 8, and 11 of every 21 days) with thalidomide 150 mg/d from cycle 2 forward. Dexamethasone (20 mg) was added on the day of and day after each bortezomib dose from cycle 4 forward, in the absence of PR. Among 82 evaluable patients, 63% achieved at least PR, and 22% achieved CR/nCR. Median durations of OS and event-free survival were 22 and 6 months. Sensory neuropathy was the most common adverse event leading to study discontinuation. Other grade 3 to 4 toxicities of note were thrombocytopenia and neutropenia.

More recently, Anderson et al[58] have published their experience with the combination of bortezomib (1 mg/m$^2$ IV days 1, 4, 8, 11)

with lenalidomide 15 mg orally on days 1 to 14 and dexamethasone (cycles 1–4/5–8: 40 or 20 mg on the day of and day after bortezomib). After a median of 2 prior lines of therapy, the ORR among 62 evaluable patients was 68% including 21% CR/nCR. The most common adverse event was grade 1 to 2 myelosuppression; other toxicities of particular interest include the development of deep vein thrombosis in 2 patients despite aspirin prophylaxis, atrial fibrillation in 2 patients, and grade 3 peripheral neuropathy in 1 patient. One patient died of a fungal pneumonia while on study.

Bortezomib has also been combined with thalidomide and PLD. In studies by Chanan-Khan et al[59] and Ciolli et al[60], rates of overall response were high (56%–74%) with 22% to 24% of patients obtaining CR. Median OSs in these studies were 15.7 and 19 months, respectively. The most common grade 3 or 4 toxicities noted were lymphopenia, neutropenia, infections, fatigue, and peripheral neuropathy.

Finally, Colado et al,[61] evaluated a regimen of bortezomib 1.3 mg/m$^2$ IV, days 1, 4, 8, and 11; melphalan 9 mg/m$^2$ orally, days 1 to 4; prednisone 60 mg/m$^2$ orally, days 1 to 4; and conventional or liposomal adriamycin 40 or 30 mg/m$^2$ on day 1 of a 28-day cycle (VAMP) alternating with thalidomidomide-cyclophosphamide-dexamethasone

## TABLE 6. Bortezomib + IMiD Combinations

| Author | Regimen | No. Evaluable Patients | ORR (%) | CR (%) | TTP/PFS/EFS (mo) | Median OS (mo) | Zoster (%) | VTE (%) |
|---|---|---|---|---|---|---|---|---|
| Anderson et al[58] | L 15 mg PO, d 1–14<br>Bz 1 mg/m$^2$ IV d 1, 4, 8, 11<br>D 40 mg (cycles 1–4), 20 mg (cycles 5–8) days of/after Bz<br>After cycle 8: L 15 mg PO, d 1–14 Bz 1 mg/m$^2$ IV d 1, 8; Dex 10 mg, d 1, 2, 8, 9 | 62 | 68 | 21 (Cr + nCR) | NR | NR | NR | 3.1 |
| Terpos et al[75] | B 1 mg/m$^2$/d IV, d 1, 4, 8, 11<br>M 0.15 mg/kg/d PO, d 1–4<br>D 12 mg/m$^2$/d PO, d 1–4, 17–20<br>T 100 mg/d PO, d 1–28 | 62 | 66 | 13 | 9.3 TTP | NR | 8.1 | 0 |
| Colado et al[61] | B 1.3 mg/m$^2$/d IV, d 1, 4, 8, 11<br>M 9 mg/m$^2$/d PO, d 1–4<br>P 60 mg/m$^2$/d PO, d 1–4<br>Do 40 mg/m$^2$/d IV, d 1 or PLD 30 mg/m$^2$/d IV, d 1<br>Alternating with T 200 mg/d PO, d 1–28; C 50 mg/d PO, d 1–28; D 40 mg/d PO, d 1–4 | 20 | 94.7 | 42 | NR | NR | NR | NR |
| Pineda-Roman et al[57] | B 1–1.3 mg/m$^2$/d IV, d 1, 4, 8, 11<br>T 50–200 mg/d PO, d 1–21<br>D 20 mg PO d 1, 2, 4, 5, 8, 9, 11, 12 | 82 | 63 | 22 (CR/nCR) | 6 EFS | 22 | NR | NR |
| Ciolli et al[60] | B 1 mg/m$^2$/d IV, d 1, 4, 8, 11<br>PLD 30–50 mg/m$^2$/d IV, d 4<br>D 24 mg/d PO, d 1, 2, 4, 5, 8, 9, 11, 12<br>T 100 mg/d PO, 1–28 | 42 | 74 | 24 | 15 PFS | 19 | 2 | 2 |
| Chanan-Khan et al[59] | T 200 mg/d PO, d 1–28<br>B 1.3 mg/m$^2$/d IV, d 1, 4, 15, 18<br>PLD 20 mg/m$^2$/d IV, d 1, 15 | 18 | 56 | 22 | 10.9 PFS | 15.7 | NR | 0 |

PFS indicates progression-free survival; VTE, venous thromboembolism; NR, not reached; nCR, near complete remission; PO, orally; IV, intravenous; and EFS, event-free survival.

(thalidomide 200 mg/d orally day 1–28; cyclophosphamide 50 mg/d orally, days 1–28; and dexamethasone 40 mg/d orally, days 1–4) in an effort to overcome drug resistance without increased toxicity. After 6 cycles, responding patients received thalidomidomide-cyclophosphamide-dexamethasone every other month for consolidation. Among 20 evaluable patients, the ORR was 94.7%, including 47% CR. Interestingly, CR/nCR was achieved in 4 of 7 patients who presented with high-risk cytogenetic abnormalities [t(4;14) and/or del *RB*], allowing for subsequent allogeneic stem-cell transplantation in 2 of these patients. Grade 3 to 4 toxicities included thrombocytopenia (30%), neutropenia (30%), and infection (16%) Peripheral neuropathy was developed in 3 patients (15%), but all were grade 2 or lower in severity.

## Considerations in Novel Agent Combinations

Among previously untreated patients with multiple myeloma, 50% have evidence of both small and large fiber neuropathy on nerve conduction studies, and nearly 40% of the 221 patients who received bortezomib on the APEX trial experienced either development or progression of neuropathy.[62,63] The rate of developing peripheral neuropathy is also high (75%) with long-term use of thalidomide.[64] By contrast, fewer than 2% of patients who received lenalidomide on the phase III lenalidomide-dexamethasone versus placebo-dexamethasone studies experienced grade 3 to 4 neuropathy, and only 10% reported neuropathy of any grade.[20,21] Thus, for patients with diabetes mellitus, amyloidosis, or other comorbid conditions predisposing them to develop peripheral neuropathy, lenalidomide may be preferable to the other available novel agents.

Renal function is another important treatment consideration for patients with multiple myeloma. Approximately, 20% of patients will develop renal impairment during the course of their disease.[65] In subanalysis of the phase III lenalidomide-dexamethasone studies, patients treated with lenalidomide-dexamethasone who had a CrCl <30 mL/min had a shorter median TTP and OS than those whose CrCl exceeded 30 mL/min.[66] These patients also had higher rates of ≥3 grade thrombocytopenia (18.8% vs. 5.5%, $P < 0.05$), but no significant difference was noted in rates of ≥3 grade neutropenia. The effect noted on platelet count, together with pharmacokinetic studies performed in patients without myeloma who had varied degrees of renal dysfunction, led to recommendations for dose adjustments of lenalidomide in patients with a CrCl below 60 mL/min (10 mg/d for CrCl 30–60 mL/min, 15 mg every 48 hours for CrCl <30 mL/min not requiring dialysis; 5 mg once daily for CrCl <30 mL/min—requiring dialysis, taken after dialysis on days of dialysis).[67] It should be noted that regardless of CrCl, patient outcomes remained superior among those treated with lenalidomide-dexamethasone compared with those who received placebo-dexamethasone.[66] Close monitoring of blood counts and appropriate dose modifications during lenalidomide therapy is essential to improve the tolerability and maintaining patients on therapy.

While lenalidomide undergoes renal excretion, bortezomib undergoes metabolism by the liver and thalidomide by nonenzymatic hydrolysis, thus dose modifications of bortezomib or thalidomide in patients with impaired renal function are not required. Among patients with a CrCl ≤50 mL/min compared with those having a CrCl >50 mL/min, there were no significant differences in ORR, median TTP, or median OS on subset analysis of the APEX study.[46] Likewise, in a retrospective study of relapsed patients with CrCL <60 mL/min treated with thalidomide-dexamethasone, ORR was 45%, and 80% of patients had improvement of their renal function with treatment.[68] However, unexplained hyperkalemia has been reported in some patients with renal dysfunction who have received thalidomide.[69]

Consideration must also be given to the use of dexamethasone in treatment combinations. Although it is an integral part of myeloma therapy (ORR 45% in previously untreated patients), dexamethasone can be difficult to tolerate and may exacerbate diabetes, hypertension, fluid retention, and steroid-induced psychosis. In patients with these complicating factors, a steroid-free treatment regimen, such as bortezomib and PLD or bortezomib-lenalidomide, may provide improved tolerability. However, in those patients who require quick response due to impaired renal function, hypercalcemia, or cord compression, high-dose steroids are instrumental in achieving rapid tumor reduction.

In patients receiving lenalidomide or thalidomide in combination with high-dose dexamethasone or who have a high-risk comorbidity, low molecular weight heparin or warfarin should be instituted. However, in a selected group of patients receiving low-dose dexamethasone in combination with lenalidomide-thalidomide therapy, low-dose aspirin may be sufficient to prevent VTE. Care should be taken to consider comorbidities, particularly dose reductions for renal impairment, before initiating low-molecular-weight heparin. Because bortezomib has not been associated with an increased risk of thrombosis, a bortezomib-based regimen may be a prudent choice for patients with a prior history or otherwise increased risk for VTE.

High-risk cytogenetic disease is characterized by hypodiploidy or deletion of chromosome 13 (del [13]) with conventional cytogenetics or the presence of t(4;14), t(14;16), or del(17p) by FISH. These features are seen in approximately 25% of patients with symptomatic multiple myeloma and have been associated with a median OS between 12 and 30 months in retrospective studies.[24,70] Because available outcome data comes from patients whose cytogenetic profiles have been determined by various methods, it is somewhat difficult to make extrapolations to larger cohorts of patients. Therefore, until prospective studies are performed, a combination of bortezomib/lenalidomide may be ideal in this group of patients.

Finally, while at times it may be necessary to change therapy altogether, patients relapsing after extended treatment-free remissions (>6 months) often benefit from receiving their last line of therapy and may also benefit from combining prior therapies, even after resistance has developed to one or more of the component agents.[71]

## CONCLUSIONS

With approval of 4 new drugs in the last decade, many treatment combinations exist for the relapsed/refractory patient. Although this has expanded the breadth of therapeutic options for patients with multiple myeloma, it has also complicated the choice of therapy for any given patient. Treatment algorithms should give consideration to comorbidities, prior VTE, pre-existing neuropathy, organ function, chromosomal abnormalities, and prior treatment history. However, randomized studies evaluating the sequencing of agents after induction therapy are also needed to clarify an optimal treatment plan.

With the next generation of novel agents, including the proteasome inhibitor, carfilzomib, and the IMiD, pomalidomide, we look for continued improvement in duration of response and OS, together with a more favorable side effect profile, so that both quantity and quality of life may be improved for patients with multiple myeloma.

## REFERENCES

1. Singhal S, Mehta J, Desikan R, et al. Antitumor activity of thalidomide in refractory multiple myeloma [see comment]. *N Engl J Med.* 1999;341:1565–1571; erratum in *N Engl J Med.* 2000;342:364.
2. Anagnostopoulos A, Weber D, Rankin K, et al. Thalidomide and dexamethasone for resistant multiple myeloma. *Br J Haematol.* 2003;121:768–771.
3. Garcia-Sanz R, Gonzalez-Porras JR, Hernandez JM, et al. The oral combination of thalidomide, cyclophosphamide and dexamethasone (ThaCyDex) is

effective in relapsed/refractory multiple myeloma. *Leukemia.* 2004;18:856–863.

4. Kyriakou C, Thomson K, D'Sa S, et al. Low-dose thalidomide in combination with oral weekly cyclophosphamide and pulsed dexamethasone is a well tolerated and effective regimen in patients with relapsed and refractory multiple myeloma. *Br J Haematol.* 2005;129:763–770.

5. Palumbo A, Avonto I, Bruno B, et al. Intravenous melphalan, thalidomide and prednisone in refractory and relapsed multiple myeloma. *Eur J Haematol.* 2006;76:273–277.

6. Roussou M, Anagnostopoulos A, Kastritis E, et al. Pulsed cyclophosphamide, thalidomide and dexamethasone regimen for previously treated patients with multiple myeloma: long term follow up and disease control after subsequent treatments. *Leuk Lymphoma.* 2007;48:754–758.

7. Reece DE, Leitch HA, Atkins H, et al. Treatment of relapsed and refractory myeloma. *Leuk Lymphoma.* 2008;49:1470–1485.

8. Weber DM, Gavino M, Delasalle K, et al. Thalidomide alone or with dexamethasone for multiple myeloma. *Blood.* 1999;94(suppl 1):604a.

9. Lee CK, Barlogie B, Munshi N, et al. DTPACE: an effective, novel combination chemotherapy with thalidomide for previously treated patients with myeloma. *J Clin Oncol.* 2003;21:2732–2739; erratum in *J Clin Oncol.* 2008;26:2066.

10. Ponisch W, Rozanski M, Goldschmidt H, et al. Combined bendamustine, prednisolone and thalidomide for refractory or relapsed multiple myeloma after autologous stem-cell transplantation or conventional chemotherapy: results of a Phase I clinical trial. *Br J Haematol.* 2008;143:191–200.

11. Suvannasankha A, Fausel C, Juliar BE, et al. Final report of toxicity and efficacy of a phase II study of oral cyclophosphamide, thalidomide, and prednisone for patients with relapsed or refractory multiple myeloma: a Hoosier Oncology Group Trial, HEM01–21. *Oncologist.* 2007;12:99–106.

12. Hussein MA, Baz R, Srkalovic G, et al. Phase 2 study of pegylated liposomal doxorubicin, vincristine, decreased-frequency dexamethasone, and thalidomide in newly diagnosed and relapsed-refractory multiple myeloma [see comment]. *Mayo Clin Proc.* 2006;81:889–895.

13. Offidani M, Bringhen S, Corvatta L, et al. Thalidomide-dexamethasone plus pegylated liposomal doxorubicin vs. thalidomide-dexamethasone: a case-matched study in advanced multiple myeloma. *Eur J Haematol.* 2007;78:297–302.

14. Mileshkin L, Stark R, Day B, et al. Development of neuropathy in patients with myeloma treated with thalidomide: patterns of occurrence and the role of electrophysiologic monitoring. *J Clin Oncol.* 2006;24:4507–4514.

15. Palumbo A, Rajkumar SV, Dimopoulos MA, et al. Prevention of thalidomide-and lenalidomide-associated thrombosis in myeloma. *Leukemia.* 2007;22:414–423.

16. Vallet S, Palumbo A, Raje N, et al. Thalidomide and lenalidomide: mechanism-based potential drug combinations. *Leuk Lymphoma.* 2008;49:1238–1245.

17. Richardson PG, Schlossman RL, Weller E, et al. Immunomodulatory drug CC-5013 overcomes drug resistance and is well tolerated in patients with relapsed multiple myeloma. *Blood.* 2002;100:3063–3067.

18. Zangari M, Barlogie B, Jacobson J, et al. VTD regimen comprising Velcade (V) + thalidomide (T) and added DEX (D) for non-responders to V + T effects a 57% PR rate among 56 patients with myeloma (M) relapsing after autologous transplant. *Blood.* 2003;102:236a. Abstract.

19. Richardson P, Jagannath S, Hussein M, et al. Safety and efficacy of single-agent lenalidomide in patients with relapsed and refractory multiple myeloma. *Blood.* 2009;114:772–778.

20. Dimopoulos M, Spencer A, Attal M, et al. Lenalidomide plus dexamethasone for relapsed or refractory multiple myeloma [see comment]. *N Engl J Med.* 2007;357:2123–2132.

21. Weber DM, Chen C, Niesvizky R, et al. Lenalidomide plus dexamethasone for relapsed multiple myeloma in North America [see comment]. *N Engl J Med.* 2007;357:2133–2142.

22. Weber D, Knight R, Chen C, et al. Prolonged overall survival with lenalidomide plus dexamethasone compared with dexamethasone alone in patients with relapsed or refractory multiple myeloma. *ASH Annu Meet Abstr.* 2007;110 (Abstract 412).

23. Wang M, Knight R, Dimopoulos M, et al. Lenalidomide in combination with dexamethasone was more effective than dexamethasone in patients who have received prior thalidomide for relapsed or refractory multiple myeloma. *ASH Annu Meet Abstr.* 2006;108 (Abstract 3553).

24. Kapoor P, Kumar S, Fonseca R, et al. Impact of risk stratification on outcome among patients with multiple myeloma receiving initial therapy with lenalidomide and dexamethasone. *Blood.* 2009;114:518–521.

25. Reece D, Song KW, Fu T, et al. Influence of cytogenetics in patients with relapsed or refractory multiple myeloma treated with lenalidomide plus dexamethasone: adverse effect of deletion 17p13. *Blood.* 2009;114:522–525.

26. Barlogie B, Attal M, Crowley J, et al. Long-term follow-up of autotransplant (AT)-supported high-dose melphalan (hdm) for multiple myeloma (MM): update of Intergroup Francophone du Myelome (IFM), Southwest Oncology Group (SWOG), and Arkansas (ARK) Total Therapy (TT) trials. *J Clin Oncol.* 2009;27(15s, Abstract 8519).

27. Lonial S. Risky business in myeloma. *Blood.* 2009;114:496–497.

28. Hideshima T, Chauhan D, Shima Y, et al. Thalidomide and its analogs overcome drug resistance of human multiple myeloma cells to conventional therapy. *Blood.* 2000;96:2943–2950.

29. Knop S, Gerecke C, Liebisch P, et al. Lenalidomide, adriamycin, and dexamethasone (RAD) in patients with relapsed and refractory multiple myeloma: a report from the German Myeloma Study Group DSMM (Deutsche Studiengruppe Multiples Myelom). *Blood.* 2009;113:4137–4143.

30. Schey S, Morgan GJ, Ramasamy K, et al. CRD: a phase 1 dose escalation study to determine the maximum tolerated dose of cyclophosphamide in combination with lenalidomide and dexamethasone in relapsed/refractory myeloma. *Blood (ASH Ann Meet Abstr).* 2008;112 (Abstract 3707).

31. Palumbo A, Bringhen S, Caravita T, et al. Oral melphalan and prednisone chemotherapy plus thalidomide compared with melphalan and prednisone alone in elderly patients with multiple myeloma: randomised controlled trial [see comment]. *Lancet.* 2006;367:825–831.

32. Palumbo A, Bringhen S, Liberati AM, et al. Oral melphalan, prednisone, and thalidomide in elderly patients with multiple myeloma: updated results of a randomized controlled trial [see comment]. *Blood.* 2008;112:3107–3114.

33. Palumbo A, Falco P, Corradini P, et al. Melphalan, prednisone, and lenalidomide treatment for newly diagnosed myeloma: a report from the GIMEMA—Italian Multiple Myeloma Network. *J Clin Oncol.* 2007;25:4459–4465.

34. Palumbo A, Falco P, Sanpaolo G, et al. Combination of lenalidomide, melphalan, prednisone and thalidomide (RMPT) in relapsed/refractory multiple myeloma: results of a multicenter phase II clinical trial. *Blood (ASH Annu Meet Abstr).* 2008;112 (Abstract 868).

35. Adams J. Development of the proteasome inhibitor PS-341. *Oncologist.* 2002;7:9–16.

36. Hideshima T, Chauhan D, Richardson P, et al. NF-kappa B as a therapeutic target in multiple myeloma. *J Biol Chem.* 2002;277:16639–16647.

37. Hideshima T, Richardson P, Chauhan D, et al. The proteasome inhibitor PS-341 inhibits growth, induces apoptosis, and overcomes drug resistance in human multiple myeloma cells. *Cancer Res.* 2001;61:3071–3076.

38. Richardson PG, Mitsiades C, Hideshima T, et al. Bortezomib: proteasome inhibition as an effective anticancer therapy. *Annu Rev Med.* 2006;57:33–47.

39. Roccaro AM, Hideshima T, Richardson PG, et al. Bortezomib as an antitumor agent. *Curr Pharm Biotechnol.* 2006;7:441–448.

40. Chauhan D, Hideshima T, Anderson KC. Proteasome inhibition in multiple myeloma: therapeutic implication. *Annu Rev Pharmacol Toxicol.* 2005;45:465–476.

41. Ciechanover A, Schwartz AL. The ubiquitin-proteasome pathway: the complexity and myriad functions of proteins death. *Proc Natl Acad Sci USA.* 1998;95:2727–2730.

42. Orlowski RZ, Stinchcombe TE, Mitchell BS, et al. Phase I trial of the proteasome inhibitor PS-341 in patients with refractory hematologic malignancies. *J Clin Oncol.* 2002;20:4420–4427.

43. Jagannath S, Barlogie B, Berenson J, et al. A phase 2 study of two doses of bortezomib in relapsed or refractory myeloma. *Br J Haematol.* 2004;127:165–172.

44. Richardson PG, Barlogie B, Berenson J, et al. A phase 2 study of bortezomib in relapsed, refractory myeloma [see comment]. *N Engl J Med.* 2003;348:2609–2617.

45. Richardson PG, Sonneveld P, Schuster MW, et al. Bortezomib or high-dose dexamethasone for relapsed multiple myeloma [see comment]. *N Engl J Med.* 2005;352:2487–2498.

46. San-Miguel JF, Richardson PG, Sonneveld P, et al. Efficacy and safety of bortezomib in patients with renal impairment: results from the APEX phase 3 study. *Leukemia.* 2008;22:842–849.

47. Jagannath S, Richardson PG, Sonneveld P, et al. Bortezomib appears to overcome the poor prognosis conferred by chromosome 13 deletion in phase 2 and 3 trials. *Leukemia.* 2006;21:151–157.

48. Chanan-Khan AA, Sonneveld P, Schuster MW, et al. Analysis of varicella zoster virus reactivation among bortezomib-treated patients in the APEX study. *Blood (ASH Annu Meet Abstr).* 2006;108 (Abstract 3535).

49. Mitsiades N, Mitsiades CS, Richardson PG, et al. The proteasome inhibitor PS-341 potentiates sensitivity of multiple myeloma cells to conventional chemotherapeutic agents: therapeutic applications. *Blood.* 2003;101:2377–2380.

50. Orlowski RZ, Nagler A, Sonneveld P, et al. Randomized phase III study of pegylated liposomal doxorubicin plus bortezomib compared with bortezomib alone in relapsed or refractory multiple myeloma: combination therapy improves time to progression. *J Clin Oncol.* 2007;25:3892–3901.

51. Palumbo A, Gay F, Bringhen S, et al. Bortezomib, doxorubicin and dexamethasone in advanced multiple myeloma. *Ann Oncol.* 2008;19:1160–1165.

52. Berenson JR, Yang HH, Sadler K, et al. Phase I/II trial assessing borte-zomib and melphalan combination therapy for the treatment of patients with relapsed or refractory multiple myeloma. *J Clin Oncol.* 2006;24:937–944.

53. Berenson JR, Yang HH, Vescio RA, et al. Safety and efficacy of bortezomib and melphalan combination in patients with relapsed or refractory multiple myeloma: updated results of a phase 1/2 study after longer follow-up. *Ann Hematol.* 2008;87:623–631.

54. Davies FE, Wu P, Jenner M, et al. The combination of cyclophosphamide, velcade and dexamethasone induces high response rates with comparable toxicity to velcade alone and velcade plus dexamethasone. *Haematologica.* 2007;92:1149–1150.

55. Popat R, Oakervee H, Williams C, et al. Bortezomib, low-dose intravenous melphalan, and dexamethasone for patients with relapsed multiple myeloma. *Br J Haematol.* 2009;144:887–894.

56. Reece DE, Rodriguez GP, Chen C, et al. Phase I-II trial of bortezomib plus oral cyclophosphamide in relapsed and refractory multiple myeloma. *J Clin Oncol.* 2008;26:4777–4783.

57. Pineda-Roman M, Zangari M, van Rhee F, et al. VTD combination therapy with bortezomib-thalidomide-dexamethasone is highly effective in advanced and refractory multiple myeloma. *Leukemia.* 2008;22:1419–1427.

58. Anderson KC, Jagannath S, Jakubowiak A, et al. Lenalidomide, bortezomib, and dexamethasone in relapsed/refractory multiple myeloma (MM): encour-aging outcomes and tolerability in a phase II study. *J Clin Oncol.* 2009;27 (15 suppl; Abstract 8536).

59. Chanan-Khan A, Miller KC, Musial L, et al. Bortezomib in combination with pegylated liposomal doxorubicin and thalidomide is an effective steroid in-dependent salvage regimen for patients with relapsed or refractory multiple myeloma: results of a phase II clinical trial. *Leuk Lymphoma.* 2009;50:1096–1101.

60. Ciolli S, Leoni F, Casini C, et al. The addition of liposomal doxorubicin to bortezomib, thalidomide and dexamethasone significantly improves clini-cal outcome of advanced multiple myeloma. *Br J Haematol.* 2008;141:814–819.

61. Colado E, Mateos M-V, Moreno M-J, et al. VAMP/ThaCyDex: velcade(R) (bortezomib), adriamycin, melphalan and prednisone alternating with thalido-mide, cyclophosphamide and dexametason as a salvage regimen in relapsed multiple myeloma patients. *Blood (ASH Annu Meet Abstr).* 2008;112 (Abstract 3694).

62. Richardson PG, Xie W, Mitsiades C, et al. Single-agent bortezomib in pre-viously untreated multiple myeloma: efficacy, characterization of peripheral neuropathy, and molecular correlations with response and neuropathy. *J Clin Oncol.* 2009;27:3518–3525.

63. Richardson PG, Sonneveld P, Schuster MW, et al. Reversibility of symptomatic peripheral neuropathy with bortezomib in the phase III APEX trial in relapsed multiple myeloma: impact of a dose-modification guideline. *Br J Haematol.* 2009;144:895–903.

64. Tosi P, Zamagni E, Cellini C, et al. Neurological toxicity of long-term (>1 yr) thalidomide therapy in patients with multiple myeloma. *Eur J Haematol.* 2005;74:212–216.

65. Goldschmidt H, Lannert H, Bommer J, et al. Multiple myeloma and renal failure. *Nephrol Dial Transplant.* 2000;15:301–304.

66. Weber D, Wang M, Chen C, et al. Lenalidomide plus high-dose dexametha-sone provides improved overall survival compared to high-dose dexamethasone alone for relapsed or refractory multiple myeloma (MM): results of 2 phase III studies (MM-009, MM-010) and subgroup analysis of patients with impaired renal function. *Blood (ASH Annu Meet Abstr).* 2006;108 (Abstract 3547).

67. Chen N, Lau H, Kong L, et al. Pharmacokinetics of lenalidomide in subjects with various degrees of renal impairment and in subjects on hemodialysis. *J Clin Pharmacol.* 2007;47:1466–1475.

68. Tosi P, Zamagni E, Cellini C, et al. Thalidomide alone or in combination with dexamethasone in patients with advanced, relapsed or refractory multiple myeloma and renal failure. *Eur J Haematol.* 2004;73:98–103.

69. Harris E, Behrens J, Samson D, et al. Use of thalidomide in patients with myeloma and renal failure may be associated with unexplained hyperkalaemia. *Br J Haematol.* 2003;122:159–167.

70. Smadja NV, Bastard C, Brigaudeau C, et al. Hypodiploidy is a major prognostic factor in multiple myeloma. *Blood.* 2001;98:2229–2238.

71. Alexanian R, Weber DM, Anagnostopoulos A, et al. Thalidomide with or with-out dexamethasone for refractory or relapsing multiple myeloma. *Semin Hema-tol.* 2003;40:3–7.

72. Reece DE, Masih-Khan E, Khan A, et al. Phase I-II trial of oral cyclophos-phamide, prednisone and lenalidomide (revlimid(R)) (CPR) for the treatment of patients with relapsed and refractory multiple myeloma. *Blood (ASH Annu Meet Abstr).* 2008;112 (Abstract 1723).

73. Baz R, Walker E, Karam MA, et al. Lenalidomide and pegylated liposomal doxorubicin-based chemotherapy for relapsed or refractory multiple myeloma: safety and efficacy. *Ann Oncol.* 2006;17:1766–1771.

74. Di Raimondo F, Romano A, Gorgone A, et al. Salvage therapy with intravenous liposomal adryamicin (A), bortezomib (B), cyclophosphamide (C), and dex-amethasone (D) (ABCD) in previously treated myeloma patients. *ASH Annu Meet Abstr.* 2008;112 (Abstract 2779).

75. Terpos E, Kastritis E, Roussou M, et al. The combination of bortezomib, mel-phalan, dexamethasone and intermittent thalidomide is an effective regimen for relapsed/refractory myeloma and is associated with improvement of abnormal bone metabolism and angiogenesis. *Leukemia.* 2008;22:2247–2256.

# Evolving Role of Novel Agents for Maintenance Therapy in Myeloma

Valeria Magarotto • Antonio Palumbo

Multiple myeloma (MM) is an incurable malignant plasma cell disorder. In the last 2 decades, with the introduction of autologous stem cell transplantation (ASCT) and, more recently, with the new drugs (thalidomide, lenalidomide, and bortezomib) has been possible to improve the response rate (RR), to prolong the progression free survival (PFS) and the overall survival (OS). Unfortunately, despite these recent advances, myeloma relapses and, often, subsequent salvage treatment options are limited.

The median duration of response (DOR) after the most recent chemotherapeutic protocols and ASCT does not exceed 3 years. To prolong the DOR and survival, maintenance therapy is an interesting approach, but its role in myeloma remains unclear. Corticosteroids prolonged the DOR, but the effects on survival were controversial.[1,2]

Berenson et al[1] showed a significant benefit in term of event-free survival (EFS) and OS derived from high-dose prednisone (50 mg every other day) versus physiologic dose (10 mg/d) in patients who received conventional chemotherapy (CC). After a median follow-up of 44 months, EFS was 14 months versus 5 months, respectively ($P = 0.003$), and OS was 37 months for high-dose prednisone versus 26 months for low dose. The therapy was well tolerated, using an alternate prednisone regimen. More recently, another study failed to show a survival benefit from steroids used in maintenance.[2] The median PFS was slightly elevated in patients who received dexamethasone (40 mg on days 1–4 every 28 days till progression) versus no maintenance: 2.8 and 2.1 years, respectively ($P = 0.0002$). But the median OS was 4.1 years in the dexamethasone arm versus 3.8 years in no maintenance group ($P = 0.4$). As expected, patients who received dexamethasone experienced more nonhematologic toxicity, in particular hyperglycemia and infection.

Interferon-$\alpha$ (IFN-$\alpha$) represented a great hope, especially after ASCT, because the tumor burden is lower. The preliminary data of a randomized clinical trial showed an advantage of IFN-$\alpha$ after high-dose treatment, but after a longer follow-up, there were a modest increased of PFS and OS, with important side effects.[3] The final results of the phase III US intergroup trial S9321 decreed the definitive failure of interferon used in maintenance therapy after both ASCT and CC for patients who achieved >75% tumor reduction.[4]

The introduction of the novel agent and the promising results obtained in the up-front and relapsed MM, led to explore the role of thalidomide, bortezomib, and lenalidomide in maintenance setting.

## Maintenance Therapy With Thalidomide

Different studies showed that thalidomide plays a role as consolidation and maintenance treatment both in newly diagnosed and in relapsed/refractory MM (Table 1).

The French IFM-99 trial showed that the association of thalidomide and pamidronate, given after double ASCT, is better in terms of OS and EFS than no maintenance or pamidronate alone.[5] The effect of thalidomide on EFS did not differ according to the $\beta$2-microglobulin dosage, LDH level, Durie-Salmon stage, or age, but patients with deletion of chromosome 13 (del13) had not benefit from thalidomide ($P < 0.006$). Moreover, thalidomide improves the quality of response in patients who achieved less than a very good partial remission (VGPR) showing a consolidation rather than a maintenance activity, by reducing tumor mass after high-dose therapy (HDT).

The Arkansas group scheduled thalidomide in both the induction treatment and in the maintenance therapy post tandem-ASCT in the experimental arm of total therapy II trial (Table 1).[6] After a median follow-up of 72 months, they observed that thalidomide increasing the frequency of complete remission (CR) and VGPR, reaching the level of 50% and 72%, respectively, at 3 years from randomization. The EFS was prolonged in thalidomide arm, regardless the presence of cytogenetic abnormalities (CA), but OS was superior on experimental arm only in patients with CA. Moreover, in 351 patients was available the gene expression profiling that revealed a survival benefit from thalidomide in those with low-risk disease. Estimate 5-years OS in patients enrolled in the experimental arm and with CA was 70% versus 51% in patients with CA treated with standard chemotherapy ($P = 0.01$). In contrast, the estimate 5-years OS in patients without CA was 71% versus 80% in patients treated with or without thalidomide, respectively ($P = 0.42$). Postrelapse survival was longer in the control arm, except for patients with CA, who benefit from thalidomide maintenance also in the subsequent line of treatment. Reiterative landmark analyses revealed that the duration and cumulative dose of thalidomide administration did not impact on clinical outcome, meaning that it is possible to limit thalidomide exposure, reducing toxicity, without compromising the efficacy. This result has been recently confirmed by a phase II trial that enrolled 100 patients for maintenance treatment post-ASCT, in 5 different thalidomide dose cohorts (50, 100, 200, 250 and 300 mg/d).[7] Median PFS was 34 months and 3-years OS was 76%, without differences among the 5 courts, unless toxicity, that increases at dose of 200 mg/d or above. Fifteen patients improved their disease status from a partial remission (PR) to a CR, confirming the consolidation role given to thalidomide by the IFM-99 trial.

The English MCR Myeloma IX study evaluated maintenance with thalidomide (100 mg/d) versus no maintenance in patients treated with HDT and in those treated with nonintensive chemotherapy.[8] There was no significant difference in OS, whereas thalidomide improved PFS, but only in patients who achieved less than VGPR (Table 1). Moreover, thalidomide may be detrimental in terms of OS and EFS for patients with deletion of chromosome 17.

Three different studies evaluated the association of thalidomide with corticosteroids as maintenance therapy both after HDT[9,10] and after noninvasive-chemotherapy.[11]

An Australian study compared maintenance with alternate day prednisolone alone versus alternate day prednisolone plus thalidomide

**TABLE 1.** Maintenance Therapy With Thalidomide in Patient Candidates to High-Dose Therapy (HDT) and Autologous Stem Cell Transplantation (ASCT)

| Study | Therapy | Schedule Sf Maintenance | PFS | EFS | OS | Toxicities Thal Related |
|---|---|---|---|---|---|---|
| IFM-99–02[5] | Double ASCT Maintenance: none (A) vs. pamidronate (B) vs. thalidomide (C) | Thal 50–400 mg/d | | At 3 yr = A, 36%; B, 37%; C, 52% | At 4 yr = A, 77%; B, 74%; C, 87% | Neuropathy, fatigue, constipation, neutropenia, cardiotox |
| MRC myeloma IX[8] | Young/fit pt: CTD or CVAD-> HDM Maintenance: no vs. thal Elderly/unfit pt: induction: MP vs. reduced CTD Maintenance: no vs. thal | Starting dose 100 mg/d | In young and elderly: benefit from maintenance in < VGPR | | No difference | NA |
| Australian study[9] | Single ASCT Maintenance: TP vs. P | Thal 200 mg/d, Pdn 50 mg AD (for maximum 12 mo) | At 3 yr 42% vs. 23% | | At 3 yr 86% vs. 75% | Neuropathy, infection, constipation, fatigue, skin rash |
| S0204[10] | Double ASCT (induction with TD) Maintenance: TP | Thal 200 mg/d Pdn 50 mg AD (till undue toxicity or progression) | | At 4 yr 50% | At 4 yr 64% | Neuropathy, infection, thrombosis |
| TT2[6] | Induction therapy: chemo vs. chemo plus thal Double ASCT Consolidation: chemo vs. chemo + thal Maintenance: IFN + Thal vs. IFN alone | Thal in maintenance phase: 100 mg/d (1st yr) 50 mg/d (2nd yr) | | Median 6 yr thal arm vs. 4.1 yr no thal arm | At 8 yr 57% (thal arm) 44% (no thal arm) | Thrombosis, neutropenia, peripheral neuropathy, syncope, bowel obstruction |
| Feyler S et al[7] | Single ASCT Maintenance with thal | Five dose cohorts: 50, 100, 200, 250, 300 mg/d thal | At 3 yr 41% | | At 3 yr 76% | Peripheral neuropathy, skin, shortness of breath, dizziness, DVT |

CTD indicates cyclophosphamide, thalidomide, dexamethasone; CVAD, cyclophosphamide, vincristine, adriamycin, dexamethasone; DVT, deep vein thrombosis; HDM, high-dose melphalan; prednisone; P, prednisone; TD, thalidomide, dexamethasone; and TP, thalidomide, prednisone.

(TP) given after ASCT.[9] Thalidomide induced a highly significant improvement in term of response (63% versus 40% at 1 year from the beginning of maintenance therapy) and an evident prolonged PFS and OS (Table 1). Moreover in TP arm, PFS was not affected by response to ASCT (CR/VGPR versus PR) or by level of $\beta$2-microglobulin. In contrast with Arkansan group study, thalidomide maintenance did not affect postrelapse survival, with an estimated 1-year postrelapse survival of 79% and 77% in thalidomide and control arm, respectively ($P = 0.237$).

Hussein et al[10] combined thalidomide and dexamethasone (TD) both as induction treatment, before tandem ASCT and in the subsequent maintenance therapy. The study confirmed the consolidation role of thalidomide that improved the response achieved with tandem ASCT. After the second transplantation, the VGPR and CR rate were 53% and 12%, respectively, but at the end of first year of thalidomide maintenance, they increased to 72% for VGPR and 22% for CR. The estimate 4-year EFS and OS were 50% and 64%, respectively, with a superior survival outcome for patients in stage I ISS, with low-LDH level and if received the second ASCT in a timely fashion.

Thal-dex (TD) combination has been also compared with IFN-$\alpha$ plus dexamethasone (ID) as maintenance treatment after *Tha*DD (thalidomide-dexamethasone-liposomal doxorubicin) in

newly diagnosed not candidate to ASCT and in relapsed MM.[11] After a median follow-up of 30 months, 60% of patients in ID arm relapsed versus 33% of patients who received TD ($P = 0.024$) with a 2-years PFS of 32% and 63%, respectively. The advantage was evident both in newly diagnosed and in relapsed MM. A significant benefit in terms of PFS was seen in patients with ISS score I, favorable cytogenetic, and in patients not achieving VGPR with induction treatment. Two-years OS was better in TD than in ID arm (84% versus 68%; $P = 0.030$). Peripheral neuropathy (PN), neutropenia, fatigue, constipation, infection, and skin rash were the most frequently thalidomide-related adverse events (Table 1).

Considering that the cumulative dose of thalidomide, does not influence the efficacy of maintenance therapy and that patients with a response to induction regimen $\geq$ VGPR did not benefit from the treatment, stopping thalidomide when a VGPR has been reached and do not exceed the dose of 200 mg/d, may reduce the side effect (in particular PN) avoiding thalidomide resistance in case of relapse.

Maintenance with thalidomide has been also used after induction treatment of elderly or unfit patients, not candidates to ASCT. The results are controversial, because different studies showed that thalidomide did not prolong OS.

In the GIMEMA study,[12] newly diagnosed patients with MM (aged 65–85 years), or younger patients not eligible for ASCT, were

**TABLE 2.** Maintenance With Thalidomide in Patient Candidates to Conventional Chemotherapy

| Study | Therapy | Schedule of Maintenance | PFS | OS |
|---|---|---|---|---|
| GIMEMA[12] | MP vs. MPT: mel 4 mg/m² days 1–7; pdn 40 mg/m² days 1–7; thal 100 mg continuously every 4 wk | 100 mg thal/d until disease progression | 14.5 vs. 21.8 mo | 47.6 vs. 45 mo |
| IFM 99–06[14] | MP vs. MPT vs. Mel100 mel 0.25 mg/kg days 1–4; pdn 2 mg/kg days 1–4; thal 400 mg continuously every 4 wk | No maintenance | | 33.2 vs. 51.6 vs. 38.3 mo |
| IFM 01–01[15] | MP vs. MPT mel 0.2 mg/kg days 1–4; pdn 2 mg/kg days 1–4; thal 100 mg continuously every 4 wk | No maintenance | 18.5 vs. 24.1 mo | 29.1 vs. 44 mo |
| HOVON 49 study[13] | MP vs. MPT Mel: 0.25 mg/kg; pdn 1 mg/kg on 1–5 d every 4 wk Thalidomide 200 mg/d | Thalidomide 50 mg/d until disease progression | PFS at 2 yr 19% vs. 33% | Median OS 30 vs. 37 mo |
| Ludwig et al[16] | MP vs. TD Mel 0.25 mg/kg days 1–4; pdn 2 mg/kg days 1–4 Thal 200 mg/d; dex 40 mg/d on days 1–4, 15–18 | Thal 100 mg/d + IFN 3 MU 3 times/wk vs. IFN 3 MU 3 times/wk only | 20.7 vs. 16.7 mo | 49.5 vs. 41.5 mo |
| Offidani et al[11] | Induction: ThaDD (6–28 d cycles): Thalidomide 100 mg/d continuously; dexamethasone 40 mg days 1–4, 9–12; doxorubicin 40 mg/m² on day 1 Maintenance: IFNα-D vs. TD | Thal maintenance 100 mg/d<br><br>Prednisone 20 mg on days 1–4 every month vs. IFN 3 MU × 3/wk Prednisone 20 mg on days 1–4 every month | At 2 yr: 32% vs. 63% | At 2 yr: 68% vs. 84% |

randomly assigned to melpahalan (MP) or to MP plus thalidomide (MPT). At the end of induction therapy, patients in MPT arm, received maintenance with thalidomide (100 mg/d) until recurrence of disease (Table 2). After a median follow-up of 38.1 months, the median PFS was 21.8 months for MPT and 14.5 months for MP, whereas the median OS was 45 months and 47.6 months respectively. Oral MPT, followed by thalidomide as maintenance showed a better RR and DOR than did standard MP, but failed to show a benefit in OS.

The HOVON group presented a similar study (Table 2). The addiction of thalidomide to MP resulted in a significant better RR (66% in MPT versus 47% in MP) and a significantly better EFS and PFS. But even this study was unable to confirm the positive effect of Thalidomide on OS.[13]

In contrast, the French IFM 99-06 and IFM-01-01 trials showed the advantage of MPT combination in terms of OS and PFS, over MP or ASCT[14] and in patients older than 75 years[15] without including maintenance with thalidomide (Table 2).

Ludwig et al[16] compared MP with TD in elderly newly diagnosed MM. Patients achieving stable disease or better were randomly assigned to maintenance therapy with either thalidomide (100 mg/d) plus IFN-α 2b (3 MU 3 times a week) or to 3 MU interferon α-2b (IFN-a) only at the same dose (Table 2). Thalidomide arm resulted in higher proportion of overall response rate (included a higher CR/VGPR rate) but TTP and PFS were similar (Table 2). The OS was significantly shorter in TD group, partly due to increased toxicity of this combination. Moreover, maintenance with thalidomide and interferon induced similar survival than did interferon alone. Because the randomization was sequential to induction treatment, half of patients had already received TD, which could explain the similar survival in both maintenance groups. Moreover, maintenance with IFN-α is associated with a shorter OS after relapse,[17] contributing to

the shorter survival of TD group. Also thalidomide could contribute to the shorter survival after relapse, inducing a sort of resistance, as shown in the GIMEMA study.[12]

It's difficult to compare these clinical trials, because the difference between population and schedules but what emerged is that thalidomide has not a consolidated role as maintenance after CC. One of the main topics is the toxicity, in particular PN. These kinds of patients tolerate a lower dose of thalidomide and for a limited period. Moreover, a prolonged exposure to thalidomide seems to induce resistance to the after treatment, reducing the OS.

Thalidomide has a consolidation role rather than maintenance, in the context of HDT, inducing benefit when used after ASCT and in patients with low-risk MM who achieved less than VGPR. In the context of CC, the role is controversial, because thalidomide increased PFS/EFS, without a clear prolongation of OS and a potential induction of resistance to following treatment.

## Maintenance Therapy With Lenalidomide

Lenalidomide is an effective and safe analogue of thalidomide, with a consolidated role for the treatment of MM. Giving to its high antimyeloma activity and low toxicity profile, especially in term of PN, it is a valid alternative to thalidomide both in newly diagnosed and in relapsed MM. As maintenance therapy, the role of lenalidomide is still under evaluation.

In a phase I/II study, lenalidomide has been combined to melphalan and prednisone for the treatment of newly diagnosed, not candidates to ASCT myeloma patients (Table 3).[18] The schedule included nine 28 day cycles of induction, followed by continuous maintenance with lenalidomide (10 mg/d) till relapsed or intolerance. Eighty-one percent of patients achieved at least a PR, 47.6% achieved a VGPR and 23.8% achieved an immunofixation-negative CR. In all patients,

**TABLE 3.** Maintenance Therapy With Lenalidomide

| | Lenalidomide | Schedule | Response | Survival Analysis | Main Toxicities |
|---|---|---|---|---|---|
| San Miguel et al[20] | RD in relapsed/ refractory | Rev: 25 mg on days 1–21 | See MM-009 | RD <10 mo after best response vs. RD >10 mo | Neutropenia, thrombocytopenia, fatigue, infection, DVT |
| | MM | Dex: 40 mg on days 1–4, 9–12, 17–20 | MM-010[18,19] | Median OS = 29.5 mo vs. NR | |
| | | | | Median TTP= 13.6 moths vs. NR | |
| Palumbo et al[24] | RMPT for 6 cycles Lenalidomide maintenance | Induction (6 cycles): RMPT (2 different thal dose) | Arm A: PR = 93.3% (included VGPR = 46.7%) vs. arm B: PR = 64.7% | At 1 yr PFS = 48.6% | Neutropenia, thrombocytopenia, anemia, infection, neuropathy, fatigue |
| | In relapsed/refractory MM | Maintenance: lenalidomide 10 mg/d on days 1–21 with 7 d rest | | At 1 yr OS = 30% | |
| Palumbo et al[22] | PAD as induction | Induction (4–21 d cycles) PAD | After induction: PR 94% (VGPR 59%, CR 13%) | At 1 y PFS 92% | Thrombocytopenia, neutropenia, infections, gastrointestinal, peripheral neuropathy, DVT |
| | RP as consolidation R as maintenance | SCM and double ASCT Consolidation: (4–28 d cycles): RP Lenalidomide: 25 mg/d on days 1–21 | After double ASCT: CR + VGPR = 41% | At 1 y TTP 97% | |
| | | Prednisone: 50 mg every other days Maintenance: lenalidomdie 10 mg/d on days 1–21 | After LP consolidation: 100% PR, 88% VGPR, 53% CR | At 1 y OS 92% | |
| Palumbo et al[21] | MPR as induction R as maintenance | Induction: MPR Maintenance: Lenalidomide 10 mg/d | 81% at least a PR, 47.6% VGPR 23.8% immunofixation-negative CR | At 1-yr EFS 92% At 1 yr OS 100% | Neutropenia thrombocytopenia febrile neutropenia vasculitis thromboembolism |

RMPT indicates lenalidomide 10 mg/d on days 1–21, melphalan 0.18 mg/kg on days 1–4, prednisone 2 mg/kg on days 1–4; thalidomide, 50 mg/d (arm A) vs. 100 mg/d (arm B) on days 1–28; PAD Bortezomib, 1.3 mg/m² on days 1, 4, 8, and 11; Doxil, 30 mg/m² on day 4; Dex 40 mg on days 1–4, 8–11, 15–18; MPR, melphalan doses ranging from 0.18 to 0.25 mg/kg on days 1–4; prednisone, 2 mg/kg dose on days 1–4 lenalidomide ranging from 5 mg to 10 mg on days 1 to 21 every 28 (9 cycles).

1-year EFS and OS were 92% and 100% respectively. Remarkable is the 1-year OS of 100% that is unprecedented in a newly diagnosed MM trial.

Lenalidomide has been used also as consolidation/maintenance in elderly untreated patients with MM candidate to ASCT (Table 3).[19] One-hundred and 2 patients received bortezomib, pegylated doxorubicin and dexamethasone (PAD) as induction, followed by reduced intensity autologous transplantation (Mel 100). The schedule included also four 28-days of consolidation cycles with lenalidomide (25 mg/d on days 1–21) and prednisone (50 mg every other days) followed by lenalidomide alone maintenance (10 mg on days 1–21 every 28 days). RR increased progressively: after PAD the PR rate was 94%, including 59% VGPR, and 13% CR; after tandem Mel 100, 88% of patients received at least a VGPR and 41% CR; after LP consolidation all patients obtained a PR, 88% at least VGPR and 53% CR. With a median follow-up of 14 months, 1 year OS and PFS were 92%. Moreover, PFS was not significantly affected by $\beta$2-microglobulin levels and presence of chromosome 13 deletion.

A French double blind clinical trial is ongoing for evaluating the relevance of maintenance therapy using lenalidomide after ASCT. Patients under 65 years receive a double ASCT and, if they do not present sign of progression, are subsequently randomized for receiving placebo or lenalidomide as maintenance, till progression.[20]

In the relapse/refractory setting, lenalidomide combined with dexamethasone (RD) showed a significantly improved RR and prolonged median TTP and OS compared with dexamethasone alone.[21,22] In a recent substudy, has been demonstrated that patients who prolonged the treatment with RD for $\geq$10 months after achieving their best response has a longer OS and TTP than patients who discontinued treatment for emerging side effects.[23] At 24 months after achieving their best response, 93.8% of patients who continued the treatment were alive versus 48.4% of patients who interrupted TD ($P = 0.0001$). Median time to progression has been not reached in patients who continued the treatment vs13.6 month in patients who stopped RD ($P = 0.0001$). Prolonging the treatment of relapsed/refractory MM with RD till the recurrence of disease or intolerance seems to ensure one of the best TTP, even compared with bortezomib alone which showed a TTP of 6.2 months (APEX study).[24]

Lenalidomide has also been combined with melphalan, prednisone, and thalidomide (RMPT) as induction, followed by maintenance with single agent lenalidomide, for the treatment of relapsed/refractory MM[25] (Table 3). Forty-four patients has been enrolled,

26 patients received melphalan, prednisone, and thalidomide as second line of therapy, 18 as third line. After a median of 2 courses, 75.8% of patients achieved at least a PR, included 30% of VGPR. The 1-year PFS from study entry was 90%. The main adverse events were hematologic (neutropenia 66.6%, thrombocytopenia 36.3%, and anemia 30.2%). PN rate was only 6%, and no thromboembolic events were reported.

The most frequent adverse event lenalidomide related included fatigue, thrombocytopenia, neutropenia, infection, and deep vein thrombosis (especially in combination with steroids). PN is significantly reduced, usually grade 1–2 and in case of pre-existing PN, exacerbation is less frequent as consequence of lenalidomide treatment.

Lenalidomide is an effective and safety drug, also in maintenance setting. As shown by these studies, it can be used for longer time, without important toxicity or resistance to after treatment and in high-risk MM (high b2-microglobulin or deletion chromosome13) prolonging OS and PFS. These make lenalidomide one of the best choices in term of maintenance. The recommended dose of lenalidomide for the induction is 25 mg/d which can be used for up to 6 months and generally, till the achievement of the best response.[21,22] For maintenance purpose, the suggested dose is 10 mg/d,[18,19] which ensures a prolonged TTP, without intolerable toxicity, like cytopenias and fatigue.

## Maintenance Therapy With Bortezomib

Bortezomib is the first proteasome inhibitor to enter the clinic and to be approved for the treatment of MM. It showed to be very active and safe for the treatment of both newly diagnosed and relapsed MM. Different studies are on going for evaluating bortezomib as maintenance. The data are preliminary and often in form of abstract, but it seems that bortezomib is helpful to postpone the disease relapse and to increase the RR obtained with induction.

Schiller et al[26] evaluated the impact of bortezomib used as maintenance therapy, beginning 3 to 4 months after ASCT. At the moment of analysis, they enrolled 29 patients in 3 different bortezomib dose levels (Table 4). The maximum tolerated dose was established 1.3 mg/m$^2$. Five patients stopped the treatment (2 for disease progression, 2 for side effects, and 1 for personal reasons). After a median follow-up of 17.1 months, 6 patients have been relapsed, 13 continue to be followed every 3 months for evidence of disease recurrence, and 4 continue on treatment. The median relapse-free survival was 15.5 months.

In another recent study, bortezomib has been used as induction therapy, before ASCT transplantation and after, as maintenance (Table 4). Forty newly diagnosed patients have been enrolled.[27] Response assessment before ASCT included: CR + VGPR 15%, PR 55%, >75% reduction in monoclonal protein in 19% of patients and 25% to 75% paraprotein reduction in 10% of patients. Twenty-eight patients received bortezomib in the posttransplant phase: 1 patient improved from VGPR to CR and another improved form PR to VGPR. After a median follow-up of 838 days, VGPR + CR rate was 43%. Three-year estimate EFS and OS were 32.3% and 62.2%, respectively.

The HOVON-65/GMMG-HD4 phase III clinical trial compared bortezomib-contain regimen (PAD-B) given in induction, before ASCT and in the subsequent maintenance phase with anthracyclin-contain regimen as induction, followed by maintenance with thalidomide (VAD-T), as therapy for newly diagnosed MM.[28] The preliminary data showed a superiority of bortezomib, with overall complete RR included maintenance of 27% versus 5% of VAD-T arm. Chromosome abnormalities, in particular deletion of chromo-

some 13, did not impact on efficacy. PN and constitutional symptoms were the major adverse events.

The Mayo Clinic group evaluated the role of single agent bortezomib given in induction, maintenance and reinduction in patients with high-risk MM, with $\beta$2-microglobulin $\geq 5.5$, plasma cell labeling index $\geq 1$ or deletion chromosome 13 (Table 4).[29] Forty patients has been enrolled, 19 completed the induction phase achieving a RR of 40% (PR or better, no CR achieved). During the maintenance phase, one's patient response was upgraded to CR. Median PFS was 16.3 months, increased to 19.8 months for patients who entered in maintenance phase.

Another clinical trial is ongoing, comparing induction treatment with bortezomib plus MPT (VMPT) versus bortezomib plus MP (VMP) in newly diagnosed patients with MM not candidate to ASCT.[30] After induction, only for VMPT arm has been scheduled a maintenance treatment with bortezomib at reduced dose (1.3 mg/m$^2$ every other week) till recurrence of disease or intolerable toxicity. The results of this trial will help to clarify the role of bortezomib in induction treatment and the benefit derived from a prolonged, but reduced dose of bortezomib in maintenance phase.

Bortezomib (1.3 mg/m$^2$ every other week) combined with dexamethasone has evaluated as maintenance therapy in relapsed/refractory myeloma patients, after the achievement of their best response.[31] Forty patients have been enrolled. After a median follow-up of 13 months, in 5 patients there was an improvement of response, with 5 PR converted in 1 CR and 4 VGPR and a remarkable reduction of monoclonal component was evident in 11 patients. Median time to progression was 23 months, with a 1-year PFS of 69%. The 1 year OS was 63%. Toxicities were low, with only cases of grade 1 PN, gastrointestinal affection and zoster reactivation.

In the context of relapsed/refractory MM, the association of bortezomib with lenalidomide and dexamethasone, given in induction and subsequently in maintenance at lower doses seems to be an effective and safety treatment (Table 4).[32] The preliminary data showed an ORR of 84% $\geq$ MR, including 21% CR/nCR and 68% of PR, independently from high-risk features and previous treatment. Toxicity were manageable, with only 1 case over 64 patients enrolled of grade 3 PN.

As shown in these studies, the most common bortezomib-related adverse events are fatigue, PN, gastrointestinal problems, herpes virus infection reactivation, thrombocytopenia, and neutropenia (Table 4).

The role of bortezomib as consolidation/maintenance is still under evaluation. Probably, as thalidomide, plays more a consolidation role, but only a longer follow-up of the ongoing studies will clarify this aspect. Like lenalidomide it is effective for patients with high-risk MM. The major problem derived from a prolonged administration is the potential irreversible PN. Reducing the dose of Bortezomib to 1.3 mg/m$^2$ once every other week in consolidation/maintenance setting,[30–32] would allow the advantage derived from a prolonged administration of bortezomib, without compromising the safety.

## DISCUSSION

The role of maintenance therapy in MM is still controversial corticosteroids[1,2] and IFN-$\alpha$[3,4] showed only a modest increase in PFS and OS. Novel agents, such as IMiDS (thalidomide and lenalidomide) and proteasome inhibitors (bortezomib) induce a superior CR rate and a prolonged PFS and OS, replacing CC both in newly diagnosed and in relapsed/refractory MM.

These promising results led to explore the role of novel agent in the maintenance setting. Almost all the studies presented, showed

**TABLE 4.** Maintenance Therapy With Bortezomib

| Study | Bortezomib | Schedule | Response | Survival Analysis | Main Toxicities |
|---|---|---|---|---|---|
| Schiller et al (ongoing study)[26] | Bortezomib maintenance<br><br>After single ASCT | Three cohort (1.0, 1.3, 1.6 mg/m² q wk for 3 wk, followed by 1 wk rest period<br><br>MTD 1.3 mg/m² | 13 patients disease recurrence<br><br>6 patients relapsed 4 patients on treatment | Median relapse-free survival 15.5 mo | Thrombocytopenia, neuropathy, anemia, fatigue, neutropenia, musculoskeletal, zoster, gastrointestinal |
| Uy et al[27] | Induction chemotherapy Bortezomib given before ASCT and in maintenance | Induction: chemotherapy<br><br>Pretransplant + bortezomib 1.3 mg/m² on days 1, 4, 8, 11 of 28 d cycles (2 cycles) and ASCT<br><br>Maintenance: bortezomib 1.3 mg/m² weekly for 4 of every 5 wk for up to 6 cycles | Induction: CR + VGPR = 15% PR = 55%<br><br>Posttransplant bortezomib: ORR = 73% CR + VGPR = 43% | EFS @ 3 y 32% from start of pretransplant Bortezomib OS at 3 yr 62.2% from start of pretransplant bortezomib OS at 1 yr 88.1% | Peripheral neuropathy, fatigue, Herpes virus reactivation |
| Dispenzieri et al[29] | Bortezomib given in induction, maintenance and reinduction after relapse | Induction: bortezomib 1.3 mg/m² on days 1, 4, 8, 11 every 21 d for 8 cycles<br><br>After 4 cycles, allowed SCM<br><br>After 8 cycles, maintenance: bortezomib 1.3 mg/m² every other week | Induction: 2 VGPR, 17 PR, 3 MR<br><br>Maintenance: 1 CR | Median PFS 16.3 mo for patients in maintenance (15 pts): 19.8 mo | Peripheral neuropathy |
| HOVON-65/GMMG-HD4 (ongoing study)[28] | PAD vs. VAD (induction) ASCT<br><br>Bortezomib vs. thalidomide (mainteinance) | Induction: PAD vs. VAD<br><br>Maintenance: PAD arm: bortezomib 1.3 mg/m² every other week<br><br>VAD arm: thalidomide 50 mg/d | Overall CR included maintenance 27% vs. 5% | NA | Peripheral neuropathy, DVT, constitutional symptoms |
| Benevolo et al (ongoing study)[31] | Bortezomib maintenance after salvage therapy with bortezomib or thelidomide | Maintenance: bortezomib: 1.3 mg/m² on days 1, 15<br><br>Dexamethasone: 20 mg on days 1–2, 15–16<br><br>In a 28 cycles x a total of 6 cycles | Conversion in 1 CR and 4 VGPR, the PR after salvage therapy | Median TTP 23 mo | Neuropathy, zoster reactivation, gastrointestinal |
| Anderson et al (ongoing study)[32] | RVD induction in patients with relapsed/refractory MM and RV in maintenance | Induction: 8–21 d cycles RVD<br><br>Maintenance: lenalidomide 15 mg on days 1–14<br><br>Bortezomib 1 mg/m² on days 1–8<br><br>Dexamethasone 10 mg day of and day after bortezomib | ORR 84% ≥ MR (21% CR/nCR) | OS at yr: 63%<br><br>Median duration of response 24 wk | Myelosuppression, DVT, neuropathy |

PAD indicates Bortezomib 1.3 mg/m² on days 1, 4, 8, and 11, Adriamycine 9 mg/m² on days 1–4, dexamethasone 40 mg on days 1–4, 9–12, 17–20; VAD, vincristine 0.4 mg and adriamycine 9 mg/m² on days 1–4; dexamethasone, 40 mg on days 1–4, 9–12, 17–20 ASCT; RVD, lenalidomide 15 mg/d on days 1–14, bortezomib 1 mg/m² on days 1, 4, 8, and 11, dexamethasone 20/40 mg: day of and day after bortezomib.

the consolidation role of thalidomide, with an improved quality of response for patients who reached less than VGPR after induction therapy. PFS is generally prolonged in all patients who received thalidomide, but OS is implemented in patients with stage I ISS, with gene expression profiling-defined low-risk MM (eg, absence of deletion of chromosome 13 or 17) or low LDH level.[6] The effect on postrelapse survival is controversial, because the Australian study showed no difference in postrelapse survival between patients who received thalidomide in maintenance or not.[9] In contrast, the Arkansas group[6] showed a shorter postrelapse survival for patients who received thalidomide, except those with CA, who benefited. The GIMEMA study (MP versus MPT) confirmed the shorter postrelapse survival in patients who receive thalidomide at diagnosis and during maintenance, probably caused by a certain drug resistance, derived from the prolonged administration of the drug.[12]

The duration and cumulative dose of thalidomide administration do not impact on clinical outcome, but has important consequences on toxicity, especially on PN. Moreover, considering that the major benefit is for patients with less than VGPR as postinduction response, maintenance regimen should be administered at a dose less than 200 mg/d, till the achievement of VGPR and only in patients who can really benefit from thalidomide, like patients without or with low risk CA. All these data, led to conclude that, probably, thalidomide is a good choice for consolidation treatment, since it has limited duration, without compromising safety and avoiding resistance to after treatment.

The role of bortezomib and lenalidomide in maintenance is still under investigation. Lenalidomide is an effective and less toxic derivative of thalidomide. Used as maintenance therapy, prolongs OS and PFS, even in patients with CA or high $\beta$2-microglobulin,[19] representing a valid alternative to thalidomide for these kinds of patients. It plays a role also as consolidation regimen, since it increased the CR/VGPR rate.[19] In contrast with thalidomide it seems that continuing lenalidomide after the achievement of best response prolongs PFS and OS without inducing resistance to after treatment.[21–23] No data are available about the cumulative toxicity related to prolonging exposure of lenalidomide. The reduction of the dose from 25 mg/d (used in induction) to 10 mg/d (used in maintenance) is suggested, because it allows continuing lenalidomide treatment without intolerant toxicities. Bortezomib showed a more pronounced consolidation role, particularly in patients with less than VGPR. The data are still preliminary to evaluate the effects on survival, but they are encouraging. Like lenalidomide, bortezomib is a valid choice for patients with high-risk MM, as those with high plasma cell labeling index or with chromosome 13 deletion.[26–28] Actually, there are limited data on the impact of duration and cumulative dose on outcome, when bortezomib is used for long period. The reduction of the dose to 1.3 mg/m² every other week in maintenance treatment is under investigation and could be a good choice for balancing efficacy and safety.

In conclusion, thalidomide seems to have more a consolidation role, because improves the response obtained with induction regimen. Moreover, its toxicity profile and the potential induction of resistance to postrelapse treatment, suggests the use of thalidomide for a limited period of time, as the consolidation requires. Low-toxicity profile and the potential longer PFS/OS derived from lenalidomide prolonged administration, makes it one of the best drug for maintenance treatment. Bortezomib seems to have both consolidation and maintenance role. Since the main toxicity is the potential irreversible PN, a reduced schedule (1.3 mg/m² every other week) for maintenance treatment could be a solution for balancing efficacy and safety.[30–32]

Probably in the next future we will have a more clear idea about the role of lenalidomide and bortezomib as consolidation/maintenance therapy. The preliminary data are encouraging but, actually we have no data about the superiority of a drug over another and a longer follow-up needed before making any conclusion. The goal will be to determine the best maintenance strategy for each category of patients, taking into account distinct variables such as tolerability, efficacy, cytogentic, age, or comorbidity.

## REFERENCES

1. Berenson JR, Crowley JJ, Grogan TM, et al. Maintenance therapy with alternate day prednisone improves survival in multiple myeloma patients. *Blood.* 2002;99:3163–3168.
2. Shustik C, Belch A, Robinson S, et al. A randomised comparison of melphalan with prednisone or dexamethasone as induction therapy and dexamethasone or observation as maintenance therapy in multiple myeloma. *Br J Hematol.* 2006;136:203–211.
3. Cunnigham D, Powles R, Malpas JS, et al. A randomized trial of maintenance therapy with intron A following high dose melphalan and ABMT in myeloma. *Br J Haematol.* 1998;102:195–202.
4. Barlogie B, Kyle RA, Anderson KC, et al. Standard chemotherapy compared with high-dose chemoradiotherapy for multiple myeloma: final results of phase III US intergroup trial S9321. *J Clin Oncol.* 2006;24:929–936.
5. Attal M, Harousseau JL, Leyvraz S, et al. Maintenance therapy with thalidomide improves survival in multiple myeloma patients. *Blood.* 2006;15:3289–3294.
6. Barlogie B, Pineda-Roman M, van Rhee F, et al. Thalidomide arm of Total Therapy II improves complete remission duration and survival in myeloma patients with metaphase cytogenetic abnormalities. *Blood.* 2008;112:3115–3121.
7. Feyler S, Rawstron A, Jackson G, et al. Thalidomide maintenance following high-dose therapy in multiple myeloma: a UK myeloma forum phase II. *Br J Hematol.* 2007;139:429–433.
8. Morgan GJ, Jackson GH, Davies FE, et al. Maintenance thalidomide may improve progression free but not overall survival; results form the myeloma IX maintenance randomisation. *Blood.* 2008;112:656.
9. Spencer A, Prince HM, Roberts AW, et al. Consolidation therapy with low-dose thalidomide and prednisolone prolongs the survival of multiple myeloma patients undergoing a single autologous stem-cell transplantation procedure. *J Clin Oncol.* 2009;27:1788–1793.
10. Hussein MA, Bolejack V, Zonder JA. Phase II study of thalidomide plus dexamethasone induction followed by tandem melphalan-based autotransplantation and thalidomide-plus-prednisone maintenance for untreated multiple myeloma: a Southwest Oncology group trial (S0204). *J Clin Oncol.* 2009;27:1–8.
11. Offidani M, Corvatta L, Polloni C, et al. Thalidomide-dexamethasone versus Interferon-alphadexamethasone as maintenance treatment after ThaDD induction for multiple myeloma: a prospective, multicentre, randomised study. *Br J Hematol.* 2008;144:653–659.
12. Palumbo A, Bringhen S, Liberati AM, et al. Oral melphalan, prednisone and thalidomide in elderly patients with multiple myeloma: updated results of a randomized control trial. *Blood.* 2008;112:3107–3114.
13. Wijermans P, Schaafsma P, van Norden P, et al. Melphalan + prednisone versus melphalan + prednisone + thalidomide in induction therapy for multiple myeloma in elderly patients: final analysis of the dutch cooperative group HOVON 49 study. *Blood.* 2008;112:649.
14. Facon T, Mary JY, Hulin C, et al. Melphalan and prednisone plus thalidomide versus melphalan and prednisone alone or reduced-intensity autologous stem cell transplantation in elderly patients with multiple myeloma (IFM99–06) a randozmized trial. *Lancet.* 2007;370:1209–1218.
15. Hulin C, Facon T, Rodon P, et al. Efficacy of melphalan and prednisone plus thalidomide in patients older than 75 years with newly diagnosed multiple myeloma: IFM 01/01 trial. *J Clin Oncol.* 2009;27:3664–3670.
16. Ludwig H, Hajek R, Tothova E, et al. Thalidomide-dexamethasone compared with melphalan-prednisone in elderly patients with multiple myeloma. *Blood.* 2009;113:3435–3442.
17. Drayson MT, Chapman CE, Dunn JA, et al. MRC trial of alpha-2b-interferon maintenance therapy in first plateau phase of multiple myeloma. MRC working party on leukemia in adults. *Br J Hematol.* 1998;101:195–202.
18. Palumbo A, Falco P, Corradini P, et al. Melphalan, prednisone, and lenalidomide treatment for newly diagnosed myeloma: a report from the GIMEMA Italian Multiple Myeloma Network. *J Clin Oncol.* 2007;25:4459–4465.

19. Palumbo A, Falco P, Gay F, et al. Bortezomib-doxorubicin-dexamethasone as induction prior to reduced intensity autologous transplantation followed by lenalidomide as consolidation/maintenance in elderly untreated myeloma patients. *Blood.* 2008;112:159.

20. Maintenance therapy using lenalidomide in myeloma (IFM 2005–02). NCT00430365. Available at http://clinicaltrial.gov. Accessed January 31, 2007.

21. Weber D, Chen C, Niesvizky R, et al. Lenalidomide plus Dexamethasone for relapsed multiple myeloma in North America. *N Engl J Med.* 2007;357:2133–2142.

22. Dimopoulos M, Spencer A, Attal M, et al. Lenalidomide plus dexamethasone for relapsed ore refractory multiple myeloma. *N Engl J Med.* 2007;357:2123–2132.

23. San Miguel JF, Dimopoulos MA, Stadtmauer EA, et al. Longer duration of treatment and maintenance of best response with lenalidomide and dexamethasone prolongs overall survival in patients with relapsed or refractory multiple myeloma. *Blood.* 2008;112:3702.

24. Richardson PG, Sonneveld P, Schuster M, et al. Extended follow-up of a phase 3 trial in relapsed multiple myeloma: final time-to-event results of the APEX trial. *Blood.* 2007;110:3557–3560.

25. Palumbo A, Falco P, Sanpaolo G, et al. Combination of lenalidomide, melphalan, prednisone and thalidomide (RMPT) in relapsed/refractory multiple myeloma: results of a Multicenter Phase II clinical trial. *Blood.* 2008;112:868.

26. Schiller GJ, Liao M, Sohn JP, et al. Phase I/II trial of bortezomib maintenance in order to prolong remission duration following autologous peripheral blood progenitor cell transplantation as treatment for intermediate and advanced-stage multiple myeloma. *Blood.* 2007;110:3617.

27. Uy GL, Goyal SD, Fisher NM, et al. Bortezomib administered pre-auto-SCT and as maintenance therapy post-transplant for multiple myeloma: a single institution phase II study. *Bone Marrow Transpl.* 2009;43:793–800.

28. Sonneveld P, van der Holt B, Schimdt-Wolf GH, et al. First analysis of HOVON-65/GMMG-HD4 randomized phase III trial comparing bortezomib, adriamycine, dexamethasone (PAD) vs VAD as induction treatment prior to high dose melphalan (HDM) in patients with newly diagnosed multiple myeloma (MM). *Blood.* 2008;112:653.

29. Dispenzieri A, Jacobus S, Vesole D, et al. Primari therapy with bortezomib-the role of induction, maintenance and re-induction in patients with high-risk myeloma. Update of results from E2A02. *Blood.* 2008;112:1738.

30. Palumbo A, Bringhen S, Rossi D, et al. A prospective, randomized, phase iii study of bortezomib, melphalan, prednisone and thalidomide (VMPT) versus bortezomib, melphalan and prednisone (VMP) in elderly newly diagnosed myeloma patients. *Blood.* 2008;112:652.

31. Benevolo G, Larocca A, Pregno P, et al. Bortezomib and dexamethasone as maintenance therapy in relapsed/refractory multiple myeloma patients. *Blood.* 2008;112:2771.

32. Anderson KC, Jagannath S, Jakubowiak A, et al. Lenalidomide, bortezomib and dexamethasone in relapsed/refractory multiple myeloma (MM): encouraging outcomes and tolerability in phase II study. *J Clin Oncol.* 2009;27:15s (abstract 8536).

# Novel Immunotherapies

Qing Yi

Multiple myeloma (MM), characterized by the clonal expansion of malignant plasma cells, remains a fatal disease, and nearly 11,000 Americans die of the disease each year.[1] MM constitutes 10% of hematologic malignancies in the United States and is more prevalent than lymphocytic leukemia, myelocytic leukemia, or Hodgkin disease. Despite advances in the treatment of MM by using conventional and novel therapeutics in combination with transplantation,[2] long-term survival is rare and most patients will relapse and die of the disease.[2,3] Thus, novel therapeutic approaches that have a mode of action different from and noncross-resistant with cytotoxic chemotherapy are required to eradicate myeloma cells that have become multidrug resistant. Immunotherapy is an appealing option for this purpose.[4,5]

Results from recent research have indicated that myeloma cells are susceptible to T-cell–mediated cytolysis. In the postallograft relapse setting in which patients with myeloma are chemotherapy refractory, long-lasting disease remission has been achieved after infusion of donor lymphocytes, a phenomenon termed graft-versus-myeloma effect.[6,7] This graft-versus-myeloma effect is closely associated with graft-versus-host disease (GVHD), and donor-derived alloreactive and tumor-specific T cells are believed to mediate these effects.[6,7] These observations strongly suggest that chemotherapy and immunotherapy kill myeloma cells by different modes of action that are noncross resistant; therefore, they should work synergistically.

Clonogenic myeloma cells, either preplasmacytic or plasma cells, may include postswitch B cells. These cells are present in the bone marrow and peripheral blood of patients with MM. Myeloma B cells may express monoclonal immunoglobulin (Ig) on their cell surface, in addition to major histocompatibility complex (MHC) class I and class II molecules and are sensitive to regulatory signals provided by cellular and humoral components of the idiotype-specific immune network.[4,8,9] Plasma cells compose the major tumor burden and constitute at least 10%, but can be greater than 90%, of the total bone marrow cell count.[1,10] Myeloma plasma cells secrete the monoclonal M-component and express cytoplasmic Ig.[11–13] Moreover, myeloma plasma cells may express MHC class-I antigens[14–16]; adhesion molecules, such as CD44, CD56, CD54, and VLA-4[17–19]; signaling or costimulatory molecules CD40 and CD28[19,20]; and the Fas antigen (CD95).[21,22] Some of the plasma cells also express HLA-DR, CD80, and CD86.[15,23] Our study showed that myeloma plasma cells were able to activate alloreactive T cells and present the recalled antigens, purified protein derivative, and tetanus toxoid to autologous T cells.[15] Therefore, myeloma plasma cells may also be subject to immune regulation, at least by the cellular components of the immune system.

## TUMOR ANTIGENS FOR IMMUNE TARGETING IN MM

### Idiotype Proteins and Idiotype-Specific T Cells

Idiotype proteins are tumor-specific antigens, and active immunization against idiotypic determinants on malignant B cells has produced resistance to tumor growth in transplantable murine B-cell lymphoma and plasmacytoma.[24–28] The presence of idiotype-specific T cells in the peripheral blood of patients with MM or with the benign form of the disease, monoclonal gammopathy of undetermined significance (MGUS), has been studied by detecting idiotype-induced T-cell proliferation and cytokine secretion by using the enzyme-linked immunospot (ELISPOT) assay.[29]

Idiotype-specific T cells at a low frequency were detected in 90% of patients with MM or MGUS.[30–32] Consistent with these results, we and others have shown that T cells in patients with myeloma responded to peptides corresponding to complementarity-determining regions I to III of heavy and light chains of the autologous M-component.[16,33–35] We found that idiotype-induced T-cell stimulation was mainly confined to the $CD4^+$ subset in most of the patients examined and was MHC class II restricted. Idiotype-specific $CD8^+$ T cells were also demonstrated but at a lower frequency. Idiotype-specific $CD4^+$ and $CD8^+$ T cells were mainly of the type 1 subsets, as judged by their secretion of interferon (IFN)-$\gamma$ and interleukin (IL)-2.[36,37] Moreover, the proportion of individuals who had an idiotype-specific response of the T helper-1 ($T_H1$)-type (IFN-$\gamma$- and/or IL-2-secreting cells)[38,39] was significantly higher in patients with indolent disease (MGUS and MM stage I) compared with those with advanced MM (stage II/III). In contrast, cells secreting the $T_H2$-subtype cytokine profile (IL-4 only)[38,39] were seen more frequently in patients with advanced MM (stage II/III).[31] A similar pattern of cytokine secretion was also reported by others.[40] Collectively, these findings indicate that the existing idiotype-specific immune response is too weak to control the growth of myeloma cells in vivo and that a shift from an idiotype-specific type 1 response, ie, $T_H1$ and T cytotoxic-1 (Tc1),[41] in early MM to a type 2 response ($T_H2$ and probably Tc2[41]) in advanced disease may have occurred. These studies provide indirect evidence that idiotype-specific T cells may have a regulatory impact on human tumor B cells.

To examine whether idiotype-specific T cells can recognize and kill myeloma cells, we generated idiotype-specific cytotoxic T lymphocyte (CTL) lines from patients with myeloma.[42] To enhance the immunogenicity of idiotype proteins, we used dendritic cells (DCs) as antigen-presenting cells. After repeated rounds of in vitro T-cell stimulation with idiotype-pulsed autologous DCs, idiotype-specific T-cell lines, which consisted of both $CD4^+$ and $CD8^+$ T cells, were generated and propagated from the peripheral blood mononuclear cells (PBMCs) of patients with myeloma. Idiotype-specific proliferative responses were observed when these T cells were rechallenged with the autologous, but not allogeneic, idiotype-pulsed DCs. By using a standard [51]chromium-release assay, our results showed that idiotype-specific CTLs not only recognized and lysed autologous idiotype-pulsed DCs but also significantly killed autologous primary myeloma cells. The cytotoxicity was MHC class I, and to a lesser extent, class II restricted, suggesting that myeloma cells could process idiotype protein and present idiotype peptides in the context of their surface MHC molecules. Taken together, these findings provide direct evidence that myeloma plasma cells express idiotype peptides-MHC molecules on their surface and are susceptible to idiotype-specific T-cell–mediated lysis.

## Myeloma Plasma Cells and Myeloma-Specific T Cells

Myeloma tumor cells may contain a multitude of tumor antigens that can stimulate an increased repertoire of antitumor T cells and lead to an induction of stronger antimyeloma responses. To explore the possibility of using myeloma cells as the source of tumor antigens for immunotherapy, myeloma cell lysate-specific CTLs were generated from patients by culturing T cells with autologous DCs pulsed with freeze-thaw lysate from myeloma cells.[43] After 4 to 6 cycles of antigen stimulation, specific CTL lines containing both CD4+ and CD8+ T cells were obtained from 4 patients. These cell lines proliferated in response to autologous primary myeloma cells and DCs pulsed with autologous but not allogeneic, tumor lysate, and secreted predominantly IFN-$\gamma$ and tumor necrosis factor (TNF)-$\alpha$, indicating that they are type 1 T cells ($T_H1$ and Tc1). The CTLs had strong cytotoxic activity against autologous tumor lysate-pulsed DCs and primary myeloma cells.

Myeloma-specific CTLs can also be induced and propagated by using myeloma-DC fusion cells as antigen-presenting cells. The heterokaryons generated by cancer-DC fusion cells combine the machinery needed for immune stimulation with presentation of a large repertoire of antigens. In murine plasmacytoma models, vaccination with DCs fused with mouse 4TOO plasmacytoma cells[44] or J558 myeloma cells[45] was associated with induction of antitumor humoral and CTL responses. Immunization with the fusion cells protected mice against tumor challenge and extended the survival of tumor-established mice without eradication of the tumor cells. In a more recent study, human myeloma cells, either primary myeloma cells from patients or a myeloma cell line (U266), were fused to human DCs.[46] Fusions with mature, when compared with immature, DCs induced higher levels of T-cell proliferation and activation, as assessed by intracellular IFN-$\gamma$ expression and stronger cytotoxic T-cell activity against the tumor cells. Alternatively, myeloma-specific CTLs could be generated in vitro by stimulating T cells with tumor-derived RNA-transfected autologous DCs.[47]

## DKK1 as a Universal Myeloma Antigen

Dickkopf-1 (DKK1) is a secreted protein that specifically inhibits the Wnt/$\beta$-catenin signaling by interacting with the coreceptor Lrp-6.[48,49] Previous studies have shown that the *DKK1* gene has restricted expression in placenta and mesenchymal stem cells (MSCs) and not in other normal tissues.[50,51] Recent studies demonstrated that DKK1 in patients with myeloma was associated with the presence of lytic bone lesions.[52] Immunohistochemical analysis of bone marrow biopsy specimens showed that only myeloma cells contain detectable DKK1. Recombinant human DKK1 or bone marrow serum containing an elevated level of DKK1 inhibited the differentiation of osteoblast precursor cells in vitro. Furthermore, anti-DKK1 antibody

treatment was associated with reduced tumor growth in myeloma mouse models.[53-55] These results indicate that DKK1 is an important player in myeloma bone disease.

The identification of novel tumor-associated antigens, particularly those shared among patients, is urgently needed to improve the efficacy of immunotherapy for MM. For this purpose, we examined whether DKK1 could be a good candidate. We identified and synthesized DKK1 peptides for HLA-A*0201 and confirmed their immunogenicity by in vivo immunization of HLA-A*0201 transgenic mice. We detected low frequencies of DKK1 peptide-specific CD8+ T cells in patients with myeloma by using peptide tetramers and generated peptide-specific T-cell lines and clones from HLA-A*0201+ blood donors and patients with myeloma. These T cells efficiently lysed peptide-pulsed but not unpulsed T2 or autologous DCs, DKK1+/HLA-A*0201+ myeloma cell lines U266 and IM-9 and, more importantly, HLA-A*0201+ primary myeloma cells from patients. No killing was observed on DKK1+/HLA-A*0201− myeloma cell lines and primary myeloma cells or HLA-A*0201+ normal lymphocytes, including B cells (Fig. 1). These T cells were also therapeutic in vivo against established myeloma in SCID-hu mice after adoptive transfer. These results indicate that these T cells were potent CTLs and recognized DKK1 peptides naturally presented by myeloma cells in the context of HLA-A*0201 molecules. Hence, our study identified DKK1 as a potentially important antigen for immunotherapy in MM.

## Other Antigens

Recent studies have shown that the cancer-testis antigens MAGE-3 and NY-ESO-1 may be expressed by myeloma cells.[56-58] DNA microarray analysis of gene expression of >95% pure myeloma cells

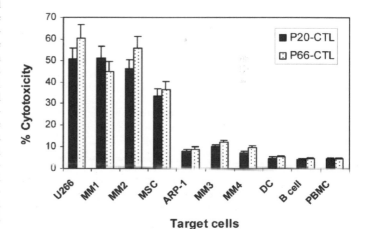

**FIGURE 1.** Cytotoxicity of DKK1 peptide-specific T-cell clones. P20-specific or P66-specific T-cell clones against human myeloma cell lines U266 (DKK1+/HLA-A*0201+) and ARP-1 (DKK1+/HLA-A*0201−) and primary myeloma cells from 4 patients with MM (MM1–MM4). Control target cells include normal mesenchymal stem cells (MSCs), DCs, B cells and PBMCs from HLA-A*0201+ healthy donors. Patients 1 and 2 were HLA-A*0201+ and patients 3 and 4 were HLA-A*0201−. All primary myeloma cells expressed DKK1 protein. P20 and P66 are 2 DKK1 peptides that have high affinity for HLA-A*0201. An effector:target (*E:T*) ratio of 10:1 was used. Results of 4 independent experiments with 2 CTL clones generated from a patient with MM are shown.

from more than 300 patients showed that the genes of these antigens were expressed in the tumor cells, particularly from patients with relapsed disease or abnormal cytogenetics (in 7%–20% of MGUS and newly diagnosed MM and in 40% to 50% of relapsed patients or in patients with cytogenetic abnormalities).[59,60] With the use of specific monoclonal antibodies (mAbs) against MAGE-3 or NY-ESO-1, it was evident that the proteins of these antigens were also expressed in the tumor cells of patients with positive gene expression. We then generated MAGE-3- and NY-ESO-1-specific CTLs from healthy individuals by using HLA-A1-restricted or HLA-A2-restricted MAGE-3-derived and NY-ESO-1-derived synthetic peptides as the antigens with which to pulse autologous DCs. MAGE-3-specific CTLs killed peptide-pulsed autologous target cells and MAGE-3- and HLA-A1-postive myeloma cells (line ARK-RS). No killing was observed with K562 cells, unpulsed target cells, or myeloma cell lines that were HLA-A1 positive but MAGE-3 negative.[61] Similar results were obtained with NY-ESO-1-specific CTLs.[62]

Furthermore, other antigens, such as MUC-1,[63–65] sperm protein 17 (Sp17),[66,67] and HM1.24,[68–70] may also be expressed on myeloma cells, and MHC-restricted antigen (MUC-1[71] and Sp17[72])-specific CTLs have been generated from patients with myeloma that were able to lyse myeloma cells. Recently, a phase I/II clinical trial has been initiated to examine the safety and efficacy of Sp17-pulsed DC vaccination in patients with myeloma.[67] However, there is evidence that Sp17 is also expressed on normal T and B cells[73]; hence, although these antigens may be potential targets, further research is warranted to examine their applicability for immunotherapy in MM.

## T CELL-BASED IMMUNOTHERAPY IN MM

### Idiotype-Based Protein Vaccines for Myeloma

Our group at the Karolinska Institute, Stockholm, Sweden, was the first to introduce active immunization of patients with myeloma with Id proteins.[74,75] Considering that immunotherapy may work better in immunocompetent patients with a low tumor burden, we targeted untreated patients with early disease. In our first pilot study, we recruited and immunized 5 previously untreated patients with stages I to III MM with the autologous Id protein precipitated in an aluminum phosphate suspension.[74] In 3 patients, an anti-Id T-cell response, detected by enumeration of IFN-$\gamma$- and IL-2-secreting cells by ELISPOT assay, was amplified 1.9- to 5-fold during the immunization. The number of B cells secreting anti-Id antibodies also increased in these 3 patients, and 2 of the 3 patients had a gradual decrease of blood CD19$^+$ B cells. However, the induced T-cell response was transient and was eliminated during repeated immunization. The disease was stable in all patients, and no side effects or clinical response were noted. In our second series of the study, immunization was performed by subcutaneous or intradermal injection of Id protein and granulocyte-monocyte colony-stimulating factor (GM-CSF).[75] Five patients with IgG myeloma were treated and an Id-specific type 1 T-cell response developed in all of them. The response involved both CD8$^+$ and CD4$^+$ subsets and was mainly MHC class I restricted. There was a transient rise in B cells producing IgM antiidiotypic antibodies in all patients. One patient had a clinical response, defined by a significant decrease in serum Id protein (from 20 to 7 g/L) and normalization of serum Ig levels, which lasted for >1 year after immunization was started. Although these studies involved a limited number of patients, the results clearly indicated that Id protein vaccination, particularly in combination with GM-CSF, was able to induce specific anti-Id cellular and humoral immune responses, which were occasionally accompanied by a clinical response in treated patients. Furthermore, idiotype vaccination

combined with IL-12 also was efficient at inducing myeloma-specific immune responses in patients with myeloma.[76]

Other clinical settings for immunotherapy could be minimal residual disease status achieved by high-dose chemotherapy and early host immunologic recovery after stem-cell transplantation. These are supported by a study from Massaia et al[77] showing that Id vaccination of patients with myeloma with minimal residual disease was able to induce a strong Id-specific cellular immunity in many of the patients. In their study, 12 patients who had been treated with high-dose chemotherapy followed by stem cell support received Id-keyhole limpet hemocyanin (KLH) vaccines and a low dose of GM-CSF or IL-2. In most of the patients, the interval between the completion of prior high-dose therapy and vaccination was only 2 to 3 months. Generation of Id-specific T-cell proliferative responses was documented in only 2 cases; however, a positive, Id-specific, delayed-type hypersensitivity (DTH) skin test reaction was observed in 8 of the 10 patients studied. The induction of humoral and cellular immune responses to KLH was observed in 100% and 80% of the patients, respectively, suggesting that the majority of patients were already able to mount immune responses to KLH shortly after high-dose therapy and stem-cell transplantation. Collectively, these results indicate that immunization of patients with myeloma with the autologous Id protein, together with GM-CSF, might be a promising method of immunotherapy.[78]

## DC-Based Vaccines for Myeloma

Preclinical studies have shown that DCs generated from patients with myeloma were functional and could efficiently present Id determinants to autologous T cells.[79,80] Compared with their progenitor monocytes, Id-pulsed DCs induced not only a stronger Id-specific T-cell response but also a predominant type 1 (IFN-$\gamma$) T-cell response.[79] Both type 1 and type 2 (IFN-$\gamma$ and IL-4) T-cell responses were noted when monocytes were used as the APCs. These results indicate that DCs pulsed with Id protein can be used to induce the type 1 anti-Id response in patients with myeloma.

Wen et al[81] reported vaccinating a patient with MM with autologous Id protein-pulsed DCs generated from blood adherent cells. Enhanced Id-specific cellular and humoral responses were observed in the patient. The immune responses were associated with a transient minor decrease in the serum Id protein level. In their subsequent study, 6 additional patients were treated according to the same protocol.[82] An immune response against Id was demonstrated in many of the patients. A minor clinical response (25% reduction in the M component) was observed in 1 patient and stable disease in the remaining patients. Reichardt et al[83] reported their experience with Id-pulsed DC vaccination in 12 patients with myeloma after autologous peripheral blood stem-cell transplantation. Their results were less compelling because only 2 of 12 patients mounted cellular Id-specific proliferative responses as the sole evidence for effective vaccination. Nevertheless, all patients with myeloma could mount a strong anti-KLH response despite recent high-dose therapy. Similar results were also obtained in their subsequent study involving 26 patients treated on the same protocol.[84] Although 24 of 26 patients generated a KLH-specific cellular proliferative immune response, an Id-specific proliferative immune response developed in only 4 patients. No clinical benefit was observed. These results suggest that DC-based Id vaccination is feasible after transplantation and can induce an Id-specific T-cell response in certain patients.

Other clinical trials of Id-pulsed DC vaccination in patients with myeloma have been reported. Cull et al[85] reported on their experience of vaccinating 2 patients with advanced refractory MM with Id-pulsed DCs combined with GM-CSF. An anti-Id T-cell proliferative response was detected in both patients, which was associated with

IFN-$\gamma$ production by the T cells. One patient also had an anti-Id humoral response. Titzer et al[86] treated 11 patients with advanced MM with Id-pulsed, CD34$^+$ stem cell-derived DCs and GM-CSF. After vaccination, 3 of 10 analyzed patients showed an increased anti-Id antibody titer, and 4 of the 10 patients had an Id-specific T-cell response measured by ELISPOT assay.

To improve the efficacy of DC vaccination in myeloma, we investigated the use of Id-pulsed mature DCs administered subcutaneously. In our study, 5 patients with stable partial remission after high-dose chemotherapy were vaccinated at least 4 months posttransplantation.[87] After 4 DC vaccinations, Id-specific T-cell responses, detected by ELISPOT assays (4 patients) and proliferation assays (2 patients), were elicited in 4 patients and anti-Id B-cell responses in all 5 patients. The cytokine-secretion profile of activated T cells demonstrated a type 1 T-cell response. A 50% reduction in serum Id protein was observed in 1 immunologically responding patient and persisted for more than 1 year; stable disease was noted in the other 3 patients. The remaining patient without an immune response to the vaccination experienced disease relapse. Similar results were recently reported by Curti et al.[88] In their study, 15 patients received DCs pulsed with Id proteins or their peptides, and an Id-specific IFN-$\gamma$ response was seen in 8 patients. Clinically, 7 of the 15 patients had stable disease after a median follow-up of 26 months, 1 patient achieved durable partial remission after 40 months and 7 patients progressed. Alternatively, Id-pulsed allogeneic DCs could also be used to vaccinate patients with myeloma.[89] Taken together, these results indicate that subcutaneous DC vaccination indeed induces better antimyeloma responses than intravenous DC vaccination.

DC vaccines can also be made in the form of fusion of tumor cells with DCs. The heterokaryons generated by tumor-DC fusion cells combine the machinery needed for immune stimulation with presentation of a large repertoire of antigens. Vaccination with fusions of tumor cells and DCs is an effective treatment in animal tumor models[90,91] and possibly in patients with metastatic renal carcinoma.[92] In a murine plasmacytoma model, vaccination with DCs fused with mouse 4TOO plasmacytoma cells was associated with induction of antitumor humoral and CTL responses.[44] Immunization with the fusion cells protected mice against tumor challenge and extended the survival of tumor-established mice without eradication of the tumor cells. Addition of IL-12 helped eradicate the established tumor. In a more recent study, human myeloma cells, either primary myeloma cells from patients or a myeloma cell line, U266, were fused to human DCs.[93] Fusions with mature rather than immature DCs induced higher levels of T-cell proliferation and activation, as assessed by intracellular IFN-$\gamma$ expression, and stronger CTL activity against the tumor cells. Similar results were also obtained by other investigators.[94,95] Based on these results, a clinical trial was designed to evaluate the efficacy of vaccinating patients with myeloma with a fusion of myeloma cells and autologous mature DCs.[93]

## DNA Vaccines for Myeloma

Various approaches to antitumor therapy that use both antigen-encoding DNA and noncoding nucleotides as components of genetic vaccination are currently being explored.[96] These strategies include the construct that fuses an scFv incorporating both variable-region genes necessary to encode the Id determinants with fragment C of tetanus toxin[28] and gene transfer of cytokines or costimulatory molecules into myeloma cells by nonviral and viral vectors.[97] In animal studies, DNA vaccination promoted specific immune responses and induced strong protection against B-cell lymphoma and myeloma.[28,98] These strategies may have implications for immunotherapy in human diseases.

A phase I study has been completed to evaluate the feasibility and safety of vaccinating patients with MM after high-dose chemotherapy with adenovector-engineered, IL-2-expressing autologous plasma cells.[99] Eight patients were enrolled, and vaccines were successfully made in 6 patients, who received 1 to 5 subcutaneous injections of 3.5 to $9.0 \times 10^7$ cells/injection. Vaccines were well tolerated, with only minor systemic symptoms reported. Vaccination induced a local inflammatory response consisting predominantly of CD8$^+$ T cells. However, no specific antitumor immune or clinical responses were noted. Hence, further studies of immunologic and clinical efficacy are needed to examine the applicability of this approach to the treatment of patients.

## Combined Donor Vaccination and Allogeneic Stem-Cell Transplantation

Allogeneic stem-cell transplantation showed efficacy in MM but was accompanied by severe GVHD.[100-103] One strategy for enhancing antimyeloma effects without aggravating GVHD is to target an immune response selectively against a defined tumor-specific antigen. This could be accomplished by eliciting an antimyeloma immune response in allogeneic HSCT donors by active immunization before allogeneic HSCT and/or DLI. This strategy was pioneered by Kwak et al.[104] An HLA-matched donor received 2 subcutaneous immunizations of patient-derived idiotype conjugated to KLH at a 1-week interval before marrow harvest. The recipient patient demonstrated no preexisting antiidiotype immunity pretransplantation. Thirty and 60 days after conditioning with busulfan and cyclophosphamide and transfer of unmanipulated donor bone marrow, significant lymphocyte proliferative responses against the idiotype were detected in the recipient. A CD4$^+$, idiotype-specific T-cell line was generated from the recipient's blood, which was, unequivocally, of donor origin because in situ hybridization assay demonstrated the presence of Y chromosome in more than 95% of the T cells. By day 220, a greater than 90% reduction in serum M-protein was observed, which persisted for over 3 years.

On the basis of this encouraging result from the single patient mentioned above, the investigators, then at the National Cancer Institute, opened a clinical trial of donor immunization in MM under the Food and Drug Administration-approved Investigational New Drug application in collaboration with the Arkansas myeloma research group at the University of Arkansas. The clinical protocol was designed to explore whether a booster immunization of the recipient might improve the potency and duration of the transferred idiotype-specific response. Five additional donor-recipient pairs were enrolled and vaccinated with idiotype-KLH protein plus GM-CSF. Two recipients succumbed to early postallogeneic stem-cell transplantation complications, unrelated to vaccination. The 3 remaining recipients achieved and remained in continuous complete remission 3.5, 4, and 5 years after transplantation. One recipient suffered from chronic GVHD and was on chronic steroid therapy, whereas the other 2 recipients and all the donors were medically well, without any significant complications. In all 3 recipients, transfer of T-cell responses to the KLH carrier protein has been documented. Analysis and serial monitoring of idiotype-specific T-cell responses in the donors and recipients have been in progress.[105]

Taken together, these proof-of-principle studies demonstrate a direct transfer of myeloma idiotype-specific T-cell immunity from donor to recipient after allogeneic stem-cell transplantation or donor lymphocyte infusion. These results also suggest that the donor-derived T-cell response was not blocked by circulating myeloma idiotype protein in recipient during and after transplantation or inhibited by the immunosuppressive medication used for GVHD prophylaxis in the patients. Furthermore, GVHD did not seem to be exacerbated secondary to this immunotherapeutic maneuver.

## Immunotherapy With Donor-Derived or Patient-Derived, Tumor-Specific Lymphocytes

Successful immunotherapy of patients with tumors requires the in vivo generation of large numbers of highly reactive antitumor lymphocytes that are not restrained by normal tolerance mechanisms and are capable of sustaining immunity against tumor cells. Immunizing patients with MM with myeloma antigens such as the idiotype proteins or tumor lysate can increase the number of circulating antigen-specific T cells. To date, this has not correlated with clinical tumor regression, suggesting that the numbers of these T cells, particularly those of the CTLs, are still insufficient to cause major tumor damage, and/or there are defects in function or activation of these T cells.

Falkenburg et al[106] reported the first successful treatment of a hematological malignancy with donor-derived tumor-specific CTL lines. A patient with accelerated phase chronic myeloid leukemia (CML) received infusions of 3 donor-derived leukemia-reactive CTL lines at 5-week intervals at a cumulative dose of $3.2 \times 10^9$ CTLs after allogeneic HSCT. The CTLs were selected based on their ability to inhibit the in vitro growth of CML progenitor cells and to lyse the leukemic cells from the patient. Shortly after the third infusion, complete eradication of the leukemic cells was observed, as shown by cytogenetic analysis, fluorescence in situ hybridization, molecular analysis of BCR/ABL mRNA, and chimerism studies. Thus, these results show that in vitro cultured leukemia-reactive CTLs can be successfully applied to treat accelerated phase CML after allogeneic HSCT.

In addition to obtaining tumor-specific CTLs from donors, these cells can also be obtained from patients themselves, ex vivo expanded, and used adoptively to eradicate tumor cells. In patients with metastatic melanoma refractory to treatment with high-dose IL-2 and to chemotherapy, the transfer of in vitro-activated and expanded autologous antitumor lymphocytes plus IL-2 into lymphodepleted patients mediated objective cancer regression in 6 of 13 patients. Persistence of the transferred cells was seen for up to 4 months after cell administration.[107] The number of patients enrolled on this protocol was expanded, and the investigators have observed objective cancer regression in 18 of 35 patients (51%), many of whom have bulky disease.[108] These studies demonstrate that adoptive transfer of tumor-reactive lymphocytes after nonmyeloablative conditioning can be an effective treatment for patients with metastatic cancers.

## ANTIBODY-BASED IMMUNOTHERAPY IN MM

Within the past decade, mAbs have broadened the therapeutic armamentarium in oncology.[109] Hematological malignancies are recognized as particularly promising targets, reflected by the current list of Food and Drug Administration-approved mAbs that are used to treat patients.[110,111] The mAbs exert their in vivo effect largely through the immunologic effector mechanisms of complement-mediated lysis (CDC) and/or antibody-dependent cell-mediated cytotoxicity (ADCC). Thus, their efficacy depends on intact immunologic mechanisms in the treated patients. Although the molecules targeted by these mAbs are usually widely expressed on normal lymphoid and myeloid cells in addition to malignant cells, the therapeutic efficacy of these mAbs has been promising.[109–111] Nevertheless, it will be useful to develop mAbs with an inherent capability to kill tumor cells, ie, independent of complement and ADCC, and with selectivity toward neoplastic cells.

## Targeting Surface $\beta_2$-Microglobulin to Induce Apoptosis in Myeloma Cells

$\beta_2$-microglobulin ($\beta_2$M) is an 11.6-kDa nonglycosylated polypeptide composed of 100 amino acids. It is part of the MHC class I molecule on the cell surface of nucleated cells. Its best characterized function is to interact with and stabilize the tertiary structure of the MHC class I $\alpha$-chain.[112] Because it is noncovalently associated with the $\alpha$-chain and has no direct attachment to the cell membrane, $\beta_2$M on the cell surface can exchange with free $\beta_2$M present in serum-containing medium.[113] Free $\beta_2$M is found in body fluids under physiological conditions as a result of intracellular release. Elevated levels of serum $\beta_2$M are present in hematological malignancies, including lymphomas,[114] leukemias,[115,116] and MM[2,117] and correlate with a poor prognosis regardless of a patient's renal function.[117,118] This observation suggests an important, yet unidentified, role of this protein in these malignancies. Although examining the effects of $\beta_2$M on myeloma cells, we made a novel and exciting discovery, namely that mAbs against $\beta_2$M have a remarkably strong apoptotic effect on myeloma cells and on other hematological tumor cells.[119] Anti-$\beta_2$M mAbs induced apoptosis in up to 90% of cells in a 48-hour culture in all tested human myeloma cell lines (n = 8) and primary myeloma cells from patients (n = 10). The mAbs also kill $\beta_2$M/MHC class I-bearing lymphoma and leukemia cells. Anti-MHC class I mAbs (LY5.1, IgG1 or W6/32, and IgG2a), purified mouse IgG and IgG1 had no effect. Cell death occurred rapidly, without the need for exogenous immunologic effector mechanisms (eg, complement or NK cells) or secondary crosslinking. Anti-$\beta_2$M mAb-induced apoptosis in myeloma cells were not blocked by soluble $\beta_2$M (10–100 $\mu$g/mL, 3- to 30-fold higher than the levels in most patients with MM), IL-6, or other myeloma growth and survival factors and was stronger than apoptosis observed with chemotherapy drugs currently used to treat MM (eg, dexamethasone).

Although the expression of $\beta_2$M on normal hematopoietic cells is a potential safety concern, the mAbs were selective to tumor-transformed cells and did not induce apoptosis of normal cells, including T and B lymphocytes, plasma cells, and purified CD34$^+$ stem cells. Furthermore, the mAbs selectively and effectively killed myeloma cells without damaging osteoclasts (OCs) or PBMCs in their cocultures with myeloma cells. More importantly, anti-$\beta_2$M mAbs are therapeutic in vivo in xenograft SCID (Fig. 2) and SCID-hu mouse models,[119] and in the HLA-A2-transgenic NOD-SCID (A2-NOD-SCID) models of myeloma, in which every mouse tissue expresses human MHC class I/$\beta_2$M molecules and circulating human $\beta_2$M could reach the levels seen in most patients with myeloma without causing damage to normal human hematopoiesis or murine organs.[120] Interestingly, after our publication, others have reported similar results using anti-MHC class single-chain Fv diabody or anti-$\beta_2$M antibodies, respectively, in human myeloma,[121] renal cell carcinoma,[122] and prostate cancer.[123] Therefore, such mAbs offer the potential for a therapeutic approach to hematological malignancies.

The mAbs induced apoptosis in myeloma cells by recruiting MHC class I to lipid rafts, activated JNK, and inhibited PI3K/Akt and ERK pathways.[119] Growth and survival cytokines such as IL-6 and IGF-I, which could protect myeloma cells from dexamethasone-induced apoptosis, did not affect mAb-mediated cell death. We elucidated the mechanisms underlying anti-$\beta_2$M mAb-induced PI3K/Akt and ERK inhibition and the inability of IL-6 and IGF-I to protect myeloma cells from mAb-induced apoptosis. We focused on lipid rafts and confirmed that these membrane microdomains are required for IL-6 and IGF-I signaling. By recruiting MHC class I into lipid rafts, anti-$\beta_2$M mAbs excluded IL-6 and IGF-I receptors and their

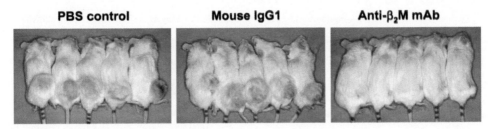

**PBS control**      **Mouse IgG1**      **Anti-β₂M mAb**

**FIGURE 2.** In vivo therapeutic effects of $\beta_2$M-specific mAbs on established human myeloma in a SCID mouse model. Mice were xenografted subcutaneously with ARP-1, and tumor burdens were monitored as tumor volumes. Mice received intraperitoneal injections every 3 days for a total of 4 injections of 250 $\mu$L ascites containing about 500 $\mu$g D1 $\beta_2$M-specific mAb, 500 $\mu$g mouse IgG1, or an equal volume of PBS. Results (image of tumor burdens in the mice) from 1 representative experiment of 3 performed using D1 mAb with 5 mice per group are shown.

substrates from the rafts. The mAbs were not only redistributed the receptors in cell membrane but also abrogated IL-6- or IGF-I-mediated JAK/STAT3, PI3K/Akt, and Ras/Raf/ERK pathway signaling, which are otherwise constitutively activated in myeloma cells.[124] Thus, our study further defines the tumoricidal mechanism of the mAbs and provides strong evidence to support the potential of these mAbs as therapeutic agents for myeloma.

## Anti-CS1 Antibodies

CS1, a glycoprotein and a member of the Ig gene superfamily, has been found to be highly expressed on tumor cells from patients with myeloma, and soluble serum CS1 correlates with active disease in patients with myeloma.[125] However, CS1 is also expressed by NK cells, NKT cells, and CD8+ T cells.[125] Recent studies demonstrated that CS1 promotes myeloma cell adhesion, clonogenic growth, and tumorigenicity through c-maf-mediated interactions with bone marrow stromal cells.[126]

As the above data suggest that CS1 could be a novel target for therapy, a humanized mAb against CS1, HuLuc63, was generated.[125] HuLuc63 inhibited myeloma cell binding to bone marrow stromal cells and induced ADCC against myeloma cells in dose-dependent and CS1-specific manners. Furthermore, the mAb mediated autologous ADCC against primary myeloma cells resistant to conventional or novel therapies and pretreatment with conventional or novel antimyeloma drugs markedly enhanced HuLuc63-induced myeloma cell lysis. In vivo injection of the mAb significantly induced tumor regression in xenograft myeloma mouse models.[127] Based on these results, phase I clinical trials are underway to evaluate the safety and toxicity of the mAb in patients with myeloma.

## Other Antibodies

Inhibiting DKK1 activity by using specific mAbs to treat MM and myeloma-associated bone disease is a novel approach because DKK1 has been shown to contribute to osteolytic bone disease in MM by inhibiting the differentiation of osteoblasts.[52] A humanized DKK1-neutralizing mAb, BHQ880 has been developed by Novartis and tested in preclinical studies.[53–55] In both murine[54] and xenograft human[53,55] myeloma mouse models, this mAb was shown to sustain or increase the numbers of osteoblasts, protect myeloma-induced bone loss, and reduce the development of osteolytic bone lesions. Furthermore, the mAb was also shown to inhibit the growth of xenografted human myeloma cells in SCID-hu[55] or SCID-rab[53] mouse models. These results provide the rationale for clinical evaluation of BHQ880 to improve bone disease and to inhibit myeloma growth.

Another potential target is CD40, which is expressed on B-cell tumors including MM. Two humanized anti-CD40 mAbs, SGN-40 and HCD122, have been developed and tested in preclinical studies.[128,129] These mAb induced modest cytotoxicity in myeloma cell lines and primary myeloma cells from patients but can effectively kill myeloma cell through mediating ADCC. Furthermore, the immunomodulatory drug lenalidomide further augmented anti-CD40 mAb-induced cytotoxicity in human myeloma cells.[130] In addition to anti-CD40 mAbs, other mAbs currently in clinical trials include anti-CD74, anti-CD56, and anti-HM1.24.[131]

## CONCLUSIONS

Various clinical immunotherapy treatment strategies have been tested in B-cell malignancies, including MM. Most of these have focused on targeting idiotype-specific immunity. Idiotype-based vaccines have been shown to induce or enhance idiotype-specific immunity, indicating that the vaccines are able to elicit a specific immune response. However, clinical response is still a rare event, occurring only in a minority of treated patients, suggesting that the elicited or enhanced immunity is still too weak to cause significant tumor destruction. Alternatively, a nonbeneficial immune response (such as the type 2 T-cell response) may also be generated by immunization, which may enhance tumor B-cell growth and facilitate differentiation into plasma cell tumors.

Ideally, a tumor-specific immunotherapy should induce or expand only the beneficial immune responses mediated by CTLs ($T_H1$ and Tc1 subsets) that have sufficient cytotoxic effects toward tumor cells but not normal cells. Further studies are warranted so that we can better understand the immune regulation mechanism in MM.

## ACKNOWLEDGMENTS

*The author thanks Ms. Alison Woo for providing editorial assistance.*

## REFERENCES

1. Kyle RA, Rajkumar SV. Multiple myeloma. *N Engl J Med.* 2004;351:1860–1873.
2. Barlogie B, Jagannath S, Desikan KR, et al. Total therapy with tandem transplants for newly diagnosed multiple myeloma. *Blood.* 1999;93:55–65.
3. Desikan R, Barlogie B, Sawyer J, et al. Results of high-dose therapy for 1000 patients with multiple myeloma: durable complete remissions and superior survival in the absence of chromosome 13 abnormalities. *Blood.* 2000;95:4008–4010.
4. Yi Q. Immunotherapy in multiple myeloma: current strategies and future prospects. *Expert Rev Vaccines.* 2003;2:391–398.
5. Yi Q. *Vaccines for Hematological Malignancies.* Totowa, NJ: Humana Press; 2004.

6. Tricot G, Vesole DH, Jagannath S, et al. Graft-versus-myeloma effect: proof of principle. *Blood.* 1996;87:1196–1198.

7. Verdonck LF, Lokhorst HM, Dekker AW, et al. Graft-versus-myeloma effect in two cases. *Lancet.* 1996;347:800–801.

8. Yi Q. *Immunoregulatory Mechanisms and Immunotherapy.* London: Martin Dunitz; 2002.

9. Sze DM, Giesajtis G, Brown RD, et al. Clonal cytotoxic T cells are expanded in myeloma and reside in the CD8(+)CD57(+)CD28(−) compartment. *Blood.* 2001;98:2817–2827.

10. Alexanian R, Dimopoulos MA, Hester J, et al. Early myeloablative therapy for multiple myeloma. *Blood.* 1994;84:4278–4282.

11. San Miguel JF, Garcia-Sanz R, Gonzalez M, et al. Immunophenotype and DNA cell content in multiple myeloma. *Baillieres Clin Haematol.* 1995;8:735–759.

12. San Miguel JF, Almeida J, Mateo G, et al. Immunophenotypic evaluation of the plasma cell compartment in multiple myeloma: a tool for comparing the efficacy of different treatment strategies and predicting outcome. *Blood.* 2002;99:1853–1856.

13. Wearne AJ, Joshua DE, Young GA, et al. Multiple myeloma: light chain iso-type suppression—a marker of stable disease at presentation. *Eur J Haematol.* 1987;38:43–49.

14. Duperray C, Klein B, Durie BG, et al. Phenotypic analysis of human myeloma cell lines. *Blood.* 1989;73:566–572.

15. Yi Q, Dabadghao S, Osterborg A, et al. Myeloma bone marrow plasma cells: evidence for their capacity as antigen-presenting cells. *Blood.* 1997;90:1960–1967.

16. Szea DM, Brown RD, Yang S, et al. Prediction of high affinity class I-restricted multiple myeloma idiotype peptide epitopes. *Leuk Lymphoma.* 2003;44:1557–1568.

17. Leo R, Boeker M, Peest D, et al. Multiparameter analyses of normal and ma-lignant human plasma cells: CD38++, CD56+, CD54+, cIg+ is the common phenotype of myeloma cells. *Ann Hematol.* 1992;64:132–139.

18. Barker HF, Hamilton MS, Ball J, et al. Expression of adhesion molecules LFA-3 and N-CAM on normal and malignant human plasma cells. *Br J Haematol.* 1992;81:331–335.

19. Pellat-Deceunynck C, Bataille R, Robillard N, et al. Expression of CD28 and CD40 in human myeloma cells: a comparative study with normal plasma cells. *Blood.* 1994;84:2597–2603.

20. Westendorf JJ, Ahmann GJ, Armitage RJ, et al. CD40 expression in malignant plasma cells. Role in stimulation of autocrine IL-6 secretion by a human myeloma cell line. *J Immunol.* 1994;152:117–128.

21. Hata H, Matsuzaki H, Takeya M, et al. Fas/Apo-1 (CD95)-mediated and CD95-independent apoptosis of malignant plasma cells. *Leuk Lymphoma.* 1996;24:35–42.

22. Silvestris F, Cafforio P, Tucci M, et al. Negative regulation of erythroblast mat-uration by Fas-L(+)/TRAIL(+) highly malignant plasma cells: a major patho-genetic mechanism of anemia in multiple myeloma. *Blood.* 2002;99:1305–1313.

23. Pope B, Brown RD, Gibson J, et al. B7–2-positive myeloma: incidence, clin-ical characteristics, prognostic significance, and implications for tumor im-munotherapy. *Blood.* 2000;96:1274–1279.

24. Sirisinha S, Eisen HN. Autoimmune-like antibodies to the ligand-binding sites of myeloma proteins. *Proc Natl Acad Sci USA.* 1971;68:3130–3135.

25. Stevenson FK, Gordon J. Immunization with idiotypic immunoglobulin pro-tects against development of B lymphocytic leukemia, but emerging tumor cells can evade antibody attack by modulation. *J Immunol.* 1983;130:970–973.

26. Kaminski MS, Kitamura K, Maloney DG, et al. Idiotype vaccination against murine B cell lymphoma. Inhibition of tumor immunity by free idiotype pro-tein. *J Immunol.* 1987;138:1289–1296.

27. Campbell MJ, Esserman L, Byars NE, et al. Idiotype vaccination against murine B cell lymphoma. Humoral and cellular requirements for the full expression of antitumor immunity. *J Immunol.* 1990;145:1029–1036.

28. King CA, Spellerberg MB, Zhu D, et al. DNA vaccines with single-chain Fv fused to fragment C of tetanus toxin induce protective immunity against lymphoma and myeloma. *Nat Med.* 1998;4:1281–1286.

29. Holm G, Bergenbrant S, Lefvert AK, et al. Anti-idiotypic immunity as a potential regulator in myeloma and related diseases. *Ann NY Acad Sci.* 1991;636:178–183.

30. Yi Q, Bergenbrant S, Osterborg A, et al. T-cell stimulation induced by id-iotypes on monoclonal immunoglobulins in patients with monoclonal gam-mopathies. *Scand J Immunol.* 1993;38:529–534.

31. Yi Q, Osterborg A, Bergenbrant S, et al. Idiotype-reactive T-cell subsets and tumor load in monoclonal gammopathies. *Blood.* 1995;86:3043–3049.

32. Osterborg A, Yi Q, Bergenbrant S, Holm G, et al. Idiotype-specific T cells in multiple myeloma stage I: an evaluation by four different functional tests. *Br J Haematol.* 1995;89:110–116.

33. Wen YJ, Ling M, Bailey-Wood R, et al. Idiotypic protein-pulsed adherent pe-ripheral blood mononuclear cell-derived dendritic cells prime immune system in multiple myeloma. *Clin Cancer Res.* 1998;4:957–962.

34. Fagerberg J, Yi Q, Gigliotti D, et al. T-cell-epitope mapping of the idiotypic monoclonal IgG heavy and light chains in multiple myeloma. *Int J Cancer.* 1999;80:671–680.

35. Hansson L, Rabbani H, Fagerberg J, et al. T-cell epitopes within the complementarity-determining and framework regions of the tumor-derived immunoglobulin heavy chain in multiple myeloma. *Blood.* 2003;101:4930–4936.

36. Yi Q, Eriksson I, He W, et al. Idiotype-specific T lymphocytes in monoclonal gammopathies: evidence for the presence of CD4+ and CD8+ subsets. *Br J Haematol.* 1997;96:338–345.

37. Dabadghao S, Bergenbrant S, Anton D, et al. Anti-idiotypic T-cell activation in multiple myeloma induced by M-component fragments presented by dendritic cells. *Br J Haematol.* 1998;100:647–654.

38. Romagnani S. Human TH1 and TH2 subsets: doubt no more. *Immunol Today.* 1991;12:256–257.

39. Romagnani S. Human TH1 and TH2 subsets: regulation of differentiation and role in protection and immunopathology. *Int Arch Allergy Immunol.* 1992;98:279–285.

40. Walchner M, Wick M. Elevation of CD8+ CD11b+ Leu-8− T cells is as-sociated with the humoral immunodeficiency in myeloma patients. *Clin Exp Immunol.* 1997;109:310–316.

41. Salgame P, Abrams JS, Clayberger C, et al. Differing lymphokine pro-files of functional subsets of human CD4 and CD8 T cell clones. *Science.* 1991;254:279–282.

42. Wen YJ, Barlogie B, Yi Q. Idiotype-specific cytotoxic T lymphocytes in mul-tiple myeloma: evidence for their capacity to lyse autologous primary tumor cells. *Blood.* 2001;97:1750–1755.

43. Wen YJ, Min R, Tricot G, et al. Tumor lysate-specific cytotoxic T lymphocytes in multiple myeloma: promising effector cells for immunotherapy. *Blood.* 2002;99:3280–3285.

44. Gong J, Koido S, Chen D, et al. Immunization against murine multiple myeloma with fusions of dendritic and plasmacytoma cells is potentiated by interleukin 12. *Blood.* 2002;99:2512–2517.

45. Liu Y, Zhang W, Chan T, et al. Engineered fusion hybrid vaccine of IL-4 gene-modified myeloma and relative mature dendritic cells enhances antitumor immunity. *Leuk Res.* 2002;26:757–763.

46. Raje N, Hideshima T, Davies FE, et al. Tumour cell/dendritic cell fusions as a vaccination strategy for multiple myeloma. *Br J Haematol.* 2004;125:343–352.

47. Milazzo C, Reichardt VL, Muller MR, et al. Induction of myeloma-specific cytotoxic T cells using dendritic cells transfected with tumor-derived RNA. *Blood.* 2003;101:977–982.

48. Mao B, Wu W, Li Y, et al. LDL-receptor-related protein 6 is a receptor for Dickkopf proteins. *Nature.* 2001;411:321–325.

49. Zorn AM. Wnt signalling: antagonistic Dickkopfs. *Curr Biol.* 2001;11:R592–R595.

50. Glinka A, Wu W, Delius H, et al. Dickkopf-1 is a member of a new family of secreted proteins and functions in head induction. *Nature.* 1998;391:357–362.

51. Gregory CA, Singh H, Perry AS, et al. The Wnt signaling inhibitor dickkopf-1 is required for reentry into the cell cycle of human adult stem cells from bone marrow. *J Biol Chem.* 2003;278:28067–28078.

52. Tian E, Zhan F, Walker R, et al. The role of the Wnt-signaling antagonist DKK1 in the development of osteolytic lesions in multiple myeloma. *N Engl J Med.* 2003;349:2483–2494.

53. Yaccoby S, Ling W, Zhan F, et al. Antibody-based inhibition of DKK1 sup-presses tumor-induced bone resorption and multiple myeloma growth in vivo. *Blood.* 2007;109:2106–2111.

54. Heath DJ, Chantry AD, Buckle CH, et al. Inhibiting Dickkopf-1 (Dkk1) re-moves suppression of bone formation and prevents the development of oste-olytic bone disease in multiple myeloma. *J Bone Miner Res.* 2009;24:425–436.

55. Fulciniti M, Tassone P, Hideshima T, et al. Anti-DKK1 mAb (BHQ880) as a potential therapeutic agent for multiple myeloma. *Blood.* 2009;114:371–379.

56. van Baren N, Brasseur F, Godelaine D, et al. Genes encoding tumor-specific antigens are expressed in human myeloma cells. *Blood.* 1999;94:1156–1164.

57. Pellat-Deceunynck C, Mellerin MP, Labarriere N, et al. The cancer germ-line genes MAGE-1, MAGE-3 and PRAME are commonly expressed by human myeloma cells. *Eur J Immunol.* 2000;30:803–809.

58. Dhodapkar MV, Osman K, Teruya-Feldstein J, et al. Expression of cancer/testis (CT) antigens MAGE-A1, MAGE-A3, MAGE-A4, CT-7, and NY-ESO-1 in malignant gammopathies is heterogeneous and correlates with site, stage and risk status of disease. *Cancer Immun.* 2003;3:9.

59. Gupta SK, Shaughnessy J, Droojenbroeck JV, et al. NY-ESO-1 RNA and protein expression in multiple myeloma is highest in aggressive myeloma and is correlated with chromosomal abnormalities. *Blood.* 2002;100:401a.

60. Gupta SK, Pei L, Droojenbroeck JV, et al. Intra- and intertumoral variation in the expression of cancer testis antigens, MAGE-3 and NY-ESO-1 in multiple myeloma. *Blood.* 2002;100:603a.

61. Szmania SM, Bennett G, Batchu RB, et al. Dendritic cells pulsed with NY-ESO-1 and MAGE-3 peptide stimulate myeloma cytotoxic T lymphocytes. *Blood.* 2002;100:399a.

62. van Rhee F, Szmania SM, Zhan F, et al. NY-ESO-1 is highly expressed in poor-prognosis multiple myeloma and induces spontaneous humoral and cellular immune responses. *Blood.* 2005;105:3939–3944.

63. Treon SP, Mollick JA, Urashima M, et al. Muc-1 core protein is expressed on multiple myeloma cells and is induced by dexamethasone. *Blood.* 1999;93:1287–1298.

64. Akagi J, Nakagawa K, Egami H, et al. Induction of HLA-unrestricted and HLA-class-II-restricted cytotoxic T lymphocytes against MUC-1 from patients with colorectal carcinomas using recombinant MUC-1 vaccinia virus. *Cancer Immunol Immunother.* 1998;47:21–31.

65. Moore A, Medarova Z, Potthast A, et al. In vivo targeting of underglycosylated MUC-1 tumor antigen using a multimodal imaging probe. *Cancer Res.* 2004;64:1821–1827.

66. Lim SH, Wang Z, Chiriva-Internati M, et al. Sperm protein 17 is a novel cancer-testis antigen in multiple myeloma. *Blood.* 2001;97:1508–1510.

67. Lim SH, Chiriva-Internati M, Wang Z, et al. Sperm protein 17 (Sp17) as a tumor vaccine for multiple myeloma. *Blood.* 2002;100:673a.

68. Ohtomo T, Sugamata Y, Ozaki Y, et al. Molecular cloning and characterization of a surface antigen preferentially overexpressed on multiple myeloma cells. *Biochem Biophys Res Commun.* 1999;258:583–591.

69. Ono K, Ohtomo T, Yoshida K, et al. The humanized anti-HM1.24 antibody effectively kills multiple myeloma cells by human effector cell-mediated cytotoxicity. *Mol Immunol.* 1999;36:387–395.

70. Treon SP, Raje N, Anderson KC. Immunotherapeutic strategies for the treatment of plasma cell malignancies. *Semin Oncol.* 2000;27:598–613.

71. Noto H, Takahashi T, Makiguchi Y, et al. Cytotoxic T lymphocytes derived from bone marrow mononuclear cells of multiple myeloma patients recognize an underglycosylated form of MUC1 mucin. *Intern Immunol.* 1997;9:791–798.

72. Chiriva-Internati M, Wang Z, Salati E, et al. Sperm protein 17 (Sp17) is a suitable target for immunotherapy of multiple myeloma. *Blood.* 2002;100:961–965.

73. Lacy HM, Sanderson RD. Sperm protein 17 is expressed on normal and malignant lymphocytes and promotes heparan sulfate-mediated cell-cell adhesion. *Blood.* 2001;98:2160–2165.

74. Bergenbrant S, Yi Q, Osterborg A, et al. Modulation of anti-idiotypic immune response by immunization with the autologous M-component protein in multiple myeloma patients. *Br J Haematol.* 1996;92:840–846.

75. Osterborg A, Yi Q, Henriksson L, et al. Idiotype immunization combined with granulocyte-macrophage colony-stimulating factor in myeloma patients induced type I, major histocompatibility complex-restricted, CD8- and CD4-specific T-cell responses. *Blood.* 1998;91:2459–2466.

76. Hansson L, Abdalla AO, Moshfegh A, et al. Long-term idiotype vaccination combined with interleukin-12 (IL-12), or IL-12 and granulocyte macrophage colony-stimulating factor, in early-stage multiple myeloma patients. *Clin Cancer Res.* 2007;13:1503–1510.

77. Massaia M, Borrione P, Battaglio S, et al. Idiotype vaccination in human myeloma: generation of tumor-specific immune responses after high-dose chemotherapy. *Blood.* 1999;94:673–683.

78. Coscia M, Mariani S, Battaglio S, et al. Long-term follow-up of idiotype vaccination in human myeloma as a maintenance therapy after high-dose chemotherapy. *Leukemia.* 2004;18:139–145.

79. Dabadghao S, Bergenbrant S, Anton D, et al. Anti-idiotypic T-cell activation in multiple myeloma induced by M-component fragments presented by dendritic cells. *Br J Haematol.* 1998;100:647–654.

80. Butch AW, Kelly KA, Munshi NC. Dendritic cells derived from multiple myeloma patients efficiently internalize different classes of myeloma protein. *Exp Hematol.* 2001;29:85–92.

81. Wen YJ, Ling M, Bailey-Wood R, et al. Idiotypic protein-pulsed adherent peripheral blood mononuclear cell-derived dendritic cells prime immune system in multiple myeloma. *Clin Cancer Res.* 1998;4:957–962.

82. Lim SH, Bailey-Wood R. Idiotypic protein-pulsed dendritic cell vaccination in multiple myeloma. *Int J Cancer.* 1999;83:215–222.

83. Reichardt VL, Okada CY, Liso A, et al. Idiotype vaccination using dendritic cells after autologous peripheral blood stem cell transplantation for multiple myeloma—a feasibility study. *Blood.* 1999;93:2411–2419.

84. Liso A, Stockerl-Goldstein KE, Auffermann-Gretzinger S, et al. Idiotype vaccination using dendritic cells after autologous peripheral blood progenitor cell transplantation for multiple myeloma. *Biol Blood Marrow Transplant.* 2000;6:621–627.

85. Cull G, Durrant L, Stainer C, et al. Generation of anti-idiotype immune responses following vaccination with idiotype-protein pulsed dendritic cells in myeloma. *Br J Haematol.* 1999;107:648–655.

86. Titzer S, Christensen O, Manzke O, et al. Vaccination of multiple myeloma patients with idiotype-pulsed dendritic cells: immunological and clinical aspects. *Br J Haematol.* 2000;108:805–816.

87. Yi Q, Desikan R, Barlogie B, et al. Optimizing dendritic cell-based immunotherapy in multiple myeloma. *Br J Haematol.* 2002;117:297–305.

88. Curti A, Tosi P, Comoli P, et al. Phase I/II clinical trial of sequential subcutaneous and intravenous delivery of dendritic cell vaccination for refractory multiple myeloma using patient-specific tumour idiotype protein or idiotype (VDJ)-derived class I-restricted peptides. *Br J Haematol.* 2007;139:415–424.

89. Bendandi M, Rodriguez-Calvillo M, Inoges S, et al. Combined vaccination with idiotype-pulsed allogeneic dendritic cells and soluble protein idiotype for multiple myeloma patients relapsing after reduced-intensity conditioning allogeneic stem cell transplantation. *Leuk Lymphoma.* 2006;47:29–37.

90. Gong J, Chen D, Kashiwaba M, Kufe D. Induction of antitumor activity by immunization with fusions of dendritic and carcinoma cells. *Nat Med.* 1997;3:558–561.

91. Gong J, Chen D, Kashiwaba M, et al. Reversal of tolerance to human MUC1 antigen in MUC1 transgenic mice immunized with fusions of dendritic and carcinoma cells. *Proc Natl Acad Sci USA.* 1998;95:6279–6283.

92. Kugler A, Stuhler G, Walden P, et al. Regression of human metastatic renal cell carcinoma after vaccination with tumor cell-dendritic cell hybrids. *Nat Med.* 2000;6:332–336.

93. Raje N, Hideshima T, Davies FE, et al. Tumour cell/dendritic cell fusions as a vaccination strategy for multiple myeloma. *Br J Haematol.* 2004;125:343–352.

94. Hao S, Bi X, Xu S, et al. Enhanced antitumor immunity derived from a novel vaccine of fusion hybrid between dendritic and engineered myeloma cells. *Exp Oncol.* 2004;26:300–306.

95. Walewska R, Teobald I, Dunnion D, et al. Preclinical development of hybrid cell vaccines for multiple myeloma. *Eur J Haematol.* 2007;78:11–20.

96. Stevenson FK, Link CJ Jr, Traynor A, et al. DNA vaccination against multiple myeloma. *Semin Hematol.* 1999;36:38–42.

97. Wendtner CM, Nolte A, Mangold E, et al. Gene transfer of the costimulatory molecules B7-1 and B7-2 into human multiple myeloma cells by recombinant adeno-associated virus enhances the cytolytic T cell response. *Gene Ther.* 1997;4:726–735.

98. Rice J, Elliott T, Buchan S, et al. DNA fusion vaccine designed to induce cytotoxic T cell responses against defined peptide motifs: implications for cancer vaccines. *J Immunol.* 2001;167:1558–1565.

99. Trudel S, Li Z, Dodgson C, et al. Adenovector engineered interleukin-2 expressing autologous plasma cell vaccination after high-dose chemotherapy for multiple myeloma—a phase 1 study. *Leukemia.* 2001;15:846–854.

100. Angelucci E, Polchi P, Lucarelli G, et al. Allogeneic bone marrow transplantation for hematological malignancies following therapy with high doses of busulphan and cyclophosphamide. *Haematologica.* 1989;74:455–461.

101. Angelucci E, Baronciani D, Lucarelli G, et al. Long-term complete remission after allogeneic bone marrow transplantation in multiple myeloma. *Bone Marrow Transplant.* 1991;8:307–309.

102. Bensinger WI, Buckner CD, Anasetti C, et al. Allogeneic marrow transplantation for multiple myeloma: an analysis of risk factors on outcome. *Blood.* 1996;88:2787–2793.

103. Gahrton G, Tura S, Ljungman P, et al. Allogeneic bone marrow transplantation in multiple myeloma. European Group for Bone Marrow Transplantation. [See comment.] *N Engl J Med.* 1991;325:1267–1273.

104. Kwak LW, Taub DD, Duffey PL, et al. Transfer of myeloma idiotype-specific immunity from an actively immunised marrow donor. *Lancet.* 1995;345:1016–1020.

105. Neelapu SS, Munshi NC, Jagannath S, et al. Tumor antigen immunization of sibling stem cell transplant donors in multiple myeloma. *Bone Marrow Transplant.* 2005;36:315–323.

106. Falkenburg JH, Wafelman AR, Joosten P, et al. Complete remission of accelerated phase chronic myeloid leukemia by treatment with leukemia-reactive cytotoxic T lymphocytes. *Blood.* 1999;94:1201–1208.

107. Dudley ME, Wunderlich JR, Robbins PF, et al. Cancer regression and autoimmunity in patients after clonal repopulation with antitumor lymphocytes. *Science.* 2002;298:850–854.

108. Rosenberg SA, Dudley ME. Cancer regression in patients with metastatic melanoma after the transfer of autologous antitumor lymphocytes. *Proc Natl Acad Sci USA.* 2004;101(suppl 2):14639–14645.

109. Lin MZ, Teitell MA, Schiller GJ. The evolution of antibodies into versatile tumor-targeting agents. *Clin Cancer Res.* 2005;11:129–138.

110. Owaidah TM, Aljurf MD. The evolving role of monoclonal antibodies and dendritic cell therapy in hematologic malignancies. *Hematology.* 2002;7:265–272.

111. Reff ME, Hariharan K, Braslawsky G. Future of monoclonal antibodies in the treatment of hematologic malignancies. *Cancer Control.* 2002;9:152–166.

112. Bjorkman PJ, Burmeister WP. Structures of two classes of MHC molecules elucidated: crucial differences and similarities. *Curr Opin Struct Biol.* 1994;4: 852–856.

113. Strominger JL. Human histocompatibility proteins. *Immunol Rev.* 2002;185: 69–77.

114. Cooper EH, Plesner T. Beta-2-microglobulin review: its relevance in clinical oncology. *Med Pediatr Oncol.* 1980;8:323–334.

115. Shvidel L, Hofstein R, Berrebi A. Serum beta-2 microglobulin as a marker of B-cell activation in chronic lymphoid malignancies. *Am J Hematol.* 1996;53:148–149.

116. Molica S, Levato D, Cascavilla N, et al. Clinico-prognostic implications of simultaneous increased serum levels of soluble CD23 and beta2-microglobulin in B-cell chronic lymphocytic leukemia. *Eur J Haematol.* 1999;62:117–122.

117. Bataille R, Durie BG, Grenier J. Serum beta2 microglobulin and survival duration in multiple myeloma: a simple reliable marker for staging. *Br J Haematol.* 1983;55:439–447.

118. Alexanian R, Barlogie B, Fritsche H. Beta 2 microglobulin in multiple myeloma. *Am J Hematol.* 1985;20:345–351.

119. Yang J, Qian J, Wezeman M, et al. Targeting beta(2)-microglobulin for induction of tumor apoptosis in human hematological malignancies. *Cancer Cell.* 2006;10:295–307.

120. Yang J, Cao Y, Hong S, et al. Human-like mouse models for testing the efficacy and safety of anti-beta2-microglobulin monoclonal antibodies to treat myeloma. *Clin Cancer Res.* 2009;15:951–959.

121. Sekimoto E, Ozaki S, Ohshima T, et al. A single-chain Fv diabody against human leukocyte antigen-A molecules specifically induces myeloma cell death in the bone marrow environment. *Cancer Res.* 2007;67:1184–1192.

122. Nomura T, Huang WC, Seo S, et al. Targeting beta2-microglobulin mediated signaling as a novel therapeutic approach for human renal cell carcinoma. *J Urol.* 2007;178:292–300.

123. Huang WC, Wu D, Xie Z, et al. beta2-microglobulin is a signaling and growth-promoting factor for human prostate cancer bone metastasis. *Cancer Res.* 2006;66:9108–9116.

124. Yang J, Zhang X, Wang J, et al. Anti beta2-microglobulin monoclonal antibodies induce apoptosis in myeloma cells by recruiting MHC class I to and excluding growth and survival cytokine receptors from lipid rafts. *Blood.* 2007;110:3028–3035.

125. Hsi ED, Steinle R, Balasa B, et al. CS1, a potential new therapeutic antibody target for the treatment of multiple myeloma. *Clin Cancer Res.* 2008;14:2775–2784.

126. Tai YT, Soydan E, Song W, et al. CS1 promotes multiple myeloma cell adhesion, clonogenic growth, and tumorigenicity via c-maf-mediated interactions with bone marrow stromal cells. *Blood.* 2009;113:4309–4318.

127. Tai YT, Dillon M, Song W, et al. Anti-CS1 humanized monoclonal antibody HuLuc63 inhibits myeloma cell adhesion and induces antibody-dependent cellular cytotoxicity in the bone marrow milieu. *Blood.* 2008;112:1329–1337.

128. Tai YT, Catley LP, Mitsiades CS, et al. Mechanisms by which SGN-40, a humanized anti-CD40 antibody, induces cytotoxicity in human multiple myeloma cells: clinical implications. *Cancer Res.* 2004;64:2846–2852.

129. Tai YT, Li X, Tong X, et al. Human anti-CD40 antagonist antibody triggers significant antitumor activity against human multiple myeloma. *Cancer Res.* 2005;65:5898–5906.

130. Tai YT, Li XF, Catley L, et al. Immunomodulatory drug lenalidomide (CC-5013, IMiD3) augments anti-CD40 SGN-40-induced cytotoxicity in human multiple myeloma: clinical implications. *Cancer Res.* 2005;65:11712–11720.

131. Anderson KC. New agents and approaches in the treatment of multiple myeloma. *Clin Adv Hematol Oncol.* 2003;1:151–152.

# Future Novel Single Agent and Combination Therapies

Diana Cirstea  •  Sonia Vallet  •  Noopur Raje

Multiple myeloma (MM) is a malignant neoplasm of plasma cells that accumulate in bone marrow, leading to bone destruction and marrow failure. The American Cancer Society estimates that about 20,580 new cases of multiple myeloma (11,680 in men and 8900 in women) will be diagnosed in 2009. In the United States, the lifetime risk of developing MM is 1 in 161 (0.62%).[1] The treatment of MM has dramatically improved over the past decade. The 5-year survival rate reported in the Surveillance Epidemiology and End Results database has increased from 25% in 1975 to 34% in 2003. These improvements are largely a reflection of outcomes seen in the age group younger than 50 years, leading to 5- and 10-year relative survival of 56.7% and 41.3% in 2002–2004, and in the age group 50 to 59 years, leading to 5- and 10-year relative survival of 48.2% and 28.6%.[2] This is most likely a result of recent advances in the use of novel therapies and their dissemination in clinical practice. By contrast, only modest improvement was seen in the age group 60 to 69 years, and essentially no improvement was noted among older patients. Further research into the best treatment for older patients, including greater involvement of older patients in clinical trials, improved tolerability of stem-cell transplantation (SCT), and increased understanding of how best to use novel agents in older patients is needed.

The availability of a rich pipeline of novel agents undergoing early-phase clinical trials in MM is an exciting and active area of research. Here, we will review future novel agents used either alone or in combination strategies. These strategies will help transform MM into a chronic disease in all age groups and ultimately lead to long-term survival and cure.

## NEWLY FOOD AND DRUG ADMINISTRATION-APPROVED DRUG COMBINATIONS IN MYELOMA

Over the last several years, 5 treatment strategies have received Food and Drug Administration approval either alone or in combination for MM with thalidomide (thal), lenalidomide (len), and bortezomib as important backbone drugs in these approaches. In the upfront setting, thal with dexamethasone (thal/dex) and Velcade (Vel) in combination with melphalan and prednisone (MPV) increased the overall response rate (RR) and significantly prolonged time to progression (TTP) and are Food and Drug Administration approved. The RR with thal/dex is 64%[3] and 71% with MPV.[4] In the relapsed setting, Vel alone[5,6] and the combinations of len/dexamethasone (len/dex)[7–9] and Vel and Doxil (Vel/Doxil)[10] have been approved. The addition of len to high-dose dex (40 mg 4 times/wk for 3 weeks) in patients with relapsed/refractory MM induces a 61% RR with a median TTP of 11 months.[11] Although a recent analysis based on a longer follow-up showed improved overall survival with an acceptable toxicity profile[7,8] by len/dex compared with dex alone, preliminary results of a phase III randomized trial suggest that lower doses of dex (40 mg weekly for 4 weeks) provide

a survival advantage, at least in the upfront setting, mainly due to increased toxicity with high doses of dex.[12,13] The combination of Vel/Doxil is approved in patients with relapsed refractory MM after at least 1 prior therapy and who have not received Vel previously. Although the combination of pegylated liposomal doxorubicin with Vel did not significantly increase RR, it prolonged TTP of 3 months and increased survival rates from 65% to 76%. These data resulted in approval of the combination for the treatment of relapsed and refractory MM and is now being studied as frontline therapy.[10]

The availability of these novel agents have not only provided us with several treatment options but also have importantly impacted overall survival of our patients. To improve on current outcomes, optimal combinations of Vel, thal, and len are currently under evaluation in phase II/III clinical trials. Promising combination strategies include MPV with thal and melphalan and prednisone with len in elderly patients and Vel with len/dex and Vel with thal/dex in both patients with relapsed/refractory MM and as frontline therapy.

## NOVEL SINGLE AGENTS

### Carfilzomib and Other Novel Proteasome Inhibitors

Although bortezomib or Vel is an effective agent in MM, about 20% of newly diagnosed patients are resistant to bortezomib, and ultimately, all patients relapse and develop resistance. To this end, novel proteasome inhibitors have been studied. Carfilzomib irreversibly blocks chymotrypsin-like and immunoproteasome activities and in phase I studies achieved more than 80% proteasome inhibition. Preclinical data confirmed caspase-mediated apoptosis and demonstrated greater efficacy compared with bortezomib and potent cytoxicity in primary cells from bortezomib-resistant patients. Carfilzomib induced at least stable disease in heavily pretreated patients with MM, most of them relapsing after use of novel agents and responses occurred rapidly, often after the first cycle.[14,15] Importantly, the overall RR increased up to 50% in bortezomib-naive patients.[16] The toxicity profile was manageable, consisting mainly of myelosuppression and with strikingly very little neuropathy. Other than single agent activity, Carfilzomib has shown promising activity in combination strategies with len/dex with limited toxicity.[17] Future studies with longer follow-up will define the patient population benefiting from therapy with Carfilzomib and identify safe combination strategies to improve RR and survival.

Early data with other second-generation proteasome inhibitors, NPI-0052[18] and CEP-18770,[19] are promising, and ongoing phase I clinical trials are evaluating these drugs in patients with relapsed or refractory MM and previous resistance to Vel. Mechanistically, CEP-18770 more potently inhibits the chymotryptic-like activity of the proteosome compared with bortezomib, whereas NPI0052 inhibits the chymotryptic-like activity and the tryptic-like and caspase-like activities; all overcome bortezomib resistance in preclinical studies

**TABLE 1.**    Novel Agents and Combinations in Clinical Trials for Multiple Myeloma

| Novel Agent | Trial Phase | No. Patients (n) | Response Rate (RR) | References |
|---|---|---|---|---|
| Carfilzomib (PR-171) | I | n = 29 (MM:6) | ≥ MR: 50% | Orlowski et al[93] |
| Carfilzomib (PR-171) | I | n = 37 (MM:13) | ≥ MR: 30% | Alsina et al[94] |
| Carfilzomib (PR-171) | II | n = 46 refractory to bortezomib and IMiDs | ORR: 26% (PR 13%, MR 13%) | Jagannath et al[14] |
| Carfilzomib (PR-171) | II | n = 31 bortezomib treated (n = 16) bortezomib naïve (n = 13) | ORR: 25% (PR: 19%, MR: 6%) ORR: 54% (CR 8%, PR 46%) | Vij et al[16] |
| Carfilzomib + len + dex | I | 8/11 evaluable | PR: 50%, MR: 12.5% | Niesvizky et al[17] |
| Pomalidomide (CC-4047) + low dose Dex | II | n = 37 (62% previous IMiDs treatment) | Very good partial response (VGPR): 24%, PR: 38%, RR: in len-refractory patients 29% | Lacy et al[29] |
| Tanespimycin (KOS-953/17-AAG) + bortezomib | II | n = 63 | ORR 35% (CR 5%, PR 22%, 16% in bortezomib refractory patients) | Richardson et al[95] |
| Vorinostat (SAHA) + bortezomib | I | n = 57, 2 trials: n = 34 and n = 23 | ORR: 47% and 43% | Weber et al[96] |
| Vorinostat (SAHA) + len + dex | I | n = 7 | ORR: 28% (PR 14%, MR 14%) | Siegel et al[39] |
| Panobinostat (LBH) + bortezomib ± dex | Ib | n = 14 | ORR: 35% (VGPR: 7%, CR: 7%, PR: 21%) | Siegel et al[97] |
| Romidepsin (depsipeptide) + bortezomib ± dex | I/II | n = 25 | ORR: 67% (VGPR: 22%, CR: 22%, PR: 22%) | Harrison et al[38] |
| Temsirolimus (CCI-779) + bortezomib | I | n = 20 (all previous bortezomib) | ORR: 33% (nCR: 7%, MR: 27%) | Ghobrial et al[72] |

VGPR indicates very good partial response.

and are undergoing clinical evaluation. Importantly, according to preliminary data from a phase I study in patients with relapsed/refractory MM, NPI-0052 has not seemed to induce peripheral neuropathy or myelosuppression, was well tolerated, and demonstrated unique safety profiles compared with bortezomib despite up to 100% proteasome inhibition.[20] Excitingly, combining bortezomib with NPI-0052 results in even greater activity in both in vitro and in vivo MM preclinical models.[21] Additionally, novel combination approaches and novel agents targeting processes upstream of the proteasome are in development (Table 1; Figure 1).

## Pomalidomide

The promising results of thal in advanced relapsed and refractory MM[22] established thal as an effective therapy in the relapsed and upfront settings.[23,24] However, the dose-related and duration-related adverse effects including sedation, neuropathy, constipation, and deep vein thrombosis[25] have significantly limited its clinical use. This led to the development of thal-derived immunomodulatory analogs (IMiDs), in particular CC-4047 [Pomalidomide (Pom)] and CC-5013 (len), which demonstrated up to 50,000 times more potent inhibition of tumor necrosis factor (TNF)-$\alpha$ than the thal parent compound in vitro.[26] Preclinical evidence suggest IMiDs induce caspase-8–dependent apoptosis, repress nuclear factor (NF)-$\kappa$B transcriptional activity, and sensitize MM cells to apoptosis induced by Fas crosslinking, TNF-related apoptosis-inducing ligand/Apo-2L (TRAIL/Apo-2L), Dex, and Vel.[27] Moreover, the antiproliferative and proapoptotic effects were complemented with antiangiogenic activity, inhibition of cytokine synthesis and secretion triggered by MM cell adhesion to bone marrow stromal cells (BMSCs), inhibition of TNF-$\alpha$ signaling, and stimulation of patients' natural killer cell anti-MM immunity.[28] Recent data on Pom, the newest IMiD has shown single-agent activity in phase I studies and was subsequently tested in a phase II trial in

combination with low-dose dex (Pom/dex) in patients with relapsed or refractory MM. Pom/dex was found to be highly active and well tolerated with RR of 62%, including a 29% RR among patients who were len refractory. No grade 3 neuropathy was seen, and there have been no thromboembolic events.[29] Therefore, Pom seems to be a promising agent in the therapy for MM and provides an alternative to patients who have received both len and Vel-based treatments.

## FUTURE AGENTS AS COMBINATION STRATEGIES

### Histone Deacetylase Inhibitors

Histone deacetylase inhibitors (HDACi) are a novel class of anticancer agents. Although their antitumor effects have been extensively proven in vitro, in vivo, and in the clinical setting, their mechanism of action remains unclear. Four classes of histone deacetylase have been identified with different functions. Indeed, the acetylation process involves several other substrates other than histones. Therefore, not only DNA transcription is affected by histone deacetylase and histone acetylase but also posttranslation modifications of protein. The latter affects protein stability, interactions, localization, and DNA bindings.

Several HDACi have been developed, and some are already in the clinical setting, including suberoylanilide hydroxamic acid or vorinostat (SAHA), LBH589, and romidepsin. These are generally nonselective inhibitors, except for tubacin that specifically targets HDAC6. They have been considered epigenetic drugs for their global effects on gene transcription. However, because of the pleiotropic effects of HDACs, the inhibitors have additional effects. They mediate tumor cell death through caspase-dependent and nondependent apoptosis and autophagy. They induce cell cycle arrest through p21 upregulation. They also block the aggresome complex, a scavenger pathway linked to the proteasome degradation pathway, and induce cell death through accumulation of ubiquinated proteins.

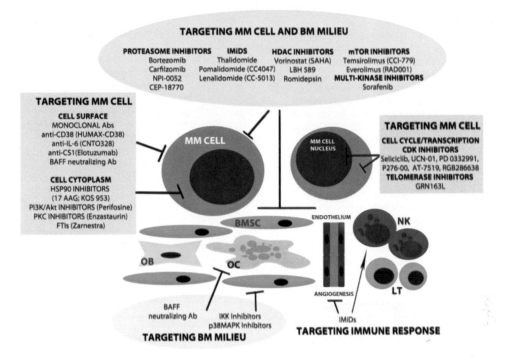

**FIGURE 1.** Novel agents targeting the multiple myeloma (MM) cell and its bone marrow (BM) microenvironment in clinical trials tested either alone or in combination for the treatment of MM. The interaction of MM cells with BM stromal cells (BMSCs) and other components in the BM milieu [ie, osteoblast (OB), OC, and vascular endothelial cells] plays a crucial role in MM cell pathogenesis and drug resistance. Thus, future novel MM therapies can be categorized as (1) agents targeting both MM cell and its BM microenvironment [proteasome inhibitors, IMiDs, HDACi, mTOR, and multikinase (ie, Ras/Raf/MEK/Erk) inhibitors]; (2) agents acting at MM cell surface (anti-IL-6, anti-CD38, anti-Cs1, and anti-BAFF monoclonal antibodies) or on signaling and protein dynamics (PI3K/Akt and PKC inhibitors, HSP90, and FTIs); (3) agents targeting cell cycle and transcriptional inhibitors (CDKIs and telomerase inhibitors), (4) agents targeting BM microenvironment: BMSCs (p38 mitogen-activated protein kinase and IKK inhibitors), tumor vasculature (mTOR and multikinase inhibitors and IMiDs), bone components (anti-BAFF Ab); and finally, (5) agents improving anti-MM immune responses (IMiDs).

In the setting of MM, HDACi are effective anticancer agents in both in vitro and in vivo studies. The transcriptional signature of the HDACi SAHA reveals downregulation of insulin-like growth factor (IGF)-1R/AKT and interleukin (IL)6R/STAT3 signaling pathways and DNA synthesis and repair enzymes.[30] Cell death induced by HDACi is associated with upregulation of p21 and requires inhibition of antiapoptotic factors BCL2 and BCXL. No caspase activation has been observed in the MM setting with SAHA; however, other HDACi such as NVP-LAQ824 and LBH589 induced caspase activation in vitro. Several xenograft models confirmed the anti-MM effects of HDACi, resulting in reduced tumor burden and increased survival.[31] In the clinical setting, single-agent HDACi differ in their effects and toxicities according to the specific compound, the formulation, and schedule of administration. Toxicities of oral formulation of SAHA were limited to fatigue, diarrhea, and dehydration, whereas intravenous doses induced mainly myelosuppression and thrombocytopenia. SAHA demonstrated significant activity in the lymphoma setting but only modest activity in MM.[32,33] Similarly, adverse effects of oral LBH589 consisted of thrombocytopenia and neutropenia, and clinical responses were observed mainly in patients with lymphoma.[34,35] Therefore, single-agent HDACi treatment requires optimization of the dosing schedules to limit toxicity and enhance clinical response. HDACi have been assessed also in combination strategies with novel anti-MM agents, mainly bortezomib and len. In vitro evidence suggests that HDACi sensitizes MM cell to death receptor–mediated apoptosis and dex and actimid-induced cytotoxicity.[30] Particularly promising is the synergistic activity with the proteasome inhibitor, bortezomib. HDACis suppress proteasome activity, expression of proteasome subunits, and inhibit aggresome. Aggresome represents a protein-scavenger system that mediates protein degradation in case of proteasome overload or inhibition. The high protein turnover characteristic of plasma cells and MM cells requires aggresome formation. Inhibition of this pathway through tubacin, a specific HDAC6 inhibitor, synergizes with proteasome inhibition achieved with bortezomib. Interestingly, in vivo combination of HDACi and bortezomib not only effectively reduced tumor burden but also improved osteolytic lesions in a mouse model of bone disease.[36] Based on these promising preclinical data, several HDACi have been studied in combination with bortezomib in patients with advanced MM. The combination was well tolerated and effective even in bortezomib-pretreated patients.[37–40] Promising results in terms of safety profile and clinical activity have also been noted with the combination of HDACi and len.[41,42] Ongoing studies are also evaluating SAHA in combination with doxorubicin or melphalan-prednisone regimes. Conclusive results on efficacy of these combinations require randomized, placebo-controlled, phase III trials, which are ongoing in some settings.

## Heat-Shock Protein 90 Inhibitors

Heat-shock protein 90 (HSP90) is a chaperone protein that regulates protein folding and translocation into the different cellular compartments. A promising HSP90 inhibitor is KOS-953, a novel formulation of 17-AAG. As a single agent, KOS-953 produced durable responses in patients with relapsed/refractory MM and demonstrated a manageable toxicity profile, mainly consisting of transaminase elevation and anemia. Profiling of gene and protein expression provided the preclinical rationale for clinical protocols combining HSP90 inhibitors with bortezomib. Studies demonstrate that bortezomib treatment of MM cells in vitro induces death signaling, downregulates survival signaling, and upregulates both ubiquitin/proteasome and stress response gene transcripts.[43] Specifically, bortezomib induces HSP90, which not only is a stress response protein but also plays a major role in protein unfolding required before proteins can be degraded by the proteasome. In vitro studies show that HSP90 inhibitor 17AAG can block the Hsp90 stress response induced by bortezomib and thereby increase MM cell apoptosis. Therefore, these gene microarray studies provided the framework for a clinical trial coupling these agents in MM, which shows that HSP90 inhibitor KOS953 can sensitize to and even overcome resistance to Bortezomib.[44] KOS-953 is currently undergoing studies in combination with Vel in patients with relapse/refractory myeloma and a phase III clinical trial of bortezomib versus bortezomib with KOS953 in relapsed MM is ongoing.

## Phosphatidylinositol 3-Kinase/Protein Kinase B (PI3K/Akt) Inhibitors

The relevance of molecular targeted therapy for PI3K/Akt pathway in MM has been demonstrated in cell line and xenograft models. Cytokine-induced activation of Akt has been reported to induce growth and survival advantage to MM cells through phosphorylation of glycogen synthase kinase (GSK)-3$\beta$ and mammalian target of rapamycin (mTOR).[45] Moreover, in the context of BM microenvironment, besides the various downstream antiapoptotic effects, PI3K/Akt cascade has been found to mediate dex-resistance in MM cells.[46] Finally, the correlation between constitutively activated Akt with advanced stage and poor prognosis in patients with MM[47] confirmed the rational of PI3K/Akt inhibitors evaluation in the treatment of MM. Consequently, agents targeting PI3K/Akt network directly, in particular Akt inhibitor perifosine, the protein kinases C (PKC) inhibitor enzastaurin, and the mTOR inhibitors, RAD001 and CCI-779, or acting on PI3K/Akt pathway indirectly through IL-6, IGF-1, or HSP90 inhibitors have been examined in MM preclinical models.

Targeting Akt in MM cells with the novel oral Akt inhibitor perifosine (NSC 639966; Keryx Biopharmaceuticals) triggered cytotoxicity against MM cells, both in vitro and in vivo.[48] Molecular studies revealed that perifosine-induced inhibition of Akt phosphorylation and its downstream molecules forkhead (Drosophila) homolog (rhabdomyosarcoma) like 1 (FKHRL1) and GSK-3$\beta$ associated with c-jun NH$_2$-terminal kinase activation. Additionally, perifosine treatment triggered the formation of the death-inducing signaling complex and the recruitment of TRAIL-R1/DR4, TRAIL-R2/DR5,[49] ultimately resulting in complementary extrinsic and intrinsic apoptosis.[48] Preclinical data has been reported on bortezomib-induced activation of Akt, which has been completely blocked by perifosine, whereas bortezomib successfully abrogated perifosine-induced extracellular signal-related kinase (ERK) phosphorylation.[48] This blockade by perifosine and bortezomib of both Akt and ERK signaling cascades enhances c-Jun N-terminal kinases (JNK) phosphorylation, caspase/poly(ADP) ribose polymerase (PARP) cleavage, and apoptosis.[48] This combination in vitro anti-MM activity served as

strong rationale for the evaluation of bortezomib and perifosine combination with or without dex to overcome clinical proteasome resistance. In fact, promising preliminary data presented demonstrate that perifosine in combination with bortezomib ($\pm$dex) was well tolerated and active in heavily pretreated, bortezomib-exposed patients with MM, with an overall response of 40%, including an overall response of 37% and a median TTP of 9.25 months in responding but previously bortezomib-refractory population.[50] In the meantime, preliminary data reported on the phase I study of the safety and efficacy of perifosine (peri) in combination with len and dex for patients with relapsed or refractory MM demonstrated that patients have tolerated peri + len + dex well with manageable toxicity and with encouraging clinical activity as confirmed by an overall response rate (ORR) of 50%.[51]

Potent suppression of PI3K/Akt signaling, through PKC-Akt interaction was demonstrated with the PKC inhibitor Enzastaurin (LY317615; Eli Lilly and Company). Dual PKC and PI3K/Akt signaling inhibition by enzastaurin has been reported to abrogate tumor growth, survival, and angiogenesis in in vitro and in vivo models of MM.[52] The latter advanced enzastaurin to a phase II clinical trial ongoing in patients with previously treated MM or Waldenstrom's Macroglobulinemia.

## mTOR Inhibitors

Among the major pathways mediating cytokine-induced MM cell growth and survival, PI3K/Akt/mTOR kinase cascade plays a critical role in cell proliferation, survival, and development of drug resistance.[53–55] Identifying mTOR as a key kinase acting downstream of Akt led to the prediction that rapamycin, a universal inhibitor of mTORC1-dependent S6K1 phosphorylation may be useful in the treatment of MM.[56–58] Cumulative evidence supports the hypothesis that rapamycin-induced cytotoxicity is predominantly triggered as a consequence of autophagy (programmed cell death type II) through excessive cell digestion. Therefore, activated Akt can be a key upstream inhibitor of 2 cell death-inducing events: autophagy through mTOR activation and apoptosis through phosphorylation of BCL2-associated agonist of cell death (BAD) and inhibition of the catalytic subunit of caspase-9. In vitro and in vivo preclinical studies have demonstrated anti-MM activity of rapamycin and its analogs (CCI-779 and RAD001),[59–63] and yet first-generation mTOR inhibitors when used as single agents have had only modest efficacy in clinical trials,[64–67] paving the way for combination approaches.

A growing body of evidence indicates that resistance to rapamycin results from a strong positive feedback loop from mTOR/S6K1 to Akt with a consequent Akt activation.[68–70] This effect in some cancer types is due to rapamycin activity only on mTORC1 complex, whereas mTORC2, the one responsible for Akt activation, remains unaffected. The latter finding served as rationale for preclinical examination of rapamycin combinations with PI3K/Akt inhibitors, ie, perifosine to enhance rapamycin-induced toxicity in MM cells.[71] Promising data reported on combined targeting of mitogen-activated protein kinase and PI3K/mTOR pathways by rapamycin with len[59] and of Raf/VEGFR and mTOR kinases through rapamycin with sorafenib have recently been translated to clinical trials. Parallel ongoing phase I studies of mTOR inhibitors, RAD001 and CCI-779, in combination with len for the treatment of relapsed and relapsed/refractory MM, and phase I/II study of RAD001 in combination with sorafenib for hematological malignancies including MM are ongoing. Similarly, the in vitro success of combining rapamycin with HDACi to enhance mTOR-targeted therapy has translated into phase I/II study of RAD001 in combination with LBH589 (Panobinostat) in patients with relapsed MM. Similarly, the combination of CCI-779 and bortezomib is being tested in a phase I/II study in patients with relapsed and/or relapsed, refractory MM, and preliminary data reported in 15 evaluable patients demonstrate an overall RR (complete remission + partial response + minimal response) of 33%; all responses occurred in patients who had received prior bortezomib. Minimal peripheral neuropathy was observed.[72] Additionally, an ongoing phase I study of CCI-779 and dexamethasone combination will conclude if mTOR inhibition potentiates dex-induced MM cytotoxicity as demonstrated in preclinical MM settings.[60]

## CDK Inhibitors

Numerous CDK inhibitors with differing mechanistic profiles are currently being preclinically and clinically evaluated for MM therapy. The rationale for targeting the cell cycle and, in particular, the CDKs in MM originated from comprehensive cytogenetic studies finding that dysregulated and/or increased expression of cyclin D1, D2, or D3, occurred as an early, unifying event in MM pathogenesis, predisposing MM cells to proliferative stimuli, and are frequent seen in relapsed patients with poor prognosis.[73] Specific inhibition of CDK4/6 by PD 0332991, an orally bioavailable small molecule CDK inhibitor, has demonstrated only growth arrest in MM cells,[74] suggesting that selective CDK inhibition may not be sufficient in inducing MM cell death. Rather, effective MM cytotoxicity may be best achieved when multiple CDKs are inhibited concurrently, as demonstrated in preclinical studies with multitargeted cyclin dependent kinase inhibitors (multi-CDKIs) such as Seliciclib,[75] UCN-01, P276-00,[76] AT7519, and RGB 286638. These drugs target several CDKs, which may be 1 of the mechanisms by which they preferentially resulted in apoptosis, as opposed to growth arrest of MM cells. Moreover in addition to their effect against the cyclins and CDKs, they target CDK complexes that phosphorylate RNA pol II resulting in inhibition of RNA pol II phosphorylation and transcriptional inhibition. Another interesting feature found through preclinical screening of multi-CDKIs in MM was the modulation of expression/activity of multiple signaling pathways critical for MM cell proliferation and survival in the context of the bone marrow microenvironment. In particular, the inhibition of Janus kinase/signal transducers and activators of transcription (JAK/STAT) pathway is a common feature of Seliciclib, P276-00, and RGB 286638 and plays an important role in MM survival.[77–79] Alternatively, AT7519 independent of its potent inhibitory effects on CDKs effectively induces the dephosphorylation of GSK-3$\beta$,[80] another important target in MM therapy, again demonstrating the multifaceted mechanism by which this class of drugs promotes MM cell death. Promising data from preclinical work has translated into evaluation of CDKIs as monotherapy and in combination strategies in clinical trials for patients with MM. P276-00 recently entered a phase I/II open label, multicenter study in subjects with relapsed and refractory MM. Ongoing is the evaluation of PD 0332991 in combination with bortezomib and dexamethasone in patients with refractory MM and clinical trials with RGB 286638 and AT 7519 are in development.

## MONOCLONAL ANTIBODIES

### IL-6 Targeting Antibodies

IL-6 is an inflammatory cytokine that plays a key role in MM as both an autocrine and paracrine survival factor for malignant plasma cells. IL-6 activates the STAT3 pathway, promoting cell survival through induction of the antiapoptotic protein Mcl-1. Myeloma cells directly secrete IL-6 and, more importantly, stimulate its production in the tumor niche by BMSCs and osteoclasts (OC). In addition, IL-6 stimulates osteoclastogenesis, therefore contributing to the development of osteolytic lesions.[81] Therefore, IL-6 represents an appealing target

in the treatment of MM. Among the antibodies against IL-6 studied in the preclinical setting, only CNTO328 is currently undergoing clinical assessment. CNTO328 is a novel human-mouse chimeric monoclonal antibody against IL-6. It derives from the fusion of the murine variable IL-6-binding region with human IgG1k constant domain. Preclinical in vivo data using the severe combined immunodeficiency (SCID)-hu mouse model suggest a dual inhibitory effect on tumor burden and OC differentiation. Moreover, CNTO328 enhanced bortezomib-induced cytotoxicity on MM cells increasing the activation of the proapoptotic caspases 8, 9, and 3.[82] In the clinical setting, the activity of anti-IL-6 antibody therapy is assessed by C-reactive protein levels. CNTO328 decreased C-reactive protein levels below detection limits, and therapy-associated adverse effects consisted mainly of infections and myelosuppression. Stable disease and partial responses were observed in patients with MM treated with single-agent CNTO328. More promising are the results of the combination with bortezomib in patients with relapsed-refractory MM, with an overall RR of 57% and manageable side effects. Currently, a phase II randomized trial with bortezomib and either CNTO328 or placebo is accruing.

### CD38 and CS1-Targeting Antibodies

After the excellent results of the anti-CD20 monoclonal antibody, Rituximab, several attempts have been made to identify MM-cell surface targets and design specific antibodies with cytotoxic properties. CD38 and CS-1 are multifunctional glycoproteins widely and highly expressed on MM cell surface. Two antibodies against CD38 are being tested in clinical trials, HUMAX-CD38, and MOR202. In vitro, they both induce antibody-dependent cell cytotoxicity and complement dependent cytotoxicity (CDC) against MM cells. Elotuzumab (HuLuc63) is a CS1-targeting monoclonal antibody exerting antibody-dependent cell cytotoxicity-mediated cell death in vitro and effectively reducing tumor growth in vivo in MM model.[83] In patients with relapsed/refractory MM, elotuzumab has a manageable toxicity profile and stable disease was observed on a low dose schedule. Ongoing studies are assessing the safety and efficacy of elotuzumab in combination with bortezomib.

### B-Cell Activating Factor Targeting Antibody

B-cell activating factor (BAFF) is an OC-derived MM growth factor and its inhibition reduces tumor burden and OCs and lytic lesions in in vivo models of bone disease.[84] Because the neutralizing BAFF antibody impairs MM-BMSCs interactions, the anti-OC activity observed in vivo may be mediated by reduction in MM burden or decreased secretion of pro-OC cytokines.[85] Based on these promising in vitro data, clinical trials of BAFF neutralizing antibody in combination with Vel are currently ongoing to confirm the effects on bone lesions and tumor burden.

## OTHER NOVEL SMALL MOLECULES

### Telomerase Inhibitors (GRN163L)

Human telomerase is a reverse transcription that protects chromosome endings and therefore expands cell life span. It is expressed at high levels in cancer cells, including MM, whereas almost no expression is detected in normal somatic cells. Targeting telomerase through a novel inhibitor, GRN163L, results in MM cell death in vitro. In vivo studies demonstrated that GRN163L impaired tumor growth and enhanced animal survival.[86] Data from a phase I dose escalation study of the telomerase inhibitor GRN163L in 12 heavily pretreated patients with relapsed and refractory MM revealed a minimum tolerated dose (MTD) of $\geq 4.8$ and $< 7.2$ mg/kg, with thrombocytopenia and a partial thromboplastin time prolongation as dose limiting toxicities.[87] In the meantime, ongoing phase I study of GRN163L is exploring its combination activity with bortezomib and dexamethasone in patients with relapsed or refractory MM.

## Farnesyl Transferase Inhibitors

The small guanosine triphosphatase (GTP-ase) Ras is an important target in MM as mutations of this gene are commonly encountered and are associated with disease progression and decreased survival.[88] Because Ras and other proteins require farnesylation, a lipid post-translational modification, for malignant transformation activity, farnesyl transferase inhibitors (FTIs) were studied as potential anticancer drugs. In fact, disease stabilization was achieved in 64% of patients with advanced MM treated with FTI5777 (Zarnestra) in a phase II clinical trial.[89] Preclinical evaluation of the combination of the FTI, tipifarnib, and bortezomib in microenvironment models of MM revealed synergistic anti-MM activity. This combination has been shown to enhance the endoplasmic reticulum-stress-induced apoptosis and overcome the cell adhesion-mediated drug resistance phenotype, therefore delineating a treatment strategy that specifically targets microenvironment-mediated drug resistance.[90] A parallel study has suggested that the mechanism responsible for this profound synergy is due to inhibition of HDAC6 with a resultant inhibition of both the proteasome and aggresome pathway.[91] Based on these observations, a phase I trial combining escalating doses of tipifarnib (100–400 mg/BID) with bortezomib (1.0 mg/m$^2$) in patients with relapsed MM was initiated, and encouraging preliminary data reported stabilization of disease or better seen among 7 of 16 patients with 2 of the 7 achieving an MR; no serious drug-related toxicities were noted including cardiac events or DVT.

## Small Molecule Multikinase Inhibitors

Because the Ras/Raf/mitogen-activated protein kinase/extracellular signal-regulated kinase (MEK) kinase/Erk pathway is critical for the proliferation of MM cells and is often upregulated, multikinase inhibitors that act predominantly through inhibition of Raf-kinase and vascular endothelial growth factor receptor-2 have been studied. The novel multikinase inhibitor sorafenib exhibited potent in vitro anti-MM activity, overcoming the proliferative advantage of coculture with stromal cells or with IL-6, vascular endothelial growth factor, or IGF. Examination of cellular signaling pathways demonstrated downregulation of induced myeloid leukemia cell differentiation protein and decreased phosphorylation of the STAT3 and MEK/ERK, as potential mechanisms of sorafenib antitumor effect, complemented by its antiangiogenic activity. Promising preclinical data have resulted in the clinical evaluation and development of novel sorafenib combinations. However, data have been recently presented from a phase II study, which concluded that single-agent sorafenib did not show activity in heavily pretreated patients with MM previously exposed to bortezomib.[92] Nevertheless, because the frequency of Ras oncogene mutations increases resulting in resistance to traditional chemotherapeutic agents, sorafenib is being studied in combination therapy with bortezomib in relapsed/refractory MM. Similarly, an ongoing phase I/II study will test whether sorafenib and len have anti-MM activity in patients with relapsed/refractory MM.

## CONCLUSIONS AND FUTURE DIRECTIONS

There is unanimous agreement that novel therapies have increased responses and prolonged survival in patients with MM. Our understanding of genomics and proteomics has provided us with insights into rationally designed clinical trials of both single agents and combination strategies. The next several years will provide us with opportunities to use these novel drug combinations based on patient profiles

and risk stratification allowing us to maximize efficacy without compromising quality of life with special attention to the toxicities of these agents.

## REFERENCES

1. Jemal A, Siegel R, Ward E, et al. Cancer statistics, 2008. *CA Cancer J Clin.* 2008;58:71–96.
2. Brenner H, Gondos A, Pulte D. Recent major improvement in long-term survival of younger patients with multiple myeloma. *Blood.* 2008;111:2521–2526.
3. Rajkumar SV, Rosiñol L, Hussein M, et al. Multicenter, randomized, double-blind, placebo-controlled study of thalidomide plus dexamethasone compared with dexamethasone as initial therapy for newly diagnosed multiple myeloma. *J Clin Oncol.* 2008;26:2171–2177.
4. San Miguel JF, Schlag R, Khuageva NK, et al; VISTA Trial Investigators. Bortezomib plus melphalan and prednisone for initial treatment of multiple myeloma. *N Engl J Med.* 2008;359:906–917.
5. Richardson PG, Barlogie B, Berenson J, et al. A phase 2 study of bortezomib in relapsed, refractory myeloma. *N Engl J Med.* 2003;348:2609–2617.
6. Richardson PG, Sonneveld P, Schuster MW, et al; Assessment of Proteasome Inhibition for Extending Remissions (APEX) Investigators. Bortezomib or high-dose dexamethasone for relapsed multiple myeloma. *N Engl J Med.* 2005;352:2487–2498.
7. Dimopoulos MA, Chen C, Spencer A, et al. Long-term follow-up on overall survival from the MM-009 and MM-010 phase III trials of lenalidomide plus dexamethasone in patients with relapsed or refractory multiple myeloma. *Leukemia.* In press.
8. Weber DM, Chen C, Niesvizky R, et al; Multiple Myeloma (009) Study Investigators. Lenalidomide plus dexamethasone for relapsed multiple myeloma in North America. *N Engl J Med.* 2007;357:2133–2142.
9. Chen C, Reece DE, Siegel D, et al. Expanded safety experience with lenalidomide plus dexamethasone in relapsed or refractory multiple myeloma. *Br J Haematol.* 2009;146:164–170.
10. Orlowski RZ, Nagler A, Sonneveld P, et al. Randomized phase III study of pegylated liposomal doxorubicin plus bortezomib compared with bortezomib alone in relapsed or refractory multiple myeloma: combination therapy improves time to progression. *J Clin Oncol.* 2007;25:3892–3901.
11. Dimopoulos M, Spencer A, Attal M, et al; Multiple Myeloma (010) Study Investigators. Lenalidomide plus dexamethasone for relapsed or refractory multiple myeloma. *N Engl J Med.* 2007;357:2123–2132.
12. Rajkumar SV, Jacobus S, Callander N, et al. Phase III trial of lenalidomide plus high-dose dexamethasone versus lenalidomide plus low-dose dexamethasone in newly diagnosed multiple myeloma (E4A03): a trial coordinated by the Eastern Cooperative Oncology Group. *J Clin Oncol.* Annual Meeting Abstracts 2007;25(suppl 18):LBA8025.
13. Rajkumar SV, Jacobus S, Callander N, et al. A randomized trial of lenalidomide plus high-dose dexamethasone (RD) versus lenalidomide plus low-dose dexamethasone (Rd) in newly diagnosed multiple myeloma (E4A03): a trial coordinated by the Eastern Cooperative Oncology Group. *Blood.* 2007;110:31a. [Abstract 74].
14. Jagannath S, Vij R, Stewart AK, et al. Initial results of PX-171-003, an open-label, single-arm, phase II study of carfilzomib (CFZ) in patients with relapsed and refractory multiple myeloma (MM). *Blood.* 2008;112:Abstract 864.
15. Jagannath S, Vij R, Stewart AK, et al. Final results of PX-171-003-A0, part 1 of an open-label, single-arm, phase II study of carfilzomib (CFZ) in patients (pts) with relapsed and refractory multiple myeloma (MM). *J Clin Oncol.* 2009;27(suppl 15):Abstract 8504.
16. Vij R, Wang M, Orlowski RZ, et al. Initial results of PX-171-04, an open-label, single-arm, phase II study of carfilzomib (CFZ) in patients with relapsed myeloma (MM). *Blood.* 2008;112:Abstract 865.
17. Niesvizky R, Bensinger W, Vallone M, et al. PX-171-006: phase Ib multicenter dose escalation study of carfilzomib (CFZ) plus lenalidomide (LEN) and low-dose dexamethasone (loDex) in relapsed and refractory multiple myeloma (MM): preliminary results. *J Clin Oncol.* 2009;27:15s (suppl; Abstract 8541).
18. Chauhan D, Catley L, Li G, et al. A novel orally active proteasome inhibitor induces apoptosis in multiple myeloma cells with mechanisms distinct from bortezomib. *Cancer Cell.* 2005;8:407–419.
19. Piva R, Ruggeri B, Williams M, et al. CEP-18770: a novel, orally active proteasome inhibitor with a tumor-selective pharmacologic profile competitive with bortezomib. *Blood.* 2008;111:2765–2775.
20. Hofmeister CC, Richardson P, Zimmerman T, et al. Clinical trial of the novel structure proteasome inhibitor NPI-0052 in patients with relapsed and relapsed/refractory multiple myeloma (r/r MM). *J Clin Oncol.* 2009;27:15s (suppl; Abstract 8505).

21. Chauhan D, Singh A, Brahmandam M, et al. Combination of proteasome inhibitors bortezomib and NPI-0052 trigger in vivo synergistic cytotoxicity in multiple myeloma. *Blood.* 2008;111:1654–1664.

22. Singhal S, Mehta J, Desikan R, et al. Antitumor activity of thalidomide in refractory multiple myeloma. *N Engl J Med.* 1999;341:1565–1571.

23. Rajkumar SV, Hayman S, Gertz MA, et al. Combination therapy with thalidomide plus dexamethasone for newly diagnosed myeloma. *J Clin Oncol.* 2002;20:4319–4323.

24. Weber D, Rankin K, Gavino M, et al. Thalidomide alone or with dexamethasone for previously untreated multiple myeloma. *J Clin Oncol.* 2003;21:16–19.

25. Richardson P, Schlossman R, Jagannath S, et al. Thalidomide for patients with relapsed multiple myeloma after high-dose chemotherapy and stem cell transplantation: results of an open-label multicenter phase 2 study of efficacy, toxicity, and biological activity. *Mayo Clin Proc.* 2004;79:875–882.

26. Bartlett JB, Dredge K, Dalgleish AG. The evolution of thalidomide and its IMiD derivatives as anticancer agents. *Nat Rev Cancer.* 2004;4:314–322.

27. Mitsiades N, Mitsiades CS, Poulaki V, et al. Apoptotic signaling induced by immunomodulatory thalidomide analogs in human multiple myeloma cells: therapeutic implications. *Blood.* 2002;99:4525–4530.

28. Gupta D, Treon SP, Shima Y, et al. Adherence of multiple myeloma cells to bone marrow stromal cells upregulates vascular endothelial growth factor secretion: therapeutic applications. *Leukemia.* 2001;15:1950–1961.

29. Lacy MQ, Hayman SR, Gertz MA, et al. Pomalidomide (CC4047) plus low-dose dexamethasone (pom/dex) is highly effective therapy in relapsed multiple myeloma. *Blood.* 2008;112:Abstract 866.

30. Mitsiades CS, Mitsiades NS, McMullan CJ, et al. Transcriptional signature of histone deacetylase inhibition in multiple myeloma: biological and clinical implications. *Proc Natl Acad Sci USA.* 2004;101:540–545.

31. Catley L, Weisberg E, Tai YT, et al. NVP-LAQ824 is a potent novel histone deacetylase inhibitor with significant activity against multiple myeloma. *Blood.* 2003;102:2615–2622.

32. O'Connor OA, Heaney ML, Schwartz L, et al. Clinical experience with intravenous and oral formulations of the novel histone deacetylase inhibitor suberoylanilide hydroxamic acid in patients with advanced hematologic malignancies. *J Clin Oncol.* 2006;24:166–173.

33. Richardson P, Mitsiades C, Colson K, et al. Phase I trial of oral vorinostat (suberoylanilide hydroxamic acid, SAHA) in patients with advanced multiple myeloma. *Leuk Lymphoma.* 2008;49:502–507.

34. Wolf JL, Siegel D, Matous J, et al. A phase II study of oral panobinostat (LBH589) in adult patients with advanced refractory multiple myeloma. *Blood.* 2008;112:Abstract 2774.

35. Ottmann OG, Spencer A, Prince HM, et al. Phase IA/II study of oral panobinostat (LBH589), a novel pan-deacetylase inhibitor (DACi) demonstrating efficacy in patients with advanced hematologic malignancies. *Blood.* 2008;112:Abstract 958.

36. Deleu S, Lemaire M, Arts J, et al. Bortezomib alone or in combination with the histone deacetylase inhibitor JNJ-26481585: effect on myeloma bone disease in the 5T2MM murine model of myeloma. *Cancer Res.* 2009;69:5307–5311.

37. Badros AZ, Philip S, Niesvizk R, et al. Phase I trial of vorinostat plus bortezomib (bort) in relapsed/refractory multiple myeloma (mm) patients (pts). *J Clin Oncol.* 2008;26:Abstract 8548.

38. Harrison S, Quach H, Yuen K, et al. High response rates with the combination of bortezomib, dexamethasone and the pan-histone deacetylase inhibitor romidepsin in patients with relapsed or refractory multiple myeloma in a phase I/II clinical trial. *Blood.* 2008;112:Abstract 3698.

39. Siegel D, Weber D, Mitsiades CS, et al. A phase I study of vorinostat in combination with lenalidomide and dexamethasone in patients with relapsed or refractory multiple myeloma. *Blood.* 2008;112:Abstract 3705.

40. Weber D, Jagannath S, Mazumder A, et al. Phase I trial of oral vorinostat (suberoylanilide hydroxamic acid, SAHA) in combination with bortezomib in patients with advanced multiple myeloma. *Blood.* 2007;110:Abstract 1172.

41. Siegel DS, Weber DM, Mitsiades CS, et al. Vorinostat in combination with lenalidomide and dexamethasone in patients with relapsed/refractory multiple myeloma: a phase I study. *J Clin Oncol.* 2009;27:15s (suppl; Abstract 8586).

42. Spencer A, Taylor K, Lonial S, et al. Panobinostat plus lenalidomide and dexamethasone phase I trial in multiple myeloma (MM). *J Clin Oncol.* 2009;27:15s (suppl; Abstract 8542).

43. Mitsiades N, Mitsiades CS, Poulaki V, et al. Molecular sequelae of proteasome inhibition in human multiple myeloma cells. *Proc Natl Acad Sci USA.* 2002;99:14374–14379.

44. Chanan-Khan A, Richardson P, Alsina M, et al. Phase 1 clinical trial of KOS-953 + bortezomib (BZ) in relapsed refractory multiple myeloma (MM). *J Clin Oncol.* 2006;24:18S (suppl; Abstract 3066).

45. Hideshima T, Catley L, Raje N, et al. Inhibition of Akt induces significant downregulation of survivin and cytotoxicity in human multiple myeloma cells. *Br J Haematol.* 2007;138:783–791.

46. Tai YT, Podar K, Catley L, et al. Insulin-like growth factor-1 induces adhesion and migration in human multiple myeloma cells via activation of beta1-integrin and phosphatidylinositol 3′-kinase/AKT signaling. *Cancer Res.* 2003;63:5850–5858.

47. Hsu J, Shi Y, Krajewski S, et al. The AKT kinase is activated in multiple myeloma tumor cells. *Blood.* 2001;98:2853–2855.

48. Hideshima T, Catley L, Yasui H, et al. Perifosine, an oral bioactive novel alkylphospholipid, inhibits Akt and induces in vitro and in vivo cytotoxicity in human multiple myeloma cells. *Blood.* 2006;107:4053–4062.

49. Gajate C, Mollinedo F. Edelfosine and perifosine induce selective apoptosis in multiple myeloma by recruitment of death receptors and downstream signaling molecules into lipid rafts. *Blood.* 2007;109:711–719.

50. Richardson P, Wolf J, Jakubowiak A, et al. Phase I/II results of a multicenter trial of perifosine (KRX-0401) + bortezomib in patients with relapsed or relapsed/refractory multiple myeloma who were previously relapsed from or refractory to bortezomib. *Blood.* 2008;112:Abstract 870.

51. Jakubowiak A, Richardson P, Zimmerman TM, et al. Phase I results of perifosine (KRX-0401) in combination with lenalidomide and dexamethasone in patients with relapsed or refractory multiple myeloma (MM). *Blood.* 2008;112:Abstract 3691.

52. Podar K, Raab MS, Zhang J, et al. Targeting PKC in multiple myeloma: in vitro and in vivo effects of the novel, orally available small-molecule inhibitor enzastaurin (LY317615.HCl). *Blood.* 2007;109:1669–1677.

53. Hideshima T, Chauhan D, Richardson P, et al. Identification and validation of novel therapeutic targets for multiple myeloma. *J Clin Oncol.* 2005;23:6345–6350.

54. Hideshima T, Raje N. Akt as a therapeutic target in multiple myeloma. *Haematologica.* 2007;92[suppl 2]:abstract n. S8.3.

55. Anderson KC. Future perspectives in the management of myeloma. *Haematologica.* 2007;92[suppl. 2]:abstract n.S13.4.

56. Shi Y, Hsu JH, Hu L, et al. Signal pathways involved in activation of p70S6K and phosphorylation of 4E-BP1 following exposure of multiple myeloma tumor cells to interleukin-6. *J Biol Chem.* 2002;277:15712–15720.

57. Shi Y, Gera J, Hu L, et al. Enhanced sensitivity of multiple myeloma cells containing PTEN mutations to CCI-779. *Cancer Res.* 2002;62:5027–5034.

58. Hu L, Shi Y, Hsu JH, et al. Downstream effectors of oncogenic ras in multiple myeloma cells. *Blood.* 2003;101:3126–3135.

59. Raje N, Kumar S, Hideshima T, et al. Combination of the mTOR inhibitor rapamycin and CC-5013 has synergistic activity in multiple myeloma. *Blood.* 2004;104:4188–4193.

60. Strömberg T, Dimberg A, Hammarberg A, et al. Rapamycin sensitizes multiple myeloma cells to apoptosis induced by dexamethasone. *Blood.* 2004;103:3138–3147.

61. Yan H, Frost P, Shi Y, et al. Mechanism by which mammalian target of rapamycin inhibitors sensitize multiple myeloma cells to dexamethasone-induced apoptosis. *Cancer Res.* 2006;66:2305–2313.

62. Frost P, Moatamed F, Hoang B, et al. In vivo antitumor effects of the mTOR inhibitor CCI-779 against human multiple myeloma cells in a xenograft model. *Blood.* 2004;104:4181–4187.

63. Mitsiades N, McMullan C, Poulaki V, et al. The mTOR inhibitor RAD001 (everolimus) is active against multiple myeloma cells in vitro and in vivo. ASH Annual Meeting Abstracts. 2004;104:1496.

64. Easton JB, Houghton PJ. mTOR and cancer therapy. *Oncogene.* 2006;25:6436–6446.

65. Faivre S, Kroemer G, Raymond E. Current development of mTOR inhibitors as anticancer agents. *Nat Rev Drug Discov.* 2006;5:671–688.

66. Guertin DA, Sabatini DM. Defining the role of mTOR in cancer. *Cancer Cell.* 2007;12:9–22.

67. Farag SS, Zhang S, Jansak BS, et al. Phase II trial of temsirolimus in patients with relapsed or refractory multiple myeloma. *Leuk Res.* 2009;33:1475–1480.

68. Wan X, Harkavy B, Shen N, et al. Rapamycin induces feedback activation of Akt signaling through an IGF-1R-dependent mechanism. *Oncogene.* 2007;26:1932–1940.

69. Sun SY, Rosenberg LM, Wang X, et al. Activation of Akt and eIF4E survival pathways by rapamycin-mediated mammalian target of rapamycin inhibition. *Cancer Res.* 2005;65:7052–7058.

70. O'Reilly KE, Rojo F, She QB, et al. mTOR inhibition induces upstream receptor tyrosine kinase signaling and activates Akt. *Cancer Res.* 2006;66:1500–1508.

71. Cirstea D, Hideshima T, Pozzi S, et al. Combination of Nab-rapamycin and perifosine induces synergistic cytotoxicity and antitumor activity via autophagy and apoptosis in multiple myeloma (MM). *Blood.* 2008;112:Abstract 3663.

72. Ghobrial IM, Munshi N, Schlossman R, et al. Phase I trial of CCI-779 (temsirolimus) and weekly bortezomib in relapsed and/or refractory multiple myeloma. *Blood.* 2008;112:Abstract 3696.

73. Bergsagel PL, Kuehl WM. Molecular pathogenesis and a consequent classification of multiple myeloma. *J Clin Oncol.* 2005;23:6333–6338.

74. Baughn LB, Di Liberto M, Wu K, et al. A novel orally active small molecule potently induces G1 arrest in primary myeloma cells and prevents tumor growth by specific inhibition of cyclin-dependent kinase 4/6. *Cancer Res.* 2006;66:7661–7667.

75. Raje N, Kumar S, Hideshima T, et al. Seliciclib (CYC202 or R-roscovitine), a small-molecule cyclin-dependent kinase inhibitor, mediates activity via down-regulation of Mcl-1 in multiple myeloma. *Blood.* 2005;106:1042–1047.

76. Raje N, Hideshima T, Mukherjee S, et al. Preclinical activity of P276-00, a novel small-molecule cyclin-dependent kinase inhibitor in the therapy of multiple myeloma. *Leukemia.* 2009;23:961–970.

77. Puthier D, Bataille R, Amiot M. IL-6 up-regulates mcl-1 in human myeloma cells through JAK/STAT rather than ras/MAP kinase pathway. *Eur J Immunol.* 1999;29:3945–3950.

78. Puthier D, Derenne S, Barillé S, et al. Mcl-1 and Bcl-xL are co-regulated by IL-6 in human myeloma cells. *Br J Haematol.* 1999;107:392–395.

79. Cirstea D, Hideshima T, Pozzi S, et al. RGB 286638, a novel multi-targeted small molcecule inhibitor, induces multiple myeloma (MM) cell death through abrogation of CDK-dependent and independent survival mechanisms. *Blood.* 2008:112:Abstract 2759.

80. Santo L, Vallet S, Hideshima T, et al. ASH 2008-AT7519, a novel small molecule multi-cyclin dependent kinase inhibitor, induces apoptosis in multiple myeloma VIA GSK3β. *Blood.* 2008;112:Abstract 251.

81. Kurihara N, Bertolini D, Suda T, et al. IL-6 stimulates osteoclast-like multinucleated cell formation in long term human marrow cultures by inducing IL-1 release. *J Immunol.* 1990;144:4226–4230.

82. Voorhees PM, Chen Q, Kuhn DJ, et al. Inhibition of interleukin-6 signaling with CNTO 328 enhances the activity of bortezomib in preclinical models of multiple myeloma. *Clin Cancer Res.* 2007;13:6469–6478.

83. Tai YT, Dillon M, Song W, et al. Anti-CS1 humanized monoclonal antibody HuLuc63 inhibits myeloma cell adhesion and induces antibody-dependent cellular cytotoxicity in the bone marrow milieu. *Blood.* 2008;112:1329–1337.

84. Neri P, Kumar S, Fulciniti MT, et al. Neutralizing B-cell activating factor antibody improves survival and inhibits osteoclastogenesis in a severe combined immunodeficient human multiple myeloma model. *Clin Cancer Res.* 2007;13:5903–5909.

85. Tai YT, Li XF, Breitkreutz I, et al. Role of B-cell-activating factor in adhesion and growth of human multiple myeloma cells in the bone marrow microenvironment. *Cancer Res.* 2006;66:6675–6682.

86. Shammas MA, Koley H, Bertheau RC, et al. Telomerase inhibitor GRN163L

87. Chanan-Khan AA, Munshi NC, Hussein MA, et al. Results of a phase I study of GRN163L, a direct inhibitor of telomerase, in patients with relapsed and refractory multiple myeloma (MM). *Blood.* 2008;112:Abstract 3701.

88. Bezieau S, Devilder MC, Avet-Loiseau H, et al. High incidence of N and K-Ras activating mutations in multiple myeloma and primary plasma cell leukemia at diagnosis. *Hum Mutat.* 2001;18:212–224.

89. Alsina M, Fonseca R, Wilson EF, et al. Farnesyltransferase inhibitor tipifarnib is well tolerated, induces stabilization of disease, and inhibits farnesylation and oncogenic/tumor survival pathways in patients with advanced multiple myeloma. *Blood.* 2004;103:3271–3277.

90. Yanamandra N, Colaco NM, Parquet NA, et al. Tipifarnib and bortezomib are synergistic and overcome cell adhesion-mediated drug resistance in multiple myeloma and acute myeloid leukemia. *Clin Cancer Res.* 2006;12:591–599.

91. Lonial S, Francis D, Karanes C, et al. A phase i mmrc clinical trial testing the combination of bortezomib and tipifarnib in relapsed/refractory multiple myeloma. *Blood.* 2008;112:Abstract 3706.

92. Srkalovic G, Hussein M, Bolejack V, et al. A phase II trial of sorafenib in patients with relapsing and resistant multiple myeloma (MM) previously treated with bortezomib (S0434). *J Clin Oncol.* 2009;27(suppl):Abstract e19517.

93. Orlowski RZ, Stewart K, Vallone M, et al. Safety and antitumor efficacy of the proteasome inhibitor carfilzomib (PR-171) dosed for five consecutive days in hematologic malignancies: phase 1 results. *Blood (ASH Annual Meeting Abstracts).* 2007;110:409.

94. Alsina M, Trudel S, Vallone M, et al. Phase 1 single agent antitumor activity of twice weekly consecutive day dosing of the proteasome inhibitor carfilzomib (PR-171) in hematologic malignancies. *Blood (ASH Annual Meeting Abstracts).* 2007;110:411.

95. Richardson P, Chanan-Khan AA, Lonial S, et al. A multicenter phase 1 clinical trial of tanespimycin (KOS-953) + bortezomib (BZ): encouraging activity and manageable toxicity in heavily pre-treated patients with relapsed refractory multiple myeloma (MM). *Blood (ASH Annual Meeting Abstracts).* 2006;108:406.

96. Weber D, Badros AZ, Jagannath S, et al. Vorinostat plus bortezomib for the treatment of relapsed/refractory multiple myeloma: early clinical experience. *Blood.* 2008;112:Abstract 871.

97. Siegel D, Sezer O, San Miguel JF, et al. A phase IB, multicenter, open-label, dose-escalation study of oral panobinostat (LBH589) and I.V. bortezomib in patients with relapsed multiple myeloma. *Blood.* 2008;112:Abstract 2781.

inhibits myeloma cell growth in vitro and in vivo. *Leukemia.* 2008;22:1410–1418.

# Index